MW01078137

A Sonographer's Guide to the Assessment of Heart Disease

Bonita Anderson

Diploma in Medical Ultrasonography (Cardiac),
Master of Applied Science (Medical Ultrasound),
Accredited Medical Sonographer.

Echotext Pty Ltd
AUSTRALIA.
www.echotext.info

Copyright © 2014 Murray Anderson, trading as MGA Graphics.
Copyright © 2016 Echotext Pty Ltd

Sixth printing August, 2022

All rights reserved. No part of this publication may be reproduced or transmitted in
any form or by any means, electronic or mechanical, including photocopy, recording,
or any information storage and retrieval system, without permission in writing from
the publisher.

Printed in the U.S.A.

National Library of Australia Cataloguing-in-Publication entry:

Author:	Anderson, Bonita, author.
Title:	A sonographer's guide to the assessment of heart disease / Bonita Anderson.
ISBN:	9780992322205 (hardback)
Notes:	Includes index.
Subjects:	Echocardiography.
	Heart Diseases--Ultrasonic imaging.
Dewey Number:	616.07543

Disclaimer
This document is produced by Echotext Pty Ltd. Copyright in the whole and every
part of this document belongs to Echotext Pty Ltd and may not be used, sold,
transferred or reproduced in whole or in part in any manner or form in or in media, to
any persons other than by agreement with Echotext Pty Ltd.
To the extent permitted by law, Echotext Pty Ltd and the author exclude liability for
any loss suffered by any person resulting in any way from the use or alliance on this
publication.
Every effort has been made to ensure that the information in this publication
is accurate. However, the author expressly disclaims all warranties, express or
implied, including, but not limited to, the implied warranty of fitness for a particular
purpose. To the extent permitted by law, the author does not warrant or make any
representations regarding the use or the results of the use of the information provided
within the publication in terms of its correctness, accuracy, reliability, or otherwise,
no oral or written information or advice given by the author shall create a warranty
or in any way increase the scope of this warranty. Some jurisdictions do not allow the
exclusion of implied warranties, so the above exclusion may not apply to you.
It is also advised that readers seek other sources of information and remain up to date
with any new developments on the subjects discussed within this book.

For updates, information and availability please visit: **www.echotext.info**

for
Lucy, Madeleine
and Oscar

Preface

My first textbook, "Echocardiography: The Normal Examination and Echocardiographic Measurements" was published in 2000 with the second edition being published in 2007. Since its publication, I have been asked on a number of occasions if I was planning to write another textbook regarding the role of echocardiography in the assessment of cardiac diseases. I was always reluctant to do this for two main reasons: (1) there were already many excellent textbooks on echocardiography available which covered pathology, and (2) the amount of work involved in accomplishing such a task would be immense! However, over time, I came to realise that a sonographer-orientated textbook on echocardiography which covered pathology might be useful for students studying echocardiography, for echocardiography educators and for cardiac sonographers working in routine clinical practice. So I decided that it was time that I 'bit the bullet' and took on the task.

The primary goal of the resulting text is to provide a comprehensive review of transthoracic echocardiography in the assessment of various cardiac pathologies. Refresher notes on cardiac anatomy and the relevant cardiac physiology are included as I believe that it is crucial that the cardiac sonographer has a detailed knowledge of cardiac anatomy, cardiac physiology and cardiac pathophysiology to improve their understanding of various diseases, disease processes and associated findings. In particular, the cardiac pathological photos generously provided by Dr William Edwards are intended to further enhance the cardiac sonographer's recognition and understanding of cardiac diseases.

Within this text, I have deliberately not included what I refer to as 'advanced technologies'. This is because I wanted to write a textbook for the 'everyday' cardiac sonographer, many of whom either do not have access to these advanced technologies or do not have time to utilise them. Therefore, advanced technologies such as 3D echocardiography, strain and strain rate imaging are not included within this text. Should the reader be interested in these 'newer' techniques, I would encourage them to seek out some of the excellent textbooks available on these specialised areas of echocardiography. In addition, the chapter on congenital heart disease is intended as a brief introduction to this extensive topic; there are many excellent textbooks devoted to congenital heart disease and I would encourage readers to seek out these textbooks as well, should they require further information.

BA

Acknowledgements

This textbook could not have been written without the support of family, friends and other work colleagues. Firstly, words cannot express the appreciation that I have for the support and dedication of my husband, Murray, who has produced and published this book. I could not have completed this mammoth task without his help.

I am especially thankful for the contributions of two very prominent pathologists: Dr William (Bill) Edwards, MD, Cardiac Pathologist at the Mayo Clinic, Rochester, Minnesota, USA and Dr Robert (Bob) Anderson, BSc MD FRCPath. I have been privileged to attend several of Bill Edward's presentations on cardiac pathology and I have also seen the many pathological photos that he has contributed to numerous textbooks and journal articles. I am extremely fortunate that Bill was willing to provide photos for use in this book. As readers will note, Bill has provided the majority of cardiac pathology photos within this text. Bill's meticulous attention to detail is evident in these exceptional photos and I believe that they will be a major highlight of this book. Bob Anderson has also allowed me to reproduce pathological photos from his out-of-print textbook, *Cardiac Anatomy: An Integrated Text and Color Atlas* (authors Robert H. Anderson and Anton E. Becker). Bob also provided expert advice on how I should describe various areas of cardiac anatomy, such as the mitral valve complex.

Two prominent cardiologists from The Prince Charles Hospital (TPCH) have also been vital to the information provided within this book: Dr Darryl Burstow, MBBS, Senior Staff Cardiologist and Clinical Director of the Echocardiography Laboratory and Dr Dorothy Radford, MBBS, Senior Staff Cardiologist, Director of Adult Congenital Heart Disease and founder of the Echocardiography Laboratory at TPCH. I am tremendously fortunate that Darryl and Dorothy both agreed without hesitation to review, edit and proof-read various chapters of this book. Darryl's tasks included the extensive review of Chapters 1-14 while Dorothy offered her specialist advice on the congenital heart disease sections of this book (Chapter 15 and Appendices 5-6). The expert advice from Darryl and Dorothy has reinforced my confidence in the accuracy of the information shared in this book. So I must thank them both for their support and the donation of their valuable time to this project.

A special acknowledgment must go to Margo Gill (formerly Senior Lecturer and Coordinator of Ultrasound programs at the Queensland University of Technology) and her husband Dr Robert Gill PhD (formerly Principal Research Scientist at the Ultrasonics Institute and Deputy Chief of the Division of Applied Physics, CSIRO). Both Margo and Rob committed an enormous amount of their time to the meticulous proofreading of this entire text. Twice! Their frequent words of encouragement and expert knowledge have kept me focused over the years that it has taken to finish this book.

Further, I am always grateful for the support and encouragement that I receive from my colleagues at TPCH Echocardiography Laboratory and across Australia. I would especially like to extend my appreciation to Mrs Susan Boucaut (former Director of Cardiac Sciences) and Dr Darren Walters (Executive Director) at TPCH for their flexibility and willingness to allow me to take extended leaves of absence to enable me to write this book. Also special thanks to Dr Greg Scalia, Dr Helen Thomson, Dr Tau Boga, Tony Forshaw and Karen Hillcoat for their contributions to this book.

Finally, to my family: thanks for your patience and willingness to take a 'back-seat' while I have spent most weekends and any other spare time devoted to writing this book. So to my family, please accept my apologies for all the 'absences'.

BA

Table of Contents

Abbreviations

ΔP	pressure difference/gradient	IMH	intramural haematoma	PR	pulmonary regurgitation
2D	two dimensional	IAP	intraabdominal pressure	PS	pulmonary stenosis
3D	three dimensional	IAS	interatrial septum	P-V	pressure-volume
AAS	acute aortic syndrome	ICP	intracavity pressure	PV	pulmonary valve
ACS	acute coronary syndrome	IPP	intrapericardial pressure	PVR	pulmonary vascular resistance
APE	acute pulmonary embolism	IPV	intrapericardial volume	Q	volumetric flow rate
AR	aortic regurgitation	ITP	intrathoracic pressure	QP:QS	ratio of pulmonary venous and
AS	aortic stenosis	IVC	inferior vena cava		systemic venous volumetric flow
ASD	atrial septal defect	IVS	interventricular septum		rates
ASE	American Society of	L/min	litres per minute	R	resistance
	Echocardiography	LA	left atrium	RA	right atrium
AVA	aortic valve area	LAD	left anterior descending coronary	RAP	right atrial pressure
AVR	aortic valve replacement		artery	RBCs	red blood cells
BAV	bicuspid aortic valve	LAP	left atrial pressure	RCA	right coronary artery
BP	blood pressure	LAV	left atrial volume	RV	right ventricle
bpm	beats per minutes	LCA	left coronary artery	RVAcT	right ventricular acceleration time
BSA	body surface area	LMCA	left main coronary artery	RVEDP	right ventricular end-diastolic
CFI	colour flow imaging	LV	left ventricle		pressure
CHD	congenital heart disease	LVEDP	left ventricular end-diastolic	RVOT	right ventricular outflow tract
CI_{IVC}	collapsibility index for inferior		pressure	RVSP	right ventricular systolic pressure
	vena cava	LVH	left ventricular hypertrophy	RWT	relative wall thickness
CMRI	cardiac magnetic resonance	LVM	left ventricular mass	SAM	systolic anterior motion
	imaging	LVOT	left ventricular outflow tract	SBP	systolic blood pressure
CO	cardiac output	LVSP	left ventricular systolic pressure	SV	stroke volume
CoAo	coarctation of the aorta	MIPG	maximum instantaneous pressure	SVA	sinus of Valsalva aneurysm
COPD	chronic obstructive airways	mL	millilitres	SVC	superior vena cava
	disease	mm Hg	millimetres of mercury	SVR	systemic vascular resistance
CSA	cross-sectional area	mPAP	mean pulmonary artery pressure	TAPSE	tricuspid annular plane systolic
CW	continuous-wave	mPG	mean pressure gradient		excursion
Cx	circumflex coronary artery	MPI	myocardial performance index	TGA	transposition of the great
DBP	diastolic blood pressure	MR	mitral regurgitation		arteries
DSI	dimensionless severity index	MS	mitral stenosis	TMFP	transmural filling pressure
DTI	Doppler tissue imaging	MVA	mitral valve area	TOE	transoesophageal echocardiograph
DVI	Doppler velocity imaging	MVR	mitral valve replacement	TOF	tetralogy of Fallot
ECG	Electrocardiogram	PA	pulmonary artery	TR	tricuspid regurgitation
EF	ejection fraction	PAH	pulmonary arterial hypertension	TTE	transthoracic echocardiography
EFG	effective filling gradient	PAEDP	pulmonary artery end diastolic	TVA	tricuspid valve atresia
ELI	energy loss index		pressure	TVR	tricuspid valve replacement
EOA	effective orifice area	PASP	pulmonary artery systolic pressure	UAV	unicuspid aortic valve
EROA	effective regurgitant orifice area	PAU	penetrating aortic ulcer	VC	vena contracta
F	frequency	PCWP	pulmonary capillary wedge	VC-W	vena contracta-width
FAC	fractional area change		pressure	VSD	ventricular septal defect
FS	fractional shortening	PDA	patent ductus arteriosus	VTI	velocity time integral
g	grams	PFO	patent foramen ovale	WHO	World Health Organization
HTN	hypertension	PHTN	pulmonary hypertension	WMSI	wall motion score index
HV	hepatic vein	PISA	proximal isovelocity surface area		

Introduction to Basic Haemodynamic Calculations

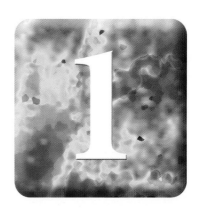

Essentially Doppler haemodynamic calculations can be divided into three groups based on the: (1) determination of pressure gradients, (2) estimation of volumetric flow, and (3) application of the continuity principle. Each of these concepts is discussed in detail below.

Determination of Pressure Gradients

One of the fundamental applications of Doppler echocardiography is the determination of pressure differences or pressure gradients based on velocities derived by the application of the Doppler principle.

Doppler Principles

The Doppler effect describes the assumed change in frequency (f) or wavelength (λ) that occurs due to relative motion between the wave source, the receiver of the wave, and the reflector of the wave. In diagnostic ultrasound, the reflectors of the wave are the red blood cells (RBCs) while the wave

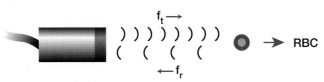

Figure 1.1 When the RBCs are stationary compared to the transducer the transmitted frequency will be the same as the received frequency ($f_r = f_t$) and there is no Doppler shift (*top*).
When RBCs are moving toward the transducer the received frequency is greater than the transmitted frequency ($f_r > f_t$) so there is a positive Doppler shift (*middle*).
When RBCs are moving away from the transducer the received frequency is less than the transmitted frequency ($f_r < f_t$) so there is a negative Doppler shift (*bottom*).
f_r = received frequency; f_t = transmitted frequency; RBC = red blood cells.

source and receiver of the wave is the ultrasound transducer. When the ultrasound beam is directed toward moving RBCs, there are two separate frequencies detected by the ultrasound transducer: (1) the transmit frequency of the transducer (f_t), and (2) the received frequency (f_r). The difference between f_r and f_t is the Doppler shift or frequency shift (Δf). This Doppler shift may be non-existent, positive or negative depending upon the motion and direction of blood flow in relation to the ultrasound beam (Fig. 1.1).

> Positive Doppler shifts occur when blood flow is toward the transducer while negative Doppler shifts occur when blood flow is away from the transducer.

The degree of Doppler shift (that is, how much this shift increases or decreases) is determined by five variables: (1) the transducer frequency, (2) the speed of sound in soft tissue, (3) blood flow velocity, (4) the angle of intercept between the direction of blood flow and the ultrasound beam and (5) the "double Doppler shift" (Fig. 1.2 and 1.3). The relationship between these variables and the Doppler shift is expressed by the Doppler equation:

Equation 1.1

$$\pm\Delta f = \frac{2\,f_t\,V\,\cos\,\theta}{c}$$

where Δf = Doppler shift ($f_r - f_t$) (Hz)
f_t = known transmitted frequency of the transducer (Hz)
V = velocity of blood flow (m/s)
c = assumed speed of sound in soft tissue (m/s)
θ = incident angle between the ultrasound beam and blood flow direction
2 = the "double Doppler shift" (see Fig. 1.3)

In clinical practice, the velocity of blood flow rather than the Doppler shift is more meaningful; hence, this equation can be rearranged to solve for the velocity of blood flow:

Equation 1.2

$$V\cos\theta = \frac{c\,(\pm\Delta f)}{2\,f_t}$$

Furthermore, assuming that the angle of intercept between the ultrasound beam and the direction of blood flow is zero and because the value of cos at 0 degrees is 1, this equation can be further simplified:

Equation 1.3

$$V = \frac{c\ (\pm \Delta f)}{2\ f_t}$$

> The ultrasound system does not measure blood flow velocity, it determines the Doppler shift. From the Doppler shift and assuming that flow is parallel to the ultrasound beam, the ultrasound system then uses equation 1.3 to display velocity.

The Bernoulli Equation

There is an indirect relationship between velocity, which can be derived via the Doppler equation, and pressure; this relationship is described by the Bernoulli principle. This principle simply states that as the velocity of a moving fluid increases, the pressure within the fluid decreases.

In the presence of a narrowing, the pressure at the narrowing drops, and since velocity and pressure are inversely related, the velocity distal to the narrowing accelerates or increases (Fig. 1.4). This drop in pressure creates a pressure difference

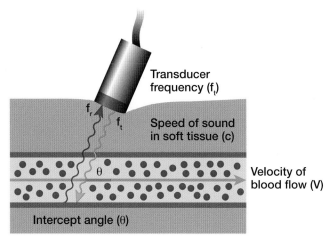

Figure 1.2 The Doppler shift is determined by the transducer frequency (f_t), the received frequency (f_r) the speed of sound in soft tissue (c), blood flow velocity (V) and the angle of intercept between the direction of blood flow and the ultrasound beam (θ).

Doppler Shift 1:
Stationary source (Tx) ⇒ *Moving receiver (RBCs)*

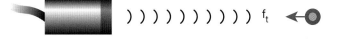

Doppler Shift 2:
Moving source (RBCs) ⇒ Stationary receiver (Tx)

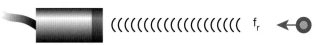

Figure 1.3 This schematic illustrates the "double Doppler shift" between the transducer (Tx) and the red blood cells (RBCs). The first Doppler shift results when there is a change in the frequency between the stationary source (the Tx) and the moving receivers (the RBCs). The second Doppler shift results when there is a change in frequency between the moving source (the RBCs) and the stationary receiver (the Tx).

between the region proximal to the narrowing and the region at the narrowing. The relationship between velocity and the pressure difference between two points is expressed by the Bernoulli Equation:

Equation 1.4

$$\Delta P = \tfrac{1}{2}\rho\ (V_2^2 - V_1^2) + \rho \int^2 \frac{d\vec{v}}{dt} \times d\vec{s} + R(\vec{\eta})$$

| pressure difference | = | convective acceleration | + | flow acceleration | + | viscous friction |

where ΔP = the pressure difference between 2 points
$\quad\quad V_1$ = velocity at proximal location
$\quad\quad V_2$ = velocity at distal location
$\quad\quad \rho$ = mass density of blood
$\quad\quad dv/dt$ = change in velocity over the change in time
$\quad\quad ds$ = distance over which pressure decreases
$\quad\quad R$ = viscous resistance in the vessel
$\quad\quad \eta$ = viscosity

There are three important components to this complex equation: (1) convective acceleration which refers to the rate of change of velocity due to the change of position of fluid particles in a fluid flow, (2) flow acceleration which refers to the pressure drop required to overcome inertial forces between two points and (3) viscous friction which refers to the loss of velocity due to friction between blood cells and vessel walls between two points.

In most clinical situations, the following assumptions can be made: (1) flow acceleration can be ignored as at peak velocities acceleration is zero, (2) viscous friction is negligible as the flow profile within the centre of the lumen is generally flat and losses are minimal toward the centre of the vessel, (3) the mass density ($\tfrac{1}{2}\rho$) for normal blood approximates 4. Therefore, accounting for these assumptions, the Bernoulli equation can be modified to:

Equation 1.5

$$\Delta P = 4\left(V_2^2 - V_1^2\right)$$

Furthermore, assuming that flow velocity proximal to a narrowed orifice (V_1) is insignificant, this equation can be further simplified to:

Equation 1.6

$$\Delta P = 4V^2$$

where ΔP = the pressure difference between 2 points (mm Hg)
$\quad\quad V$ = peak velocity between 2 points (m/s)

Clinical applications of this equation include the estimation of: (1) maximum instantaneous pressure gradients, (2) mean pressure gradients, and (3) intracardiac pressures.

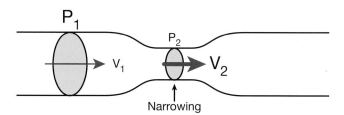

Figure 1.4 According to the Bernoulli principle in order to maintain energy through a narrowing, the velocity through that narrowing must accelerate or increase (V_2). Since pressure and velocity are inversely related, this means that the pressure at the narrowing (P_2) must drop. This creates a pressure difference between the region proximal to the narrowing (P_1) and the region at the narrowing (P_2). This pressure difference is determined by application of the Bernoulli equation.

Measurements of Pressure Gradients

Pressure gradients that are commonly determined by Doppler echocardiography include: (1) the maximum instantaneous pressure gradient and (2) the mean pressure gradient (Fig. 1.5).

Maximum Instantaneous Pressure Gradient

From the peak velocity, the maximum instantaneous pressure gradient (MIPG) is calculated using the simplified Bernoulli equation:

Equation 1.6

$$\Delta P = 4V^2$$

where ΔP = maximum instantaneous pressure gradient
(mm Hg)
V = peak velocity (m/s)

Mean Pressure Gradient

The mean pressure gradient can be determined from the calculation of the arithmetic mean of derived instantaneous pressure gradients obtained at regular intervals throughout the period of flow. Thus, the mean pressure gradient (mPG) is calculated from the following equation:

Equation 1.7

$$mPG = \frac{4\left[\sum (V_1)^2 + (V_2)^2 + (V_3)^2 + \ldots\ldots (V_n)^2\right]}{n}$$

where mPG = mean pressure gradient (mm Hg)
V_1 to V_n = peak velocity measured at various intervals (m/s)
n = number of intervals measured

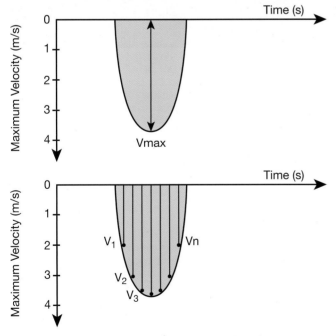

Figure 1.5 From the peak velocity (Vmax) the maximum instantaneous pressure gradient is derived by the application of Equation 1.6 *(top)*. By tracing the spectral Doppler signal, the peak velocities at various intervals throughout the Doppler spectrum are derived (V₁ to Vₙ); from these velocities the mean pressure gradient is then derived by application of Equation 1.7 *(bottom)*.

Limitations of Pressure Gradient Estimations

The most common pitfall encountered in estimating pressure gradients is the underestimation of velocities, and thus pressure gradients, due to suboptimal alignment of the ultrasound beam with blood flow direction. The accuracy of pressure gradients is also dependent on the various assumptions associated with the simplified Bernoulli equation. Confusion can also occur when comparing Doppler derived pressure gradients with the invasively measured pressure gradients.

Underestimation of Doppler Velocities

When there is a large incident angle (poor alignment) between the ultrasound beam and blood flow direction, a significant underestimation of the true velocity occurs. Recall the Doppler equation rearranged to calculate velocity (Eq. 1.2):

$$V\cos\theta = \frac{c\,(\pm \Delta f)}{2\,f_t}$$

From this equation, it can be appreciated that in order for the velocity to be accurately determined, the value of $\cos\theta$ needs to be 1. Cos at zero degrees is equal to 1; a zero degree angle means that there must be parallel alignment between the ultrasound beam and flow direction. Table 1.1 lists the cosine values for various angles and the percentage error at these angles. Note that angles of less than 20^0 will underestimate the true velocity by 6% or less, whereas, greater angles will significantly underestimate the true velocity. It is important to note, however, that even though an angle of 20^0 only slightly underestimates the true velocity, pressure is proportional to the velocity squared; thus, the error in the estimation of the pressure gradient will be much higher.

Significant Flow Acceleration

In most clinical situations, flow acceleration (inertial force) is usually ignored. However, under some conditions, flow acceleration becomes relevant and may significantly contribute to the overall result of the Bernoulli equation. Flow acceleration becomes significant when evaluating certain types of prosthetic valves where a greater increase in the momentum of blood flow is required to open the valve. Flow acceleration cannot be measured by echocardiography. Therefore, in the above conditions, the use of the simplified Bernoulli equation may lead to an underestimation of the true pressure gradient.

Table 1.1 **Cosines for Various Angles and Percentage Error.**

Angle θ (degrees)	Cos θ	Percentage Error (%)
0	1.00	0
10	0.98	2
20	0.94	6
30	0.87	13
40	0.77	23
50	0.64	36
60	0.50	50
70	0.34	66
80	0.17	83
90	0.00	100

Significant Viscous Forces

As for flow acceleration, viscous friction is considered to be negligible in most clinical situations. However, viscous friction may be significant in the presence of long, tubular stenoses. In particular, it has been shown that viscous friction becomes important when the cross-sectional area is less than or equal to 0.1 cm² and when the length of the stenosis is greater than 10 mm. Eccentric wall jets can also result in viscous losses, due to increased viscous friction. As for flow acceleration, viscous friction cannot be measured but by ignoring viscous friction the simplified Bernoulli equation will lead to an underestimation of the true pressure gradient.

Increased Proximal Velocities

The simplified Bernoulli equation also assumes that the velocity proximal to a narrowing is insignificant. When the proximal velocity (V_1) becomes significantly elevated, calculation of the pressure gradient will be overestimated as this proximal velocity is not accounted for in the simplified Bernoulli equation. In these instances, V_1 can no longer be ignored and this value should be taken into account. Hence, the pressure gradient should be "corrected" for the increased V_1 by using the "expanded" Bernoulli equation (Eq. 1.5) (Fig. 1.6).

Clinical situations where V_1 may be significantly increased include aortic stenosis with: (1) an associated high output state such as anaemia, sepsis, and coexistent arteriovenous fistulas, (2) significant aortic regurgitation, or (3) a coexistent subvalvular obstruction (such as hypertrophic obstructive cardiomyopathy). Other situations in which V_1 may be increased include coarctation of the aorta, and stenoses in series such as long coarctations and tunnel-like ventricular septal defects.

> V_1 is considered to be significantly elevated when this velocity is ≥1.2 m/s. Therefore, when the velocity proximal to a narrowing is ≥1.2 m/s the maximum and mean pressure gradients should be corrected using the expanded Bernoulli equation (Eq. 1.5).

Doppler versus Invasively Measured Pressure Gradients

An apparent overestimation of Doppler-derived pressure gradients may occur when instantaneous Doppler gradients are compared with non-instantaneous invasively derived pressure gradients. This is particularly relevant in the presence of aortic valve stenosis and due to a phenomenon called "rapid pressure recovery".

Figure 1.7 illustrates the difference between the invasively measured and the Doppler-derived pressure gradients in aortic stenosis. The invasively-derived pressure gradient is measured as the difference between the peak left ventricular (LV) and the peak aortic pressures; this is referred to as the "peak-to-peak gradient". The peak-to-peak gradient is a non-simultaneous measurement as the peak aortic pressure occurs *after* the peak LV pressure.

The Doppler-derived pressure gradient, on the other hand, is measured as the maximum *instantaneous* pressure gradient obtained from application of the simplified Bernoulli equation. In mild-moderate aortic stenosis, the Doppler-derived pressure gradient is greater than the invasive peak-to-peak pressure gradient. This is because this gradient is derived as the difference between the peak LV pressure and the aortic pressure at this same point in systole and at this point in systole

the aortic pressure is yet to peak (Fig. 1.7, left). In patients with critical aortic stenosis, the Doppler-derived pressure gradient and the invasively-derived peak-to-peak pressure gradient may be very similar due to damping and 'flattening' of the aortic pressure trace (Fig. 1.7, right).

"Rapid pressure recovery" is an important and complex concept that may result in an apparent overestimation of pressure gradients when derived by Doppler and when compared with the invasively measured pressure gradients.

As the name suggests, pressure recovery refers to the recovery of pressure, which occurs downstream from a narrowing. When flow passes through a narrowed orifice, the velocity at the narrowest point (the vena contracta) increases and the pressure at this point drops; once flow has passed through the narrowed orifice, the pressure gradually 'recovers' so that the pressure increases towards its original value (Fig. 1.8, left).

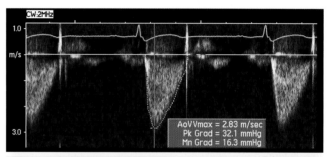

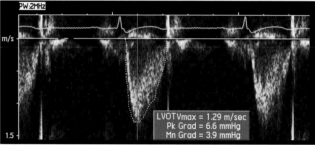

Figure 1.6 The signal on the top is the aortic valve (AV) signal recorded via continuous-wave Doppler; the signal on the bottom was recorded using pulsed-wave Doppler with the sample volume placed within the left ventricular outflow tract (LVOT). When the LVOT velocity is ≥ 1.2 m/s then the maximum and mean AV gradients must be corrected. The corrected maximum pressure gradient (ΔPc) can be calculated from the expanded Bernoulli equation (Eq. 1.5) where V_2 is the peak aortic velocity and V_1 is the peak LVOT velocity:

$$
\begin{aligned}
\Delta Pc &= 4\,(V_2^2 - V_1^2) \\
&= 4\,(2.83^2 - 1.29^2) \\
&= 4\,(8.01 - 1.59) \\
&= 4\,(6.42) \\
&= 25.68 \\
&= 26 \text{ mmHg}
\end{aligned}
$$

Note that the corrected maximum aortic pressure gradient (ΔPc) can also be derived as the difference between the peak AV pressure gradient and the peak LVOT pressure gradient. This is because ΔP = 4 $(V_2^2 - V_1^2)$ is mathematically the same as ΔP = $(4\,V_2^2) - (4\,V_1^2)$; therefore,

$$
\begin{aligned}
\Delta Pc &= (4\,V_2^2) - (4\,V_1^2) \\
&= 32.1 - 6.6 \\
&= 25.5 \\
&= 26 \text{ mmHg}
\end{aligned}
$$

The corrected mean pressure gradient (ΔmPc) can be derived as the difference between the mean AV pressure gradient and the mean LVOT pressure gradient:

$$
\begin{aligned}
\Delta mPc &= (4\,V_2^2) - (4\,V_1^2) \\
&= 16.3 - 3.9 \\
&= 12.4 \\
&= 12 \text{ mmHg}
\end{aligned}
$$

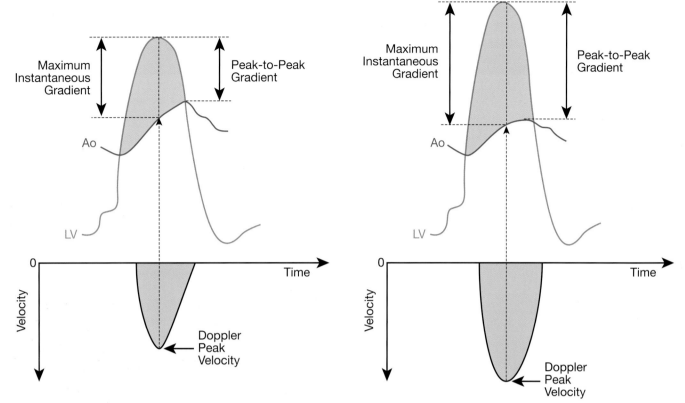

Figure 1.7 The peak left ventricular (LV) and aortic (Ao) pressures occur at different points in systole with the aortic pressure peaking after the LV pressure. The invasive pressure gradient is a non-simultaneous measurement of the difference between the peak LV and peak aortic pressures; thus is termed the "peak-to-peak" gradient. The Doppler-derived pressure gradient measures the maximal **instantaneous** pressure gradient between the peak LV pressure and the aortic pressure at that same point in systole. As a result, in patients with mild-moderate aortic stenosis *(left)*, the Doppler-derived pressure gradient is higher than the peak-to-peak invasively-derived gradient. However, in patients with critical aortic stenosis *(right)*, the Doppler-derived pressure gradient and the invasively-derived peak-to-peak pressure gradient may be very similar due to damping and 'flattening' of the aortic pressure trace. Also observe that the mean pressure gradients *(shaded areas)* derived invasively and via Doppler are comparable and have correlated well in comparative studies.

Figure 1.8 The schematic on the left shows normal pressure recovery while the schematic on the right shows rapid pressure recovery. In the case of aortic stenosis, the invasively measured pressure gradient across the aortic valve is measured from the left ventricle (LV) to the proximal ascending aorta.

In the example of normal pressure recovery (left), the pressure in the LV proximal to the stenotic aortic valve is 170 mm Hg (point A), the pressure drops at the stenotic aortic valve to 90 mm Hg (point B) and the pressure increases slightly to 100 mm Hg in the ascending aorta (point C) and then the pressure recovers somewhat to 120 mm Hg further downstream (point D). In this situation, the pull-back gradient from the LV to the ascending aorta (from points A to C) will be 70 mm Hg and this gradient would be similar to the gradient that would be measured at the aortic valve itself (from points A to B).

In the example of rapid pressure recovery (right), the pressure in the LV proximal to the stenotic aortic valve

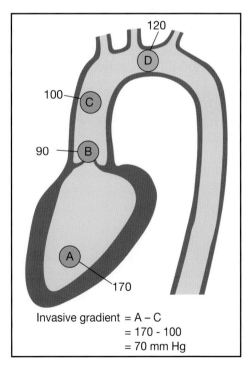

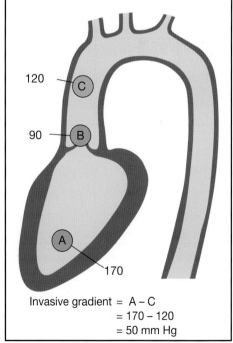

Invasive gradient = A – C
= 170 - 100
= 70 mm Hg

Invasive gradient = A – C
= 170 – 120
= 50 mm Hg

is 170 mm Hg (point A), the pressure drops at the stenotic aortic valve to 90 mm Hg (point B) but now the pressure within the ascending aorta has rapidly recovered to 120 mm Hg (point C). Therefore, the pull-back gradient from the LV to the ascending aorta (from points A to C) is only 50 mm Hg and this gradient is NOT the same as the gradient that would be measured at the aortic valve itself (from points A to B). The Doppler-derived pressure gradient measures the pressure difference between the LV and the aortic valve (points A to B). So in cases where there is rapid pressure recovery, there may be a large discrepancy between the Doppler-derived pressure gradient and the invasively measured pressure gradient.

Table 1.2 **Estimation of Intracardiac Pressures from the Doppler Velocities**

Doppler Signal	Reflects ΔP between the	Intracardiac pressure estimated	Other pressure required	Formula	Additional comments
AR	Aorta and the LV during diastole	LVEDP	AoDP	$LVEDP = AoDP - 4V_{AR}^2$	To estimate the LVEDP, the AR velocity is measured at end diastole.
MR	LV and the LA during systole	LAP	LVSP	$LAP = LVSP - 4V_{MR}^2$	A low velocity MR signal indicates either an elevated LAP or a low LVSP (i.e. hypotension).
				$LAP = AoSP - 4V_{MR}^2$	In the absence of LV outflow tract obstruction or aortic stenosis, the LVSP can be assumed to be the same as the AoSP.
		LVSP	LAP	$LVSP = 4V_{MR}^2 + LAP$	Calculation of the LVSP can be useful in cross-checking gradients across the LVOT (see Chapter 6 – Hypertrophic Cardiomyopathy).
PDA	Aorta and the PA throughout the cardiac cycle	PASP	AoSP	$PASP = AoSP - 4V_{PDA}^2$	Because the pressure in the aorta is greater than the PA pressure throughout the cardiac cycle, the PDA signal is continuous. To estimate the PASP, the PDA velocity is measured at peak systole.
PR	PA and RV during diastole	PAEDP	RVEDP or RAP	$PAEDP = 4V_{PR-ED}^2 + RVEDP$	To estimate the PAEDP, the PR velocity is measured at end diastole (PR-ED).
				$PAEDP = 4V_{PR-ED}^2 + RAP$	In the absence of tricuspid stenosis, the RVEPD can be assumed to be the same as the RAP.
		mPAP	RAP*	$mPAP = 4V_{PR-peak}^2 + RAP$	To estimate the mPAP, the PR velocity is measured at its peak in early diastole (PR-peak) – refer to Chapter 4 for a further explanation of this pressure estimation.
TR	RV and the RA during systole	RVSP	RAP *	$RVSP = 4V_{TR}^2 + RAP$	This is the most common method for estimating the RVSP.
		PASP		$RVSP = PASP$	In the absence of RV outflow tract obstruction or pulmonary stenosis, the RVSP is the same as the PASP.
VSD	LV and the RV during systole	RVSP	LVSP	$RVSP = LVSP - 4V_{VSD}^2$	In the absence of RV outflow tract obstruction or pulmonary stenosis, the RVSP is the same as the PASP.
				$RVSP = AoSP - 4V_{VSD}^2$	In the absence of LV outflow tract obstruction or aortic stenosis, the LVSP can be assumed to be the same as the AoSP.

* Methods of estimating right atrial pressure are described in Chapter 4.
AR = aortic regurgitation; AoDP = aortic diastolic blood pressure; AoSP = aortic systolic blood pressure; LA = left atrium; LAP = left atrial pressure; LV = left ventricle; LVEDP = left ventricular end diastolic pressure; LVSP = left ventricular systolic pressure; mPAP = mean pulmonary artery pressure; MR = mitral regurgitation; PA = pulmonary artery; PAEDP = pulmonary artery end diastolic pressure; PASP = pulmonary artery systolic pressure; PDA = patent ductus arteriosus; PR = pulmonary regurgitation; PR-ED = pulmonary regurgitant velocity at end diastole; PR-peak = pulmonary regurgitant peak velocity; RA = right atrium; RAP = right atrial pressure; RV = right ventricle; RVEDP = right ventricular end diastolic pressure; RVSP = right ventricular systolic pressure; TR = tricuspid regurgitation; VSD = ventricular septal defect.

"Rapid" pressure recovery refers to the rapid recovery of pressure downstream from a narrowed orifice (Fig. 1.8, right). Rapid pressure recovery may become an issue when comparing the invasively measured pressure gradients with the Doppler-derived pressure gradients in certain clinical situations; for example, rapid pressure recovery and apparent overestimation of pressure gradients by Doppler may occur in: (1) patients with aortic stenosis who have a small aortic root, (2) tunnel-like narrowings such as subpulmonary tunnels, subaortic membranes, coarctation of the aorta and hypertrophic obstructive cardiomyopathies and (3) small-sized, mechanical prosthetic valves (also see Chapter 10: Prosthetic Valves).

Intracardiac Pressure Estimation

Doppler echocardiography can be used to noninvasively estimate pressures within the heart. In the presence of a regurgitant valve or a shunt lesion, the peak velocity through these lesions reflects the pressure gradient between two chambers (or great vessels); thus, if the pressure is known or assumed within one of these chambers (or great vessels), then the unknown pressure in the second chamber (or great vessel) can be estimated (Fig. 1.9).

Table 1.2 summarises the basic concepts and measurements needed to estimate various intracardiac pressures. Normal intracardiac pressures are illustrated in Figure 1.10.

Limitations of Intracardiac Pressure Estimation

The accuracy of intracardiac pressure estimation is dependent upon many variables, many of which have already been discussed in the limitations of pressure gradient estimations. In particular, accurate pressure estimation relies on accurate velocity measurements. Other limitations of intracardiac pressure estimation are described below.

Absolute Pressure versus Estimated Pressure

Intracardiac pressures estimated via Doppler calculations provide an estimation of the true intracardiac pressure. Although correlations between the Doppler-derived and the invasively measured intracardiac pressures are excellent, Doppler-derived intracardiac pressures are not exact due to numerous potential sources of errors. Therefore, Doppler-derived intracardiac pressures cannot be substituted for actual intracardiac pressures.

Inaccurate Velocity Measurements

As previously mentioned, poor alignment of the Doppler beam with the direction of blood flow will lead to an underestimation of the peak velocity which will, in turn, underestimate or overestimate the Doppler-derived intracardiac pressure. Underestimation of intracardiac pressures due to underestimation of the Doppler velocity occurs when summing the Doppler-derived pressure with another pressure; for example, in estimating the right ventricular systolic pressure (RVSP) from the tricuspid regurgitant velocity. Overestimation of intracardiac pressures due to underestimation of the Doppler velocity occurs when the Doppler-derived pressure is subtracted from another pressure; for example, in estimating the left ventricular end diastolic pressure (LVEDP) from the aortic regurgitant velocity. Therefore, to minimise error in both the velocity measurement and intracardiac pressure estimation, parallel alignment of the ultrasound beam with blood flow is essential.

This is accomplished by careful Doppler interrogation utilising multiple transducer positions and/or off-axis imaging. Colour Doppler imaging can be extremely valuable in ensuring that there is parallel alignment of the ultrasound beam with flow direction (Fig. 1.11).

In the presence of right ventricular outflow tract (RVOT) obstruction or pulmonary stenosis, the RVSP will be higher than the PASP. Estimation of the PASP in this instance can be determined based on the peak pressure gradient across the RVOT/pulmonary valve. Details regarding the calculation of the PASP in this situation are explained in Chapter 9 – Pulmonary Stenosis.

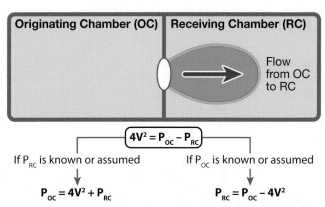

Figure 1.9 When there is flow from one chamber (or great vessel) to another the pressure difference between these two chambers ($P_{OC} - P_{RC}$) is reflected by the Doppler velocity. Thus, using the simplified Bernoulli equation, this velocity can be converted to pressure:

$$4V^2 = P_{OC} - P_{RC}$$

To estimate the pressure in the originating chamber (P_{OC}) the peak Doppler velocity and the pressure in the receiving chamber at the same phase of the cardiac cycle (P_{RC}) are required. Then by simply rearranging the above equation, P_{OC} can be estimated:

$$P_{OC} = 4V^2 + P_{RC}$$

To estimate the pressure in the receiving chamber (P_{RC}) the peak Doppler velocity and the pressure in the originating chamber at the same phase of the cardiac cycle (P_{OC}) are required. Then by simply rearranging the above equation, P_{RC} can be estimated:

$$P_{RC} = P_{OC} - 4V^2$$

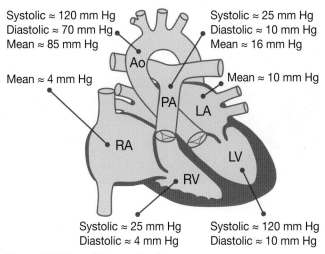

Figure 1.10 Normal Intracardiac Pressures.
Ao = aorta; LA = left atrium; LV = left ventricle; PA = pulmonary artery; RA = right atrium; RV = right ventricle.

Non-simultaneous Measurements

Measurement of the peak systolic velocity across a ventricular septal defect estimates the MIPG between the LV and the right ventricle (RV) during systole. However, the RV and the LV do not contract simultaneously as the RV begins to contract slightly before the LV. Therefore, the MIPG may not equal the true systolic pressure difference between these two ventricles.

Blood Pressure Measurement Errors

Sphygmomanometer errors are typically ± 5 - 10 mmHg; this may therefore result in overestimation or underestimation of intracardiac pressures. In the presence of left ventricular outflow (LVOT) obstruction (such as aortic stenosis), the systolic blood pressure is not the same as the systolic LV pressure, therefore, estimation of intracardiac pressures based on the assumption that the LVSP is the same as the aortic systolic blood pressure will be erroneous.

Estimation of Low Pressures

Estimates of the left atrial pressure (LAP) and the LVEDP are derived from the subtraction of two significantly higher pressures. An elevated LVEDP or LAP is considered to be around 12-15 mm Hg; hence, any small errors in measurement of peak velocity or blood pressure can result in an overestimation or underestimation of these relatively low pressures.

Misinterpretation of Doppler Signals

Differentiating between the tricuspid regurgitant (TR) and mitral regurgitant (MR) signals is crucial if they are to be accurately used in the estimation of intracardiac pressures. 2D guidance and colour flow imaging will help to overcome this problem. Other factors that aid in the differentiation of these two signals include: (1) the peak velocity of the MR signal is usually greater than 4 m/s, (2) the TR signal duration is longer than the MR signal, and (3) the tricuspid inflow velocities are usually lower than the mitral inflow velocities.

Arrhythmias

Multiple Doppler velocity measurements are required to minimise measurement inaccuracies that may occur due to beat-to-beat variation. In sinus rhythm, an average of 2 to 3 beats is recommended. Arrhythmias such as atrial fibrillation require additional averaging (3 to 5 beats) due to increased variation in the R-R interval. It should also be noted that due to cyclic variations in the TR velocity with respiration, the TR velocity should be averaged over a full respiratory cycle.

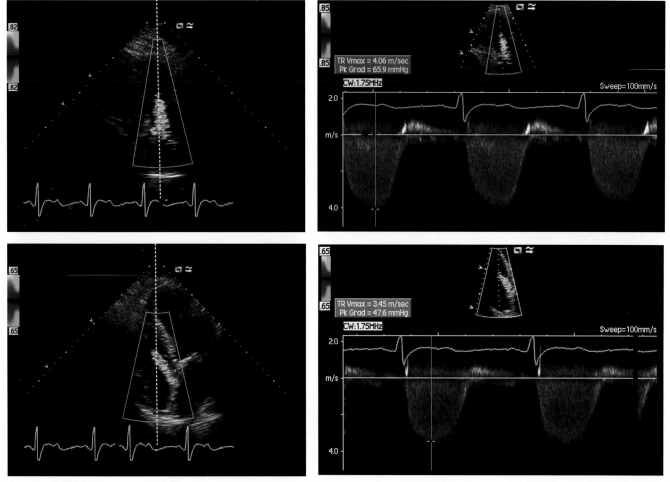

Figure 1.11 The image on the top left was recorded from a parasternal long axis view of the right ventricle. From this image it can be appreciated that the alignment of the Doppler beam (yellow dashed line) is close to parallel with the tricuspid regurgitant (TR) jet. From the resultant continuous-wave Doppler trace shown to the top right, the peak velocity (TR Vmax) is measured at 4.06 m/s.
The image on the bottom left was recorded from an apical 4-chamber view. From this image it can be appreciated that there is a large incident angle between the Doppler beam (yellow dashed line) and the TR jet. From the resultant continuous-wave Doppler trace shown to the bottom right, the peak velocity (TR Vmax) is underestimated at 3.45 m/s.
The velocity that should be reported and used in any subsequent calculations should be the velocity that is obtained with the Doppler beam aligned parallel with flow (that is, the velocity recorded from the top trace); velocities recorded from non-parallel alignments should be ignored.

Volumetric Flow Calculations

Spectral Doppler velocity measurements, in conjunction with 2D echocardiographic imaging, can be reliably used to noninvasively measure volumetric flow at specific locations within the heart and great vessels.

Basic Concepts

Volumetric flow rate calculations are based on simple hydraulic principles which state that the volumetric flow rate (Q) through a tube of a constant diameter is equal to the product of the cross-sectional area (CSA) of the tube and the mean velocity of fluid moving through the tube ($\overline{V}$) providing that the CSA is fixed and that the velocity is constant. Hence, the calculation of volumetric flow rate is expressed by the following equation:

Equation 1.8

$$Q = \overline{V} \times CSA$$

where   Q   = volumetric flow rate (mL/s)
          $\overline{V}$ = mean velocity (cm/s)
          CSA = cross-sectional area (cm²)

However, within the heart blood flow is pulsatile and is, therefore, constantly changing over the cardiac cycle as well as throughout the flow period. In this situation, volumetric flow, rather than flow rate, can be derived as the product of the "integrated" velocity over time and the CSA. The integrated velocity over time or the velocity time integral (VTI) is equal to the area under the spectral Doppler curve (Fig. 1.12):

Equation 1.9

$$VTI = \int_{t_1}^{t_2} v \, dt$$

where   VTI = velocity time integral (cm)
          v   = velocity (cm/s)
          t   = time (s)

So rather than calculating volumetric flow rate, by substituting the VTI for mean velocity, the volumetric flow or stroke volume (SV) is calculated:

Equation 1.10

$$SV = CSA \times VTI$$

where   SV   = stroke volume (mL)
          CSA = cross-sectional area (cm²)
          VTI = velocity time integral (cm)

The most common analogy used to describe SV calculations is that of a volume of a cylinder where the volume of a cylinder is the SV, the height of the cylinder is the VTI and the CSA is derived from the radius or the diameter of the cylinder (Fig. 1.13).

> The CSA is typically derived from πr^2. In the heart the diameter rather than the radius is measured. The CSA can be calculated from the diameter (D) assuming that $\pi = 3.14$ and that the radius = D ÷ 2:
>
> CSA $= 3.14 \times (D \div 2)^2$
> $= 3.14 \times (D^2 \div 4)$
> $= (3.14 \div 4) \times D^2$
> $= 0.785 \times D^2$

Theoretically the SV be calculated from any cardiac site where CSA and VTI can be measured (refer to Chapter 2 for more details).

Clinical applications of SV calculations include: (1) the estimation of the SV and cardiac output, (2) calculation of regurgitant volumes and regurgitant fractions, (3) the calculation of intracardiac shunt ratios and (4) calculation of the stenotic, prosthetic and/or regurgitant orifice areas. This latter application of SV calculations will be discussed separately under the Continuity Principle.

Stroke Volume and Cardiac Output

Stroke volume (SV) is defined as the volume of blood pumped by the heart with each beat. As previously mentioned, SV can be calculated from Equation 1.10 as:

$$SV = CSA \times VTI$$

where   SV   = stroke volume (mL)
          VTI = distance a column of blood travels with each stroke (cm)
          CSA = cross-sectional area (cm²)

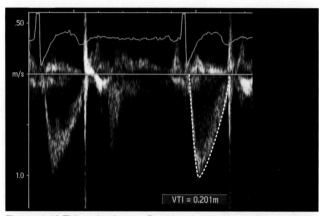

Figure 1.12 This pulsed-wave Doppler signal was recorded with the sample volume within the left ventricular outflow tract (LVOT). The velocity time integral (VTI) is derived by tracing the area under the spectral Doppler curve from the beginning to the end of flow. In this example the VTI is 0.201 m (or 20.1 cm); this means that for each time the heart beats, the column of blood within the LVOT moves 0.201 m (or 20.1 cm).

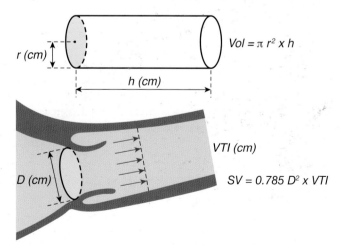

Figure 1.13 Stroke volume calculations are analogous to the calculations of a volume of a cylinder. The volume of a cylinder (V) is derived from the radius (r) and the height (h) of the cylinder *(top)*. Because the VTI is a measure of distance, the stroke volume (SV) can be derived from the VTI and the diameter (d) of a valve annulus or great vessel *(bottom)*.

Cardiac output (CO) is defined as the volume of blood pumped by the heart each minute. Therefore, CO is a product of the SV and the heart rate:

Equation 1.11

$$CO = (SV \times HR) \div 1000$$

where   CO   = cardiac output (L/min^2)
        SV   = stroke volume (mL)
        HR   = heart rate (bpm)
        1000 = conversion of millilitres (mL) to litres (L)

> SV and CO are most commonly estimated from the LVOT (see Chapter 2). This is because the geometry of the LVOT is almost circular and because the flow profile through the LVOT is laminar and flat.

Regurgitant Volumes and Regurgitant Fractions

In the normal heart when there is no valvular regurgitation and no intracardiac shunt, the SV across all four valves will be the same (Fig. 1.14). In the presence of valvular regurgitation, the SV across the leaky (regurgitant) valve will be greater than the SV through a non-leaking (competent) valve. This is because the SV through the regurgitant valve is equal to the volume of blood that leaked through this valve (the regurgitant volume (RV)) plus the usual SV across this valve (Fig. 1.15).

Therefore, the SV across the regurgitant valve can be expressed as:

Equation 1.12

$$SV_{RV} = SV_{CV} + RV$$

where SV_{RV} = stroke volume across the regurgitant valve (mL)
      SV_{CV} = stroke volume through a competent valve (mL)
      RV   = regurgitant volume (mL)

If the SV across the regurgitant valve and across the competent valve can be estimated, the RV can be derived by rearranging Equation 1.12:

Equation 1.13

$$RV = SV_{RV} - SV_{CV}$$

where   RV   = regurgitant volume (mL)
      SV_{RV} = stroke volume across the regurgitant valve (mL)
      SV_{CV} = stroke volume through a competent valve (mL)

The regurgitant fraction (RF) is equal to the percentage of blood that regurgitates back through the leaky valve and this is calculated as:

Equation 1.14

$$RF = RV \div SV_{RV}$$

where   RF   = regurgitant fraction (%)
      RV   = regurgitant volume (mL)
      SV_{RV} = stroke volume across the regurgitant valve (mL)

Theoretically, the RV and RF can be estimated across any incompetent valve. However, most commonly these calculations are performed for aortic and mitral regurgitation only (see Chapters 7 and 8, respectively).

Intracardiac Shunt Ratios

Using the basic principles of SV calculations, it is possible to calculate the ratio of pulmonary venous flow (QP) to systemic venous flow (QS). QP estimates the volume of blood flow to the lungs or returning from the lungs while QS estimates the volume of blood flow travelling to the body or returning from the body (Fig. 1.16).

In the absence of a shunt, QP equals the QS so that the ratio (QP:QS) equals 1. In the presence of an intracardiac shunt, the SV through one side of the heart will be greater than that through the other side of the heart. Whether flow is greater through the left or right sides of the heart is dependent upon the direction of the shunt which is determined by intracardiac pressures. As the pressures in the left heart are usually higher than the pressures in the right heart, shunting is usually left-to-right. The QP:QS shunt ratio is simply derived from the QP and the QS:

Equation 1.15

$$QP{:}QS = SV_{pulmonary} \div SV_{systemic}$$

where $SV_{pulmonary}$ = pulmonary stroke volume (mL)
      $SV_{systemic}$ = systemic stroke volume (mL)

The locations selected for the determination of the QP and the QS will depend upon the location of the shunt. Most commonly, the LVOT and RVOT are used to derive the QP and QS. The calculation of the QP:QS shunt ratios through various shunt lesions is discussed in Chapter 15.

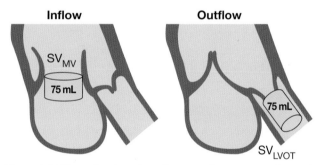

Figure 1.14 Normally when the valves are all competent, the stroke volume through each valve will be the same. In this illustration, during diastole the stroke volume across the mitral valve (SV_{MV}) is 75 mL; this will be the same as the stroke volume across the left ventricular outflow tract (SV_{LVOT}) during systole.

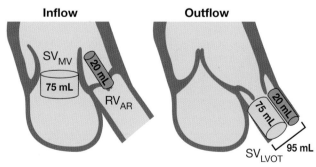

Figure 1.15 This schematic illustrates the regurgitant volume in the case of aortic regurgitation (AR). During diastole, the AR regurgitant volume (RV_{AR}) enters the left ventricle to combine with the normal inflow stroke volume across the mitral valve (SV_{MV}). Therefore during systole, the stroke volume across the left ventricular outflow tract (SV_{LVOT}) is the sum of the mitral inflow stroke volume (SV_{MR}) the AR regurgitant volume (RV_{AR}).

Limitations of Stroke Flow Calculations

Assumptions of Stroke Flow Calculations

As described above, SV calculations are based on a simple hydraulic formula that determines the volumetric flow rate through a cylindrical tube under steady flow conditions. Therefore, in applying this concept to the heart, the following assumptions are made: (1) flow is occurring in a rigid, circular tube, (2) there is a uniform velocity across the vessel, (3) the derived CSA is circular, (4) CSA remains constant throughout the period of flow, and (5) the pulsed-wave (PW) Doppler sample volume remains in a constant position throughout the period of flow. However, blood vessels are elastic (not rigid) and annular diameters may change throughout the period of flow. Furthermore, while the left and right ventricular outflow tracts assume a circular configuration, the same may not be said for the atrioventricular valves, which are more elliptical in shape.

Error in VTI Measurements

Technical errors in the VTI measurements may also occur. For example, non-parallel alignment between the ultrasound beam and blood flow direction will lead to an underestimation of the velocities.

Failure to correctly trace the VTI through the modal velocity can also lead to an overestimation of the VTI. The VTI should be traced along the modal velocity which represents the velocity at which the majority of RBCs are travelling (Fig. 1.17).

Incorrect placement of the PW sample volume for VTI measurement (the sample volume must be placed at the same location as the diameter measurement), incorrect gain settings (overgain often leads to 'overtracing' of signals), and incorrect filter settings (if the filter setting is too high low velocity signals may be missed) will also result in erroneous VTI measurements.

Furthermore, measurement of too few beats can also produce inaccuracies. For sinus rhythm it is recommended that 2-3 beats are measured and averaged while for atrial fibrillation, 3-5 beats should be measured and averaged.

Error in Diameter Measurement

Erroneous measurement of the diameter will be reflected in the accuracy of the calculated CSA and, hence, the SV. Commonly encountered technical errors in the diameter measurement include: (1) measurement of the diameter during the wrong phase of the cardiac cycle (measurements must be performed at the time of flow through that site), (2) inconsistent annulus measurements, and (3) difficulty in measuring the RVOT. In particular, as axial resolution is superior to lateral resolution annular measurements should be performed in the axial plane; however, measurement of the RVOT in the axial plane is not possible due to the orientation of the RVOT in the views used to image this structure. When calculating the CSA from the diameter measurement it is assumed that the valve annulus has a circular geometry and that the annular area remains constant throughout the flow period.

QP = pulmonary venous volume *to* +/- from lungs

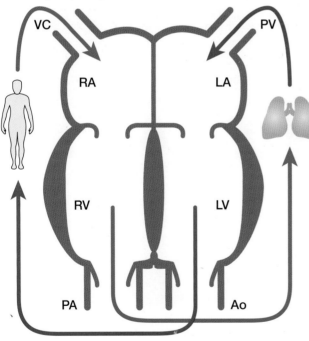

QS = systemic volume *to* +/- from body

Figure 1.16 Pulmonary venous flow (QP) is the flow to or returning from the lungs while the systemic venous flow (QS) is the flow to or returning from the body.
Ao = aorta; LA = left atrium; LV = left ventricle; PA = pulmonary artery; PV = pulmonary veins; RA = right atrium; RV = right ventricle; VC = vena cava.

Area of an Ellipse
The area of an ellipse can be determined by the following equation:

Equation 1.16: $$Area = (\pi\, a\, b) \div 4$$

where Area = area of an ellipse (cm²)
    a   = diameter in one plane (cm)
    b   = diameter in the plane orthogonal to a (cm)

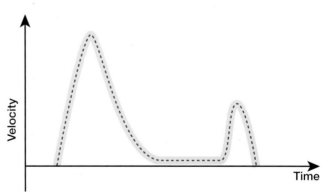

Figure 1.17 This schematic demonstrates where the modal velocity would be traced on a transmitral PW Doppler profile. The modal velocity (*red dotted line*) is traced through the centre of the PW Doppler spectral band (*blue line*). The modal velocity represents that velocity at which the majority of red blood cells are travelling.

Continuity Principle

Basic Concepts

The continuity principle is based on the conservation of mass principle which can be applied to any specified region of flow. This principle states that providing there is no loss of fluid from the system, whatever mass flows in must also flow out. Therefore, the continuity principle states that when the volumetric flow rate (Q) is maintained, volumetric flow rate proximal to the narrowing (Q_1) is equal to the volumetric flow rate through the narrowed orifice (Q_2):

Equation 1.17

$$Q_1 = Q_2$$

where Q_1 = volumetric flow rate proximal to narrowing (mL/s)
        Q_2 = volumetric flow rate through narrowing (mL/s)

As per Equation 1.8, Q is equal to the product of the mean velocity ($\overline{V}$) and the CSA:

$$Q = \overline{V} \times CSA$$

So if $Q_1 = Q_2$ then:

Equation 1.18

$$CSA_1 \times \overline{V}_1 = CSA_2 \times \overline{V}_2$$

where CSA_1 = cross-sectional area proximal to the narrowing (cm^2)
        $\overline{V}_1$ = mean velocity proximal to the narrowing (cm/s)
        CSA_2 = cross-sectional area of the narrowing (cm^2)
        $\overline{V}_2$ = mean velocity across the narrowing (cm/s)

It can be appreciated that as the CSA decreases, the mean velocity must increase to maintain a constant flow rate.

There are two methods that can be used to calculate the area of a narrowed orifice using the continuity principle in echocardiography: (1) the SV method and (2) the proximal isovelocity surface area (PISA) method.

Stroke Volume Method

As the name suggests, the SV method is based on the calculation of the SV using the CSA and the VTI. If volumetric flow is maintained, the SV proximal to the narrowing (SV_1) is equal to the SV through the narrowed orifice (SV_2):

Equation 1.19

$$SV_1 = SV_2$$

where SV_1 = stroke volume proximal to the narrowing (mL)
        SV_2 = stroke volume through the narrowing (mL)

So if $SV_1 = SV_2$ then:

Equation 1.20

$$CSA_1 \times VTI_1 = CSA_2 \times VTI_2$$

where CSA_1 = cross-sectional area proximal to the narrowing (cm^2)
        VTI_1 = velocity time integral proximal to the narrowing (cm)
        CSA_2 = cross-sectional area of the narrowing (cm^2)
        VTI_2 = velocity time integral across the narrowing (cm)

Therefore, as the CSA decreases, the VTI must increase to maintain a constant flow rate (Fig. 1.18).

Proximal Isovelocity Surface Area (PISA) Method

The PISA method is based on the calculation of the volumetric flow rate using colour Doppler imaging and spectral Doppler velocities.

Based on this principle, the volumetric flow rate proximal to a narrowed orifice can be determined by assuming that as flow converges toward this narrowed orifice, it accelerates in a laminar manner forming a flow convergence zone. This flow convergence zone is comprised of a series of concentric

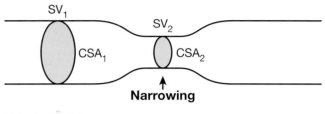

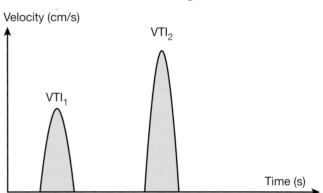

Figure 1.18 When volumetric flow is maintained, the volumetric flow on each side of the narrowing is equal ($SV_1 = SV_2$). Stroke volume (SV) is the product of the cross-sectional area (CSA) and the velocity time integral (VTI). Therefore, $CSA_1 \times VTI_1 = CSA_2 \times VTI_2$. Hence, as the CSA decreases, the VTI must increase to maintain a constant volumetric flow.

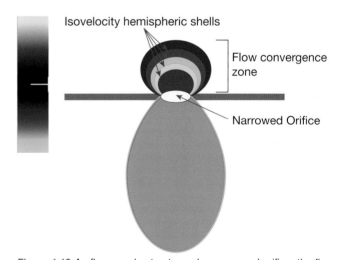

Figure 1.19 As flow accelerates towards a narrowed orifice, the flow convergence zone proximal to the narrowing is comprised of a series of isovelocity hemispheric shells of increasing velocity and decreasing surface area. Each hemispheric shell will have a particular velocity relative to its surface area and via colour Doppler imaging the different velocities of these hemispheric shells is depicted by different colours. Note that the proximal flow convergence dome is not truly hemispherical in shape; there is an area of 'drop-out' of colour at the sides of the dome close to the narrowed orifice. This is explained by the Doppler equation and the angle of intercept between the Doppler beam and flow direction. When flow is at 90^0 to the Doppler beam, no Doppler shift will be detected (cos at 90^0 = 0). As flow occurring at the side of the dome is aligned perpendicular to the ultrasound beam no flow is displayed in this region.

hemispheric shells of uniform velocity (isovelocities). As flow advances closer to the narrowed orifice, the area of each hemispheric shell decreases and the velocity of each shell increases. These isovelocity hemispheric shells are identified using colour Doppler imaging (Fig. 1.19). The flow rate at any hemispheric shell proximal to the narrowed orifice is derived as a product of its surface area and the velocity at this hemispheric shell. The surface area of the hemispheric shell is derived from the proximal flow convergence radius (r) which is identified as the distance from the first aliased velocity (the blue-red interface) to the narrowed orifice. The velocity at this proximal flow convergence radius is identified by the Nyquist limit as depicted on the colour velocity bar (V_N) (Fig. 1.20). Thus, flow rate proximal to a narrowed orifice (Q_1) is expressed by the following equation:

Equation 1.21

$$Q_1 = 2\pi\, r^2 \times V_N$$

where Q_1 = volumetric flow rate (mL/s)

$2\pi\, r^2$ = surface area of a hemispheric shell derived from the proximal flow convergence radius [r] (cm²)

V_N = velocity at the radial distance of the hemispheric shell (colour aliased velocity or Nyquist limit) (cm/s)

Based on the continuity principle, blood passing through a given hemispheric shell must ultimately pass through the narrowed orifice. In other words, the flow rate through any given hemispheric shell must equal the flow rate through the narrowed orifice; this relationship can be expressed by the following equation:

Equation 1.22

$$2\pi\, r^2 \times V_N = EOA \times V_{max}$$

where $2\pi r^2$ = surface area of a hemispheric shell derived from the proximal flow convergence radius [r] (cm²)

V_N = velocity at the radial distance of the hemispheric shell (colour aliased velocity or Nyquist limit) (cm/s)

EOA = effective orifice area (cm²)

V_{max} = peak velocity through the narrowed orifice (cm/s)

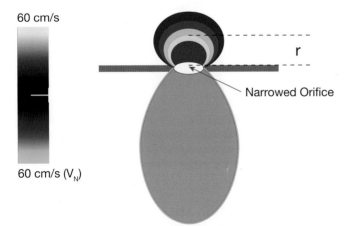

60 cm/s

r

Narrowed Orifice

60 cm/s (V_N)

Figure 1.20 In this schematic, flow is away from the transducer. The first aliased velocity is identified as the velocity at which flow changes from blue to red. By measuring the radial distance (r) from the narrowed orifice to this first aliased velocity, the surface area of this hemispheric shell can be derived using $2\pi r^2$. The velocity of this hemispheric shell is identified as the colour Nyquist limit (V_N) at the bottom of the colour bar. Thus, the flow rate proximal to the narrowed orifice can be derived using Equation 1.21: $Q_1 = 2\pi r^2 \times V_N$.

Clinical applications of the continuity principle include the calculation of the stenotic, prosthetic and/or regurgitant orifice areas.

Calculation of Valve Areas

Stroke Volume Method

Based on Equation 1.20, if the CSA proximal to the valve (CSA_1), the VTI proximal to the valve (VTI_1) and the VTI across the valve (VTI_2) are measured, the unknown valve area (CSA_2) can be derived by simply rearranging this equation:

Equation 1.23

$$CSA_2 = (CSA_1 \times VTI_1) \div VTI_2$$

where CSA_2 = cross-sectional area of the stenotic/prosthetic valve (cm²)

CSA_1 = cross-sectional area proximal to the stenotic/prosthetic valve (cm²)

VTI_1 = velocity time integral proximal to the stenotic/prosthetic valve (cm)

VTI_2 = VTI across the stenotic/prosthetic valve (cm)

To simplify this concept even further, by assuming that the stroke volume through the LVOT and across a stenotic or prosthetic valve is the same, the area of the stenotic or prosthetic valve can then be derived as:

Equation 1.24

$$EOA = (CSA_{LVOT} \times VTI_{LVOT}) \div VTI_V$$

where EOA = effective orifice area of the stenotic/prosthetic valve (cm²)

CSA_{LVOT} = cross-sectional area of the LVOT (cm²)

VTI_{LVOT} = velocity time integral of the LVOT (cm)

VTI_V = VTI across the stenotic/prosthetic valve (cm)

PISA Method

The PISA principle is most commonly used to calculate regurgitant orifice areas. However, in theory, this principle can also be used to calculate the effective orifice area (EOA) of a stenotic valve, a ventricular septal defect or a patent ductus arteriosus.

Based on Equation 1.22, if the radius (r), the velocity at the Nyquist limit (V_N) and the peak velocity across the valve (V_{max}) are measured, the unknown valve area (EOA) can be derived by simply rearranging this equation:

Equation 1.25

$$EOA = (2\pi r^2 \times V_N) \div V_{max}$$

where EOA = effective orifice area (cm²)

$2\pi r^2$ = surface area of the hemispheric shell derived from the flow convergence radius [r] proximal to the stenotic valve (cm²)

V_N = colour Nyquist limit at the radial distance of the hemispheric shell (cm/s)

V_{max} = peak velocity across the stenotic valve (cm/s)

Technical Tip

Most errors arising from the calculations using the PISA principle occur due to failure to convert velocity units from m/s to cm/s.

Calculation of the Regurgitant Orifice Area

The effective regurgitant orifice area (EROA) can be derived by application of the PISA principle. Based on Equation 1.22, if the radius (r), the velocity at the Nyquist limit (V_N) and the peak velocity of the regurgitant jet (V_{max}) are measured, the EROA can be derived by simply rearranging this equation:

Equation 1.26

$$EROA = (2\pi r^2 \times V_N) \div V_{max}$$

where EROA = effective regurgitant orifice area (cm²)

$2\pi r^2$ = surface area of the hemispheric shell derived from the flow convergence radius [r] proximal to the regurgitant valve (cm²)

V_N = colour Nyquist limit at the radial distance of the hemispheric shell (cm/s)

V_{max} = peak velocity of the regurgitant jet (cm/s)

Limitations of the Continuity Principle for Area Calculations

Stroke Volume Method

Determination of CSA

Estimation of valve areas via the SV method requires the calculation of the CSA proximal to the valve. CSA is derived from diameter measurements. Therefore, any error in this measurement will affect the accuracy of both the CSA and the derived valve area.

Technical errors which may occur in the diameter measurement include: (1) measurement of the diameter during the wrong phase of the cardiac cycle (measurements must be performed at the time of flow through that site), (2) inconsistent annulus measurements, and (3) difficulty in measuring the RVOT. In particular, as axial resolution is superior to lateral resolution annular measurements should be performed in the axial plane; however, measurement of the RVOT in the axial plane is not possible due to the orientation of the RVOT with respect to 2D echocardiographic images. As previously mentioned, it is also assumed that the valve annulus has a circular geometry which remains constant throughout the period of flow.

Errors in VTI Measurements

Technical errors in the VTI measurements may also occur. For example, non-parallel alignment between the ultrasound beam and blood flow direction will lead to an underestimation of the velocities.

Failure to correctly trace the VTI through the modal velocity can also lead to an overestimation of the VTI. The VTI should be traced along the modal velocity which represents the velocity at which the majority of RBCs are travelling (refer to Fig. 1.17).

Incorrect placement of the PW sample volume for VTI measurement (the sample volume must be placed at the same location as the diameter measurement), incorrect gain settings (overgain often leads to 'overtracing' of signals), and incorrect filter settings (if the filter setting is too high low velocity signals may be missed) will also result in erroneous VTI measurements.

Furthermore, measurement of too few beats can also produce inaccuracies. For sinus rhythm it is recommended that 2-3 beats are measured and averaged while for atrial fibrillation, 3-5 beats should be measured and averaged.

Inaccurate Peak Velocity Measurements

As previously mentioned, non-parallel alignment of the Doppler beam with the direction of blood flow will lead to an underestimation of the peak velocity which will, in turn, overestimate the EOA. Therefore, ensuring parallel alignment of the ultrasound beam with the direction of blood flow is essential. This is accomplished by careful Doppler interrogation utilising multiple transducer positions and/or off-axis imaging. Colour Doppler imaging can be extremely valuable in ensuring that there is parallel alignment of the ultrasound beam with flow direction.

Differential Flow

Calculation of the EOA via the SV method requires that the SV proximal to the valve and the SV across the valve are equal. Therefore, when using the SV from the LVOT in the EOA calculation, the SV across the LVOT must be the same as the SV across a stenotic or prosthetic valve. For example, the EOA of a prosthetic mitral valve replacement (MVR) cannot be calculated via this method when there is coexistent MR. In this situation, the stroke volume across the LVOT and across the MVR are no longer equal; the stroke volume across the MVR includes the mitral regurgitant volume as well as the forward stroke volume.

PISA Method

Radius Measurements

Accurate calculations of a narrowed orifice area by the PISA technique are dependent upon the precise measurement of the radial distance between the narrowed orifice and the first aliased velocity.

As the EOA and EROA are derived by squaring the radius (Equations 1.25 and 1.26, respectively), failure to measure the correct radius may result in a significant underestimation or overestimation of the EOA and EROA.

In addition, the relatively small size of the proximal convergence region to the field of view may limit the accuracy of this measurement. Methods that may be employed to overcome this potential limitation include magnification or 'zooming' of the proximal flow convergence region and reduction of the aliasing velocity. Reduction of the aliased velocity effectively increases the radius; decreasing the aliased velocity can be achieved by shifting the colour baseline toward the direction of flow. This baseline shift results in the magnification of the proximal flow convergence region, a reduction of the aliasing velocity, and an increase in the radial distance (Fig. 1.21), which will improve measurement accuracy. However, it should also be noted that reducing the aliased velocity also has limitations of its own. At very low aliasing velocities, overestimation of the mean velocity displayed by the colour Doppler may result due to suppression of low velocities by colour wall filters; this will result in an overestimation of the radius measurement.

Inaccurate Peak Velocity Measurements

As previously mentioned, non-parallel alignment of the Doppler beam with the direction of blood flow will lead to an underestimation of the peak velocity which will, in turn, overestimate the EOA and EROA.

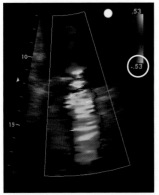 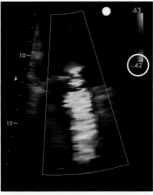 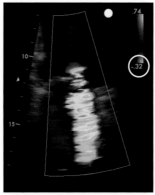 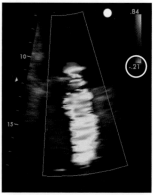

Figure 1.21 These still frame images were obtained from a patient with mitral regurgitation (MR). In the far left image, the baseline is set in the centre of the colour bar and the colour Nyquist limit is 0.53 m/s. As the colour baseline in shifted downwards in the direction of flow (middle and right images), the colour Nyquist limit decreases leading to a magnification of the proximal flow convergence region (PISA dome). As a result, the PISA radius is also magnified and this will improve measurement accuracy.

Multiple Jets

When there are multiple regurgitant jets, the EROA is usually calculated for the largest jet. It is important to note that in the case of multiple jets, the calculated values of the EROA are not additive.

Flow Constraint

In mitral stenosis and with eccentric regurgitant jets, constraint of flow may occur due to structures encroaching on the proximal flow convergence region which prohibits the formation of hemispheric contours by effectively pushing the contours out from the orifice (Fig. 1.22). As a result, the PISA dome is no longer hemispherical and measurement of the PISA radius in this situation will lead to an overestimation of the EOA or EROA.

When proximal flow is constrained the true flow can be obtained by correcting for the angle (α) between the two structures encroaching on the flow region. Specifically, an angle correction factor of α/180 has been derived to account for the altered shape of the constrained flow profile. Angle α is measured as the minimum angle between the two sides of the proximal flow region. Thus, calculation of the corrected EOA (or EROA) when there is flow constraint is derived as the product of the EOA (or EROA) and α/180:

Equation 1.27

$$EOAc = EOA \times (\alpha \div 180)$$

where EOAc = corrected effective orifice area [or EROA] (cm²)

EOA = effective orifice area [or EROA] (cm²) calculated using equations 1.25 [or 1.26]

α = minimum angle between the two sides of the proximal flow convergence field

Assumption of Concentric Hemispheric Shells

The PISA theory is based upon the assumption that the isovelocity surface areas appear as concentric hemispheric shells. In fact, the configuration of the PISA dome changes as the aliasing velocity changes. For example, the convergence zone is flatter with higher aliasing velocities and becomes more elliptical with lower aliasing velocities. Therefore, calculation of the flow rate proximal to a narrowed orifice (based on the assumption that flow converges towards the regurgitant orifice in hemispheric shells) may result in the underestimation or overestimation of the EOA or EROA.

Regurgitant Valve Motion through the Regurgitant Flow Period

The mitral and tricuspid valve orifices are not static throughout systole. Therefore, dynamic changes in the location of the regurgitant orifice may occur during systole resulting in changes to the proximal convergence region. In addition, the movement of the regurgitant orifice relative to the ultrasound beam may affect the calculation of the proximal flow convergence area. This concept is based on the fact that movement of the regurgitant orifice relative to the transducer occurs at a detectable velocity (the orifice velocity). For example, when the regurgitant orifice moves away from the transducer, the orifice velocity is added to the actual blood flow velocity resulting in a falsely large flow convergence region proximal to the regurgitant orifice; thus, a larger radius is created resulting in the overestimation of the EROA. Conversely, when the regurgitant orifice moves toward the transducer, the orifice velocity is subtracted from the actual flow velocity resulting in a smaller radius and an underestimation of the EROA. This effect may be enhanced by low aliasing velocities and further emphasises the importance of the correct selection of the aliasing velocity for the radius measurement.

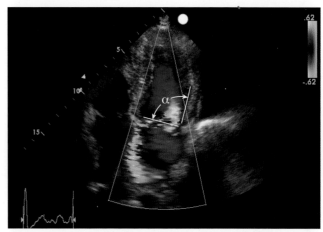

Figure 1.22 From this apical 4-chamber view it can be appreciated that the proximal convergence zone of the mitral regurgitant jet is not hemispherical. This effect is produced by the constraint of proximal flow convergence by the anterolateral wall of the left ventricle. Flow constraint prevents the formation of concentric hemispheres and pushes the contours outwards from the regurgitant orifice. From the measurement of angle α, the corrected EROA can be calculated as the product of the EROA and α/180.

α = proximal convergence angle.

Mitral Valve Prolapse

Erroneous calculation of the EROA may also occur in patients with mitral valve prolapse (MVP). For example, the PISA radius may increase progressively over the systolic period. Hence, calculation of the EROA using the largest PISA radius measured at late systole and the peak MR velocity which occurs at mid-late systole will result in an overestimation of the EROA. To avoid overestimation of the EROA, measurement of the PISA radius should be performed at the same time as the peak MR velocity; that is, in mid-late systole.

In addition, with MVP regurgitation may be confined to the latter half of systole. Calculation of the EROA assumes that the EROA is consistent throughout the systolic period. Therefore, in the case of mid-late systolic mitral regurgitation (MR), the EROA will overestimate the MR severity (see Chapter 8).

Left Ventricular Outflow Tract Flow

The position selected for measurement of the PISA radius is crucial to the accurate calculation of the EOA and EROA. This is especially relevant in the assessment of MR where systolic flow through the LVOT into the aorta may contaminate the flow field. Therefore, if a distance too great from the proximal flow convergence region is selected; contribution of LVOT flow may exaggerate the flow convergence region proximal to the MR orifice. Furthermore, the close proximity of the LVOT to the MR orifice may also alter the overall shape of the flow convergence region.

Effective Orifice Area versus Anatomical Orifice Area

Finally, it is important to remember that valve areas and regurgitant orifice areas calculated via the SV or PISA methods are measurements of the **"effective orifice area"** and this EOA will be smaller than the true anatomical area (Fig. 1.23). This is because the EOA is calculated downstream from the anatomical valve area at the vena contracta. The vena contracta is the narrowest part of the jet downstream from the narrowed orifice; this narrowing of the jet is created as blood streamlines through the narrowed orifice.

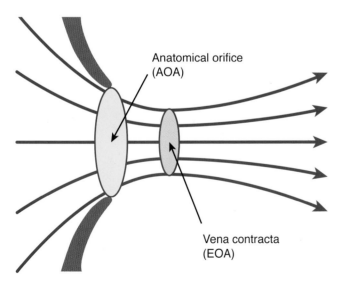

Figure 1.23 This schematic illustrates flow through a narrowed orifice. The vena contracta refers to the narrowest region of the jet which is located downstream from the true anatomical orifice. The area at the vena contracta, which is the area derived via the stroke volume and PISA methods, correlates with the effective orifice area (EOA). Note that the EOA area is smaller than the true anatomical orifice area (AOA).

> ### Key Points
>
> **Pressure Estimation and Pressure Gradients**
> - The simplified Bernoulli equation ($\Delta P = 4\,V^2$) is used to estimate the maximum and mean pressure gradients and intracardiac pressures.
> - Intracardiac pressures can be estimated when the velocity between two chambers is measured and when the pressure within one of those chambers is known or estimated.
> - The main limitation of pressure gradient estimation is non-parallel alignment of the ultrasound beam with flow.
>
> **Volumetric Flow Calculations**
> - Stroke volume (SV) can be estimated from the product of the CSA and VTI measured at the valve annulus.
> - From this calculation cardiac output, regurgitant volumes and shunt ratios can be estimated.
> - The primary limitations of these calculations include technical limitations relating to the measurement of annular diameters which are used to calculate the CSA and the measurement of the VTI.
>
> **Continuity Principle**
> - Based on the "what goes in must come out" concept.
> - By comparing the SV or volumetric flow rate (Q) between two sites the effective orifice area (EOA) of stenotic, prosthetic or regurgitant valves can be estimated.
> - Two methods can be used to determine the EOA: (1) SV method and (2) proximal isovelocity surface area (PISA) method.
> - The major limitations of the SV method are listed above. The primary limitations of the PISA method include technical factors such as measurement error of the proximal flow convergence radius and inaccurate peak velocity measurements. Other limitations of this method include flow constraint assumptions relating to the PISA principle.

Further Reading (listed in alphabetical order)

Determination of Pressure Gradients

Baumgartner H, Khan S, DeRobertis M, Czer L, Maurer G. Discrepancies between Doppler and catheter gradients in aortic prosthetic valves in vitro. A manifestation of localized pressure gradients and pressure recovery. *Circulation.* 1990; Oct; 82(4):1467-75.

Baumgartner H, Stefenelli T, Niederberger J, Schima H, Maurer G. 'Overestimation' of catheter gradients by Doppler ultrasound in patients with aortic stenosis: a predictable manifestation of pressure recovery. *J Am Coll Cardiol.* 1999; May; 33(6):1655-61.

Levine RA, Jimoh A, Cape EG, McMillan S, Yoganathan AP, Weyman AE. Pressure recovery distal to a stenosis: potential cause of gradient "overestimation" by Doppler echocardiography. *J Am Coll Cardiol.* 1989; Mar 1; 13(3):706-15.

Teirstein PS, Yock PG and Popp RL. The accuracy of Doppler ultrasound measurement of pressure gradients across irregular, dual, and tunnel-like obstructions to blood flow. *Circulation.* 1985; Sep;72(3):577-84.

Yoganathan AP, Valdes-Cruz LM, Schmidt-Dohna J, Jimoh A, Berry C, Tamura T, Sahn DJ. Continuous-wave Doppler velocities and gradients across fixed tunnel obstructions: studies in vitro and in vivo. Circulation. 1987; Sep;76(3):657-66.

Yoganathan AP, Cape EG, Sung HW, Williams FP, Jimoh A. Review of hydrodynamic principles for the cardiologist: applications to the study of blood flow and jets by imaging techniques. *J Am Coll Cardiol.* 1988; Nov; 12(5):1344-53.

Intracardiac Pressure Estimation

Ge Z, Zhang Y, Fan D, Zhang M, Duran CM. Simultaneous measurement of left atrial pressure gradients by Doppler echocardiography and catheterization. *Int J Cardiol.* 1992; Nov; 37(2):243-51.

Ge Z, Zhang Y, Kang W, Fan D, An F. Noninvasive evaluation of interventricular pressure gradient across ventricular septal defect: a simultaneous study of Doppler echocardiography and cardiac catheterization. *Am Heart J.* 1992; Jul; 124(1):176-82.

Ge Z, Zhang Y, Fan D, Kang W, Hatle L, Duran C. Simultaneous measurement of pulmonary artery diastolic pressure by Doppler echocardiography and catheterization with patent ductus arteriosus. *Am Heart J.* 1993; Jan;125(1):263-6

Ge ZM, Zhang Y, Fan DS, Zhang M, Fan JX, Zhao YX. Quantification of left-sided intracardiac pressures and gradients using mitral and aortic regurgitant velocities by simultaneous left and right catheterization and continuous-wave Doppler echocardiography. *Clin Cardiol.* 1993; Dec;16(12):863-70.

Lei MH, Chen JJ, Ko YL, Cheng JJ, Kuan P, Lien WP. Reappraisal of quantitative evaluation of pulmonary regurgitation and estimation of pulmonary artery pressure by continuous wave Doppler. *Cardiology.* 1995; 86(3):249-56.

Continuity Principle (Valve Stenosis)

Baumgartner H, Hung J, Bermejo J, Chambers JB, Evangelista A, Griffin BP, Iung B, Otto CM, Pellikka PA, Quiñones M; American Society of Echocardiography; European Association of Echocardiography. Echocardiographic assessment of valve stenosis: EAE/ASE recommendations for clinical practice. *J Am Soc Echocardiogr.* 2009; Jan; 22(1):1-23

Proximal Isovelocity Surface Area (PISA) Principles

Enriquez-Sarano M, Tajik AJ, Bailey KB and Seward JB. Color flow imaging compared with quantitative Doppler assessment of severity of mitral regurgitation: influence of eccentricity of jet and mechanism of regurgitation. *J Am Coll Cardiol.* 1993; Apr;21(5):1211-9.

Enriquez-Sarano M, Miller FA Jr, Hayes SN, Bailey KR, Tajik AJ, Seward JB. Effective mitral regurgitant orifice area: Clinical use and pitfalls of the proximal isovelocity surface area method. *J Am Coll Cardiol.* 1995; Mar 1;25(3):703-9.

Enriquez-Sarano M, Sinak LJ, Tajik AJ, Bailey KR, Seward JB. Changes in effective regurgitant orifice throughout systole in patients with mitral valve prolapse. A clinical study using the proximal isovelocity surface area method. *Circulation.* 1995; Nov 15; 92(10):2951-8.

Eren M, Dagdeviren B, Bolca O, Polat M, Gürlertop Y, Norgaz T, Tezel T. Proximal Isovelocity Surface Area (PISA) as a noninvasive method for the estimation of the shunt quantification in perimembranous ventricular septal defects. *Echocardiography.* 2001 Feb;18(2):137-47.

Francis DP, Willson K, Ceri Davies L, Florea VG, Coats AJ, Gibson DG. True shape and area of proximal isovelocity surface area (PISA) when flow convergence is hemispherical in valvular regurgitation. *Int J Cardiol.* 2000 May 31;73(3):237-42.

Kronzon I, Tunick PA and Rosenzweig BP. Quantification of left-to-right shunt in patent ductus arteriosus with the PISA method. *J Am Soc Echocardiogr.* 2002; Apr;15(4):376-8.

Lancellotti P, Tribouilloy C, Hagendorff A, Moura L, Popescu BA, Agricola E, Monin JL, Pierard LA, Badano L, Zamorano JL; European Association of Echocardiography recommendations for the assessment of valvular regurgitation. Part 1: aortic and pulmonary regurgitation (native valve disease). *Eur J Echocardiogr.* 2010; Apr;11(3):223-44.

Vandervoort PM, Rivera JM, Mele D, Palacios IF, Dinsmore RE, Weyman AE, Levine RA, Thomas JD. Application of color Doppler flow mapping to calculate effective regurgitant orifice area. *Circulation.* 1993; Sep;88(3):1150-6.

Yamachika S, Reid CL, Savani D, Meckel C, Paynter J, Knoll M, Jamison B, Gardin JM. Usefulness of color Doppler proximal isovelocity surface area method in quantitating valvular regurgitation. *J Am Soc Echocardiogr.* 1997; Mar; 10(2):159-68.

Zoghbi WA, Enriquez-Sarano M, Foster E, Grayburn PA, Kraft CD, Levine RA, Nihoyannopoulos P, Otto CM, Quiñones MA, Rakowski H, Stewart WJ, Waggoner A, Weissman NJ; American Society of Echocardiography. Recommendations for evaluation of the severity of native valvular regurgitation with two-dimensional and Doppler echocardiography. *J Am Soc Echocardiogr.* 2003; Jul;16(7):777-802.

Ventricular Systolic Function

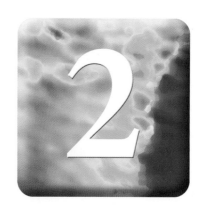

Ventricular Anatomy

Ventricular Geometry

The shape of the left ventricle (LV) is considered to approximate that of an ellipsoid while the shape of the right ventricle (RV) is more complex (Fig. 2.1). When viewed from the side, the RV appears triangular and when viewed in cross-section it appears more crescent-shaped. The interventricular septum (IVS) is the most important determinant of the shape of the RV. Under normal loading and electrical conditions, the IVS is concave toward the LV in both systole and diastole due to the higher pressures in the LV compared to the RV.

Even though the RV appears smaller than the LV on the echocardiographic examination, the RV volume is actually larger than the LV volume. Based on cardiac magnetic resonance imaging (CMRI), the normal range of RV end-diastolic volume (RVEDV) is 49–101 mL/m^2 whereas the normal range of LV end-diastolic volume (LVEDV) is 44–89 mL/m^2 [2.1].

Ventricular Components

The ventricles can be described in terms of three components or portions: (1) the inlet, (2) apical, and (3) outlet components. For the LV, the inlet consists of the mitral valve and its supporting apparatus; the apical component consists of fine apical trabeculations with a smooth septal surface; and the outlet supports the aortic valve (Fig. 2.2, top).

For the RV, the inlet consists of the tricuspid valve and its supporting apparatus; the apical component consists of coarse muscular trabeculations; and the outlet component consists of the smooth myocardial outflow region of the infundibulum which supports the pulmonary valve (Fig. 2.2, bottom). Importantly, the inlet portion of the RV is separated from the outlet component by the supraventricular crest, which is formed by a muscular band (the parietal band) and the infundibular septum. Two other prominent muscular bands are found within the RV, namely the septal band and the moderator band. The septal band courses along the IVS while the moderator band extends from the base of the anterior papillary muscle to the IVS. The anatomic separation of the inlet and outlet portions of the RV is an important differentiator between the morphological right and left ventricles as the LV inlet and outlet components are in fibrous continuity.

Atrioventricular Valves

The atrioventricular (AV) valves are specifically related to each ventricle. As such the mitral valve is always associated with the LV and the tricuspid valve is always associated with the RV. Therefore, identifying the AV valves also identifies the ventricles. Detailed anatomy of the mitral and tricuspid valves is discussed in Chapters 8 and 9, respectively.

Papillary Muscles

The papillary muscles are located within the LV and RV. They attach to the AV valves via the tendinous chords (chordae tendinae). The primary aim of the papillary muscles is to contract during ventricular systole, thus tightening the

Figure 2.1 The geometry of the left and right ventricles is shown in this three dimensional reconstruction of the right ventricle (**RV**). This illustrates its complex shape compared with the left ventricle (**LV**). Observe how the RV wraps around the LV.
P = pulmonary valve; **T** = tricuspid valve.
Reproduced from Sheehan F and Redington A, The right ventricle: anatomy, physiology and clinical imaging, *Heart,* Vol. 94(11), page 1511,© 2008 with permission from BMJ Publishing Group Ltd.

[2.1] Haddad F, Couture P, Tousignant C, Denault AY. The right ventricle in cardiac surgery, a perioperative perspective: I. Anatomy, physiology, and assessment. *Anesth Analg.* 2009 Feb;108(2):407-21.

tendinous chords to prevent the AV valves from prolapsing back into the atria during systole.

In the normal LV there are two prominent groups of papillary muscles located within the ventricle (Fig. 2.3, top). These papillary muscles are commonly referred to as the posteromedial and anterolateral papillary muscles. The anterolateral group is often has a single pillar (base) whereas the posteromedial group may have more than one pillar. Each pillar may have one head or multiple heads into which the tendinous chords insert (Fig. 2.3, middle).

The papillary muscles of the RV are also relatively constant, with an anterior papillary muscle located on the anterior wall near its junction with the IVS and a small posterior papillary muscle arising under the supraventricular crest at the inferior border of the RV outflow tract. In addition, there is an inconstant group of posterior papillary muscles that arise from the diaphragmatic wall of the RV (Fig. 2.3, bottom).

> **Papillary Muscle Terminology**
> The two papillary muscles in the LV are commonly referred to as anterolateral and posteromedial. This terminology is a consequence of anatomists taking the heart out and sitting it on its apex when describing the orientation of the structures within. However, new technologies such as CMRI and 3D echocardiography, now show the heart as it lies in the chest. Based on these technologies, the true orientation of the papillary muscles is really inferoseptal and posterolateral.

> **Cordal Attachments**
> Not all tendinous chords arise from the papillary muscles. In the RV, chords can also arise directly from the ventricular walls and IVS. In fact, a characteristic feature of the tricuspid valve is that there are multiple cordal attachments from the septal leaflet directly to the IVS.

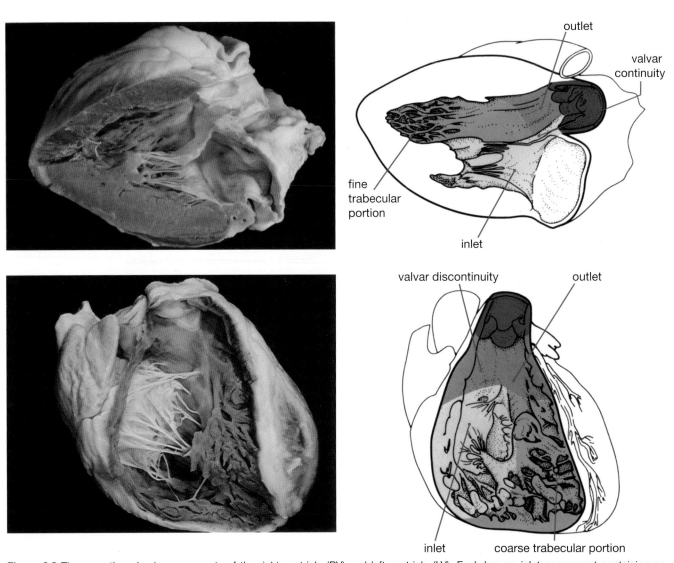

Figure 2.2 There are three basic components of the right ventricle (RV) and left ventricle (LV). Each has an inlet component containing an atrioventricular valve and its supporting apparatus, an apical trabecular zone, and an outlet component supporting an arterial valve. Components of the LV are shown at the top; on the left is an anatomic section of the opened LV and on the right is the corresponding schematic illustration. Components of the RV are shown at the bottom; on the left is an anatomic section of the heart in its situ position with the anterior wall removed and on the right is the corresponding schematic illustration.

Note that the inlet and outlet components of the RV are separated by the supraventricular crest (coloured orange in the cartoon, and labelled as valvar discontinuity); while in contrast, in the LV the aortic and mitral valves are in fibrous continuity. Also note that the apical component of the LV is less trabeculated compared with the apical component of the RV.

Adapted from Anderson RH and Becker AE. 1980, Cardiac Anatomy. An Integrated Text and Color Atlas, Gower Medical Publishing Ltd, pp 3.1, 3.12 & 4.3. Reproduced with permission from Robert H. Anderson, M.D., FRCPath. University College London and Anton E. Becker, M.D., University of Amsterdam.

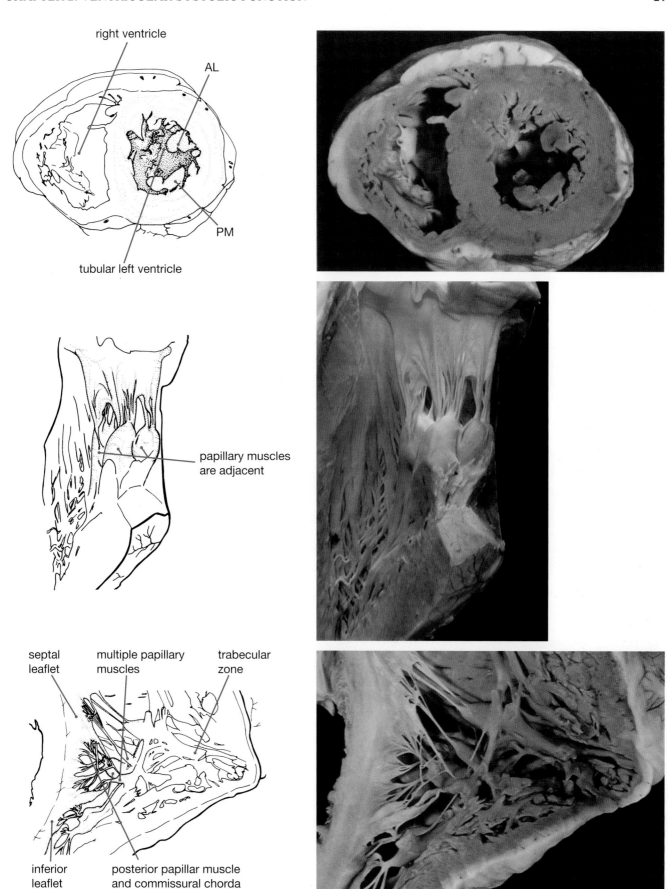

Figure 2.3 The short axis cut on the top shows the two prominent anterolateral (AL) and posteromedial (PM) papillary muscles of the left ventricle. Also observe the comparative wall thickness of the left and right ventricles in this example. The middle images show an overall view of the mitral valve and its supporting apparatus; observe how the papillary muscles arise adjacent to each other. Multiple heads to the lateral papillary muscle are also noted. The inlet part of the right ventricle is displayed at the bottom; observe the multiple papillary muscles supporting the septal and inferior (posterior) leaflets.

Adapted from Anderson RH and Becker AE. 1980, *Cardiac Anatomy. An Integrated Text and Color Atlas*, Gower Medical Publishing Ltd, pp. 3.21, 4.2 and 4.8. Reproduced with permission from Robert H. Anderson, M.D., FRCPath. University College London and Anton E. Becker, M.D., University of Amsterdam.

Ventricular Wall Layers

Heart walls, including those of the ventricles, consist of three major layers: (1) the endocardium, (2) the myocardium and (3) the epicardium (Fig. 2.4).

The endocardium is the innermost lining of the chamber wall. It is a smooth membrane of endothelial cells which also cover the cardiac valves. Endocardial cells are similar to the endothelial cells that line blood vessels.

The myocardium is the thick, middle layer of the chamber wall and is primarily responsible for contraction. The myocardium is composed almost completely of interlacing bundles of cardiac myocytes (Fig. 2.5).

The epicardium is the outer layer of the ventricle. This thin layer consists mostly of connective tissue and fat. The epicardium is also considered as a layer of the pericardium and is therefore also referred to as the visceral pericardium.

In the normal heart the walls of the LV are thicker than the walls of the RV (Fig. 2.3, top). This is because the pressures within the LV exceed the pressures within the RV, especially during ventricular systole. The overall wall thickness of the RV, excluding trabeculations, is normally 3–5 mm. The normal thickness of the LV, excluding trabeculations, is 10–12 mm when measured approximately 1.5 cm below the mitral

annulus. LV walls are thickest at the base and gradually become thinner towards the apex. In both ventricles, the wall at the very tip of the apex is very thin with only 1-2 mm of muscle separating the ventricular cavity from the epicardium (Fig. 2.6). Due to the significant difference between LV and RV wall thicknesses, the RV mass is approximately one-sixth of that of the LV.

Ventricular Wall Myofibre Architecture

Transmurally through the ventricular wall, the myocardium is composed of a complex helical arrangement of myofibrils in three layers: (1) superficial (subepicardial), (2) middle, and (3) deep (subendocardial) layers. The distinction between these layers is based on the orientation of the muscle fibres through the ventricular wall.

The superficial or subepicardial layer in the normal heart consists of muscle fibres which pass from the base of the heart toward the apex, extending from one ventricle to the other to form one common layer. At the apex, the superficial layer invaginates in a spiral pattern to continue into the deep (subendocardial) layer. The fibres on the sternocostal aspect run obliquely, crossing the anterior interventricular groove (Fig. 2.7A), while on the diaphragmatic aspect they cross the posterior interventricular groove (Fig. 2.7B). The fibres in the superficial layer of the RV are arranged more circumferentially than in the LV. The superficial layer occupies approximately 25% of the LV wall thickness.

The middle layer, which is only present in the LV, occupies approximately 53–59% of the LV wall thickness. The fibres of the middle layer are oriented more horizontally (circumferentially) than those of the superficial layer (Fig. 2.8A). This layer is thickest at the mid LV level, thinning out towards both the basal and apical ends. At the apical end, the middle layer encloses a small aperture through which the superficial muscle fibres invaginate to become subendocardial fibres (Fig. 2.8B).

The deep (subendocardial) layer is composed of longitudinal fibres which pass through the vortices toward the papillary muscles to the AV orifices and the arterial orifices, and to the ventricular septum (Fig. 2.8C). This is the thinnest layer, accounting for less than 20% of the LV wall thickness.

In respect to LV contraction, the middle layer fibres contribute to the circumferential contraction while the epicardial and subendocardial fibres contribute to the longitudinal contraction of the ventricle. In particular, the myofibril geometry changes smoothly from a right-handed helix in the subendocardium to a left-handed helix in the subepicardium. Due to the helical arrangement of the myocardial geometry, during systole epicardial fibres will rotate the apex in a counterclockwise direction and the base in a clockwise direction, while contraction of the subendocardial region will rotate the LV apex and base in exactly the opposite directions. The 'twist' and 'untwist' motion of the myocardium along with the circumferential and longitudinal contraction combine to contribute to the stroke volume during systole. In the RV, longitudinal shortening accounts for the majority of RV contraction.

Distinguishing Anatomic Features between the Left and Right Ventricles

The anatomic features that differentiate the RV from the LV are summarised in Table 2.1.

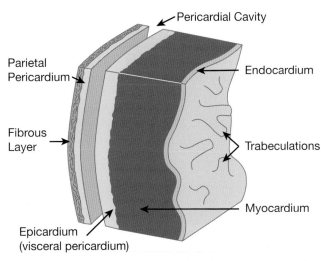

Figure 2.4 The heart walls consist of three layers: the endocardium (innermost layer); the myocardium (middle layer) and the epicardium (outer layer which is also known as the visceral pericardium).

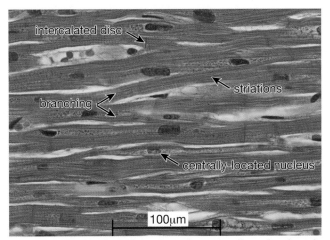

Figure 2.5 This histological specimen (haematoxylin and eosin stain at x 150 objective) shows the characteristic features of cardiac muscle. By permission of Mayo Foundation for Medical Education and Research. All rights reserved. Courtesy of William D. Edwards, MD.

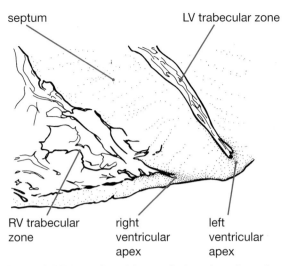

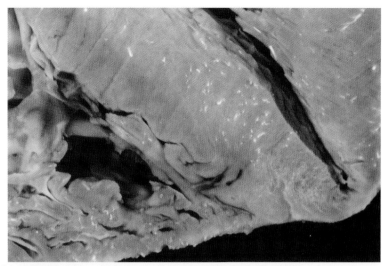

septum

LV trabecular zone

RV trabecular zone

right ventricular apex

left ventricular apex

Figure 2.6 This section of the ventricular apices shows how thin both the right and left ventricular myocardia are at this point. From Anderson RH and Becker AE. 1980, *Cardiac Anatomy. An Integrated Text and Color Atlas*, Gower Medical Publishing Ltd, pp. 3.14. Reproduced with permission from Robert H. Anderson, M.D., FRCPath. University College London and Anton E. Becker, M.D., University of Amsterdam.

Figure 2.7 These photos show the arrangement of the ventricular fibres of the superficial (subepicardial) layer of a normal heart. Observe that on the sternocostal surface (A) and on the diaphragmatic surface (B), the fibres run obliquely across the interventricular grooves (*arrows*).
LV = left ventricle; **P** = pulmonary trunk; **RV** = right ventricle.
Reproduced from Sanchez-Quintana D, Climent V, Ho SY, Anderson RH, Myoarchitecture and connective tissue in hearts with tricuspid atresia, *Heart,* Vol. 81(2), page number 185, © 1999 with permission from BMJ Publishing Group Ltd.

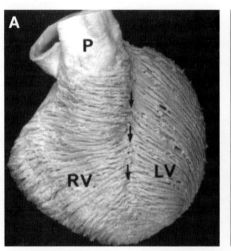

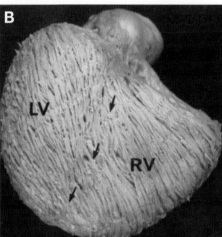

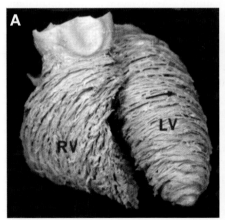

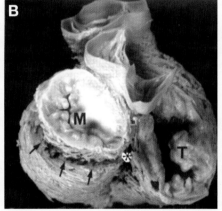

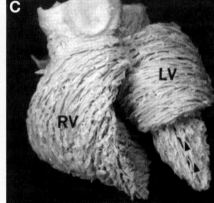

Figure 2.8 These photos show the arrangement of the ventricular fibres in the middle and deep (subendocardial) layers of a normal heart. The sternocostal aspects (A and C) show the circular arrangement (*arrow*) of the left ventricular fibres, in contrast to the oblique arrangement of the right ventricular fibres in the normal heart. The basal view (**B**) shows the distinct invagination at the crux (*asterisk*) and the basal aperture (*arrows*) in the normal heart. The deep layers (arrowheads) are revealed by removing the apical half of the middle layer (C).
LV = left ventricle; **M** = mitral valve; **RV** = right ventricle; **T** = tricuspid valve.x
Reproduced from Sanchez-Quintana D, Climent V, Ho SY, Anderson RH, Myoarchitecture and connective tissue in hearts with tricuspid atresia, *Heart*, Vol. 81(2), page number 186, © 1999 with permission from BMJ Publishing Group Ltd.

> **Ventricular Interdependence**
> While the deeper layers of myocardial fibres of the LV and RV are separated, superficial fibres encircle both the LV and RV. The function of the two ventricles is therefore linked. As a result the size, shape, and compliance of one ventricle affects the size, shape, pressure and volume of the other ventricle; this is referred to as ventricular interdependence. In particular, normal RV contractile performance is significantly dependent on the contractile performance of the LV with approximately 20% to 40% of the RV systolic pressure and stroke volume resulting from LV contraction.

Table 2.1 Distinguishing Anatomic Features of the Left and Right Ventricles

	Right Ventricle	Left Ventricle
Geometry	Complex shape From the side it appears triangular; in cross-section it appears crescent-shaped	Ellipsoid shape Interventricular septum convexes into the RV cavity
Ventricular Components	Inlet and outlet components are separated by a muscular arch	Continuity between the inlet and outlet components
Trabeculations	Heavily trabeculated at the apex; Moderator band	Fine trabeculations at the apex
Atrioventricular valves	Trileaflet configuration of the tricuspid valve with septal papillary attachments Apical displacement of the septal tricuspid leaflet relative to anterior mitral leaflet	Bileaflet mitral valve with no attachments to the interventricular septum
Papillary muscles	Multiple (> 3) papillary muscles	2 prominent papillary muscles
Tendinous chords	Multiple attachments of chords from the septal leaflet to the interventricular septum	No cordal attachments to the interventricular septum
Wall thickness	3-5 mm base to mid (RV mass 1/6 of LV mass)	10-12 mm at base Gradual thinning from base to apex
Myofibre Architecture	2 layers only: 1. superficial (subepicardial) 2. deep (subendocardial)	3 layers: 1. superficial (subepicardial) 2. middle 3. deep (subendocardial)

Basic Cardiac Physiology

Ventricular systole is defined from closure of the AV valves to the closure of the semilunar valves (Fig. 2.9). On the electrocardiogram (ECG), systole is defined from the R wave to the end of the T wave. Ventricular systole is comprised of: (1) an isovolumetric contraction phase, (2) a rapid ejection phase and (3) a reduced ejection phase.

Phases of Systole

Isovolumic Contraction

Isovolumic contraction is the period between AV valve closure and semilunar valve opening. During this phase of the cardiac cycle, the ventricular volumes at end-diastole are maximal and the ventricular pressure rises rapidly without a change in the end-diastolic volume (EDV).

The EDV does not change during this phase of the cardiac cycle because all valves are closed so there is no blood entering or leaving the ventricles. Therefore, contraction at this stage of the cardiac cycle is isovolumic ("iso" meaning equal and "volumic" meaning volume). So even though the pressure is rapidly rising within the ventricles, there is no ejection of blood from the ventricles. The rate of pressure rise in the ventricles during isovolumic contraction is determined by the rate of contraction of the muscle fibres.

Rapid Ejection (Acceleration) Phase

When the pressure within the ventricles exceeds the pressure within the respective great arteries, the semilunar valves snap open. This results in the rapid ejection of blood from the ventricles into the aorta and pulmonary artery. As a result, ventricular volumes also rapidly decline. Rapid ejection occupies approximately the first half of systole.

Reduced Ejection (Deceleration) Phase

Approximately 200 ms after the onset of ventricular contraction, ventricular repolarization occurs. Repolarization leads to a decline in the rate of ejection and ventricular emptying. Ventricular pressure falls slightly below the pulmonary artery and aortic pressures; however, some ejection still occurs due to kinetic (or inertial) energy of the blood flow. During this phase of the cardiac cycle, the ventricular volumes continue to decline but at a slower rate than during rapid ejection. The ventricular volume at the end of ejection (end-systole) is the smallest ventricular volume.

Pressure-Volume Loops

By combining the ventricular pressure and ventricle volumes, a pressure-volume (P-V) loop can be derived to more precisely describe the relationship between pressure and volume over the cardiac cycle. To generate a P-V loop for the

LV, the LV pressure (LVP) is plotted against LV volume at multiple points throughout a single cardiac cycle (Fig. 2.10). The P-V loop for the LV is rectangular in shape. The point

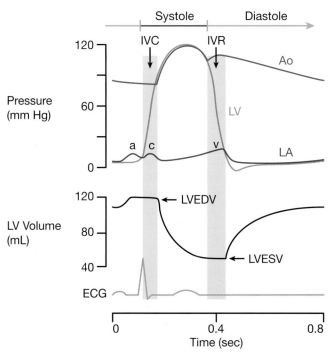

Figure 2.9 This schematic illustrates the various phases of the cardiac cycle for the left heart with respect to pressures and LV volumes (see text for details).

a = atrial pressure following atrial contraction; Ao = aorta; c = atrial pressure due to bulging of mitral valve leaflets back into left atrium; IVC = isovolumic contraction; IVR = isovolumic relaxation; LA = left atrium; LV = left ventricle; LVEDV = left ventricular end-diastolic volume; LVESV = left ventricular end-systolic volume; v = atrial pressure at the end of ventricular contraction.

at mitral valve closure (MC) illustrates the LV pressure and LV volume at the end of ventricular filling (end-diastole); this correlates to the LV end-diastolic pressure (LVEDP) and the LVEDV.

The vertical line between MC and aortic valve opening (AO) represents isovolumic contraction. During isovolumic contraction, the LV begins to contract and the LV pressure increases but the LV volume remains the same because all valves are closed (no blood is entering the LV and no blood is leaving the LV).

When the LV pressure exceeds the aortic pressure, the aortic valve opens (AO) and systolic ejection begins. During the ejection phase the LV volume decreases as blood is ejected from the LV; at the same time the LV pressure continues to increase slightly to its peak systolic pressure and then LV pressure declines as the ventricle begins to relax.

At the end of ejection, when the pressure in the LV falls below the aortic pressure, the aortic valve closes (AC). The LV volume at this point in the cardiac cycle is the LV end-systolic volume (LVESV).

The vertical line between AC and mitral valve opening (MO) represents isovolumic relaxation (IVR). During IVR, the LV continues to relax and the LV pressure falls but the LV volume remains unchanged as all valves are closed (no blood is leaving the LV and no blood is entering the LV).

MO occurs when the pressure in the LV falls below the pressure in the left atrium (LA). At this point the LV begins to fill. Initially, the LV pressure continues to fall even as the ventricle fills because the ventricle is still relaxing. Once the LV is fully relaxed, the LV pressure gradually increases as the LV volume increases.

The maximal pressure that can be developed by the ventricle at any given LV volume is defined by the end-systolic pressure-volume relationship (ESPVR), which represents the contractile state of the ventricle.

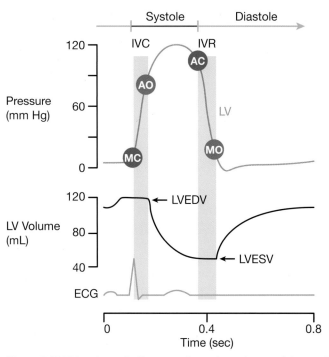

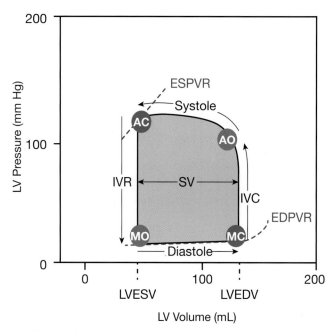

Figure 2.10 This schematic illustrates the various phases of the cardiac cycle for the left heart with respect to left ventricular pressure and left ventricular volumes *(left)* and the corresponding pressure-volume loop *(right)* (see text for details).

AC = aortic valve closure; AO = aortic valve opening; EDPVR = end-diastolic pressure-volume relationship; ESPVR = end-systolic pressure-volume relationship; IVC = isovolumic contraction; IVR = isovolumic relaxation; LVEDV = left ventricular end-diastolic volume; LVESV = left ventricular end-systolic volume; MC = mitral valve closure; MO = mitral valve opening; SV = stroke volume.

The diastolic filling phase of the LV moves along the end-diastolic pressure-volume relationship (EDPVR) and this reflects the passive filling curve for the ventricle. The slope of the EDPVR is the reciprocal of ventricular compliance. The width of the P-V loop represents the stroke volume (SV) which is the difference between the LVEDV and the LVESV.

The normal P-V relationship for the RV is more triangular or trapezoidal than that of the LV, with poorly defined periods of isovolumic contraction and IVR (Fig. 2.11).

The difference in the P-V loops between the LV and the RV can be explained by the lower pressures in the right heart and the lower impedance characteristics of the pulmonary vascular bed. In particular, in the right heart, the pulmonary valve remains open for some time even after the RV pressure equalises with the pulmonary artery pressure at end-systole. As a result there may be continued end-systolic flow in the presence of a negative ventricular-arterial pressure gradient. This is referred to as the "hangout interval" (Fig. 2.12). The "hangout interval" is explained by the low pulmonary vascular resistance (PVR). Blood continues to flow until it is halted by a resistance and since the PVR is low, it takes some time for the blood flow from the RV to stop. This "hangout interval" is negligible in the left heart due to high systemic vascular resistance (SVR) so the aortic valve closes as soon as the LV pressure equalises with the aortic pressure at end-systole.

Determinants of Stroke Volume

SV is defined as the volume of blood pumped out by the RV or LV in one systolic contraction. SV is the difference between the volume of the ventricle immediately prior to contraction (end-diastolic volume [EDV]) and the residual volume remaining in the ventricle after ejection (end-systolic volume [ESV]):

Equation 2.1

$$SV = EDV - ESV$$

where SV   = stroke volume (mL)
      EDV = end-diastolic volume (mL)
      ESV   = end-systolic volume (mL)

On the P-V loop SV is represented by the width of the P-V loop (Fig. 2.10). Three primary mechanisms regulate EDV and ESV and therefore the SV. These mechanisms include: (1) preload, (2) afterload and (3) contractility (inotropy).

Preload

Preload is described as the muscle length (or muscle stretch) immediately prior to contraction at end-diastole. Muscle length cannot be determined in the intact heart, and therefore other indices are used to describe preload. The most commonly used indices to describe preload of the left heart include LVEDV, LVEDP and/or LA pressure. The most commonly used indices to describe preload of the right heart include RVEDV, RVEDP and/or right atrial (RA) pressure.

Changes in preload alter SV by essentially changing the EDV. For example, an increase in venous return to the heart increases the EDV which stretches the muscle fibres thereby increasing preload. This will result in an increase in SV. Conversely decreasing preload results in a decrease in EDV which leads to a decrease in SV.

It should also be noted that breathing has a major impact on right heart haemodynamics including preload. In a spontaneously breathing patient, during inspiration venous return (preload) is increased and during expiration it is decreased. This leads to corresponding fluctuations in the RV SV over the respiratory cycle.

Afterload

Afterload is the tension or load that the heart must eject against or the tension that myocytes must overcome before shortening occurs. Afterload is related to ventricular wall stress and can be expressed by Laplace's law for a thin-walled sphere as:

Equation 2.2

$$\sigma = (Pr) \div 2h$$

where σ = tension or wall stress (dynes/cm^2)
      P = intracavity pressure (dynes/cm^2)
      r = radius at the endocardial surface of a thin-walled sphere (cm)
      h = wall thickness (cm)

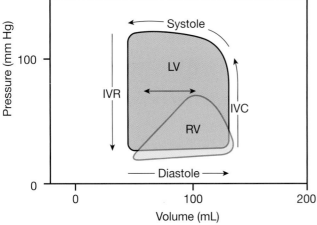

Figure 2.11 This schematic illustrates the P-V loops for the normal left ventricle (LV) and the normal right ventricle (RV). Note that the P-V loop of the LV is rectangular while the P-V loop for the RV is more triangular with poorly defined isovolumic periods. Also observe the continued ejection from the RV during pressure decline *(double-ended arrow)*, correlating with the hangout period (see text for details).

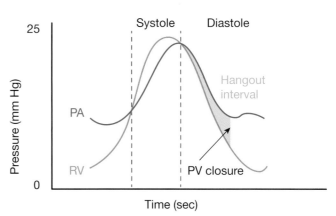

Figure 2.12 This schematic illustrates the pressure traces of the right ventricle (RV) and the pulmonary artery (PA). Note the continued flow between the RV and the PA at end-systole in the presence of a negative ventricular-arterial pressure gradient (blue fill). This is referred to as the "hangout interval". This interval terminates at the closure of the pulmonary valve (PV).

From this equation it can be appreciated that afterload is directly related to pressure and radius and inversely related to wall thickness. Therefore changes in ventricular volume, wall thickness, and vascular resistance affect the afterload. For the LV afterload is most commonly determined by the SVR which is reflected by the systemic (aortic) blood pressure. For the RV afterload is determined by the PVR which is reflected by the pulmonary artery pressures.

Changes in afterload affect the ability of the ventricle to eject blood and thereby alter ESV and SV. For example, an increase in afterload decreases SV and increases ESV. Conversely a decrease in afterload increases SV and decreases ESV.

Contractility (Inotropy)

Contractility or inotropy refers to the inherent strength of cardiac muscle and its ability to shorten with ventricular systole. In particular, contractility is the ability of muscle to contract at a given force for a given stretch, independent of preload or afterload. Changes in ventricular inotropy alter the rate of ventricular pressure rise, thereby affecting ESV and SV. For example, an increase in inotropy increases SV and decreases ESV. Conversely a decrease in inotropy reduces SV and increases ESV.

Interdependence of Preload, Afterload and Contractility

It is important to note that preload, afterload and inotropy do not remain constant and that changes to any one of these variables also changes another variable. For example, changing preload is accompanied by a change in afterload, changing afterload is accompanied by a change in preload, and a change in inotropy is accompanied by a change in preload. As a result changes in SV are based on this complex interdependence.

The relationship between preload and SV is described by the Frank-Starling principle (Fig. 2.13). This principle simply describes the ability of the heart to change its force of contraction, and hence SV, in response to changes in venous return. For example, an increase in venous return to the heart increases the EDV which stretches the muscle fibres thereby increasing preload. This increase in EDV, with no change in ESV, will result in an increase in SV. The overall result of increased preload, within a physiological limit, is an increase in the force of ventricular contraction. However, increasing SV also leads to an increase in afterload (due to an increase in cardiac output and arterial pressure). Therefore as afterload increases the ESV the increased SV is slightly counteracted by the increasing ESV.

Decreasing preload has the opposite effects. A decrease in venous return results in a decrease in preload (EDV) which leads to a decrease in SV and a decrease in the force of ventricular contraction. This reduction in SV, however, is partially counteracted by the decreased afterload (due to reduced aortic pressure) so that the ESV decreases slightly.

Afterload of the LV can be increased by increasing aortic pressure and SVR. This effect can be explained by the relationship between afterload and myocardial fibre shortening velocity (Fig. 2.14). An increase in afterload decreases the shortening velocity and this decrease in shortening velocity reduces the rate of volume ejection so that more blood remains within the ventricle at end-systole. It would then be expected that increased afterload, which increases ESV, would result in a decreased SV. However, increased ESV also results in a secondary increase in EDV because more blood remains within the ventricle following ejection and this extra blood volume is added to the venous return, thereby increasing preload. This secondary increase in preload partially counteracts the reduction in SV caused by increased afterload. Therefore, in the normal LV SV is not strongly influenced by afterload. However it should be noted that the RV exhibits a heightened sensitivity to changes in afterload. As a result, a modest increase in total PVR leads to a significant decrease in RV SV.

Decreasing afterload (by reducing aortic pressure) has the opposite effects. A decrease in afterload results in increased shortening velocity which augments the volume ejection rate so that less blood remains within the ventricle at the end of systole. Therefore decreasing afterload decreases ESV which increases SV. In addition, a decrease in ESV results in a secondary decrease in EDV (preload) because less blood remains within the ventricle following ejection. Thus, SV can be significantly increased by reducing afterload.

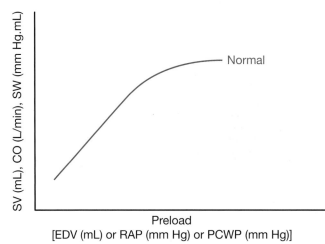

Figure 2.13 The Frank-Starling curve plots the stroke volume (SV), stroke work (SW), or cardiac output (CO) on the vertical axis against preload (end-diastolic volume [EDV], right atrial pressure [RAP], or pulmonary capillary wedge pressure [PCWP]) on the horizontal axis. For a given degree of contractility there is a curvilinear relationship between these variables; therefore, increasing preload results in an increase in SV (SW or CO).

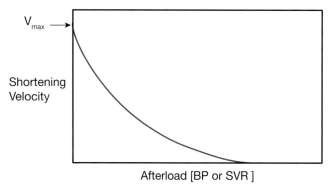

Figure 2.14 Myocardial fibre shortening velocity is plotted on the vertical axis and afterload (blood pressure [BP] or systemic vascular resistance [SVR]) is plotted on the horizontal axis. For a given degree of contractility there is an inverse relationship between these variables; therefore, increasing afterload results in a decrease in shortening velocity.

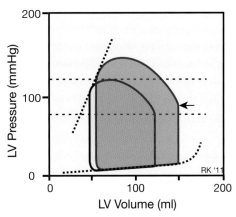

Increased preload (increased EDV; red loop) at constant inotropy. SV increases; ESV increases slightly because afterload (aortic pressure - arrow) increases. Horizontal dashed lines represent normal aortic systolic and diastolic pressures.

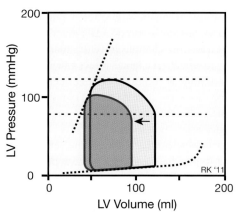

Decreased preload (decreased EDV; red loop) at constant inotropy. SV decreases; ESV decreases slightly because afterload (aortic pressure - arrow) decreases. Horizontal dashed lines represent normal aortic systolic and diastolic pressures.

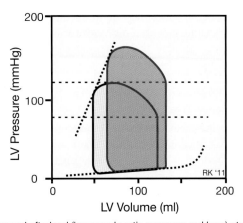

Increased afterload (increased aortic pressure; red loop) at constant inotropy. SV slightly decreases (ESV increases and EDV slightly increases secondarily). Horizontal dashed lines represent normal aortic systolic and diastolic pressures.

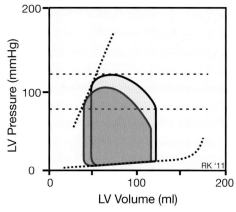

Decreased afterload (decreased aortic pressure; red loop) at constant inotropy. SV slightly increases (ESV decreases and EDV slightly decreases secondarily). Horizontal dashed lines represent normal aortic systolic and diastolic pressures.

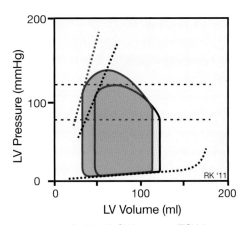

Increased inotropy (red loop). SV increases (ESV decreases, and EDV decreases secondarily a small amount); EF increases. Horizontal dashed lines represent normal aortic systolic and diastolic pressures.

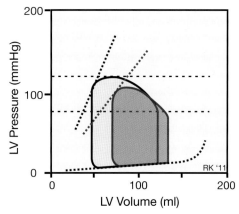

Decreased inotropy (red loop). SV decreases (ESV increases, and EDV increases secondarily a small amount); EF decreases. Horizontal dashed lines represent normal aortic systolic and diastolic pressures.

Figure 2.15 The interdependent effects of preload, afterload and inotropy using left ventricular pressure-volume loops is illustrated on this series of schematics. Observe the interdependent changes that can occur as preload, afterload and inotropy are altered.
Reproduced from Cardiovascular Physiology Concepts with permission from Richard Klabunde, Ph.D. Ohio University, Athens, Ohio. Accessed on 10 August 2011, http://www.cvphysiology.com/Cardiac%20Function/CF026.htm

Increasing inotropy (contractility) allows the ventricle to generate more pressure at a given ventricular volume. Increased inotropy also increases the rate of pressure development and ejection velocity, which increases SV and ejection fraction, and decreases ESV. The secondary consequence of decreasing ESV is a decrease in EDV (preload) because less blood remains within the ventricle following ejection.

Decreasing inotropy (contractility) has the opposite effects whereby decreasing inotropy results in an increase in ESV which decreases SV and ejection fraction. This is accompanied by a small secondary increase in EDV (preload).

In summary, this interdependence between preload and afterload, and preload and inotropy can be illustrated on the P-V loops (Fig. 2.15) and the Frank-Starling curves (Fig. 2.16). The overall effect of these variables on SV are summarised in Figure 2.17.

Measurements of the Left Ventricle

M-Mode Measurements of the LV

The M-mode examination of the LV can be performed from the parasternal long axis view of the LV, the parasternal short axis view at the level of the papillary muscles, and from the subcostal 4-chamber and short axis views. The M-mode cursor is positioned perpendicular to the long or short axis of the LV just distal to the tips of the open mitral valve leaflets (Fig. 2.18).

Linear Dimensions

From the M-mode trace, LV dimensions can be measured at end-diastole and end-systole (Fig. 2.19). End-diastolic measurements are performed at the onset of the QRS complex of the ECG. The interventricular septal thickness (IVST) is measured between the anterior and posterior endocardial surfaces of the IVS; that is, from leading edge of the IVS to the trailing edge of the IVS. The LV end-diastolic dimension (LVEDD) is measured from the posterior endocardial surface of the IVS to the endocardial surface of the posterior wall (PW); that is, from trailing edge of the IVS to the leading edge of the PW. The posterior wall thickness (PWT) is measured from endocardial surface to epicardial surface of the posterior wall of the LV.

End-systole is identified based on the motion of the IVS. When IVS motion is normal, end-systole is identified at the peak posterior point of the IVS; when the IVS motion is abnormal, end-systole is identified as the most anterior point of the PW (Fig. 2.20). The LV end-systolic dimension (LVESD) is measured from the posterior endocardial surface of the IVS to the endocardial surface of the PW; that is, from trailing edge of the IVS to the leading edge of the PW.

Volume Estimation

LV volumes can be estimated from M-mode linear dimensions based on the geometric assumptions of the LV shape. The most commonly used method for estimating LV volumes from linear measurements is the Teichholz method. This method is based on a regression equation that describes the changes in LV geometry as the LV dilates and is expressed as:

Equation 2.3

$$LVV = (7.0 \div [2.4 + D]) (D^3)$$

where LVV = left ventricular volume (mL)
 D   = left ventricular dimension (cm)

Using this equation, the LVEDV and LVESV can be estimated from the LVEDD and the LVESD, respectively.

LV Mass

LV mass can be calculated from the M-mode end-diastolic measurements of the LV, IVS and PW. M-mode LV mass calculations are described in detail in Chapter 4 (Systemic Hypertension).

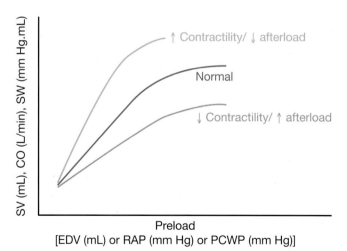

Figure 2.16 Frank Starling curves can be used as an indicator of muscle contractility. However, there is no single Frank-Starling curve on which the ventricle operates, but rather a 'family' of curves. Each curve is defined by the afterload and contractility. Increased afterload or decreased contractility shifts the curve down and to the right while decreased afterload or increased contractility shifts the curve up and to the left.

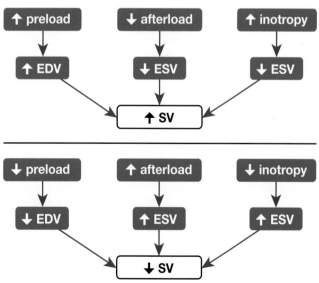

Figure 2.17 Stroke volume (SV) can be increased by increasing preload and/or inotropy and by decreasing afterload. SV is decreased when preload and/or inotropy are decreased and when the afterload is increased (see text for further details).

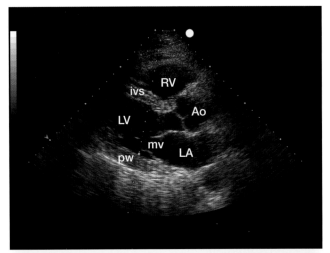

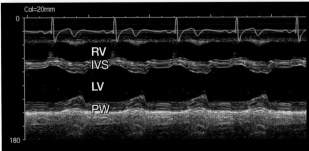

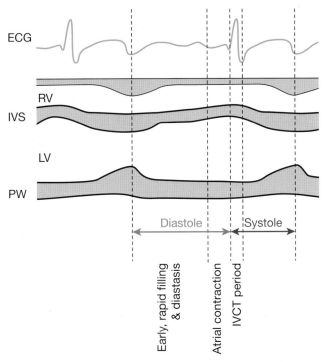

2D Measurements of the LV

Linear Dimensions

LV linear dimensions can also be measured from the parasternal long axis view of the LV at end-diastole and at end-systole. Via 2D imaging, end-diastole and end-systole are identified based on the motion of the mitral valve.

End-diastole is identified as the frame at initial coaptation of the mitral leaflets, or the frame immediately prior to initial coaptation of the mitral leaflets following the P wave of the ECG when the patient is in sinus rhythm; the frame chosen is the one in which the LV cavity size is largest (Fig. 2.21). End-systole is identified as the frame immediately preceding the initial descent of the mitral annulus towards the LV apex; this frame usually coincides with the end of the T wave of the ECG and the smallest LV cavity size.

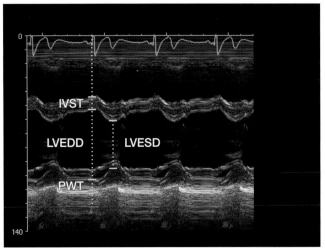

Figure 2.19 M-mode measurements of the left ventricle are shown. End-diastole is identified at the onset of the QRS complex of the ECG while end-systole is identified based on the motion of the interventricular septum (**IVS**). When IVS motion is normal, end-systole is identified at the peak posterior point of the IVS. All measurements are performed at the blood-tissue interfaces (see text for details and abbreviations).

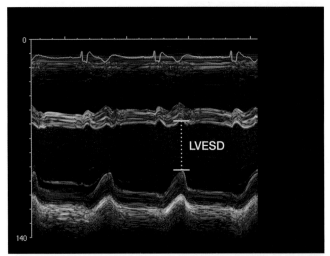

Figure 2.20 In the presence of abnormal interventricular septal motion, the end-systole is identified as the most anterior point of the posterior wall of the left ventricle. The left ventricular end-systolic dimension (LVESD) is then measured from the leading edge of the posterior wall back up to the trailing edge of the IVS.

Figure 2.18 The top image shows the imaging plane, M-mode cursor position and structures transected by the M-mode cursor from the parasternal long axis of the left ventricle (**LV**). The corresponding M-mode trace is displayed below. The M-mode cursor is aligned parallel with the mitral annulus (perpendicular to the LV long axis) and just distal to the mitral tips in diastole.

Ao = aorta; IVS = interventricular septum; LA = left atrium; LV = left ventricle; mv = mitral valve; PW = posterior wall of the left ventricle; RV = right ventricle.

From the end-diastolic and end-systolic frames, linear measurements of the LV can be performed in a similar manner as to M-mode measurements (Fig. 2.22). The IVST is measured between the anterior and posterior endocardial surfaces of the IVS; that is, from leading edge of the IVS to the trailing edge of the IVS. The LVEDD is from the posterior endocardial surface of the IVS to the endocardial surface of the PW; that is, from trailing edge of the IVS to the leading edge of the PW. The PWT is measured from endocardial surface to epicardial surface of the posterior wall of the LV. The LVESD is measured from the posterior endocardial surface of the IVS to the endocardial surface of the PW; that is, from trailing edge of the IVS to the leading edge of the PW.

Volume Estimation

LV volumes can be estimated from linear measurements via the Teichholz method as described for M-mode. However, due to pitfalls of geometric assumptions of this technique, the preferred methods for estimating LV volumes are the Simpson's method of discs (disc summation method) and the area-length method.

Simpson's Method

The Simpson's method of discs or the disc summation method calculates the total volume of a structure based on the calculation of volumes derived from a series of elliptical discs stacked one upon another (Fig. 2.23).

In applying this concept to the LV, the biplane LV volume is derived by dividing the ventricle into a series of discs of equal height in the apical 4-chamber view and in the apical 2-chamber view. This is achieved by tracing the total area of the LV cavity and by measuring the overall length of the LV in both of these views. The volume of each disc is then calculated from the area of the disc, which is derived from the diameter of the ventricle at a particular point, and the height of the disc, which is derived from the total LV length divided by

---

Electrical versus Mechanical Events

It is important to be aware that electrical events and mechanical events do not occur simultaneously; there is a short phasic delay following an electrical event before the mechanical event occurs. For example, via 2D imaging end-diastole will usually occur after the onset of the QRS complex rather than right at the onset of the QRS complex of the ECG. This effect is less notable on M-mode traces due to the superior sampling rate of M-mode compared with 2D imaging.

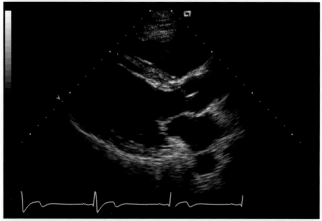
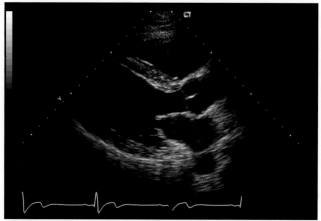

Figure 2.21 End-diastole is identified as the frame at *(left)* or immediately prior to *(right)* mitral valve closure following the P wave of the ECG when the patient is in sinus rhythm. In the normal heart, end-diastole usually corresponds to the largest LV cavity dimension.

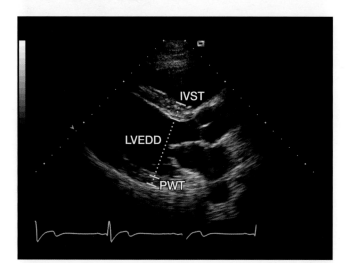
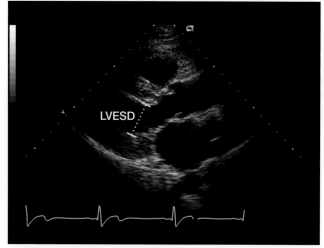

Figure 2.22 From the parasternal long axis of the left ventricle (**LV**), 2D measurements of the LV can be performed at end-diastole *(left)* and end-systole *(right)*. All measurements are performed at the blood-tissue interfaces (see text for details and abbreviations).

the number of discs (usually 20 discs). The volume is then derived from the equation:

Equation 2.5

$$Vol = \sum \pi \, (D_1 \div 2) \, (D_2 \div 2) \, (L \div n)$$

where Vol = biplane ventricular volume (mL)

D_1 = diameter at various points in the apical 4-chamber view (cm)

D_2 = diameter at various points in the apical 2-chamber view (cm)

L = long axis length of the ventricle (cm)

n = number of discs

LV volumes are measured in the apical 4-chamber and apical 2-chamber views at end-diastole and end-systole (Fig. 2.24). The primary advantage of the Simpson's biplane method in the estimation of LV volumes is that this calculation accounts for LV distortion so when there are significant regional wall motion abnormalities, the estimated LV volumes are theoretically more accurate.

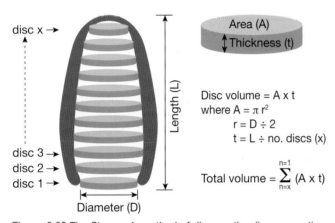

Figure 2.23 The Simpson's method of discs or the disc summation method calculates total volume from a series of discs of equal height that are stacked one upon another. The volume of each disc is calculated from the area of the disc (A), which is derived from the disc diameter (D), and the disc thickness (t), which is derived from the total length (L) of the stack discs divided by the number of discs (x) in the stack.

Area-Length Method

The area-length method is an alternative method for calculating LV volumes when the LV endocardium cannot be well defined from the apical views. This method is based on the assumption that the LV is bullet-shaped; that is, the basal half of the ventricle is assumed to be cylindrical in shape while the apical half of the ventricle is assumed to be shaped as a prolate ellipse.

Using this method, LV volumes are estimated by measuring the mid LV cross-sectional area from the parasternal short axis view at the level of the papillary muscles and by measuring the long axis (length) of the LV from the apical 4-chamber view (Fig. 2.25). Measurements are performed at end-diastole and end-systole with end-diastole and end-systole being identified based on the motion of the mitral valve as described previously. Ventricular volume can then be calculated as:

Equation 2.6

$$Vol = (5 \, AL) \div 6$$

where Vol = ventricular volume (mL)

A = endocardial area of the ventricle from the parasternal short axis (cm²)

L = long axis length of the ventricle from the apical 4-chamber (cm)

LV Mass

LV mass can be calculated from the 2D end-diastolic measurements of the LV, IVS and PW and from 2D myocardial areas. 2D LV mass calculations are described in detail in Chapter 4 (Systemic Hypertension).

The reference limits and various partition values of LV dimensions and volumes are listed in Table 2.2.

Indexing to Body Surface Area

The body surface area (BSA) is the most widely used parameter for indexing cardiac chambers and other cardiac parameters. Indexing a value to the BSA is performed by dividing a particular parameter by the BSA. The recommended and best validated values for identifying normal LV size is the LV volume indexed to the BSA (see Table 2.2).

Table 2.2 Reference Limits and Partition Values of Left Ventricular Size

	WOMEN				MEN			
	Reference range	Mildly abnormal	Moderately abnormal	Severely abnormal	Reference range	Mildly abnormal	Moderately abnormal	Severely abnormal
LV dimension								
LV diastolic diameter, cm	3.9–5.3	5.4–5.7	5.8–6.1	≥6.2	4.2–5.9	6.0–6.3	6.4–6.8	≥ 6.9
LV diastolic diameter/BSA, cm/m²	2.4–3.2	3.3–3.4	3.5–3.7	≥3.8	2.2–3.1	3.2–3.4	3.5–3.6	≥ 3.7
LV diastolic diameter/height, cm/m	2.5–3.2	3.3–3.4	3.5–3.6	≥3.7	2.4–3.3	3.4–3.5	3.6–3.7	≥ 3.8
LV volume								
LV diastolic volume, mL	56–104	105–117	118–130	≥131	67–155	156–178	179–201	≥201
LV diastolic volume/BSA, mL/m²	*35–75*	*76–86*	*87–96*	*≥97*	*35–75*	*76–86*	*87–96*	*≥97*
LV systolic volume, mL	19–49	50–59	60–69	≥ 70	22–58	59–70	71–82	≥83
LV systolic volume/BSA, mL/m²	*12–30*	*31–36*	*37–42*	*≥43*	*12–30*	*31–36*	*37–42*	*≥43*

BSA = body surface area; **LV** = left ventricular. **Bold italic values:** Recommended and best validated.
Reprinted from Lang RM, Bierig M, Devereux RB, et al., Chamber Quantification Writing Group; American Society of Echocardiography's Guidelines and Standards Committee; European Association of Echocardiography. Recommendations for Chamber Quantification: A Report from the American Society of Echocardiography's Guidelines and Standards Committee and the Chamber Quantification Writing Group, Developed in Conjunction with the European Association of Echocardiography, a Branch of the European Society of Cardiology, *J Am Soc Echocardiogr*, Vol. 18(12), page 1448, © 2005 with permission from Elsevier.

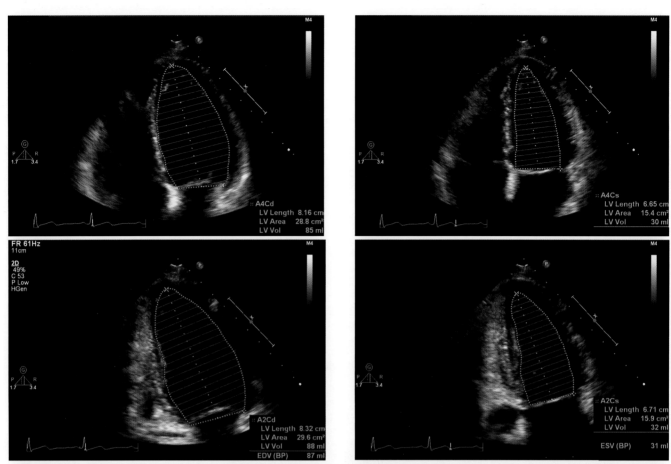

Figure 2.24 Calculation of the ventricular volumes from the Simpson's biplane method is based on the summation of discs (see text for details). The discs are derived from the apical 4-chamber and apical 2-chamber views. The apical 4-chamber end-diastolic volume is shown to the top left; the apical 4-chamber view end-systolic volume is shown to the top right; the apical 2-chamber end-diastolic volume is shown at the bottom left and the apical 2-chamber end-systolic volume is shown at the bottom right. End-diastole and end-systole are identified based on the motion of the mitral valve (see text for details). Observe that the length of the left ventricle at end-diastole in the apical 4-chamber view is 8.16 cm and in the apical 2-chamber view is 8.32 cm. Hence, the apical 4-chamber length is approximately 2% shorter than the apical 2-chamber length. Because the difference between the lengths of the two views is minimal, this suggests that these two views are closely orthogonal to one another.

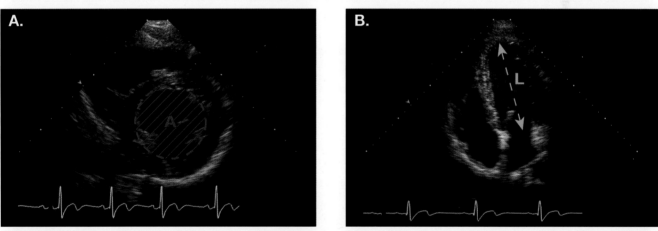

Figure 2.25 Estimation of the left ventricular volume via the area-length method can be performed when the endocardial definition is suboptimal from the apical images. From the parasternal short axis at the level of the papillary muscles *(left)*, the endocardial area (**A**) is determined by tracing around the ventricular endocardium. From the apical 4-chamber view *(right)*, the long axis of the ventricle (**L**) is measured from a line drawn from the middle of the mitral annulus to the apical endocardium, perpendicular to the mitral annulus. The volume is calculated using Equation 2.6

Technical Tips for Simpson's Biplane Volumes

Imaging Depth

Decrease imaging depth so that the ventricle fills the image display. The aim of this is to display the LV as large as is possible on the screen. The same imaging depth should be used for both the 4-chamber and 2-chamber views.

Image Optimisation

Ensure that the 2D image is optimised appropriately: for example, use harmonic imaging to improve contrast resolution and endocardial borders, position the focal zone at the centre of the cavity, optimise the 2D gain, TGC and dynamic range settings.

Foreshortening

Foreshortening of the ventricle is probably the biggest source of error in estimating LV volumes. Foreshortening leads to the LV appearing wider and shorter; thus, making the slices wider and thinner. Foreshortening is easily recognised: (1) when the ventricle appears short and squat rather than elongated, and (2) when the apex moves "downwards" in systole rather than squeezing in "sideways". The most common cause of foreshortening is having the transducer too high on the chest wall.

Identifying End-diastole and End-systole

End-diastolic (ED) and end-systolic (ES) measurements should be performed from the same beat (that is, do not measure end-diastole on one beat and then end-systole on a different beat).

As mentioned the mitral valve motion rather than the ECG is used to identify ED and ES. However, the ECG can be very useful in comparing ED and ES frames between the apical 4-chamber and apical-2 chamber views. In the example below, both images are supposedly ED frames. Note that the yellow vertical line of the ECG identifies the frame chosen for ED. The apical 2- chamber view frame *(right)* is correct but the apical 4-chamber view frame *(left)* is at a different point in the cardiac cycle; that is, the apical 4-chamber frame is not at the same point on the ECG as the apical 2-chamber frame.

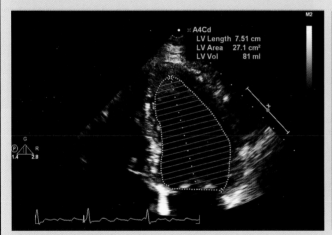 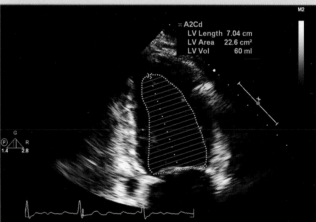

Trace Blood-Tissue Border

The endocardial border at the blood-tissue interface should be traced excluding trabeculations and papillary muscles from the LV myocardium (that is, trabeculations and papillary muscles are included in the ventricular volume).

LV Length

The LV length should be measured from the centre of the mitral annulus to the ventricular apex. To ensure that the centre of the annulus is correctly identified, commence the trace at the lateral or medial mitral annulus and then end the trace at the opposite annulus; the machine will then automatically default to the centre of the annulus. The distal point of the LV length can then be moved to ensure that the true long axis of the LV is measured. In the example below, the machine has automatically measured the LV length perpendicular to the mitral annulus *(lbelow left)*. However, this is not a true measure of the LV length *(see below right)*. Underestimation of the LV length will result in an underestimation of LV volume.

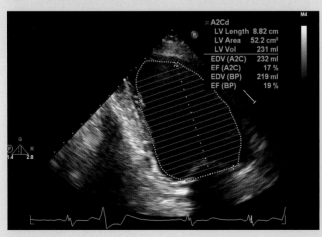 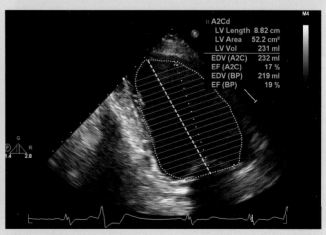

Technical Tips for Simpson's Biplane Volumes (continued)

Comparing the LV length between the apical 4-chamber and apical 2-chamber views is important to ensure that these views are orthogonal to one another. The difference in length between these views should be less than 10%. From the apical 4-chamber view *(below left image)*, the LV length is 8.4 cm while from the apical 2-chamber view *(below right image)*, the LV length is 6.4 cm; this is a difference of 24%. The most common source of error is foreshortening of the apical 2-chamber. **Note:** Do not compare LV volumes - these should not be the same between the 2 views as the LV is not spherical.

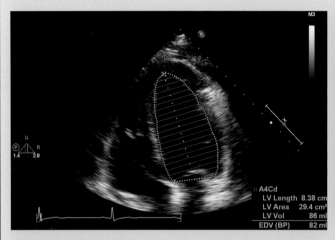
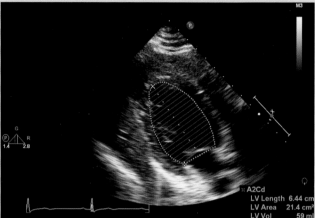

Do Not Extrapolate
When the entire LV cannot be encompassed within the 2D sector width, it is recommended that the tracing of the LV cavity be terminated at the limits of the 2D sector *(below left)* rather than extrapolated to an imagined endocardial boundary *(below right)*.

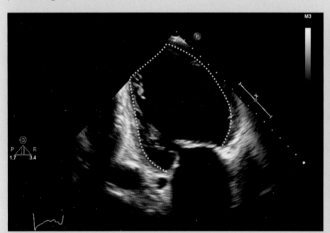
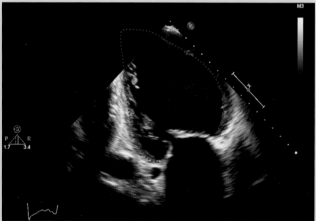

Suboptimal Endocardial Definition
When there is suboptimal visualisation of endocardial borders of 2 or more LV segments in an apical view, an intravenous contrast agent can be used to improve endocardial borders. The use of contrast agents opacifies the LV cavity which improves the recognition of the endocardial borders.

In the example below, the image on the left was recorded without a contrast agent while the image on the right was recorded following the injection of a contrast agent. Observe the improved endocardial border definition following the opacification of the LV cavity in the contrast image.

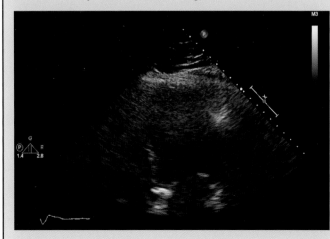
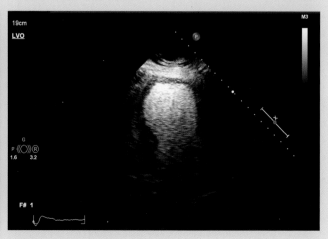

Measurements of LV Systolic Function

Many methods for assessing LV systolic function via 2D echocardiography have been described (Table 2.3). Only the methods most commonly employed in routine clinical practice are described in the following section (**bold, italic** indices in Table 2.3). The regional wall motion score index is discussed in Chapter 5. The normal values for these selected indices of LV systolic function are listed in Table 2.4.

Fractional Shortening

Fractional shortening (FS) or shortening fraction is the percentage of change in the LV cavity dimension with systole. The FS can be calculated from the M-mode or 2D measurements of the LVEDD and the LVESD (Fig. 2.26). FS is calculated from the equation:

Equation 2.7

$$FS = [(LVEDD - LVESD) \div LVEDD] \times 100$$

where FS   = fractional shortening (%)
       LVEDD = left ventricular end-diastolic dimension (cm)
       LVESD = left ventricular end-systolic dimension (cm)

The reference limits and various partition values of the FS with respect to LV systolic function are listed in Table 2.5.

Limitations of FS

The principal limitation of the FS is that this measurement is performed in one dimension, usually at the base of the LV. Therefore, when there are regional wall motion abnormalities, in particular apical abnormalities, this one-dimensional measurement can overestimate the overall LV systolic function.

Therefore, the FS as an indicator of LV systolic function is only reliable when the function is normal or globally reduced. Other limitations of this technique relate to errors in linear measurements such as the overestimation of LV dimensions due to oblique M-mode measurements and underestimation of the LV dimensions by confusing cordal structures for the endocardium of the posterior LV wall.

Ejection Fraction

The ejection fraction (EF) is the percentage of the LV diastolic volume that is ejected with systole. In other words, the EF is a measure of the ability of the ventricle to empty. The EF can be calculated from the M-mode or 2D derived LV volumes (Fig. 2.26 and 2.27). EF is calculated from the equation:

Equation 2.8

$$EF = [(LVEDV - LVESV) \div LVEDV] \times 100$$

where EF   = ejection fraction (%)
       LVEDV = left ventricular end-diastolic volume (mL)
       LVESV = left ventricular end-systolic volume (mL)

Recall that SV is derived as the difference between the LVEDV and LVESV (Eq. 2.1). Therefore, the EF can also be described as the ratio of the SV to the end-diastolic volume:

Equation 2.9

$$EF = (SV \div LVEDV) \times 100$$

where EF   = ejection fraction (%)
       LVEDV = left ventricular end-diastolic volume (mL)
       SV   = stroke volume (mL)

Simplified Quiñones's Method for EF

An alternative method for calculating the EF from 2D or M-mode linear LV measurements is the simplified Quiñones's method. This method is based on the diameter-length estimation of volumes. Volumes derived via the diameter-length method are expressed as:

Equation 2.10

$$Vol = (\pi/6)\,(D^2\,L)$$

where Vol = volume (mL)
      D   = minor axis of the chamber (cm)
      L   = major or long axis of the chamber (cm)

Table 2.3 Echocardiographic Methods for Assessing Left Ventricular Systolic Function

• Aortic acceleration time	• Mitral annular descent
• Aortic deceleration time	• Mitral EPSS
• Aortic root systolic excursion	• ***Myocardial performance index***
• ***Cardiac index***	• Myocardial velocities (Doppler tissue imaging)
• ***Cardiac output***	• Pre-ejection wall stress
• Circumferential fibre shortening	• Regional wall motion score index
• ***dP/dt***	• Strain and strain rate imaging
• ***Doppler tissue imaging systolic velocity***	• ***Stroke volume***
• ***Ejection fraction***	• Systolic time intervals
• ***Fractional shortening***	• Systolic wall tension
• Isovolumic contraction time	• Tissue displacement
• Mean systolic ejection rate	• Tissue tracking
• Mean wall stress	• Velocity Vector Imaging
• Mid wall fractional shortening	• Wall stress (circumferential & meridional)

Bold, italic indices represent commonly employed methods for assessing LV systolic function in routine clinical practice.

Table 2.4 Normal Values for Commonly Used Indices of Left Ventricular Systolic Function

Index of LV Systolic Function	Normal Value
Cardiac Index (CI)	$2.4 - 4.2$ L/min/m^2
Cardiac Output (CO)	$4 - 8$ L/min
Doppler tissue imaging systolic velocity (s')	> 9 cm/s
dP/dt	> 1200 mm Hg/s
Ejection Fraction (EF)	$\geq 55\%$
Fractional Shortening (FS)	$27 - 45\%$
Myocardial Performance Index (MPI) [conventional method]	< 0.4
Myocardial Performance Index (MPI) [DTI method]	< 0.6
Stroke Volume (SV)	$70 - 100$ mL

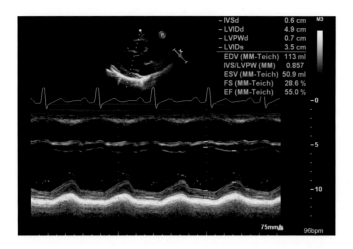

Figure 2.26 From this M-mode trace of the left ventricle, the LVEDD (**LVIDd**) is 4.9 cm and the LVESD (**LVIDs**) is 3.5 cm. The FS in this example is calculated as:

$$FS\ (\%) = (LVEDD - LVESD) \div LVEDD \times 100$$
$$= (4.9 - 3.5) \div 4.9 \times 100$$
$$= 29\%$$

From the LVIDd and LVIDs, the LVEDV (EDV (MM-Teich)) and the LVESV (ESV (MM-Teich)) are derived via the Teichholz equation:

$$LVEDV = (7.0 \div [2.4 + LVEDD]) \times LVEDD^3$$
$$= 7.0 \div [2.4 + 4.9]) \times 4.9^3$$
$$= (7.0 \div 7.3) \times 117.649$$
$$= 113\ mL$$

$$LVESV = (7.0 \div [2.4 + LVESD]) \times LVESD^3$$
$$= 7.0 \div [2.4 + 3.5]) \times 3.5^3$$
$$= (7.0 \div 5.9) \times 42.875$$
$$= 51\ mL$$

The EF is then derived from the LVEDV and the LVESV:

$$EF\ (\%) = (LVEDV - LVESV) \div LVEDV \times 100$$
$$= (113 - 51) \div 113 \times 100$$
$$= 55\%$$

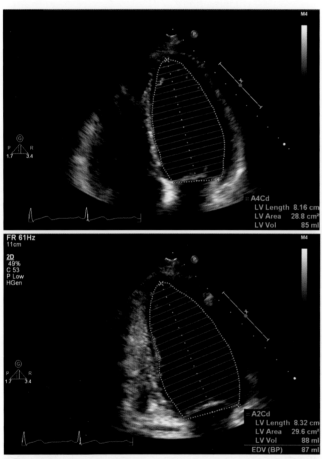

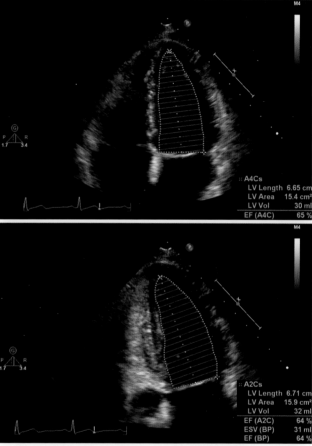

Figure 2.27 LV volumes are derived from the Simpson's biplane method. The EF is then derived from the LVEDV and LVESV. In the apical 4-chamber view the LVEDV (LV Vol) is 85 mL *(top left)* and the LVESV (LV Vol) is 30 mL *(top right)*. In the apical 2-chamber view the LVEDV (LV Vol) is 88 mL *(bottom left)* and the LVESV (LV Vol) is 32 mL *(bottom right)*. The biplane LVEDV (EDV(BP)) is 87 mL *(bottom left)* and the biplane LVESV (ESV(BP)) is 31 mL *(bottom right)*. The apical 4-chamber EF (A4C), apical 2-chamber EF (A2C) and the biplane EF (BP) in this example are calculated as:

$$EF\ (A4C)\ (\%) = (LVEDV - LVESV) \div LVEDV \times 100$$
$$= (85 - 30) \div 85 \times 100$$
$$= 65\%$$

$$EF\ (A2C)\ (\%) = (LVEDV - LVESV) \div LVEDV \times 100$$
$$= (88 - 32) \div 88 \times 100$$
$$= 64\%$$

$$EF\ (BP)\ (\%) = (LVEDV - LVESV) \div LVEDV \times 100$$
$$= (87 - 31) \div 87 \times 100$$
$$= 64\%$$

By combining equations 2.8 and 2.10, the EF can then be calculated as:

Equation 2.11

$$EF = \frac{(\pi/6)\,[(LVEDD^2 \times LVEDL) - (LVESD^2 \times LVESL)] \times 100}{(\pi/6)\,(LVEDD^2 \times LVEDL)}$$

where EF   = ejection fraction (%)
LVEDD = left ventricular end-diastolic dimension (cm)
LVEDL = left ventricular end-diastolic length (cm)
LVESD = left ventricular end-systolic dimension (cm)
LVESL = left ventricular end-systolic length (cm)

This equation can be algebraically converted to:

Equation 2.12

$$EF = \left[\frac{LVEDD^2 - LVESD^2}{LVEDD^2}\right] + \left[1 - \frac{LVEDD^2 - LVESD^2}{LVEDD^2}\right] \times \left[\frac{LVEDL - LVESL}{LVEDL}\right] \times 100$$

Thus, Equation 2.12 expresses the EF as a function of the fractional shortening of the square of the minor axis ($\%\Delta D^2$) and the fractional shortening of the long axis ($\%\Delta L$) and, therefore, can be simplified further to:

Equation 2.13

$$EF = \{\%\Delta D^2 + [(1 - \%\Delta D^2)\,(\%\Delta L)]\} \times 100$$

Using this method, the EF can be derived from the LVEDD, LVESD and the contractility of the LV apex. Thus, the calculation of the EF via this simplified method is a two-step process.

Step 1:
Calculate the fractional shortening of the square of the minor axis ($\%\Delta D^2$) from the LVEDD and LVESD measurements performed via 2D or M-mode:

Equation 2.14

$$\%\Delta D^2 = (LVEDD^2 - LVESD^2) \div LVEDD^2$$

Step 2:
Correct for apical contractility by observing the apical contractility of the LV from the apical views:

Equation 2.15

$$EF = (\%\Delta D^2) + [(1 - \%\Delta D^2)\,(\%\Delta L)]$$

where $\%\Delta L$ = 0.15 (15% for normal apical contraction)
         = 0.05 (5% for hypokinetic apical contraction)
         = 0 (0% for akinetic apical contraction)
         = -0.05 (-5% for slightly dyskinetic apical contraction)
         = -0.10 (-10% for frankly dyskinetic apical contraction)

The reference limits and various partition values of the EF with respect to LV systolic function are listed in Table 2.5.

> The recommended method of estimating the EF is the Simpson's biplane method as this method does not rely on geometric assumptions to convert linear measurements into volumes.

M-mode versus 2D Linear Measurements

When comparing M-mode and 2D linear LV measurements, it must be emphasised that M-mode is measuring slightly different levels of the ventricle between end-diastole (ED) and end-systole (ES). This is because the M-mode cursor remains stationary but during systole the base of the heart moves towards the LV apex; as such the M-mode cursor will be positioned a little closer to the mitral annulus in systole. Therefore, when measuring the LV via M-mode LV shortening is not being measured at the same level. 2D measurements on the other hand can be performed at the same level of the ventricle at ED and ES. The images below demonstrate the location of M-mode and 2D LV measurements at ED and ES. M-mode measurements are performed along the stationary M-mode cursor while 2D measurements are performed at the yellow circles.

Note that there is no difference between the M-mode and 2D measurement sites at ED *(left)*. However at ES the M-mode measurements would be performed a little closer to the mitral annulus compared with 2D measurements which are performed at the base of the LV *(right)*.

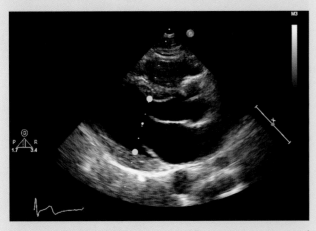 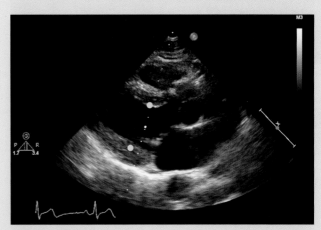

The advantages of M-mode over 2D measurements are its superior temporal resolution and interface definition. Hence, when the M-mode assessment of the LV can be correctly performed from on-axis images of the LV, M-mode measurements tend to be more accurate than 2D measurements.

Limitations of EF

Limitations of EF calculations include the technical factors which prohibit accurate linear measurements of the LV, as previously described, as well as the obvious limitations of converting these linear measurements into 3-dimensional (3D) volumes. Limitations to the biplane Simpson's EF relate to limitations of obtaining accurate LV volumes (refer to Technical Tips for Simpson's Biplane Volumes).

It is also important to note that the EF does not just reflect ventricular contractility as the EF is highly dependent upon loading conditions as well as contractility. Recall that the EF is derived from SV and the LVEDV, and that the SV is determined by preload, afterload and contractility (refer to Determinants of Stroke Volume). The effect of loading conditions on EF can be illustrated by cases of mitral regurgitation (MR) and aortic stenosis (AS). In MR, increased preload and decreased afterload increases EF and may cause an overestimation of contractility; that is, because EF is "normal", contractility may be misleadingly assumed to also be normal when it is in fact abnormal. In AS, excess afterload may cause the EF to be reduced and may cause an underestimation of contractility; that is, because EF is reduced contractility may also be mistakenly assumed to be reduced when it is in fact normal.

Stroke Volume, Cardiac Output and Cardiac Index

Stroke Volume

SV refers to the amount of blood pumped by the heart on each single beat. As previously mentioned SV is calculated as the difference between the EDV and the ESV (Refer to Equation 2.1). LVEDV and LVESV can be derived from 2D and M-mode measurements as described above.

SV can also be determined via the 2D/Doppler method as described in Chapter 1. Recall that the SV via 2D/Doppler is calculated from the cross-sectional area (CSA) and velocity time integral (VTI):

Equation 2.16

$$SV = CSA \times VTI$$

where SV = stroke volume (mL)
      VTI = distance a column of blood travels with each stroke (cm)
      CSA= cross-sectional area (cm^2)

Theoretically, the SV can be calculated from any cardiac site where CSA and VTI can be measured, assuming that the flow profile at the site is flat and flow is laminar. Generally the sites used to calculate the SV are the valve annuli and the outflow tracts (Table 2.6). Of these, the SV is most commonly calculated from the left ventricular outflow tract (LVOT) (Fig. 2.28).

Cardiac Output

Cardiac output (CO) is the volume of blood pumped by the heart per minute. CO is derived from the SV and the heart rate and is expressed as:

Equation 2.17

$$CO = (SV \times HR) \div 1000$$

where CO = cardiac output (L/min)
    SV = stroke volume (mL)
    HR = heart rate (bpm)
    1000 = conversion of millilitres (mL) to litres (L)

Myocardial Contractility versus Ventricular Function

"Myocardial contractility" refers to the contractile or inotropic state of the myocardium; myocardial contractility is independent of loading conditions and remodelling. "Ventricular function" relates LV performance (i.e. SV) to preload based on the Frank-Starling mechanism. The term ventricular function also includes shortening indices such as the FS and EF. These indices are often mistakenly referred to as measurements of ventricular contractility. However, these indices are sensitive to changes in loading conditions as well as contractility.

Practical Pointer

The LVOT is the most common site for the calculation of the SV and CO because: (1) in most patients, the LVOT can be measured with greater ease and accuracy than other areas of the heart, (2) the LVOT can be measured in the axial plane of the transducer (axial resolution is generally better than the lateral resolution), (3) the LVOT diameter is nearly circular so that calculation of the CSA is more accurate and closer to the true area, (4) the CSA of the LVOT is constant throughout systole (AV valve areas are constantly changing during diastole), and (5) flow within the entrance of the LVOT has a flat flow profile.

Caveat

In the presence of aortic regurgitation (AR), the CO cannot be estimated from the LVOT SV. In the case of AR, not all of the SV into the LVOT travels to the body, some leaks back through the aortic valve during diastole. Therefore, the CO will be overestimated in this setting.

Table 2.5 **Reference Limits and Partition Values of Left Ventricular Systolic Function**

	WOMEN				MEN			
	Reference range	Mildly abnormal	Moderately abnormal	Severely abnormal	Reference range	Mildly abnormal	Moderately abnormal	Severely abnormal
Linear method								
Endocardial fractional shortening, %	27–45	22–26	17–21	≤ 16	25–43	20–24	15–19	≤ 14
2D Method								
Ejection fraction, %	*≥ 55*	*45–54*	*30–44*	*< 30*	*≥ 55*	*45–54*	*30–44*	*< 30*

Bold italic values: Recommended and best validated.

Reprinted from Lang RM, Bierig M, Devereux RB, et al., Chamber Quantification Writing Group; American Society of Echocardiography's Guidelines and Standards Committee; European Association of Echocardiography. Recommendations for Chamber Quantification: A Report from the American Society of Echocardiography's Guidelines and Standards Committee and the Chamber Quantification Writing Group, Developed in Conjunction with the European Association of Echocardiography, a Branch of the European Society of Cardiology, *J Am Soc Echocardiogr*, Vol. 18(12), page 1448, © 2005 with permission from Elsevier.

Table 2.6 **Methods for Estimating the Stroke Volume from Various Sites**

Site	Diameter (CSA) Measurement		VTI Measurement	
Ascending aorta	Echo View	PLAX (LV) at or above sinotubular junction	Echo View	Suprasternal view
	Phase of cardiac cycle	Mid-systole	Technique	2-4 mm PW sample volume is placed 3-5 cm above aortic valve and within ascending aorta Signal traced at edge of modal velocity
	Technique	Measure perpendicular to aortic root Calipers are placed from inner edge of anterior aortic wall to inner edge posterior aortic wall		
LVOT (Fig. 2.28)	Echo View	PLAX (LV) – zoom of the LVOT	Echo View	Apical 5-chamber or apical long axis view
	Phase of cardiac cycle	Mid-systole	Technique	2-4 mm PW sample volume is placed 0.5 cm proximal to the aortic valve Signal traced at edge of modal velocity
	Technique	Measure perpendicular to aortic root Calipers are placed from inner edge of junction between anterior aortic wall and IVS to inner edge of junction between posterior aortic wall and anterior mitral valve leaflet		
Main pulmonary artery	Echo View	PSAX (RVOT)	Echo View	PSAX (RVOT)
	Phase of cardiac cycle	Mid-systole	Technique	2-4 mm PW sample volume is placed at same level as diameter measurement Signal traced along modal velocity
	Technique	Measure perpendicular to pulmonary annulus Calipers are placed from inner edge to inner edge of main pulmonary artery		
Mitral annulus	Echo View	Apical 4-chamber (zoom of mitral valve)	Echo View	Apical 4-chamber (zoom of mitral valve)
	Phase of cardiac cycle	Early diastole (2-3 frames post end-systole)	Technique	1-2 mm PW sample volume is placed at mitral annulus Signal traced along modal velocity
	Technique	Calipers are placed from inner edge to inner edge of mitral leaflets where leaflets insert into ventricular myocardium		
RVOT	Echo View	PLAX (RVOT) or PSAX (RVOT)	Echo View	PSAX (RVOT)
	Phase of cardiac cycle	Mid-systole	Technique	2-4 mm PW sample volume is placed 0.5 cm proximal to pulmonary valve (RVOT side of valve) Signal traced at edge of modal velocity
	Technique	Perpendicular to pulmonary annulus Calipers are placed from inner edge to inner edge of RVOT at cuspal insertions		
Tricuspid annulus	Echo View	Apical 4-chamber (zoom of tricuspid valve)	Echo View	Apical 4-chamber (zoom of tricuspid valve)
	Phase of cardiac cycle	Early diastole (2-3 frames post end-systole)	Technique	1-2 mm PW sample volume is placed at tricuspid annulus Signal traced along modal velocity
	Technique	Calipers are placed from inner edge to inner edge of tricuspid leaflets where leaflets insert into ventricular myocardium		

All measurements should be averaged: sinus rhythm average 2-3 consecutive cardiac cycles; atrial fibrillation average 3-5 consecutive cardiac cycles.

CSA = cross-sectional area; IVS = interventricular septum; LVOT = left ventricular outflow tract; PLAX (LV) = parasternal long axis view of the left ventricle; PLAX (RVOT) = parasternal long axis view of the right ventricular outflow tract; PSAX (RVOT) = parasternal short axis view at the level of the aorta; PW = pulsed-wave Doppler; RVOT = right ventricular outflow tract; VTI = velocity time integral.

The CO can be derived from 2D and M-mode measurements of LVEDV and LVESV or from the 2D/Doppler method (Fig. 2.28).

Cardiac Index

The cardiac index (CI) is simply the CO divided by the BSA:

Equation 2.18

$$CI = CO \div BSA$$

where CI   = cardiac index (L/min/m^2)
     CO   = cardiac output (L/min)
     BSA = body surface area (m^2)

Indexing the CO to the BSA relates the heart performance to the size of an individual which allows the direct comparison of this index between large and small patients.

Relationship between EF, SV and CO

EF and CO are important indices for assessing the overall LV systolic function. However, it is important to note that the EF and CO are not the same. That is, while both are indices

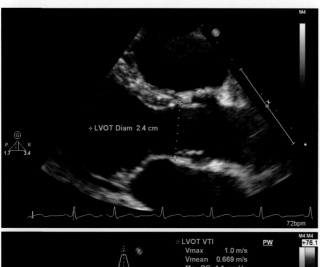

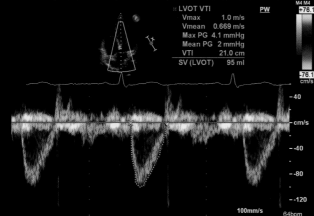

Figure 2.28 The left ventricular outflow tract diameter (LVOT Diam) is measured at 2.4 cm *(top)* and the LVOT velocity time integral (VTI) is 21 cm *(bottom)*. The SV in this example is calculated as:

SV (mL)   = LVOT CSA x LVOT VTI
           = 0.785 x LVOT Diam^2 x VTI
           = 0.785 x 2.4^2 x 21
           = 95 mL

The heart rate (HR) is 64 bpm (recorded on the VTI trace at the bottom right corner). The CO is then calculated as:

CO (L/min) = SV x HR ÷ 1000
             = 95 x 64 ÷ 1000
             = 6.1 L/min

of the LV systolic performance, they are actually measuring different elements of LV performance.

As discussed, CO is derived from the SV and heart rate (Eq. 2.17), and the SV is derived from the LVEDV and LVESV (Eq. 2.1). Therefore, the CO is a measure of the *integrated* pumping function of the heart. Furthermore, SV is related to EF and LVEDV (Eq. 2.9). Therefore, the overall output of the LV (SV and CO) is determined by: (1) the degree of LV filling (LVEDV), and (2) the percentage of LV emptying (EF) (Fig. 2.29).

Importantly, increases and decreases in EF are not paralleled by reciprocal changes in SV. This is because SV is the combined result of many factors such as the LVEDV and EF. LVEDV is dependent upon the diastolic function of the LV which is determined by a number of extrinsic and intrinsic factors such as LV compliance, LV relaxation, LA volume and pressure, the mitral valve structure, and the pericardium. The EF reflects the systolic function of the LV and this is dependent upon factors such as LV contractility, afterload (impedance to LV emptying), preload (LVEDV) and heart rate. Furthermore, the forward SV and CO are also affected by the competency of the mitral and aortic valves. Any changes to these determining factors can alter the LVEF, the CO or both variables. Clinical examples illustrating the relationship between EF and CO are shown in Table 2.7.

Limitations of SV, CO and CI

Limitations of these calculations when derived from M-mode and 2D methods include the technical factors which prohibit accurate linear measurements of the LV as well as the pitfalls of obtaining accurate biplane Simpson's LV volumes as previously described. It is also a well-recognised fact that the biplane Simpson's volumes underestimate LV volumes when compared with 3D echocardiographic volumes and volumes derived via the CMRI.

Pitfalls of 2D/Doppler SV calculations are described in Chapter 1. In particular, when using the LVOT for calculation of the SV, CO and CI, the most common errors relate to inaccurate measurement of LVOT diameter, overtracing of the LVOT VTI, suboptimal positioning of the pulsed-wave Doppler sample volume within the LVOT, and non-parallel alignment of the Doppler beam with LVOT flow (Fig. 2.30).

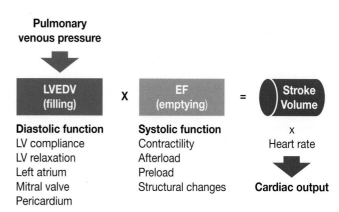

Figure 2.29 This figure illustrates the relationship between filling (LVEDV), emptying (EF) and output (SV and CO). See text for further details.

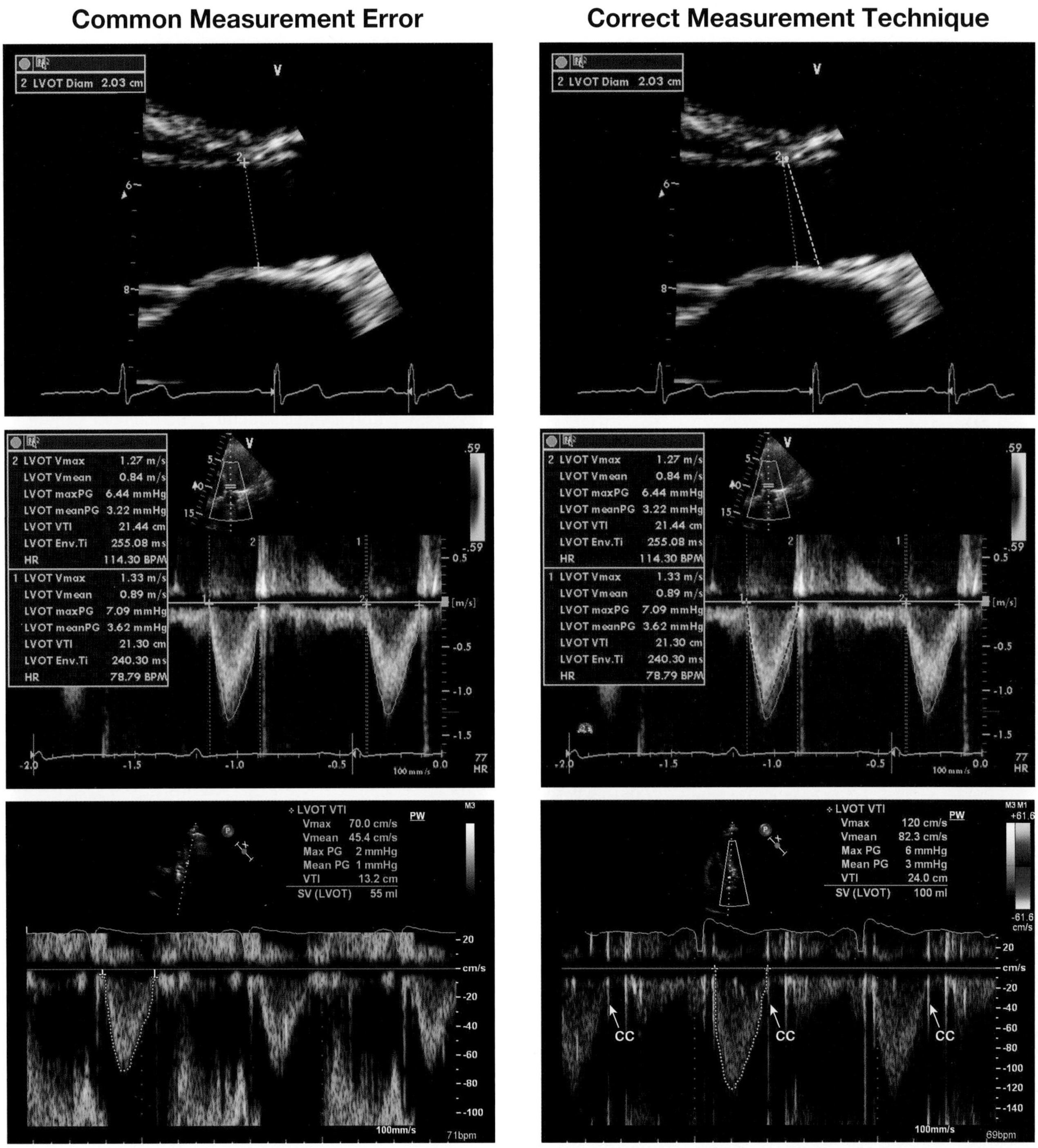

Common Measurement Error

Correct Measurement Technique

Figure 2.30 Common errors in 2D/Doppler calculation of LVOT stroke volume are shown in the images on the left; correct measurements are shown in the adjacent images on the right. **Top:** When measuring the LVOT diameter ensure that the LVOT is measured perpendicular to the aortic root. Use the cuspal insertion points as anatomical landmarks for the LVOT. **Middle:** When tracing the LVOT VTI be sure to trace along the edge of the most solid line (red dashed line on right trace); this is the modal velocity. The "fluffy" component of the signal represents spectral broadening. **Bottom:** On the left trace, the sample volume is positioned too far from the LVOT so the VTI is underestimated at 13 cm. On the right trace, the sample volume is correctly placed and the VTI is now 24 cm. To determine the correct sample volume position, look for a closing click (cc) on the spectral Doppler LVOT trace. Also in the presence of normal LV systolic function, the LVOT VTI should be greater than 18 cm. If VTI is less than 18 cm, in the setting of normal LV systolic function, consider that the sample volume may be positioned too low into the LV. Zooming on the LVOT will also assist with precise sample volume placement.

While it is feasible to calculate the SV, CO and CI from ventricular volumes derived via linear dimensions and 2D volumes, the preferred method of estimating these indices is the 2D/Doppler method. This is due to the limitations of linear measurements in determining LV volumes and the significant underestimation of LV volumes via the Simpson's biplane method.

Table 2.7 Clinical Examples Illustrating the Relationship between EF and CO

	LVEDV (mL)	EF (%)	SV (mL)	HR (bpm)	CO (L/min)	Comment
Normal Heart	120	65	78	70	5.5	Good correlation between the LV size, EF and CO (i.e. all values within normal range)
DCM with normal CO	200 (↑)	35 (↓)	70 (-)	80	5.6 (-)	LVEDV increases due to Frank-Starling mechanism and within certain limits, increased LVEDV increases contractility and SV. Therefore, despite a decreased EF, SV and CO can still be within the normal range.
DCM with low CO	250 (↑)	20 (↓)	50 (↓)	60	3.0 (↓)	The Frank-Starling mechanism also shows that the ability of the LV to dilate and increase its SV to increase its contractility is limited. In other words, further increases in LVEDV do not increase the SV or contractility. So in this instance, the EF, SV and CO are all reduced.
RCM	80 (↓)	60 (-)	48 (↓)	70	3.4 (↓)	LVEDV is decreased due to increased myocardial stiffness which impedes diastolic filling. In these cases, even though the EF is normal, the SV and CO are reduced because of a decreased LVEDV.
Severe MR (RV 56mL)	180 (↑)	60 (-)	52 (↓)	75	3.6 (↓)	The LVEDV is increased due to the combination of normal forward SV returning from the lungs plus the regurgitant volume (RV). In the example illustrated, total LV SV is 108 mL (LVSV = LVEDV x EF = 180 x 0.60 = 108 mL). Forward SV to the body is equal to the difference between the total LV SV and the RV (forward SV = 108 – 56 = 52 mL). Therefore, even though the EF is normal CO is reduced. The 'effective' EF (EEF) is equal to forward SV divided by LVEDV (EEF = 52 ÷ 180 x 100 = 29%).

DCM = dilated cardiomyopathy; **MR** = mitral regurgitation; **RCM** = restrictive cardiomyopathy; **RV** = regurgitant volume; - = no change

dP/dt

Indices obtained during the ejection phase of the cardiac cycle such as the EF, SV and CO are commonly used to assess LV systolic function. However, these indices are influenced by loading conditions. Indices obtained during the non-ejection phase of the cardiac cycle are relatively independent of load and are considered better measures of intrinsic contractility compared with ejection phase indices. The dP/dt is one such measurement.

The dP/dt is a measurement of the rate of LV pressure rise during isovolumic contraction, where dP is the change in LV pressure and dt is the time taken for the change to develop. The dP/dt can be measured in the presence of MR. The MR Doppler velocity reflects the pressure difference between the LV and LA during systole; assuming that the LAP remains relatively constant then the rate of rise of the Doppler velocity reflects the rate of LV pressure rise.

The dP/dt is performed by measuring the time interval between two arbitrary points on the MR velocity spectrum (usually between 1 and 3 m/s). Using the simplified Bernoulli equation, the velocity at these points can be converted to pressure and, hence, the pressure difference between these two points can be determined. For example, the pressure difference between 1 m/s (4 mm Hg) and 3 m/s (36 mm Hg) is 32 mm Hg. Therefore, the dP/dt,may be defined as the time it takes for the LV to generate 32 mm Hg of pressure during the isovolumic contraction (Fig. 2.31):

Equation 2.19

$$dP/dt = 32 \div \Delta t$$

where dP/dt = rate of pressure rise over time (mm Hg/s)

    32   = the pressure difference between 1 m/s and 3 m/s using the simplified Bernoulli equation: $[4 (3)^2] – [4 (1)^2] = 32$ mm Hg

    Δt = time interval between 1 m/s and 3 m/s (s)

With normal LV systolic function, the ventricle is able to generate 32 mm Hg of pressure during the isovolumic contraction phase very rapidly while in the setting of LV systolic dysfunction there is prolongation of the dP/dt (Fig. 2.32). Values indicating the relationship between the dP/dt and LV systolic function are listed in Table 2.8.

> **Usefulness of the dP/dt**
> Significant MR with impaired contractility may show a "normal" EF due to increased preload (increased LVEDV) and decreased afterload (ejection into a low-resistance LA) . Therefore, measurement of the dP/dt is especially valuable in this setting to avoid the overestimation of LV contractility based on a "normal" EF.

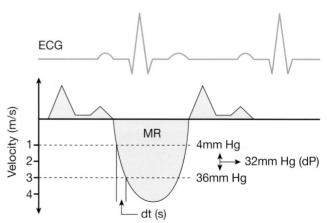

Figure 2.31 From the continuous-wave Doppler signal of the mitral regurgitant (MR) jet, the time interval between 1 m/s and 3 m/s is measured (dt). Using the simplified Bernoulli equation, the velocity can be converted to pressure so that the change in pressure (**dP**) between 1 and 3 m/s can be determined: $[4 (3)^2] – [4 (1)^2] = 32$ mm Hg. Therefore, the dP/dt, the change in pressure over time, is derived from the time it takes for the LV to generate 32 mmHg of pressure during the isovolumic contraction phase of the cardiac cycle.

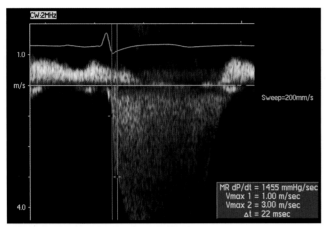

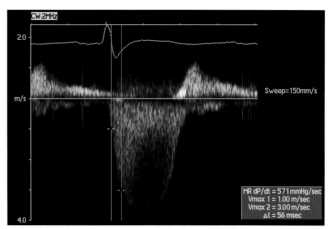

Figure 2.32 On the left is a measurement of the dP/dt in a patient with normal LV systolic function. The time interval (Δt) between 1 m/s and 3 m/s is 22 ms or 0.022 s. Thus, the dP/dt in this example is equal to 32 ÷ 0.022 which is 1455 mm Hg/s. On the right is a measurement of the dP/dt in a patient with severe LV systolic dysfunction. Observe the obvious prolongation of the ascending limb of the MR signal compared with the image on the left. The time interval (Δt) between 1 m/s and 3 m/s is 56 ms or 0.056s. Thus, the dP/dt in this example is equal to 32 ÷ 0.056 or 571 mm Hg/s. Also observe that a fast sweep speed is used for these measurements to improve measurement accuracy.

Limitations of dP/dt

As mentioned, the MR velocity signal reflects the instantaneous pressure gradient between the LV and the LA during systole. The dP/dt is calculated based on the assumption that the LA pressure remains relatively constant during the isovolumic contraction phase, and this assumption is based on a compliant LA. That is, it is assumed that the LA is able to accept the MR volume without a significant increase in its pressure during isovolumic contraction. However, in acute MR, the LA is relatively noncompliant and, therefore, the pressure in the LA during isovolumic contraction may be significantly elevated. In this instance the dP/dt is not a measure of LV pressure rise alone.

Suboptimal MR signals may occur when there is poor alignment of the Doppler beam with the regurgitant jet. This is particularly problematic with eccentric jets. Another problem which may affect the accuracy of this measurement is valve click artefact which may obscure the early regurgitant Doppler profile.

Systolic Myocardial Velocities

The arrangement of myocardial muscle fibres is very complex. Fibres are orientated in the oblique, circumferential and longitudinal directions with all fibres acting together to maintain a normal EF. In particular, longitudinal fibres contribute to the long-axis shortening of the ventricle during systolic contraction; therefore long-axis LV shortening can be used as measure of LV systolic function.

Doppler tissue imaging (DTI) enables the measurement of the longitudinal myocardial velocities and therefore provides an estimation of LV systolic function.

Longitudinal myocardial velocities via DTI can be measured from the apical views. Measurement of the peak systolic velocity of myocardial tissue reflects the systolic longitudinal shortening of the ventricle.

The myocardial velocity profile obtained by pulsed DTI from the apical views is characterised by three distinct waveforms: (1) an apically directed systolic myocardial velocity (s'), (2) an early diastolic atrially directed myocardial velocity (e'), and (3) a late diastolic atrially directed myocardial velocity (a'). In addition to these three distinct velocities, less prominent biphasic velocities may be seen between the s' and e' waves during the isovolumic relaxation period and between the a' and s' waves during the isovolumic contraction period (Fig. 2.33).

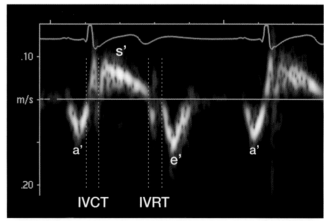

Figure 2.33 From the apical views, the systolic myocardial velocity (s') is apically directed and is, therefore, displayed above the zero baseline. The early diastolic myocardial velocity (e') and the late diastolic myocardial velocity (a') are both atrially directed velocities and, therefore, are displayed below the zero baseline. The time interval between the end of the s' velocity and the beginning of the next e' velocity is the isovolumic relaxation time (IVRT) while the interval between the end of the a' velocity and the beginning of the next s' velocity is the isovolumic contraction time (IVCT).

Table 2.8 Reference Limits and Partition Values for the dP/dt

	Normal	Mild-Moderate LV Systolic Dysfunction	Severe LV Systolic Dysfunction
dP/dt Values (mm Hg/s)*	> 1200	800 – 1200	< 800
Time for LV to generate 32 mm Hg	< 27 ms	27 – 40 ms	> 40 ms

* Source: Nishimura, R.A. and Tajik, A.J. Quantitative hemodynamics by Doppler echocardiography: A noninvasive alternative to cardiac catheterization. *Prog Cardiovasc Dis.* 1994 Jan-Feb;36(4):309-42

Limitations of s' Velocities

DTI is a pulsed Doppler technique which measures localised velocities within one segment of the ventricular wall as indicated by the sample volume position. Measurement of the s' velocity at this localised segment is then assumed to reflect the systolic function of the entire ventricle. This is one of the primary disadvantages of DTI in the evaluation of systolic ventricular function.

It is important to note that DTI velocities are influenced not only by myocardial function, but also by myocardial tethering and cardiac translational motion. In particular, DTI is not able to distinguish between actively contracting myocardium and passive myocardial motion. For example, normal s' velocities may be detected when a hypocontractile or akinetic myocardial segment is being 'pulled on' by normally contracting myocardium; this effect is referred to as myocardial tethering. Likewise, s' velocities can be affected by the normal translational motion of the heart within the thorax during the cardiac cycle.

It is also important to remember that normally the s' velocities progressively decrease from the base to the apex; thus, sample volume positioning is important when using this variable in the assessment of systolic function.

DTI is a Doppler technique and, therefore, the accuracy of velocity measurements is dependent upon the incident angle between the sampling site and myocardial motion. Furthermore, myocardial velocities from the apical views do not detect radial and circumferential myocardial motion, which significantly contribute to overall systolic function.

While it is possible to measure myocardial velocities from stored colour encoded DTI images it is important to note that colour-coded tissue Doppler yields lower velocities than pulsed DTI. This is because the encoded data represents the *mean* instantaneous velocities. Therefore, the normal cut-off values via pulsed-wave DTI cannot be applied to the colour-coded tissue Doppler velocities.

DTI Terminology
The terminology for DTI velocities is variable. Early diastolic annular velocities have been termed Ea (a for annular), Em (m for myocardial), E', or e'. Likewise late diastolic velocities have been referred to as Aa, Am, A' or a' and systolic velocities called Sa, Sm, S', or s'. Ea is commonly used to refer to arterial elastance and the 'm' may be confused with the acquisition of the velocity from the medial annulus; therefore, this text uses the terms e', a' and s' when referring to myocardial velocities.

Myocardial Performance Index

There are many parameters that can be used to assess either systolic or diastolic ventricular function; however, systolic and diastolic dysfunction may coexist. Systolic ventricular dysfunction is evident when there is a decreased EF, prolongation of the pre-ejection period (IVCT) and a shortening of the ejection phases of the cardiac cycle. Diastolic ventricular dysfunction is evident by impaired myocardial relaxation and increased ventricular filling pressures.

The myocardial performance index (MPI) reflects the "global" myocardial performance and incorporates both the elements of systole and diastole. This index is particularly useful in the assessment of conditions where systolic and diastolic dysfunction coexist such as in patients with: (1) dilated cardiomyopathy, (2) cardiac amyloidosis, (3) pulmonary hypertension, (4) right ventricular infarction, and (5) right ventricular dysplasia. In addition, the MPI may be particularly valuable in the echocardiographic evaluation of RV function in patients with congenital heart disease because of the complex geometry of the RV.

The MPI is simply the ratio between the isovolumic contraction time (IVCT) plus the isovolumic relaxation time (IVRT), and the ejection time (ET):

Equation 2.20

$$MPI = (IVCT + IVRT) \div ET$$

where MPI = myocardial performance index (unitless)
IVCT = isovolumic contraction time (ms)
IVRT = isovolumic relaxation time (ms)
ET = ejection time (ms)

Several methods have been described for the calculation of the MPI; the most common methods used are described in Figure 2.34.

The MPI has a moderate inverse relationship with the EF; therefore, the higher the value of the MPI, the lower the EF and the lower the value of the MPI, the higher the EF.

Limitations of MPI

In the calculation of the MPI via conventional Doppler, measurements are not performed simultaneously and, therefore, the accuracy of this calculation may be affected by changes in the cycle lengths between each measurement.

In particular, arrhythmias such as atrial flutter/fibrillation and AV heart block affect the mitral inflow profiles; hence, accurate measurement of the MPI may be hindered under these circumstances.

Calculation of the MPI via DTI may overcome the above limitation as the DTI allows the calculation of the MPI from a single cardiac cycle. However, as previously mentioned, calculation of the MPI via this method is only measuring the MPI at one site of the ventricle. Therefore, this is a measurement of the *regional* MPI which may not reflect the overall ventricular function. It has also been noted that the systolic intervals are longer and the diastolic intervals are shorter via DTI. Therefore the normal values obtained via the conventional MPI cannot be applied to the MPI derived via DTI. In particular, the cut-off values for normal are higher for the DTI method.

Clinical Considerations
Measurement of the MPI via DTI provides a measurement of the MPI at one site of the ventricle only. Hence, this is measurement of the regional MPI and this index, therefore, may not reflect the overall ventricular function. In addition, it has been noted that the systolic intervals are longer and the diastolic intervals are shorter via the DTI method; as such, the normal MPI values obtained via conventional Doppler should not be extrapolated to DTI.

Conventional Doppler Method

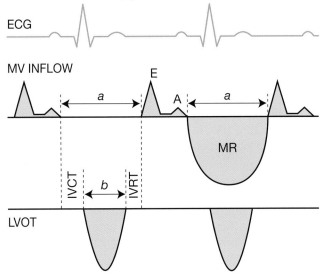

Doppler Tissue Imaging Method

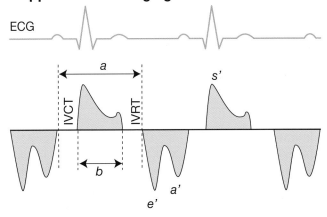

Figure 2.34 The myocardial performance index (MPI) is the ratio between the isovolumic contraction time (IVCT) plus the isovolumic relaxation time (IVRT), and the ejection time (ET): MPI = (IVCT + IVRT) ÷ ET. This index can be derived via conventional Doppler or via Doppler tissue imaging (DTI).

Conventional Doppler Method: Using spectral Doppler, two intervals are measured: (1) Interval a is measured from the mitral inflow trace as the interval between the end of the mitral A wave to the beginning of the next mitral E wave or as the duration of mitral regurgitation (MR); (2) Interval b is the ET which is measured from the left ventricular outflow tract (LVOT) trace from the beginning to end of flow. Observe that interval a incorporates the IVCT, ET and IVRT. Therefore, the sum of the IVCT and IVRT can be simply derived by subtracting the ET (interval b) from interval a: (IVCT + IVRT) = a - b. Therefore: *MPI = (a - b) ÷ b.*

DTI Method: DTI of the mitral annulus is used to calculate two intervals: (1) Interval a is measured from the end of the a' velocity to the beginning of the next e' velocity; and (2) Interval b is measured from the beginning to the end of the s' velocity. Observe that interval a incorporates the IVCT, IVRT plus interval b. Therefore, the sum of the IVCT and IVRT can be simply derived by subtracting the interval b from interval a: (IVCT + IVRT) = a - b. Therefore: *MPI = (a - b) ÷ b.*

> **SV, CO, dP/dt, s' and MPI**
> Unlike the EF, Doppler indices such as the SV, CO, dP/dt, s' and MPI are not dependent on image quality. Therefore, these indices may be especially useful in determining LV systolic function when an estimation of the EF is not possible.

Measurements of Right Ventricular Size

Echocardiographic Views for the RV

The geometry of the RV is quite complex and therefore comprehensive assessment of the RV needs to be performed from a number of echocardiographic views, including the parasternal long axis of the LV, the parasternal long axis of the RV inflow, the parasternal short axis views, the apical 4-chamber, and the subcostal views (Fig. 2.35).

Qualitative Estimates of RV Size

RV size can be qualitatively estimated by using the echocardiographic views above and by comparing the RV size to the LV size.

When the LV is a normal size and when imaged from the standard apical 4-chamber view, the RV should be less than two-thirds the size of the LV with the LV being the "apex-forming" ventricle and the RV apex being closer to the base of the heart. Therefore, when assessing the degree of RV dilatation qualitatively, consideration is made based on the RV cavity size compared with the normal LV cavity size and on which ventricle is the apex-forming ventricle (Fig. 2.36):

- A normal RV size is when the RV is smaller than the LV and the RV apex is more basal than the LV apex with the LV as the apex forming ventricle,
- Mild RV dilatation is when the RV cavity area is greater than two-thirds of the LV but it is still smaller than the LV and the RV apex more basal than the LV apex with the LV as the apex forming ventricle,
- Moderate RV dilatation is when the RV cavity area is similar to that of the LV and the RV shares the apex,
- Severe RV dilatation is when the RV cavity area exceeds that of the LV and the RV forms the apex.

The obvious limitation of this qualitative estimation of RV size is that it is based on comparing the RV with a normal-sized LV. Therefore, when the LV is dilated, qualitative estimation of RV size becomes more difficult.

Quantitative Measurements of the RV

Linear Dimensions of the RV

Linear dimensions of the RV are performed from an RV-focused apical 4-chamber view. Measurements from this RV-focused view are preferred over the standard apical 4-chamber view. This is because of potential variations in RV measurements that may occur from the standard apical 4-chamber view and because the RV-focused view provides improved imaging of the RV lateral wall.

The RV-focused apical 4-chamber view is simply a variation of the standard apical 4-chamber view. This view is obtained by angling the transducer medially from the standard apical 4-chamber view (Fig. 2.37).

Linear measurements of RV dimensions are performed at end-diastole. End-diastole is identified as the frame at initial coaptation of the tricuspid leaflets, or the frame immediately prior to initial coaptation of the tricuspid leaflets following the P wave of the ECG when the patient is in sinus rhythm; the frame chosen is the one in which the RV cavity size is largest. Linear RV measurements performed include: (1) the basal RV cavity diameter, (2) the mid RV cavity diameter, and (3) the RV length (Fig. 2.38).

Linear Dimensions of the RVOT

Linear dimensions of the RVOT can be measured from the parasternal views at end-diastole. End-diastole is based on the motion of the tricuspid valve as previously described. When the tricuspid valve is not seen, end-diastole can be identified as the onset of the QRS complex of the ECG.

The proximal RVOT can be measured from the parasternal long axis view of the LV while the distal RVOT can be measured from the parasternal short-axis views (Fig. 2.39).

The reference limits for RV and RVOT dimensions are listed in Table 2.9.

> **Practical Pointer**
> When measuring the RVOT diameter for the calculation of the SV, this measurement is performed during mid-systole rather than at end-diastole. Recall that the calculation of the SV is performed during the flow period so all measurements should be performed when flow is occurring.
>
> Furthermore, to improve measurement accuracy, the RVOT diameter should be measured from a zoomed view of the RVOT and measurements should be averaged over 2-3 consecutive cardiac cycles.

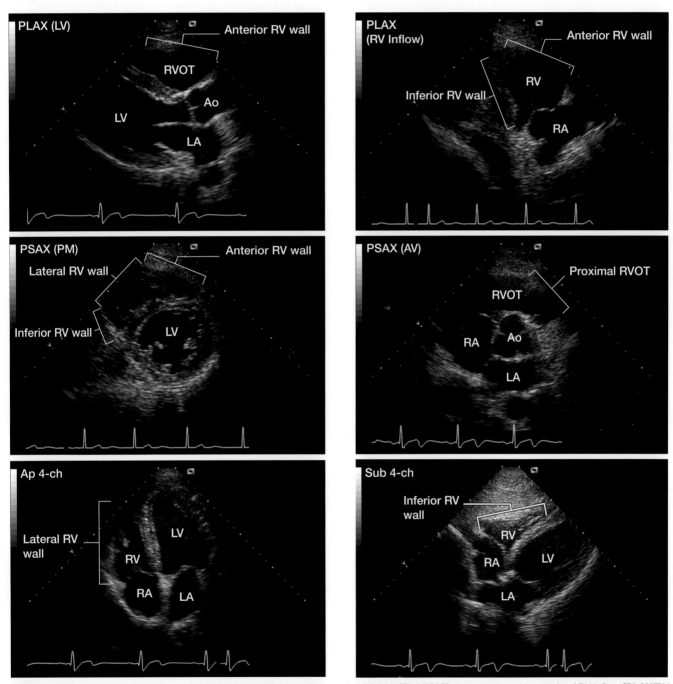

Figure 2.35 The right ventricle can be viewed from the parasternal long axis of the LV [**PLAX(LV)**], the parasternal long axis of RV inflow [**PLAX(RV Inflow)**], the parasternal short axis at the level of the papillary muscles [**PSAX(PM)**], the parasternal short axis at the level of the aortic valve [**PSAX(AV)**], the apical 4-chamber view [**Ap 4-ch**] and the subcostal 4-chamber [**sub 4-ch**] views.
Ao = aorta; LA = left atrium; LV = left ventricle; RA = right atrium; RV = right ventricle; RVOT = right ventricular outflow tract.

Limitations of Linear Dimensions

Image orientation tends to be based on the appearance of the LV rather than the RV. As such there can be a wide variation in the appearance of the RV. For example, the RV can appear dilated in one view and normal in another. This occurs due to the complex shape of the RV and because it wraps around the LV (refer to Fig. 2.1). As a result RV dimensions are highly dependent on the image orientation. For this reason, the RV-focused apical 4-chamber view is recommended for all linear

measurements of the RV.

RVOT measurements from the parasternal long axis view of the LV are not reproducible due to the variable position of the RV based on patient and transducer positioning. As a result oblique imaging of the RVOT can result in an underestimation or overestimation of the RVOT. In addition, the endocardial definition of the RV anterior wall from the parasternal views is often suboptimal because this wall is very close to the transducer; as a result the anterior border of this wall is often obscured by reverberation and/or near field artefacts.

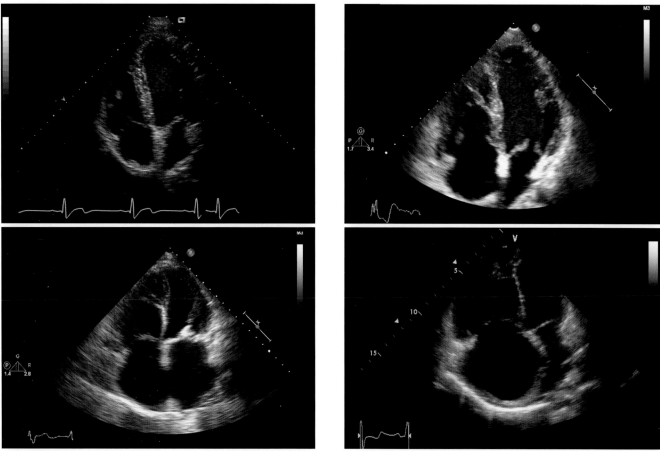

Figure 2.36 Qualitative evaluation of right ventricular size is achieved from the apical 4-chamber view. Normal RV size is when the RV area or mid-cavity diameter is smaller than that of the LV and the apex is formed by the LV *(top left)*. Mild RV dilatation is when the RV cavity area appears increased (greater than 2/3 of the LV but it is still smaller than the LV) and the apex is still formed by the LV *(top right)*. Moderate RV dilatation is when the RV cavity area appears similar to the LV cavity area and the RV shares the apex *(bottom left)*. Severe RV dilatation is when the RV cavity area exceeds the LV cavity area and the RV forms the apex *(bottom right)*.

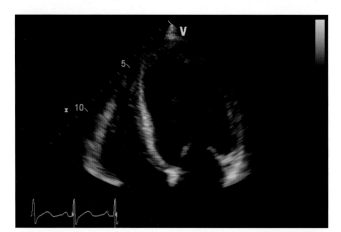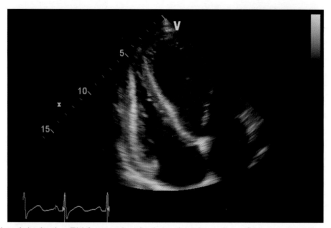

Figure 2.37 To the left is the standard apical 4-chamber view while to the right is the RV-focused apical 4- chamber view. Observe that the RV-focused view optimises imaging of the RV lateral wall. This view is obtained by angling the transducer medially from the standard apical 4-chamber view. It is recommended that RV measurements are performed from the RV-focused view.

In addition, the normal values for linear dimensions are absolute (that is, normal values are not indexed to the BSA) and the partition values for the classification of mild, moderate, and severe RV dilatation have not been defined. Hence, an arbitrary judgment in determining the degree of dilatation for any given measurement is required.

Right Ventricular Volumes

Estimation of RV volumes is difficult via 2D echocardiography because there is no simple geometric shape that approximates the complex shape of the RV.

While the Simpson's method of discs has been used to estimate RV volumes from the apical 4-chamber view the RVOT is not incorporated into this calculation so RV volumes are underestimated.

Table 2.9 **Normal Values for Right Ventricular Dimensions**

RV Dimension	Imaging View	Cut-off for Normal
Basal cavity diameter	RV focussed view	≤ 4.2 cm
Mid cavity diameter	RV focussed view	≤ 3.5 cm
RV Length (long axis)	RV focussed view	≤ 8.6 cm
RVOT diameter (proximal)	PLAX (LV) &/or PSAX (RVOT)	≤ 3.3 cm
RVOT diameter (distal)	PSAX (RVOT)	≤ 2.7 cm

Source: Rudski LG, Lai WW, Afilalo J, Hua L, Handschumacher MD, Chandrasekaran K, Solomon SD, Louie EK, Schiller NB. Guidelines for the echocardiographic assessment of the right heart in adults: a report from the American Society of Echocardiography endorsed by the European Association of Echocardiography, a registered branch of the European Society of Cardiology, and the Canadian Society of Echocardiography. *J Am Soc Echocardiogr.* 2010 23(7):685-713. **PLAX (LV)** = parasternal long axis view of the left ventricle; **PLAX (RVOT)** = parasternal long axis view of the right ventricular outflow tract; **RV** = right ventricle; **RVOT** = right ventricular outflow tract.

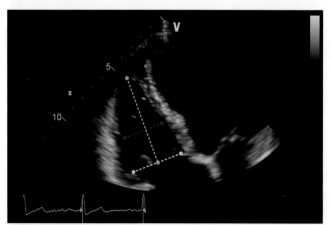

Figure 2.38 RV linear dimension measurements are performed from the RV focused apical 4-chamber view at end-diastole. The RV longitudinal diameter (long axis) is measured perpendicular to the tricuspid annulus and from the centre of the tricuspid annulus to RV apex *(green line)*. The RV cavity diameter (minor axis) is measured at the base and the mid-cavity level, parallel with the tricuspid valve annulus. The basal diameter is measured within the basal third of RV just inferior to the tricuspid annulus *(blue line)*. The mid cavity diameter is measured at the middle third of RV at level of LV papillary muscles *(pink line)*.

Interventricular Septal Motion

The motion of the IVS can be used to differentiate RV volume overload from RV pressure overload.

The normal IVS curvature is convex to the RV and concave to the LV throughout the cardiac cycle. Therefore, from the parasternal short axis views of the LV, the LV appears circular in shape and the RV appears crescent-shaped, wrapping over the LV (Fig. 2.40, top).

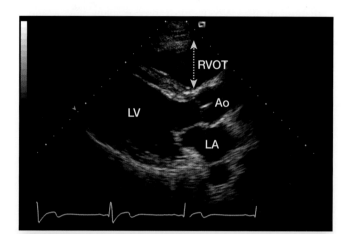

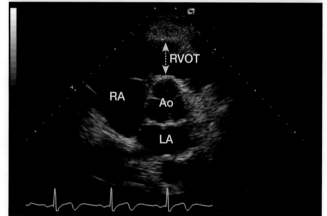

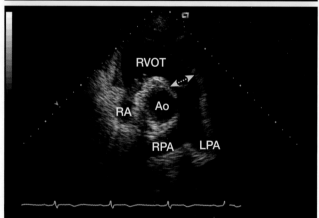

Figure 2.39 From the parasternal long axis view of the LV, the proximal RVOT is measured at end-diastole from the inner edge of the anterior aortic wall to the inner edge of the RV free wall above the aortic valve *(top)*. From the parasternal short-axis view at the level of the aortic valve, the proximal RVOT is measured at end-diastole from the inner edge of the anterior RVOT to the inner edge of the anterior aortic wall *(middle)*. From the parasternal short-axis view at the level of the pulmonary artery bifurcation, the distal RVOT is measured at end-diastole from the inner edge to the inner edge of the RVOT *(bottom)*. Ao = aorta; LA = left atrium; LPA = left pulmonary artery; LV = left ventricle; RA = right atrium; RV = right ventricle; RPA = right pulmonary artery; RVOT = right ventricular outflow tract.

RV volume overload and RV pressure overload both result in RV dilatation. RV dilatation leads to a more spherical RV cavity. In addition, increased RV pressure results in paradoxical (reversed) IVS motion; that is, the normal IVS curvature becomes reversed. Therefore, from the parasternal short axis views of the LV, the LV appears "D-shaped" due to the flattening of the IVS.

RV volume overload can be differentiated from RV pressure overload based on the phase of the cardiac cycle in which flattening of the IVS is most predominant. RV volume overload results in increased RV diastolic filling pressures due to an increase in the RV SV. When the RV diastolic pressure approaches or exceeds LV diastolic pressures, the IVS motion reverses during diastole. Therefore, from the parasternal short axis views of the LV the IVS shifts leftwards towards the centre of the LV during diastole (Fig. 2.40, middle).

RV pressure overload results in increased RV pressures during diastole and systole. When the RV diastolic and systolic pressures approach or exceed LV pressures, the IVS motion reverses over the entire cardiac cycle. Therefore, from the

parasternal short axis views of the LV the IVS shifts leftwards towards the centre of the LV during systole and diastole (Fig. 2.40, bottom).

Measurements of RV Systolic Function

Accurate assessment of RV systolic function by 2D echocardiography is challenging due to the complex geometry of the RV. In particular, the RV outflow and RV inflow tracts cannot be viewed together in any 2D imaging plane. A further limitation of RV systolic function measurements is that partition values for the classification of mild, moderate, and severe RV systolic dysfunction have not been defined. Therefore, an arbitrary judgment in determining the degree of dilatation for any given measurement is required.

Despite these limitations, several methods for assessing RV systolic function via 2D echocardiography have been described (Table 2.10). Only the methods currently recommended by the American Society of Echocardiography for routine clinical use are described in the following section (bold, italic indices in Table 2.10). The normal values for these indices are listed in Table 2.11.

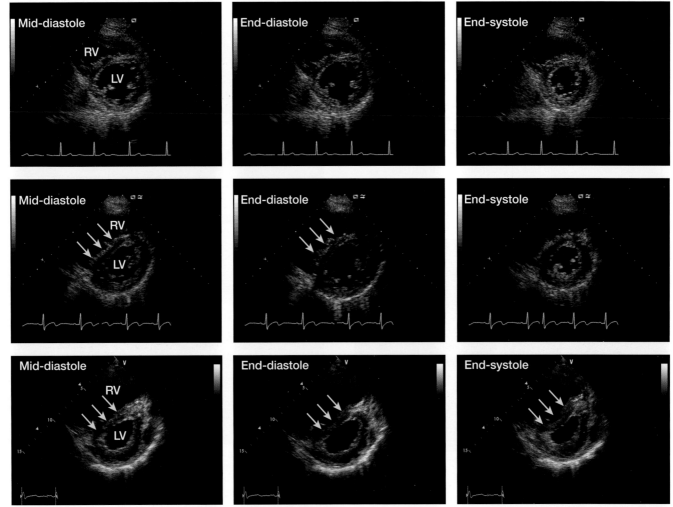

Figure 2.40 Each series of images was recorded from the parasternal short axis view at the level of the papillary muscles at mid-diastole, end-diastole and end-systole. The top images show normal IVS motion; observe that the LV cavity maintains a circular shape throughout the cardiac cycle. The middle images show the IVS motion in a patient with RV volume overload due to severe pulmonary regurgitation; observe that leftward IVS shift and flattening of the IVS occurs predominantly in mid to late diastole with the normalisation of IVS curvature by end-systole. The bottom images show the IVS motion in a patient with RV pressure overload due to pulmonary hypertension secondary to severe mitral stenosis; observe that the leftward shift of the IVS and reversal of IVS curvature occurs throughout systole and diastole with the IVS deformity being greatest at end-systole.

Fractional Area Change

The fractional area change (FAC) is the percentage of change in the RV cavity area between end-diastole and end-systole. This measurement is similar in principle to the LV calculations of the FS and EF. The FAC is calculated from 2D measurements of the RV area at end-diastole (RVAED) and the RV area at end-systole (RVAES), measured from an RV-focused apical 4-chamber view (Fig. 2.41). End-diastole is identified based on the motion of the tricuspid valve as previously described. The end-systolic frame is identified as the frame immediately preceding the initial descent of the tricuspid annulus towards the RV apex; this frame usually coincides with the end of the T wave of the ECG and the smallest RV cavity size. The FAC is calculated from the equation:

Equation 2.21

$$FAC = [(RVAED - RVAES) \div RVAED] \times 100$$

where FAC = fractional area change (%)
RVAED = right ventricular area at end-diastole (cm²)
RVAES = left ventricular area at end-systole (cm²)

FAC measured by 2D echocardiography has been shown to correlate well with the CMRI-derived RV EF.

Limitations of FAC

The primary limitation of this method in the assessment of RV systolic function is that it relies on good quality images which allow optimal visualisation of endocardial borders. Difficult delineation of the RV lateral wall is especially problematic when the RV is dilated; in these cases, dilatation of the RV often results in 'drop-out' of the lateral wall. Heavy trabeculations of the RV also pose a significant limitation of this measurement; when the RV is heavily trabeculated it is difficult to identify the true endocardial border. In addition, the FAC does not take into account the outflow region of the RV.

Tricuspid Annular Plane Systolic Excursion

The tricuspid annular plane systolic excursion (TAPSE), also known as tricuspid annular motion (TAM), is a measure of RV longitudinal fibre shortening during ventricular systole. Normally during ventricular contraction the tricuspid annulus descends toward the cardiac apex as the RV shortens. The degree of systolic descent of the tricuspid annulus is a reflection of RV longitudinal fibre shortening and overall RV systolic function; therefore, the greater the descent of the base in systole, the better the RV systolic function. TAPSE has shown

Table 2.10 Echocardiographic Methods for Assessing Right Ventricular Systolic Function

• 2D strain
• *Doppler tissue imaging systolic velocity*
• dP/dt
• Ejection fraction
• *Fraction area change*
• Myocardial isovolumic acceleration time
• *Myocardial performance index*
• RVOT shortening fraction
• Strain and strain rate imaging (Doppler)
• *Tricuspid annular plane systolic excursion*

Bold, italic indices represent commonly employed methods for assessing RV systolic function in routine clinical practice as recommended by the American Society of Echocardiography (Rudski LG, Lai WW, Afilalo J, Hua L, Handschumacher MD, Chandrasekaran K, Solomon SD, Louie EK, Schiller NB. Guidelines for the echocardiographic assessment of the right heart in adults: a report from the American Society of Echocardiography endorsed by the European Association of Echocardiography, a registered branch of the European Society of Cardiology, and the Canadian Society of Echocardiography. *J Am Soc Echocardiogr.* 2010 Jul;23(7):685-713).

Table 2.11 Normal Values for Commonly Used Indices of Right Ventricular Systolic Function.

Index of RV Systolic Function	Normal Value
Doppler tissue imaging systolic velocity (s')	≥ 10 cm/s
Fractional Area Change (FAC)	≥ 35%
Myocardial Performance Index (MPI) [conventional method]	≤ 0.4
Myocardial Performance Index (MPI) [DTI method]	≤ 0.55
Tricuspid Annular Plane Systolic Excursion (TAPSE)	≥ 1.6 cm

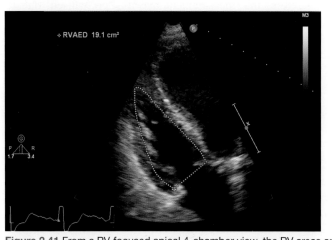 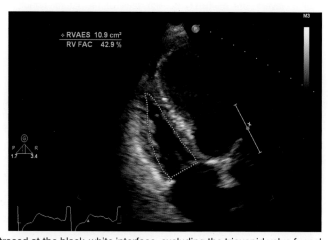

Figure 2.41 From a RV-focused apical 4-chamber view, the RV areas are traced at the black-white interface, excluding the tricuspid valve funnel and papillary muscles, at end-diastole *(left)* and end-systole *(right)*. The FAC in this example is calculated as:

FAC (%) = (RVAED – RVAES) ÷ RVAED × 100
= (19.1 – 10.9) ÷ 19.1 × 100
= 42.9%

good correlation with other estimates of RV systolic function such as the radionuclide-derived RV EF and the RV FAC.

TAPSE can be measured via 2D imaging or via M-mode. The preferred method is M-mode due to its superior interface definition. Via M-mode TAPSE is measured by placing the M-mode cursor at the lateral tricuspid annulus from the apical 4-chamber view. From the M-mode trace, TAPSE is measured as the vertical distance of the lateral annulus between end-diastole and end-systole (Fig. 2.42).

Limitations of TAPSE

While TAPSE is a relatively easy measurement for assessing longitudinal RV systolic function, it remains a one-dimensional measurement of RV function that is also angle-dependent. Therefore, when the M-mode cursor is not placed parallel to annular motion underestimation of TAPSE, and RV systolic function, will occur.

TAPSE is also a measure of *regional* RV systolic function as it is measuring the motion of the basal lateral annulus of the RV. Assumptions that this localised motion of the RV reflects overall RV function may be erroneous when there are regional abnormalities. In particular, this measurement may be 'normalised' due to tethering of an akinetic segment by actively contracting myocardium. Rotational and translational

movements of the whole heart may also affect this parameter. TAPSE is also a load-dependent parameter so in the case of significant tricuspid regurgitation TAPSE may be exaggerated and will, therefore, overestimate RV contractility.

A reduction in the TAPSE has also been observed in patients following cardiac surgery despite the presence of a normal RV EF. Possible explanations for this reduction in RV longitudinal function relate to geometrical rather than functional changes in the RV; examples include geometrical changes of the RV chamber in association with paradoxical IVS motion, and extra-myocardial causes such as post-operative adherence of the RV to the thoracic wall.

Furthermore, TAPSE is not only determined by RV systolic function but also appears to be dependent on LV systolic function. For example, TAPSE may be reduced when there is LV systolic dysfunction despite normal RV systolic function.

Technical limitations include poor alignment of the M-mode cursor with the lateral RV annulus, poor optimisation of the M-mode trace, and failure to measure the correct borders of the annulus between end-diastole and end-systole (Fig. 2.43).

Systolic Myocardial Velocities

As for the LV, measurement of the peak systolic myocardial velocity via DTI can be used in the assessment of longitudinal systolic shortening of the RV.

The DTI myocardial velocity profile of the RV is the same as the LV in that this profile is characterised by three distinct waveforms (s', e' and a') with biphasic velocities seen during the isovolumic relaxation and isovolumic contraction phases. For the purpose of RV systolic function, the peak s' velocity is measured (Fig. 2.44).

Limitations of s' Velocities

The limitations of s' velocities in the assessment of RV systolic function are similar to those limitations described for the s' velocity in the assessment of LV systolic function and for those descibed for TAPSE measurements.

In particular, DTI measures localised velocities within one segment of the ventricular wall and measurement of the s' velocity at this localised segment is then assumed to reflect the systolic function of the entire ventricle. DTI velocities are influenced not only by myocardial function, but also by myocardial tethering and cardiac translational motion.

Therefore, this measurement may be 'normalised' due to tethering of an akinetic segment by actively contracting

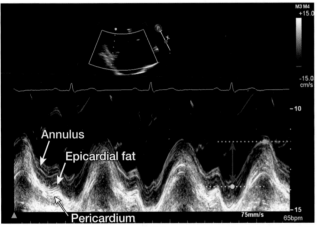

Figure 2.42 TAPSE is measured from a zoomed, standard apical 4-chamber view, the M-mode cursor is positioned parallel to the lateral tricuspid annulus *(top)*. From the M-mode trace *(bottom)*, TAPSE is measured as the vertical distance of the lateral annulus between end-diastole and end-systole. Also observe on this trace that 3 'layers' are seen: (1) the interface of the lateral annulus, (2) the pericardium and (3) epicardial fat between the annulus and the pericardium.

TAPSE Tip

At times the lateral wall definition is not very clear. In these situations, colour-coded DTI may improve both the definition of the lateral annulus as well as assisting in the identification of end-diastole and end-systole. End-diastole and end-systole are easily identified by the blue/red and red/blue interfaces, respectively.

Compare the standard M-mode trace *(top)* with the colour-coded DTI M-mode trace *(bottom)*. The border of the lateral annulus can be better appreciated on the colour-coded DTI M-mode trace. End-diastole is easily identified as the blue-red interface and end-systole is easily identified as the blue-red interface.

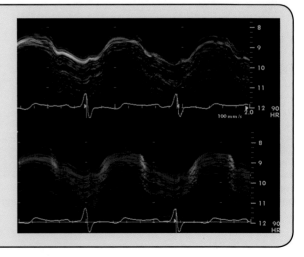

myocardium. Rotational and translational movements of the whole heart may also affect this measurement.

As mentioned for TAPSE limitations, a reduction in the s' has also been observed in patients following cardiac surgery despite the presence of a normal RV EF.

DTI is not a valid measurement of RV systolic function in the presence of tricuspid valve disease (tricuspid valve stenosis, significant tricuspid regurgitation, and significant tricuspid annular calcification), or following tricuspid annulo-plasty or where there are prosthetic tricuspid valves in-situ.

DTI is a Doppler technique and, therefore, the accuracy of velocity measurements is highly dependent upon the incident angle between the sampling site and myocardial motion. Failure to align the ultrasound beam parallel to myocardial motion will result in an underestimation of the DTI velocities. In the apical 4-chamber view, the Doppler cursor should be aligned parallel with the RV lateral wall; if this is not feasible, angle correction can be used (Fig. 2.45).

Another technical limitation is mistaking the isovolumic contraction spike for the s' velocity (Fig. 2.46). This spike coincides with the QRS complex of the ECG while the s' velocity occurs after the QRS complex.

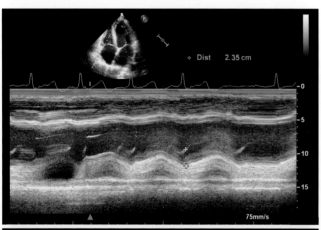

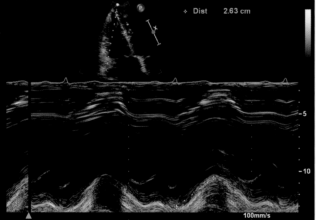

Figure 2.43 These examples show technical measurement errors for TAPSE. The trace on the top shows a poorly optimised M-mode trace and an inaccurate measurement of TAPSE. This trace could have been improved by: (1) zooming on the lateral RV annulus, (2) ensuring that the M-mode cursor is aligned parallel with the lateral RV annulus and (3) decreasing the M-mode gain. The trace on the bottom shows another inaccurate measurement of TAPSE; in this example, the end-diastolic caliper is placed too deep so this measurement is overestimated. As for all M-mode measurements, calipers should be placed by following the most continuous line.

While it is possible to measure myocardial velocities from stored colour encoded DTI images, as mentioned for the LV, it is important to note that colour-coded tissue Doppler yields lower velocities than pulsed DTI because the colour-coded DTI represents the mean instantaneous velocities.

Myocardial Performance Index

As for the LV, measurement of the MPI can be used in the assessment of global RV function. As previously stated, the MPI is the ratio of the sum of the isovolumic times and the ejection time:

Equation 2.20

$$MPI = (IVCT + IVRT) \div ET$$

where MPI = myocardial performance index (unitless)
IVCT = isovolumic contraction time (ms)
IVRT = isovolumic relaxation time (ms)
ET = ejection time (ms)

RV MPI has shown a significant inverse relationship with RV EF by nuclear ventriculography; that is, the higher the value of the MPI, the lower the RV EF and visa versa.

The MPI can be measured via conventional spectral Doppler using the tricuspid inflow trace (or tricuspid regurgitation (TR) trace) and the RVOT trace (Fig. 2.47). The ET is measured from the RVOT tract from the beginning to the end of the RVOT signal (Fig. 2.47, left). From the tricuspid inflow trace, the time interval between tricuspid valve closure and the tricuspid valve opening (TVc-TVo) is measured from the end of the tricuspid A wave to the beginning of the next tricuspid E wave. This interval is the sum of IVRT + ET + IVCT (refer to Fig. 2.34). By subtracting the ET from this interval, the sum of IVCT + IVRT can be derived. In the presence of TR, the TVc-TVo interval can be measured as the duration of the TR signal (Fig. 2.47, right). Measurements should be averaged over at least 2 cardiac cycles.

Via DTI, all intervals required for the measurement of the MPI can be measured from a single beat (Fig. 2.48). From the DTI trace of the lateral tricuspid annulus, the ET is measured from the beginning to the end of the s' signal (that is, the duration of the s' signal). The IVCT can be measured as the interval from the end of the a' velocity to the beginning of s' velocity and the IVRT can be measured as the interval between the

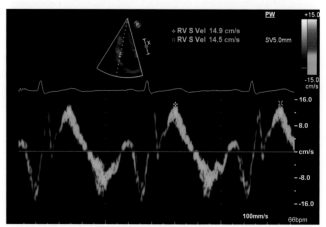

Figure 2.44 From the apical 4 chamber view and ensuring parallel alignment with the RV myocardium, a 5 mm pulsed-wave Doppler sample volume is placed within the basal RV myocardium *(top)*. The peak systolic myocardial velocity (s') is measured from the spectral DTI trace *(bottom)*.

end of s' velocity to the beginning of the e' velocity (Fig. 2.48, left). Alternatively, the time interval from the end of the a' velocity to the beginning of the next e' velocity can be measured (*interval a*); this interval incorporates the IVRT, the ET and the IVCT (Fig. 2.48, right). By subtracting the ET from *interval a*, the sum of IVCT + IVRT can be derived. As stated for the LV MPI, it is important to note that the correlation between the conventional Doppler MPI and the MPI via DTI are only modest and that normal values differ on the basis of the method employed.

Limitations of MPI

The limitations described for the MPI in the assessment of LV systolic function also apply to the RV MPI.

In particular, the accuracy of the MPI calculation via conventional Doppler is compromised as the required measurements are not performed simultaneously.

Furthermore, arrhythmias such as atrial flutter/fibrillation and AV heart block affect the tricuspid inflow profiles; hence, accurate measurement of the MPI may be hindered under these circumstances.

While calculation of the MPI via DTI may overcome these

limitations, the DTI MPI is only measuring the MPI at one site of the ventricle. Therefore, this is a measurement of the *regional* MPI which may not reflect the overall RV function. In addition, the normal P-V relationship for the RV shows that isovolumic contraction and isovolumic relaxation periods are poorly defined (see Fig. 2.11). Therefore, the relevance of the index is considered controversial.

The RV MPI is load dependent and has proven to be unreliable when RA pressure is elevated. Specifically, it has been noted that shortening of the isovolumic contraction occurs following a severe RV infarction. In these circumstances, the isovolumic contraction is shortened due to highly elevated RV diastolic pressures secondary to decreased RV compliance, and this may lead to a pseudonormalisation of the RV MPI.

> Due to significant errors in each parameter for the assessment of RV systolic function, no one parameter can be reliably used to evaluate RV systolic function. Therefore, more than one measure of RV function should be used to distinguish between normal and abnormal RV systolic function.

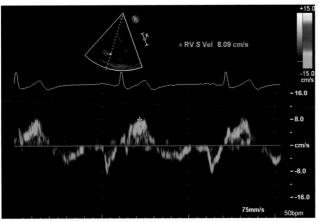
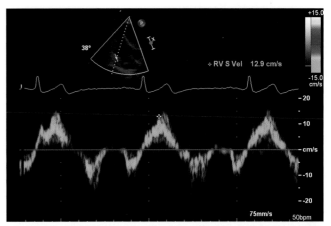

Figure 2.45 In order to measure the most accurate velocity, the ultrasound beam must be aligned parallel with myocardial motion. As seen in the example to the left, there is a significant incident angle between the ultrasound beam and the RV lateral wall; the peak s' velocity at this angle is underestimated at 8 cm/s. The trace on the right is recorded in the same patient. Observe that the DTI velocities are higher; this is because angle correction (38°) has been used. As such the DTI velocities are accurately calculated and the s' is now measured at 13 cm/s.

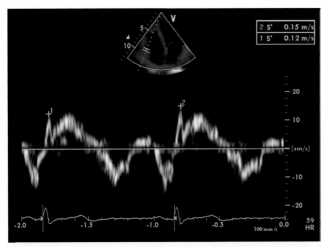
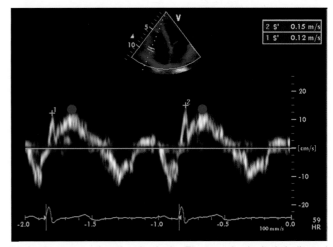

Figure 2.46 In the example on the left the isovolumic contraction spike is mistakenly measured as the s' velocity. The true s' velocity is indicated by the pink dots on the right image.

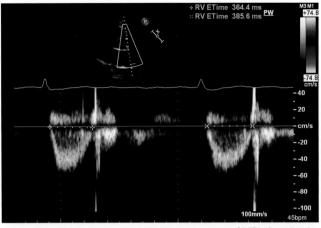
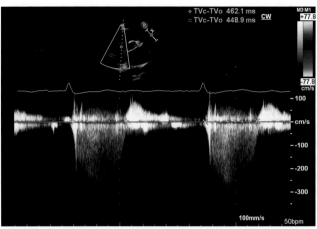

Figure 2.47 These traces show the measurement of MPI via pulsed-wave Doppler (conventional method). The pulsed-wave Doppler trace on the left shows the RVOT signal. The right ventricular ejection time (**RV ETime**) is measured as the time interval from the onset of flow to the end of flow. The averaged RV ETime is 375 ms. The continuous-wave Doppler trace on the right shows the tricuspid regurgitant (**TR**) signal. From this signal the TVc-TVo interval is measured as the duration of the TR signal; this interval is the sum of the IVCT + ET + IVRT. The averaged TVc-TVo interval is 455.5 ms. By subtracting the ET from this interval, the sum of IVCT + IVCT is derived. From these values, the RV MPI in this example is calculated as:

$$RVMPI = (IVCT + IVRT) \div ET$$
$$= (TVc\text{-}TVo - ET) \div ET$$
$$= (455.5 - 375) \div 375$$
$$= 0.21$$

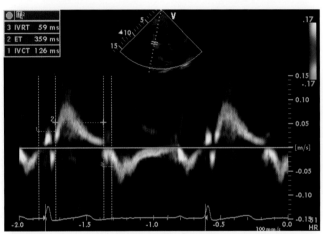
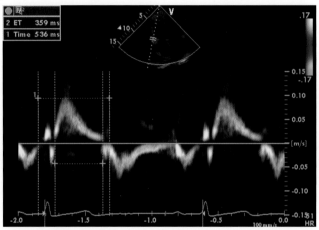

Figure 2.48 These traces show the measurement of MPI via the DTI method. The left trace shows how the individual time intervals of the IVCT, ET and IVRT can be measured. On the right trace, the interval from the end of the a' velocity to the beginning of the next e' velocity has been measured (Time). This interval is the sum of IVCT + ET + IVRT; by subtracting ET from this interval, the sum of IVCT + IVCT is derived. In this example, the RV MPI is calculated as:

$$RVMPI = (IVCT + IVRT) \div ET$$
$$= (Time - ET) \div ET$$
$$= (536 - 359) \div 359$$
$$= 0.49$$

Key Points

Ventricular Anatomy
- LV shape is ellipsoidal; RV shape is complex (triangular when viewed from the side and crescent-shaped when viewed in cross-section).
- Each ventricle consists of three components: (1) the inlet, (2) apical, and (3) outlet components. The inlet and outlet portions of the RV are anatomically separate while the inlet and outlet components of the LV are in fibrous continuity.
- Ventricular myocardium is composed of a complex arrangement of myofibrils in three layers: (1) superficial (subepicardial), (2) middle, and (3) deep (subendocardial) layers. Middle layer fibres contribute to the radial contraction while the epicardial and subendocardial fibres contribute to the longitudinal contraction. The middle layer is absent in the RV so the majority of RV contractility is due to longitudinal shortening.

Basic Cardiac Physiology
- The relationship between pressure and volume over the cardiac cycle is described by P-V loops. The P-V loop of the LV is rectangular in shape while the P-V loop of the RV is triangular in shape with poorly defined isovolumic periods.
- Stroke volume (SV) is measured as the width of the P-V loop. SV is determined by three primary mechanisms: (1) preload, (2) afterload and (3) contractility (inotropy). These three variables have interdependent relationships.

(continued over...)

Key Points (continued)

Measurements of the Left Ventricular Size
- Linear measurements of the LV can be performed via M-mode or 2D imaging. From these linear measurements LV volumes can be estimated based on geometric assumptions of LV shape (not recommended).
- 2D volume estimates of LV volumes can be determined via the Simpson's biplane method of discs or the area-length method.

Measurements of the Left Ventricular Systolic Function
- 2D/M-mode methods for estimating LV systolic function include the fractional shortening (FS) and the ejection fraction (EF).
- Doppler methods for estimating LV systolic function include cardiac output, cardiac index, dP/dt, DTI s' velocity and the MPI.
- Doppler measurements of LV systolic function are especially useful when an estimation of the EF is not possible and when the EF is influenced by loading conditions.

Measurements of the Right Ventricular Size
- Qualitative assessment of RV size is based on comparing the RV with the LV and on determining the apex-forming ventricle as imaged from the apical 4-chamber view.
- Quantitative measurements include linear measurements of the RV from an RV-focused apical 4-chamber view and linear measurements of the RVOT from the parasternal views.
- IVS motion, viewed from the parasternal short axis images, can be used to differentiate RV volume overload from RV pressure overload.

Measurements of the Right Ventricular Systolic Function
- 2D and M-mode measurements of RV systolic function include the fractional area change (FAC) and the TAPSE.
- Doppler methods for estimating RV systolic function include the DTI s' velocity and the MPI.
- Because of significant errors in each RV systolic function parameter more than one measure of RV function should be used to distinguish between normal and abnormal RV systolic function.

Further Reading (listed in alphabetical order)

Ventricular Anatomy

Haddad F, Hunt SA, Rosenthal DN, Murphy DJ. Right ventricular function in cardiovascular disease, part I: Anatomy, physiology, aging, and functional assessment of the right ventricle. *Circulation.* 2008 Mar 18;117(11):1436-48.

Ho SY. Anatomy and myoarchitecture of the left ventricular wall in normal and in disease. *Eur J Echocardiogr.* 2009 Dec; 10(8):iii3-7.

Ho SY, Nihoyannopoulos P. Anatomy, echocardiography, and normal right ventricular dimensions. *Heart.* 2006 Apr; 92 Suppl 1:i2-13.

Sanchez-Quintana D, Climent V, Ho SY, Anderson RH. Myoarchitecture and connective tissue in hearts with tricuspid atresia. *Heart.* 1999 Feb;81(2):182-91.

Sheehan F, Redington A. The right ventricle: anatomy, physiology and clinical imaging. *Heart.* 2008. Nov;94(11):1510-5.

Cardiac Physiology

Haddad F, Hunt SA, Rosenthal DN, Murphy DJ. Right ventricular function in cardiovascular disease, part I: Anatomy, physiology, aging, and functional assessment of the right ventricle. *Circulation.* 2008 Mar 18;117(11):1436-48.

Klabunde RE. Cardiovascular Physiology Concepts. http://www.cvphysiology.com/index.html

Sheehan F, Redington A. The right ventricle: anatomy, physiology and clinical imaging. *Heart.* 2008. Nov;94(11):1510-5.

LV Measurements and Systolic Function

Gaibazzi N, Petrucci N, Ziacchi V. Left ventricle myocardial performance index derived either by conventional method or mitral annulus tissue-Doppler: a comparison study in healthy subjects and subjects with heart failure. *J Am Soc Echocardiogr.* 2005 Dec;18(12):1270-6.

Lang RM, Bierig M, Devereux RB, et al. Chamber Quantification Writing Group; American Society of Echocardiography's Guidelines and Standards Committee; European Association of Echocardiography. Recommendations for Chamber Quantification: A Report from the American Society of Echocardiography's Guidelines and Standards Committee and the Chamber Quantification Writing Group, Developed in Conjunction with the European Association of Echocardiography, a Branch of the European Society of Cardiology. *J Am Soc Echocardiogr.* 2005 Dec;18(12): 1440-1463.

Rojo EC, Rodrigo JL, Pérez de Isla L, Almería C, Gonzalo N, Aubele A, Cinza R, Zamorano J, Macaya C. Disagreement between tissue Doppler imaging and conventional pulsed wave Doppler in the measurement of myocardial performance index. *Eur J Echocardiogr.* 2006 Oct;7(5):356-64.

Schiller NB, Shah PM, Crawford M, DeMaria A, Devereux R, Feigenbaum H, et al. Recommendations for quantitation of the left ventricle by two-dimensional echocardiography: American Society of Echocardiography committee on standards, subcommittee on quantitation of two-dimensional echocardiograms. *J Am Soc Echocardiogr* 1989; 2:358–67

St John Sutton MG, Plappert T, Rahmouni H. Assessment of left ventricular systolic function by echocardiography. *Heart Fail Clin.* 2009 Apr;5(2):177-90.

Tei C, Ling LH, Hodge DO, Bailey KR, Oh JK, Rodeheffer RJ, Tajik AJ, Seward JB. New index of combined systolic and diastolic myocardial performance: a simple and reproducible measure of cardiac function--a study in normals and dilated cardiomyopathy. *J Cardiol.* 1995 Dec;26(6):357-66.

RV Measurements and Systolic Function

Anavekar NS, Gerson D, Skali H, Kwong RY, Yucel EK, Solomon SD. Two-dimensional assessment of right ventricular function: an echocardiographic-MRI correlative study. *Echocardiography.* 2007 May;24(5):452-6.

Horton KD, Meece RW, Hill JC. Assessment of the right ventricle by echocardiography: a primer for cardiac sonographers. *J Am Soc Echocardiogr.* 2009 Jul;22(7):776-92

Jurcut R, Giusca S, La Gerche A, Vasile S, Ginghina C, Voigt JU. The echocardiographic assessment of the right ventricle: what to do in 2010? *Eur J Echocardiogr.* 2010 Mar;11(2):81-96.

López-Candales A, Rajagopalan N, Saxena N, Gulyasy B, Edelman K, Bazaz R. Right ventricular systolic function is not the sole determinant of tricuspid annular motion. *Am J Cardiol.* 2006 Oct 1;98(7):973-7.

Rudski LG, Lai WW, Afilalo J, Hua L, Handschumacher MD, Chandrasekaran K, Solomon SD, Louie EK, Schiller NB. Guidelines for the echocardiographic assessment of the right heart in adults: a report from the American Society of Echocardiography endorsed by the European Association of Echocardiography, a registered branch of the European Society of Cardiology, and the Canadian Society of Echocardiography. *J Am Soc Echocardiogr.* 2010 Jul;23(7):685-713.

Tei C, Dujardin KS, Hodge DO, Bailey KR, McGoon MD, Tajik AJ, Seward SB. Doppler echocardiographic index for assessment of global right ventricular function. *J Am Soc Echocardiogr.* 1996 Nov-Dec;9(6):838-47.

Yoshifuku S, Otsuji Y, Takasaki K, Yuge K, Kisanuki A, Toyonaga K, Lee S, Murayama T, Nakashima H, Kumanohoso T, Minagoe S, Tei C. Pseudonormalized Doppler total ejection isovolume (Tei) index in patients with right ventricular acute myocardial infarction. *Am J Cardiol.* 2003 Mar 1;91(5):527-31.

Ventricular Diastolic Function

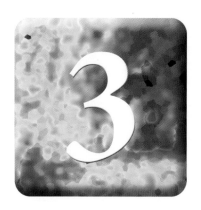

Basic Principles of Diastole

Phases of Diastole

Diastole refers to the period in the cardiac cycle that relates to filling of the ventricle. It is begins at the closure of the semilunar valves at the end of ventricular ejection and terminates at the closure of the atrioventricular (AV) valves at the end of ventricular filling. There are four phases incorporated within the period of diastole, these are: (1) isovolumic relaxation (IVR), (2) early, rapid filling, (3) diastasis and (4) atrial contraction (Fig. 3.1).

Isovolumic Relaxation

IVR is the period between aortic valve closure and mitral valve opening. During the IVR phase, the left ventricle (LV) is relaxing and the LV pressure falls but the LV volume remains unchanged as all valves are closed (no blood is leaving the LV and no blood is entering the LV). When the LV pressure falls below the pressure in the left atrium (LA), the mitral valve opens. This represents the end of the IVR phase and the beginning of the early, rapid filling phase.

The duration of IVR or the isovolumic relaxation time (IVRT) is determined by several factors including: (1) cessation of excitation-contraction coupling, (2) loading conditions of the LV (preload or LA pressure [LAP]), and (3) age (relaxation lengthens with advancing age).

Early, Rapid Filling

The early, rapid filling phase commences at the end of IVR when the pressure in the LV falls below the LAP. During early, rapid filling the LV fills and both the LV volume and LV pressure increase. LV filling during this phase is augmented by the elastic recoil of the ventricle following LV relaxation which effectively results in suction of the blood into the LV. At the same time as the LV is filling, the LA is emptying; as a result both the LA volume and LAP decrease so the diastolic pressure gradient between the LA and LV also decreases. The rate of decline of the LV-LA pressure gradient reflects the rate of LV filling and the rate of LA emptying.

This phase of diastole is primarily determined by four factors: (1) the rate of LV relaxation, (2) the elastic recoil of the ventricle, (3) chamber compliance, and (4) the LAP.

Normally, this phase of diastole contributes to 70-80% of LV filling.

Diastasis

During diastasis, the LV and LA pressures are almost equal. Pressure equalisation occurs due to the simultaneous decrease in the LAP as the atrium empties and the rise in the LV pressure as the ventricle fills. A small amount of blood continues to flow across the mitral valve during diastasis due to inertia. The duration of diastasis is determined by the heart rate; with slower heart rates diastasis is longer while at faster heart rates diastasis is shortened or it may be totally absent.

Atrial Contraction

With atrial contraction there is a small increase in the LAP which results in a further bolus of blood being propelled into the LV. Normally, this phase of diastole contributes approximately 20% of total LV filling. At the end of atrial contraction and when the pressure in the LV exceeds the LAP, the mitral valve closes.

Diastolic Function

Simplistically, diastolic function refers to the ability of the ventricles to fill to an adequate volume at end-diastole to ensure that there is an adequate stroke volume (SV) during systole. When there is normal diastolic function, the ventricle is able

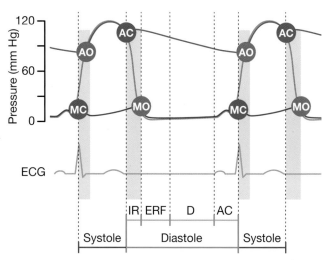

Figure 3.1 This schematic illustrates the phases of the cardiac cycle for the left heart. Diastole begins at the closure of the aortic valve (AC) and ends at the closure of the mitral valve (MC). Included within diastole is the isovolumic relaxation phase (IR), the early, rapid filling phase (ERF), diastasis (D) and atrial contraction (AC). See text for details.
AO = aortic valve opening; MO = mitral valve opening

to fill to an adequate end-diastolic volume at low ventricular filling pressures during rest or exercise, ensuring an adequate SV during systole.

Diastolic dysfunction means that in order for the ventricle to fill to an adequate end-diastolic volume during rest or exercise, there is an abnormal increase in ventricular filling pressures. For example, when there is primarily LV diastolic dysfunction, the heart maintains its normal end-diastolic volume by increasing LV filling pressures.

The factors that affect diastolic function are very complex with several interrelated events affecting ventricular filling.

> **Diastolic Dysfunction versus Increased LV Filling Pressures**
> It is important to note that "diastolic dysfunction" and "increased LV filling pressures" are not the same. Diastolic dysfunction refers to changes in LV filling properties while increased LV filling pressures occur as a *secondary* consequence of diastolic dysfunction.

Left Ventricular Filling Pressures

LV filling pressures (LVFP) include the LV end-diastolic pressure (LVEDP) and the mean LAP (mLAP) (Fig. 3.2). The LVEDP is defined as the LV pressure immediately following LA contraction. It is important to note that LVEDP and mLAP are not the same. For example, three situations may exist: (1) a *normal* mLAP and a *normal* LVEDP; (2) a *normal* mLAP and an *elevated* LVEDP; and (3) an *elevation of both* the mLAP and the LVEDP.

Direct measurement of the mLAP requires a trans-septal puncture of the interatrial septum. However, there are other correlates of mLAP which can be determined from the LV pressure trace. These include the LV pre-A wave pressure and the mean LV diastolic pressure (Fig. 3.3). Other pressures that correlate with the mLAP include the pulmonary capillary wedge pressure (PCWP), or pulmonary artery occlusion pressure (PAOP), which is defined as the pressure measured in a pulmonary artery distal to an occlusion of that artery. Although these pressures are different in absolute terms, they are closely related.

Diastolic Filling Properties

Diastolic filling properties include LV stiffness and compliance, and myocardial relaxation. Stiffness and compliance determine the pressure and volume that result from LV filling while myocardial relaxation is the process by which the myocardium returns to its initial length and tension.

Chamber Compliance and Stiffness

As the ventricle fills with blood, the resultant pressure and volume within the ventricle are determined by the compliance or the stiffness of the ventricle.

Compliance (dV/dP or $\Delta V/\Delta P$) is measured as the change in volume (dV or ΔV) over the change in pressure (dP or ΔP). A compliant ventricle means that it is able to increase its volume without a significant increase in pressure.

Stiffness is the reciprocal of compliance and, therefore, is a measure of the change in pressure over the change in volume (dP/dV or $\Delta P/\Delta V$). A stiff ventricle means that for an increase in diastolic volume there is a concurrent and relatively larger increase in diastolic pressure. Therefore, a stiff ventricle equals a less compliant ventricle.

From the end-diastolic pressure-volume relationship (EDPVR), the diastolic filling phase of the LV can be appreciated. The slope of the EDPVR reflects the passive filling curve for the ventricle and this can be used to measure ventricular stiffness (Fig. 3.4).

When there is increased ventricular stiffness (decreased ventricular compliance), the pressure–volume curve is shifted upwards and to the left; therefore, the tangent is steeper. This means that the LVEDP is higher at any given end-diastolic volume.

Myocardial Relaxation

Myocardial relaxation is an active and energy dependent process during which the myocardium returns to its initial pre-systolic length and tension. Relaxation largely regulates ventricular filling during early diastole. Following myocardial relaxation, due to the elastic recoil of the LV and at low LA-LV pressure gradients, blood is effectively 'sucked' into the ventricle.

Measurement of the peak *negative* dP/dt can be used to identify the rate of LV relaxation. This is achieved by measuring the rate of LV pressure decline during the IVR phase. The 'gold standard' for the measurement of LV relaxation is determined from the calculation of the time constant of relaxation or tau (τ) (Fig. 3.5). When the LV pressure decline during the IVR phase is slowed tau is prolonged and, therefore, the numerical value

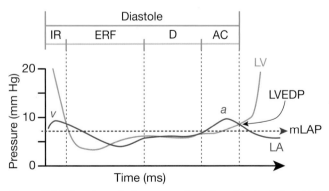

Figure 3.2 This schematic focuses on the left ventricular (LV) and left atrial (LA) pressure traces during diastole. LV filling pressures include: (1) the LV end-diastolic pressure (LVEDP) which is defined as the pressure after LA contraction and just prior to LV systolic pressure rise and (2) the mean left atrial pressure (mLAP). a = LA pressure following atrial contraction; AC = atrial contraction; D = diastasis; ERF = early rapid filling; IR = isovolumic relaxation; v = LA pressure at the end of ventricular contraction.

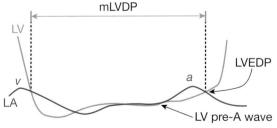

Figure 3.3 From the left ventricular (LV) pressure trace, the LV pre-A wave pressure and the mean LV diastolic pressure (mLVDP) can be used as surrogates for the mean left atrial (LA) pressure. The LV pre–A wave pressure is defined as the LV pressure midway through diastole and just prior to the *a* wave of the LA pressure trace. The mLVDP is measured from 5 mm Hg above the LV pressure during LV isovolumic relaxation to the LVEDP by digitizing the range of the LV pressure tracing. LVEDP = LV end-diastolic pressure.

of tau increases. A normal tau is approximately 30 to 40 ms. In addition to relaxation and stiffness, there are a number of other extrinsic and intrinsic factors that contribute to diastolic function. Extrinsic factors that can lead to a reduction in ventricular compliance include pericardial constraint (e.g. constrictive pericarditis, pericardial tamponade), acute right ventricular (RV) overload and increased pleural pressures. Examples of intrinsic factors that alter ventricular compliance include myocardial stiffness due to diffuse fibrosis and/or infiltrative diseases, and chamber stiffness resulting from increases in chamber size and/or wall thickness.

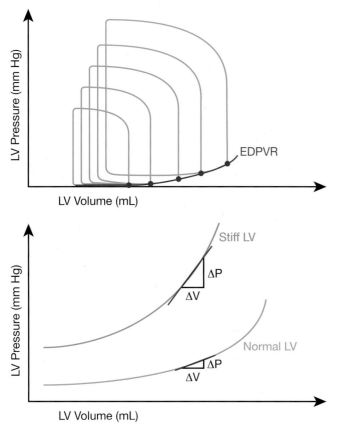

Figure 3.4 Stiffness, defined as the change in ventricular pressure relative to a change in volume of the ventricular chamber (ΔP/ΔV), can be measured from slope of the end-diastolic pressure-volume relationship (EDPVR). The schematic on the top illustrates how the EDPVR is derived by connecting the single end-diastolic pressure-volume points from a 'family' of pressure-volume (P-V) loops. Each loop is reproduced following an intervention such as altering preload while keeping contractility and afterload constant; this allows the observation of the relationship between ventricular pressure and volume during diastole. Observe that at lower ventricular volumes, the P-V loops shift leftward and downward towards lower diastolic filling pressures while at higher ventricular volumes the loops shift rightward and upwards towards higher diastolic filling pressures. In particular, observe that the slope of the EDPVR is non-linear indicating that stiffness increases at higher levels of end-diastolic volume.

The schematic on the bottom demonstrates the EDPVR slopes from two different hearts: a normal heart (blue line) and a stiff heart (green line). Chamber stiffness is the change in ventricular pressure relative to a change in volume of the ventricular chamber (ΔP/ΔV). Therefore, stiffness is measured from the EDPVR slope by a tangent (red line) drawn between two volumes (ΔV) and two pressures (ΔP). Observe that, in a normal LV, for a given increase in diastolic volume (ΔV) there is only a small increase in pressure (ΔP); this means that the ventricle fills easily to a normal diastolic volume without a significant increase in LV diastolic pressure. By comparison, in a stiff LV, the EDPVR slope is much steeper so that for a similar change in diastolic volume (ΔV), there is a significantly greater increase in the diastolic pressure (ΔP). Therefore, this ventricle is harder to fill to an adequate diastolic volume and is accompanied by high LV diastolic pressures.

Echocardiographic Parameters for Assessing Left Ventricular Diastolic Function

The comprehensive evaluation of LV diastolic function incorporates a number of 2D morphological and Doppler echocardiographic parameters. 2D morphological parameters for assessing LV diastolic function include LV wall thickness and LA volume; Doppler parameters include LV and LA filling profiles, the IVRT, myocardial velocities and flow propagation into the LV. These parameters provide information regarding impaired myocardial relaxation, increased ventricular stiffness and increased LVFP (Table 3.1).

Left Ventricular Wall Thickness

LV wall thickness and LV mass can be measured via M-mode or 2D echocardiography (see Chapters 2 and 4). The normal LV wall thickness in men is 0.6 to 1.0 cm and is 0.6 to 0.9 cm in women; the normal indexed LV mass derived via 2D methods in men is 50–102 g/m^2 and is 44–88 g/m^2 in women (see Table 4.8). In the presence of left ventricular hypertrophy (LVH), LV relaxation is slowed. LVH can be identified by an increase in LV wall thickness and/or an increase in LV mass.

Left Atrial Volume

The LA volume can be measured via the biplane area-length method at end-systole (Fig. 3.6). From the apical 4-chamber and apical 2-chamber views, the LA area is traced at the

> *"No one parameter clearly defines diastolic dysfunction and predicts elevated filling pressure. Thus, integration of multiple Doppler parameters with 2D echocardiography findings is required for a comprehensive assessment of diastolic function."*
>
> From: Modern evaluation of left ventricular diastolic function using Doppler echocardiography by Gabriel RS, Klein AL. *Curr Cardiol Rep.* 11(3):232, © 2009, reproduced with kind permission from Springer Science + Business Media.

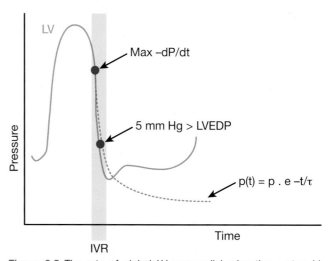

Figure 3.5 The rate of global LV myocardial relaxation or tau (τ) can be measured from the LV pressure trace during the isovolumic relaxation period. Tau (τ) is derived from a monoexponential equation that is fitted between two points on the LV pressure curve. The first point is at the maximum negative dP/dt, which occurs around aortic valve closure and the second point is at 5 mm Hg above the LVEDP, which occurs around mitral valve opening.

e = base of the natural logarithm; p = pressure; t = time and τ = tau.

blood-tissue interface from the lateral to the medial mitral annulus, being sure to exclude the pulmonary venous confluence, LA appendage and the area between the leaflets and the annulus. The LA length is then measured from the centre of the mitral annulus to the superior aspect of the LA, perpendicular to the mitral annulus. From these measurements, the biplane LA volume is calculated as:

Equation 3.1

$$LAV = (0.85 \times A_1 \times A_2) \div L$$

where LAV = left atrial volume (mL)
     A_1 = left atrial area from apical 4-chamber view (cm^2)
     A_2 = left atrial area from apical 2-chamber view (cm^2)
     L = shortest long axis (length) of left atria (cm)

The LA volume is then indexed for body surface area:

Equation 3.2

$$ILAV = LAV \div BSA$$

where ILAV = indexed left atrial volume (mL/m^2)
     BSA = body surface area (m^2)

Important elements and common pitfalls for accurate, reproducible measurement of LA volumes are outlined in Table 3.2. In patients with diastolic dysfunction and associated increased LVFP, the LA is usually enlarged to at least a moderate degree. In particular, an indexed LA volume (ILAV) ≥ 34 mL/m^2 has been defined as one of the variables that identifies increased LV filling pressures[3.1].

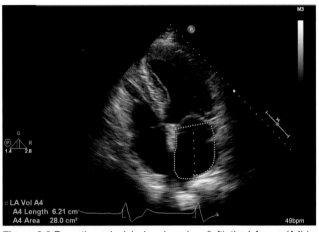
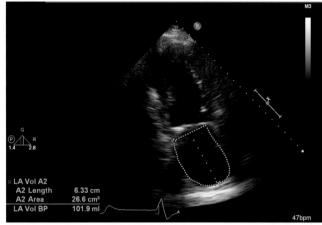

Figure 3.6 From the apical 4-chamber view *(left)*, the LA area (A4) is measured by tracing around the blood-tissue interface at end-systole. The long axis (length) of the atrium is measured from a line drawn perpendicularly from the centre of the mitral annulus to the superior aspect of the left atrium. From the apical 2-chamber view *(right)*, the atrial area (A2) is measured by tracing around the blood-tissue interface at end-systole. The long axis (L) of the atrium is measured from a line drawn perpendicularly from the centre of the mitral annulus to the superior aspect of the left atrium. The LA volume (LA Vol BP) in this example is:

LAV = (0.85 x A4 x A2) ÷ L
     = (0.85 x 28 x 26.6) ÷ 6.21
     = 101.9 mL

Table 3.1 Relationship between Echocardiographic Parameters and Diastolic Properties.

Diastolic Property	Echocardiographic Parameter	Relevance
Increased LV Stiffness	Mitral deceleration time	↓ DT
Impaired Myocardial Relaxation	LV wall thickness	↑ LV wall thickness
	Isovolumic relaxation time	↑ IVRT
	Transmitral inflow profile	↓ E velocity, ↑ DT, ↑ A velocity
	Pulmonary venous flow profile	↓ D velocity
	DTI early myocardial velocity (e')	↓ e' velocity, ↑ a' velocity
	Flow propagation velocity (Vp)	↑ Vp
Left Ventricular Filling Pressures (LVFP)	Left atrial volume (LAV)	↑ LAV
	Transmitral inflow profile	↑ E/A ratio, ↓ DT
	Pulmonary venous flow profile	↓ S, ↑ AR
	Mitral E to DTI e' ratio (E/e')	↑ E/e'
	Mitral E to Vp ratio (E/Vp)	↑ E/Vp
	Pulmonary artery end-diastolic pressure (PAEDP)	↑ PAEDP

A = transmitral velocity with atrial contraction; a' = myocardial velocity with atrial contraction; AR = pulmonary venous atrial reversal velocity; DT = transmitral deceleration time; E = transmitral early diastolic velocity; e' = early myocardial velocity; LV = left ventricle; S = pulmonary venous systolic velocity.

[3.1] Tsang TS, Barnes ME, Gersh BJ, Bailey KR, Seward JB. Left atrial volume as a morphophysiologic expression of left ventricular diastolic dysfunction and relation to cardiovascular risk burden. *Am J Cardiol.* 2002 Dec 15;90(12):1284-9.

Transmitral Inflow

The transmitral Doppler signal reflects the pressure gradient between the LA and LV during diastole (Fig. 3.7).

The transmitral inflow signal is acquired via pulsed-wave (PW) Doppler signal recorded from the apical 4-chamber view. A 1-3 mm sample volume size is placed at the tips of the mitral valve (Fig. 3.8). From the spectral Doppler trace, several measurements are performed (Fig. 3.9).

The transmitral peak E velocity reflects the early diastolic pressure gradient between the LA and LV (Fig. 3.9, A). Following the peak E velocity, the diastolic LA-LV pressure gradient quickly decreases and this results in a corresponding decrease in the Doppler velocity. The rate of decline between LA and LV pressures reflects the rapidity of LV filling and/or LA emptying. The rate of this pressure decline between these two chambers and, thus, Doppler velocities, is reflected by the deceleration rate or slope. From the deceleration slope, the deceleration time (DT) is measured as the time interval between the peak E velocity and the point of deceleration extrapolated to the zero baseline (Fig. 3.9, B). The transmitral peak A velocity is measured as the second peak on the transmitral inflow trace (Fig. 3.9, C). This velocity reflects forward blood flow from the LA to the LV following atrial contraction. Measurement of the duration of the mitral A velocity, when compared with the atrial reversal duration of the pulmonary venous signal, is also a useful parameter for the evaluation of diastolic function. The mitral A duration is simply measured from the beginning to the end of the A velocity (Figure 3.9, D). In addition, the transmitral E/A ratio can be derived as the peak E velocity divided by the peak A velocity.

All measurements should be performed at a sweep speed of 100 mm/s, at end-expiration, and averaged over 3 consecutive cardiac cycles.

The normal values for these measurements are dependent on the patient's age (Table 3.3). For example, in the young there is

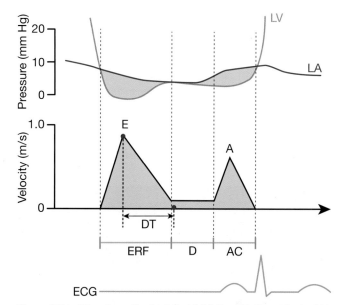

Figure 3.7 In this schematic, the left atrial (LA) and left ventricular (LV) pressure traces are shown at the top and the transmitral inflow profile is shown at the bottom. The peak transmitral E velocity correlates with the early, rapid filling gradient (*ERF*). The deceleration time (*DT*) reflects the rate of LV filling and LA emptying. The mid diastolic signal reflects diastasis (*D*) and the peak transmitral A velocity reflects the pressure gradient between the LA and LV with atrial contraction (*AC*).

Table 3.2 Critical Elements and Common Pitfalls for Accurate Measurement and Interpretation of Maximum LA Volume

Step	Common Limitations/Errors	Suggestions
A. Optimize LA image quality	Atria are located in the far field of the apical views. Reduction of lateral resolution may result in apparently thicker LA walls.	Not improved by modifying the gain settings: • Increase in gain will further reduce LA lumen size • Decrease in gain may lead to image "drop out" and difficulties in planimetry of LA area Use high resolution sample box to increase pixel density and facilitate accurate tracing of the endocardial border Capture at least five beats for each cine loop to maximize likelihood of obtaining adequate image quality
B. Obtain maximal LA size	LA is foreshortened	Modify transducer angulation or location (place the transducer one intercostal space lower) until LA image is optimized and not foreshortened If discrepancy in the two lengths measured from the orthogonal planes is 5 mm, acquisition should be repeated until the discrepancy is reduced
C. Timing of maximum LA size	Correct frame for measurement is not selected	Choose frame just before mitral valve opening
D. LA area planimetry	LA border is inconsistently defined	Consistently adhere to convention: • Inferior LA border—plane of mitral annulus (not the tip of leaflets) • Exclude atrial appendage and confluences of pulmonary veins
E. Long-axis LA length	LA long axis is inconsistently delineated	Consistently adhere to convention: • Inferior margin—midpoint of mitral annulus plane • Superior (posterior) margin—midpoint of posterior LA wall
F. Interpretation	Qualitative categorization of LA size	LA volume indexed to body surface area is optimally interpreted as a continuous variable (using a reference point of 22 ± 5 ml/m^2 as "normal")

Reprinted from Abhayaratna WP, Seward JB, Appleton CP, Douglas PS, Oh JK, Tajik AJ, et al. Left atrial size: physiologic determinants and clinical applications, *J Am Coll Cardiol*, Vol 47, page 2358, © 2006, with permission from Elsevier.

vigorous elastic recoil and rapid myocardial relaxation; this leads to rapid filling in early diastole with only a small amount of filling with atrial contraction. The resultant transmitral inflow profile displays a large E velocity, small A velocity and a short DT. In the elderly, there is a decline in elastic recoil and myocardial relaxation; this leads to "slow" early diastolic filling with compensatory increase in filling with atrial contraction. The resultant transmitral inflow profile displays small E velocity, large A velocity and a prolonged DT.

Transmitral Inflow Patterns

As the transmitral inflow profile reflects the pressure gradient between the LA and LV over diastole, the pattern of this profile provides important information regarding LV relaxation and LV filling pressures. There are essentially three transmitral inflow patterns that relate to varying and worsening stages of diastolic dysfunction: (1) impaired relaxation, (2) pseudonormalisation, (3) restrictive filling. Restrictive filling can be further categorised as being reversible or fixed (irreversible).

Normal

In a normal transmitral inflow profile, the majority of LV filling occurs during early diastole. Therefore, the mitral E velocity is greater than the mitral A velocity with the subsequent E/A ratio falling between 1 and 2. In addition, due to rapid suction of blood into the LV during early diastole, the DT is short and is usually between 150 and 200 ms (Fig. 3.10, A).

Impaired Relaxation

An impaired LV relaxation pattern occurs when there is delayed myocardial relaxation with normal LA pressures. With impaired relaxation, the early diastolic filling gradient

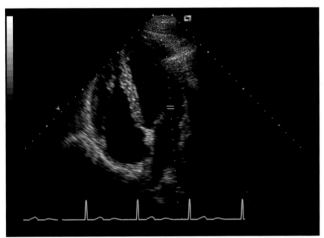
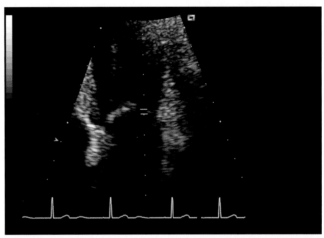

Figure 3.8 Transmitral signals are obtained via PW Doppler from the apical four chamber view; a 1-3 mm sample volume is positioned centrally at the tips of the open mitral valve leaflets (*left*). Zooming on the mitral valve further assists with precise sample volume placement (*right*).

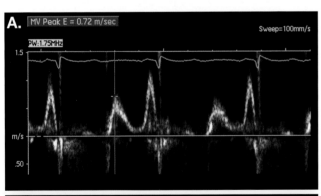
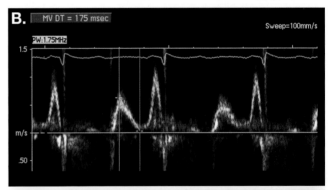
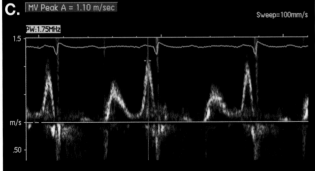
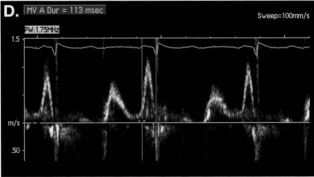

Figure 3.9 Measurements derived from the transmitral inflow trace include: measurement of the peak E velocity (*panel A*); measurement of the deceleration time (*panel B*); measurement of the peak A velocity (*panel C*); and measurement of the mitral A duration (*panel D*). The E/A ratio is derived from the peak E velocity divided by the peak A velocity.

is decreased so the transmitral E velocity is decreased. There is also a longer early diastolic filling gradient so the DT is prolonged. In addition, because of decreased LV filling in early diastole, there is a compensatory increase in LV filling with atrial contraction which results in an increased A velocity (Fig. 3.10, B). This pattern is characterised by E/A ratio less than 0.8 and a DT greater than 200 ms.

Impaired relaxation may be associated with an increased LVEDP. In this situation, the A duration is shortened because the increase in the LVEDP results in an early crossover between the LV and LA pressures which terminates mitral inflow prematurely (recall that the mitral valve closes when the pressure in the LV exceeds the pressure in the LA). As there are no defined values for the A duration, recognition of A duration shortening requires the additional investigation of pulmonary venous flow (see Pulmonary Venous Flow Patterns below).

Pseudonormal

"Normalisation" or pseudonormalisation of the transmitral inflow profile occurs when there is impaired relaxation in conjunction with a moderate reduction in LV compliance which results in a moderate increase in LAP. As the name suggests, pseudonormalisation refers to the fact that the transmitral inflow profile mimics a normal transmitral flow profile. This

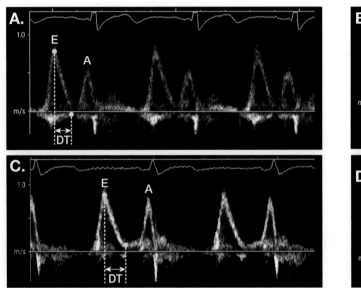
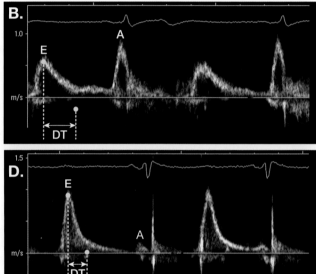

Figure 3.10 Patterns of transmitral inflow profiles are shown. Panel A shows an example of a normal transmitral inflow profile; observe that the E velocity is greater than A velocity (E/A = 1.5) and the deceleration time *(DT)* is reasonably steep (157 ms). Panel B is an example of a transmitral inflow profile that is seen with impaired LV relaxation; observe that the E velocity is less than the A velocity (E/A = 0.72) and that the DT is prolonged (286 ms). Panel C is an example of a pseudonormal profile; observe that this profile appears similar to the normal transmitral flow profile (E/A = 1.15, DT = 172 ms). Panel D is an example of a transmitral inflow profile that is seen with restrictive filling; observe that the E velocity is much higher than the A velocity, which is almost non-existent in this example (E/A = 6.2). The DT is also very short (100 ms). See text for further details.

Table 3.3 Normal Values for Doppler-Derived Diastolic Measurements.

Measurement	Age group (y)			
	16-20	21-40	41-60	>60
IVRT (ms)	50 ± 9 (32-68)	67 ± 8 (51-83)	74 ± 7 (60-88)	87 ± 7 (73-101)
E/A ratio	1.88 ± 0.45 (0.98-2.78)	1.53 ± 0.40 (0.73-2.33)	1.28 ± 0.25 (0.78-1.78)	0.96 ± 0.18 (0.6-1.32)
DT (ms)	142 ± 19 (104-180)	166 ± 14 (138-194)	181 ± 19 (143-219)	200 ± 29 (142-258)
A duration (ms)	113 ± 17 (79-147)	127 ± 13 (101-153)	133 ± 13 (107-159)	138 ± 19 (100-176)
PV S/D ratio	0.82 ± 0.18 (0.46-1.18)	0.98 ± 0.32 (0.34-1.62)	1.21 ± 0.2 (0.81-1.61)	1.39 ± 0.47 (0.45-2.33)
PV Ar (cm/s)	16 ± 10 (1-36)	21 ± 8 (5-37)	23 ± 3 (17-29)	25 ± 9 (11-39)
PV Ar duration (ms)	66 ± 39 (1-144)	96 ± 33 (30-162)	112 ± 15 (82-142)	113 ± 30 (53-173)
Septal e' (cm/s)	14.9 ± 2.4 (10.1-19.7)	15.5 ± 2.7 (10.1-20.9)	12.2 ± 2.3 (7.6-16.8)	10.4 ± 2.1 (6.2-14.6)
Septal e'/a' ratio	2.4*	1.6 ± 0.5 (0.6-2.6)	1.1 ± 0.3 (0.5-1.7)	0.85 ± 0.2 (0.45-1.25)
Lateral e' (cm/s)	20.6 ± 3.8 (13-28.2)	19.8 ± 2.9 (14-25.6)	16.1 ± 2.3 (11.5-20.7)	12.9 ± 3.5 (5.9-19.9)
Lateral e'/a' ratio	3.1*	1.9 ± 0.6 (0.7-3.1)	1.5 ± 0.5 (0.5-2.5)	0.9 ± 0.4 (0.1-1.7)

Data are expressed as mean ± SD (95% confidence interval). Note that for e' velocity in subjects aged 16 to 20 years, values overlap with those for subjects aged 21 to 40 years. This is because e' increases progressively with age in children and adolescents. Therefore, the e' velocity is higher in a normal 20-year-old than in a normal 16-year-old, which results in a somewhat lower average e' value when subjects aged 16 to 20 years are considered. *Standard deviations are not included because these data were computed, not directly provided in the original articles from which they were derived. Reprinted from Nagueh SF, Appleton CP, Gillebert TC, Marino PN, Oh JK, Smiseth OA, Waggoner AD, Flachskampf FA, Pellikka PA, Evangelista A. Recommendations for the evaluation of left ventricular diastolic function by echocardiography, *J Am Soc Echocardiogr*, Vol. 22 (2), page 112 © 2009 with permission from Elsevier.

pattern is, therefore, characterised by E/A ratio between 1 and 1.5 and a DT between 150 and 200 ms (Fig. 3.10, C). In addition, the A duration is shortened as the LVEDP is elevated so there is an early crossover between the LV and LA pressures which terminates mitral inflow prematurely.

> **LVEDP and LAP**
> When the LAP is increased the LVEDP must also be increased. That is, the LVEDP cannot be normal when the LAP is elevated. Note, however, that there can be an elevated LVEDP with a normal LAP.

Pseudonormalisation of the transmitral inflow profile occurs when the LAP is increased. In this situation, despite the presence of impaired relaxation, elevated LAP increases the driving pressure across the mitral valve. Therefore, the abnormally low transmitral E velocity that is typical of impaired relaxation will increase so the transmitral E velocity returns to the normal range. Furthermore, when there is decreased compliance of the ventricle, ventricular pressure rises more rapidly in early diastole and the abnormally long DT that is typically seen with impaired relaxation shortens so the DT also returns to the normal range.

A pseudonormal transmitral flow profile can be differentiated from a normal transmitral profile by decreasing the preload, which effectively decreases LAP. Preload reduction can be accomplished by asking the patient to perform the Valsalva manoeuvre. During the strain phase of this manoeuvre, intrathoracic pressure exceeds the pressure in the great veins which decreases venous return and, thus, preload. The effect of decreased preload on a normal transmitral trace is a similar reduction in both the mitral E and A velocities; as a result the E/A ratio is essentially unchanged (Fig. 3.11, top). In a pseudonormal flow profile, preload reduction unmasks the

underlying abnormal relaxation pattern; that is, the E velocity decreases and the DT prolongs with the A velocity increasing or remaining unchanged (Fig. 3.11, bottom).

A triphasic mitral inflow profile with mid-diastolic flow is also suggestive of pseudonormalisation (Fig. 3.12). The proposed mechanism for this mid-diastolic flow (or an L-wave) relates to markedly abnormal LV relaxation; that is, LV relaxation is markedly prolonged such that it continues into mid diastole and as a result there is a continued LA-LV pressure gradient over diastasis (Fig. 3.13). It is important to differentiate this triphasic profile from IVR flow. IVR flow may be seen in hyperdynamic or hypertrophic ventricles. In these instances, flow during IVR occurs because of the earlier than normal relaxation of the LV apex relative to the LV base; this effectively creates an intraventricular pressure gradient between these two regions (Fig. 3.14). Careful attention to the timing of flow with the ECG will distinguish IVR flow from a triphasic mitral flow profile.

Other parameters can also be used to differentiate between pseudonormal and normal transmitral patterns by either identifying the underlying abnormality in myocardial relaxation or by providing other evidence of increased LVFP (Table 3.4).

> The Valsalva manoeuvre is performed by instructing the patient to strain down without breathing at expiration. Statements that may help the patient to understand what is required include: "Hold your nose and try to pop your ears as you would do on an airplane" or "Pretend that you have a belt around your tummy and try to bust this" or "Place your thumb in your mouth and try to blow it up as though it is a balloon".
>
> An adequate Valsalva attempt, in patients without restrictive filling, is a decrease of 20 cm/s and/or a 10% reduction in the peak E velocity from the baseline value.

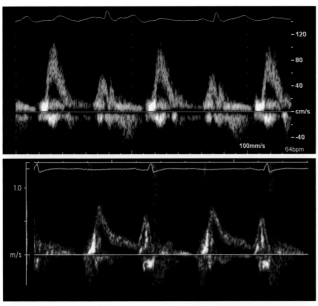
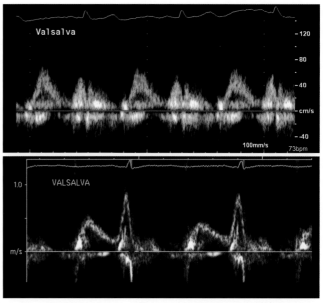

Figure 3.11 The two resting transmitral inflow profiles displayed to the left show characteristic features of a normal filling profile. Following the Valsalva manoeuvre, the transmitral inflow profile on the top right shows a reduction in both the E and A velocities; this response is characteristic for a normal flow profile. The transmitral inflow profile on the bottom right reverts to an impaired relaxation pattern (note the reduction in the E velocity, an increase in the A velocity and prolongation of the DT); this response is a characteristic finding of pseudonormalisation.

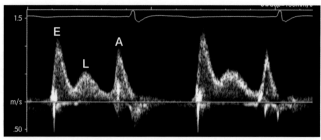

Figure 3.12 This mitral inflow profile displays a triphasic pattern with an early diastolic *(E)*, a mid-diastolic *(L)* and late diastolic *(A)* waves. In the presence of associated LVH this flow profile is a marker of pseudonormal LV filling.

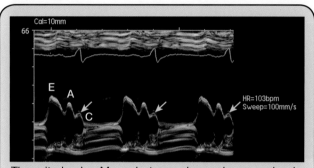

The mitral valve M-mode trace above shows a classic example of a "B-notch" or "B-bump" interrupting the AC slope of the anterior mitral leaflet *(arrows)*. A B-bump is a very specific sign for an elevated LVEDP (> 20 mm Hg).

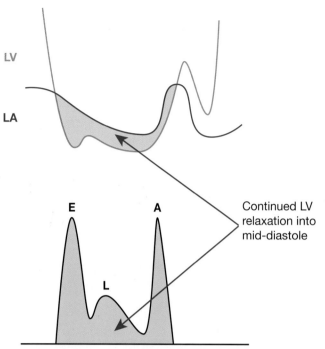

Figure 3.13 The top schematic shows the left ventricular *(LV)* and left atrial *(LA)* pressure curves and the bottom schematic shows the resultant mitral inflow profile. Marked prolongation of LV relaxation into mid-diastole in conjunction with an elevated LA pressure leads to a continued LA-LV pressure gradient over the period of diastasis. This continued LA-LV pressure gradient appears as mid-diastolic flow on the mitral inflow profile (L-wave).

Table 3.4 Clues to Pseudonormalisation of the Transmitral Inflow Profile

Clue to Pseudonormalisation	Explanation/Justification
Advanced age	With advancing age, an impaired relaxation pattern is expected. Therefore, the presence of a 'normal' transmitral inflow profile in a person older than 60 years is suggestive of pseudonormalisation.
Dilated LA	A dilated LA suggests chronic elevation in LAP. Therefore, a moderate increase in LA volume (ILAV $\geq$ 34 mL/m²), in the absence of other causes for LA dilatation*, is suggestive of pseudonormalisation.
Increased LV size and/or LV wall thickness	An impaired relaxation pattern is expected when there is LVH while increased LVFP are expected when the LV is dilated. Therefore, a 'normal' transmitral inflow profile in these circumstances is suggestive of pseudonormalisation.
LV systolic dysfunction	Diastolic dysfunction precedes systolic dysfunction. Therefore, the presence of systolic dysfunction (ejection fraction < 40%) infers diastolic dysfunction.
Reversal of the transmitral profile with the Valsalva manoeuvre	Pseudonormal = impaired relaxation + ↑ LAP. Therefore, by decreasing preload and the LAP via the Valsalva manoeuvre, the underlying abnormal relaxation will be unmasked.
Triphasic mitral inflow (L-wave)	The presence of mid-diastolic flow on the mitral profile reflects a marked abnormality in LV relaxation which is associated with pseudonormalisation.
Increased AR velocity (> 35 cm/s) and/or AR_{dur}-$A_{dur} \geq$ 30 ms	Increase AR velocities on the pulmonary venous flow profile and/or AR_{dur}-$A_{dur} \geq$ 30 ms is associated with an elevated LVEDP; patients with pseudonormalisation have elevated LVFP which includes an elevated LVEDP.
Decreased DTI e' +/- delayed onset to e'	e' is inversely related to LV relaxation; therefore, when LV relaxation is impaired, the e' is decreased. In addition, with impaired LV relaxation, the onset of the e' velocity is delayed when compared to the onset of the mitral E velocity.
Slow flow propagation velocity (< 45 cm/s)	The flow propagation velocity (Vp) is inversely related to LV relaxation; therefore, when LV relaxation is impaired, the Vp is slowed.
Other evidence of increased LVFP	Increased E/e' ratio is consistent with increased LVFP (E/e'$\geq$15 (medial); $\geq$12 (lateral); $\geq$13 average)# Presence of a B-bump on the mitral valve M-mode trace indicates an elevation in the LVEDP.

* Other causes of LA dilatation include atrial arrhythmias such as atrial fibrillation and atrial flutter, bradycardia, mitral valve disease and increased cardiac output states such as anaemia and sepsis.

Medial, lateral and average refers to location of the e' measurement; that is, medial annulus, lateral annulus or an average of medial and lateral annuli.

Technical Tips for Transmitral Inflow

Correct Sample Volume Alignment and Position

As for all Doppler measurements, parallel alignment with flow is crucial to ensuring that the velocities are accurately displayed; off-axis imaging may be required to achieve parallel alignment with transmitral inflow. For the PW Doppler assessment of transmitral inflow it is important that the sample volume is placed at the tips of the mitral valve which corresponds to the vena contracta. One way of ensuring that the sample volume is correctly placed is to first check the velocities across the valve via continuous-wave (CW) Doppler (*below left*); CW Doppler will detect the highest velocity at the vena contracta. Then via PW Doppler, the peak E and peak A velocities should be similar to those recorded with CW Doppler (*below right*).

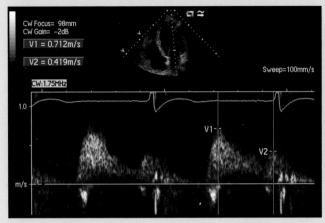 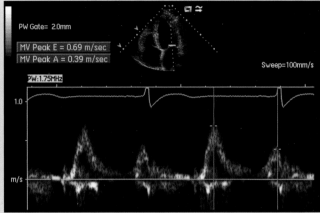

Sample Volume Size

The sample volume size significantly affects the appearance of the transmitral flow profile. To the left is a mitral inflow profile with the sample volume set at 12 mm – observe that there is significant spectral broadening of this signal. To the right, the sample volume has been set at 1.5 mm, observe that there is less spectral broadening and the profile appears crisper. Measurements from the trace with the smaller sample volume will be more accurate.

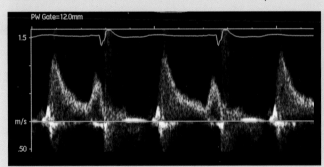 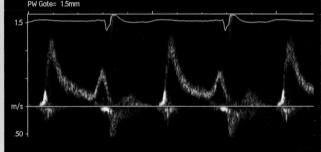

Common Measurement Errors

The example below and left illustrates common transmitral measurement errors. Firstly, the sweep speed is set too slow at only 66.67 mm/s; as a result the accuracy of time-related intervals such as the DT and A duration may be compromised. Secondly, the DT, A velocity and A duration are all overestimated. The example below and right shows where these measurements should have been performed. The DT should be measured along the modal velocity (centre of the brightest spectral line) and the A velocity should also be measured at the modal velocity. The end of the A duration is also earlier; in fact, the A duration should not have been attempted from this trace (see Technical Tip below on Unclear A Durations).

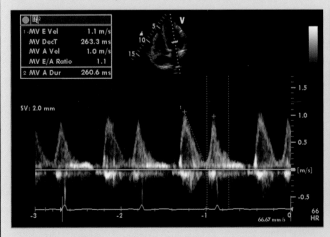 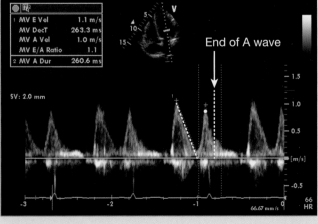

Technical Tips for Transmitral Inflow

Unclear A Durations

Low wall filters are required to ensure that the beginning and end of the mitral A velocity is clearly seen. Another limitation to accurate A duration measurement occurs when there is flow around the zero baseline at the end of the A velocity so the end of this velocity is not clear. The sample volume is usually placed at the tips of the mitral valve in early diastole (*position A* on the adjacent schematic). However, when there is a large increase in the LV early diastolic volume, the mitral annulus and leaflet tips move superiorly with the atrioventricular (AV) groove so that the sample volume is actually in the ventricle by the time of atrial contraction; this results in flow eddies at the end of the A velocity. By moving the sample volume *towards* the mitral annulus (*position B* on the adjacent schematic), these flow eddies are avoided.

Observe on the image below and left, the end of A velocity is not clear because of flow around the zero baseline at the end of the A velocity. On the image below and right, the sample volume was moved a little towards the mitral annulus; as a result the end of the A velocity is now more apparent and accurate measurement of the A duration is now possible.

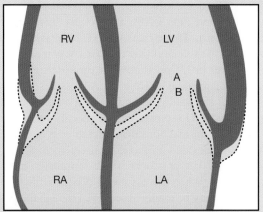

Adapted from Appleton CP, Jensen JL, Hatle LK, Oh JK. Doppler evaluation of left and right ventricular diastolic function: a technical guide for obtaining optimal flow velocity recordings. *J Am Soc Echocardiogr,* Vol. 10(3), page 281, © 1997 with permission from Elsevier.

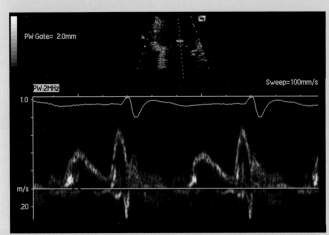

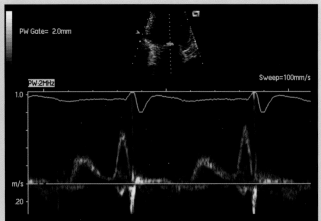

Measurement of the DT in Atrial Fibrillation

Measurement of the DT in atrial fibrillation is only useful when the DT ends *before* the onset of the next QRS complex of the ECG. When the diastolic filling period is very short and the DT is terminated early by the onset of the next cardiac cycle, the DT is shorter than it would be at longer diastolic filling periods. On the adjacent example, observe that the DT is very short on the beats where the DT is 'prematurely' terminated by the onset of the next QRS complex. The DT should only be averaged when the DT ends *before* the onset of the next QRS complex. Averaging from R-R intervals corresponding to a heart rate of 70-80 bpm is also recommended.

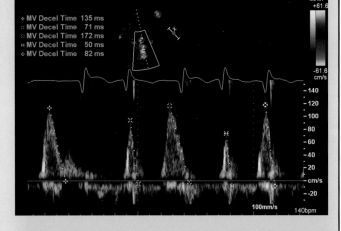

E-A Fusion

The E and A velocities are often fused when the diastolic filling period shortens such as occurs with sinus tachycardia and first-degree heart block (see example opposite). In particular, when the E velocity at the onset of the A velocity ("E at A") is greater than 20 cm/s, the A velocity is higher than it would be at slower heart rates. In these cases, the E/A ratio will be decreased and is not comparable with that which would be derived when the "E at A" is less than 20 cm/s. In these situations, other Doppler parameters are required to evaluate diastolic function.

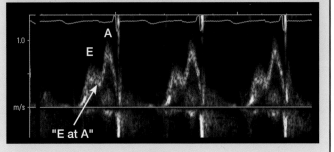

Restrictive Filling

When there is poor LV compliance (or increased LV stiffness), with LV filling there is a marked and early increase in LVFP (and thus LAP); this results in a restrictive LV filling pattern. The increased LAP results in an increased transmitral E velocity. Due to poor LV compliance, there is a rapid rise in LV pressure with early diastolic filling with a rapid equalization of LV and LA pressures. This results in significant shortening of the DT. With atrial contraction, due to the very high LV pressures, there is only a small transmitral A velocity. In addition, the A duration is shortened as the LVEDP is elevated so there is an early crossover between the LV and LA pressures which terminates mitral inflow prematurely. When there is poor LA contractile function, the A velocity may be totally absent even though the patient is in sinus rhythm. This restrictive filling pattern is characterised by E/A ratio ≥ 2 and a DT less than 160 ms (Fig. 3.10, D).

The restrictive filling profile can be further classified as reversible restrictive filling or irreversible (fixed) restrictive filling. A reversible restrictive filling can be differentiated from an irreversible restrictive filling by decreasing preload; for example, by asking the patient to perform the Valsalva manoeuvre. When there is a reversible restrictive filling, preload reduction will result in a reversal of this filling profile to either a pseudonormal filling profile or even to an impaired relaxation filling profile (Fig. 3.15, top). In an irreversible restrictive filling, preload reduction will not change the pattern of this profile; that is, it maintains the characteristic features of a restrictive profile (E/A ratio ≥ 2 and a DT <160 ms) (Fig. 3.15, bottom).

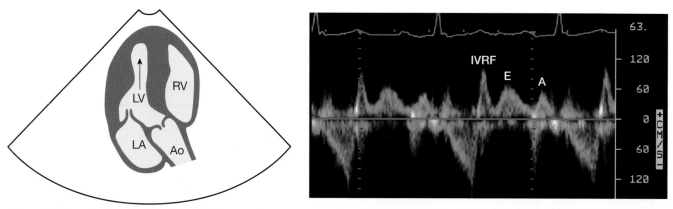

Figure 3.14 Isovolumic relaxation flow *(IVRF)* occurs between two regions of the left ventricle *(LV)* due to marked asynchrony in ventricular relaxation *(left)*. This flow is most commonly directed from the base of the heart to the apex during the isovolumic relaxation flow period *(right)*. IVRF may be seen in patients with intracavity gradients caused by LV hypertrophy and vigorous LV systolic function with near cavity obliteration in systole. It is important to recognise IVRF and not to confuse this flow pattern with that of a triphasic mitral flow profile. Ao = aorta; LA = left atrium; LV = left ventricle; RV = right ventricle.

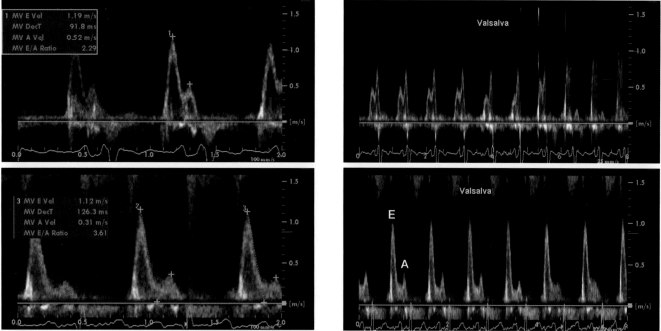

Figure 3.15 The two resting transmitral inflow profiles displayed to the left show characteristic features of a restrictive filling profile: E/A ratio > 2.0, a DT (DecT) < 160 ms. Following the Valsalva manoeuvre the transmitral inflow pattern on the top reverts to an impaired relaxation pattern *(top right)*; this is characteristic of reversible restrictive filling. Following the Valsalva manoeuvre the transmitral inflow pattern on the bottom does not change *(bottom right)*; that is, the profile maintains the characteristic features of a restrictive filling profile (high E/A ratio and short DT). This is characteristic of irreversible restrictive filling.

Isovolumic Relaxation Time

As mentioned, the IVRT is the interval between aortic valve closure and mitral valve opening. The IVRT can therefore be measured by displaying both the transmitral signal and the left ventricular outflow tract (LVOT) signal on the same spectral trace. This is accomplished by aligning either the PW or continuous-wave (CW) Doppler beam so that it intercepts flow between these two regions (Fig. 3.16). The IVRT is optimally displayed when the closing click of the aortic valve is depicted both above and below the zero baseline. Measurements should be performed at a sweep speed of 100 mm/s, at end-expiration, and averaged over 3 consecutive cardiac cycles.

In the normal heart, the IVRT is between 50-100 ms. However, as for the transmitral measurements, the normal value for the IVRT is dependent on the patient's age (Table 3.3). For example, with advancing age there is a decline in elastic recoil and myocardial relaxation; this leads to prolongation of the IVRT.

Factors Affecting IVRT

The IVRT is influenced by a number of factors including LV relaxation and LAP (Fig. 3.17). When there is impaired LV relaxation, the LV pressure decline during IVR is slowed

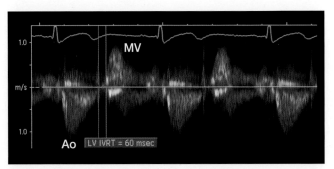

Figure 3.16 The isovolumic relaxation time (*IVRT*) is measured as the time interval between aortic valve closure and mitral valve opening. This is achieved by aligning the Doppler beam so that is intercepts flow between the aorta (*Ao*) and mitral valve (*MV*).

so there is a longer time before the LV pressure falls below (crosses over) the LAP which means that mitral valve opening is delayed; this results in prolongation of the IVRT. An IVRT ≥ 100 ms is consistent with impaired LV relaxation (Fig. 3.17, B). IVRT is also dependent on preload or LAP. Therefore, as for the transmitral inflow profile, pseudonormalisation of the IVRT can also occur. Recall that pseudonormalisation occurs when there is impaired relaxation with a moderate increase in LAP. So even though the LV pressure decline is slower because the LAP is elevated the crossover between the LA and LV pressures now occurs within a normal timeframe and, thus, the IVRT is within the normal range (Fig. 3.17, C). When there is a marked increase in LAP, as seen with restrictive filling, the crossover between the LV and LA pressures occurs earlier than normal; this results in earlier than normal mitral valve opening and shortening of the IVRT. An IVRT ≤ 60 ms is consistent with restrictive filling (Fig. 3.17, D).

Pulmonary Venous Flow

The pulmonary venous signal reflects the pressure gradient between the pulmonary veins and the LA over the cardiac cycle (Fig. 3.18).

The pulmonary venous signal is acquired via PW Doppler from the apical 4-chamber view. A 3-5 mm sample volume is positioned approximately 1 cm into the right upper pulmonary vein (Fig. 3.19). From the spectral Doppler trace, several measurements are performed (Fig. 3.20).

Systolic forward flow reflects the systolic pressure gradient between the pulmonary vein and the LA and is identified as the peak systolic (S) velocity on the pulmonary venous trace (Fig. 3.20, A). The S velocity may appear biphasic with S1 and S2 components. S1 occurs in early systole and represents the increase in pulmonary venous flow secondary to LA relaxation. S2 occurs in mid to late systole and is produced predominately by the increase in pulmonary venous pressure that occurs with transpulmonary propagation of flow after RV systole.

Diastolic forward flow reflects the diastolic pressure gradient between the pulmonary vein and the LA and is identified as the peak diastolic (D) velocity on the pulmonary venous

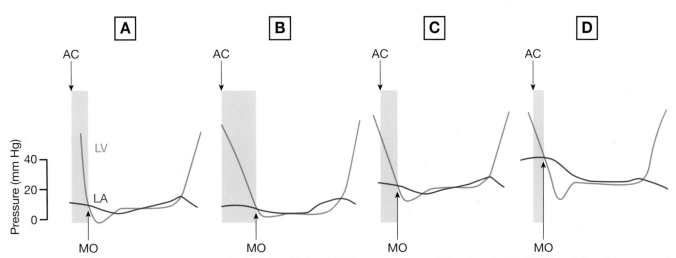

Figure 3.17 This schematic shows the left ventricular (LV) and left atrial (LA) pressure traces during diastole. The IVRT (shaded area) is measured from aortic valve closure (AC) to mitral valve opening (MO); MO occurs when the LV pressure falls below the LA pressure. **A** = an example of a normal IVRT. **B** = an example of an IVRT seen with impaired LV relaxation; observe that due to delayed LV relaxation, the LV pressure decline is slower than normal and crosses over the LA pressure later resulting in prolongation of the IVRT. **C** = an example of a pseudonormal profile; observe that the IVRT is normal. Pseudonormalisation of the IVRT occurs when there is impaired LV relaxation plus an increase in the LA pressure; therefore, LV pressure crosses over the elevated LA pressure within a normal timeframe. **D** = an example of an IVRT seen with restrictive filling; observe that the IVRT is very short even though there is impaired LV relaxation. Shortening of the IVRT occurs due to a marked increase in the LA pressure so that crossover between the LV and LA pressures occurs earlier than normal.

Doppler trace (Fig. 3.20, B). Pulmonary venous diastolic flow essentially parallels that of the transmitral E velocity. For example, when the transmitral peak E velocity is decreased, the peak diastolic velocity of the pulmonary venous trace is also decreased.

Atrial flow reversal into the pulmonary vein reflects the pressure gradient between the LA and the pulmonary vein following atrial contraction. Atrial flow reversal (AR) is identified as a retrograde velocity on the pulmonary venous Doppler trace occurring just after the P wave on the ECG (Fig. 3.20, C). The AR duration is measured from the beginning of the AR velocity to the end of the AR velocity (Figure 3.20, D).

The S/D ratio is derived from the peak S velocity divided by the peak D velocity. In the presence of a biphasic S velocity, S2 should be measured and used in the calculation of the S/D ratio.

The difference between the mitral A duration and the pulmonary venous AR duration (AR_{dur}-A_{dur}) is also a useful parameter for the evaluation of diastolic function.

Measurements should be performed at a sweep speed of 100 mm/s, at end-expiration, and averaged over at least 3 consecutive cardiac cycles.

As for the transmitral and IVRT measurements, the normal values for pulmonary venous measurements are dependent on the patient's age (Table 3.3). In particular, with advancing age the D velocity decreases and S velocity increases (S/D ratio increases), and the AR increases slightly.

Pulmonary Venous Flow Patterns

Pulmonary venous flow profiles are influenced by LV filling pressures. Pulmonary venous flow patterns correspond to the transmitral inflow patterns; therefore, abnormal pulmonary venous patterns include: (1) impaired relaxation, (2) pseudonormalisation, (3) restrictive filling.

Normal

In the normal pulmonary venous flow profile, the S velocity is higher than the D velocity and when biphasic the S2 velocity is higher than S1 velocity. The S/D ratio is approximately 1.0. The AR velocity is less than 35 cm/s and the AR_{dur}-A_{dur} is less than 20 ms (Fig. 3.21, A).

In young patients (less than 40 years of age), the S/D may be less than 1; this occurs when there is an increased D velocity caused by enhanced LV suction and filling.

Impaired Relaxation

The pulmonary venous D velocity parallels the transmitral E velocity. As such when there is impaired LV relaxation, the pulmonary venous D velocity is decreased (Fig. 3.21, B). A decrease in the D velocity occurs because the early diastolic filling gradient is decreased so there is also less filling of the atrium via the pulmonary veins during early diastole.

The AR velocity is influenced by LVEDP, preload and LA contractility. When the LVEDP is normal the AR velocity is less than 35 cm/s and the AR_{dur}-A_{dur} is less than 30 ms (Fig. 3.22, A). However, when LVEDP is elevated, both the amplitude and the duration of AR velocity increase and the duration of mitral inflow A velocity also decreases. As a result, the AR_{dur}-A_{dur} increases (Fig. 3.22, B). An increase in the AR_{dur}-A_{dur} by 30 ms or more is consistent with an elevated LVEDP.

Pseudonormal

As mentioned, pseudonormalisation is associated with impaired relaxation in conjunction with a moderate reduction

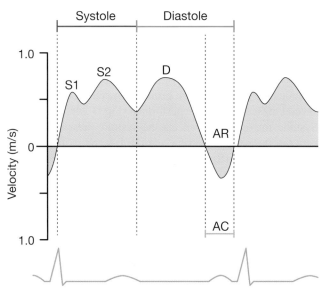

Figure 3.18 This schematic illustrates the pulmonary venous signal. Normal pulmonary venous flow consists of three primary velocities: (1) systolic forward flow *(S)*, (2) diastolic forward flow *(D)* and (3) retrograde flow or flow reversal with atrial contraction *(AR)*. The S velocity may be biphasic: the early peak (S1) is related to left atrial relaxation while the later peak (S2) corresponds with an increase in pulmonary venous pressure after right ventricular systole.

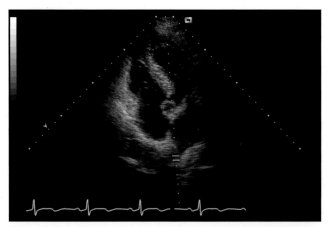
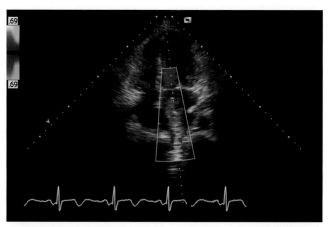

Figure 3.19 Pulmonary venous signals are obtained via PW Doppler from the apical four chamber view; a 3-5 mm sample volume is positioned 1 cm into the right upper pulmonary vein *(left)*. Colour flow Doppler imaging is useful in identifying pulmonary venous flow and may assist with precise sample volume placement *(right)*.

in LV compliance which results in a moderate increase in LAP. On the transmitral inflow trace, this results in an increased E velocity into the normal range; as the pulmonary venous D velocity parallels the mitral E velocity, there is also an increase in the pulmonary D velocity into the normal range with pseudonormalisation. In addition, systolic filling from the pulmonary veins is reduced as the LAP is increased so there is also a reduction in the pulmonary S velocity and, therefore, a reduction in the S/D ratio (Fig. 3.21, C). As the LVEDP is elevated, the AR velocity and the AR_{dur}-A_{dur} are usually increased. An increase in the AR velocity of more than 35 ms and an increase in the AR_{dur}-A_{dur} by 30 ms or more are consistent with an elevated LVEDP.

Restrictive Filling

When there is poor LV compliance there is associated rapid ventricular filling in diastole and this is associated with a concurrent increase in LA filling via the pulmonary veins. As a result the pulmonary venous D velocity is increased. In addition, due to the marked elevation in LAP there is a corresponding marked reduction in the pulmonary S velocity; therefore, the S/D ratio in reduced (Fig. 3.21,D). When LA function is preserved, an increase in both the velocity and duration of the AR velocity is expected. However, when there is LA enlargement and reduced LA contractile function, as seen with worsening LV diastolic function, the AR velocity may be reduced or even absent.

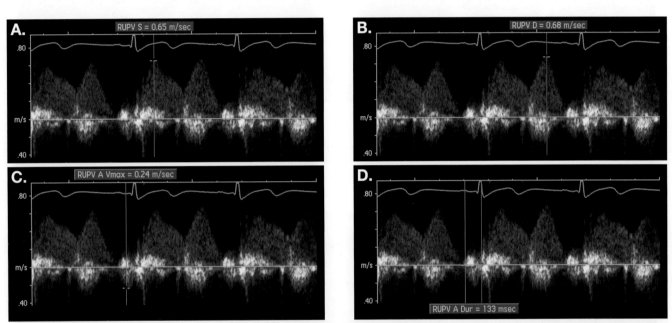

Figure 3.20 Measurements derived from the pulmonary venous trace include measurement of the peak S velocity *(panel A)*; measurement of the peak D velocity *(panel B)*; measurement of the peak AR velocity *(panel C)* and measurement of the AR duration *(panel D)*. The S/D ratio is derived from the peak S velocity divided by the peak D velocity.

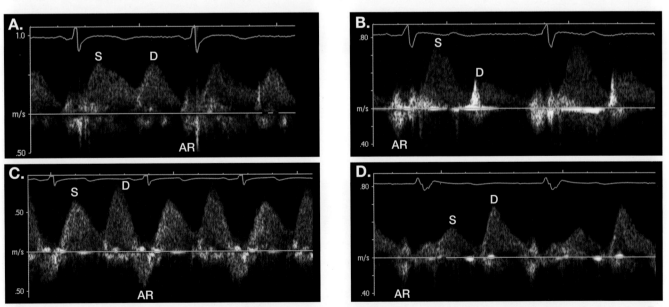

Figure 3.21 Patterns of pulmonary venous flow profiles are shown. Panel A shows an example of a normal pulmonary venous flow profile; observe that the S velocity and the D velocity are equal (S/D = 1) and the AR velocity is small (30 cm/s). Panel B is an example of a pulmonary venous flow profile seen with impaired LV relaxation; observe that the D velocity is decreased and the S/D ratio is increased (S/D = 2.3); the AR velocity is 35 cm/s. Panel C is an example of a pulmonary venous flow profile seen with pseudonormalisation; observe that the D velocity > S velocity (S/D = 0.8); the AR velocity is also increased (47 cm/s), consistent with an elevated LVEDP. Panel D is an example of a pulmonary venous flow profile seen with restrictive filling; observe that the S velocity is significantly decreased (S/D = 0.6); AR velocity is only 23 cm/s which is consistent with poor LA function. See text for further details.

Technical Tips for Pulmonary Venous Flow

Correct Sample Volume Position

The sample volume should be placed at least 1 cm into the pulmonary vein. In the example below and left, the sample volume (*larger white dot along the cursor*) is placed at the entrance of the pulmonary vein into the LA. The sample volume should be placed further into the pulmonary vein as indicated on the example below and right (*larger yellow dot along the cursor*).

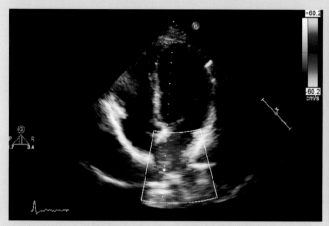 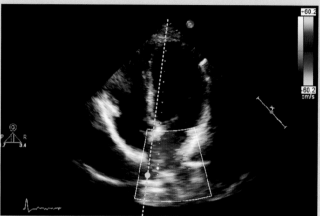

Sample Volume Size

The sample volume size may significantly affect the quality of the pulmonary venous trace. The trace below and left shows a signal acquired with a 1 mm sample volume size; the trace below and right shows the signal acquired with a 3.5 mm sample volume. Observe that the signal obtained with the larger sample volume significantly improves the signal quality. It should be noted, however, that larger sample volume sizes may contaminate the signal due to pulmonary venous wall motion artefacts.

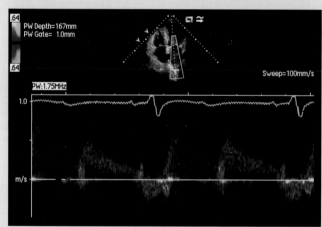 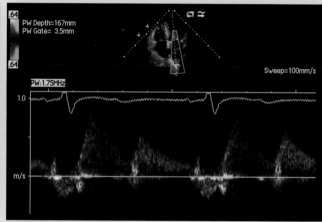

Wall Filters

As pulmonary venous velocities are relatively low, low wall filters are required to ensure that the beginning and end of flow are clearly seen. This is especially important when measuring the AR duration or the velocity time integrals of the pulmonary venous signals. On the example below and left the wall filter is set too high, as such the beginning and end of the D, S and AR velocities are unclear; accurate measurement of the AR duration is not possible from this trace. The example below and right shows the same signal with lower wall filters; the AR duration can be clearly seen and can be accurately measured from this trace.

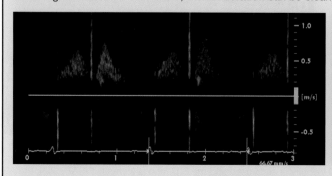 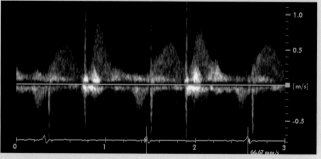

Technical Tips for Pulmonary Venous Flow

AR Duration Measurements

Underestimation of the AR duration can occur when the end of the AR velocity is not correctly identified as shown in the example below and left. In the example below and right, the actual end of the AR duration is indicated (*dashed yellow line*). Remember that venous flow is continuous so the end of the AR velocity will coincide with the onset of the S velocity.

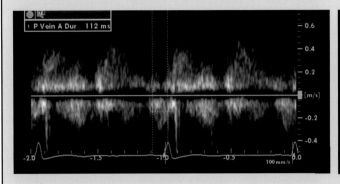 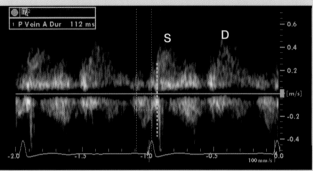

Atrial Contraction against a Closed Mitral Valve

When the atria contract against a closed mitral valve, there will be an 'artificial' increase in the AR velocity. This may occur in the presence of ventricular ectopics (*see example below, left*), pacemaker rhythms and junctional rhythms (*see example below, right*). Observe on the traces below that the labelled AR velocity is markedly increased. This is because atrial contraction has occurred during ventricular systole against the closed mitral valve (observe the timing of the AR velocity compared to the ECG). Measurement of these AR velocities will be overestimated when compared with the AR velocities on the sinus beats (*yellow asterisks*). Careful attention to the timing of flow with the ECG will avoid these measurement errors.

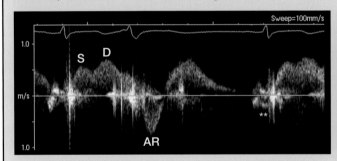 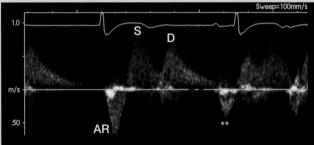

High PRF

In order to increase the maximum velocity that can be displayed via PW Doppler, the ultrasound machine will employ High PRF mode. This is achieved by increasing the number of PW Doppler sample volumes. In the case of pulmonary venous interrogation, a second sample volume is often coincidentally placed at the level of the mitral valve and, therefore, the signals from both the pulmonary vein and the mitral inflow will return to the transducer at the same time. As a result, both signals are simultaneously displayed (superimposed one on top of one another). The signal below and left is acquired at High PRF. Note that there are two sample volumes, one in the pulmonary vein (SV$_1$) and another at the mitral valve (SV$_2$); the displayed signal is therefore the 'sum' of the pulmonary venous and the transmitral inflow signals. The signals displayed below and right were recorded with a single sample volume in the pulmonary vein and at the tips of the mitral valve.

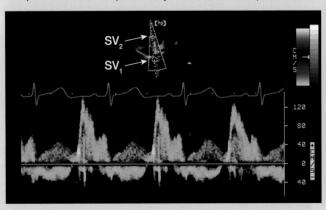 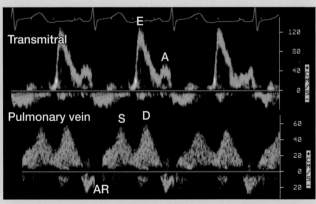

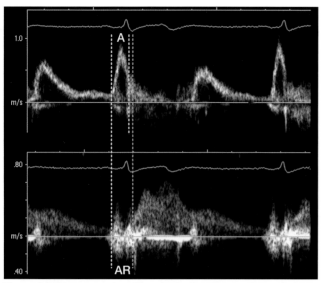
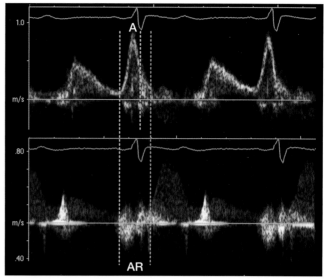

Figure 3.22 Two examples of impaired relaxation are shown. In the example on the left, the AR velocity is 24 cm/s and the AR_{dur}-A_{dur} is 8 ms (note that the end of the A and AR signals occur almost at the same time); these findings suggest that the LVEDP is normal. In the example on the right, the AR velocity is 36 cm/s and the AR_{dur}-A_{dur} is 32 ms (note that the end of the A signals occurs earlier than the end of the AR signal); these findings suggest that the LVEDP is elevated.

Doppler Tissue Imaging

As discussed in Chapter 2, the myocardial velocity profile obtained by DTI is characterised by three distinct velocities: (1) an apically directed systolic myocardial velocity (s'), (2) an early diastolic atrially directed myocardial velocity (e'), and (3) a late diastolic atrially directed myocardial velocity (a'). In addition to these three distinct velocities, less prominent biphasic velocities may be seen during the isovolumic periods (see Fig. 2.33). The e' velocity, which coincides with the mitral E velocity, reflects the longitudinal expansion or lengthening of the LV in early diastole as blood rapidly fills the LV.

DTI velocities are recorded via PW Doppler by placing the 5-10 mm sample volume at the medial (septal) and lateral corner of the mitral annulus from the apical 4-chamber view, ensuing that the sample volume covers the annulus over both systole and diastole (Fig. 3.23). From the spectral Doppler trace, the e' and a' velocities are measured (Fig. 3.24). Measurements should be performed at a sweep speed of 50-100 mm/s, and the e' and a' velocities from the medial annulus and lateral anulus should be averaged to account for regional dysfunction.

As for the transmitral, IVRT and pulmonary venous measurements, the normal values for DTI measurements are dependent on the patient's age (Table 3.3). In particular, with advancing age the e' velocity decreases and the a' velocity increases; as a result the e'/a' ratio also increases.

The terminology for DTI velocities is variable. Early diastolic annular velocities have been termed Ea (a for annular), Em (m for myocardial), E', or e'. Likewise late diastolic velocities have been referred to as Aa, Am, A' or a' and systolic velocities called Sa, Sm, S', or s'. Ea is commonly used to refer to arterial elastance and the 'm' may be confused with the acquisition of the velocity from the medial annulus; therefore, this text uses the terms e', a' and s' when referring to myocardial velocities.

The e' velocity from the lateral annulus is usually higher than the medial e' velocity. While an average of the medial and lateral e' velocities is recommended, when there are no basal regional wall motion abnormalities (RWMAs), using the e' from either the medial or lateral annulus is reasonable providing that the same annulus is always sampled in serial studies. However, when there are basal RWMAs, it is crucial that an average of the medial and lateral e' velocities is obtained.

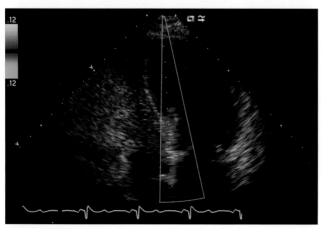
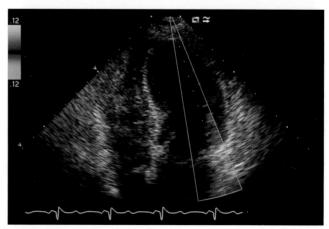

Figure 3.23 DTI signals are acquired from the apical four chamber view; a 5-10 mm sample volume is positioned over the medial *(left)* and lateral mitral annulus *(right)* ensuring that the sample volume covers the annulus over systole and diastole.

Factors Affecting DTI Diastolic Velocities

The e' is inversely related to the time constant of isovolumic relaxation (tau); therefore, when there is prolongation of LV relaxation (a longer tau) there is a lower e' velocity (< 8 cm/s). The a' velocity is directly related to LA systolic function and inversely related to the LVEDP; therefore, an increase in LA contractility leads to increased a' velocity, while an increase in LVEDP leads to a decrease in a' velocity.

During all stages of diastolic dysfunction, there is an underlying impairment of LV relaxation; as a result the e' velocity is reduced and remains reduced across all diastolic dysfunction stages. In addition, the e' velocity is a less preload-dependent measure of myocardial relaxation compared with the transmitral E velocity. This means that the e' velocity does not normalise with increasing LAP. Therefore, the presence of a decreased e' velocity is useful in identifying those patients who have a pseudonormal transmitral inflow profile. The e' velocity however may also be reduced in patients with significant mitral annular calcification, mitral stenosis, surgical rings and prosthetic mitral valves.

Furthermore, with slower LV relaxation, the onset of the e' is delayed, occurring after the transmitral E velocity. Therefore, the time interval between the onset of the transmitral E velocity and the DTI e' velocity ($T_{e'-E}$) may be useful in identifying patients with pseudonormalisation.

This interval is measured as the difference between time intervals from: (1) the onset of the QRS complex on the ECG

to the transmitral E velocity and (2) the onset of the QRS complex to the DTI e' velocity (Fig. 3.25). Because these time intervals are measured from different traces, matching the same cardiac cycle length, with an R-R interval difference less than 5 ms, is important.

Annulus Reversus

In normal subjects the lateral e' velocity is normally higher than the medial e' velocity; however, in patients with constrictive pericarditis this relationship is reversed. A possible explanation for "annulus reversus" is the tethering effect of the adjacent fibrotic and scarred pericardium on the lateral mitral annulus.

Flow Propagation Velocities

Colour M-mode Doppler can be used to measure intraventricular pressure gradients over time as blood flow propagates from the mitral annulus toward the LV apex (Fig. 3.26). In sinus rhythm, two waves are seen. The first wave corresponds to early diastolic filling and is determined by the rate of relaxation and the diastolic suction of the LV; the second wave corresponds to atrial contraction.

Several methods for measuring the flow propagation velocities (Vp) have been described. One such method is the Garcia method [3.2]; this is the method that is referred to in this text. From an apical 4-chamber view, using colour flow

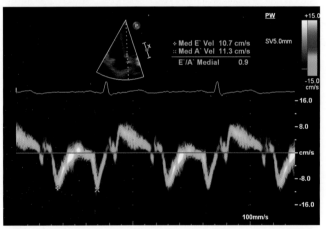 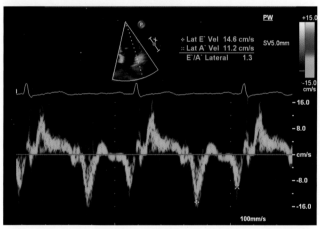

Figure 3.24 Measurements derived from the DTI trace include measurements of the peak e' velocity and the peak a' velocity from the medial annulus (*left*) and measurement of the peak e' velocity and the peak a' velocity from the lateral annulus (*right*). From the e' and a' velocities the e'/a' ratio can be derived.

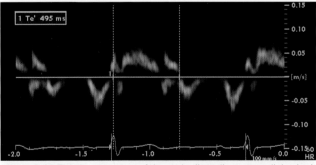 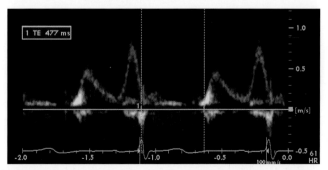

Figure 3.25 The time to onset of the early diastolic myocardial velocity (e') is measured as the time interval from the onset of the QRS complex on the ECG to the commencement of the e' signal (*left*). The time to onset of the transmitral inflow signal is measured as the time interval from the onset of the QRS complex on the ECG to the commencement of the transmitral E velocity (*right*). The $T_{e'-E}$ is calculated as the difference between these two intervals: $T_{e'-E} = 495 - 477 = 18$ ms.

[3.2] Garcia MJ, Ares MA, Asher C, Rodriguez L, Vandervoort P, Thomas JD. An index of early left ventricular filling that combined with pulsed Doppler peak E velocity may estimate capillary wedge pressure. J Am Coll Cardiol. 1997 Feb;29(2):448-54

Doppler imaging, an M-mode cursor is placed along the path of transmitral inflow. The colour Nyquist limit is lowered by decreasing the colour velocity scale or by moving the colour baseline upwards in the direction of flow; this creates aliasing and enhances the demarcation of the Vp slope. The Vp slope is measured along the aliased velocity, during early diastole, from the level of the mitral annulus to a distance of at least 4 cm into the LV cavity (Fig. 3.27). The normal Vp is greater than 50 cm/s.

Factors Affecting Vp

The Vp is inversely related to the time constant of relaxation (tau); therefore, when there is prolongation of LV relaxation (a longer tau) there is a slower Vp (less than 45 cm/s).

As mentioned, during all stages of diastolic dysfunction there is an underlying impairment of LV relaxation, as a result Vp is slowed and will remain slowed across all diastolic dysfunction stages.

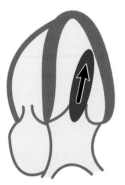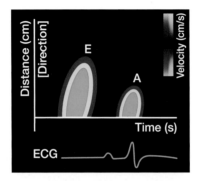

Figure 3.26 This schematic illustrates the information displayed via colour Doppler M-mode of transmitral inflow. The 2D colour Doppler image (*left*) displays the maximum mean velocity of blood flow into the LV during diastole. The colour Doppler M-mode trace (*right*) displays time along the X-axis, spatial distance (and direction of flow) along the Y-axis and velocity which is represented by a colour Doppler bar. When the patient is in sinus rhythm, two first distinct waves are seen during diastole: (1) an early filling wave (*E*) as blood propagates from the LA to the LV apex and (2) a second wave which follows atrial contraction (*A*).

Echocardiographic Parameters for Left Ventricular Filling Pressures

As already discussed, there are essentially four stages of diastolic dysfunction: (1) impaired relaxation, (2) pseudonormalisation, (3) reversible restrictive filling and (4) irreversible restrictive filling. These stages of diastolic function may also be graded and based on the stage/grade of diastolic dysfunction the LVFP can be assumed (Table 3.5). Therefore, if the pattern or stage of diastolic function can be clearly recognised then the LVFP can also be estimated.

Ratios and LVFP

Besides recognition of the pattern or grade of diastolic dysfunction, various Doppler ratios can be used to estimate LV filling pressures. These include: (1) the E/e' ratio which is the ratio between the transmitral peak E velocity and the DTI peak e' velocity, (2) the E/Vp ratio which is the ratio between the transmitral peak E velocity and the Vp, and (3) the IVRT/$T_{e'-E}$ ratio which is the ratio between the IVRT and the time interval between the onset of the transmitral E velocity and the DTI e' velocity ($T_{e'-E}$). The cut-off values for these ratios in identifying elevated LVFP are listed in Table 3.6.

E/e' ratio

Measuring the E/e' ratio allows the estimation of the LAP. As discussed, when the LAP is elevated, the transmitral E velocity is increased. However, the DTI e' velocity, which is inversely related to myocardial relaxation, remains reduced and delayed across all stages of diastolic dysfunction and does not normalise with increasing LAP. Therefore, a high transmitral E and a low e' (or an increased E/e' ratio) indicates an elevation of LAP. In particular, the E/e' ratio has been found to correlate with the PCWP, the mLVDP and the pre-A wave pressure.

The cut-off values for E/e' ratio in identifying elevated LAP are dependent on the sampling location for the DTI e' velocity (Table 3.6). When sampled at the medial annulus, an E/e' ≥15 has been found to clearly indicate elevated mean LV diastolic pressures, whereas an E/e' <8 is associated with normal LV filling pressures. In the intermediate range (E/e' 9-14) other clues for elevated LAPs should be considered; for example, LA volume, transmitral inflow profile, and the IVRT.

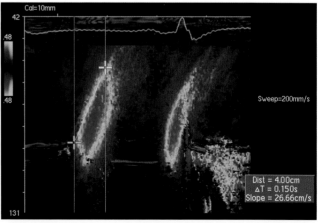

Figure 3.27 On the colour Doppler image from the apical 4-chamber view, the M-mode cursor is positioned along the transmitral inflow path (*left*). Vp is measured along the early diastolic slope of the first aliased velocity (red-blue interface) from the level of the mitral annulus to 4 cm into the LV cavity (*right*). The Vp is derived from the distance (Dist) and the time interval (ΔT) between the two points: in this example the slope = 4.00 ÷ 0.150 = 26.66 cm/s. Observe that the colour Nyquist limit has been decreased to create aliasing to enhance the visualisation of the Vp slope.

Table 3.5 Grading of Diastolic Function and Associated LVFP

Stage of LV Diastolic Dysfunction	Grade	LVFP
Impaired relaxation	Grade 1a	Normal
	Grade 1b	Elevated LVEDP *
Pseudonormalisation	Grade 2	Moderate increase in LAP
Reversible restrictive filling	Grade 3a	Marked increase in LAP
Irreversible restrictive filling	Grade 3b	Marked increase in LAP

* An elevated LVEDP should be suspected when the $AR_{dur}-A_{dur} \geq 30$ ms and/or when the AR velocity exceeds 35 cm/s.

Because the e' velocity from the lateral annulus is usually higher than the medial e' velocity the cut-off value for E/e' ratio in identifying an elevated LAP is ≥ 12. Using an average of the medial and lateral annular velocities, the cut-off value for E/e' ratio in identifying elevated LAP is ≥ 13.

It should be noted that there are several situations when E/e' may not provide an accurate estimate of LAP. The E/e' ratio in the estimation of LVFP is based on the assumption that the e' is independent of preload; however, in normal hearts e' is preload-sensitive. In particular, the e' velocity increases with increasing preload. This means that the E/e' ratio is also preload-sensitive in normal hearts. As such the E/e' ratio cannot be reliably used to estimate increased LAP in normal hearts. However, since an elevation in LAP is rarely seen in a normal heart the E/e' ratio in these patients is not clinically important.

In patients with significant mitral annular calcification, mitral stenosis, surgical rings and prosthetic mitral valves, the e' velocity is usually reduced because the longitudinal excursion of the annulus during diastole is impeded. In patients with moderate to severe mitral regurgitation the E/e' ratio is increased as the transmitral E velocity is augmented by increased flow across the regurgitant valve.

In patients with hypertrophic cardiomyopathy, the E/e' ratio is not a reliable indicator of LAP. This may be due to the less sensitive relationship between e' and LV relaxation in these patients. In patients with constrictive pericarditis, an inverse relationship between the E/e' ratio and LVFP has been shown. In other words, the E/e' ratio actually decreases, rather than increases, when there is increased LVFP. This is referred to as annulus paradoxus.

E/Vp ratio

The E/Vp ratio also allows the estimation of the LAP. As discussed, when the LAP is elevated, the transmitral E velocity is increased. However, as for the DTI e' velocity, the Vp which is also inversely related to myocardial relaxation, remains slowed across all stages of diastolic dysfunction and does not normalise with increasing LAP. Therefore, a high transmitral E and a slow Vp (or an increased E/Vp ratio) indicates an elevation of LAP. In particular, the E/Vp ratio has been found to correlate with the PCWP; for example, an

Table 3.6 Significance of Ratios in Identifying Increased LVFP

Ratio	Increased LVFP
E/e' (medial)	≥ 15
E/e' (lateral)	≥ 12
E/e' (average)	≥ 13
E/Vp	≥ 2.5
IVRT/ $T_{e'-E}$ ratio	< 2

$E/Vp \geq 2.5$ is consistent with an elevated $PCWP \geq 15$ mm Hg. In patients with concentric hypertrophy and small hyperdynamic ventricles, however, this ratio does not reliably predict LVFP. In these patients with small LV volumes there is little room for flow propagation to occur so the Vp may be normal even when there is impaired relaxation; therefore, the E/Vp ratio may also be normal despite elevated LV filling pressures.

IVRT/ $T_{e'-E}$ ratio

Normally, the transmitral E and DTI e' velocities have a simultaneous onset while with delayed LV relaxation, the onset of e' is also delayed (Fig. 3.28). Therefore a positive $T_{e'-E}$ infers impaired relaxation. The IVRT is directly related to LV relaxation and is inversely related to LAP; therefore, the longer the relaxation the longer the IVRT and the higher the LAP the shorter the IVRT. Therefore, the IVRT/$T_{e'-E}$ ratio is inversely related to the LAP (Fig. 3.29). This means that as the LAP increases the IVRT/$T_{e'-E}$ ratio decreases. In particular, the IVRT/$T_{e'-E}$ ratio has been found to correlate with the PCWP; for example, a IVRT/$T_{e'-E}$ less than 2 is consistent with an elevated PCWP greater than 15 mm Hg.

The major limitation in determining this ratio is based on the requirement to measure three separate time intervals from three different cardiac cycles.

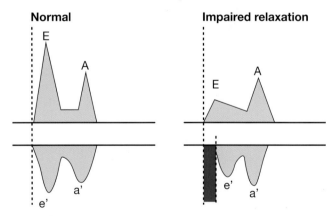

Figure 3.28 Normally, the transmitral E and DTI e' velocities have a simultaneous onset *(left)*. When there is delayed LV relaxation the onset of e' is delayed *(right)*.

Annulus Paradoxus

This term refers to an inverse (or paradoxical) relationship between the E/e' ratio and LVFP in patients with constrictive pericarditis. In these patients, medial e' increases and the E/e' decreases as LVFP increases. This paradoxical relationship is thought to occur due to the presence of a 'supranormal' e' velocity that results from exaggerated longitudinal motion of the mitral annulus, despite high LVFP, secondary to lateral constraint of the heart by the constricting pericardium.

Relationship between Pulmonary Artery Pressures and LVFP

Elevated LAP is usually associated with some degree of pulmonary hypertension due to the backward transmission of an elevated LAP to the lungs. Therefore, in the presence of diastolic

---

Value of the IVRT

The IVRT provides a valuable clue to the presence of normal or significantly elevated LAP. An IVRT greater than 100 ms suggests that the LAP is not elevated; recall that delayed mitral valve opening with impaired relaxation occurs because longer time passes before the LV pressure falls below, and crosses over, the LAP. A short IVRT ($\leq$ 60 ms) reflects a significant elevation in the LAP; recall that early mitral valve opening occurs because there is an earlier than normal crossover between the LV and LAPs due to an increase in the LAP.

IVRT is directly related to LV relaxation inversely related to LAP:

$$IVRT \approx \frac{LV\ relaxation}{LAP}$$

$T_{e'-E}$ is directly related to LV relaxation:

$$T_{e'-E} \approx LV\ relaxation$$

Therefore, IVRT/Te'-E ratio is related to the inverse of LAP:

$$\frac{\cancel{LV\ relaxation}}{LAP} \div \cancel{LV\ relaxation}$$

Therefore:

$$\downarrow IVRT/T_{e'-E} \approx \uparrow LAP$$

Figure 3.29 This schematic illustrates the relationship between the IVRT and $T_{e'-E}$. IVRT is directly related to LV relaxation and inversely related to LAP while $T_{e'-E}$ is directly related to LV relaxation. Therefore, by dividing the IVRT by $T_{e'-E}$, LV relaxation is "cancelled out" so now the IVRT/$T_{e'-E}$ratio reflects an inverse relationship with LAP. Therefore, the IVRT/$T_{e'-E}$ ratio decreases as the LAP increases.

dysfunction with increased LAP an increase in pulmonary artery (PA) pressures is expected. In particular, it has been noted that there is a relationship between the pulmonary artery systolic pressure (PASP) and noninvasively derived LVFP such that a PASP of 30 mm Hg or less indicates a normal PCWP while a PASP greater than 40 mm Hg is associated with elevated PCWP. Furthermore, the PA end-diastolic pressure (PAEDP) has been found to correlate well with the PCWP. Therefore, the PAEDP may be used as a surrogate for PCWP. The methods for estimation of various PA pressures are detailed in Chapter 4 (Pulmonary Hypertension).

Pulmonary Artery Pressures and Arrhythmias

Sinus tachycardia and first-degree heart block can result in partial or complete fusion of the mitral E and A velocities; other problematic arrhythmias include atrial flutter, second-degree AV heart block and complete heart block. In these cases, the transmitral inflow profile in the assessment of LVFP is compromised. However, in these patients, estimation of the pulmonary artery pressures, in the absence of lung disease, may be useful in assessing LVFP.

Assessment of LV Filling Pressures in Special Populations

There are various patient populations in which the assessment of diastolic function and the estimation of LVFP is difficult. An explanation for why assessment is hampered, as well as clues to the presence of increased LVFP in these populations, is summarised in Table 3.7.

Figure 3.30 provides a summary of the variables used in the assessment of LV diastolic function including the characteristic features of each parameter as associated with the different stages and grades of diastolic dysfunction.

Table 3.7 Assessment of LV Filling Pressures in Special Populations

Population	Assessment is hampered by ...	Clues to Increased LVFP *
Atrial Fibrillation	• Absence of synchronised atrial contraction (no mitral A or pulmonary venous AR velocities, blunted pulmonary venous S velocity) • Variability in cycle lengths • Associated LA dilatation irrespective of LAP	• IVRT $\leq$ 65 ms • DT of pulmonary venous D $\leq$ 65 ms • E/Vp ratio $\geq$ 1.4 • E/e' (medial) $\geq$ 11
Hypertrophic Cardiomyopathy	• Poor correlation of conventional Doppler variables with LVFP	• Lateral E/e' $\geq$ 10 • AR_{dur}-$A_{dur} \geq$ 30 ms • PASP > 35 mm Hg • ILAV $\geq$ 34 mL/m^2
Mitral Regurgitation (MR)	• LAP elevation and LA dilatation related to MR regurgitant volume: therefore, difficulty in determining whether the increase in LAP is due to the valve lesion or diastolic dysfunction	Normal ejection fraction (EF): • AR_{dur}-$A_{dur} \geq$ 30 ms • IVRT < 65 ms • IVRT/Te'-E < 3 Depressed EF (< 45%): • E/e' (average) > 15

Sinus Tachycardia	• Shortening of the diastolic filling period which results in either:
	  - increased "E at A" (see Technical Tips for Transmitral Inflow) or
	  - complete E-A fusion
		• E/e' (lateral) $\geq$ 10 #
		• IVRT $\leq$ 70 ms

* Source: Nagueh SF, Appleton CP, Gillebert TC, Marino PN, Oh JK, Smiseth OA, Waggoner AD, Flachskampf FA, Pellikka PA, Evangelista A. Recommendations for the evaluation of left ventricular diastolic function by echocardiography. *J Am Soc Echocardiogr.* 2009 Feb;22(2):122.
# When there is E-A and e'/a' fusion, measure the combined single velocity as E and e' to determine this ratio.

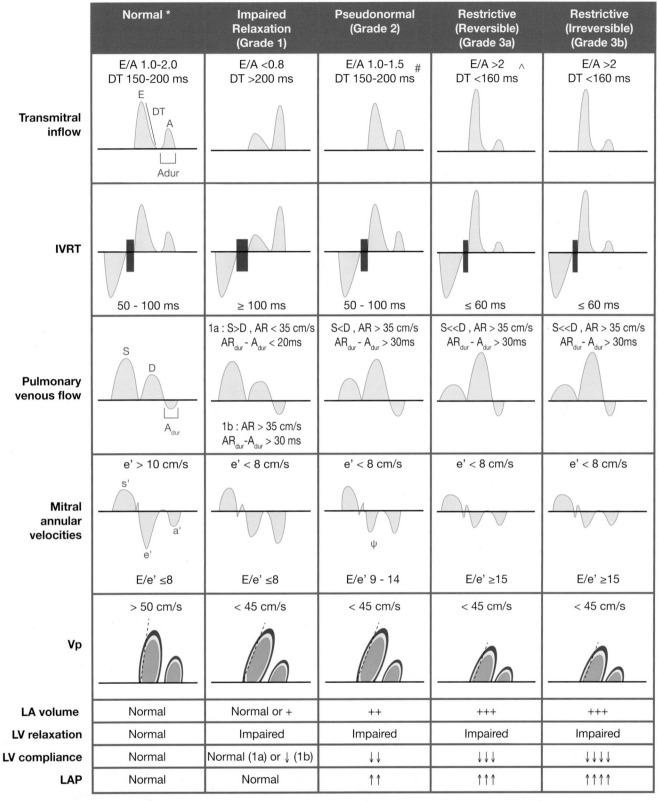

	Normal *	Impaired Relaxation (Grade 1)	Pseudonormal (Grade 2)	Restrictive (Reversible) (Grade 3a)	Restrictive (Irreversible) (Grade 3b)
Transmittal inflow	E/A 1.0-2.0 DT 150-200 ms	E/A <0.8 DT >200 ms	E/A 1.0-1.5 # DT 150-200 ms	E/A >2 ^ DT <160 ms	E/A >2 DT <160 ms
IVRT	50 - 100 ms	≥ 100 ms	50 - 100 ms	≤ 60 ms	≤ 60 ms
Pulmonary venous flow		1a : S>D , AR < 35 cm/s AR$_{dur}$ - A$_{dur}$ < 20ms / 1b : AR > 35 cm/s AR$_{dur}$ -A$_{dur}$ > 30 ms	S<D , AR > 35 cm/s AR$_{dur}$ - A$_{dur}$ > 30ms	S<<D , AR > 35 cm/s AR$_{dur}$ - A$_{dur}$ > 30ms	S<<D , AR > 35 cm/s AR$_{dur}$ - A$_{dur}$ > 30ms
Mitral annular velocities	e' > 10 cm/s ... E/e' ≤8	e' < 8 cm/s ... E/e' ≤8	e' < 8 cm/s ... E/e' 9 - 14	e' < 8 cm/s ... E/e' ≥15	e' < 8 cm/s ... E/e' ≥15
Vp	> 50 cm/s	< 45 cm/s	< 45 cm/s	< 45 cm/s	< 45 cm/s
LA volume	Normal	Normal or +	++	+++	+++
LV relaxation	Normal	Impaired	Impaired	Impaired	Impaired
LV compliance	Normal	Normal (1a) or ↓ (1b)	↓↓	↓↓↓	↓↓↓↓
LAP	Normal	Normal	↑↑	↑↑↑	↑↑↑↑

Figure 3.30 This schematic provides a simplistic guide to the identification of various grades of diastolic dysfunction.
Note: It should be noted that not all variables will meet the criteria as indicated. The presence of ≥ 2 abnormal measurements increases the confidence in identifying the grade of diastolic dysfunction. Grade 1a refers to impaired relaxation with normal LVFP; Grade 1b refers to impaired relaxation with an elevated LVEDP.
* Normal values of all indices vary according to age (see Table 3.3)
\# Transmitral inflow profile reverts to impaired relaxation pattern following the Valsalva manoeuvre
^ Transmitral inflow profile reverts to impaired relaxation or pseudonormalisation following the Valsalva manoeuvre
ψ Onset of the DTI e' is delayed compared with onset of mitral E.
A$_{dur}$ = mitral A duration; AR$_{dur}$ = pulmonary venous AR duration; AR$_{dur}$-A$_{dur}$ = difference between the mitral A duration and the pulmonary venous AR duration DT = deceleration time; DTI = Doppler tissue imaging; E/e' = mitral E to DTI e' ratio; IVRT = isovolumic relaxation time; LA = left atrial; LAP = left atrial pressure; LV = left ventricular; LVEDP = left ventricular end-diastolic pressure; Vp = flow propagation velocity.

Echocardiographic Parameters for Assessing Right Ventricular Diastolic Function

Diastolic function of the RV can be assessed in a similar manner as for the LV. In particular, RV diastolic function can be evaluated via interrogation of RV and right atrial (RA) filling profiles and myocardial velocities of the lateral tricuspid annulus.

Tricuspid Inflow

The tricuspid Doppler signal reflects the pressure gradient between the RA and RV during diastole (Fig. 3.31).

The tricuspid inflow signal is acquired via PW Doppler signal from an off-axis apical 4-chamber view; the transducer is moved medially and superiorly on the chest wall to ensure parallel alignment with tricuspid inflow. A 2-3 mm sample volume size is placed at the tips of the tricuspid valve and from the spectral Doppler trace, several measurements are performed (Fig. 3.32). The tricuspid peak E velocity reflects the early diastolic

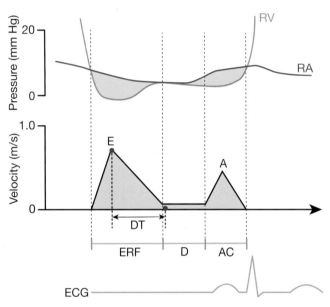

Figure 3.31 In this schematic, the right atrial (RA) and right ventricular (RV) pressure traces are shown at the top and the tricuspid inflow profile is shown at the bottom. The peak tricuspid E velocity correlates with the early, rapid filling gradient (*ERF*). The deceleration time (*DT*) reflects the rate of RV filling and RA emptying. The mid diastolic signal reflects diastasis (*D*) and the peak tricuspid A velocity reflects the pressure gradient the RA and RV with atrial contraction (*AC*).

pressure gradient between the RA and RV. Following the peak E velocity, the diastolic RA-RV pressure gradient quickly decreases and this results in a corresponding decrease in the Doppler velocity. From the deceleration slope, the DT is measured as the time interval between the peak E velocity and the point of deceleration extrapolated to the zero baseline. The tricuspid peak A velocity is measured as the second peak on the tricuspid inflow trace and this velocity reflects forward blood flow from the RA to the RV following atrial contraction. In addition, the tricuspid E/A ratio can be derived as the peak E velocity divided by the peak A velocity.

Due to augmentation of systemic venous return to the right heart during inspiration, tricuspid inflow velocities increase with inspiration. Therefore, measurements should be either averaged over 5-7 consecutive cardiac cycles or measured at end-expiratory apnoea[3.3]. Measurements of the DT should be performed at a sweep speed of 100 mm/s to improve measurement accuracy.

As for transmitral inflow velocities, assessment of diastolic function based on the tricuspid inflow profile is hampered in patients with AF and/or significant tricuspid regurgitation. The most common limitation to recording adequate tricuspid inflow signals is failure to align tricuspid flow parallel to

---

Important Differences between LV and RV Filling

- **RV inflow velocities vary with respiration:** the negative intrapleural pressures during inspiration increases venous return to the RA which produces a corresponding increase in RA volume and pressure as well as a transient increase in RV filling. As a result the RV inflow velocities vary over the respiratory cycle (velocities with inspiration increase up to 20% compared with end-expiratory values).

- **RV inflow velocities are lower:** the continuity principle states that in the absence of regurgitant or intracardiac shunts, flow through all four valves is the same. Thus, the SV through the mitral valve equals the SV through the tricuspid valve. SV is derived from the annular diameter (cross-sectional area) and the velocity time integral (VTI) (see Chapter 1). Therefore, as the tricuspid annulus is larger than the mitral annulus it follows that the VTI (and velocities) must be lower.

- **RV diastolic filling time is longer:** the tricuspid valve opens before and closes after the mitral valve.

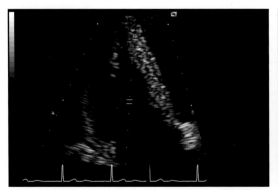
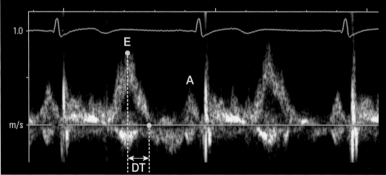

Figure 3.32 Tricuspid signals are obtained via PW Doppler from an off-axis apical four chamber view; a 2-3 mm sample volume is positioned centrally at the tips of the tricuspid valve (*left*). Measurements derived from the tricuspid inflow trace include measurement of the peak E and peak A velocities and the deceleration time (*right*). The E/A ratio is derived from the peak E velocity divided by the peak A velocity.

[3.3] Measurements of Doppler parameters averaged over 5-7 consecutive beats is nearly identical to measurements obtained during apnoea. Zoghbi WA, Habib JB, Quiñones MA. Doppler assessment of right ventricular filling in a normal population: comparison with left ventricular filling dynamics. *Circulation.* 1990;82:1316-1324.

the Doppler beam. Other technical limitations of acquiring and measuring tricuspid inflow signals are similar to those discussed for transmitral inflow signals (see Technical Tips for Transmitral Inflow).

Tricuspid Inflow Patterns

Tricuspid inflow patterns are similar to transmitral inflow patterns. Therefore the tricuspid inflow profile can show: (1) impaired relaxation, (2) pseudonormalisation, (3) restrictive filling. Pattern recognition for tricuspid profiles is mostly based on the E/A ratio (see Grading of Right Ventricular Diastolic Function Table 3.8).

Hepatic Venous and Superior Vena Caval Flow

Hepatic venous (HV) and superior vena caval (SVC) flow can be used to assess RA filling. HV flow, rather than inferior vena cava (IVC) flow is used to assess RA filling as it is not possible to align IVC flow parallel with the Doppler beam. HV flow, therefore, reflects the pressure gradient between the hepatic veins and RA while SVC flow reflects the pressure gradient between the SVC and RA.

The HV signal is acquired via PW Doppler signal from the subcostal view demonstrating the long axis of the IVC (Fig. 3.33). From this view, a 3-5 mm sample volume size is positioned into the middle hepatic vein, approximately 1-2 cm proximal to its entrance into the IVC. From the spectral Doppler trace, four distinct waveforms are seen: (1) systolic

forward flow, (2) ventricular (systolic) flow reversal, (3) diastolic forward flow, and (4) atrial reversal of flow.

Systolic forward flow reflects the systolic pressure gradient between the hepatic vein and the IVC/RA and is identified as the peak systolic (S) velocity on the HV trace. As flow is directed away from the transducer it is displayed below the zero baseline. Diastolic forward flow reflects the diastolic pressure gradient between the hepatic vein and the IVC/RA and is identified as the peak diastolic (D) velocity on the HV Doppler trace. The D velocity is usually slightly lower that the S velocity. As for systolic forward flow, diastolic forward flow is directed away from the transducer and, therefore, is displayed below the zero baseline.

Atrial flow reversal (AR) refers to the retrograde flow of blood back into the hepatic veins following atrial contraction. The AR velocity is directed towards the transducer and therefore appears above the baseline just after the P wave on the ECG. Ventricular flow reversal (VR) refers to the retrograde flow of blood back into the hepatic vein in late systole; this flow corresponds to the atrial V wave on the RA pressure trace. This flow is directed toward the transducer and therefore it is displayed above the zero baseline just after the T wave on the ECG. The AR and VR velocities are low with the VR velocity being slightly lower than the AR velocity.

The SVC signal is acquired via PW Doppler from the suprasternal notch or from the right supraclavicular fossa (Fig. 3.34). A 3-5 mm sample volume is placed 5 to 7 cm into

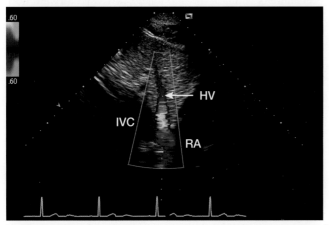
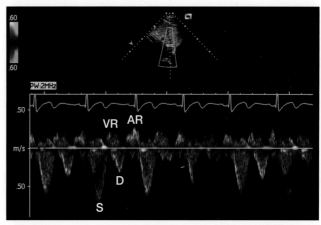

Figure 3.33 From the subcostal view, a 3-5 mm PW Doppler sample volume is placed1-2 cm into the middle hepatic vein (*left*). From the HV trace, 4 waveforms are seen: (1) systolic forward flow (S), (2) ventricular flow reversal (VR), (3) diastolic forward flow (D), (4) atrial flow reversal (AR) (*right*). The peak systolic velocity (S) and the peak diastolic velocity (D) can be averaged over 5-7 beats or measured at end-expiratory apnoea.

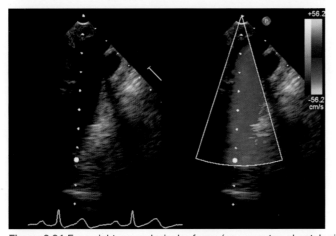
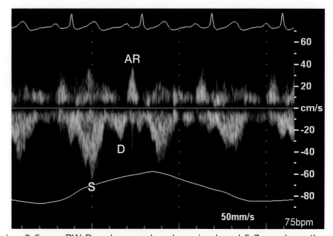

Figure 3.34 From right supraclavicular fossa (or suprasternal notch view), a 3-5 mm PW Doppler sample volume is placed 5-7 cm down the SVC (*left*). From the SVC trace, 3 waveforms are seen: (1) systolic forward flow (S), (2) diastolic forward flow (D), and (3) atrial flow reversal (AR) (*right*). The peak systolic velocity (S) and the peak diastolic velocity (D) can be averaged over 5-7 beats or measured at end-expiratory apnoea.

the SVC. Identification of the SVC may be aided by the use of colour Doppler imaging; the SVC can be identified by the appearance of blue laminar flow down the vessel. From the spectral Doppler trace, three distinct waveforms are seen: (1) systolic forward flow, (2) diastolic forward flow, and (3) atrial reversal of flow.

Systolic forward flow reflects the systolic pressure gradient between the SVC and the RA and is identified as the peak systolic (S) velocity on the SVC trace. As flow is directed away from the transducer it is displayed below the zero baseline. Diastolic forward flow reflects the diastolic pressure gradient between the SVC and the RA and is identified as the peak diastolic (D) velocity on the SVC Doppler trace. The D velocity is usually slightly lower than the S velocity. As for systolic forward flow, diastolic forward flow is directed away from the transducer and, therefore, is displayed below the zero baseline. Atrial flow reversal (AR) refers to the retrograde flow of blood back up the SVC following atrial contraction. The AR velocity is directed towards the transducer and therefore it appears above the baseline just after the P wave on the ECG.

As for RV filling, augmentation of systemic venous return to the right heart during inspiration leads to increased inspiratory forward flow velocities. Therefore, measurements should be either averaged over 5-7 consecutive cardiac cycles or measured at end-expiratory apnoea.

The most common limitation to recording adequate HV signals is movement of the hepatic vein across the imaging view due to normal respiration; as a result maintaining the sample volume within this vessel is very difficult. Other technical limitations of acquiring adequate HV and SVC signals are similar to those discussed for pulmonary venous signals (see Technical Tips for Pulmonary Venous Flow). In particular, due to the low velocity of HV and SVC flow, low velocity scales and low wall filters should be utilized to optimise these signals.

Doppler Tissue Imaging

As previously discussed, the myocardial velocity profile obtained by DTI is characterised by three distinct velocities (e', a' and s') and two less prominent biphasic velocities occurring during the isovolumic periods (see Fig. 2.33). The e' velocity, which coincides with the tricuspid E velocity, reflects the longitudinal expansion or lengthening of the RV in early diastole as blood rapidly fills the RV.

DTI velocities are recorded via PW Doppler by placing the 5-10 mm sample volume at the lateral corner of the tricuspid annulus from the apical 4-chamber view, ensuring that the sample volume covers the annulus over both systole and diastole. From the spectral Doppler trace, the e' and a' velocities can be measured (Fig. 3.35). Measurements should be performed at a sweep speed of 50-100 mm/s.

Echocardiographic Parameters for Identifying Increased Right Atrial Pressures

Right atrial pressures (RAP) can be estimated using the IVC, HV Doppler parameters and via Doppler tissue imaging (DTI) of the RV lateral annulus. Estimation of the RAP via these methods is discussed in detail in Chapter 4 (Pulmonary Hypertension).

Using the IVC, elevated RAP is indicated when the IVC diameter is greater than 2.1 cm and collapses less than 50% with inspiration (Fig. 3.36).

The HV flow profile can also been used for identifying increased

RAP. The HV forward systolic flow velocity is reflective of the RAP whereby the higher the RAP the lower the pressure gradient between the HV and the RA and, thus, the lower the forward systolic flow velocity. Therefore, diastolic flow predominance in the hepatic veins is a clue to elevated RAP (Fig. 3.37). Measurement of the systolic filling fraction (SFF) is also useful in estimation of RAP (see Fig. 4.20). In particular, SFF of less than 55% is useful for predicting a mean RAP greater than 8 mm Hg.

Calculation of the tricuspid E to RV e' ratio can be used to estimate RAP (Fig. 3.38). An E/e' ratio greater than 6 has a high sensitivity and specificity for predicting a mean RAP greater than or equal to 10 mm Hg.

Grading of Right Ventricular Diastolic Function

RV diastolic dysfunction may be graded as impaired relaxation, pseudonormal and restrictive filling by considering the tricuspid E/A ratio, the tricuspid E to e' ratio and the HV flow profiles (Table 3.8).

Impaired relaxation is suggested by a tricuspid E/A ratio less than 0.8. Pseudonormal filling is suspected when the tricuspid E/A ratio is 0.8 to 2.1 in conjunction with either an E/e' ratio greater than 6 or diastolic flow predominance in the hepatic veins. Restrictive filling is indicated when the tricuspid E/A ratio is greater than 2.1 with a DT less than 120 ms. Another clue to the presence of restrictive RV filling is antegrade flow into the PA following atrial contraction which leads to premature opening of the pulmonary valve and forward flow into the PA. Evidence of late diastolic antegrade flow can be seen on the CW Doppler recording across the pulmonary valve (Fig. 3.39).

Table 3.8 Grading of RV Diastolic Function

Stage of RV Diastolic Dysfunction	Criteria
Impaired relaxation	E/A < 0.8
Pseudonormalisation	E/A 0.8 – 2.1 + E/e' > 6 (or HV diastolic flow predominance)
Restrictive filling	E/A > 2.1 + DT < 120 ms

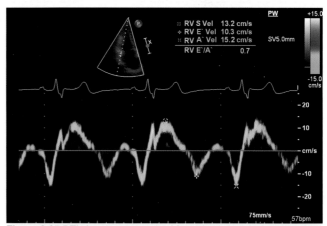

Figure 3.35 DTI signals are acquired from the apical 4-chamber view; a 5-10 mm sample volume is positioned over the lateral tricuspid annulus ensuring that the sample volume covers the annulus over systole and diastole (*top*). Measurements derived from the DTI trace include measurements of the peak e' and the peak a' velocities (*bottom*). The peak systolic myocardial velocity (s') can also be measured from this trace for the assessment of RV systolic function (see Chapter 2).

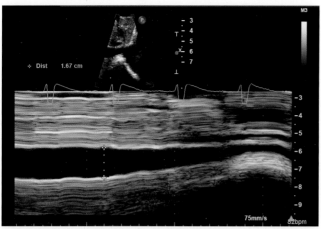
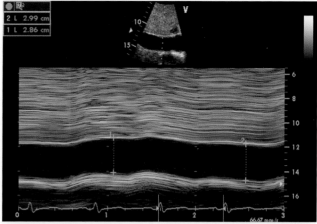

Figure 3.36 When the RAP is normal, the IVC diameter is less than 2.1 cm and the IVC collapses more than 50% (*left*). When the RAP is elevated, the IVC diameter is greater than 2.1 cm and the IVC collapses less than 50% with inspiration (*right*).

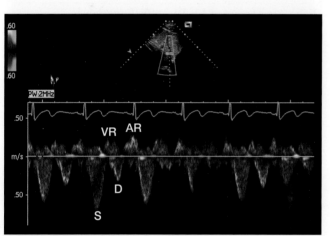
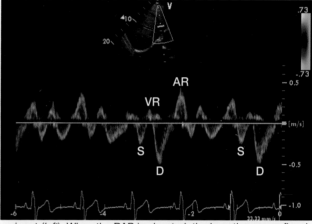

Figure 3.37 When the RAP is normal, the hepatic venous flow is systolic dominant (*left*). When the RAP is elevated, the hepatic venous flow is diastolic dominant (*right*).

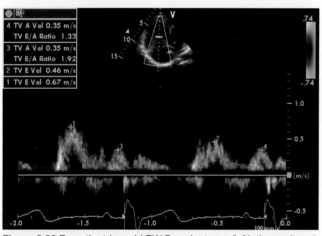
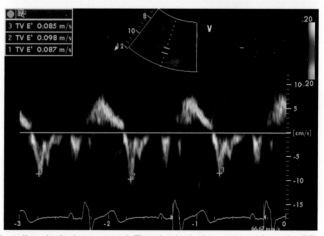

Figure 3.38 From the tricuspid PW Doppler trace *(left)*, the peak early (E) diastolic velocity is measured. The e' velocity is measured from the DTI trace with the sample volume placed at the lateral tricuspid annulus *(right)*. The E/e' ratio, which reflects the RA pressure, is calculated as the tricuspid E velocity divided by the DTI e' velocity. In this example, the E/e ratio is 6.3.

> When calculating the TV E/e' ratio, measurements should be averaged over 5 or more consecutive beats comprising 1 or more respiratory cycles.

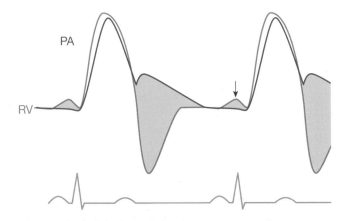

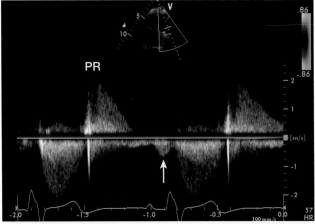

Figure 3.39 The schematic at the top shows the right ventricular (RV) and pulmonary artery (PA) pressure traces. When there is restrictive filling, there is a marked and rapid rise in the RV diastolic pressures. As a result, there is a rapid pressure decline between the PA and RV during diastole with pressure equalization occurring in mid-diastole. Following atrial contraction, the additional bolus of blood ejected into the RV increases the RV pressure above the PA pressure resulting in antegrade flow into the PA at end-diastole (*arrow*). A CW Doppler trace recorded across the pulmonary valve is shown at the bottom. This signal shows pulmonary regurgitation (PR) above the zero baseline. Observe that the velocity slope of the PR signal is very steep and terminates in mid-diastole; this reflects the rapid pressure decline between the PA and RV in early diastole and pressure equalization in mid-diastole. In addition antegrade flow is noted below the zero baseline following atrial contraction (*arrow*). This indicates that the RV pressure has exceeded the PA pressure resulting in forward flow across the pulmonary valve at end-diastole.

| Key Points |

Basic Principles of Diastole
- 4 phases of diastole include (1) IVR, (2) early, rapid filling, (3) diastasis and (4) atrial contraction.
- Normal diastolic function refers to the ability of the ventricles to fill to an adequate end-diastolic volume, at low filling pressures, to ensure an adequate SV during systole.
- Diastolic dysfunction means that for the ventricle to fill to an adequate end-diastolic volume to ensure an adequate SV during systole there is an abnormal increase in filling pressures.
- Elevated LVFP is defined as a PCWP > 12 mm Hg and/or a LVEDP > 16 mm Hg.
- Diastolic filling properties include myocardial relaxation and compliance or stiffness.

Echo Assessment of LV Diastolic Function
- Comprehensive evaluation incorporates 2D and Doppler parameters:
  - 2D parameters include LV wall thickness and LA volume
  - Doppler parameters include mitral and pulmonary venous flow profiles, IVRT, DTI e' and the Vp
- Patterns (grades) of diastolic dysfunction include:
  - Abnormal relaxation (Grades 1a & 1b)
  - Pseudonormalisation (Grade 2)
  - Restrictive filling, either reversible or fixed (Grades 3a and 3b, respectively)
- LVFP is based on pattern (grade) of diastolic dysfunction:
  - Abnormal relaxation: LVFP normal (Grade 1a) or ↑ LVEDP (Grade 1b)
  - Pseudonormalisation (Grade 2): moderate ↑ LAP
  - Restrictive filling (Grades 3a and 3b): marked ↑ LAP
- Increased LVFP also recognised from various ratios:
  - E/e' (medial) ≥ 15, E/e' (lateral) ≥ 12, or E/e' (average) ≥ 13
  - E/Vp ≥ 2.5
  - IVRT/$T_{e'-E}$ < 2

Echo Assessment of RV Diastolic Function
- Assessed via tricuspid inflow profile, DTI e', and HV and/or SVC flow profiles
- Patterns (grades) of diastolic dysfunction include:
  - Abnormal relaxation (E/A < 0.8)
  - Pseudonormalisation (E/A 0.8-2.1 + E/e' > 6)
  - Restrictive filling (E/a > 2.1 + DT < 120 ms)
- Increased RAP identified when:
  - IVC diameter > 2.1 cm & collapses < 50% with inspiration
  - Hepatic venous diastolic predominance or SFF < 55%
  - E/e' ratio > 6
  - Restrictive filling profile

Further Reading (listed in alphabetical order)

Physiology

Nishimura RA, Housmans PR, Hatle LK and Tajik AJ. Assessment of diastolic function of the heart: Background and current applications of Doppler echocardiography. Part 1. Physiologic and pathologic features. *Mayo Clin Proc.* 1989 Jan;64(1):71-81

Paulus WJ, Tschöpe C, Sanderson JE, Rusconi C, Flachskampf FA, Rademakers FE, Marino P, Smiseth OA, De Keulenaer G, Leite-Moreira AF, Borbély A, Edes I, Handoko ML, Heymans S, Pezzali N, Pieske B, Dickstein K, Fraser AG, Brutsaert DL. How to diagnose diastolic heart failure: a consensus statement on the diagnosis of heart failure with normal left ventricular ejection fraction by the Heart Failure and Echocardiography Associations of the European Society of Cardiology. *Eur Heart J.* 2007 Oct;28(20):2539-50

Shub C. Heart failure and abnormal ventricular function. Pathophysiology and clinical correlation (Part 2). *Chest.* 1989 Oct;96(4):906-14.

LA Volume

Abhayaratna WP, Seward JB, Appleton CP, Douglas PS, Oh JK, Tajik AJ, Tsang TS. Left atrial size: physiologic determinants and clinical applications. *J Am Coll Cardiol.* 2006 Jun 20;47(12):2357-63.

Tsang TS, Barnes ME, Gersh BJ, Bailey KR, Seward JB. Left atrial volume as a morphophysiologic expression of left ventricular diastolic dysfunction and relation to cardiovascular risk burden. *Am J Cardiol.* 2002 Dec 15;90(12):1284-9.

LV Diastolic Function

Appleton CP, Jensen JL, Hatle LK, Oh JK. Doppler evaluation of left and right ventricular diastolic function: a technical guide for obtaining optimal flow velocity recordings. *J Am Soc Echocardiogr.* 1997 Apr;10(3):271-92.

Gabriel RS, Klein AL. Modern evaluation of left ventricular diastolic function using Doppler echocardiography. Curr Cardiol Rep. 2009 May;11(3):231-8.

Garcia MJ, Ares MA, Asher C, Rodriguez L, Vandervoort P, Thomas JD. An index of early left ventricular filling that combined with pulsed Doppler peak E velocity may estimate capillary wedge pressure. *J Am Coll Cardiol.* 1997 Feb;29(2):448-54

Geske JB, Sorajja P, Nishimura RA, Ommen SR. Evaluation of left ventricular filling pressures by Doppler echocardiography in patients with hypertrophic cardiomyopathy: correlation with direct left atrial pressure measurement at cardiac catheterization. *Circulation.* 2007 Dec 4;116(23):2702-8.

Ha JW, Oh JK, Ling LH, Nishimura RA, Seward JB, Tajik AJ. Annulus Paradoxus Transmitral Flow Velocity to Mitral Annular Velocity Ratio Is Inversely Proportional to Pulmonary Capillary Wedge Pressure in Patients With Constrictive Pericarditis. *Circulation.* 2001 Aug 28;104(9):976-8.

Lam CS, Han L, Ha JW, Oh JK, Ling LH. The mitral L wave: A marker of pseudonormal filling and predictor of heart failure in patients with left ventricular hypertrophy. *J Am Soc Echocardiogr.* 2005 Apr;18(4):336-41.

Nagueh SF, Appleton CP, Gillebert TC, Marino PN, Oh JK, Smiseth OA, Waggoner AD, Flachskampf FA, Pellikka PA, Evangelista A. Recommendations for the evaluation of left ventricular diastolic function by echocardiography. *J Am Soc Echocardiogr.* 2009 Feb;22(2):107-33

Oh JK, Appleton CP, Hatle LK, Nishimura RA, Seward JB, Tajik AJ. The noninvasive assessment of left ventricular diastolic function with two-dimensional Doppler echocardiography. *J Am Soc Echocardiogr.* 1997 Apr;10(3):246-70.

Oh JK, Park SJ, Nagueh SF. Established and novel clinical applications of diastolic function assessment by echocardiography. *Circ Cardiovasc Imaging.* 2011 Jul 1;4(4):444-55.

Mid-diastolic Flow

Keren G, Meisner JS, Sherez J, Yellin EL, Laniado S. Interrelationship of mid-diastolic mitral valve motion, pulmonary venous flow, and transmitral flow. *Circulation.* 1986 Jul;74(1):36-44.

Lam CS, Han L, Ha JW, Oh JK, Ling LH. The mitral L wave: A marker of pseudonormal filling and predictor of heart failure in patients with left ventricular hypertrophy. *J Am Soc Echocardiogr.* 2005 Apr;18(4):336-41.

RV Diastolic Function

Appleton CP, Jensen JL, Hatle LK, Oh JK. Doppler evaluation of left and right ventricular diastolic function: a technical guide for obtaining optimal flow velocity recordings. *J Am Soc Echocardiogr.* 1997 Apr;10(3):271-92.

Nageh MF, Kopelen HA, Zoghbi WA, Quiñones MA, Nagueh SF. Estimation of Mean Right Atrial Pressure Using Tissue Doppler Imaging. *Am J Cardiol.* 1999 Dec 15;84(12):1448-51, A8.

Nagueh SF, Kopelen HA, Zoghbi WA. Relation of mean right atrial pressure to echocardiographic and Doppler parameters of right atrial and right ventricular function. *Circulation.* 1996 Mar 15;93(6):1160-9.

Rudski LG, Lai WW, Afilalo J, Hua L, Handschumacher MD, Chandrasekaran K, Solomon SD, Louie EK, Schiller NB. Guidelines for the echocardiographic assessment of the right heart in adults: a report from the American Society of Echocardiography endorsed by the European Association of Echocardiography, a registered branch of the European Society of Cardiology, and the Canadian Society of Echocardiography. *J Am Soc Echocardiogr.* 2010 Jul;23(7):685-713.

Zoghbi WA, Habib GB, Quiñones MA. Doppler assessment of right ventricular filling in a normal population. Comparison with left ventricular filling dynamics. *Circulation.* 1990 Oct;82(4):1316-24.

Hypertensive Heart Disease

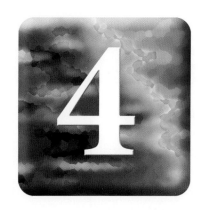

Systemic Hypertension

Definition and Classification of Systemic Hypertension

The diagnosis of systemic hypertension (HTN) is based upon the average blood pressure (BP) readings recorded at two or more separate visits. The diagnostic categories of HTN are based on these BP recordings (Tables 4.1 – 4.3).

HTN may also be classified as either essential or secondary. Essential HTN is typically defined as HTN without a known cause. Essential HTN, also known as primary or idiopathic hypertension, accounts for approximately 90 - 95% of patients with systemic HTN. Secondary HTN, as the name suggests, is caused secondary to an identifiable underlying disease.

Aetiology of Hypertension

The definitive cause of essential HTN remains unknown; however, a number of risk factors have been identified (Table 4.4). A number of identifiable disorders are also associated with secondary HTN, and the pathogenesis of HTN is related to the underlying condition (Table 4.5).

Pathophysiology of Hypertension

To understand the pathophysiology of HTN, it is first important to understand how BP is determined. Determinants of BP can be explained by Ohm's Law which describes the relationship between voltage, current and resistance:

Equation 4.1

$$R = V \div I$$

where R = resistance (Ohms)
      V = voltage difference (volts)
      I = current (amps)

In translating Ohm's Law to haemodynamics, the following substitutions are made: (1) resistance becomes the resistance to blood flow; (2) voltage difference becomes the pressure difference and (3) current becomes flow rate. This haemodynamic relationship can then be expressed as:

Equation 4.2

$$R = \Delta P \div Q$$

where R = resistance (mmHg/L/min)
     ΔP = pressure difference (mm Hg)
     Q = flow rate (L/min)

By: (1) defining the pressure difference as the change in pressure across the systemic circulation from its beginning to its end (the difference between mean arterial pressure [mAP] and central venous pressure [CVP]), (2) substituting the resistance with systemic vascular resistance (SVR), and (3) substituting flow rate with cardiac output (CO), this equation becomes:

Equation 4.3

$$SVR = (mAP - CVP) \div CO$$

where SVR = systemic vascular resistance (mm Hg/L/min)
     mAP = mean arterial pressure (mm Hg)
     CVP = central venous pressure (mm Hg)
     CO = cardiac output (L/min)

Therefore, to derive the mAP, Equation 4.3 is rearranged to:

Equation 4.4

$$mAP = (CO \times SVR) + CVP$$

Because CVP is usually at or near 0 mm Hg, this equation can be further simplified to:

Equation 4.5

$$mAP = (CO \times SVR)$$

There is also a direct relationship between the mAP and the systolic and diastolic BP. At normal resting heart rates it can be assumed that diastole accounts for approximately two-thirds of the cardiac cycle while systole accounts for approximately one-third of the cardiac cycle, hence the mAP can also be derived from the systolic and diastolic BP as:

Equation 4.6

$$mAP = [(2 \times P_D) + P_S] \div 3$$

where mAP = mean arterial pressure (mm Hg)
     P_D = diastolic blood pressure (mm Hg)
     P_S = systolic blood pressure (mm Hg)

Importantly, it can be appreciated from Equation 4.5 that two factors determine mAP. These factors are the CO and the SVR. It can also be appreciated that an increase in the mAP, which increases BP and results in HTN, is caused by either an increase in SVR or an increase in CO. There are a number of factors that can lead to an increase in SVR and/or CO and these are illustrated in Figure 4.1.

Table 4.1 **Classification of Blood Pressure Levels in Adults (Australian Classification)**

Diagnostic Category *	Systolic (mm Hg)	Diastolic (mm Hg)
Normal	< 120	< 80
High Normal	120-139	80–89
Grade 1 (mild) HTN	140–159	90–99
Grade 2 (moderate) HTN	160–179	100–109
Grade 3 (severe) HTN	≥ 180	≥ 110
Isolated systolic HTN	≥ 140	< 90
Isolated systolic HTN with widened pulse pressure	≥ 160	≤ 70

* When a patient's systolic and diastolic blood pressure levels fall into different categories, the higher diagnostic category should apply for the classification of HTN.
Source: Heart Foundation Guide to Management of Hypertension, 2008. Assessing and managing raised blood pressure in adults. Updated August 2009. Web version.

Table 4.2 **Classification of Blood Pressure Levels in Adults (American Classification)**

Diagnostic Category	Systolic (mm Hg)	Diastolic (mm Hg)
Normal	< 120	and < 80
Prehypertension *	120-139	or 80–89
Stage 1 HTN	140–159	or 90–99
Stage 2 HTN	≥ 160	or ≥ 100
Isolated systolic HTN	≥ 140	and < 90

*Prehypertension refers to an elevation in the blood pressure above normal but not to the level considered to be HTN; this classification identifies individuals at high risk of developing HTN.
Source: Chobanian AV, Bakris GL, Black HR, Cushman WC, Green LA, Izzo JL Jr, Jones D Wet al. Joint National Committee on Prevention, Detection, Evaluation, and Treatment of High Blood Pressure. *Hypertension.* 2003 Dec;42(6):1206-52.

Table 4.3 **Classification of Blood Pressure Levels in Adults (European Classification)**

Diagnostic Category *	Systolic (mm Hg)	Diastolic (mm Hg)
Optimal	< 120	and < 80
Normal	120–129	and/or 80–84
High Normal	130–139	and/or 85–89
Grade 1 HTN	140–159	and/or 90–99
Grade 2 HTN	160–179	and/or 100–109
Grade 3 HTN	≥ 180	and/or ≥ 110
Isolated systolic HTN	≥ 140	and < 90

* When a patient's systolic and diastolic blood pressures fall into different categories the higher category should apply for the classification of HTN.
Source: Mancia G, De Backer G, Dominiczak A, Cifkova R, Fagard R, Germano G, et al. 2007 Guidelines for the management of arterial hypertension: The Task Force for the Management of Arterial Hypertension of the European Society of Hypertension (ESH) and of the European Society of Cardiology (ESC). *Eur Heart J.* 2007 Jun;28(12):1462-536.

Table 4.4 **Identifiable Risk Factors for Essential Hypertension**

Identifiable Risk Factors of Essential Hypertension
Older age
Race/Ethnicity (higher incidence in African Americans)
Male gender
Obesity (especially abdominal obesity)
Dyslipidemia (independent of obesity)
Diabetes mellitus
Insulin resistance
Emotional or work-related stress
Unhealthy Lifestyle Habits: • Excessive sodium intake • Excess alcohol intake • Inadequate dietary intake of potassium and calcium • Lack of physical activity • Smoking

Table 4.5 **Identifiable Causes of Secondary Hypertension**

Category	Cause/disease
Endocrine/ Hormonal causes	Acromegaly
	Congenital adrenal hyperplasia
	Cushing syndrome
	Exogenous hormones (e.g. corticosteroids, oestrogens)
	Hyperparathyroidism
	Hypothyroidism / hyperthyroidism
	Monoamine oxidase inhibitors (antidepressants)
	Pheochromocytoma
	Primary hyperaldosteronism
	Sympathomimetic drugs (e.g. cocaine)
Renal causes	Chronic renal disease / failure
	Intrarenal vasculitis
	Polycystic kidney disease
	Renal artery stenosis
	Renal parenchymal disease
Vascular	Coarctation of aorta
	Collagen vascular disease
	Intracranial hypertension
	Renovascular disease
	Vasculitis
Other	Obstructive sleep apnoea
	Pregnancy-induced HTN
	Isolated systolic HTN (due to increased stiffness of the vasculature; observed in elderly people)
	Isolated systolic HTN (due to increased cardiac output secondary to a hyperdynamic circulation; examples include atrioventricular fistulas, aortic regurgitation, and patent ductus arteriosus)

Complications of Hypertension

There are a number of complications associated with HTN (Table 4.6). The likelihood of developing complications varies with the grade or severity of HTN.

Table 4.6 **Complications of Hypertension**

Organ / Vessels	Complication
Brain	Dementia Encephalopathy Intracerebral haemorrhage Stroke Transient ischemic attack
Eye	Choroidopathy Optic neuropathy Retinopathy
Heart	Angina / ischaemic heart disease Arrhythmias Coronary artery disease Heart failure Left ventricular hypertrophy Myocardial infarction
Kidney	Glomerulosclerosis Nephrosclerosis Renal failure
Vascular	Aneurysm Arteriosclerosis and atherosclerosis Aortic dissection

Role of Echocardiography in Hypertension

Echocardiography is not used in the diagnosis of HTN but rather in the assessment of the secondary complications of HTN to the heart. The role of echocardiography in the assessment of HTN includes:
• Determining the presence and degree of LVH
• Assessing LV systolic and diastolic function
• Excluding identifiable causes of hypertension
• Identifying other cardiac anomalies associated with hypertensive heart disease.

In particular, echocardiography has the ability to determine the presence and degree of left ventricular hypertrophy (LVH) and to assess left ventricular (LV) systolic and diastolic function. Identifiable causes of HTN and other findings associated with hypertensive heart disease may also be detected via echocardiography.

Left Ventricular Hypertrophy
1. LV Wall Thickness
The development of concentric LVH is an adaptive response to increased afterload that is caused by an elevation in the BP (Fig. 4.2). The presence and severity of LVH can be identified based on measurements of the LV wall thickness. LV wall thickness can be measured via M-mode (Fig. 4.3) or 2D echocardiography (Fig. 4.4). The reference limits and various partition values of LV wall thickness are listed in Table 4.7.

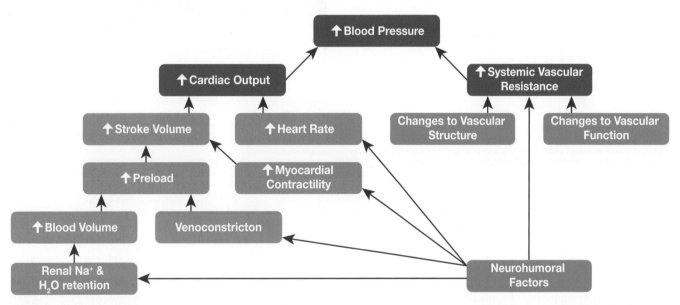

Figure 4.1 Increased blood pressure (BP) is caused by either an increase in systemic vascular resistance (SVR) or an increase in cardiac output (CO). CO is determined by the product of stroke volume and heart rate. Therefore, an increase in heart rate will increase CO and, therefore, BP. Likewise, an increase in stroke volume, as occurs when there is an increase in myocardial contractility or preload will increase CO and, therefore, BP. Increased preload may occur when there is a decrease in venous compliance as occurs when the veins constrict or when there is an increase in total blood volume. Blood volume is regulated by renal function including the management of sodium (Na^+) and water (H_2O). Retention of sodium causes water to be retained, thus increasing blood volume and blood pressure. SVR (also known as total peripheral resistance) is determined by vascular structure and function. The most important mechanism for changing SVR involves changes in vessel luminal diameter. A decrease in vessel luminal diameter may occur due to thickening of the vessel wall or due to a number of other mechanisms. Importantly, heart rate, contractility, venous compliance, renal function and SVR are also strongly influenced by neurohumoral factors.

2. Left Ventricular Mass

LVH is caused by the response of myocytes to an elevated BP and this ultimately results in an increase in the mass of the LV. LV mass is calculated as the LV muscle volume multiplied by the specific gravity of muscle which is often quoted as 1.04 g/mL (although 1.05 g/mL is also sometimes used). LV muscle volume is derived as the difference between the LV epicardial volume and the LV endocardial volume (Fig. 4.5). M-mode and/or 2D imaging can be employed to estimate LV muscle volume and, therefore, LV mass.

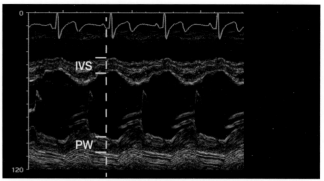

Figure 4.3 Via M-mode LV wall thickness is measured at end-diastole which is identified at the onset of the QRS complex of the ECG. Measurements are performed at the blood-tissue interfaces so the interventricular septum (IVS) is measured from the leading edge of the IVS to the trailing edge of the IVS and the posterior LV wall (PW) is measured from the leading edge of the PW to the pericardial interface.

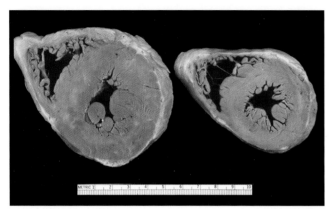

Figure 4.2 These gross pathological specimens show a cross section of the ventricles. The heart on the right is normal. The heart on the left shows marked concentric left ventricular hypertrophy (LVH) which is characterised by increased wall thickness and a reduced cavity size. Concentric LVH occurs as an adaptive response to an increased resistance (afterload) against which the left ventricle must contract to expel blood out of the ventricle.
By permission of Mayo Foundation for Medical Education and Research. All rights reserved. Courtesy of William D. Edwards, MD.

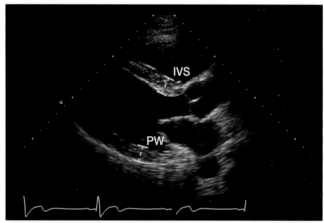

Figure 4.4 Via 2D echo LV wall thickness is measured at end-diastole which is identified as the frame at or immediately prior to mitral valve coaptation following the P wave of the ECG when the patient is in sinus rhythm. Measurements are performed at the blood-tissue interfaces such that the interventricular septum (IVS) is measured from the leading edge of the IVS to the trailing edge of the IVS and the posterior wall (PW) is measured from the leading edge of the PW to the pericardial interface.

Table 4.7 Reference Limits and Partition Values of Left Ventricular Mass and Geometry

	WOMEN				MEN			
	Reference range	Mildly abnormal	Moderately abnormal	Severely abnormal	Reference range	Mildly abnormal	Moderately abnormal	Severely abnormal
Linear Method								
LV mass, g	67–162	163–186	187–210	≥211	88–224	225–258	259–292	≥293
LV mass/BSA, g/m²	*43–95*	*96–108*	*109–121*	*≥122*	*49–115*	*116–131*	*132–148*	*≥149*
LV mass/height, g/m	41–99	100–115	116–128	≥ 129	52–126	127–144	145–162	≥163
LV mass/height²·⁷, g/m²·⁷	18–44	45–51	52–58	≥ 59	20–48	49–55	56–63	≥64
Relative wall thickness, cm	0.22–0.42	0.43–0.47	0.48–0.52	≥ 0.53	0.24–0.42	0.43–0.46	0.47–0.51	≥0.52
Septal thickness, cm	*0.6–0.9*	*1.0–1.2*	*1.3–1.5*	*≥1.6*	*0.6–1.0*	*1.1–1.3*	*1.4–1.6*	*≥1.7*
Posterior wall thickness, cm	*0.6–0.9*	*1.0–1.2*	*1.3–1.5*	*≥1.6*	*0.6–1.0*	*1.1–1.3*	*1.4–1.6*	*≥1.7*
2D Method								
LV mass, g	66–150	151–171	172–182	≥193	96–200	201–227	228–254	≥ 255
LV mass/BSA, g/m²	*44–88*	*89–100*	*101–112*	*≥113*	*50–102*	*103–116*	*117–130*	*≥131*

BSA = Body surface area; LV = left ventricular; 2D = 2-dimensional. ***Bold italic values***: Recommended and best validated.
Reprinted from Lang RM, Bierig M, Devereux RB, et al., Chamber Quantification Writing Group; American Society of Echocardiography's Guidelines and Standards Committee; European Association of Echocardiography. Recommendations for Chamber Quantification: A Report from the American Society of Echocardiography's Guidelines and Standards Committee and the Chamber Quantification Writing Group, Developed in Conjunction with the European Association of Echocardiography, a Branch of the European Society of Cardiology, *J Am Soc Echocardiogr*, Vol. 18(12), page 1448, © 2005 with permission from Elsevier.

a. Linear Method

LV mass can be estimated from linear measurements of the LV performed via M-mode or 2D imaging. Linear measurements required include end-diastolic measurements of the interventricular septum (IVS), the LV cavity and the posterior wall (PW) (Fig. 4.6). From these measurements, the LV mass is calculated as:

Equation 4.7

$$LVM = 1.04 \left([LVEDD + PW + IVS]^3 - LVEDD^3 \right) \times 0.8 + 0.6$$

where LVM = left ventricular mass (g)
LVEDD = left ventricular end-diastolic dimension (cm)
PW = left ventricular posterior wall thickness (cm)
IVS = interventricular septal thickness (cm)
1.04 = specific gravity of muscle (g/mL)

To help simply this complex equation, consider that $[LVEDD + PW + IVS]^3$ determines the LV epicardial volume while $LVEDD^3$ determines the LV endocardial volume and 1.04 is the specific gravity of muscle with (x 0.8 + 0.6) as a 'correction' factor.

b. 2D Method

LV mass can also be estimated via 2D echo based on the area-length method (Fig. 4.7) and the truncated ellipsoid method (Fig. 4.8). 2D measurements required include the total epicardial area, the total LV cavity area and the LV length; all measurements are performed at end-diastole. The total epicardial area and the LV cavity area are traced from the parasternal short axis view at the level of the papillary

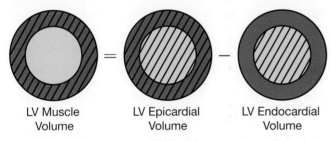

LV Muscle Volume = LV Epicardial Volume − LV Endocardial Volume

Figure 4.5 LV muscle volume is estimated as the difference between the LV epicardial volume and the LV endocardial volume.

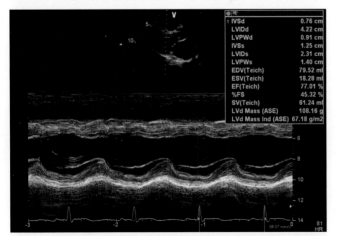

Figure 4.6 For the linear method for estimating LV mass, measurements of the interventricular septum (IVSd), the LV cavity (LVIDd) and the posterior wall (LVPWd) are performed at end-diastole and at the blood-tissue interfaces. In this example the LV mass is calculated as:
LVM (g) = 1.04 ([LVIDd + LVPWd + IVSd]³ − LVIDd³) × 0.8 + 0.6
= 1.04 ([4.22 + 0.91 + 0.76]³ − 4.22³) × 0.8 + 0.6
= 108 g

muscles. The LV length (long axis) is measured from the apical 4-chamber view from the mitral annulus to the LV apex. From these measurements the 2D LV mass can be derived via area-length method or the truncated ellipsoid method:

Area-Length Method

Equation 4.8

$$LVM = 1.05 \left[\tfrac{5}{6} A_1 (L + t) \right] - \tfrac{5}{6} A_2 L]$$

where LVM = left ventricular mass (g)
A_1 = epicardial area at end diastole (cm²)
A_2 = endocardial area at end diastole (cm²)
L = ventricular length at end diastole (cm)
t = average wall thickness (cm)
1.05 = specific gravity of muscle (g/ml)

Truncated Ellipse Method

Equation 4.9

$$LVM = 1.05 \, \pi \, (b + t)^2 \left[\tfrac{2}{3} (a + t) + d - d^3/3(a + t)^2 \right] - b^2 \left[\tfrac{2}{3} a + d - d^3 / 3a^2 \right]$$

where LVM = left ventricular mass (g)
a = semi-major axis length (cm)
b = short axis radius (cm)
d = truncated semi-major axis length (cm)
t = average wall thickness (cm)
1.05 = specific gravity of muscle (g/ml)

LV mass values should then be "normalised". The manner in which LV mass measurements should be normalised in adults is controversial. Most commonly LV mass is indexed to the body surface area (BSA) by simply dividing the LV mass by the BSA:

Equation 4.10

$$LVMi = LV\ mass \div BSA$$

where LVMi = left ventricular mass index (g/m²)
LV mass = left ventricular mass (g)
BSA = body surface area (m²)

It can be appreciated that indexing the LV mass for BSA in obese individuals will underestimate the degree of LVH. Therefore, in these individuals, height-based adjustment is recommended so the LV mass is indexed to the individual's height (LV mass divided by the height) or to an allometric power of the individual's height (LV mass divided by the height²·⁷). The reference limits and various partition values of LV mass are listed in Table 4.7.

3. Relative Wall Thickness

The relative wall thickness (RWT) is calculated from the LV posterior wall thickness and the LVEDD:

Equation 4.11

$$RWT = (2\ PW) \div LVEDD$$

where RWT = relative wall thickness (unitless)
LVEDD = left ventricular end diastolic dimension (cm)
PW = left ventricular posterior wall thickness at end diastole (cm)

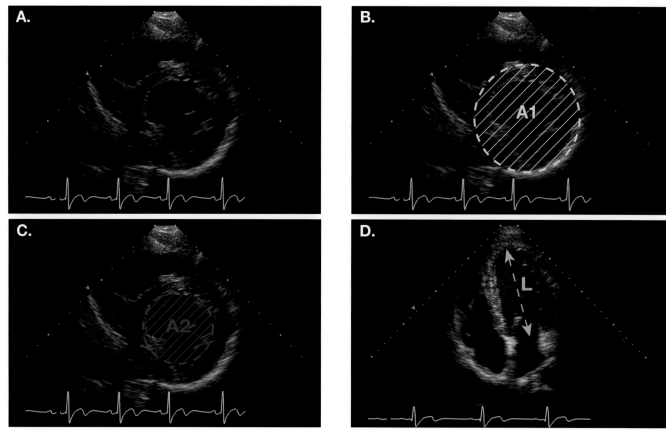

Figure 4.7 To calculate the LV mass via the area-length method a parasternal short axis of the left ventricle (LV) at the papillary muscle level is acquired at end-diastole **(A)**. Because the mitral valve cannot be seen from this view, end-diastole is identified as the onset of the QRS complex of the ECG. From this image the total epicardial area (A_1) and the total endocardial area (A_2) are traced **(B** and **C)**. The endocardial area trace includes the papillary muscles; that is, the papillary muscles are included in the cavity area. From these traces and assuming a circular area, the radius (b) is derived as $\sqrt{(A_2 \div \pi)}$ and the mean wall thickness (t) is calculated as $\sqrt{(A_1 \div \pi)} - b$. From an end-diastolic frame acquired from the apical 4-chamber view, the LV length (long axis) is measured from the mitral annulus to the LV apex **(D)**. The LV mass can then be calculated via the area-length equation: *LVM (g) = 1.05 [5/6 A_1 (L + t)] – 5/6 A_2 L]*.

Based on the LV mass and the RWT the pattern of LV geometry can be classified into the four groups: concentric hypertrophy, eccentric hypertrophy, concentric remodelling and normal geometry (Fig. 4.9). The normal geometric pattern is defined as a normal LV mass and normal RWT. The concentric hypertrophy pattern, which is the "typical" hypertensive concentric hypertrophy pattern, is defined as both an increase in LV mass and RWT. The eccentric hypertrophy pattern is defined as an increased LV mass with normal RWT; in this group, the LV mass is increased due to chamber dilatation rather than increased wall thickness. The concentric remodelling pattern is defined as having increased RWT with normal LV mass.

Limitations

Measurement accuracy of LV wall thickness is highly dependent upon image quality and the technical skill of the operator. In addition, M-mode may overestimate LV wall thickness if the M-mode cursor transects the LV walls at an oblique angle. There is also the potential that measurements performed via second harmonic imaging may overestimate LV wall thickness when compared to fundamental imaging; however this limitation has become less of a problem due to the improved spatial resolution at the harmonic frequency.

As linear LV mass calculations rely on accurate measurements of LV walls, the limitations described above will also apply to these LV mass calculations. In particular, because the linear LV mass is estimated by the cubing of these measurements, small measurement errors will be amplified to the third power (refer to Equation 4.7).

2D LV mass calculations rely on accurate tracing of endocardial and epicardial borders so suboptimal image quality, the inability to identify these borders and off axis images will compromise the accuracy of these calculations. For example, overestimation of LV wall thickness due to oblique cuts through the LV will result in an overestimation of LV mass while underestimation of the LV length due to foreshortening of the apical views will lead to an underestimation of the 2D LV mass. Furthermore, LV mass calculations are based on geometrical assumptions that represent obvious limitations to these calculations.

LV Systolic and Diastolic Function

LV systolic and diastolic function in patients with HTN is important due to the structural changes that occur within and surrounding cardiac myocytes which may inhibit normal LV contraction and relaxation. In particular, with long-term HTN heart failure and subsequent LV systolic dysfunction may develop. LV systolic function is assessed in the usual manner (see Chapter 2).

LV systolic function is often hyperdynamic in patients with HTN and this in conjunction with LVH may result in dynamic left ventricular outflow tract (LVOT) obstruction. On the continuous-wave (CW) Doppler signal dynamic LVOT obstruction is identified as a late-peaking systolic, dagger-shaped signal (Fig. 4.10).

The diastolic filling profile in HTN typically reveals an impaired relaxation pattern (Fig. 4.11). A triphasic mitral inflow profile with mid-diastolic flow may also be seen in

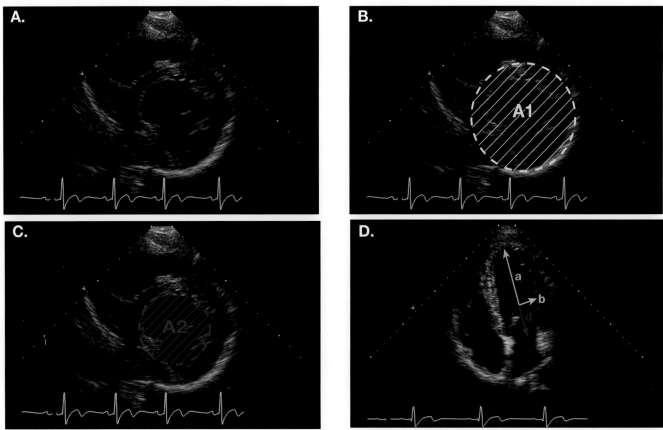

Figure 4.8 To calculate the LV mass via the truncated ellipse method a parasternal short axis of the left ventricle (LV) at the papillary muscle level is acquired at end-diastole **(A)**. Because the mitral valve cannot be seen from this view, end-diastole is identified as the onset of the QRS complex of the ECG. From this image the total epicardial area (A_1) and the total endocardial area (A_2) are traced (**B** and **C**). The endocardial area trace includes the papillary muscles; that is, the papillary muscles are included in the cavity area. From these traces and assuming a circular area, the radius (b) is derived as $\sqrt{(A_2 \div \pi)}$ and the mean wall thickness (t) is calculated as $\sqrt{(A_1 \div \pi)} - b$. From an end-diastolic frame acquired from the apical 4-chamber view, the LV length is divided into a semi-major axis (a) and a truncated semi-major axis (d) **(D)**. The radius (b) or minor axis, derived from the parasternal short axis view, is used to divide the LV length into semi-major axis (measured from the radius b to the LV apex) and a truncated semi-major axis (measured from the radius b to the mitral annulus). From these measurements the LV mass can then be calculated via the truncated ellipse equation:

$$LVM\ (g) = 1.05\ \pi\ (b + t)^2\ [\ ^2/_3\ (a + t) + d - d^3/3(a + t)^2\ ] - b^2\ [\ ^2/_3\ a + d - d^3/3a^2\ ]$$

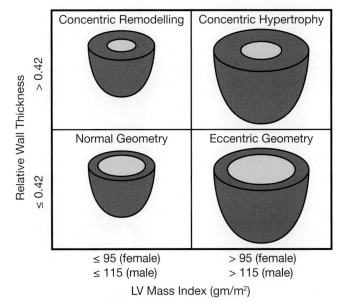

Figure 4.9 The patterns of LV geometry and LVH are based on the LV mass and the RWT. A normal RWT is defined as ≤0.42 and a normal LV mass is defined as ≤95 g/m^2 for females and ≤115 g/m^2 for males. An increased LV mass and an increased RWT is classified as concentric hypertrophy while an increased LV mass and a normal RWT is classified as eccentric hypertrophy. A normal LV mass and an increased RWT is classified as concentric remodelling while a normal LV mass and a normal RWT is classified as normal geometry.

patients with LVH (Fig. 4.12). When present in the setting of LVH, the L-wave appears to be a marker of pseudonormal LV filling. The proposed mechanism for this mid-diastolic flow (or the L-wave) relates to markedly abnormal LV relaxation. The comprehensive assessment of LV diastolic function is performed in the usual manner (see Chapter 3).

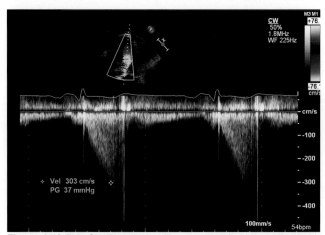

Figure 4.10 This CW Doppler profile was recorded in a patient with concentric LVH secondary to HTN. This profile is consistent with dynamic LVOT obstruction as evident by the characteristic systolic late-peaking and dagger-shaped profile of this signal. The peak velocity is 3 m/s yielding a gradient of 37 mm Hg.

Identifying Causes of Hypertension

As listed in Table 4.5, there are a number of identifiable disorders that may be associated with secondary HTN. Of these secondary causes the one that can be identified via echocardiography is coarctation of the aorta. On 2D imaging, coarctation of the aorta may be identified from the suprasternal view (Fig. 4.13). The presence of turbulent flow revealed via colour flow Doppler imaging and characteristic spectral Doppler flow profiles within the descending and abdominal aorta are also valuable in identifying this lesion (Fig. 4.14).

Identifying Cardiac Anomalies associated with Hypertension

Cardiac anomalies associated with HTN that can be detected by echocardiography include: (1) mitral annular calcification, (2) aortic valve sclerosis, (3) dilatation of the ascending aorta, (4) mild degrees of aortic regurgitation (secondary to aortic

sclerosis and/or aortic root dilatation), and (5) atherosclerosis of the aorta (Fig. 4.15).

LVH versus Increased LV Wall Thickness

LVH is identified on echocardiography as an increase in the LV wall thickness. However, it is important to note that there are a number of other causes of increased LV wall thickness other that LVH (Table 4.8). Therefore, when LV walls are thickened and LVH cannot be confirmed, "increased LV wall thickness" rather than "left ventricular hypertrophy" should be reported.

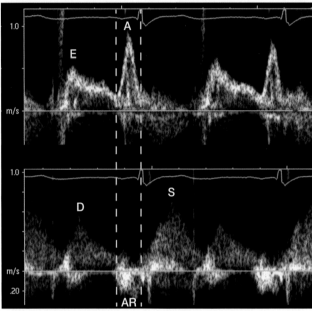

Figure 4.11 This mitral inflow signal *(top)* shows an impaired relaxation pattern which is evident by an E/A ratio < 1 and prolongation of the deceleration time (430 ms). On the pulmonary venous trace *(bottom)*, the D velocity is < S velocity which is also consistent with impaired relaxation. The atrial reversal velocity (AR) is < 35 cm/s and the mitral A duration and pulmonary AR duration are equal indicating that the left ventricular end diastolic pressure is normal.

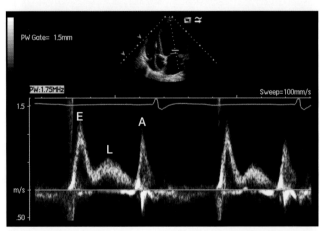

Figure 4.12 This mitral inflow profile displays a triphasic pattern with an early diastolic *(E)*, a mid-diastolic *(L)* and late diastolic *(A)* waves. In the presence of associated LVH, this flow profile is a marker of pseudonormal LV filling.

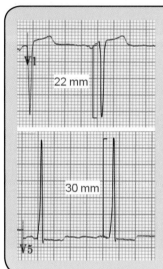

A 12 lead ECG is useful in determining if increased LV wall thickness is due to LVH. ECG evidence of LVH includes deep S waves in V1 and tall R waves in V5/V6. When the sum of the S wave in V1 and R wave in V5 or V6 (whichever is taller) exceeds 35 mm then there is LVH. In the example opposite, the sum of S ι R = 52 mm; therefore LVH is present. When inverted T waves in V5 and V6 are seen there is associated significant LV 'strain'.

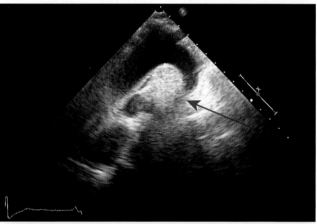

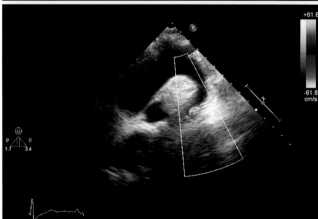

Figure 4.13 The 2D image recorded from the suprasternal long axis of the aorta *(top)* shows a narrowing or pinched appearance of the aortic lumen *(arrow)*. This appearance is consistent with a coarctation of the aorta. The corresponding colour flow Doppler image confirms the presence of turbulent flow across this narrowed region *(bottom)*.

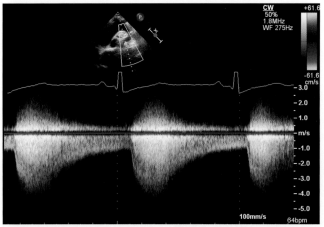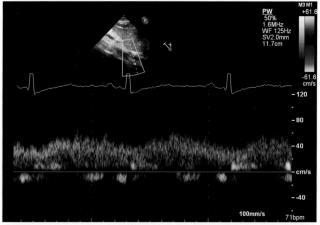

Figure 4.14 The spectral Doppler traces above show the characteristic features associated with a significant coarctation of the aorta. The CW Doppler trace on the left was recorded from the suprasternal window; observe the prominent "diastolic tail" following the systolic velocity. This "diastolic tail" reflects a continued pressure gradient across the coarctation into diastole and is a marker of a severe coarctation. The trace on the right is a pulsed-wave Doppler signal recorded from the abdominal aorta; observe the 'flat' and continuous flow profile. This profile is consistent with damped flow within the abdominal aorta; the presence of continued flow again reflects the continued pressure gradient across the coarctation into diastole. Also note that due to a large angle of incidence between the ultrasound beam and blood flow, the velocities in the abdominal aorta seem to be lower than expected.

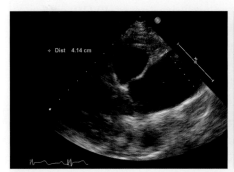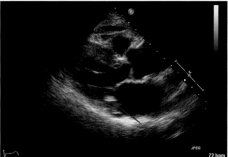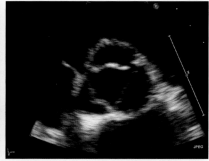

Figure 4.15 These images were recorded from a 71 year old female patient with longstanding HTN. The image on the left, recorded from a high parasternal long axis view, shows dilatation of the upper ascending aorta; the middle image, recorded from the standard parasternal long axis view, shows posterior mitral annular calcification *(arrow)* and the image on the right, recorded from the parasternal short axis, shows aortic valve sclerosis.

Table 4.8 Disorders other than Hypertension causing Increased Left Ventricular Wall Thickness

Disorder	Cause of Increased LV Wall Thickness
Cardiac Amyloidosis Amyloidosis is an infiltrative, systemic disorder characterised by interstitial deposits of amyloid fibrils in multiple organs, including the heart.	Deposition of amyloid proteins between the cardiac myocytes
Oxalosis Primary oxalosis is a rare infiltrative, hereditary, metabolic disorder in which an enhanced production of oxalic acid leads to hyperoxalemia and a deposition of calcium oxalate in different body organs such as the kidneys and the heart.	Excess accumulation of calcium oxalate crystals between myocardial fibres
Haemochromatosis* Haemochromatosis is usually a hereditary storage disease where there is excess absorption of iron from the digestive tract; excess iron accumulates in tissues throughout the body, including the heart.	Excessive iron deposition within the heart
Fabry's Disease* Fabry's disease (or Anderson-Fabry disease) is a rare X-linked lysosomal storage disorder leading to an accumulation of glycosphingolipids in all tissues and organs, including the heart.	Intracellular accumulation of glycolipids within the heart
Acute Myocarditis Myocarditis is an inflammatory disease of the myocardium. The most common causes for myocarditis include viral infections, toxins, drugs, and autoimmune reactions.	Myocardial oedema

* These disorders may also result in LVH.

Pulmonary Hypertension

Definition and Classification of Pulmonary Hypertension

Pulmonary hypertension (PHTN) is characterised by elevated pulmonary arterial pressures and secondary right ventricular (RV) failure. The haemodynamic definition of PHTN is defined as a mean pulmonary artery pressure (mPAP) greater than 25 mm Hg at rest.

Over the years the classification of PHTN has changed and evolved. The earliest classification of PTHN was based the presence or absence of identifiable causes or risk factors. Thus, primary PHTN was defined as PHTN due to unknown causes while secondary PHTN was defined as PHTN due to identifiable causes or risk factors. Subsequent classifications of PHTN from the World Health Organisation (WHO) have attempted to group together different manifestations of disease based upon similarities in pathophysiologic mechanisms, clinical presentation, and therapeutic options. This has led to a much broader, more encompassing clinical classification, with 5 major categories now used (Table 4.9). In particular, it should be noted that the term primary PHTN has now been abandoned.

Another classification of PHTN is based on the haemodynamic consequence of vascular changes in the pulmonary circulation. Vascular changes on the arterial side of the pulmonary circulation are referred to as precapillary while vascular changes on the venous side of the pulmonary circulation are referred to as postcapillary (Fig. 4.16). Precapillary PHTN results from increased pulmonary blood flow as seen with left-to-right shunts, or increased resistance to flow in the pulmonary arteries and arterioles as seen in pulmonary arterial hypertension (PAH). Postcapillary PHTN is caused by back pressure from left heart lesions and/or increased resistance to flow at the level of the pulmonary veins. Therefore, precapillary PHTN includes clinical classification groups 1, 3, 4, and 5 while post-capillary PHTN includes clinical classification group 2.

Pulmonary Arterial Hypertension (PAH) versus "Non-PAH" or Pulmonary Hypertension (PHTN)

PAH may be defined as a condition brought on by a wide range of causes characterised by structural changes in small pulmonary arteries. These changes restrict flow through the pulmonary arterial (PA) circulation and produce a progressive increase in PA pressure and pulmonary vascular resistance (PVR) which leads to RV failure. The haemodynamic definition of PAH is a mPAP > 25 mm Hg at rest with a pulmonary capillary wedge pressure (PCWP), left atrial pressure (LAP), or left ventricular end-diastolic pressure (LVEDP) ≤ 15 mm Hg and a PVR > 3 mm Hg/L/min (Wood units).

"Non-PAH PHTN" or PHTN refers to those forms of pulmonary hypertension that are found in groups 2 to 5 of the clinical classification of PHTN (Table 4.9). For example, PHTN occurs as a result of left heart disease, chronic lung disease, and recurrent venous thromboembolism. The haemodynamic definition of PHTN is a mPAP > 25 mm Hg at rest, irrespective of the PCWP, LAP, LVEDP or PVR.

Table 4.9 Clinical Classification of Pulmonary Hypertension (Dana Point, 2008)

1. Pulmonary arterial hypertension (PAH)

1.1. Idiopathic PAH

1.2. Heritable

    1.2.1. BMPR2

    1.2.2. ALK1, endoglin (with or without hereditary hemorrhagic telangiectasia)

1.2.3. Unknown

1.3. Drug- and toxin-induced

1.4. Associated with:

    1.4.1. Connective tissue diseases

    1.4.2. HIV infection

    1.4.3. Portal hypertension

    1.4.4. Congenital heart diseases

    1.4.5. Schistosomiasis

    1.4.6. Chronic haemolytic anaemia

1.5 Persistent pulmonary hypertension of the newborn

1'. Pulmonary veno-occlusive disease (PVOD) and/or pulmonary capillary haemangiomatosis (PCH)

2. Pulmonary hypertension owing to left heart disease

2.1. Systolic dysfunction

2.2. Diastolic dysfunction

2.3. Valvular disease

3. Pulmonary hypertension owing to lung diseases and/or hypoxia

3.1. Chronic obstructive pulmonary disease

3.2. Interstitial lung disease

3.3. Other pulmonary diseases with mixed restrictive and obstructive pattern

3.4. Sleep-disordered breathing

3.5. Alveolar hypoventilation disorders

3.6. Chronic exposure to high altitude

3.7. Developmental abnormalities

4. Chronic thromboembolic pulmonary hypertension (CTEPH)

5. Pulmonary hypertension with unclear multifactorial mechanisms

5.1. Hematologic disorders: myeloproliferative disorders, splenectomy

5.2. Systemic disorders: sarcoidosis, pulmonary Langerhans cell histiocytosis: lymphangioleiomyomatosis, neurofibromatosis, vasculitis

5.3. Metabolic disorders: glycogen storage disease, Gaucher disease, thyroid disorders

5.4. Others: tumoral obstruction, fibrosing mediastinitis, chronic renal failure on dialysis

ALK1 = active in receptor-like kinase 1 gene; BMPR2 = bone morphogenetic protein receptor, type 2; HIV = human immunodeficiency virus.
Reprinted from Simonneau G, Robbins I, Beghetti M, Channick RN, Delcroix M, Denton CP, Elliott CG, Gaine S, Gladwin MT, Jing ZC, Krowka MJ, Langleben D, Nakanishi N, Souza R. Updated clinical classification of pulmonary hypertension, *J Am Coll Cardiol*, Vol 54, page S45, © 2009; with permission from Elsevier.

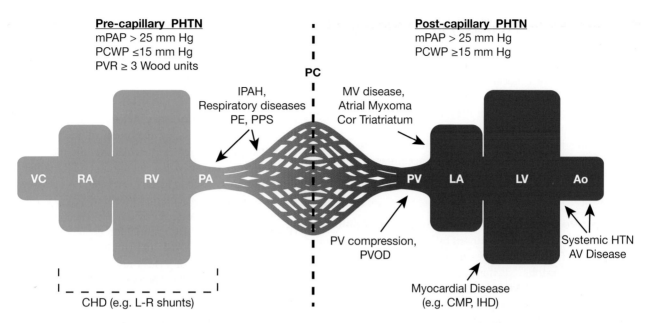

Figure 4.16 Precapillary causes of PHTN include the clinical groups 1, 3, 4 and 5 (i.e. PAH, PHTN due to lung diseases, chronic thromboembolic PHTN and PHTN with unclear and/or multifactorial mechanisms). Postcapillary PHTN includes the clinical group 2 (i.e. PHTN due to left heart disease). AV = aortic valve; CHD = congenital heart disease; CMP = cardiomyopathies; COPD = chronic obstructive pulmonary disease; HTN = hypertension; IHD = ischaemic heart disease; IPAH = idiopathic pulmonary arterial hypertension; mPAP = mean pulmonary pressure; MV = mitral valve; PCWP = pulmonary capillary wedge pressure; PE = pulmonary emboli; PHTN = pulmonary hypertension; PPS = peripheral pulmonary stenosis; PVOD = pulmonary venous occlusive disease.

Pathophysiology of Pulmonary Hypertension

Normally, pulmonary artery (PA) pressures are much lower than systemic pressures. These low pressures are due to the large cross-sectional area of the pulmonary circulation, which results in low resistance to blood flow.

PAH occurs when there is an increase in the pulmonary vascular resistance (PVR). The pathophysiology of PAH is complex and multifactorial but essentially increased PVR is caused by the loss of vascular luminal cross section due to vascular remodeling or excessive vasoconstriction.

As for systemic HTN, the basic pathophysiology of PHTN due to secondary causes can be appreciated by considering the relationship between volumetric flow rate, resistance to flow and the pressure difference (refer to Equation 4.2).

In the case of PHTN, PVR is derived from the change in pressure across the pulmonary circulation from its beginning to its end (the difference between mPAP and PCWP) and the cardiac output (CO):

Equation 4.12

$$PVR = (mPAP - PCWP) \div CO$$

where PVR = pulmonary vascular resistance (mm Hg/L/min)
mPAP = mean pulmonary arterial pressure (mm Hg)
PCWP = pulmonary capillary wedge pressure (mm Hg)
CO = cardiac output (L/min)

It can be appreciated from this equation that an abnormal increase in the mPAP or PCWP will lead to an increased PVR and PHTN. Note, however, that an increased PCWP will only lead to an increased PVR if there is a secondary increase in the mPAP. For example, a patient with PHTN secondary to left heart disease may have a mPAP > 25 mm Hg but if the PCWP is also increased, then the PVR may not that high. Some of the more common causes of secondary PHTN and the associated mechanism for the development of PHTN are briefly described in Table 4.10.

Table 4.10 Selected Secondary Causes and Mechanisms of Pulmonary Hypertension (PHTN)

2° causes of PHTN	Mechanism of PHTN
Left-to-right shunts	Shunt lesions cause pulmonary vascular injury and therefore PHTN due to volume overload and/or pressure overload.
Left heart disease	Increased pulmonary pressures may occur in any condition that impedes pulmonary venous drainage or results in an increase in the LA pressure (LAP). PHTN that occurs in LV dysfunction and left-sided valve disease is the result of an increase in resistance to pulmonary venous drainage and backward transmission of an elevated LAP to the lungs.
Acute pulmonary embolism	PHTN occurs when blood flow through large pulmonary arteries is hindered. In acute pulmonary embolism, there is usually only a mild to moderate elevation in pulmonary artery (PA) pressures because in the acute setting, the RV is unable to generate a systolic pressure greater than 50 mm Hg. Hence, PA pressures exceeding 50 mmHg suggest a chronic process.
Chronic obstructive pulmonary disease (COPD)	COPD can cause PHTN via hypoxemia-induced vasoconstriction which leads to an increase in PVR. Other disorders, such as obstructive sleep apnea, neuromuscular disorders, and disorders of the chest wall, may also lead to hypoxic pulmonary vasoconstriction and eventually PHTN.
Scleroderma	PHTN in these patients occurs due to obliteration of pulmonary vasculature.

Role of Echocardiography in PHTN

Echocardiography has a very important role in the diagnosis of PHTN as well as in the assessment of patients with known PHTN. The role of echocardiography in the assessment of PHTN includes:

- Identifying potential causes of PHTN
- Estimating pulmonary pressures
- Recognising increased pulmonary vascular resistance
- Assessing the functional and morphologic cardiac sequelae of PHTN
- Identifying prognostic variables.

Identifying Potential Cases of Pulmonary Hypertension

As mentioned, PHTN can be caused by any cardiac disorder that elevates left heart filling pressures. This includes systolic dysfunction, diastolic dysfunction, and valvular heart disease (Table 4.11). PAH can also occur as a complication of uncorrected increases in pulmonary blood flow that may occur with various congenital heart lesions with systemic-to-pulmonary shunts. The development of PAH and subsequent reversal of shunt flow (Eisenmenger's syndrome) occurs more frequently when blood flow to the lungs is extremely high

and when the pulmonary vasculature is exposed to systemic pressures; examples include ventricular septal defects, patent ductus arteriosus, or truncus arteriosus. However, PAH may also occur with low pressure-high flow abnormalities such as atrial septal defects.

Estimation of Pulmonary Artery Pressures

While the haemodynamic definition of PHTN is based on the mPAP, it is the right ventricular systolic pressure (RVSP) derived from the tricuspid regurgitant (TR) signal that is most commonly used to identify elevated PA pressures. In the absence of right ventricular outflow tract [RVOT] obstruction or pulmonary stenosis, RVSP equals PA systolic pressure [PASP]. The arbitrary criteria for detecting PHTN based on the TR velocity, PASP and additional echocardiographic variables suggestive of PHTN are listed in Table 4.12. The grading of severity of PHTN based on estimated RVSP/PASP is listed in Table 4.13.

PA pressures that can be estimated from Doppler signals are based on the assumption that the Doppler velocity reflects the pressure difference between two chambers (see Chapter 1). Table 4.14 summarizes the commonly used Doppler methods

Table 4.11 **Causes of PHTN identified via Echo**

Conditions That Predispose to Pulmonary Hypertension
- Congenital or acquired valvular disease (MR, MS, AS, prosthetic valve dysfunction)
- Left ventricular systolic dysfunction
- Impaired left ventricular diastolic function (hypertensive heart disease, HCM, Fabry's disease, infiltrative cardiomyopathies)
- Other obstructive lesions (coarctation, supravalvular AS, subaortic membrane, cor triatriatum)
- Congenital disease with shunt (ASD, VSD, coronary fistula, patent ductus arteriosus, anomalous pulmonary venous return)
- Pulmonary embolus (thrombus in IVC, right-sided cardiac chamber, or PA; tricuspid or pulmonic valve vegetation)
- Pulmonary vein thrombosis/stenosis

Findings That Suggest Specific Disease Entity
- Left-sided valve changes (SLE, anorexigen use)
- Intra-pulmonary shunts (hereditary hemorrhagic telangiectasia)
- Pericardial effusion (IPAH, SLE, systemic sclerosis)

AS = aortic stenosis; ASD = atrial septal defect; HCM = hypertrophic cardiomyopathy; IPAH = idiopathic pulmonary arterial hypertension; IVC = inferior vena cava; MR = mitral regurgitation; MS = mitral stenosis; PA = pulmonary artery; SLE = systemic lupus erythematosus; VSD = ventricular septal defect.
Reprinted from McLaughlin VV, Archer SL, Badesch DB, et al. ACCF/AHA 2009 Expert Consensus Document on Pulmonary Hypertension: A Report of the American College of Cardiology Foundation Task Force on Expert Consensus Documents and the American Heart Association Developed in Collaboration With the American College of Chest Physicians; American Thoracic Society, Inc.; and the Pulmonary Hypertension Association, *J Am Coll Cardiol,* Vol. 53, page 1590 © 2009 with permission from Elsevier.

Table 4.12 **Arbitrary criteria for estimating the presence of PHTN based on TR peak velocity and PASP at rest (assuming a normal RAP of 5 mm Hg) and on additional echocardiographic variables suggestive of PHTN.**

	Class [a]	Level [b]
Echo diagnosis: PHTN unlikely • TR velocity ≤ 2.8 m/s, PASP ≤ 36 mm Hg, and no additional echocardiographic variables suggestive of PHTN	I	B
Echo diagnosis: PHTN possible • TR velocity ≤ 2.8 m/s, PASP ≤ 36 mm Hg, but presence of additional echocardiographic variables suggestive of PHTN	IIa	C
TR velocity 2.9–3.4 m/s, PASP • 37–50 mm Hg with/without additional echocardiographic variables suggestive of PHTN	IIa	C
Echo diagnosis: PHTN likely • TR velocity > 3.4 m/s, PASP > 50 mm Hg, with/without additional echocardiographic variables suggestive of PHTN	I	B

[a] Class of recommendation. [b] Level of evidence.
PASP = pulmonary artery systolic pressure; RAP = right atrial pressure; TR = tricuspid regurgitant.
Reproduced from Galiè N, Hoeper MM, Humbert M, et al. Guidelines for the diagnosis and treatment of pulmonary hypertension: the Task Force for the Diagnosis and Treatment of Pulmonary Hypertension of the European Society of *Cardiology (*ESC) and the European Respiratory Society (ERS), endorsed by the International Society of Heart and Lung Transplantation (ISHLT). *Eur Heart J.* Vol. 30(20), page 2504, © 2009 with permission of Oxford University Press.

for estimating PA pressures. Estimation of each of these intracardiac pressures is discussed below.

1. Estimation of the RVSP/PASP from the TR Velocity

The peak systolic velocity of the TR signal reflects the systolic pressure difference between the RV and right atrium (RA). Therefore, from the TR velocity (Fig. 4.17) and from an estimation of the right atrial pressure (RAP), it is possible to estimate the RVSP using the following equation:

Equation 4.13

$$RVSP = 4\ V_{TR}^{\ 2} + RAP$$

where RVSP = right ventricular systolic pressure (mm Hg)
      V_{TR} = peak systolic TR velocity (m/s)
      RAP = right atrial pressure (mm Hg)

2. Right Atrial Pressure Estimation

The RAP can be estimated using the inferior vena cava (IVC), hepatic venous (HV) Doppler parameters and via Doppler tissue imaging (DTI) of the RV lateral annulus.

Normal Right Heart Haemodynamics
RVSP/PASP$_{Echo}$ < 36 mm Hg *
mPAP   8 - 20 mm Hg
PAEDP   4 – 12 mm Hg
RAP   0 – 5 mm Hg
PVR   < 2.0 WU

* (up to 40 mm Hg in older and obese patients)

Right Heart Haemodynamics consistent with PHTN
RVSP/PASP$_{Echo}$ > 40 mm Hg
mPAP   ≥ 25 mm Hg
PVR   > 3.0 WU

Table 4.13 Grades of Severity of PHTN based on RVSP/PASP

Severity PHTN	RVSP/PASP
Mild	40 – 54 mmHg
Moderate	55 – 64 mmHg
Severe	≥ 65 mmHg

a. RAP via IVC Size and Collapsibility

For the RAP estimation using the IVC, the IVC is measured, in its long axis, from the subcostal view via 2D imaging (Fig. 4.18) or via M-mode (Fig. 4.19). The largest diameter ($IVCD_{max}$) and the smallest diameter ($IVCD_{min}$) are measured and from these values, the collapsibility index (CI_{IVC}) is calculated:

Equation 4.14

$$CI_{IVC} = [(IVCD_{max} - IVCD_{min}) \div IVCD_{max}] \times 100$$

where CI_{IVC} = collapsibility index of the inferior vena cava (%)
      $IVCD_{max}$ = inferior vena cava diameter maximum (cm)
      $IVCD_{min}$ = inferior vena cava diameter minimum (cm)

From the IVC size and collapsibility index, the RAP can be estimated (Table 4.15).

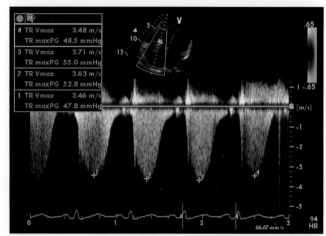

Figure 4.17 The peak systolic TR velocity is recorded via CW Doppler ensuring parallel alignment with flow. This peak systolic TR velocity reflects the pressure difference between the RV and the RA in systole. Using the simplified Bernoulli equation ($4V^2$), the TR velocity can be converted to a pressure gradient. When the RAP is estimated, then the RVSP can be estimated. Assuming a RAP of 15 mm Hg, the RVSP in this example is:

$$\begin{aligned} RVSP &= 4\ V_{TR}^{\ 2} + RAP \\ &= 4\ (3.57)^2 + 15 \\ &= 50.98 + 15 \\ &= 66\ mm\ Hg \end{aligned}$$

Note: Because the TR velocity varies during respiration, the TR velocities should be averaged over the respiratory cycle.

Table 4.14 Commonly used Doppler-estimates of Pulmonary Artery Pressures

Pressure estimated	Doppler signal	Formula
RVSP	TR peak systolic velocity	RVSP = $4\ V_{TR}^{\ 2}$ + RAP
	VSD peak systolic velocity	RVSP = SBP - $4\ V_{VSD}^{\ 2}$
PASP	PDA peak systolic velocity	PASP = SBP - $4\ V_{PDA}^{\ 2}$
	TR peak systolic velocity (in the absence of RVOT obstruction)	PASP = $4\ V_{TR}^{\ 2}$ + RAP
PAEDP	PR end-diastolic velocity	PAEDP = $4\ V_{PR\text{-}ED}^{\ 2}$ + RVEDP (RAP)
mPAP	TR signal (mean RV-to-RA systolic gradient)	mPAP = $\Delta P_{mRV\text{-}RA}$ + RAP
	RVOT acceleration time (Pulsed-wave Doppler)	mPAP = 79 – (0.45 x RVAcT)
	PR peak early diastolic velocity	mPAP = $4\ V_{PR\text{-}peak}^{\ 2}$ + RAP

mPAP = mean pulmonary artery pressure; mRV-RA = mean RV-RA pressure gradient; PAEDP = pulmonary artery end-diastolic pressure; PASP = pulmonary artery systolic pressure; PDA = patent ductus arteriosus; PR-ED = pulmonary regurgitant end-diastole; PR-peak = pulmonary regurgitation peak; RAP = right atrial pressure; RVAcT = right ventricular acceleration time; RVEDP = right ventricular end-diastolic pressure; RVOT = right ventrivular outflow tract; RVSP = right ventricular systolic pressure; SBP = systolic blood pressure; TR = tricuspid regurgitation; VSD = ventricular septal defect.

Technical Caveats: Tricuspid Regurgitation

Weak TR Signals

Weak TR signals may be enhanced by using contrast agents such as agitated saline, blood-saline contrast or commercial microbubble products. The microbubbles in intravenous contrast agents enhance the echo intensity of the TR signal by creating greater ultrasound reflections. The two traces below show an unenhanced TR signal and a contrast-enhanced TR signal.

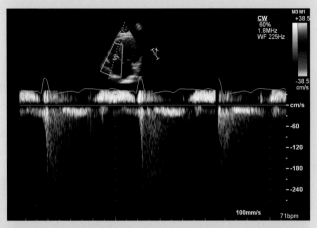

Unenhanced TR Signal

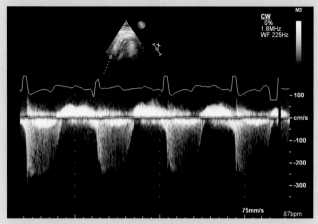

Enhanced TR Signal after Definity™ contrast agent

"Beard" versus the "Chin"

The TR signal below, left shows a "chin" *(blue line)* and a "beard" *(pink line)*. When measuring the peak TR velocity, measurements should be made at the "chin" rather than at the "beard". The "beard" is an effect of intrinsic spectral broadening and/or contribution due to non-laminar flow (e.g. there may be vortices due to mixing of the fast-moving stream of blood with slower moving blood around it). As such measurement of the "beard" will result in an overestimation of the TR velocity and the subsequent RVSP. The "beard" effect can be removed by increasing the reject *(see figure below, right)*. Observe that at a reject setting of 7 the peak TR velocity is much clearer; this velocity corresponds to the "chin" velocity on the adjacent trace.

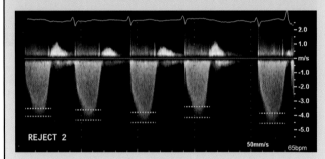

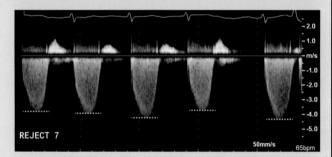

"Free TR"

The systolic still frame below, left was recorded from a parasternal long axis of the RV inflow. This colour flow Doppler image shows low velocity, laminar systolic flow which may be referred to as "free" or "wide-open" TR. The corresponding CW Doppler trace is shown to the right. This is a typical Doppler signal recorded when there is free TR. Observe that the TR velocity is low because the RA and RV are effectively functioning as a single chamber. In this situation, the RVSP cannot be accurately estimated from the peak TR velocity. This is because while the TR velocity will still reflect the pressure difference between the RV and RA in systole, the RAP is unknown and it may be as high as 40 mmHg.

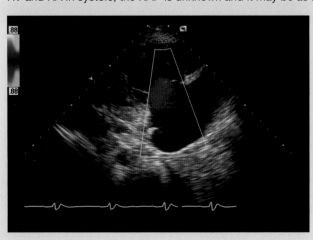

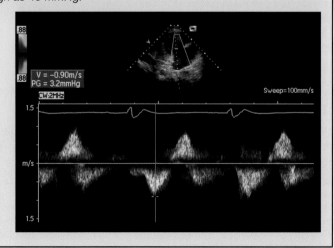

b. RAP via Hepatic Venous Doppler Parameters

The HV flow profile is obtained via pulsed-wave (PW) Doppler from the subcostal window. This flow profile can been used for the estimation of the RAP. In particular, the forward systolic flow velocity is reflective of the RAP; the higher the RAP the lower the pressure gradient between the HV and the RA and, thus, the lower the forward systolic flow velocity.

In addition, measurement of the systolic filling fraction (SFF) has been found to be useful in the estimation of RAP. In particular, a SFF of less than 55% is useful for predicting a mean RAP greater than 8 mm Hg. The SFF is simply the ratio of the systolic velocity (or velocity time integral [VTI]) with respect to the total forward flow velocity (or VTI) (Fig. 4.20):

Equation 4.15

$$SFF = S_{V/VTI} \div (S_{V/VTI} + D_{V/VTI}) \times 100$$

where SFF = systolic filling fraction (%)

$S_{V/VTI}$ = peak systolic velocity (cm/s) or velocity time integral (cm)

$D_{V/VTI}$ = peak diastolic velocity (cm/s) or velocity time integral (cm)

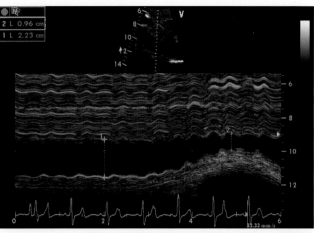

Figure 4.19 From the subcostal view, the M-mode cursor is placed perpendicular to the IVC, just proximal to the junction of IVC with hepatic veins or about 0.5–3 cm proximal to IVC entrance into the right atrium. The IVC is measured, inner edge to inner edge, at end expiration (largest - $IVCD_{max}$) and at end inspiration (smallest - $IVCD_{min}$). From these two measurements the IVC collapsibility index (CI) is calculated. In this example the CI is:

$$CI_{IVC} (\%) = [(IVCD_{max} - IVCD_{min}) \div IVCD_{max}] \times 100$$
$$= [(2.23 - 0.96) \div 2.23] \times 100$$
$$= 57\%$$

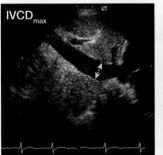
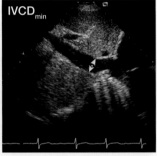

Figure 4.18 From the subcostal view, the IVC is measured perpendicular to its long axis. The IVC is measured, inner edge to inner edge, just proximal to the junction of the IVC with hepatic veins or about 0.5–3 cm proximal to the IVC entrance into the RA. The IVC is measured at end expiration ($IVCD_{max}$) and at end inspiration ($IVCD_{min}$). From these two measurements the CI_{IVC} is calculated via Equation 4.14.

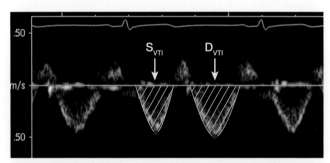

Figure 4.20 From the subcostal view, a 3-5 mm PW Doppler sample volume is placed within the medial hepatic vein. From the HV trace, the peak systolic velocity (or velocity time integral) and the peak diastolic velocity (or velocity time integral) are measured. Measurements are averaged over 5-7 beats or measured at end expiratory apnoea. The SFF is then calculated:

$$SFF = S_{V/VTI} \div (S_{V/VTI} + D_{V/VTI}) \times 100$$

Table 4.15 **Estimation of RAP based on IVC Diameter and Collapse**

Right Atrial Pressure Estimation				
	Normal RAP (0-5 [3] mm Hg)	Intermediate (5-10 [8] mm Hg)		High RAP (15 mm Hg)
IVC diameter	≤ 2.1 cm	≤ 2.1 cm	> 2.1 cm	> 2.1 cm
Collapse with sniff	> 50%	< 50%	> 50%	< 50%
Secondary indices for elevated RAP			• Restrictive filling • Tricuspid E/e' > 6 • Diastolic flow predominance in hepatic veins (SSF ratio < 55%)	

Ranges are provided for low and intermediate categories, but for simplicity, midrange values of 3 mm Hg for normal and 8 mm Hg for intermediate are suggested. Intermediate (8 mm Hg) RAP may be downgraded to normal (3 mm Hg) if no secondary indices of elevated RAP are present, upgraded to high if minimal collapse with sniff (<35%) and secondary indices of elevated RAP are present, or left at 8 mm Hg if uncertain.

IVC = Inferior vena cava; RAP = right atrial pressure; SFF = systolic filling fraction.

Reprinted from Rudski LG, Lai WW, Afilalo J, Hua L, Handschumacher MD, Chandrasekaran K, Solomon SD, Louie EK, Schiller NB. Guidelines for the echocardiographic assessment of the right heart in adults: a report from the American Society of Echocardiography endorsed by the European Association of Echocardiography, a registered branch of the European Society of Cardiology, and the Canadian Society of Echocardiography, *J Am Soc Echocardiogr*, Vol. 23 (7), page 695, © 2010 with permission from Elsevier.

c. RAP via DTI Parameters

Measurement of the tricuspid E to DTI e' ratio may be used in the estimation of the RAP (Fig. 4.21). This method is similar to that which is used in the estimation of LV filling pressures (see Chapter 3). That is, by measuring the peak early diastolic velocity (E) of the trans-tricuspid signal via PW Doppler and by measuring the peak early diastolic myocardial velocity (e') at the lateral RV annulus via DTI, estimation of RAP is possible. An E/e' ratio greater than 6 has a high sensitivity and specificity for predicting a mean RAP greater than or equal to 10 mm Hg.

3. Estimation of the RVSP from a Ventricular Septal Defect

The peak systolic velocity across a ventricular septal defect (VSD) reflects the systolic pressure difference between the LV and RV. Therefore, from the VSD velocity (Fig. 4.22) and from an estimation of the left ventricular systolic pressure (LVSP), it is possible to estimate the RVSP using the following equation:

Equation 4.16

$$RVSP = LVSP - 4\,V_{VSD}^{2}$$

where RVSP = right ventricular systolic pressure (mm Hg)
     LVSP = left ventricular systolic pressure (mm Hg)
     V_{VSD} = peak systolic VSD velocity (m/s)

In the absence of LVOT obstruction or aortic stenosis, it can be assumed that the LVSP is equal to the systolic BP. Therefore,

Equation 4.17

$$RVSP = SBP - 4\,V_{VSD}^{2}$$

where RVSP = right ventricular systolic pressure (mm Hg)
     SBP = systolic blood pressure (mm Hg)
     V_{VSD} = peak systolic VSD velocity (m/s)

4. Estimation of the PASP from a Patent Ductus Arteriosus

The peak systolic velocity across a patent ductus arteriosus (PDA) reflects the systolic pressure difference between the aorta and the PA. Therefore, from the systolic PDA velocity (Fig. 4.23) and from an estimation of the aortic systolic BP, it is possible to estimate the PASP using the following equation:

Equation 4.18

$$PASP = SBP - 4\,V_{PDA}^{2}$$

where PASP = pulmonary artery systolic pressure (mm Hg)
     SBP = systolic blood pressure (mm Hg)
     V_{PDA} = peak systolic PDA velocity (m/s)

5. Estimation of the PAEDP from the PR Signal

The pulmonary regurgitant (PR) velocity reflects the pressure gradient between the PA and the RV during diastole. Therefore, from the end-diastolic PR velocity (Fig. 4.24) and from an estimation of the RV end-diastolic pressure (RVEDP), it is possible to estimate the PAEDP using the following equation:

Equation 4.19

$$PAEDP = 4\,V_{PR\text{-}ED}^{2} + RVEDP$$

where PAEDP = pulmonary artery end-diastolic pressure (mm Hg)
     $V_{PR\text{-}ED}$ = peak end-diastolic velocity of PR signal (m/s)
     RVEDP = right ventricular end-diastolic pressure (mm Hg)

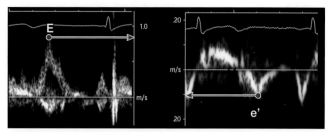

Figure 4.21 From the tricuspid PW Doppler trace *(left)*, the peak early (E) diastolic velocity is measured. The early diastolic velocity (e') is measured from the DTI trace *(right)* with the sample volume placed at the lateral tricuspid annulus. The E/e' ratio is then simply derived from the tricuspid E velocity divided by the DTI e' velocity.

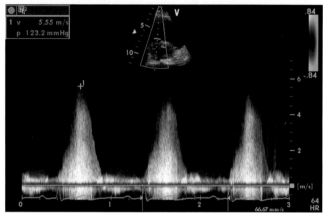

Figure 4.22 The peak systolic VSD velocity is recorded via CW Doppler ensuring parallel alignment with flow. This systolic VSD velocity reflects the pressure difference between the LV and the RV in systole. Using the simplified Bernoulli equation ($4V^2$), the VSD velocity can be converted to a pressure gradient. Therefore, if the VSD velocity is measured and the LV systolic pressure (LVSP) is known then the RVSP can be estimated. In the absence of aortic stenosis or LVOT obstruction, the LVSP can be estimated from the systolic blood pressure (SBP). Assuming a SBP of 150 mm Hg, the RVSP in this example is:

$$
\begin{aligned}
RVSP &= SBP - 4\,V_{VSD}^{2} \\
&= 150 - 4\,(5.55)^2 \\
&= 150 - 123.21 \\
&= 27 \text{ mm Hg}
\end{aligned}
$$

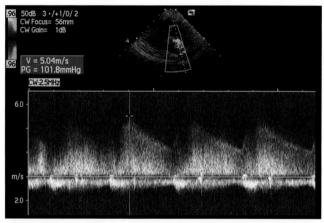

Figure 4.23 The PDA signal is recorded via CW Doppler ensuring a parallel alignment with flow. The peak systolic PDA velocity reflects the pressure difference between the aorta and the pulmonary artery in systole. Using the simplified Bernoulli equation ($4V^2$), the PDA velocity can be converted to a pressure gradient. Therefore, if the systolic PDA velocity is measured and the aortic systolic blood pressure (SBP) is known then the PASP can be estimated. Assuming a SBP of 135 mm Hg, the PASP in this example is:

$$
\begin{aligned}
PASP &= SBP - 4\,V_{PDA}^{2} \\
&= 135 - 4\,(5.04)^2 \\
&= 135 - 101.8 \\
&= 33 \text{ mm Hg}
\end{aligned}
$$

In the absence of tricuspid valve stenosis, it can be assumed that the RVEDP is equal to the RAP; therefore:

Equation 4.20

$$PAEDP = 4\ V_{PR\text{-}ED}^{2} + RAP$$

where PAEDP = pulmonary artery end-diastolic pressure (mmHg)
$V_{PR\text{-}ED}$ = peak end-diastolic velocity of PR signal (m/s)
RAP = mean right atrial pressure (mm Hg)

6. Mean Pulmonary Artery Pressure Estimation

The mPAP can be estimated from the PASP and PAEDP, the right ventricular acceleration time (RVAcT), and the PR and TR signal.

a. mPAP via the PASP and PAEDP

At normal heart rates and assuming diastole accounts for two-thirds of the cardiac cycle and systole accounts for one-third of the cardiac cycle, the mPAP can also be derived from the systolic and diastolic pulmonary pressures:

Equation 4.21

$$mPAP = [(2 \times PAEDP) + PASP] \div 3$$

where mPAP = mean pulmonary artery pressure (mm Hg)
PAEDP = pulmonary artery diastolic pressure (mm Hg)
PASP = pulmonary artery systolic pressure (mm Hg)

b. mPAP via the RVAcT

The right ventricular acceleration time (RVAcT) is measured from the PW Doppler RVOT signal as the time interval between the onset of flow to peak systolic flow (Fig. 4.25). As the PA pressure increases, there is an increase in the resistance of blood flow from the RV into the PA resulting in shortening of the RVAcT. As a general rule, an RVAcT greater than 120 ms is usually associated with normal PA pressures. At heart rates between 60–100 bpm the mPAP can be estimated from the RVAcT via one of the equations below:

Equation 4.22

$$mPAP = 79 - (0.45 \times RVAcT)$$

Equation 4.23

$$mPAP = 90 - (0.62 \times RVAcT)$$

where mPAP = mean pulmonary artery pressure (mm Hg)
RVAcT = right ventricular acceleration time (ms)

c. mPAP via the PR Signal

Estimation of the mPAP from the PR signal is based on the assumption that the PR velocity at early diastole corresponds to the dicrotic notch on the PA pressure trace. The dicrotic notch on this trace reflects the closure of the pulmonary valve and the end of RV ejection. It has been shown that the dicrotic notch pressure is a similar magnitude to mPAP. Hence, as the dicrotic notch reflects mPAP and as the peak PR pressure gradient corresponds to the pressure at the dicrotic notch (Fig. 4.26), the mPAP can be estimated from peak early diastolic PR velocity (Fig. 4.27). Furthermore, adding the RAP to this derived pressure improves the correlation between the actual mPAP and the Doppler-estimated mPAP:

Equation 4.24

$$mPAP = 4\ V_{PR\text{-}peak}^{2} + RAP$$

where mPAP = mean pulmonary artery pressure (mm Hg)
$V_{PR\text{-}peak}$ = peak early diastolic PR velocity (m/s)
RAP = right atrial pressure (mm Hg)

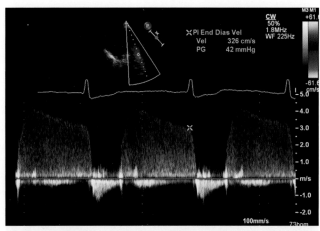

Figure 4.24 The PR velocity is recorded via CW Doppler ensuring a parallel alignment with flow. The PR velocity reflects the pressure difference between the pulmonary artery and the right ventricle in diastole. Using the simplified Bernoulli equation ($4V^2$), the PR velocity can be converted to a pressure gradient. When the PR velocity at end-diastole is measured and the RAP is known then the PAEDP can be estimated. Assuming a RAP of 3 mm Hg, the PAEDP in this example is:

$$PAEDP = 4\ V_{PR\text{-}ED}^{2} + RAP$$
$$= 4\ (3.26)^2 + 3$$
$$= 42.51 + 3$$
$$= 46\ mmHg$$

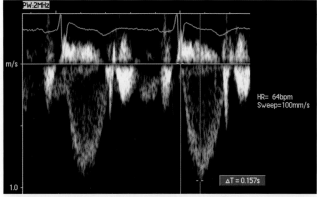

Figure 4.25 The RVAcT is derived via PW Doppler. A 3-5 mm sample volume is placed within the right ventricular outflow tract just proximal to the pulmonary valve from the parasternal short axis view or the parasternal long axis view of the RVOT. The RVAcT is measured as the time interval from the beginning of the RVOT signal to the peak velocity of this signal. From the RVAcT in this example, the mPAP is:
$$mPAP = 79 - (0.45 \times RVAcT)$$
$$= 79 - (0.45 \times 157)$$
$$= 8\ mmHg$$

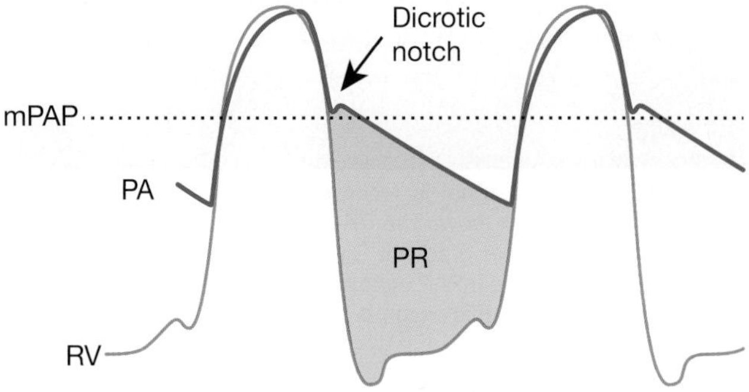

Figure 4.26 This schematic shows the right ventricular (RV) and pulmonary artery (PA) pressure curves. The dicrotic notch indicates closure of the pulmonary valve and the end of RV ejection. Pulmonary regurgitation (PR) reflects the pressure difference between the PA and RV over diastole (shaded area). The peak PR pressure difference between the PA and RV occurs in early diastole and this corresponds to the dicrotic notch.

d. mPAP via the TR Signal

The mPAP can also be estimated from the RV-to-RA mean systolic gradient. The RV-to-RA mean systolic gradient is derived by tracing the VTI of the TR jet (Fig. 4.28). The mPAP is calculated as:

Equation 4.25

$$mPAP = \Delta P_{mRV\text{-}RA} + RAP$$

where mPAP   = mean pulmonary artery pressure (mm Hg)
$\Delta P_{mRV\text{-}RA}$ = mean RV-to-RA pressure gradient (mm Hg)
RAP   = right atrial pressure (mm Hg)

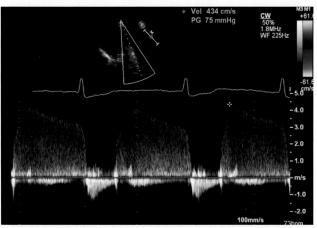

Figure 4.27 The PR velocity is recorded via CW Doppler ensuring parallel alignment with flow. The PR velocity reflects the pressure difference between the pulmonary artery and the RV in diastole. Using the simplified Bernoulli equation (4V²), the PR velocity can be converted to a pressure gradient. When the PR velocity in early diastole is measured and the RAP is known then the mPAP can be estimated. Assuming a RAP of 3 mm Hg, the mPAP in this example is:

$$mPAP = 4\,V_{PR\text{-}peak}^{2} + RAP$$
$$= 4\,(4.34)^2 + 3$$
$$= 75.34 + 3$$
$$= 78\ mmHg$$

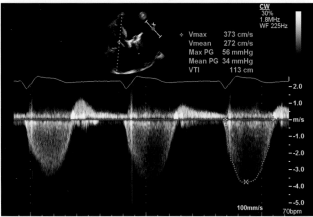

Figure 4.28 The TR signal is recorded via CW Doppler ensuring parallel alignment with flow. The TR signal is traced to derive the mean systolic RV-to-RA gradient. By adding the RAP to this mean gradient (Mean PG), the mPAP can be estimated. Assuming a RAP of 3 mm Hg, the mPAP in this example is:

$$mPAP = \Delta P_{mRV\text{-}RA} + RAP$$
$$= 34 + 3$$
$$= 37\ mmHg$$

Limitations of Estimation of Pulmonary Pressures

The accuracy of intracardiac pressure estimation is dependent upon the accurate measurement of the peak velocities. Errors in peak velocity measurements are mostly related to the intercept angle between the ultrasound beam and the direction of blood flow. The maximum velocities are measured when the ultrasound beam is aligned parallel to the direction of blood flow. Therefore, it is crucial to ensure parallel alignment with flow. This may require the use of off-axis imaging.

Underestimation of the RV-to-RA pressure gradient may also occur due to inherent limitations of the simplified Bernoulli equation. The simplified Bernoulli equation assumes that viscous friction and flow acceleration are negligible (see Chapter 1). In the case of eccentric wall jets viscous losses due to increased viscous friction may occur. In addition some clinical conditions result in increased blood viscosity. Therefore, when there is impingement of the jet by chamber walls or when viscosity is increased, the pressure gradient between the RV and RA will be underestimated.

Estimation of the RVSP from VSD velocities or the PASP from PDA signals requires the measurement of the BP and therefore, errors in BP measurement will also affect the accuracy of the RVSP/PASP estimations. In particular, BP errors of $\geq$ 5-10 mmHg are common.

The RVAcT for the estimation of the mPAP is only accurate at heart rates between 60-100 bpm.

The RAP estimation based on the IVC diameter and collapsibility may be difficult when there are suboptimal subcostal windows. Furthermore, in normal young athletes the IVC may be dilated in the presence of normal RAP; therefore, using the IVC diameter and collapsibility will result in an overestimation of the RAP. In these instances, it is recommended that the IVC diameter and collapsibility be reassessed in the left lateral position. In ventilated patients, the IVC is commonly dilated and may not collapse so it should not be used to estimate RA pressure. However, in these patients an IVC diameter $\leq$ 12 mm appears accurate in identifying patients with a RAP of less than 10 mm Hg.

Limitations to the estimation of the RAP via the SFF may also be encountered. In particular, HV Doppler signals are difficult to obtain when there are suboptimal subcostal windows. Severe TR with coexistent systolic flow reversal also limits the use of the SFF in the estimation of the RAP. In addition, in patients with atrial fibrillation reduced systolic forward flow may be seen irrespective of the RAP. HV systolic forward flow is also dependent on other factors besides RAP; for example, systolic forward flow is also dependent on RA relaxation and compliance, and tricuspid annular descent.

RAP can also be estimated from tricuspid E to DTI e' ratio. A limitation of this technique is based on the fact that the tricuspid E and DTI e' velocities are not measured simultaneously; therefore variations in the R-R interval is a limitation of this variable for the estimation of the RAP. Also this ratio is not accurate in ventilated patients and has not been validated in patients with atrial fibrillation.

Estimation of Pulmonary Vascular Resistance

PVR can be defined as the resistance offered by the pulmonary vasculature which must overcome to push blood through the lungs. In PHTN, elevated PVR occurs due to pulmonary vascular disease. It is important to note that increased PA pressures does not equal an elevated PVR as increased PA pressures can also result from high pulmonary flow. This concept can be better appreciated by the relationship between pressure, flow and resistance:

Equation 4.26

$$\Delta P = Q \times R$$

where ΔP = pressure difference (mm Hg)
    Q   = flow rate (L/min)
    R   = resistance (mm Hg/L/min)

From this equation it can be appreciated that increased PA pressures can result from high pulmonary flow rates or increased resistance to pulmonary flow (that is, increased PVR).

Several methods have been described for the calculation of the PVR using echocardiography (Table 4.16). Of these methods, the one that is most commonly employed is the ratio of the peak TR velocity (TR_V) and the VTI of the RVOT ($RVOT_{VTI}$) (Fig. 4.29). This method is based on the substitution of the TR_V for the transpulmonary gradient (mPAP – PCWP) and the $RVOT_{VTI}$ for the CO. It can be appreciated that when PVR increases, the TR_V (and RVSP) increases in order to overcome the forces opposing pulmonary valve opening and the $RVOT_{VTI}$ decreases as premature deceleration of pulmonary flow occurs; this leads to a decreased RV ejection time and ultimately reduced pulmonary blood flow. Thus, an increase in the $TR_V/RVOT_{VTI}$ ratio is expected when there is an increase in the PVR. The PVR can be estimated from the application of the following equation:

Equation 4.27

$$PVR = [(TR_V \div RVOT_{VTI}) \times 10] + 0.16$$

where PV   = pulmonary vascular resistance (mm Hg/L/min)
    TR_V = peak systolic TR velocity (m/s)
    $RVOT_{VTI}$ = right ventricular outflow tract VTI (cm)

While the estimation of the PVR by this equation is able to distinguish normal from abnormal PVR, it underestimates high PVR. Possible reasons for underestimation of a high PVR in patients with severe PHTN may include the inability of TR velocity to act as a surrogate for the transpulmonary gradient as it does not take into account the mean RAP which may be markedly elevated. Furthermore, abnormal septal displacement towards the LV due to RV dilatation may result in increased LV filling pressures so these pressures should also be considered in the estimation of PVR in patients with severe PHTN. Based on these assumptions an alternate equation has been proposed to estimate the PVR in these patients:

Equation 4.28

$$PVR = (RVSP - E/e') \div RVOT_{VTI}$$

where PVR   = pulmonary vascular resistance (mm Hg/L/min)
       RVSP   = right ventricular systolic pressure (mm Hg)
       E/e'   = mitral E to medial mitral DTI e' ratio (unitless)
       $RVOT_{VTI}$ = right ventricular outflow tract VTI (cm)

When to Estimate PVR by echo:
- Not routinely
- In patients where PASP measurements may be misleadingly low, despite increased PVR, due to low stroke volume (e.g. severe RV dysfunction)
- In patients where PASP measurements may be misleadingly high, despite a normal PVR, due to high flow rates (e.g. high cardiac output states)

How to estimate PVR:
- Use ratio ($TR_V/RVOT_{VTI}$) rather than a specific PVR value to identify normal versus abnormal PVR ($TR_V/RVOT_{VTI} > 0.2 \approx$ PVR > 2 Wood Units [WU])

Important Note:
- The echo-derived PVR should not be used as a substitute for the invasive evaluation of PVR when this value is important to guide therapy.

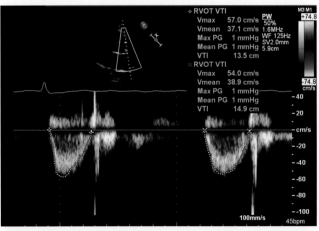 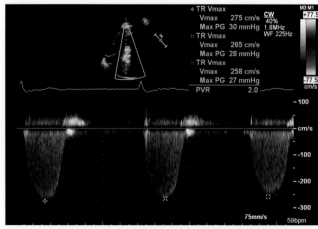

Figure 4.29 The PVR is estimated from the peak TR velocity and the RVOT signal. From the PW Doppler RVOT trace *(left)* the RVOT VTI (cm) is measured. From the CW Doppler tracing of TR *(right)* the peak TR velocity (m/s) is averaged over respiration. PVR in this example is estimated as:

$PVR = [(TR_V \div RVOT_{VTI}) \times 10] + 0.16$
    $= (2.66 \div 14.2) \times 10 + 0.16$
    $= 2.0\ WU$

Table 4.16 Selected Doppler Methods for Estimation of Pulmonary Vascular Resistance

Measurements Required	Formula for PVR (WU)	r	Pt. No.	Ref.
Functional pre-ejection period [PEP] (ms): time interval between the onset of TR and pulmonary systolic flow # **Acceleration time [AcT] (ms):** time interval between the onset of ejection to the time of peak RVOT velocity **Total systolic time [TT] (ms):** summation of PEP and ejection time (ET) where ET is the time interval between the onset and end of the systolic RVOT/PV flow	$PVR = 0.156 + 1.154 \times ([PEP \div AcT] \div TT)$	0.96	63	1
RVOT VTI (cm): traced from the PW Doppler signal **TRv (m/s):** highest TR velocity via CW Doppler	$PVR \approx TRv \div RVOT_{VTI}$ § When ratio >0.175 & <0.275: • $PVR = (TRv \div RVOT_{VTI}) \times 10$ When ratio > 0.275: • $PVR = (TRv^2 \div RVOT_{VTI}) \times 5$	0.76	150	2
Velocity propagation [Vp] (cm/s): colour M-mode flow propagation in the main pulmonary artery during systole	$PVR \approx Vp$ **Regression equation:** $PVR = -1.71 \times Vp + 26$	0.90	11	3
mPAP (mm Hg): derived from the PAEDP (estimated from the PR velocity) and PASP (estimated from the TR velocity + RAP) **Pulmonary capillary wedge pressure [PCWP] (mm Hg):** assumed to be 9 mmHg **Cardiac output [CO] (L/min):** derived from the LVOT diameter (cm²) and LVOT VTI (cm)	$PVR = (mPAP - PCWP) \div CO$	0.92 * 0.93**	52 * 15**	4
RVOT VTI (cm): traced from the PW Doppler signal **PASP (mm Hg):** estimated from TR velocity + RAP	$PVRI \approx (PASP \div [HR \times RVOT_{VTI}])$ ψ	0.86	51	5
RVOT VTI (cm): traced from the PW Doppler signal **RVSP (mm Hg):** estimated from TR velocity + RAP **E/e':** mitral E velocity divided by the medial DTI e' velocity	$PVR = (RVSP - E/e') \div RVOT_{VTI}$	0.81^ 0.88^^	42	6

Functional PEP estimated as interval between the onset of TR and the onset of pulmonary systolic flow rather than the total duration of TR. Total duration of TR may overestimate PEP in the presence of elevated PASP and PVR, as TR may continue after the premature closure of the pulmonary valve (i.e., the premature completion of the ejection period).
§ Ratio > 0.175 PVR likely > 2 WU; ratio > 0.275 PVR likely > 6 WU
* Comparison between catheter haemodynamic assessment and non-simultaneous Doppler echo data;
** Comparison between catheter haemodynamic assessment and simultaneous Doppler echo data.
ψ PVRI (WU/m²) = PVR indexed where cardiac output indexed to body surface area; threshold >0.076 PVRI likely > 15 WU/m²
^ When PCWP ≤ 15 mm Hg; ^^ when PCWP > 15 mm Hg

References: [1] Scapellato F, Temporelli PL, Eleuteri E, et al. Accurate noninvasive estimation of pulmonary vascular resistance by Doppler echocardiography in patients with chronic heart failure. *J Am Coll Cardiol* 2001;37:1813-9; [2] Abbas AE, Franey LM, Marwick T, et al. Noninvasive assessment of pulmonary vascular resistance by Doppler echocardiography. *J Am Soc Echocardiogr.* 2013 Oct;26(10):1170-7. [3] Shandas R, Weinberg C, Ivy DD, et al. Development of a noninvasive ultrasound color M-mode means of estimating pulmonary vascular resistance in pediatric pulmonary hypertension: mathematical analysis, in vitro validation, and preliminary clinical studies. *Circulation* 2001;104: 908-13; [4] Selimovic N, Rundqvist B, Bergh CH, Andersson B, Petersson S, Johansson L, Bech-Hanssen O. Assessment of pulmonary vascular resistance by Doppler echocardiography in patients with pulmonary arterial hypertension. *J Heart Lung Transplant* 2007;26:927-34; [5] Haddad F, Zamanian R, Beraud AS, Schnittger I, Feinstein J, Peterson T, Yang P, Doyle R, Rosenthal D. A Novel Non-Invasive Method of Estimating Pulmonary Vascular Resistance in Patients With Pulmonary Arterial Hypertension. *J Am Soc Echocardiogr.* 2009; 22:523-9; [6] Dahiya A, Vollbon W, Jellis C, Prior D, Wahi S, Marwick T. Echocardiographic assessment of raised pulmonary vascular resistance: application to diagnosis and follow-up of pulmonary hypertension. *Heart.* 2010 Dec;96(24):2005-9.

Other Echo Signs Suggestive of PHTN

The detection of elevated TR velocities, and the resultant elevated RVSP, is most commonly used to establish the diagnosis of PHTN. However, TR velocities can be overestimated or underestimated due to various technical and physiological factors. Therefore, it is important to identify other echocardiographic signs to support the diagnosis of PHTN.

Various 2D, M-mode and spectral Doppler signs associated with PHTN along with the likely cause of each sign are summarised in Table 4.17 and illustrated in figures 4.30 to 4.35.

RV Size and Systolic Function

RV dilatation, RV hypertrophy and RV systolic dysfunction are the most common functional and morphological changes seen in patients with chronic PHTN (Fig. 4.36).

RV dimensions can be readily measured from the parasternal, apical 4-chamber, or subcostal views (see Chapter 2). RV wall thickness can be measured from the subcostal view (Fig. 4.32). RV systolic function can be evaluated via various methods such as the RV fractional area change, tricuspid annular plane systolic excursion (TAPSE), tissue Doppler myocardial velocities (s' velocity) and the RV myocardial performance index (RV MPI) (see Chapter 2). When assessing RV systolic function, more than one measure of systolic function should be considered to more reliably distinguish normal from abnormal function.

Tricuspid Regurgitation

The aetiology of TR in PHTN includes dilatation of the tricuspid valve annulus, increased RV systolic pressures (the tricuspid valve is not "designed" to sustain high pressures) or a combination of both (Fig. 4.37).

When assessing the severity of TR, an integrated approach incorporating 2D imaging, spectral Doppler and colour flow Doppler imaging should be employed (see Chapter 9).

Table 4.17 **Various Echocardiographic Signs suggesting PHTN**

M-mode and 2D Signs of PHTN	Likely Cause
Mid-systolic notching of pulmonary valve on M-mode (Fig. 4.30)	Transient elevation of PA pressure above RV pressure causes an abrupt mid systolic deceleration of flow.
Absent *a* wave on pulmonary valve M-mode trace (Fig. 4.30)	Elevated PAEDP.
Mid-systolic notching of aortic valve on M-mode (Fig. 4.31)	A low cardiac output with normal LV size, a hyperdynamic IVS and distortion of LV geometry.
RV hypertrophy (Fig. 4.32)	Response to chronic RV pressure overload.
Dilatation of the RV (Fig. 4.33 & 4.34)	Reduced systolic function results in an increased RV size in order to increase preload in an attempt to maintain forward stroke volume.
Abnormal displacement of the interventricular septum (IVS) and a D-shaped LV with reduced diastolic and systolic volumes (Fig. 4.33 & 4.34)	Chronic elevation in systolic and diastolic RV pressures result in progressive RVH and RV dilatation. As the RV becomes more spherical, its cross-sectional area increases resulting in flattening of the IVS and subsequent distortion of the LV.
Dilatation of the RA and coronary sinus IVC dilatation with reduced or absent collapse on inspiration	Chronic RA pressure overload.
Spectral Doppler Signs of PHTN	Likely Cause
↓ RVAcT <100 ms (Fig. 4.35)	↑ PVR causes rapid acceleration of flow into the pulmonary artery in systole (also related to mPAP – see equations 4.22 & 4.23).
Mid-systolic notching or cessation of RV outflow tract flow (Fig. 4.35)	Comparable to the mid-systolic notching seen on the pulmonary valve M-mode trace.
↑PR velocity	↑ pulmonary pressures (reflects the increased pressure gradient between the PA and RV in diastole).
↑TR velocity at time of pulmonary valve opening	↑ RV diastolic pressure.

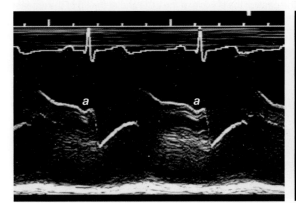 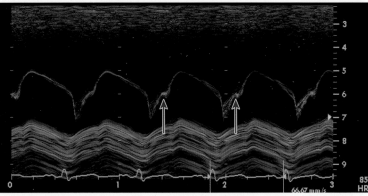

Figure 4.30 Pulmonary valve M-mode may be recorded from the parasternal short axis view. The M-mode to the left shows normal pulmonary valve motion. The *a* wave refers to the small posterior deflection following atrial contraction; this reflects the extra bolus of blood being ejected into the RV which slightly increases the RV pressure at this time and causes the pulmonary valve to move into the pulmonary root. Note that during systole, the pulmonary valve shows a gradual anterior and linear motion; this reflects the gradual decline in the RV pressure resulting in the pulmonary valve moving towards the centre of the pulmonary root. The M-mode trace on the right shows mid-systolic notching (*arrows*) of the pulmonary valve in a patient with PHTN. This mid-systolic notching is caused by an abrupt mid-systolic deceleration of flow. Also note the absence of an *a* wave on this trace. An absent *a* wave (or diminished *a* wave) occurs when the PAEDP is much greater than the RVEDP so that even with atrial contraction, the resultant increase in the RVEDP is still well below the PAEDP. Therefore, there is little or no movement of the pulmonary valve following atrial contraction and this is reflected on the M-mode trace by a very small or absent *a* wave.

Additional Echo Findings associated with PHTN
Additional 2D echo findings associated with PHTN include mitral valve prolapse (MVP) and pericardial effusions.
MVP is related to a small LV and possible involvement of leaflets affected by associated connective tissue disorders. Pericardial effusions occur due to impaired venous and lymphatic drainage secondary to elevated right heart pressures.

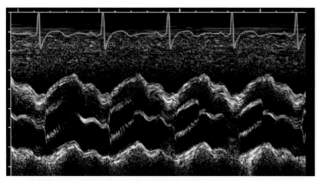 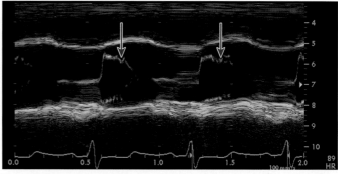

Figure 4.31 The M-mode to the left shows normal aortic valve motion. Observe that with the onset of systole, the aortic valve leaflets snap open with both leaflets remaining parallel to the aortic walls throughout systole. With the onset of diastole, the leaflets close abruptly and coapt in the centre of the aortic root. This motion of the aortic leaflets over the cardiac cycle forms a characteristic "box" within the aortic root. The M-mode trace on the right shows mid-systolic notching *(arrows)* of the aortic valve in a patient with PHTN. This mid-systolic notching may be seen when there is a low cardiac output with normal LV size, a hyperdynamic IVS and distortion of LV geometry.

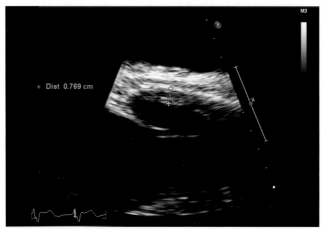 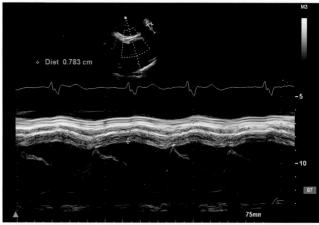

Figure 4.32 From the subcostal 4-chamber view, RV wall thickness is measured at the peak of the R wave of the ECG and at the tip of the anterior tricuspid valve leaflet. The 2D (left) and M-mode (right) measurements of the RV free wall are consistent with significant hypertrophy of the RV.

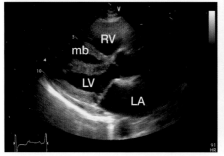 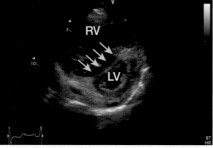 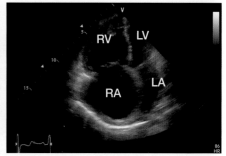

Figure 4.33 The image on the left is a parasternal long axis view of the LV: observe the hypertrophied moderator band (mb), a small pericardial effusion posterior to the LV and marked dilatation of the right ventricle (RV). The middle image is a parasternal short axis view of the LV: this image shows systolic flattening of the IVS *(arrows)* and marked dilatation of the RV; flattening of the IVS results in a D-shaped appearance of the LV in this view. The image on the right is an apical 4-chamber view: observe the marked dilatation of the RV and right atrium (RA), a small pericardial effusion superior to the RA and distortion of the LV and left atrium (LA).

Measurement of RV Wall Thickness

RV wall thickness can be measured using either M-mode or 2D imaging. RV free wall thickness can be measured from the apical and parasternal long axis views, however, measurements obtained from the subcostal view are more accurate. This is because from the subcostal views RV wall thickness is measured along the axis of the beam (axial resolution is superior to lateral resolution) and because the epicardial border is usually easier to identify from these views.

From the parasternal views, the RV is in very close proximity to the chest wall. As such reverberation artefacts in the near field may obscure the epicardial border of the anterior RV wall. In addition, the echogenicity of the chest wall and the anterior RV wall are very similar so distinction between the epicardium of the anterior RV wall and the chest wall may be very difficult. From the apical views, RV wall thickness is measured across the width of the ultrasound beam in the lateral imaging plane (lateral resolution is generally poorer than the axial resolution).

A normal RV free wall thickness is 2-3 mm; a thickness > 5 mm is considered abnormal.

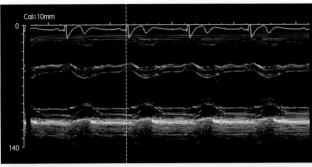
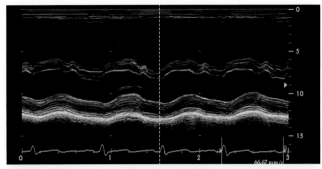

Figure 4.34 Both of the traces shown were recorded from the parasternal long axis view of the LV; the yellow line identifies end-diastole. The M-mode trace on the left was recorded from a normal heart. Observe that the IVS moves anteriorly towards the RV at end-diastole. The M-mode trace on the right was obtained from a patient with PHTN. Observe that at end-diastole the IVS is displaced posteriorly instead of moving anteriorly. This paradoxical IVS motion occurs when the RV diastolic pressure is significantly higher than the LV diastolic pressure. Also observe the marked dilatation of the RV on this trace.

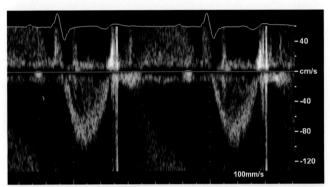
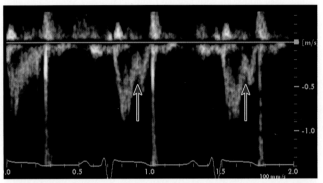

Figure 4.35 Both of these traces were recorded via PW Doppler with the sample volume placed within the RVOT. The trace on the left shows a normal RVOT trace. Observe the rounded, symmetric contour of this signal. This reflects a gradual acceleration and deceleration of flow with a rounded peak occurring in mid systole. The RVAcT was measured at 160 ms. The trace on the right was obtained from a patient with PHTN. Observe the triangular shape of this signal. This reflects a rapid acceleration of flow with the peak occurring in early systole followed by a rapid deceleration of flow which occurs because of a high afterload (PVR). The RVAcT was measured at 74 ms. Also note the presence of mid-systolic notching *(arrows)*. As for the mid-systolic notching of the pulmonary valve on the M-mode trace, mid-systolic notching of the RVOT Doppler trace is caused by an abrupt mid-systolic deceleration of flow.

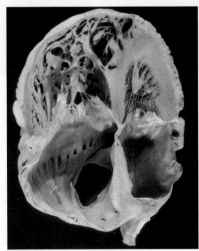
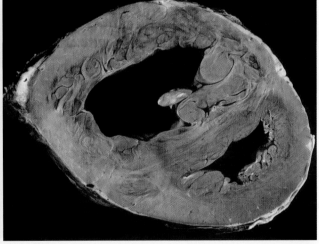

Figure 4.36 These gross pathological specimens are from two different patients with pulmonary hypertension. *Left:* This specimen shows a four-chamber orientation. *Right:* This specimen is a short axis cut through both ventricles. Marked dilatation of the right heart chambers and marked thickening of the right ventricular (RV) wall is seen in both specimens; also observe that the apex is now formed by the RV (*left*). On the short axis cut there is marked distortion of the left ventricle (LV) due to RV dilatation and increased RV mass; this creates the D-shaped LV appearance seen on 2D echocardiography. By permission of Mayo Foundation for Medical Education and Research. All rights reserved. Courtesy of William D. Edwards, MD.

LV Systolic Function in PHTN
Abnormal IVS motion secondary to PHTN is usually associated with a decrease in LV diastolic and systolic volumes. In the absence of left heart disease, LV systolic function is generally preserved. However, because of the distorted LV shape, measurements of the fractional shortening (FS) and ejection fraction (EF) by linear measurements may not accurately reflect overall LV systolic function as these measurements only account for the LV dimensions in one plane.
In patients with PHTN, the Simpson's EF should be attempted to estimate the LV EF. However, because it is often difficult to obtain an on-axis apical 2-chamber in these patients, a Simpson's EF from the apical 4-chamber view is often sufficient.

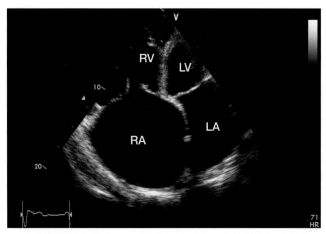
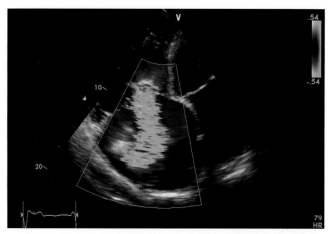

Figure 4.37 The image on the left is a mid-systolic frame recorded from an apical 4-chamber view. Observe the marked dilatation of the right atrium (RA) and right ventricle (RV) with a relatively smaller left ventricle (LV). Also observe that the tricuspid valve leaflets fail to coapt during systole; this is due to the marked dilatation of the tricuspid annulus. The interatrial septum also bows towards the left atrium (LA); this indicates a marked increase in the RAP during ventricular systole. The image on the right is the corresponding colour flow Doppler image. As expected, there is a large TR colour jet area into the RA. In addition, flow convergence on the RV side of the tricuspid valve is noted which is also consistent with signifcant TR.

Prognostic Variables

Several echocardiographic indices have been reported to offer prognostic value for patients with PAH (Table 4.18). Therefore, these indices should be assessed in the echocardiographic examination for all patients with PAH.

A frequent cause of death in PAH is RV failure (RVF). RVF occurs due to a combination of diastolic and systolic dysfunction. Systolic dysfunction occurs due to chronic pressure overload of the RV. Diastolic RV dysfunction is thought to be related to RV hypertrophy and/or chronic pressure overload. Therefore, RV dysfunction is an important variable in determining prognosis. Indices such as TAPSE and RV MPI reflect RV function and, thus, may be useful predictors of adverse outcome in patients with PAH. RV MPI is measured from the IVCT, IVRT and ET (see Chapter 2).

TAPSE has also been reported as a predictor of survival in PAH. TAPSE is measured via M-mode from the lateral tricuspid annulus (see Chapter 2). The presence of any degree of pericardial effusion has also been shown to be a predictor of mortality. Typically, patients with PAH and an associated pericardial effusion tend to have more severe PHTN with increased RAP. It is thought that pericardial effusions in patients with PAH occurs due to impaired venous and lymphatic drainage resulting from elevated RAP.

RA enlargement is another echocardiographic abnormality that reflects the severity of right heart failure and predicts adverse outcomes in patients with severe PAH. The RA area is traced from an apical 4-chamber view at end-systole; this area is then corrected (indexed) for height.

The left ventricular eccentricity index (EI) was originally described as a method of quantifying the abnormal IVS curvature in RV pressure and volume overload states. From the parasternal short axis view at the level of the papillary muscles, this index is derived from the LV cavity dimensions measured parallel and perpendicular to the IVS (Fig. 4.38). From these two measurements, the EI is derived:

Equation 4.29

$$EI = D_2 \div D_1$$

where EI = eccentricity index (unitless)

   D_1 = LV cavity dimension perpendicular to the IVS (cm)
   D_2 = LV cavity dimension parallel to the IVS (cm)

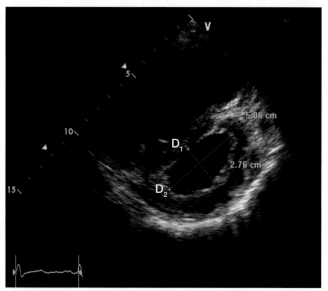

Figure 4.38 The LV diastolic eccentricity index (EI) is measured from the parasternal short axis view at the level of the papillary muscles at end-diastole. The LV cavity is measured parallel to the IVS (D_2) and perpendicular to the IVS (D_1). The diastolic EI in this example is:

$$EI = D_2 \div D_1$$
$$= 5.06 \div 2.76$$
$$= 1.83$$

Table 4.18 Echocardiographic Prognostic Variables in PAH

	Better prognosis	Worse prognosis	Ref.
RV MPI	< 0.83	≥ 0.83^	1
	< 0.98	≥ 0.98*	2
TAPSE (cm) + EI	>1.8 + <1.7	≤1.5 + ≥1.7	3
Pericardial effusion	None	Present	2, 4, 5
RA Area index (cm²/m)	< 5	> 5	4

^ patients with idiopathic PAH; * patients with PAH due to any cause.

References: [1] Yeo TC, Dujardin KS, Tei C, et al. *Am J Cardiol* 1998;81: 1157–1161; **[2]** Brierre G, Blot-Souletie N, Degano B, et al. *Eur J Echocardiogr.* 2010 Jul;11(6):516-22; **[3]** Ghio S, Klersy C, Magrini G, et al. Prognostic relevance of the echocardiographic assessment of right ventricular function in patients with idiopathic pulmonary arterial hypertension. *Int J Cardiol.* 2010 Apr 30;140(3):272-8; **[4]** Raymond RJ, Hinderliter AL, Willis PW, et al. *J Am Coll Cardiol* 2002; 39:1214–1219; **[5]** Eysmann SB, Palevsky HI, Reichek N, et al. *Circulation* 1989; 80:353–360.

Key Points

Systemic Hypertension

- Systemic hypertension (HTN) is commonly defined as a systolic BP ≥ 140 mm Hg and a diastolic BP > 90 mm Hg.
- HTN is classified as essential (unknown cause) or secondary (identifiable underlying cause).
- Role of echocardiography in HTN includes:
    1. Determining the presence and degree of LVH
    2. Assessment of LV systolic and diastolic function
    3. Excluding identifiable causes of HTN
    4. Identifying other cardiac anomalies associated with hypertensive heart disease.
- An increase in the LV wall thickness does not always relate to HTN. Other causes for increased LV wall thickness include infiltrative heart disease, various storage diseases and acute myocarditis.

Pulmonary Hypertension

- Pulmonary hypertension (PHTN) is defined as a mPAP > 25 mm Hg at rest.
- PTHN is classified based on: (1) pathophysiologic mechanisms, clinical presentation, and therapeutic options, and/or (2) haemodynamic consequences of vascular changes in the pulmonary circulation (i.e. pre-capillary versus post-capillary).
- Important cardiac causes of PHTN include left heart disease and congenital heart diseases.
- The role of echocardiography in PHTN includes:
    1. Identifying possible causes of PHTN
    2. Estimation of pulmonary pressures
    3. Recognition of elevated pulmonary vascular resistance
    4. Assessment of functional and morphologic cardiac sequelae of PHTN
    5. Identifying and determining prognostic variables

Further Reading (listed in alphabetical order)

Systemic Hypertension

Definitions and Pathophysiology

Chobanian AV, Bakris GL, Black HR, Cushman WC, Green LA, Izzo JL Jr, Jones D Wet al. Joint National Committee on Prevention, Detection, Evaluation, and Treatment of High Blood Pressure. National Heart, Lung, and Blood Institute; National High Blood Pressure Education Program Coordinating Committee. Seventh report of the Joint National Committee on Prevention, Detection, Evaluation, and Treatment of High Blood Pressure. *Hypertension.* 2003 Dec;42(6):1206-52.

Mancia G, De Backer G, Dominiczak A, Cifkova R, Fagard R, Germano G, et al. 2007 Guidelines for the management of arterial hypertension: The Task Force for the Management of Arterial Hypertension of the European Society of Hypertension (ESH) and of the European Society of Cardiology (ESC). *Eur Heart J.* 2007 Jun;28(12):1462-536.

Oparil S, Zaman MA, Calhoun DA. Pathogenesis of hypertension. *Ann Intern Med.* 2003 Nov 4;139(9):761-76.

Singh M, Mensah GA, Bakris G. Pathogenesis and clinical physiology of hypertension. *Cardiol Clin.* 2010 Nov;28(4):545-59.

Left Ventricular Mass/Hypertrophy

de Simone G, Devereux RB, Daniels SR, Koren MJ, Meyer RA, Laragh JH. Effect of growth on variability of left ventricular mass: assessment of allometric signals in adults and children and their capacity to predict cardiovascular risk. *J Am Coll Cardiol.* 1995 Apr;25(5):1056-62.

Ganau A, Devereux RB, Roman MJ, de Simone G, Pickering TG, Saba PS, Vargiu P, Simongini I, Laragh JH. Patterns of left ventricular hypertrophy and geometric remodeling in essential hypertension. *J Am Coll Cardiol.* 1992 Jun;19(7):1550-8.

Lang RM, Bierig M, Devereux RB, Flachskampf FA, Foster E, Pellikka PA, Picard MH, et al. Chamber Quantification Writing Group; American Society of Echocardiography's Guidelines and Standards Committee; European Association of Echocardiography. Recommendations for Chamber Quantification: A Report from the American Society of Echocardiography's Guidelines and Standards Committee and the Chamber Quantification Writing Group, Developed in Conjunction with the European Association of Echocardiography, a Branch of the European Society of Cardiology. *J Am Soc Echocardiogr.* 2005 Dec;18(12):1440-63.

Myerson SG, Montgomery HE, World MJ, Pennell DJ. Left ventricular mass: reliability of M-mode and 2-dimensional echocardiographic formulas. *Hypertension.* 2002 Nov;40(5):673-8.

Schiller NB, Shah PM, Crawford M, DeMaria A, Devereux R, Feigenbaum H, Gutgesell H, Reichek N, Sahn D, Schnittger I, et al. Recommendations for quantitation of the left ventricle by two-dimensional echocardiography: American Society of Echocardiography committee on standards, subcommittee on quantitation of two-dimensional echocardiograms. *J Am Soc Echocardiogr.* 1989 Sep-Oct;2(5):358-67.

Mid-diastolic Flow

Keren G , Meisner JS , Sherez J , Yellin EL , Laniado S . Interrelationship of mid-diastolic mitral valve motion, pulmonary venous flow, and transmitral flow . *Circulation.* 1986 Jul;74(1):36-44.

Lam CS, Han L, Ha JW, Oh JK, Ling LH. The mitral L wave: A marker of pseudonormal filling and predictor of heart failure in patients with left ventricular hypertrophy. *J Am Soc Echocardiogr.* 2005 Apr;18(4):336-41.

Pulmonary Hypertension

Definitions and Pathophysiology

Badesch DB, Champion HC, Sanchez MA, Hoeper MM, Loyd JE, Manes A, McGoon M, Naeije R, Olschewski H, Oudiz RJ, Torbicki A. Diagnosis and Assessment of Pulmonary Arterial Hypertension. *J Am Coll Cardiol.* 2009 Jun 30;54(1 Suppl):S55-66.

Galiè N, Hoeper MM, Humbert M, Torbicki A, Vachiery JL, Barbera JA, Beghetti M, Corris P, Gaine S, Gibbs JS, Gomez-Sanchez MA, Jondeau G, Klepetko W, Opitz C, Peacock A, Rubin L, Zellweger M, Simonneau G; ESC Committee for Practice Guidelines (CPG). Guidelines for the diagnosis and treatment of pulmonary hypertension: the Task Force for the Diagnosis and Treatment of Pulmonary Hypertension of the European Society of Cardiology (ESC) and the European Respiratory Society (ERS), endorsed by the International Society of Heart and Lung Transplantation (ISHLT). *Eur Heart J.* 2009 Oct;30(20):2493-537.

Hoeper MM, Barberà JA, Channick RN, Hassoun PM, Lang IM, Manes A, Martinez FJ, Naeije R, Olschewski H, Pepke-Zaba J, Redfield MM, Robbins IM, Souza R, Torbicki A, McGoon M. Diagnosis, Assessment, and Treatment of Non-Pulmonary Arterial Hypertension and Pulmonary Hypertension. *J Am Coll Cardiol.* 2009 Jun 30;54(1 Suppl):S85-96.

McLaughlin VV, Archer SL, Badesch DB, Barst RJ, Farber HW, Lindner JR, Mathier MA, McGoon MD, Park MH, Rosenson RS, Rubin LJ, Tapson VF, Varga J. ACCF/AHA 2009 Expert Consensus Document on Pulmonary Hypertension: A Report of the American College of Cardiology Foundation Task Force on Expert Consensus Documents and the American Heart Association Developed in Collaboration With the American College of Chest Physicians; American Thoracic Society, Inc.; and the Pulmonary Hypertension Association. *J Am Coll Cardiol.* 2009 Apr 28;53(17):1573-619

Simonneau G, Robbins IM, Beghetti M, Channick RN, Delcroix M, Denton CP, Elliott CG, Gaine SP, Gladwin MT, Jing ZC, Krowka MJ, Langleben D, Nakanishi N, Souza R. Updated Clinical Classification of Pulmonary Hypertension. *J Am Coll Cardiol.* 2009 Jun 30;54(1 Suppl):S43-54.

Pressure Estimation

Abbas AE, Fortuin FD, Schiller NB, Appleton CP, Moreno CA, Lester SJ. Echocardiographic determination of mean pulmonary artery pressure. *Am J Cardiol.* 2003 Dec 1;92(11):1373-6.

Aduen J, Castello R, Lozano MM, Hepler GN, Keller CA, Alvarez F, et al. An alternative echocardiographic method to estimate mean pulmonary artery pressure: diagnostic and clinical implications. *J Am Soc Echocardiogr.* 2009 Jul;22(7):814-9.

Chemla D, Hébert JL, Coirault C, Salmeron S, Zamani K, Lecarpentier Y. Matching dicrotic notch and mean pulmonary artery pressures: implications for effective arterial elastance. *Am J Physiol.* 1996 Oct;271(4 Pt 2):H1287-95.

Fisher MR, Forfia PR, Chamera E, Housten-Harris T, Champion HC, Girgis RE, Corretti MC, Hassoun PM. Accuracy of Doppler echocardiography in the hemodynamic assessment of pulmonary hypertension. *Am J Respir Crit Care Med.* 2009 Apr 1;179(7):615-21.

Giardini A, Tacy TA. Non-invasive estimation of pressure gradients in regurgitant jets: an overdue consideration. *Eur J Echocardiogr.* 2008 Sep;9(5):578-84.

McQuillan BM, Picard MH, Leavitt M, Weyman AE. Clinical correlates and reference intervals for pulmonary artery systolic pressure among echocardiographically normal subjects. *Circulation.* 2001 Dec 4;104(23):2797-802.

Nageh MF, Kopelen HA, Zoghbi WA, Quiñones MA, Nagueh SF. Estimation of Mean Right Atrial Pressure Using Tissue Doppler Imaging. *Am J Cardiol.* 1999 Dec 15;84(12):1448-51, A8.

Nagueh SF, Kopelen HA, Zoghbi WA. Relation of mean right atrial pressure to echocardiographic and Doppler parameters of right atrial and right ventricular function. *Circulation.* 1996 Mar 15;93(6):1160-9.

Rich JD , Shah SJ , Swamy RS , Kamp A , Rich S . Inaccuracy of Doppler echocardiographic estimates of pulmonary artery pressures in patients with pulmonary hypertension: implications for clinical practice . *Chest.* 2011 May;139(5):988-93

Rudski LG, Lai WW, Afilalo J, Hua L, Handschumacher MD, Chandrasekaran K, Solomon SD, Louie EK, Schiller NB. Guidelines for the echocardiographic assessment of the right heart in adults: a report from the American Society of Echocardiography endorsed by the European Association of Echocardiography, a registered branch of the European Society of Cardiology, and the Canadian Society of Echocardiography. *J Am Soc Echocardiogr.* 2010 Jul;23(7):685-713

Pulmonary Vascular Resistance

Abbas AE, Fortuin FD, Schiller NB, Appleton CP, Moreno CA, Lester SJ. A simple method for noninvasive estimation of pulmonary vascular resistance. *J Am Coll Cardiol.* 2003 Mar 19;41(6):1021-7.

Dahiya A, Vollbon W, Jellis C, Prior D, Wahi S, Marwick T. Echocardiographic assessment of raised pulmonary vascular resistance: application to diagnosis and follow-up of pulmonary hypertension. *Heart.* 2010 Dec;96(24):2005-9.

Haddad F, Zamanian R, Beraud AS, Schnittger I, Feinstein J, Peterson T, Yang P, Doyle R, Rosenthal D. A Novel Non-Invasive Method of Estimating Pulmonary Vascular Resistance in Patients With Pulmonary Arterial Hypertension. *J Am Soc Echocardiogr.* 2009 May;22(5):523-9.

Scapellato F, Temporelli PL, Eleuteri E, Corrà U, Imparato A, Giannuzzi P. Accurate noninvasive estimation of pulmonary vascular resistance by Doppler echocardiography in patients with chronic heart failure. *J Am Coll Cardiol.* 2001 Jun 1;37(7):1813-9.

Selimovic N, Rundqvist B, Bergh CH, Andersson B, Petersson S, Johansson L, Bech-Hanssen O. Assessment of pulmonary vascular resistance by Doppler echocardiography in patients with pulmonary arterial hypertension. *J Heart Lung Transplant.* 2007 Sep;26(9):927-34.

Shandas R, Weinberg C, Ivy DD, Nicol E, DeGroff CG, Hertzberg J, Valdes-Cruz L. Development of a noninvasive ultrasound color M-mode means of estimating pulmonary vascular resistance in pediatric pulmonary hypertension: mathematical analysis, in vitro validation, and preliminary clinical studies. *Circulation.* 2001 Aug 21;104(8):908-13..

Prognostic Variables

Brierre G, Blot-Souletie N, Degano B, Têtu L, Bongard V, Carrié D. New echocardiographic prognostic factors for mortality in pulmonary arterial hypertension. *Eur J Echocardiogr.* 2010 Jul;11(6):516-22.

Forfia PR, Fisher MR, Mathai SC, Housten-Harris T, Hemnes AR, Borlaug BA, Chamera E, Corretti MC, Champion HC, Abraham TP, Girgis RE, Hassoun PM. Tricuspid annular displacement predicts survival in pulmonary hypertension. *Am J Respir Crit Care Med.* 2006 Nov 1;174(9):1034-4.

Raymond RJ, Hinderliter AL, Willis PW, Ralph D, Caldwell EJ, Williams W, Ettinger NA, Hill NS, Summer WR, de Boisblanc B, Schwartz T, Koch G, Clayton LM, Jöbsis MM, Crow JW, Long W. Echocardiographic predictors of adverse outcomes in primary pulmonary hypertension. *J Am Coll Cardiol.* 2002 Apr 3;39(7):1214-9.

Ryan T, Petrovic O, Dillon JC, Feigenbaum HF, Conley MJ, Armstrong W. An echocardiographic index for separation of right ventricular volume and pressure overload. *J Am Coll Cardiol.* 1985 Apr;5(4):918-27.

Yeo TC, Dujardin KS, Tei C, Mahoney DW, McGoon MD, Seward JB. Value of a Doppler-derived index combining systolic and diastolic time intervals in predicting outcome in primary pulmonary hypertension. *Am J Cardiol.* 1998 May 1;81(9):1157-61.

Ischaemic Heart Disease

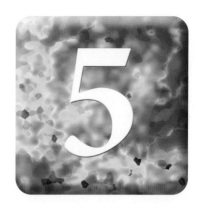

Coronary Artery Anatomy

The coronary arteries encircle or 'crown' the epicardial surface of the heart and supply blood to the myocardium and conduction system. Normally, there are two coronary arteries which originate from the aortic root: (1) the left main coronary artery (LMCA) and (2) the right coronary artery (RCA) (Fig. 5.1).

Left Main Coronary Artery (LMCA)

The LMCA arises from the aortic root at the left sinus of Valsalva; it travels a short distance along the epicardium between the pulmonary trunk and the left atrial appendage before bifurcating into the left anterior descending (LAD) and the left circumflex (Cx) arteries. The length of the LMCA ranges from 5 mm to 20 mm. In approximately 15% of individuals the LMCA trifurcates, giving rise to an additional intermediate coronary artery (ramus intermedius) which arises between the LAD and Cx. This vessel follows the course of the Cx.

Left Anterior Descending (LAD)

The LAD descends along the anterior interventricular groove towards the cardiac apex. It gives rise to several septal perforators (SP) and several diagonal (D) branches. The septal branches supply the anterior interventricular septum (IVS) while the diagonal branches course diagonally to supply the anterolateral segments of the left ventricle (LV). The first diagonal branch is used as an anatomic landmark to delineate the different segments of the LAD. The proximal LAD is between the origin of the LAD and the origin of the first diagonal branch (D1), the distal LAD is the distal 1/3 of the LAD while the mid LAD is the segment between the proximal and distal LAD. In approximately 80% of cases the LAD reaches beyond the apex to the diaphragmatic surface of the heart; in about 20% of cases the LAD terminates at or before the apex.

Left Circumflex (Cx)

The Cx courses along the left atrioventricular groove between the left atrium (LA) and the LV. It gives rise to several obtuse margin (OM) branches which supply the lateral aspect of the LV. The first obtuse marginal branch (OM1) is used as a reference point to divide the Cx into 2 segments. The proximal Cx is the segment prior to the origin of OM1 while the distal Cx is distal to OM1. The distal Cx gives rise to one or more posterolateral (PL) branches.

Right Coronary Artery (RCA)

The RCA arises from the aortic root at the right sinus of Valsalva; it courses down the right atrioventricular groove between the right atrium (RA) and right ventricle (RV). The RCA gives off several branches. The first branch is a small conus artery which courses towards the LAD to supply the right ventricular outflow tract (RVOT). Occasionally the conus artery arises from a separate ostium in the right sinus of Valsalva and less frequently arises from the LMCA. The second branch arising from the RCA is the sinoatrial (SA) nodal branch which runs

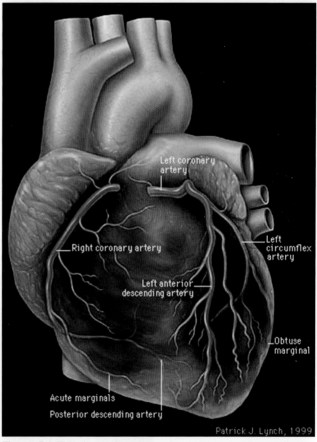

Figure 5.1 This illustration shows the coronary artery distribution viewed from the anterior aspect of the heart. This right dominant system shows the posterior descending artery arising from the right coronary artery. The left (main) coronary artery bifurcates into the left anterior descending artery and left circumflex artery.
Illustration by Patrick J. Lynch ©, Senior Digital Officer, Design, Analytics, & Social Media Office of Public Affairs & Communications, Yale University, reproduced with permission.

posteriorly to the SA node. This branch arises from the RCA in 60% of cases and from the Cx in 40% of cases. Other branches from the RCA include the RV branch which courses anteriorly to supply the anterior wall of the RV, large acute marginal (AM) branches which arise at an acute angle and course along the margin of the RV above the diaphragm, and the atrioventricular (AV) nodal artery which supplies the AV node. The AV nodal branch arises from the dominant RCA in 85% of cases and from the Cx in 15% of cases.

In a right-dominant system, the RCA bifurcates into the posterior descending artery (PDA) and the right posterolateral artery (RPLA). The PDA courses down the posterior interventricular groove and gives rise to several inferoseptal branches; this artery therefore supplies the inferior wall of the LV and the inferior IVS. The RPLA gives off one or more PL branches to the LV thus supplying the posterior and lateral aspects of the LV.

Coronary Artery Dominance

The coronary artery dominance is determined by the coronary arteries supplying the PDA and the PL branches (Fig. 5.2). In a right dominant system the PDA is a branch of the RCA and the RCA gives rise to one or more PL branches. This type of coronary system is most common and is seen in

approximately 70% of individuals. In a left dominant system the PDA is a branch of the Cx and the Cx gives rise to all PL branches. This type of coronary system is seen in about 10% of individuals. In a co-dominant system the PDA arises from the RCA, and all the PL branches arise from the Cx. This type of coronary system is seen in about 20% of individuals.

Coronary Artery Supply

The coronary artery supply to the regions of the heart varies according to the coronary artery anatomy and branching. Table 5.1 lists the typical coronary artery supply to various regions of the heart and conduction system.

Collateral Circulation

Anastomoses between the coronary arteries are present from birth and these collateral channels provide an alternative source of blood supply to the myocardium when there is significant occlusive coronary artery disease (CAD). These collateral arteries are most abundant in the IVS (between the LAD and PDA), the ventricular apex (between various LAD septal perforators), the RV anterior wall (between LAD and RCA), the anterolateral LV wall (between LAD diagonals and Cx marginals) and at the cardiac crux and atrial surfaces (between RCA and Cx).

Table 5.1 Coronary Artery Distribution to the Heart and Conduction System

Left Anterior Descending	Left Circumflex Artery	Right Coronary Artery
• His bundle and proximal left bundle branch (via SP) • Anterior LV wall (via diagonal branches) • Entire apex (including RV apex); occasionally extends as far as the mid inferior LV segment	• Left atrium • AV node in 10% of patients and SA node in 40% of patients • Inferolateral LV segments and a variable amount of anterolateral LV segments (via OM) • Inferior LV wall • Part of the anterolateral papillary muscle • Lateral LV apex (via OM) if LAD terminates before apex	• Right atrium • AV node in 90% of patients (via AV nodal artery) and SA node in 60% of patients (via sinus nodal artery), right bundle branch, posterior portion of left bundle branch • RVOT (via conus branch) • Lateral RV wall (via AM branches) • Inferior RV wall (via PDA) • Inferior LV wall (base and mid levels; via PDA - right dominant system) • Basal inferior septum; may also supply mid inferior septum (via PDA - right dominant system)

AM = acute marginal; **AV** = atrioventricular; **LV** = left ventricle; **OM** = obtuse marginals **PDA** = posterior descending artery; **RV** = right ventricle; **RVOT** = right ventricular outflow tract; **SA** = sinoatrial; **SP** = septal perforators; **LAD** = left anterior descending

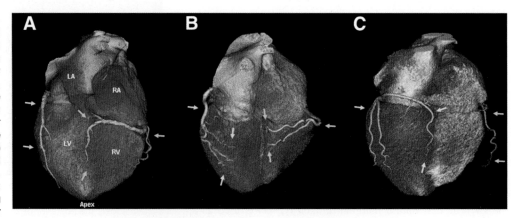

Figure 5.2 These three-dimensional, volume-rendered inferior and posterior computed tomography angiographic images show different coronary anatomy variants. **(A)** Standard, right-dominant circulation: the right coronary artery (*green arrows*) supplies the posterior descending branch; the left circumflex (*blue arrows*) supplies only the inferolateral left ventricular myocardium. **(B)** Co-dominant circulation: no clear posterior descending artery is observed; the inferior myocardium is supplied by both the right and left circumflex arteries. **(C)** Left-dominant circulation: the left circumflex supplies the posterior descending branch (*blue arrows*); the right coronary artery supplies only the right ventricular myocardium (*green arrows*).
LA = left atrium; RA = right atrium; LV = left ventricle; RV = right ventricle.
Reprinted by permission of the Society of Nuclear Medicine from Javadi MS, Lautamäki R, Merrill J, et al. Definition of Vascular Territories on Myocardial Perfusion Images by Integration with True Coronary Anatomy: A Hybrid PET/CT Analysis. *J Nucl Med.* 2010; 51(2): 198-203. Figure 1.

Coronary Artery Disease

Myocardial Ischaemia and Infarction

Ischaemia is the result of impaired vascular perfusion which deprives the affected tissue of nutrients and oxygen. Ischaemia can be reversible and this reversibility is dependent upon the duration of the ischaemic period and the metabolic demands of the tissue.

Myocardial ischaemia occurs when there is insufficient blood supply to the myocardium due to decreased or impaired coronary artery perfusion and/or increased metabolic demands of the myocardium. The most common causes of myocardial ischaemia include CAD and diseases that produce a significant increase in myocardial metabolic demands; for example, hypertrophic cardiomyopathy and severe aortic stenosis.

Infarction is death or necrosis of tissue which occurs as a result of prolonged ischaemia or total occlusion of blood flow to tissue. Unlike ischaemia, infarction is irreversible. Therefore, a myocardial infarction (MI) can be defined as myocardial cell death which occurs due to prolonged ischaemia.

Angina Pectoris

Angina pectoris is the major symptom of ischaemic heart disease. Angina refers to cardiac chest pain or discomfort resulting from a temporary imbalance between myocardial oxygen supply and demand. The major types of angina are stable, unstable, variant (Prinzmetal's), and microvascular.

- **Stable angina** (exertional or effort angina) generally occurs with exercise and is relieved by rest or medications such as glyceryl trinitrate.
- **Unstable angina** is characterised by chest pain that occurs suddenly and unexpectedly at rest and/or pain that is more severe, prolonged or frequent than previous episodes of angina.
- **Variant (Prinzmetal's) angina** is a rare type of angina thought to be caused by coronary artery spasm. This type of angina is not related to exercise and often occurs between midnight and early morning, with the attacks usually occurring at the same time each day.
- **Microvascular angina** (or "cardiac syndrome X") is characterised by angina-like pain that occurs in the absence of epicardial coronary artery disease. The cause of angina is coronary microvascular dysfunction.

Atherosclerotic Coronary Heart Disease

The most common cause of CAD is atherosclerosis which is characterized by endothelial dysfunction, vascular inflammation and the formation of atherosclerotic plaques (atheromas) within the intima of the vessel wall (Fig. 5.3). Thrombosis related to atherosclerotic plaques is the major cause for acute myocardial infarction (AMI) and unstable angina (Fig. 5.4). This thrombotic process produces epicardial coronary stenoses which reduce coronary artery flow and myocardial perfusion. Generally, the cross-sectional area of the coronary artery lumen must be reduced by 75% before there is a significant reduction in myocardial perfusion. Distal embolisation of a coronary artery thrombus may also result in obstruction of coronary flow and reduced myocardial perfusion.

A number of risk factors for the development and progression of atherosclerotic CAD have been identified and these can be classified as modifiable, non-modifiable, or non-traditional or novel risk factors (Table 5.2).

Structure of Blood Vessels

Histologically, blood vessels, including coronary arteries, consist of three concentric layers or tunics. The tunica intima is the inner lining which consists of endothelium and a relatively thin layer of supporting connective tissue. The tunica media is the middle muscular and/or elastic layer, containing smooth muscle and elastic tissue in varying proportions. The tunica adventitia is the outer, fibrous connective tissue layer.

Non-Atherosclerotic Coronary Heart Disease

While atherosclerosis is the most common cause of CAD, there are numerous non-atherosclerotic disorders that can cause myocardial ischaemia or infarction due to reduced or disrupted coronary artery flow, or due to increased myocardial metabolic demand. These disorders are summarised in Table 5.3; examples of congenital coronary artery anomalies causing myocardial ischaemia are illustrated in Figure 5.5).

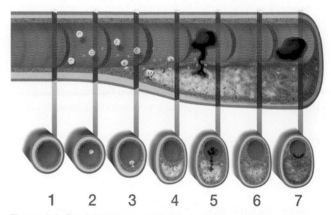

Figure 5.3 The initiation, progression, and complication of human coronary atherosclerotic plaque is illustrated in this schematic. A longitudinal section of artery depicting the "timeline" of human atherogenesis is illustrated on the top and the cross sections of the coronary artery during various stages of atheroma evolution are illustrated on the bottom.

1. Normal artery: In human arteries, the intimal layer is much better developed than in most other species. The intima of human arteries contains resident smooth muscle cells often as early as the first year of life.
2. Lesion initiation and accumulation of extracellular lipid in the intima.
3. Evolution to fibrofatty stage.
4. Lesion progression with procoagulant expression and weakening of the fibrous cap.
5. Fracture or rupture in the protective fibrous cap of the plaque causes thrombosis or nonocclusive atherosclerotic plaque.
6. Thrombus resorption may be followed by increased collagen accumulation and smooth muscle cell growth; the fibrofatty lesion can evolve into advanced fibrous and often calcified plaque which may cause significant stenosis, and produce symptoms of stable angina pectoris.
7. In some cases, occlusive thrombi arise not from fracture of the fibrous cap but from superficial erosion of the endothelial layer. Resulting mural thrombus can cause acute myocardial infarction.

Reproduced from Libby P. Current concepts of the pathogenesis of the acute coronary syndromes. *Circulation*, 104: page 366; © 2001 Lippincott, Williams & Wilkins with permission.

Table 5.2 **Risk Factors for CAD**

Modifiable	Non-modifiable	Non-traditional (Novel)
Physiological: • Hyperlipidemia, dyslipidemia • Hypertension • Type II Diabetes mellitus • Obesity • Metabolic syndrome Behavioural: • Cigarette smoking • Alcohol consumption • Lack of physical activity • Mental stress, depression	Age: • Men ≥ 45 years; women ≥ 55 years Gender: • Men > pre-menopausal women Family history of early CAD: • CAD in male 1st-degree relative < 55 years; • CAD in female 1st-degree relative < 65 years Race/ethnicity: • African or Asian ancestry	High-sensitivity C-reactive protein Elevated lipoprotein(a) Elevated homocysteine Low ankle–brachial index Impaired fasting blood glucose Periodontal disease High carotid intima–media thickness High coronary artery calcification score on electron-beam computed tomography

Table 5.3 **Nonatherosclerotic Causes of Myocardial Ischaemia or Infarction**

Nonatherosclerotic Cause	Reason for Ischaemia/Infarction	Examples
Coronary artery emboli	Obstruction of coronary flow which impairs adequate myocardial perfusion	Air embolism during coronary intervention Infective endocarditis Left heart tumours Mural thrombus from the left ventricle, mitral or aortic prosthetic valve, left atrial thrombus, or left atrial myxoma Nonbacterial thrombotic endocarditis Paradoxic embolisation (thrombi, vegetation or tumour)
Coronary artery dissection	Narrowing of coronary artery lumen and/or obstruction to lumen by dissection flap	Aortic dissection with extension into coronary artery (aortic dissection flap alone may also occlude coronary ostium) Blunt chest trauma Iatrogenic Spontaneous isolated coronary artery dissection
In-situ coronary thrombosis	Sluggish blood flow in coronary arteries with resultant thrombosis	Usually associated with underlying atherosclerosis but it may occur with certain coagulopathies such as hypercoagulable states and polycythemia and hyperviscosity syndromes
Coronary spasm	Episodic segmental stenosis	Cocaine abuse Prinzmetal angina Raynaud's disease Scleroderma
Inadequate coronary perfusion	Inadequate coronary perfusion	Anomalous coronary origin from the pulmonary trunk Aortic regurgitation Coronary fistulas
Decreased myocardial oxygen supply	Decreased coronary flow or decreased oxygen delivery of haemoglobin	Carbon monoxide poisoning Prolonged hypotension Shock
Increased myocardial oxygen demand	Increased metabolic needs of myocardium	Cocaine and amphetamine use Left ventricular hypertrophy Pheochromocytoma, Thyrotoxicosis Tetanus Thiamine deficiency (Beri Beri)
Coronary intimal proliferation	Narrowing of coronary lumen	Radiation-induced coronary artery disease (following mediastinal radiation therapy)
Inflammation of coronary arteries (coronary vasculitis)	Vascular occlusion by inflammatory thickening of coronary arteries	Kawasaki disease Polyarteritis nodosa Takayasu disease
Congenital coronary artery anomalies	Compression of artery (dependent on origin and course)	Right coronary artery arising from left sinus of Valsalva or left main coronary artery arising from right sinus of Valsalva (Fig. 5.5)

Acute Coronary Syndrome

Acute coronary syndrome (ACS) refers to a spectrum of clinical presentations related to acute myocardial ischaemia. This spectrum includes unstable angina (UA), non-ST-segment elevation myocardial infarction (NSTEMI), and ST-segment elevation myocardial infarction (STEMI). Differentiation between each group is based on the 12-lead ECG and cardiac biomarkers (Fig. 5.6). In particular, distinction between UA/NSTEMI and STEMI is crucial as STEMI requires urgent thrombolytic therapy and/or percutaneous coronary intervention (PCI) in order to prevent an AMI.

The 12-lead ECG can be used to determine the location and extent of infarction based on the anatomical relationship of ECG leads to myocardial walls. Myocardial infarctions are most commonly referred to as anterior, septal, lateral, and inferior; other types of MI include mid-anterior, apico-anterior and inferolateral. Based on the 12-lead ECG and the relationship between coronary arteries and LV walls, the coronary artery likely to be responsible for the infarct can be identified (refer to Fig. 5.13).

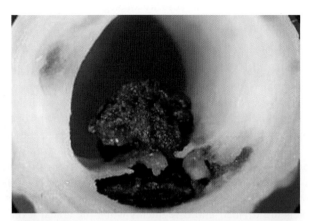

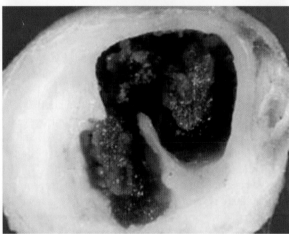

Figure 5.4 The image on the top shows a cap of a plaque that has torn and projects up into the lumen. Thrombus has formed within the original lipid core from where it projects into, but does not totally occlude, the coronary artery lumen. This is the typical lesion of unstable angina. The image on the bottom shows a cap of the plaque that has torn and thrombus within the lipid core extends into and occludes the coronary artery lumen. This is the typical lesion of acute myocardial infarction.
Reproduced from Davies MJ. The pathophysiology of acute coronary syndromes, *Heart*, Vol. 83(3), pages 362 & 363, © 2000 with permission from BMJ Publishing Group Ltd.

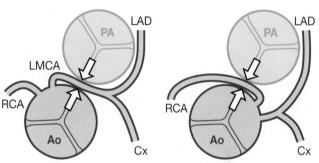

Figure 5.5 These two illustrations of anomalous coronary arteries demonstrate how myocardial ischaemia can occur. When the left main coronary artery (LMCA) arises from the right sinus of Valsalva (*left*) or when the right coronary artery (RCA) arises from the left sinus of Valsalva (*right*) the anomalous artery courses between the aorta (Ao) and pulmonary artery (PA). This interarterial course can lead to compression of the anomalous artery (*white arrows*) resulting in myocardial ischemia and/or infarction.
LAD = left anterior descending artery; Cx = left circumflex artery

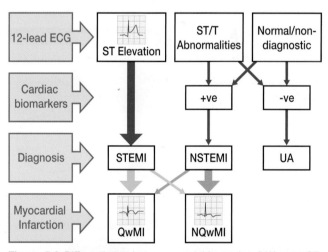

Figure 5.6 Differentiation between unstable angina (UA), non-ST-segment elevation myocardial infarction (NSTEMI) and ST-segment elevation myocardial infarction (STEMI) is based on the 12-lead ECG and cardiac biomarkers. Note that the majority of patients presenting with ST-segment elevation who do not have immediate reperfusion therapy will ultimately develop a Q-wave myocardial infarction (QwMI) (*thick blue arrow*) while a few will develop a non–Q-wave myocardial infarction (NQwMI) (*thin blue arrow*). Patients presenting without ST-segment elevation are suffering from either UA or a NSTEMI; the distinction between UA and NSTEMI is based on the presence (+) or absence (-) of cardiac biomarkers detected in the blood. The majority of patients presenting with NSTEMI ultimately develop a NQwMI (*thick pink arrow*) although a few may develop a QwMI (*thin pink arrow*).

Q-wave and non-Q-wave Myocardial Infarctions

Pathological Q waves develop when the myocardium beneath the ECG electrode is necrotic; this creates an electrical 'window' and through this window the electrical activity of myocardium opposite to the infarcted area is detected as a pathological Q wave. Therefore, a myocardial infarction can be classified as a Q-wave myocardial infarction (QwMI) or a non-Q-wave myocardial infarction (NQwMI) with a QwMI indicating a larger and more serious MI. Although pathological Q waves are often associated with transmural (full thickness) infarctions and the absence of Q waves associated with nontransmural (subendocardial) infarctions, pathological findings do not always support this. That is, pathological Q waves can be seen with nontransmural (subendocardial) infarcts while transmural infarct may occur in the absence of pathological Q waves.

Role of Echocardiography in Ischaemic Heart Disease

Echocardiography has a very important role in the assessment of patients with ischaemic heart disease (IHD). This includes the assessment of regional LV function, LV size, and LV systolic and diastolic function. In addition, echocardiography has a very important role in the assessment of complications of MI.

The advantages of 2D echocardiography in the assessment of IHD include that it is non-invasive, it can be easily performed at the bedside, it provides immediate feedback on cardiac structure and function, and it can be easily repeated on a serial basis.

Regional Analysis of the Left Ventricle

One of the most important roles of echocardiography in IHD is to identify regional variations in LV systolic function

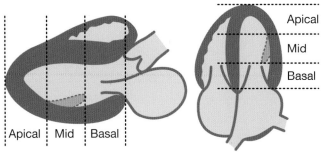

Figure 5.7 The long axis of the ventricle is divided into three equal lengths using the left ventricular papillary muscles as anatomic landmarks. The **basal** level is identified from the mitral valve annulus to the tips of the papillary muscles, the **mid** level is delineated from the tips of the papillary muscles to the base of the papillary muscles, and the **apical** level is defined as the level from the base of the papillary muscles to the apex of the left ventricle. Parasternal long axis and apical 4-chamber views are illustrated.

which occur due to myocardial ischaemia or infarction. For this purpose the LV is divided into 17 segments based on the following considerations: (1) anatomic logic, (2) easy identification of the segments using internal anatomic landmarks, (3) the relationship of the segments to known coronary artery supply, and (4) providing a uniform scoring system for grading the severity of segmental wall motion abnormalities.

The 17-Segment Model

To derive the 17-segment model of the LV, the ventricle is first divided into three levels with the LV papillary muscles providing important landmarks (Fig. 5.7). The basal level is identified from the mitral valve annulus to the tips of the papillary muscles, the mid level is delineated from the tips of the papillary muscles to the base of the papillary muscles, and the apical level is defined as the level from the base of the papillary muscles to the LV apex. At each level the ventricle is then subdivided into segments. The base and mid levels are divided into 6 segments while the apical level is divided into 4 segments plus the apical cap which is defined as the area of myocardium beyond the end of the LV cavity (Fig. 5.8 and 5.9).

Examples of the coronary distribution to each LV segment are illustrated in figure 5.10 (standard echocardiographic views) and figure 5.11 ("Bull's-eye" plot). Typically, the LAD supplies the basal and mid anterior wall segments, the anterior IVS and most of the LV apex. The RCA supplies the RV free wall, the LV inferior wall and the basal inferior IVS. The LAD and RCA supply the mid inferior IVS and the inferior apex. The Cx or LAD supplies the anterolateral segments while the Cx or RCA supply the basal and mid inferolateral segments. It is important to note that there is variability in coronary supply to myocardial segments due to variations in coronary artery branching.

Figure 5.8 The 17-segment model of the left ventricle is illustrated based on the standard parasternal and apical echocardiographic views.

Basal:
1. anterior free wall
2. anteroseptal
3. inferoseptal *
4. inferior *
5. inferolateral *
6. anterolateral

Mid:
7. anterior free wall
8. anteroseptal
9. inferoseptal *
10. inferior *
11. inferolateral *
12. anterolateral

Apical:
13. anterior (anteroapical)
14. septal (apicoseptal)
15. inferior (inferoapical)
16. lateral (apicolateral)
17. apical cap

*The basal inferolateral wall, basal inferior wall and basal inferoseptum may also be referred to as the posterobasal lateral wall, posterobasal wall and posterobasal ventricular septum, respectively.

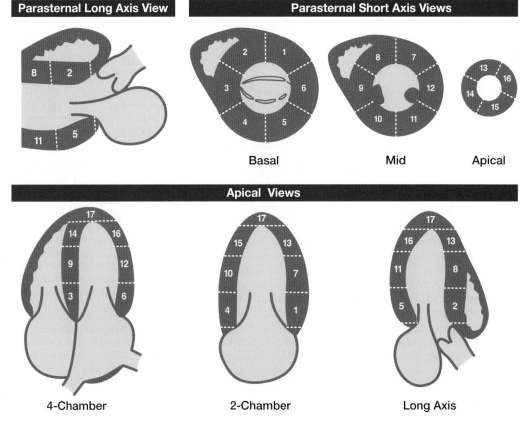

Regional Wall Motion Assessment

The principal way of detecting ischaemic or infarcted myocardium is the observation of abnormal wall motion of the ischaemic or infarcted segments. Careful scrutiny of regional wall motion is especially important in the setting of AMI or myocardial ischaemia as the movement of any given segment of the ventricle is influenced by adjacent muscle to which it is attached. For example, an abnormal wall segment may appear to 'contract' due to adjacent normally contracting myocardium 'pulling' on the abnormal segment while a normal wall segment may appear hypokinetic when attached to a dyskinetic segment.

The key to identifying regional wall motion abnormalities (RWMA) is to look for systolic myocardial *thickening*. Normal myocardium increases in thickness during systole while ischaemic tissue will show a reduction or absence of systolic wall thickening. Therefore, when looking for RWMA, it is important to assess systolic thickening by attempting to view the entire width of the segment from endocardium to epicardium.

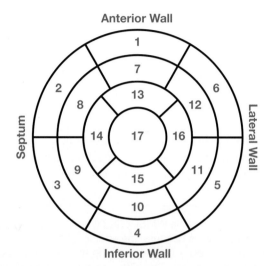

Figure 5.9 The 17-segment model of the left ventricle is displayed as a "Bull's-eye" plot.

Basal:	Mid:	Apical:
1. anterior free wall	7. anterior free wall	13. anterior (anteroapical)
2. anteroseptal	8. anteroseptal	14. septal (apicoseptal)
3. inferoseptal	9. inferoseptal	15. inferior (inferoapical)
4. inferior	10. inferior	16. lateral (apicolateral)
5. inferolateral *	11. inferolateral *	17. apical cap
6. anterolateral	12. anterolateral	

*The inferolateral wall is also commonly referred to as the posterior wall.

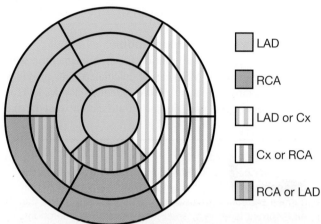

Figure 5.11 This schematic illustrates the typical distributions of the right coronary artery (RCA), the left anterior descending (LAD), and the circumflex (Cx) coronary arteries as viewed in a "bull's-eye" plot. Note that coronary arterial distribution is variable between individuals.

Figure 5.10 This schematic illustrates typical distributions of the right coronary artery (RCA), the left anterior descending (LAD), and the circumflex (Cx) coronary arteries based on the standard echocardiographic views. Note that coronary arterial distribution is variable between individuals.

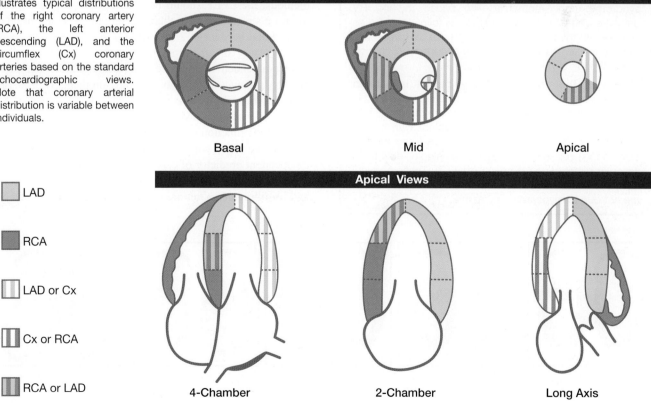

The degree of contractility for each myocardial segment may be graded and scored as follows (Fig. 5.12):

1. Normal: systolic contraction and wall thickening increasing more than 40%
2. Hypokinetic: reduced systolic wall thickening (< 40%)
3. Akinetic: diastolic wall thickness is usually thin and systolic wall thickening is absent
4. Dyskinetic: diastolic wall thickness is thin with associated outward movement or bulging in systole
5. Aneurysmal: constantly deformed segment throughout systole and diastole with outward movement bulging in systole.

Furthermore, the location of an acute or previous MI can be determined based on the distribution of RWMA (Fig. 5.13). Echocardiographic examples of RWMA associated with previous MI are shown in Figure 5.14.

Regional Wall Motion Score Index

Based on the regional wall motion for each segment, a wall motion score index (WMSI) can be calculated. This provides a semiquantitative measure of the extent of RWMA. This index has also been used in risk stratification; that is, the

---

Caveats of RWMA

The absence of a RWMA at rest does not exclude the diagnosis of IHD. For example, if ischaemia affects only a small section of myocardium and is limited to the thin endocardial layer (e.g. small non-transmural infarctions, perfusion territory of the circumflex artery) RWMA may be absent. In addition, a myocardial segment distal to an occluded coronary artery may still be adequately perfused when there are collateral vessels supplying that segment.

Abnormal IVS motion in the absence of myocardial ischaemia may be seen when there is a left bundle branch block (LBBB), Wolf–Parkinson–White (WPW) syndrome, right ventricular (RV) paced rhythm, RV pressure and/or volume overload, or following cardiac surgery. In these cases, the presence of preserved systolic thickening will confirm that abnormal IVS motion is not a result of myocardial ischaemia.

RWMA in the absence of myocardial ischaemia may be seen with a subarachnoid haemorrhage (SAH), cardiac sarcoidosis or Takotsubo cardiomyopathy (TTC). In these cases, RWMA are not consistent with known coronary artery territories (as seen in SAH and cardiac sarcoidosis) or extend beyond a single epicardial vascular distribution (as seen with TTC). These atypical RWMA provide clues that the wall motion abnormalities are not due to myocardial ischaemia.

WMSI can be used to determine the patient's risk for future cardiac events following an AMI. In particular, the higher the WMSI, the greater the size of the MI and the higher the risk of significant complications.

To calculate the WMSI, each of the LV segments is visualised from all possible views to determine its motion. Each segment is then allocated a score according to its systolic thickening/contraction. Once the segments have been scored, the individual scores are summed to produce the wall motion score. This score is then indexed by dividing the score by the number of segments visualised:

Equation 5.1

$$WMSI = \frac{\sum wall\ motion\ scores}{No.\ segments\ visualised}$$

A normal WMSI is 1. In a normal LV, each segment would receive a score of 1, the sum of all 16 segments would then be 16. 16 divided by 16 segments equals 1.

When determining the WMSI, only 16 segments of the LV are scored. This is because the additional 17th segment is the tip of the apex (apical cap) and this segment does not normally contract. The 17th segment is important in myocardial perfusion studies.

Assessment of Left Ventricular Size and Systolic and Diastolic Function

LV end-diastolic and end-systolic volumes and the LV ejection fraction (LVEF) can be used in the risk stratification and assessment of prognosis following an AMI. Measurement of LV volumes, calculation of the LVEF as well as other methods for assessing overall LV systolic function are described in Chapter 2. In particular, due to the limitations of linear methods, the LVEF should be determined from the biplane Simpson's method. When there is suboptimal visualisation of endocardial borders of 2 or more LV segments in an apical view, the use of an intravenous ultrasound contrast agent is recommended to improve endocardial border definition and the accuracy of LV volume measurements (Fig. 5.15). Echocardiography is also valuable in the assessment of LV remodelling after an AMI (Fig. 5.16).

LV diastolic function is also of prognostic value. In particular, a restrictive filling pattern has been found to be an important independent predictor of cardiovascular mortality in patients suffering an AMI. The assessment of LV diastolic function and LV filling pressures are described in detail in Chapter 3.

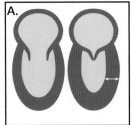 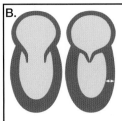 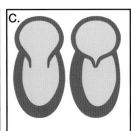 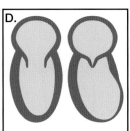 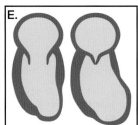

Figure 5.12 In this figure diastolic frames are shown to the left and systolic frames are shown to the right. Normal wall motion shows systolic wall thickening > 40% **(A)**. Hypokinetic wall motion shows reduced systolic wall thickening < 40% **(B)**. Akinetic wall motion is associated with a thinner diastolic wall thickness and systolic thickening is absent **(C)**. With dyskinetic wall motion the segment is thin during diastole with outward motion in systole **(D)**. Aneurysmal wall motion is identified by abnormal outward bulging and deformation during both systole and diastole **(E)**.

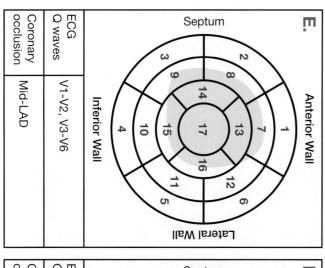

A.

ECG Q waves	V1-V2
Coronary occlusion	SP of LAD

B.

ECG Q waves	V1-V2, V4-V6, aVL
Coronary occlusion	LAD (prox. to SP and D branches)

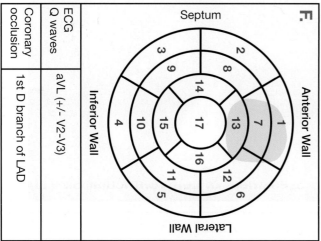

E.

ECG Q waves	V1-V2, V3-V6
Coronary occlusion	Mid-LAD

F.

ECG Q waves	aVL (+/- V2-V3)
Coronary occlusion	1st D branch of LAD

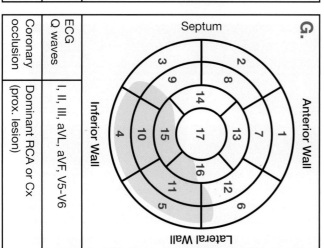

C.

ECG Q waves	I, aVL, V6
Coronary occlusion	Nondominant Cx or OM branch

D.

ECG Q waves	II, III, aVF
Coronary occlusion	Artery suppling PDA*

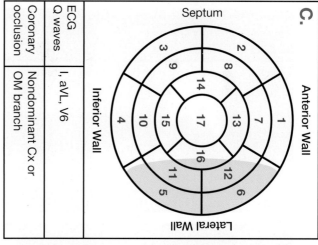

G.

ECG Q waves	I, II, III, aVL, aVF, V5-V6
Coronary occlusion	Dominant RCA or Cx (prox. lesion)

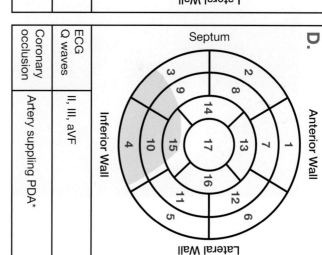

Figure 5.13 These "bulls-eye" plots illustrate the location of various myocardial infarctions: **(A)** septal, **(B)** anterior, **(C)** lateral, **(D)** inferior, **(E)** anteroapical, **(F)** mid-anterior, and **(G)** inferolateral. ECG leads showing pathological Q waves and the coronary artery that is likely occluded are also described. Note that overlap and variations between regions may exist due to variation in coronary anatomy, the presence of collateral flow and the size of the infarction.

* RCA in right dominant system or Cx in left dominant system.

Numbered segments refer to the LV segments as previously described (see Fig. 5.9). Cx = circumflex artery; D = diagonal branch; LAD = left anterior descending artery; OM = obtuse marginal branch; PDA = posterior descending artery; RCA = right coronary artery; SP = septal perforator.

Panel A

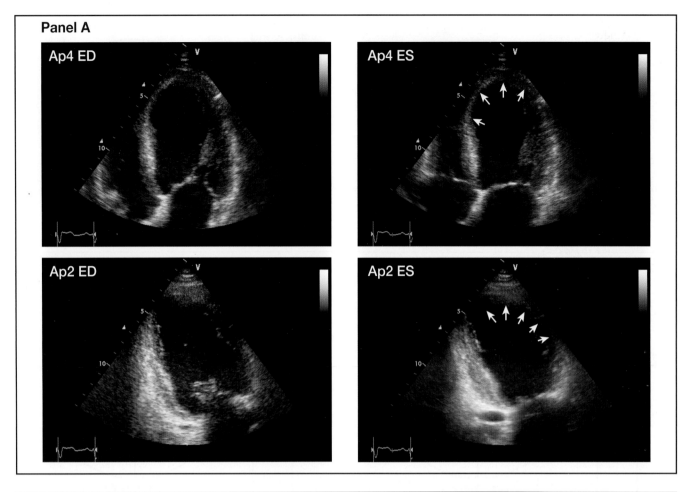

Panel B

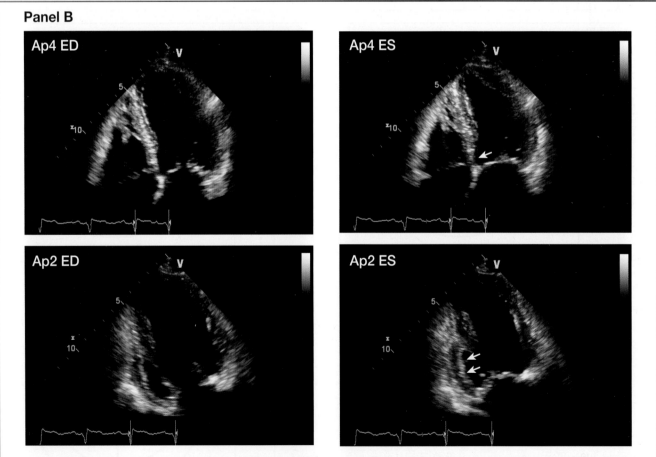

Figure 5.14 Regional wall motion abnormalities are difficult to appreciate on still frame images, however the examples shown display an obvious lack of systolic thickening in the infarcted segments (*arrows*). **Panel A** = anteroapical MI viewed from the apical 4-chamber view (Ap4) and apical 2-chamber views (Ap2) at end-diastole (ED) and end-systole (ES). **Panel B** = inferior MI viewed from the apical 4-chamber view (Ap4) and apical 2-chamber views (Ap2) at end-diastole (ED) and end-systole (ES).

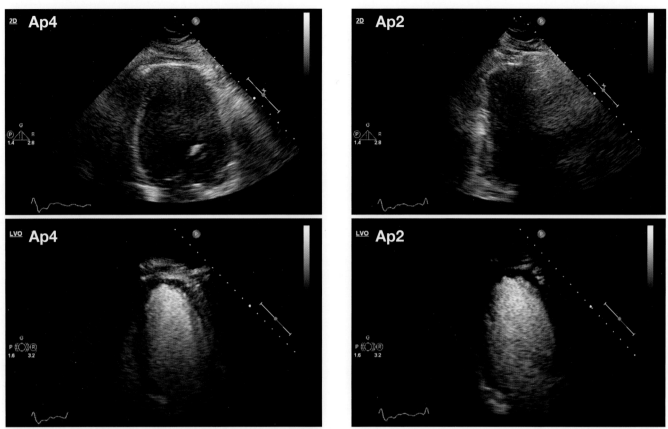

Figure 5.15 The apical 4-chamber (Ap4) and apical 2-chamber (Ap2) views on the top show suboptimal endocardial definition. The bottom images show the corresponding images following the injection of an intravenous contrast; observe the marked improved in endocardial definition on these images.

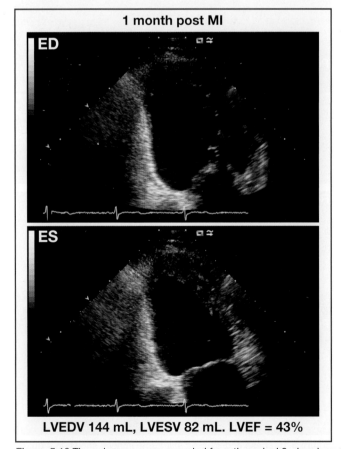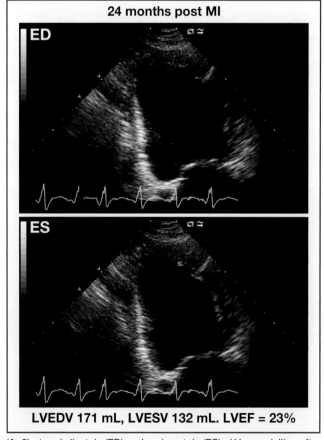

Figure 5.16 These images were recorded from the apical 2-chamber view (Ap2) at end-diastole (ED) and end-systole (ES). LV remodelling after transmural inferior myocardial infarction (MI) is evident. Compare the images recorded at 1 month post-MI *(left)* with the 24 months post-MI images *(right)*: progressive LV dilatation and LV dysfunction with increased LV sphericity are observed. LVEDV = left ventricular end-diastolic volume; LVESV = left ventricular end-systolic volume; LVEF = left ventricular ejection fraction.

Role of Stress Echocardiography in Ischaemic Heart Disease

In the presence of CAD reduced coronary blood flow will create a supply-demand mismatch resulting in myocardial ischaemia; the sequence of events that leads to the development of myocardial ischaemia is referred to as "the ischaemic cascade" (Fig. 5.17).

As mentioned, the echocardiographic identification of myocardial ischaemia due to CAD is based on the recognition of RWMA. However, patients with severe CAD may have normal LV function at rest. In these patients RWMA may be induced by increasing myocardial oxygen demand. This can be achieved by stress echocardiography which aims to increase myocardial oxygen demand in order to induce RWMA that are not present at rest.

The types of stressors used to increase myocardial oxygen demand include physical exercise (bicycle, treadmill or isometric), pharmacological stress (adrenergic stimulation [dobutamine] and vasodilation [dipyridamole and adenosine]) or rapid cardiac pacing. The normal and abnormal responses to stress are summarised in Table 5.4 and illustrated in figures 5.18-5.20.

Dobutamine stress echocardiography may also be used to differentiate between viable myocardium and irreversible myocardial necrosis (Table 5.5). Viable myocardium can be defined as dysfunctional myocardium that improves contractile function when an adequate coronary blood flow is

Table 5.4 Normal and Abnormal Responses to Stress

	Following Stress
Normal Response	• Uniform increase in regional wall motion (becomes hyperdynamic) • Decrease in LV end-systolic cavity area • Increased LVEF
Inducible ischaemia	• Development of new RWMA • Deterioration of existing RWMA • Tardokinesia (delayed systolic contraction) • Failure to augment wall thickening • Increase in LV end-systolic cavity area • Decrease in overall LVEF

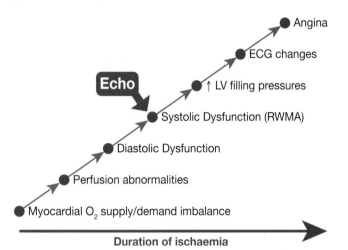

Figure 5.17 The ischaemic cascade is a series of pathophysiologic events caused by myocardial ischaemia. Coronary artery disease causes a reduction in myocardial blood flow which leads to a supply-demand imbalance. This is followed by perfusion abnormalities, diastolic dysfunction, systolic dysfunction (or regional wall motion abnormalities [RWMA]) and a subsequent rise in left ventricular (LV) filling pressures. This is then followed by ECG changes and angina. The primary role of echocardiography in this cascade is to identify RWMA.

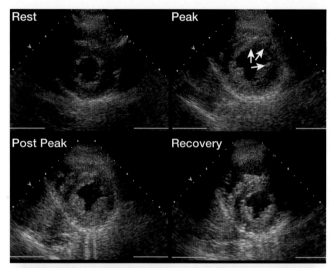

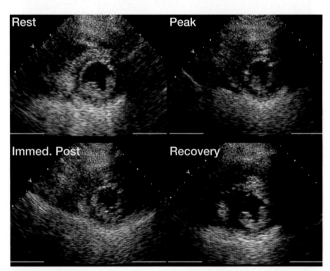

Figure 5.18 These end-systolic still frame images shown in a quad-screen format were recorded from the parasternal short axis view at the papillary muscle level. These images show a normal exercise response; observe that the LV cavity decreases in size and the walls become hyperdynamic at peak exercise *(top right)*.

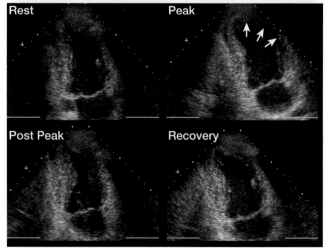

Figure 5.19 These end-systolic still frame images shown in a quad-screen format were recorded from the parasternal short axis view at the papillary muscle level *(top)* and the apical 2-chamber view *(bottom)*. These images show an abnormal exercise response; observe that at peak stress there was severe hypokinesis of the anterior wall *(arrows)*.

restored. Viable myocardium can be classified as "stunned" or "hibernating". Stunned myocardium refers to the persistence of LV regional dysfunction after transient coronary occlusion; that is, recovery of wall motion abnormalities is delayed despite adequate reperfusion therapy or restoration of normal coronary flow. Hibernating myocardium refers to chronic LV regional dysfunction when there is severe CAD and chronic ischaemia; complete or partial recovery of function occurs following coronary revascularisation.

Stress echocardiography is a specialised technique and both the reporting physician and cardiac sonographer must be highly trained in image interpretation and image acquisition. This section on stress echocardiography covers only the very basic concepts of this technique. For a more comprehensive understanding of stress echocardiography readers are advised to review other sources as listed in the Further Reading section of this Chapter.

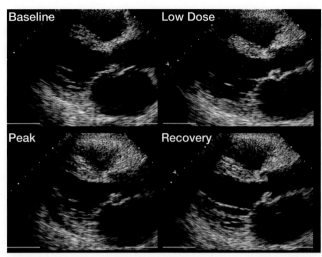

Figure 5.20 These end-systolic still frame images were recorded from a dobutamine stress echocardiogram. The quad-screen format shows images from the parasternal long axis view. These images show augmentation of all LV segments at peak dose (*bottom left*).

Table 5.5 Viable versus Non-Viable Myocardium: Responses to Dobutamine

	At Rest	Low Dose Dobutamine	High Dose Dobutamine
Stunned myocardium	Impaired wall motion	Increased wall thickening	Further increase in wall thickening
Hibernating myocardium *	Impaired wall motion	Increased wall thickening	Reduction in wall thickening
Non-viable (infarcted) myocardium	Impaired wall motion	No change in wall thickening	No change in wall thickening

* The increase in wall thickening at low dose followed by a decrease in wall thickening at high dose dobutamine is referred to as a biphasic response. This worsening of regional function at high dose occurs due to the induction of ischaemia. This biphasic response differentiates stunned from hibernating myocardium.

Complications of Myocardial Infarction

In addition to identifying acute and prior MI, echocardiography can be used to identify the complications associated with MI. Importantly, complications can be anticipated based on the location of the MI and knowledge of the incidence, risk factors and timeframe for the development of each type of complication (Table 5.6). Complications following an AMI are now less commonly encountered due to the early reperfusion and thrombolytic therapies for STEMIs.

Left Ventricular Aneurysms

As previously mentioned an aneurysm can be described as abnormal outward bulging and deformation of a myocardial segment occurring in both systole and diastole. LV aneurysms result from the weakening of an infarcted (necrotic) wall and the pulsatile force of ventricular contractions. Therefore, aneurysms occur due to stretching and thinning of the infarcted region (infarct expansion). The wall of the aneurysm is lined by myocardium and the "neck" between the ventricle and the aneurysm is wide (Fig. 5.21). Over time, the aneurysmal wall becomes thin, fibrotic and focally calcified; therefore, LV aneurysms rarely rupture.

LV aneurysms are most commonly located at the LV apex but may also been seen in the anterior, inferolateral and inferior walls. The development of LV aneurysms usually occurs within 2 to 4 weeks following an AMI.

LV aneurysms are also referred to as "true aneurysms" as opposed to the pseudoaneurysm that develops following free wall rupture (discussed below).

By echocardiography, LV aneurysms have several characteristic

features (Fig. 5.22-5.23). In particular, the neck of the aneurysm, defined as the junction between the aneurysm and the remainder of the LV, is wide with the ratio of the diameter at the neck to the maximum diameter of the aneurysm exceeding 0.5. The myocardium in the region of the aneurysm also appears thinned and echogenic; during systole the infarcted area bulges outward. Mural thrombus and/or spontaneous echo contrast (SEC) may also be seen within the aneurysm.

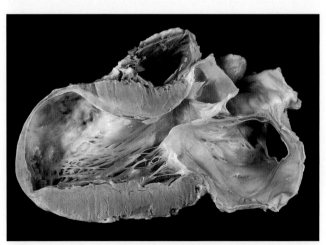

Figure 5.21 This gross pathological specimen shows the characteristic features of a post-infarction true aneurysm of the left ventricle (LV). Observe that the basal to mid septum and inferolateral LV wall are normal in thickness. The aneurysm is seen at the LV apex and apicoseptal regions. Note that the myocardium of the aneurysm is stretched and thinned and the "neck" between the ventricle and the aneurysm is wide.

By permission of Mayo Foundation for Medical Education and Research. All rights reserved. Courtesy of William D. Edwards, MD.

Table 5.6 **Complications of MI**

Complication	Approximate Incidence	Location of MI	Risk Factors	Estimated Timeline for Development Post-MI
LV aneurysm	≈ 1-5%	Apical MI Inferior MI Lateral MI	Female sex Total occlusion of the LAD artery Single vessel CAD Transmural MI	2-4 weeks (but can occur acutely) Rarely beyond 3 months post-MI
LV thrombus	≈ 20%	Anterior MI Inferior MI	Patient not treated with anticoagulant therapy	As early as 1 day
Free wall rupture (FWR)	≈ 1- 3%	Lateral MI Anterior MI	Advanced age Female sex First MI Transmural MI HTN (absence of LV hypertrophy) Poor collateral circulation	50% within 5 days 90% within 2 weeks
Ventricular septal rupture (VSR)	< 1%	Anterior MI Inferior MI	Advanced age Female sex Single vessel CAD (LAD) or multivessel CAD HTN Extensive transmural MI Poor septal collateral circulation	First 24-48 hours post reperfusion therapy 3-5 days without reperfusion therapy Rarely beyond 2 weeks post-MI
Papillary muscle rupture (PMR)	< 1%	Inferior MI Anterolateral MI	First MI (large MI) Advanced age Female sex HTN ↑ frequency of recurrent ischaemia Multivessel CAD	< 24 hrs post-thrombolysis 2-7 days without thrombolysis
RV MI	≈ 10%	Inferior MI	-	Any time
Acute pericarditis	≈ 10%	Anterior MI	Transmural MI	24-96 hrs
Dressler's syndrome	≈ 1-3%	Anterior MI	Transmural MI	1-8 weeks

CAD = coronary artery disease; HTN = systemic hypertension; LAD = left anterior descending artery; LV = left ventricular; MI = myocardial infarction; RV = right ventricle.

Left Ventricular Thrombus

LV thrombus occurs due to stasis of blood flow and may form within the first 24 hours after an AMI. Mural thrombus occurs in approximately 20% of patients with AMI who do not receive anticoagulant therapy. LV thrombus post-MI is most commonly seen with large anterior infarcts that involve the apex of the LV. LV thrombus is also commonly associated with LV aneurysms.

Identification of LV thrombus is important due to its embolic potential. Systemic emboli and/or stroke may occur in approximately 10% of patients following an AMI. Importantly, the incidence of LV thrombus has decreased due to early reperfusion and thrombolytic therapies.

Echocardiography is considered the method of choice for the diagnosis of LV thrombus. The 2D echocardiographic feature of thrombus is the appearance of echo-dense material within the LV cavity which is distinct from underlying endocardium (Fig. 5.24). Furthermore, acute thrombus, which has a greater risk of embolisation, can be differentiated from chronic thrombus. Acute thrombus appears mobile, fragile, and protrudes into the LV cavity while chronic thrombus appears organized and laminated (Fig. 5.25).

It is also important to be aware that poor image quality may mask LV thrombus (especially at the apex) while normal anatomic structures and imaging artefacts may mimic LV thrombus. Anatomic structures that mimic LV thrombus include: (1) aberrant fibrous chords or accessory bands, (2) ruptured papillary muscle and/or chords, and (3) prominent LV trabeculations. Colour flow Doppler imaging or the injection of intravenous contrast agents may be very useful in determining the presence or absence of thrombus in these situations (Fig. 5.26 and 5.27).

Value of Colour Doppler in LV Thrombus Identification
Using colour flow Doppler it is possible to 'opacify' the LV apex (see Fig. 5.26). This is accomplished by using a low colour velocity scale at a shallow imaging depth. In particular, a very low colour velocity scale enhances the sensitivity to low velocity flow; by lowering the colour velocity scale the full range of colours is set to detect small Doppler shifts. However, because the velocity of flow at the LV apex is low and because the angle of intercept between the ultrasound beam and flow direction is at 90 degrees, there may be areas of no colour filling at the apex even in the absence of an LV thrombus; this is a limitation of this technique.

Image optimisation for suspected LV thrombus

Image optimisation is crucial for the investigation of suspected LV thrombus. Therefore, when assessing regions of abnormal wall motion (especially apical aneurysms) the sonographer should:

- Use the highest possible transducer frequency (to improve spatial resolution)
- Use harmonic imaging (to improve contrast resolution)
- Use a shallow field of view (thrombus usually at the apex)
- Reposition the focal zone at the level of interest (to improve lateral resolution)
- Slowly and carefully pan through the LV (anterior to posterior) from all possible imaging planes
- Confirm the presence of thrombus in more than one imaging plane.

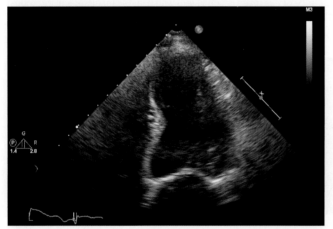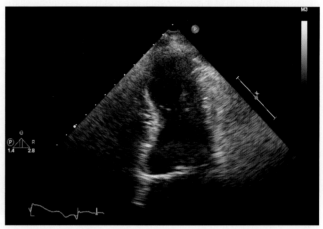

Figure 5.22 These apical 4-chamber images show thinning, dilatation and dyskinesis of the apicoseptal region of the LV. Observe that the aneurysm has an abnormal contour in diastole (*left*) and displays systolic expansion during systole (*right*).

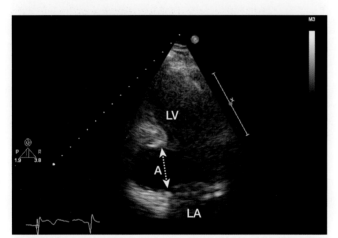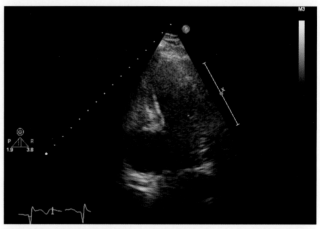

Figure 5.23 These apical 2-chamber images show an aneurysm (*A*) of the basal inferior wall. Observe that the aneurysm has an abnormal contour in diastole (*left*) which is maintained during systole (*right*). Also observe that the neck of the aneurysm (*arrow*) is wide.

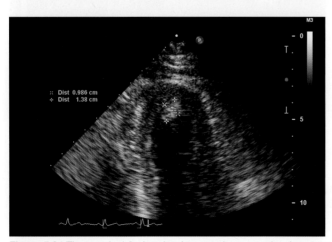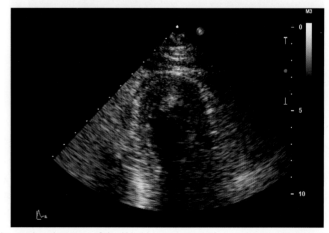

Figure 5.24 These apical 2-chamber images show an echo dense mass located at the apex of the LV; this appearance is consistent with apical mural thrombus.

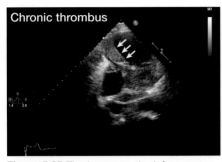
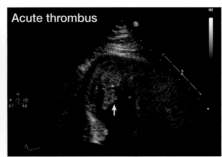
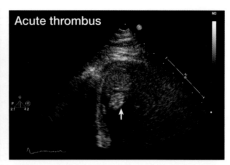

Figure 5.25 The image on the left was recorded from an apical 4-chamber view with posterior tilting; a large, crescentic echo dense mass extending the length of the apicoseptal aneurysm is seen *(arrows)*; the appearance of this mass is consistent with a large laminar apical thrombus. The middle and right images show a large echo dense mass protruding into the LV cavity *(arrows)*. Note how the shape of this thrombus varies between the two frames shown; on real-time imaging, this thrombus was highly mobile consistent with acute thrombus.

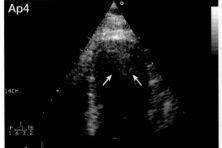
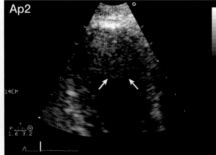
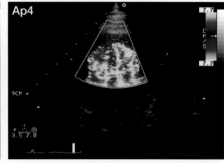

Figure 5.26 These end-systolic frames were recorded from the apical 4-chamber *(Ap4)* and the apical 2-chamber *(Ap2)* views at a shallow imaging depth. These images show an apparent echogenicity within the LV apex consistent with possible LV thrombus *(arrows)*. Colour flow Doppler at a low velocity scale (7.7 cm/s) was also used to fill the LV apex excluding the presence of LV thrombus *(right)*.

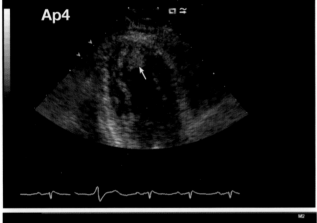
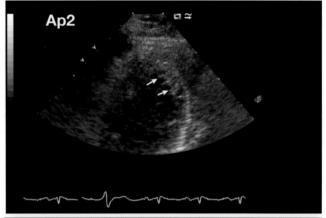
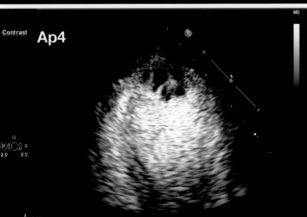
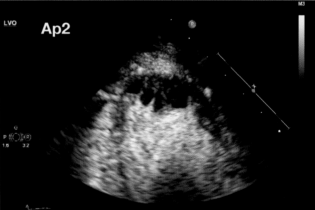

Figure 5.27 These images were recorded from the apical 4-chamber *(Ap4)* and apical 2-chamber *(Ap2)* views in the same patient. The top images show a suspicious area at the LV apex *(arrows)*. Following the administration of intravenous contrast multiple large, irregular mobile thrombi were noted in the LV apex (dark areas within the LV apex) *(bottom images)*.

Free Wall Rupture and Pseudoaneurysms

Cardiac rupture most commonly occurs in the lateral LV wall; this is commonly referred to as a free wall rupture (FWR). Approximately 50% of FWRs occur within 5 days and 90% in the first two weeks following an AMI. FWR most commonly results from a distinct tear in the myocardial wall usually between the junction of infarcted and normal muscle (Fig. 5.28). Three types of FWR have been described [5.1]:

- Type I is characterised by an abrupt, slit-like tear that is frequently associated with anterior infarcts and that occurs early (within 24 hours);
- Type II is characterised by an 'erosion' of the infarcted myocardium, indicative of a slowly progressing tear at the site of infarction (occurs 1 to 3 days post-MI);
- Type III is characterized by early aneurysm formation and occurs later in older and severely expanded infarcts.

In patients with acute FWR the echocardiogram will typically reveal a pericardial effusion or pericardial haematoma with signs of cardiac tamponade (Fig. 5.29).

Usually FWR results in acute haemopericardium (blood in pericardium), cardiac tamponade and death. However, sometimes the FWR is contained by pericardial adhesions in the vicinity of rupture and a pseudoaneurysm (false aneurysm) is formed (Fig. 5.30).

Echocardiography is extremely valuable in differentiating a pseudoaneurysm from a true aneurysm (Fig. 5.31-5.32). Characteristic features of a pseudoaneurysm include:

1. sharp discontinuity of the endocardial edge at the site of communication between the pseudoaneurysm and LV cavity;
2. a saccular or globular contour of the pseudoaneurysm chamber;
3. presence of a narrow "neck" compared with the diameter of the pseudoaneurysm (the ratio of entry diameter to maximum diameter of pseudoaneurysm is less than 0.5);
4. to-and-fro flow between the pseudoaneurysm and the LV via spectral and colour Doppler imaging; with systolic flow from the LV to the pseudoaneurysm and diastolic flow from the pseudoaneurysm back to the LV.

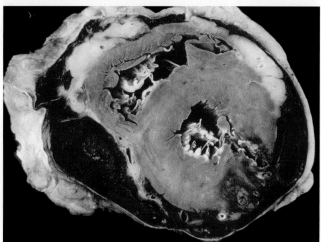

Figure 5.28 This gross pathological specimen shows a left ventricular lateral free wall rupture. This appears as a tear in the myocardium at the 4 o'clock position. Associated haemopericardium is also shown; this appears as a blood clot within the pericardial sac.
By permission of Mayo Foundation for Medical Education and Research. All rights reserved. Courtesy of William D. Edwards, MD.

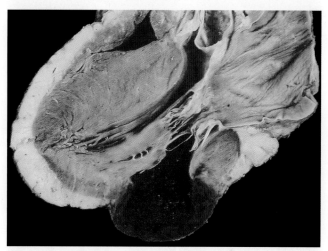

Figure 5.30 This gross pathological specimen shows a pseudo-aneurysm of the mid inferolateral wall. This free wall rupture, contained by pericardial adhesions, creates a false aneurysm; the "neck" between the ventricle and the pseudoaneurysm is narrow.
By permission of Mayo Foundation for Medical Education and Research. All rights reserved. Courtesy of William D. Edwards, MD.

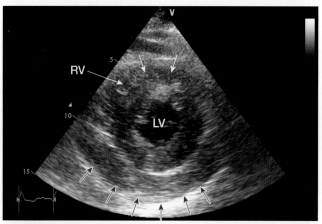

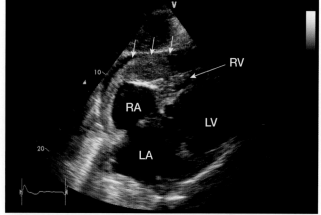

Figure 5.29 These images were recorded from a parasternal short axis view (*left*) and a subcostal 4-chamber view (*right*) in a patient with a late presentation anterior STEMI. An urgent bedside echocardiogram was requested due to sudden patient deterioration. Observe the large echodense pericardial collection (*arrows*) surrounding the heart in the parasternal short axis view. An echodense pericardial collection (*arrows*) is also seen anterior to the right ventricle (*RV*) from the subcostal view; total compression of the RV is also noted from this view. These images are consistent with acute cardiac rupture with a pericardial haematoma causing cardiac tamponade. The site of rupture is not visualised on these images.
LA = left atrium; LV = left ventricle; RA = right atrium.

[5.1] Becker AE, van Mantgem JP. Cardiac tamponade. A study of 50 hearts. *Eur J Cardiol.* 1975 Dec;3(4):349-58.

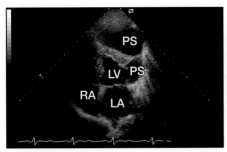 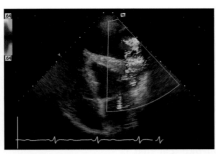 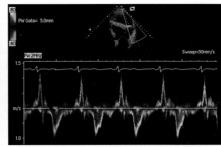

Figure 5.31 A pseudoaneurysm (PS) of the lateral LV wall is seen in this apical 4-chamber view; note that the diameter of the neck is narrow compared with the overall diameter of the body of the pseudoaneurysm (*left*). Colour flow Doppler confirms the communication between the left ventricle (LV) and the PS (*middle*). Spectral Doppler demonstrates systolic flow into the PS (flow above the zero baseline) and diastolic flow out of the PS (flow below the zero baseline) (*right*). LA = left atrium; LV = left ventricle; RA = right atrium.

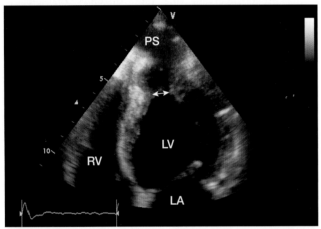 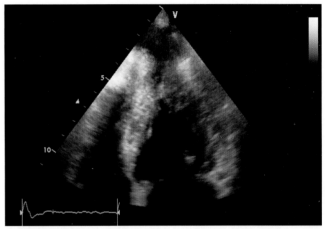

Figure 5.32 A pseudoaneurysm (*PS*) at the LV apex is seen on these apical 4-chamber views; an end-diastolic frame is shown on the left and an end-systolic frame is shown on the right. Observe the narrow neck of this pseudoaneurysm (*arrow*). LA = left atrium; LV = left ventricle; RV = right ventricle.

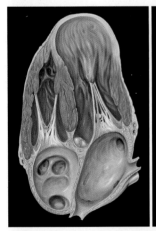 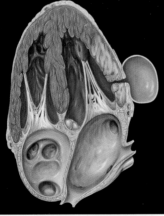

Figure 5.33 These illustrations demonstrate the difference between a true aneurysm (*left*) and a pseudoaneurysm (*right*). Observe that the true aneurysm is defined by a stretched portion of the infarcted myocardium; its wall contains all three myocardial layers and it is connected to the ventricle by a wide neck. In a pseudoaneurysm the rupture site forms a narrow neck to a false aneurysmal outpouching; communication with the LV cavity is by means of a narrow neck; the wall of a pseudoaneurysm is composed of pericardium. Organized thrombus and/or haematoma may also be associated with a pseudoaneurysm (not shown on this illustration).
Reproduced from http://commons.wikimedia.org/wiki/Category: Patrick_Lynch. Patrick J. Lynch; illustrator; C. Carl Jaffe; MD; cardiologist Yale University Center for Advanced Instructional Media Medical Illustrations by Patrick Lynch, generated for multimedia teaching projects by the Yale University School of Medicine, Center for Advanced Instructional Media, 1987-2000.

It should be noted that while pseudoaneurysms are characteristically defined as having a narrow neck, some pseudoaneurysms may have a wide neck.

Pseudoaneurysms are lined only by pericardium and the risk of rupture is very high. Therefore it is crucial that a pseudoaneurysm is differentiated from a true aneurysm (Table 5.7 and Fig. 5.33).

Ventricular Septal Rupture

Ventricular septal rupture (VSR) is a rare complication post-MI. The majority of post-MI VSRs occur within the first week and may develop as early as the first 24 hours following an acute MI; VSR rarely occurs after 2 weeks post-MI.

VRSs are most commonly located at the junction of normal and infarcted myocardium in the apical septum (anterior MI) and in the basal inferior septum (inferior MI). VSRs are characterised by the appearance of a new harsh, loud holosystolic murmur heard best at the lower left sternal border which is usually accompanied with a thrill; these clinical findings may be confused with acute mitral regurgitation (MR).

Table 5.7 Differences between True Aneurysms and Pseudoaneurysms

Parameter	True Aneurysm	Pseudoaneurysm
Cause	Infarction	Rupture
Incidence	1-5%	Rare
Neck	Wide	Narrow
Lined by	Myocardium (scar)	Pericardium +/- thrombus
Rupture	Very rare	Common

The VSR defect may be simple or complex. A simple defect results in a direct through-and-through communication between the LV and RV; these types of defects are most commonly seen at the apex following an anterior MI (Fig. 5.34). Complex defects are described as having a serpiginous (snake-like) course through the IVS with multiple defects tracking through necrotic tissue; these defects are more commonly associated with basal inferior MIs.

On 2D echocardiography, a simple VSR may be seen directly; however, due to the serpiginous nature of complex defects the actual site of VSR may not be visualised. In addition, RV trabeculations may obscure the defect.

Echocardiography can also determine the size of the defect and the extent of haemodynamic compromise. This can be achieved by measuring the anatomic size of the defect (Fig. 5.35) and by estimating the degree of left-to-right shunting via calculation of the QP:QS shunt ratio (Fig. 5.36).

Continuous-wave Doppler signal across a VSR can be used to estimate the LV-to-RV pressure gradient and the right ventricular systolic pressure (RVSP). The peak systolic velocity across the VSR reflects the systolic pressure difference between the LV and RV. In the absence of LVOT obstruction or aortic stenosis, it can be assumed that the LV systolic pressure is equal to the systolic blood pressure (SBP) (Fig. 5.37). Therefore,

Equation 5.2

$$RVSP = SBP - 4\,V_{VSR}^{2}$$

where RVSP = right ventricular systolic pressure (mm Hg)
SBP   = systolic blood pressure (mm Hg)
V_{VSR} = peak systolic VSR velocity (m/s)

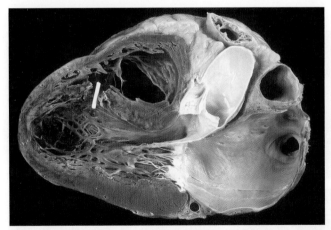

Figure 5.34 This gross pathological specimen shows a ventricular septal rupture (*white marker*) following an acute myocardial infarction. By permission of Mayo Foundation for Medical Education and Research. All rights reserved. Courtesy of William D. Edwards, MD.

Papillary Muscle Rupture

Infarction of a papillary muscle leads to papillary muscle dysfunction with varying degrees of MR. Papillary muscle infarction can also be associated with partial or incomplete rupture of the trunk of the muscle (Fig. 5.38). Papillary muscle rupture (PMR) occurs in approximately 1% of MIs. Complete rupture of the papillary muscle trunk is usually fatal due to sudden acute and severe MR, subsequent pulmonary oedema and cardiogenic shock.

PMR most commonly involves the posteromedial papillary muscle rather than the anterolateral papillary muscle; this is because the posteromedial papillary muscle is supplied by a single coronary artery (PDA) while the anterolateral papillary muscle has a dual coronary artery supply (LAD and Cx). Therefore, PMR is usually associated with an inferior MI.

Patients suffering PMR present with a new holosystolic murmur at the apex. However, the new murmur may only be heard in early-to-mid systole and it may not be loud due to the large regurgitant orifice area and the rapid rise in LA pressure which decreases the LV-to-LA pressure gradient over systole.

Echocardiography has an important role in making the early diagnosis of partial PMR as this is a potentially surgically repairable condition. Clues to the identification of PMR include:

1. a mobile mass attached to the mitral valve leaflet that prolapses into the LA in systole: this appearance is consistent with a ruptured papillary muscle head (Fig. 5.39);
2. an abnormal cut-off of one papillary muscle: the papillary muscle appears truncated and 'flat' rather than conal;
3. a flail segment of the mitral valve with ruptured chords exhibiting chaotic motion (Fig. 5.40,A);
4. severe MR on colour flow Doppler with the jet direction opposite to the flail leaflet (Fig. 5.40,B);
5. increased forward flow velocities across the mitral valve via spectral Doppler: this is indicative of increased stroke volume through the mitral valve secondary to severe MR (Fig. 5.40,C);
6. spectral Doppler of the MR signal demonstrates low velocity flow with a V cut-off sign: this is indicative of a marked elevation in the LA pressure (Fig.5.40,D);
7. small, hyperdynamic LV: the LV is contracting against a low afterload when blood is being 'ejected' into the LA.

Importantly, PMR results in acute, severe MR; hence, the typical secondary signs associated with chronic, severe MR such as dilatation of the LA and LV are not usually evident. In addition, the 2D appearance of partial PMR may mimic tumour, thrombus or vegetations; therefore, consideration of the clinical presentation of the patient and the recognition of RWMA will assist in distinguishing PMR from other pathologies.

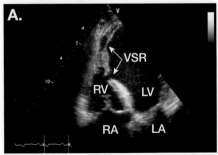
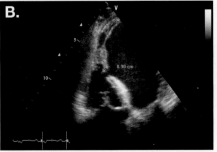
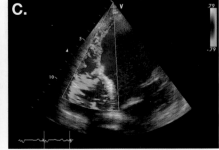

Figure 5.35 This series of images, recorded from the apical 4-chamber view, shows multiple ventricular septal ruptures **(A)**. A large simple VSR measuring approximately 0.9 cm is located in the mid septum **(B)**. Colour Doppler imaging confirms the presence of left-to-right shunting across all defects **(C)**. LA = left atrium; LV = left ventricle; RA = right atrium; RV = right ventricle.

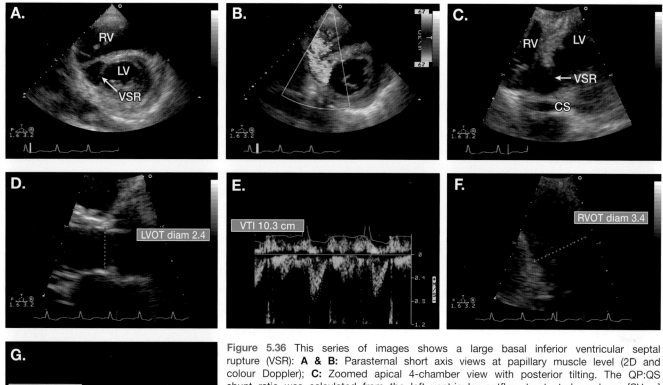

Figure 5.36 This series of images shows a large basal inferior ventricular septal rupture (VSR): **A & B:** Parasternal short axis views at papillary muscle level (2D and colour Doppler); **C:** Zoomed apical 4-chamber view with posterior tilting. The QP:QS shunt ratio was calculated from the left ventricular outflow tract stroke volume [SV_{LVOT}] (**D & E**) and right ventricular outflow tract stroke volume [SV_{RVOT}] (**F & G**):

$$SV_{LVOT} = CSA_{LVOT} \times VTI_{LVOT}$$
$$= (0.785 \times 2.4^2) \times 10.3$$
$$= 47\ mL$$

$$SV_{RVOT} = CSA_{RVOT} \times VTI_{RVOT}$$
$$= (0.785 \times 3.4^2) \times 21.4$$
$$= 194\ mL$$

$$\mathbf{QP:QS = SV_{RVOT} \div SV_{LVOT}}$$
$$\mathbf{= 194 \div 47}$$
$$\mathbf{= 4.1}$$

CS = coronary sinus; LA = left atrium; LV = left ventricle; RV = right ventricle.

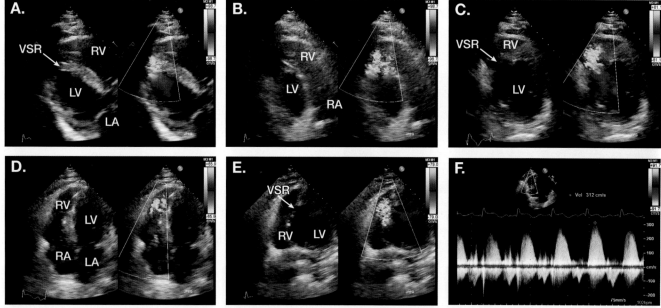

Figure 5.37 This series of systolic still frame images demonstrates an apical ventricular septal rupture *(VSR)*: **A**: Low parasternal long axis of the left ventricle; **B**: Low parasternal long axis of right ventricular inflow; **C**: Para-apical short axis view; **D**: Apical 4-chamber view; **E**: Apical 4-chamber view with posterior tilt; **F**: Continuous-wave Doppler velocity across the VSR. The peak systolic velocity across the VSR recorded via continuous-wave Doppler is 3.12 m/s; the patient's systolic blood pressure (SBP) at the time of this study was measured at 90 mm Hg. The estimated RVSP in this example is:

$$RVSP = SBP - 4\ V_{VSD}^{2}$$
$$= 90 - 4\ (3.12)^2$$
$$= 90 - 40$$
$$= 50\ mm\ Hg$$

CS = coronary sinus; LA = left atrium; LV = left ventricle; RA = right atrium; RV = right ventricle; VSR = ventricular septal rupture.

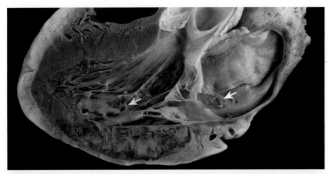

Figure 5.38 This gross pathological specimen shows a complete rupture of one of the two heads of the posteromedial papillary muscle. The white arrow shows the papillary muscle head attached to the anterior mitral leaflet, now flail in the left atrium. The papillary muscle trunk is indicated by the yellow arrow.
By permission of Mayo Foundation for Medical Education and Research. All rights reserved. Courtesy of William D. Edwards, MD.

Ischaemic Mitral Regurgitation
Ischaemic mitral regurgitation (IMR) is commonly seen in patients following an acute inferior MI. The possible mechanisms of IMR include:
• mitral annular dilatation secondary to dilatation and altered function and geometry of the papillary muscles
• papillary muscle dysfunction
• papillary muscle rupture
• acute systolic anterior motion of the mitral valve
The mechanisms and assessment of IMR are discussed in detail in Chapter 8.

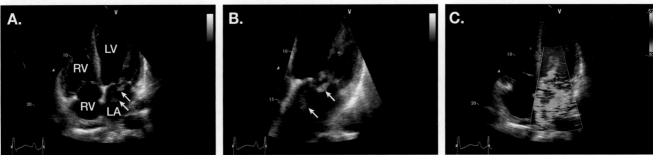

Figure 5.39 These images were recorded from the apical 4-chamber view. Observe the 'mass' attached to the mitral valve which prolapses into the left atrium (*arrows*); this appearance is consistent with a ruptured papillary muscle head. Colour flow Doppler confirms the presence of severe mitral regurgitation. LA = left atrium; LV = left ventricle; RA =right atrium; RV = right ventricle.

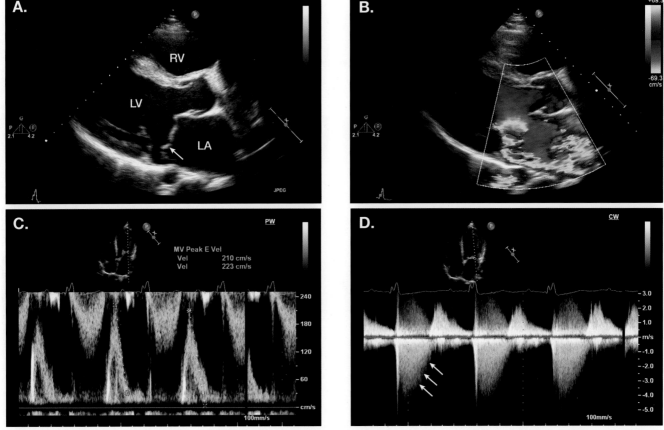

Figure 5.40 These images show some of the characteristic features associated with papillary muscle rupture: **A:** Parasternal long axis of the LV shows a flail anterior mitral valve leaflet (*arrow*); **B:** Corresponding colour Doppler image shows severe, posteriorly directed MR (also observe the large flow convergence zone on the LV side of the valve); **C:** Pulsed-wave Doppler of transmitral mitral inflow shows an increased peak E velocity; **D:** Continuous-wave Doppler signal shows a low velocity MR signal with a V cut-off sign (*arrows*). See text for further details.
LA = left atrium; LV = left ventricle; RV = right ventricle.

Right Ventricular Infarction

RV systolic dysfunction is common following an inferior or inferolateral MI. A haemodynamically significant RV myocardial infarction (RV MI) is only seen in approximately 10% of patients who have suffered an inferior MI. An isolated RV MI can occur rarely. The typical presentation of a patient with an RV MI is unexplained, persistent hypotension, clear lung fields, and elevated jugular venous pressure.

Echocardiographic findings of RV MI include:

1. Dilatation of the RV;
2. Hypokinetic, akinetic or dyskinetic segments of the RV (the RV apex is usually supplied by the LAD [Fig. 5.41]; therefore, the RV apex wall is usually normal or hyperdynamic even when there is an RV MI);
3. Paradoxical IVS motion and reversed IVS curvature due to increased RV end-diastolic pressures;
4. Tricuspid regurgitation [TR] (secondary to annular dilatation);
5. RA enlargement (secondary to TR and increased RV filling pressures);
6. Right-to-left shunting across an existing patent foramen ovale.

Pericarditis and Dressler's Syndrome

The presence of haemodynamically insignificant pericardial effusions are common following an AMI; effusions are more common with an anterior MI, with larger infarcts and when congestive heart failure is present.

Acute pericarditis associated with an AMI is seen in approximately 10% of patients and develops between 24 and 96 hours after an AMI. Acute pericarditis is a result of pericardial inflammation overlying the area of the AMI.

Late pericarditis or Dressler's syndrome is a delayed form of pericarditis that occurs 1 to 8 weeks following an AMI and has been reported in only 1 to 3% of patients with an AMI. This syndrome is characterised by a recurrent low-grade fever, pleuropericardial chest pain, pericardial friction rub and pleural effusions. The precise mechanism of this syndrome is unknown but it is thought to be related to an autoimmune process occuring in response to myocardial necrosis.

On echocardiography, pericarditis may appear as a small pericardial effusion. Cardiac tamponade is rare following MI, therefore, if a large pericardial effusion with haemodynamic compromise is detected, this should raise the possibility of cardiac rupture.

Direct Imaging of Coronary Arteries

Direct imaging of the ostium of the right and left coronary arteries is often possible via 2D echocardiography. The origins of the coronary arteries are best seen from the parasternal short axis view at the level of the aortic valve. From this view the LMCA can be seen to originate from the left coronary sinus of the aortic root at the 3-5 o'clock position (Fig. 5.42) while the RCA may be seen arising from the right coronary sinus of the aortic root at the 11-12 o'clock position approximately 1 cm superior to the origin of the LMCA (Fig. 5.43, top). The origin of the RCA may also be seen from the parasternal long axis view of the LV (Fig. 5.43, bottom). The normal luminal diameter of the LMCA is approximately 4-5 mm and the normal luminal diameter of the RCA is approximately 3-4 mm. Occasionally from the apical 4-chamber view with posterior tilting the Cx artery can be seen travelling in the posterior left AV groove (Fig. 5.44).

Coronary Artery Aneurysms

Coronary artery aneurysm (CAAN) is defined as coronary dilatation which exceeds the diameter of normal adjacent segments or the diameter of the patient's largest coronary vessel by 1.5 times. CAANs are rare lesions detected in about 1-5% of patients undergoing coronary angiography. They occur more commonly in males than females. Aneurysms are most commonly observed in the RCA (50%) followed by the LAD and the Cx (30-40%); involvement of the LMCA is least frequent (10%). The aetiologies of CAAN are listed in Table 5.8. The most common cause for CAANs in the adult is atherosclerotic CAD while Kawaski's disease is the most common cause of aneurysms in children.

While it is possible to detect CAANs at the ostium of the RCA and LMCA by transthoracic (TTX) echocardiography, coronary angiography or computed tomography are usually required to make the diagnosis.

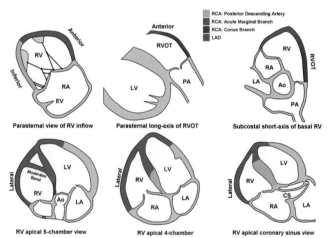

Figure 5.41 This illustration shows the coronary supply to the right ventricular walls.

Ao = aorta; CS = coronary sinus; LA = left atrium; LAD = left anterior descending artery; LV = left ventricle; PA = pulmonary artery; RA = right atrium; RCA = right coronary artery; RV = right ventricle; RVOT = right ventricular outflow tract.

Reprinted from Rudski LG, Lai WW, Afilalo J, Hua L, Handschumacher MD, Chandrasekaran K, Solomon SD, Louie EK, Schiller NB. Guidelines for the echocardiographic assessment of the right heart in adults: a report from the American Society of Echocardiography endorsed by the European Association of Echocardiography, a registered branch of the European Society of Cardiology, and the Canadian Society of Echocardiography, *J Am Soc Echocardiogr*, Vol. 23 (7), page 691, © 2010 with permission from Elsevier.

Table 5.8 Aetiology of Coronary Artery Aneurysms

Aetiology of Coronary Artery Aneurysms
• Atherosclerosis
• Congenital
• Inflammatory disorders (e.g. Kawaski's disease, Takayasu's arteritis)
• Coronary angiography (e.g. balloon, atherectomy)
• Autoimmune diseases (e.g. polyarteritis nodosa, systemic lupus erythematosus, scleroderma)
• Connective tissue disorders (Marfan's, Ehlers-Danlos syndromes)
• Mycotic coronary emboli
• Coronary artery dissection
• Trauma

Coronary Artery Anomalies

Coronary artery anomalies (CAA) are rare occurring in less than 1% of the general population. Patient presentation is variable; ranging from an incidental finding at coronary angiography to angina, myocardial infarction or a sudden death episode.

CAA can be described in terms of the variations in number, origin and/or course, and termination of the coronary arteries (Table 5.9). While it is possible to detect CAA by TTX echocardiography other imaging techniques such as transoesophageal echocardiography, coronary angiography, computed tomography and/or cardiac magnetic resonance imaging are usually required to make the diagnosis.

Coronary artery fistulas (CAF) however may be identified on TTX echocardiography by the detection of abnormal high velocity, continuous flow into a cardiac chamber, great vessel or other structure and/or by the appearance of a dilated, tortuous coronary artery (Fig. 5.45-5.46). The majority of CAF involve the RCA (40-60%) followed by the LAD (30-40%) with less than 5% of fistulas originating from both the LCA and the RCA. The most common drainage site for a CAF is the RV (45%), followed by the RA (25%) and the pulmonary artery (15%); fistula drainage into the LA or the LV is seen in less than 10% of cases. Large CAF can cause coronary artery steal phenomenon which leads to ischaemia of the myocardial segment distal to the site of the coronary artery fistula connection.

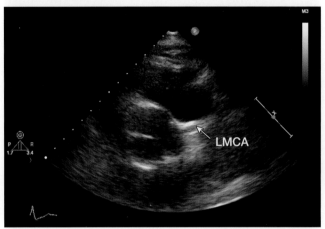

Figure 5.42 From the parasternal short axis view at the aortic valve level the origin of the left main coronary artery (*LMCA*) is seen arising from the left sinus of Valsalva at the 3 o'clock position (*arrow*).

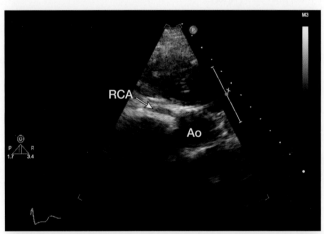

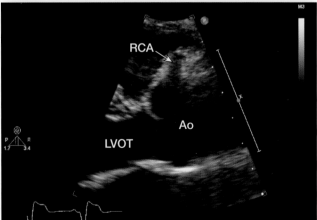

Figure 5.43 The origin of the right coronary artery (*RCA*) can be seen arising from the right sinus of Valsalva from the parasternal short axis view in the 11 o'clock position (*top*) and from the parasternal long axis view of the LV (*bottom*).
Ao = aorta; LVOT = left ventricular outflow tract.

> ### Coronary Artery Steal Syndrome
> Coronary artery steal (CAS) refers to blood being 'stolen' from one region of the coronary tree by another artery or chamber. CAS leads to myocardial ischaemia as oxygen-rich blood is diverted away from its intended myocardial segment. This phenomenon may occur:
> (1) when there are coronary stenoses in series: in this instance dilatation of normal coronary arteries (due to exercise or vasodilator therapy) "steals" blood from stenotic arteries;
> (2) post coronary artery by-pass grafting where internal mammary grafts have been used and when there is also associated left subclavian artery stenosis: in this situation there is retrograde flow from the internal mammary graft to the left subclavian artery;
> (3) when there is a coronary artery fistula: in this setting blood is being shunted away from the high pressure coronary artery system into the lower pressure 'site'.

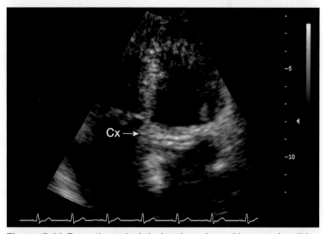

Figure 5.44 From the apical 4-chamber view with posterior tilting the left circumflex artery (*Cx*) can be seen traversing the left atrioventricular groove.

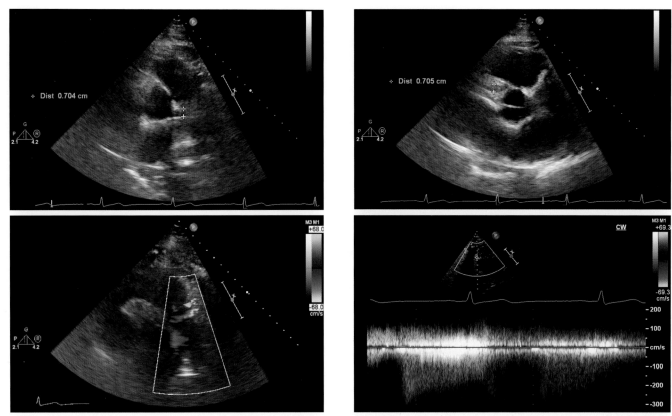

Figure 5.45 The proximal coronary arteries are dilated with both the left main coronary artery (*top left*) and the right coronary artery (*top right*) measuring 7 mm. On colour Doppler imaging multiple coronary fistulae are seen draining into the pulmonary artery distal to the pulmonary valve (*bottom left*). Continuous-wave Doppler confirms the presence of high velocity continuous flow (*bottom right*); note that due to non-parallel alignment with flow, the velocities are underestimated. Computed tomography coronary angiography confirmed the presence of an extensive complex arterial fistulae between the right and left coronary arteries and the main pulmonary artery.

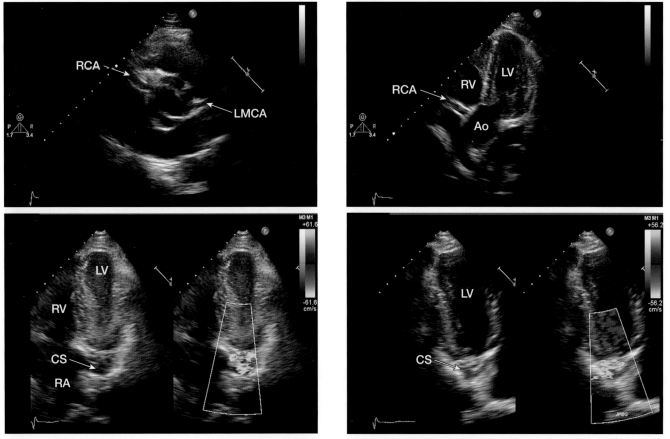

Figure 5.46 From the parasternal short axis view (*top left*) and the apical 5-chamber view (*top right*) the right coronary artery (RCA) appears dilated. The apical 4-chamber view with posterior tilting (*bottom left*) and an off-axis apical 2-chamber view (*bottom right*) show turbulent flow within the coronary sinus (CS); flow was noted to be predominantly diastolic. These findings are suggestive of a coronary artery fistula into the coronary sinus. Computed tomography coronary angiography confirmed the presence of a large tortuous RCA which emptied into the coronary sinus. Ao = aorta; LMCA = left main coronary artery; LV = left ventricle; RA = right atrium; RV = right ventricle.

Table 5.9 Coronary Artery Anomalies

Coronary Anomaly	Description
Abnormal number	Duplication of the: • LAD • RCA • Cx
Anomalous origin	Anomalous origin of coronary artery from opposite sinus of Valsalva or from NSV: • RCA arises from LSV • LCA arises from RSV • Cx or LAD artery arising from RSV • LCA or RCA (or a branch) arising from NSV Anomalous origin of coronary artery from PA: LMCA or RCA arise from: • pulmonary trunk (ALCAPA = anomalous left coronary artery from pulmonary artery) • RPA • LPA • brachiocephalic artery LCA and RCA may have a "high take-off": • arise from ascending aorta; above the sinotubular junction Multiple ostia: • Absent LMCA with separate origins of LAD and Cx Solitary coronary artery system: • entire coronary artery system originates from a single ostium or a single coronary artery Single coronary artery: • LMCA and RCA arise from a common ostium from the RSV, LSV or NSV
Anomalous course	Otherwise normal CA has an anomalous intramyocardial course (myocardial bridging)
Anomalous origin and course	Anomalous LCA arising from RSV or RCA takes 1 of 4 courses: • A (**A**nterior to right ventricular outflow tract; i.e. prepulmonic course); • B (**B**etween aorta and pulmonary trunk; i.e. interarterial course)*; • C (through the **C**rista supraventricularis; i.e. subpulmonic or septal course) • D (**D**orsal or posterior to the aorta; i.e. retroaortic course) * This interarterial course carries an increased risk for sudden cardiac death.
Anomalous termination	Fistulae: major epicardial coronary artery terminates abnormally resulting in communication between 1 or 2 coronary arteries and either: • any one of the cardiac chambers • coronary sinus • PA • SVC Coronary Arcade: • Intercoronary artery continuity between LCA and RCA Extracardiac Termination: • connections exist between coronary artery and extracardiac vessels (e.g. bronchial artery).

Cx= circumflex artery; LAD = left anterior descending artery; LCA = left coronary artery; LMCA = left main coronary artery; LPA= left pulmonary artery; LSV = left sinus of Valsalva; NSV = non-coronary sinus of Valsalva; PA = pulmonary artery; RCA = right coronary artery; RPA = right pulmonary artery; RSV = right sinus of Valsalva; SVC = superior vena cava

Non-Coronary Artery Diseases Causing Ischaemic Chest Pain

Not all ischaemic chest pain is related to CAD. Ischaemic chest pain may also be caused by aortic stenosis (AS), aortic regurgitation (AR) and hypertrophic cardiomyopathy (HCM). In the cases of significant AS and HCM, ischaemic chest pain occurs secondary to the increased oxygen demand by the hypertrophied ventricle (oxygen demand exceeds supply).

In chronic, severe AR the increased LV volume and dimensions result in increased myocardial oxygen demand and this can lead to myocardial ischaemia and chest pain. In addition, reduced diastolic perfusion pressure of the coronary arteries may lead to inadequate coronary blood flow which can also result in myocardial ischaemia and chest pain. The echocardiographic features of these lesions are discussed in detail in subsequent chapters.

Non-Ischaemic Causes of Chest Pain

Causes of non-ischaemic chest pain which can be identified by echocardiography include Takotsubo cardiomyopathy, aortic dissection, acute pericarditis, mitral valve prolapse and acute pulmonary embolism.

Takotsubo Cardiomyopathy

Takotsubo cardiomyopathy (TTC) was first described in Japan in the early 1990s due to the resemblance of the LV on ventriculography to a Japanese octopus trap, known as a Takotsubo (Fig. 5.47). TTC is a clinical syndrome that mimics ACS and is characterised by acute, transient or reversible LV dysfunction in the absence of obstructive CAD. There are four characteristic features of TTC:

1. Patients are typically post menopausal women who present with signs and symptoms mimicking ACS;
2. Symptoms are typically triggered after sudden emotional or physical stress;
3. On left ventriculography, there is hypercontractility of the basal ventricle with bulging or ballooning of the LV apex at end-systole;
4. Within days or weeks of the acute insult, on follow-up imaging, the LV systolic function returns to normal.

This syndrome is also commonly referred to as apical ballooning syndrome (due to the appearance of the LV on ventriculography and echocardiography) and/or stress cardiomyopathy (due to the link of emotional or physical triggers with this syndrome).

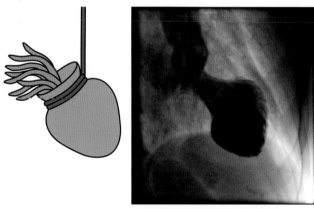

Figure 5.47 Observe the resemblance between a Takotsubo which is a Japanese octopus trap (*left*) and the left ventricle as seen on a left ventriculogram (*right*). The characteristic appearance of the LV as seen at end-systole explains the origin of the name for this cardiomyopathy.

Several mechanisms have been proposed as the pathological cause for TTC including endocrine, hormonal, neuropsychological, and microvascular factors. The most popular mechanism is considered to be catecholamine-induced myocardial stunning.

Differentiating TTC from an AMI is important. Misdiagnosing TTC for an AMI may result in the treatment of the patient with thrombolytic agents which may expose the patient to the unnecessary risk of bleeding complications. To assist in the diagnosis of TTC, the Mayo Clinic has proposed criteria that can be applied at the time of patient presentation (Table 5.10). All four criteria must be present for the diagnosis of TTC.

On the 2D echocardiographic examination typical as well as atypical morphological variants associated with TTC can be identified (Table 5.11 and Fig. 5.48-5.49). In particular, recognition of RWMA extending beyond the distribution of any single coronary artery is a characteristic feature of this condition. Echocardiography has the added advantage of being able to identify and quantify coexistent LV outflow tract

Table 5.10 Proposed Mayo Clinic criteria for TTC

Proposed Mayo Clinic criteria for TTC
1. Transient hypokinesis, akinesis, or dyskinesis of the left ventricular mid segments with or without apical involvement; the regional wall motion abnormalities extend beyond a single epicardial vascular distribution; a stressful trigger is often, but not always present.*
2. Absence of obstructive coronary disease or angiographic evidence of acute plaque rupture.†
3. New electrocardiographic abnormalities (either ST-segment elevation and/or T-wave inversion) or modest elevation in cardiac troponin.
4. Absence of: • Pheochromocytoma • Myocarditis

The diagnosis of TTC should be made with caution, and a clear stressful precipitating trigger must be sought.
* There are rare exceptions to these criteria such as those patients in whom the RWMA is limited to a single coronary territory.
† It is possible that a patient with obstructive coronary atherosclerosis may also develop TTC. However, this is very rare in the Mayo Clinic experience and in the published literature, perhaps because such cases are misdiagnosed as an acute coronary syndrome.
Reprinted from *American Heart Journal*, Vol. 155(3), Prasad A, Lerman A, Rihal CS, Apical ballooning syndrome (Tako-Tsubo or stress cardiomyopathy): a mimic of acute myocardial infarction, page 412, © 2008 with permission from Elsevier.

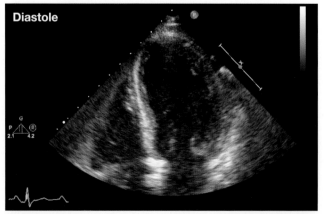
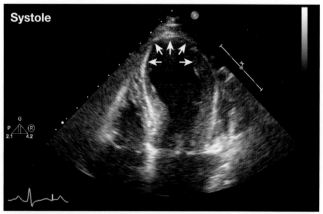

Figure 5.48 These diastolic (*left*) and systolic (*right*) freeze frames, recorded from the apical 4-chamber view, display classic apical ballooning associated with Takotsubo cardiomyopathy (*arrows*).

(LVOT) obstruction and to estimate the LVEF on the initial and follow-up studies. For diagnostic purposes, the echocardiogram must be performed early as LV function may recover within days and therefore the typical RWMA of TTC may not be observed if the examination is delayed. The LVEF should be measured in approximately 4 to 6 weeks following the initial presentation to document recovery of cardiac function.

Aortic Dissection

An aortic dissection occurs when there is a tear in the aortic intima resulting in blood entering the medial layer to create a false, blood-filled channel. Chest pain associated with an acute aortic dissection is described as severe with a sudden onset; chest pain is sometimes described as a "tearing" pain that radiates to the back. Aortic dissections are classified according to the

Table 5.11 Morphological LV Variants of TTC

Morphological Variants	Characteristic Echo Features
Apical Ballooning (most common variant) (Fig. 5.48)	• hyperdynamic basal contraction • akinesis and ballooning of the LV apex
Midventricular Ballooning (Apical Sparing)	• akinesis and ballooning of the mid-segment of the LV • preserved or hyperkinetic apical contractility
Inverted Takotsubo (rare variant)	• hypokinesis of the base of the heart • preserved apical function
LVOT Obstruction (Fig. 5.49)	• dyskinetic apical and mid-ventricular segments • hyperdynamic function of the basal LV segments • systolic anterior motion of the mitral valve (+/- mitral regurgitation) • increased and late-peaking LVOT velocities
Right Ventricular Involvement	• most frequently affected RV segments include dyskinesis, akinesis, or severe hypokinesis of the apicolateral wall, the anterolateral wall, and the inferior segment with sparing of the RV base

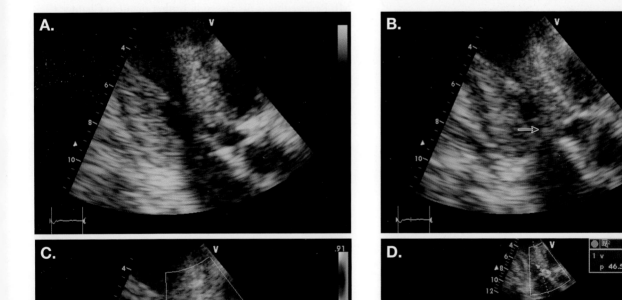

Figure 5.49 These images show left ventricular outflow tract (LVOT) obstruction in a patient with Takotsubo cardiomyopathy. The diastolic **(A)** and systolic **(B)** freeze frames were recorded from a zoomed apical 2-chamber view; the arrow in image B indicates the systolic anterior motion of the mitral valve; septal bulge is also noted in images A and B. On the colour flow Doppler image through the LVOT **(C)**, turbulent flow is noted which is consistent with LVOT obstruction. Continuous-wave Doppler across the LVOT **(D)** confirms the presence of LVOT obstruction with a recorded pressure gradient of 47 mmHg. A repeat echo performed 8 days following the initial echo showed total resolution of the LVOT gradient.

Stanford or DeBakey classifications (see Fig. 11.19). In particular, a type A aortic dissection should always be considered as a possible cause of acute chest pain due to the extremely high mortality rate associated with this condition. A type A aortic dissection can also cause an AMI and/or ischaemic chest pain due to coronary artery dissection or obstruction to the coronary artery ostium by the dissection flap. On the 2D echocardiographic examination an aortic dissection can be identified by observing an intimal flap within the aortic root. On real-time echocardiography, this flap appears as a thin, undulating structure within the aortic lumen. Visualisation of this flap in two imaging planes is required to differentiate this appearance from an imaging artefact (Fig. 5.50).

An intimal flap is not seen in all cases of aortic dissection so it is important to be aware of other clues that may indicate the presence of an aortic dissection. For example, the aortic root is usually dilated in type A dissections. In addition, associated complications with a type A aortic dissection include: (1) acute AR, (2) pericardial effusion, and/or (3) RWMA (when dissection involves a coronary artery). Therefore, when an intimal flap cannot be seen the presence of aortic root dilatation associated with acute AR and/or a pericardial effusion are highly suggestive of proximal aortic dissection. Aortic dissections are discussed in detail in Chapter 11.

> A normal TTX echocardiogram cannot exclude an aortic dissection. Therefore, if clinical suspicion for an aortic dissection is high, alternate imaging (transoesophageal echocardiography or computed tomography) is required.

Acute Pericarditis

Pericarditis is an inflammatory condition of the pericardium. The primary symptom of pericarditis is chest pain. This chest pain is characteristically increased by inspiration, coughing and in a lying position; chest pain is decreased by sitting upright and leaning forward.

Characteristic ECG changes are also noted in acute pericarditis; these changes include widespread ST-segment elevation with the ST-segments concaving upwards. In addition, an increase in cardiac troponin is frequently observed in patients with acute pericarditis, especially in younger patients and those with a recent infection. Therefore, due to the presence of chest pain, ECG changes and slightly elevated cardiac troponin levels, acute pericarditis may be confused with ACS.

Importantly, pericarditis is a clinical diagnosis. The diagnosis of acute pericarditis cannot be independently made by echocardiography as the echocardiographic findings associated with this condition are non-specific. Echocardiographic findings that may be seen with acute pericarditis include a pericardial effusion of any size (seen in approximately two-thirds of patients), and/or pericardial thickening with or without a small pericardial effusion; however, an entirely normal echocardiogram is not uncommon in this condition. Furthermore, pericardial effusions are not isolated to pericarditis. Small pericardial effusions may also be seen in patients with an AMI and in patients with a type A aortic dissection. Larger effusions may also be associated with acute myocardial rupture as a complication of a previous MI. Pericarditis is discussed in further detail in Chapter 12.

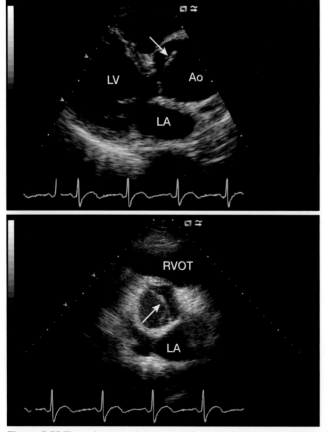
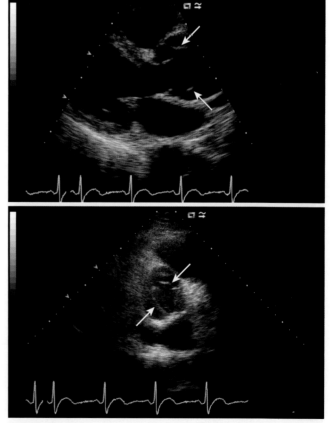

Figure 5.50 These images show a type A aortic dissection as viewed from the parasternal long axis view (*top*) and a high parasternal short axis view superior to the aortic valve (*bottom*). The left images are diastolic frames and the right images are systolic frames. Observe the linear echoes (*arrows*) within the aorta; on real-time imaging these linear echoes showed an independent and undulating motion which is characteristic of a dissection flap. Ao = aorta; LA = left atrium; LV = left ventricle; RVOT = right ventricular outflow tract.

Mitral Valve Prolapse

Chest pain is a common symptom of mitral valve prolapse (MVP). Chest pain associated with MVP is atypical and rarely resembles classic angina pectoris. The precise cause of chest pain in these patients is unknown.

MVP is diagnosed by 2D echocardiography from the parasternal long axis view of the LV. The criterion for the diagnosis of MVP is systolic displacement of one or both leaflets into the LA, below the plane of the mitral annulus, by 2 mm or more (Fig. 5.51). MVP is discussed in further detail in Chapter 8.

Acute Pulmonary Embolism

Patients with an acute pulmonary embolism (APE) may present with ischaemic-like chest pain. Associated symptoms also include severe dyspnoea, tachypnoea and intense cyanosis. The symptoms and clinical signs of APE are non-specific and may therefore be mistaken for ACS.

In patients with a large APE there is an associated acute increase in RV afterload due to blockage of the pulmonary vascular tree by the embolus. This increased afterload leads to increased RVSP, RV dilatation and impaired RV systolic function.

Echocardiography can be useful in identifying secondary pathophysiological responses of acutely elevated pulmonary artery pressures. The most common finding associated with acute RV pressure overload is dilatation of the RV with impaired systolic function (Fig. 5.52). Other findings include:

(1) dilatation of the pulmonary artery and its branches, (2) flattening and paradoxical motion of the IVS (Fig. 5.52), (3) mild-moderate elevation in RVSP (< 50 mm Hg), (4) a short RV acceleration time [RVAcT] (≤ 60 ms), (5) mid-systolic notching on the RVOT trace (Fig. 5.53, left), (6) variable degrees of tricuspid regurgitation, and (7) dilatation of the inferior vena cava.

In particular, a distinct regional pattern of RV systolic dysfunction has been described in patients with APE; this is referred to as the McConnell sign. The McConnell sign describes the presence of akinesis of the RV mid-free wall with preserved contractility or sparing of the RV apex. A suggested mechanism of this sign is localized ischaemia of the RV free wall as a result of increased wall stress. This sign has a low sensitivity for the diagnosis of APE but has a high accuracy for diagnosing massive PE. The McConnell sign is not specific for APE and may be seen in patients with RV MI. However, in patients with RV MI there are typically inferior RWMA and the RVSP is usually low.

Another sign associated with APE is the "60/60" sign (Fig. 5.53). This sign is based on the assumption that the RV is unable to generate pressures more than 40–50 mm Hg following an APE and that the marked shortening of the RVAcT occurs due to the sudden increase in afterload caused by an APE. Therefore, a short RVAcT ≤ 60 ms occurring in patients with a TR pressure gradient ≤ 60 mm Hg, the 60/60 sign, has been found to be a specific (but not sensitive) finding associated with APE.

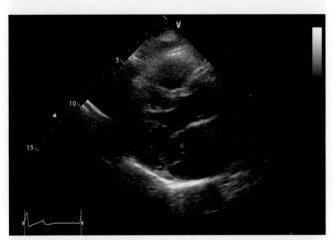
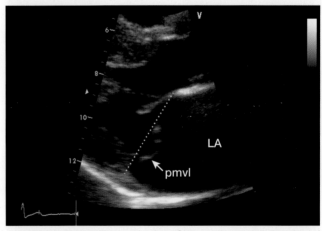

Figure 5.51 These zoomed and unzoomed systolic frames were acquired from the parasternal long axis view. Observe the systolic bowing of posterior mitral valve leaflet (*pmvl*) into the left atrium (*LA*) beyond the annular plane (*yellow dotted line*).

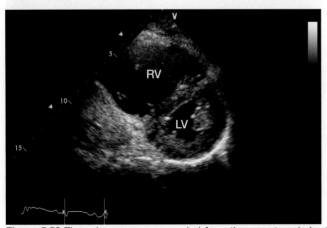
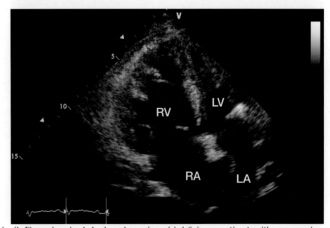

Figure 5.52 These images were recorded from the parasternal short axis (*left*) and apical 4-chamber view (*right*) in a patient with a massive pulmonary embolism confirmed by computed tomography pulmonary angiography (CTPA). Observe that there is severe dilatation of the right ventricle (RV) and the interventricular septum is flattened and displaced toward an under-filled left ventricle (LV). LA = left atrium; RA = right atrium.

Rarely, an embolism or thrombus in transit may be seen within the right heart chambers (Fig. 5.54). When seen this positively establishes the diagnosis of APE. Thrombi appear as singular or multiple echogenic and highly mobile free-floating masses trapped within the right heart chambers.

A negative transthoracic echocardiogram does not rule out an APE; however, a negative echocardiogram virtually excludes a massive pulmonary embolism.

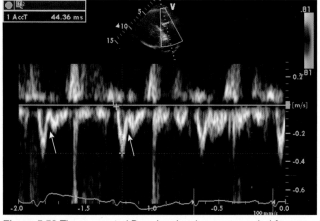
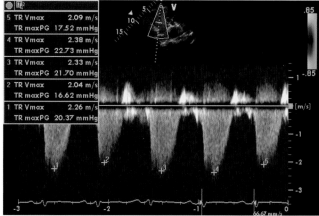

Figure 5.53 These spectral Doppler signals were recorded from a patient with acute pulmonary embolism confirmed by computed tomography angiography. The "60/60" sign is evident as the RVAcT, which is the time interval from the onset of the RVOT signal to the peak of this signal, is ≤ 60 ms (measured at 44 ms; *left*) and the TR gradient is ≤ 60 mm Hg (averaged at 18 mm Hg; *right*). Also observe the mid-systolic notching on the RVOT signal (*arrows*) which occurs when there is an acute increase in RV afterload.

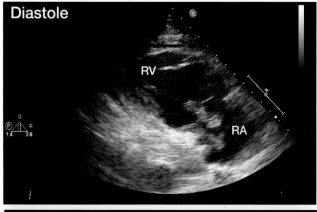
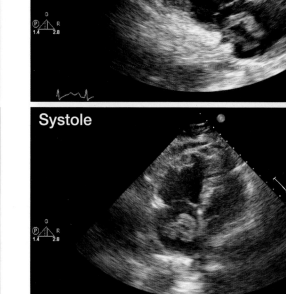
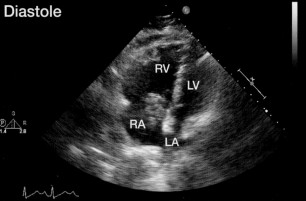

Figure 5.54 This series of images show multiple echodensities within the right atrium (RA). The top images were recorded from a parasternal long axis of RV inflow; the bottom images were recorded from an apical 4-chamber view. On real-time imaging these echodensities were noted to be highly mobile. Also note the marked dilatation of the RV which was associated with severe RV systolic dysfunction. Extensive bilateral pulmonary emboli, with extensive central pulmonary emboli, including saddle embolus were confirmed by computed tomography pulmonary angiography (CTPA). LA = left atrium; LV = left ventricle; RA = right atrium; RV = right ventricle.

Key Points
Coronary Anatomy
• LMCA arises from the left sinus of Valsalva and bifurcates into the LAD and Cx
• RCA arises from the right sinus of Valsalva
• Coronary artery dominance is determined by the artery supplying the PDA and PL branches:
- Right dominant ($\approx$ 70%) = PDA is a branch of the RCA
- Left dominant ($\approx$ 10%) = PDA branches from the Cx
- Co-dominant ($\approx$ 20%) = PDA branches from the RCA and all the PL branches arise from the Cx
Coronary Artery Disease (CAD)
• Most common cause of CAD is atherosclerosis
• There are numerous other causes of non-atherosclerotic CAD (see Table 5.3)
• Acute coronary syndrome (ACS) is a spectrum of clinical presentations related to acute myocardial ischaemia; includes unstable angina, NSTEMI and STEMI
• 12-lead ECG used to determine the location and extent of myocardial infarction
Role of Echo in Ischaemic Heart Disease
• Regional analysis of the LV function based on the 17 segment model
• RWMA determine the location and extent of myocardial infarction
• Assessment of LV size, systolic and diastolic function
• Assessment of complications of MI
• Identification of coronary artery anomalies
Stress Echo
• Useful in identifying patients with IHD when resting LV function is normal
• Dobutamine stress used to differentiate viable and non-viable myocardium
Echo can be used to identify other cases of chest pain
• Causes of ischaemic chest pain (besides CAD) include:
- Aortic stenosis
- Aortic regurgitation
- Hypertrophic cardiomyopathy
• Causes of non-ischaemic chest pain include:
- Takotsubo cardiomyopathy
- Aortic dissection
- Acute pericarditis
- Mitral valve prolapse
- Acute pulmonary embolism

Further Reading (listed in alphabetical order)

Coronary Artery Disease

American College of Cardiology/American Heart Association Task Force on Practice Guidelines (Writing Committee to Revise the 1999 Guidelines for the Management of Patients With Acute Myocardial Infarction): ACC/AHA guidelines for the management of patients with ST-elevation myocardial infarction—executive summary: A report of the American College of Cardiology/American Heart Association Task Force on Practice Guidelines (Writing Committee to Revise the 1999 Guidelines for the Management of Patients With Acute Myocardial Infarction). *Circulation*. 110: 2004; 588-636.

Bayés de Luna A, Wagner G, Birnbaum Y, Nikus K, Fiol M, Gorgels A, Cinca J, Clemmensen PM, Pahlm O, Sclarovsky S, Stern S, Wellens H, Zareba W; International Society for Holter and Noninvasive Electrocardiography. A new terminology for left ventricular walls and location of myocardial infarcts that present Q wave based on the standard of cardiac magnetic resonance imaging: a statement for healthcare professionals from a committee appointed by the International Society for Holter and Noninvasive Electrocardiography. *Circulation*. 2006 Oct 17;114(16):1755-60.

Davies MJ. The pathophysiology of acute coronary syndromes. *Heart*. 2000 Mar;83(3):361-6.

Kumar A, Cannon CP. Acute coronary syndromes: diagnosis and management, part I. *Mayo Clin Proc*. 2009 Oct;84(10):917-38.

Myocardial Infarction

Mollema SA, Nucifora G, Bax JJ. Prognostic value of echocardiography after acute myocardial infarction. *Heart*. 2009 Nov;95(21):1732-45.

Nihoyannopoulos P, Vanoverschelde JL. Myocardial ischaemia and viability: the pivotal role of echocardiography. *Eur Heart J*. 2011 Apr;32(7):810-9.

Verma A, Pfeffer MA, Skali H, Rouleau J, Maggioni A, McMurray JJ, Califf RM, Velazquez EJ, Solomon SD. Incremental value of echocardiographic assessment beyond clinical evaluation for prediction of death and development of heart failure after high-risk myocardial infarction. Am Heart J. 2011 Jun;161(6):1156-62.

Complications of MI

Brener SJ, Tschopp D. Complications of Acute Myocardial Infarction.

http://www.clevelandclinicmeded.com/medicalpubs/diseasemanagement/cardiology/complications-of-acute-myocardial-infarction/

Kondur AK, Yang EH. Complications of Myocardial Infarction. http://emedicine.medscape.com/article/164924 (Updated: Sep 15, 2011)

French JK, Hellkamp AS, Armstrong PW, Cohen E, Kleiman NS, O'Connor CM, Holmes DR, Hochman JS, Granger CB, Mahaffey KW. Mechanical complications after percutaneous coronary intervention in ST-elevation myocardial infarction (from APEX-AMI). *Am J Cardiol*. 2010 Jan 1;105(1):59-63.

Gueret P, Khalife K, Jobic Y, Fillipi E, Isaaz K, Tassan-Mangina S, Baixas C, Motreff P, Meune C; Study Investigators. Echocardiographic assessment of the incidence of mechanical complications during the early phase of myocardial infarction in the reperfusion era: a French multicentre prospective registry. *Arch Cardiovasc Dis*. 2008 Jan;101(1):41-7.

Stress Echocardiography

Nihoyannopoulos P, Vanoverschelde JL. Myocardial ischaemia and viability: the pivotal role of echocardiography. *Eur Heart J.* 2011 Apr;32(7):810-9.

Pellikka PA, Nagueh SF, Elhendy AA, Kuehl CA, Sawada SG; American Society of Echocardiography. American Society of Echocardiography recommendations for performance, interpretation, and application of stress echocardiography. *J Am Soc Echocardiogr.* 2007 Sep;20(9):1021-41.

Coronary Anomalies

Cohen P, O'Gara PT. Coronary artery aneurysms: a review of the natural history, pathophysiology, and management. *Cardiol Rev.* 2008 Nov-Dec;16(6):301-4.

Earls JP. Coronary Artery Anomalies. *Tech Vasc Interv Radiol.* 2006 Dec;9(4):210-7.

Hlavacek A, Loukas M, Spicer D, Anderson RH. Anomalous origin and course of the coronary arteries. *Cardiol Young.* 2010 Dec;20 Suppl 3:20-5.

Kim SY, Seo JB, Do KH, Heo JN, Lee JS, Song JW, Choe YH, Kim TH, Yong HS, Choi SI, Song KS, Lim TH. Coronary artery anomalies: classification and ECG-gated multi-detector row CT findings with angiographic correlation. *Radiographics.* 2006 Mar-Apr;26(2):317-33.

Takotsubo Cardiomyopathy

Akashi YJ, Nef HM, Möllmann H, Ueyama T. Stress cardiomyopathy. *Annu. Rev. Med.* 2010. 61:271–86

Bybee KA, Prasad A. Stress-related cardiomyopathy syndromes. *Circulation.* 2008 Jul 22;118(4):397-409.

Gianni M, Dentali F, Grandi AM, Summer G, Hiralal R, Loore E. Apical ballooning syndrome or Takotsubo cardiomyopathy: a systematic review. *Eur Heart J.* 2006; Dec ;27(23):2907-8.

Prasad A, Lerman A, Rihal CS. Apical ballooning syndrome (Tako-Tsubo or stress cardiomyopathy): a mimic of acute myocardial infarction. Am Heart J. 2008 Mar;155(3):408-17.

Sharkey SW, Windenburg DC, Lesser JR, Maron MS, Hauser RG, Lesser JN, Haas TS, Hodges JS, Maron BJ. Natural history and expansive clinical profile of stress (tako-tsubo) cardiomyopathy. *J Am Coll Cardiol.* 2010 Jan 26;55(4):333-41.

Acute Pulmonary Embolism

Casazza F, Bongarzoni A, Capozi A, Agostoni O. Regional right ventricular dysfunction in acute pulmonary embolism and right ventricular infarction. *Eur J Echocardiography* 2005; 6: 11-14

McConnell MV, Solomon SD, Rayan ME, Come PC, Goldhaber SZ, Lee RT. Regional right ventricular dysfunction detected by echocardiography in acute pulmonary embolism. *Am J Cardiol.* 1996; 78: 469–473

Torbicki A, Kurzyna M, Ciurzynski M, Pruszczyk P, Pacho R, Kuch-Wocial A, Szulc M. Proximal pulmonary emboli modify right ventricular ejection pattern. *Eur Respir J* 1999;13:616–621.

Cardiomyopathies

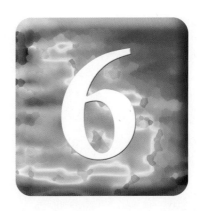

Definition and Classifications of Cardiomyopathies

In the simplest of terms, cardiomyopathy is defined as a disease of the myocardium. Many detailed definitions of cardiomyopathy have been proposed over the years (Table 6.1). Currently, there are five major categories of cardiomyopathies defined on the basis of structural and functional features; these categories include: (1) dilated cardiomyopathy (DCM), (2) hypertrophic cardiomyopathy (HCM), (3) restrictive cardiomyopathy (RCM), (4) arrhythmogenic right ventricular dysplasia or cardiomyopathy (ARVD/C), and (5) unclassified cardiomyopathies (Table 6.2).

> Secondary causes of cardiac dysfunction due to hypertension, ischaemic heart disease, or valvular disease are not strictly defined as cardiomyopathies under current American Heart Association (AHA) and European Society of Cardiology (ESC) classification systems (see Table 6.1 for references). Therefore, 'hypertensive cardiomyopathy', 'ischaemic cardiomyopathy' and 'valvular cardiomyopathy' are not referred to within this chapter.

Dilated Cardiomyopathy

Dilated cardiomyopathy (DCM) is the most common type of cardiomyopathy. DCM is characterised by dilatation and impaired systolic contraction of the left ventricle (LV) or both ventricles in the absence of other causes that can lead to global ventricular systolic impairment. In other words, DCM refers to dilatation and impaired systolic contraction of the LV or both ventricles in the absence of coronary artery disease or abnormal loading conditions caused by hypertension or significant valve disease.

Aetiology of DCM

There are a number of known causes of DCM (Table 6.3). This includes familial and genetic factors, viral myocarditis and other cytotoxic insults, and immunological abnormalities. In particular, approximately 20-30% of patients with DCM will have a first degree relative with evidence of DCM. When a specific cause for DCM cannot be identified it is referred to as idiopathic DCM.

Pathophysiology of DCM

On gross inspection of the heart, all four cardiac chambers appear dilated and the ventricular muscle mass is increased as a result (Fig. 6.1). Dilatation of the LV or both ventricles occurs in an attempt to maintain a normal cardiac output (see

Table 6.1 **Definitions of Cardiomyopathies**

Definition	Ref.
"Cardiomyopathies are heart muscle disease of unknown cause".	1
"Cardiomyopathies are defined as diseases of the myocardium associated with cardiac dysfunction."	2
"Cardiomyopathies are a heterogeneous group of diseases of the myocardium associated with mechanical and/or electrical dysfunction that usually (but not invariably) exhibit inappropriate ventricular hypertrophy or dilatation and are due to a variety of causes that frequently are genetic. Cardiomyopathies either are confined to the heart or are part of generalized systemic disorders, often leading to cardiovascular death or progressive heart failure–related disability."	3
"A myocardial disorder in which the heart muscle is structurally and functionally abnormal, in the absence of coronary artery disease, hypertension, valvular disease and congenital heart disease sufficient to cause the observed myocardial abnormality."	4

References [Ref.]: **[1]** Report of the WHO/ISFC task force on the definition and classification of cardiomyopathies. *Br Heart J*. 1980 Dec;44(6):672-3; **[2]** Richardson P, McKenna W, Bristow M, et al. Report of the 1995 World Health Organization/International Society and Federation of Cardiology Task Force on the definition and classification of cardiomyopathies. *Circulation*. 1996 Mar 1;93(5):841-2; **[3]** Maron BJ, Towbin JA, Thiene G, et al.. Contemporary definitions and classification of the cardiomyopathies: an American Heart Association Scientific Statement from the Council on Clinical Cardiology, Heart Failure and Transplantation Committee; Quality of Care and Outcomes Research and Functional Genomics and Translational Biology Interdisciplinary Working Groups; and Council on Epidemiology and Prevention. *Circulation*. 2006 Apr 11;113(14):1807-16; **[4]** Elliott P, Andersson B, Arbustini E, et al. Classification of the cardiomyopathies: a position statement from the European Society Of Cardiology Working Group on Myocardial and Pericardial Diseases. *Eur Heart J*. 2008 Jan;29(2):270-6.

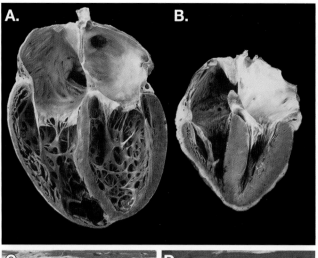
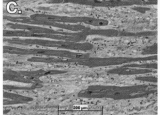
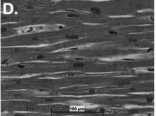

Figure 6.1 Gross and histological specimens show a heart with dilated cardiomyopathy (DCM) (A & C) and a normal heart (B & D). Observe that on the gross cardiac specimens all four cardiac chambers are markedly dilated in the DCM heart (A) when compared to a normal heart (B). In the histological examples of cardiac muscle observe that compared to the normal tissue sample (D), the DCM example (C) shows myocyte hypertrophy and interstitial fibrosis (light pink areas).
By permission of Mayo Foundation for Medical Education and Research. All rights reserved. Courtesy of William D. Edwards, MD.

the Frank-Starling mechanism in Chapter 2). However, in accordance with Laplace's law, the increased diameter of the ventricle also increases wall stress which ultimately results in a reduction in the stroke volume and contractility (see Laplace's law in Chapter 2).

Left atrial (LA) dilatation occurs secondary to elevated LV filling pressures. Dilatation of the right heart chambers also occurs due to the myopathic process or secondary to elevated pulmonary pressures. Mitral regurgitation (MR) and tricuspid regurgitation (TR) may also occur due to annular dilatation.

Clinical Manifestations of DCM

The clinical manifestations associated with DCM are related to heart failure; these symptoms include dyspnoea, peripheral oedema, fatigue and weakness, and decreased exercise tolerance. The severity or stage of heart failure can be determined according to the New York Heart Association (NYHA) functional classification system (Table 6.4). This classification system considers three parameters in patients with cardiac disease: (1) status at rest, (2) symptoms such as fatigue, palpitations, dyspnoea and/or anginal pain with ordinary physical activity, and (3) limitations on physical activity.

> Heart failure (HF) is a complex clinical syndrome that can result from any structural or functional cardiac disorder that impairs the ability of the heart to eject or fill with blood. Therefore, HF may be subdivided into either systolic HF which is caused by reduced cardiac contractility or diastolic HF where there is impaired cardiac relaxation and abnormal ventricular filling in the presence of normal or near normal contractility.

Table 6.2 Classifications of Cardiomyopathies

Type	Description	Causes
Dilated cardiomyopathy	Dilatation and impaired systolic contraction of the LV or both ventricles in the absence of abnormal loading conditions or CAD	Familial/genetic Viral Immune Alcoholic/toxic Unknown factors
Hypertrophic cardiomyopathy	Hypertrophy of the LV and/or RV in the absence of: (1) haemodynamic stresses which can produce hypertrophy and/or (2) systemic diseases such as glycogen storage disease	Familial (autosomal dominant inheritance) Mutations in sarcomeric contractile protein genes
Restrictive cardiomyopathy	Impaired ventricular filling with a reduced diastolic volume of either or both ventricles with normal or near-normal systolic function and wall thickness	Idiopathic or associated with other disease (e.g. infiltrative and glycogen storage disorders, disorders causing myocardial and/or endocardial fibrosis)
Arrhythmogenic right ventricular cardiomyopathy	Progressive fibrofatty replacement of the RV myocardium, with some LV involvement and relative sparing of the IVS	Idiopathic Familial (usually autosomal dominant inheritance with incomplete penetrance; possible autosomal recessive inheritance)
Unclassified cardiomyopathy	Diseases that do not fit readily into any other type	EFE Ion channel disorders LVNC Mitochondrial involvement Peripartum (postpartum) cardiomyopathy

CAD = coronary artery disease; EFE = endocardial fibroelastosis; IVS = interventricular septum; LV = left ventricle; LVNC = left ventricular non-compaction; RV = right ventricle.
Based on data from Richardson P, McKenna W, Bristow M, et al. Report of the 1995 World Health Organization/International Society and Federation of Cardiology Task Force on the definition and classification of cardiomyopathies. *Circulation.* 1996 Mar 1;93(5):841-2.

Role of Echocardiography in DCM

The aims and objectives of echocardiography in the assessment of patients with DCM include:
- Assessment of chamber size,
- Assessment of LV systolic function,
- Evaluation of LV diastolic function,
- Assessment of right ventricular (RV) systolic function,
- Evaluation of the degree of valvular regurgitation,
- Exclusion of LV and/or RV thrombus.

Assessment of Chamber Dimensions

As stated previously, DCM refers to dilatation of the LV or both ventricles; often all four cardiac chambers are dilated (Fig. 6.2). Measurements of chamber dimensions are performed in the standard manner. In particular, LV linear dimensions can be measured by M-mode and/or 2D echocardiography from the parasternal long or short axis views and LV volumes can be measured from the Simpson's biplane method of discs (Fig. 6.3-6.4); the LA volume can be measured from the apical 4-chamber and 2-chamber views and the right atrial (RA) area can be measured from the apical 4-chamber view (Fig. 6.5-6.6); and RV dimensions can be measured from the RV focussed, apical-4-chamber view (Fig. 6.7). The reference limits and various partition values of cardiac chamber dimensions and volumes are listed in Tables 6.5-6.6.

In addition, DCM is associated with eccentric ventricular hypertrophy. Recall that an eccentric hypertrophy pattern is defined as an increased LV mass with normal relative wall thickness (RWT) (see Fig. 4.9). In the case of DCM, LV wall thickness is thinned due to stretching of the myocytes as the ventricle dilates; however, LV mass is increased due to chamber dilatation. For example, in Figure 6.3, LV wall thickness is normal but the LV cavity is markedly dilated. Therefore, the RWT is normal (≤ 0.42) and the LV mass indexed to the body surface area (BSA) is 147 g/m^2 which is moderately abnormal (refer to Table 4.8); this is consistent with eccentric ventricular hypertrophy.

> **Degree of Dilatation**
> - *For the left heart:* when considering the degree of chamber dilatation for the left atrium and left ventricle, values should be indexed to the body surface area (BSA) (Table 6.5).
> - *For the right heart:* normal values are absolute (that is, normal values are not indexed to the BSA). In addition, the partition values for the classification of mild, moderate and severe dilatation have yet to be defined. Hence, an arbitrary judgment in determining the degree of dilatation for any given measurement is required.

Table 6.3 Selected Causes of Dilated Cardiomyopathy

Aetiology and Examples
Unknown (idiopathic):   • Accounts for ≈ 50% of cases
Familial/genetic: • Genetic transmission detectable in ≈ 25% of cases
Infectious: • viral, rickettsial, bacterial, fungal, metazoal, protozoal
Immunologic: • post vaccination, serum sickness, transplant rejection
Metabolic/nutritional: • endocrine diseases (e.g. hyperthyroidism and hypothyroidism, diabetes mellitus, phaeochromocytoma), electrolyte imbalance (e.g. potassium, phosphate, magnesium), storage diseases (e.g. glycogen storage disease, haemochromatosis)   • thiamine deficiency (beriberi), protein deficiency, starvation, carnitine deficiency
Neuromuscular disorders: • muscular dystrophies (e.g. Duchenne dystrophy), Friedreich's ataxia, myotonic dystrophy
Toxic: • alcohol, cocaine, amphetamines, chemotherapy agents (e.g. Herceptin (Trastuzumab) for breast cancer)

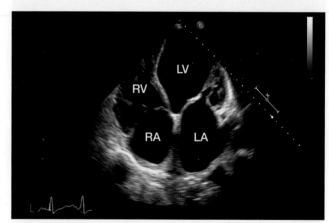

Figure 6.2 This apical 4-chamber view was recorded from a patient with a dilated cardiomyopathy. Observe that all four cardiac chambers are dilated. LA = left atrium; LV = left ventricle; RA = right atrium; RV = right ventricle.

Table 6.4 New York Heart Association (NYHA) Functional Classification System for Heart Failure*

NYHA Class	Status at Rest	Symptoms with Ordinary Physical Activity	Limitations on Physical Activity
I	Comfortable	None	None
II	Comfortable	Ordinary activities results in fatigue, palpitations, dyspnoea, or anginal pain	Slight
III	Comfortable	Less than ordinary levels of activity results in fatigue, palpitations, dyspnoea, or anginal pain	Marked
IV	Symptomatic at rest	Discomfort with any activity	Unable to perform any activity

* Cardiac disease must be present.
Based on Dolgin M, ed. Functional capacity and objective assessment. In: Nomenclature and Criteria for Diagnosis of Diseases of the Heart and Great Vessels 9th Edition. New York Little Brown and Company, pages 253-255, 1994.

Table 6.5 Reference Limits and Partition Values of Left Atrial and Left Ventricular Size

	WOMEN				MEN			
	Reference range	Mildly abnormal	Moderately abnormal	Severely abnormal	Reference range	Mildly abnormal	Moderately abnormal	Severely abnormal
LV dimension								
LV diastolic diameter, cm	3.9–5.3	5.4–5.7	5.8–6.1	≥ 6.2	4.2–5.9	6.0–6.3	6.4–6.8	≥ 6.9
LV diastolic diameter/BSA, cm/m^2	2.4–3.2	3.3–3.4	3.5–3.7	≥ 3.8	2.2–3.1	3.2–3.4	3.5–3.6	≥ 3.7
LV diastolic diameter/height, cm/m	2.5–3.2	3.3–3.4	3.5–3.6	≥ 3.7	2.4–3.3	3.4–3.5	3.6–3.7	≥ 3.8
LV volume								
LV diastolic volume, mL	56–104	105–117	118–130	≥ 131	67–155	156–178	179–201	≥ 201
LV diastolic volume/BSA, mL/m^2	*35–75*	*76–86*	*87–96*	*≥ 97*	*35–75*	*76–86*	*87–96*	*≥ 97*
LV systolic volume, mL	19–49	50–59	60–69	≥ 70	22–58	59–70	71–82	≥ 83
LV systolic volume/BSA, mL/m^2	*12–30*	*31–36*	*37–42*	*≥ 43*	*12–30*	*31–36*	*37–42*	*≥ 43*
LA								
LA area, cm^2	≤ 20	20-30	30-40	> 40	≤ 20	20-30	30-40	> 40
LA volume, mL	22-52	53-62	63-72	≥ 73	18-58	59-68	69-78	≥ 79
LA volume/BSA, mL/m^2	*22±6*	*29-33*	*34-39*	*≥ 40*	*22±6*	*29-33*	*34-39*	*≥ 40*

BSA = body surface area; LA = left atrium; LV = left ventricular. **Bold italic values:** Recommended and best validated.
Reprinted from *J Am Soc Echocardiogr,* Vol. 18(12), Lang RM, Bierig M, Devereux RB, et al., Chamber Quantification Writing Group; American Society of Echocardiography's Guidelines and Standards Committee; European Association of Echocardiography. Recommendations for Chamber Quantification: A Report from the American Society of Echocardiography's Guidelines and Standards Committee and the Chamber Quantification Writing Group, Developed in Conjunction with the European Association of Echocardiography, a Branch of the European Society of Cardiology, page 1448, © 2005 with permission from Elsevier.

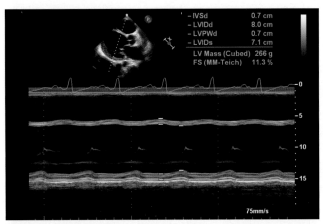

– IVSd	0.7 cm	
– LVIDd	8.0 cm	
– LVPWd	0.7 cm	
– LVIDs	7.1 cm	
LV Mass (Cubed)	266 g	
FS (MM-Teich)	11.3 %	

75mm/s

Figure 6.3 This M-mode trace was acquired from the same patient as in Fig. 6.2. Measurements are performed at the blood-tissue interfaces at end-diastole and end-systole. End-diastole is identified as the onset of the QRS complex of the ECG. As there is abnormal interventricular septal (IVS) motion, end-systole is measured from the peak anterior point of the posterior wall (PW) back up to the IVS. The LV end-diastolic dimension (LVIDd) is 8.0 cm and the LV end-systolic dimension (LVIDs) is 7.1 cm; the body surface area (BSA) for this male patient is 1.8 m^2 so the LVIDd indexed to the BSA is 4.4 cm/m^2. From the LVIDd and the LVIDs, the fractional shortening (FS) is calculated at 11%.

$$FS = ([LVIDd - LVIDs] \div LVIDd) \times 100$$
$$= ([8.0 - 7.1] \div 8.0) \times 100$$
$$= 11\%$$

From the end-diastolic measurements of the LV cavity, IVS and PW, the LV mass (LVM) is calculated at 266 g; the indexed LV mass (ILVM) is 147 g/m^2.

$$LVM = 1.04 ([LVIDd + PW + IVS]^3 - LVIDd^3) \times 0.8 + 0.6$$
$$= 1.04 ([8.0 + 0.7 + 0.7]^3 - 8.0^3) \times 0.8 + 0.6$$
$$= 266 \ g$$

$$ILVM = LVM \div BSA$$
$$= 266 \div 1.8$$
$$= 147 \ g/m^2$$

The relative wall thickness (RWT), calculated from the end-diastolic measurements of the LV cavity and PW, is 0.18.

$$RWT = (2 \times PW) \div LVIDd$$
$$= (2 \times 0.7) \div 8.0$$
$$= 0.18$$

Table 6.6 Normal Values for Right Atrial and Right Ventricular Dimensions

	Normal Values
RV	
Basal cavity diameter, cm	≤ 4.2
Mid cavity diameter, cm	≤ 3.5
Length, cm	≤ 8.6
RA	
Major dimension, cm	≤ 5.3
Minor dimension, cm	≤ 4.4
Area, cm^2	≤ 18

RA = right atrium; RV = right ventricle.
Source: Rudski LG, Lai WW, Afilalo J, Hua L, Handschumacher MD, Chandrasekaran K, Solomon SD, Louie EK, Schiller NB. Guidelines for the echocardiographic assessment of the right heart in adults: a report from the American Society of Echocardiography endorsed by the European Association of Echocardiography, a registered branch of the European Society of Cardiology, and the Canadian Society of Echocardiography. *J Am Soc Echocardiogr.* 2010 23(7):685-713.

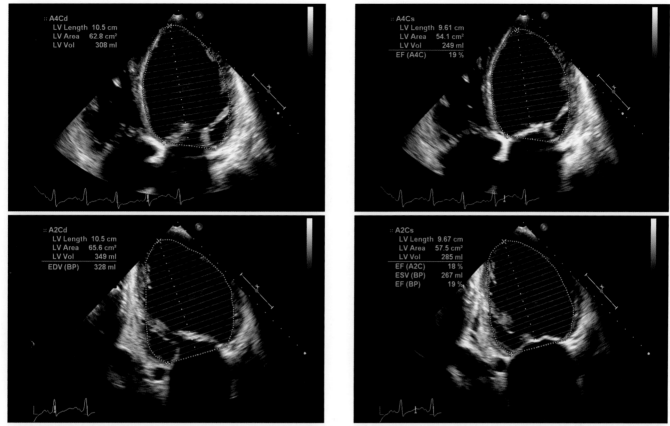

Figure 6.4 These measurements were acquired from the same patient as in Fig. 6.2. The left ventricular volumes are measured from the apical 4-chamber view at end-diastole (A4Cd) and end-systole (A4Cs) and from the apical 2-chamber view at end-diastole (A2Cd) and end-systole (A2Cs). The biplane end-diastolic volume (EDV(BP)) is 328 mL and the biplane end-systolic volume (ESV(BP)) is 267 mL; the body surface area (BSA) for this male patient is 1.8 m² so the EDV(BP) indexed to the BSA is 182 mL/m². Using the biplane volumes, the biplane left ventricular ejection fraction (EF (BP)) is calculated at 19%.

$EF\ (BP) = \{[EDV(BP) - ESV(BP)] \div EDV(BP)\} \times 100$
$\qquad\quad = \{[328 - 267] \div 328\} \times 100$
$\qquad\quad = 19\%$

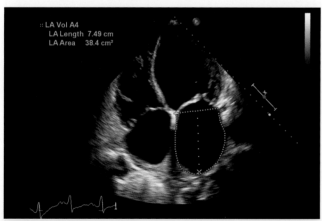

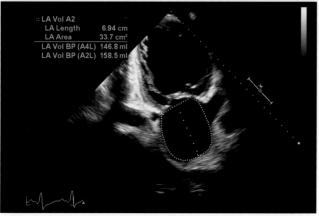

Figure 6.5 These measurements were acquired from the same patient as in Fig. 6.2. The left atrial (LA) volume is measured from the apical 4-chamber and apical 2-chamber views at end-systole. The LA area is traced at the black-white interface from the lateral mitral annulus to the medial mitral annulus, excluding the mitral funnel, LA appendage and pulmonary venous confluence; the LA length is measured from the centre of the mitral annulus to the superior aspect of the LA, perpendicular to the mitral annulus. The LA area in the apical 4-chamber view is 38.4 cm² (*top*) and the LA area in the apical 2-chamber view is 33.7 cm² (*bottom*); the shortest LA length is 6.94 cm measured from the apical 2-chamber view. Using the biplane area-length method, the LA volume (LAV) is 158.5 mL. The body surface area (BSA) for this male patient is 1.8 m² so the LA volume indexed to the BSA (ILAV) is 88 mL/m².

$LAV \quad = (0.85 \times A4\ area \times A2\ area) \div shortest\ LA\ length$
$\qquad\quad = (0.85 \times 38.4 \times 33.7) \div 6.94$
$\qquad\quad = 158.5\ mL$

$ILAV \quad = LAV \div BSA$
$\qquad\quad = 158.5 \div 1.8$
$\qquad\quad = 88\ mL/m^2$

Assessment of Left Ventricular Systolic Function

Systolic function of the LV is assessed in the traditional manner as detailed in Chapter 2. In DCM, LV systolic function is typically impaired globally; the diagnostic criteria for DCM include a LV ejection fraction (LVEF) < 45% and/or a fractional shortening (FS) < 25%. The preferred method of estimating the LVEF is the Simpson's biplane method; using this method the LVEF is calculated from the end-diastolic and end-systolic LV volumes (Fig. 6.4). When image quality is suboptimal an intravenous ultrasound contrast agent may be required to enhance endocardial border definition and improve the accuracy of LV volume measurements.

Other methods that can be used to determine the overall systolic function of the LV include calculation of the LV stroke volume (SV) and cardiac output (CO). The detailed approach for calculating these indices as well as the limitations of these techniques are described in Chapter 2.

Importantly, indices obtained during the ejection phase of the cardiac cycle such as the LVEF, SV and CO are influenced by loading conditions and, therefore, may not reflect the true intrinsic contractility of the LV. For example, when there is coexistent severe mitral regurgitation (MR), LV afterload is very low because a significant amount of blood is being ejected into the low pressure LA. As such the LVEF may seem 'better' than it would be if there was no MR. Therefore, in these circumstances, load independent indices such as the dP/dt provide a better measure of intrinsic LV contractility.

As described in Chapter 2, the dP/dt is a measurement of the rate of LV pressure rise during the isovolumic contraction (IVC) phase of the cardiac cycle. The dP/dt can be measured in the presence of MR. Recall that the MR Doppler velocity reflects the pressure difference between the LV and LA during systole. By assuming that the LA pressure (LAP) remains relatively constant then the rate of rise of the Doppler velocity reflects the rate of LV pressure rise. Therefore, by measuring the rate of the velocity increase on the ascending limb (left limb) of the MR velocity curve, a measurement of the rate of LV pressure rise during IVC can be performed (Fig. 6.8).

M-mode Signs of Reduced Cardiac Output

Indirect M-mode signs of reduced cardiac output, including the likely cause of each sign, are summarised in Table 6.7 and illustrated in figures 6.9 and 6.10.

Table 6.7 M-mode Signs suggesting a Reduced Cardiac Output

M-mode Sign	Likely Cause
Decreased mitral valve opening (Fig. 6.9)	Reduced opening due to decreased transmitral flow into the LV
Increased E point-septal separation (EPSS) (Fig. 6.9)	Increased due to: (1) anterior displacement of the IVS as the LV dilates, and (2) reduced opening of the mitral valve because of decreased transmitral flow into the LV
Decreased aortic root motion (Fig. 6.10)	Reduced motion due to decreased pulmonary venous return into the LA
Tapered aortic valve closure (Fig. 6.10)	Gradual closure of the valve during systole occurs due to an inability of the LV to maintain constant flow through the valve over systole

IVS = interventricular septum ; LA = left atrium; LV = left ventricle.

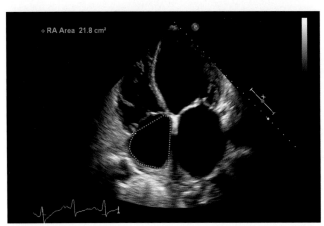

Figure 6.6 This measurement was acquired from the same patient as in Fig. 6.2. The right atrial (RA) area is measured from the apical 4-chamber view at end-systole. The RA area is traced at the black-white interface from the lateral tricuspid annulus to the medial tricuspid annulus, excluding the tricuspid funnel.

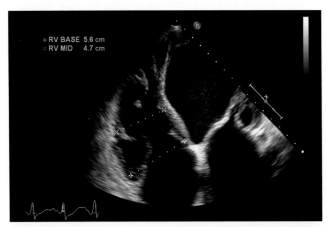

Figure 6.7 These measurements were acquired from the same patient as in Fig. 6.2. The right ventricular (RV) dimensions are measured from an RV focussed, apical 4-chamber view at end-diastole. The RV dimension is measured at the base and the mid-cavity level, parallel with the tricuspid valve annulus.

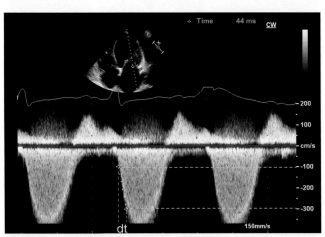

Figure 6.8 The dP/dt can be measured from the continuous-wave Doppler signal of the mitral regurgitant jet. The change in time (dt) is determined by measuring the time interval between 1 m/s and 3 m/s. In this example, this time interval is 44 ms or 0.044 s. Using the simplified Bernoulli equation to convert velocity to pressure, the change in pressure (dP) between 1 m/s and 3 m/s is 32 mmHg. The dP/dt is then derived by dividing the change in pressure (dP) by the change in time (dt); therefore, the dP/dt in this example is 32 ÷ 0.044 or 727 mm Hg/s.

Evaluation of LV Diastolic Function

The pattern of LV diastolic dysfunction in patients with DCM is an indicator of patient symptoms and is an important predictor of prognosis. In particular, two patients may have similar degrees of systolic dysfunction but different NYHA functional classifications; this can be explained by the grade of diastolic dysfunction in each patient. For example, it would be expected that the patient with a higher NYHA class would have a worse grade of diastolic dysfunction than the patient in a lower NYHA class.

The grades of diastolic dysfunction are summarized in Table 6.8. The detailed approach for the assessment of LV diastolic function is described in Chapter 3; in particular, the transmitral and pulmonary venous pulsed-wave (PW) Doppler profiles in conjunction with mitral annular Doppler tissue imaging (DTI) velocities are used to identify the pattern or grade of diastolic dysfunction (Fig. 6.11).

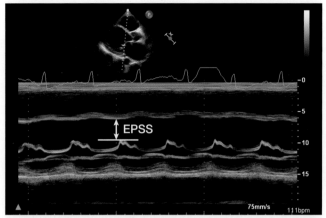

Figure 6.9 This M-mode trace recorded through the mitral valve shows decreased mitral valve opening as well as an increased mitral E-point-septal separation (EPSS). Both of these findings are consistent with a reduced cardiac output and poor left ventricular systolic function. Decreased mitral valve opening appears as a decreased separation between the anterior and posterior leaflets over diastole. The EPSS is measured as the perpendicular distance between the most posterior point of the interventricular septum during systole and the early diastolic point (E point) of the anterior mitral valve leaflet in the same cardiac cycle.

Assessment of Right Ventricular Systolic Function

RV size and systolic function are assessed in the usual manner as detailed Chapter 2. Measurements of RV systolic function include the DTI systolic velocity, the tricuspid annular plane systolic excursion (TAPSE), the fractional area change (FAC) and/or the RV myocardial performance index (MPI). Importantly, more than one measure of RV function should be considered in distinguishing between normal and abnormal RV systolic function.

Evaluation of the Degree of Valvular Regurgitation

Most patients with DCM will have some degree of functional MR secondary to mitral annular dilatation and/or malpositioning of the papillary muscles in relation to the mitral leaflets which leads to incomplete coaptation of the mitral leaflets during systole.

The degree of MR is variable and can range from mild to severe. The severity of MR is evaluated via the traditional methods which are described in detail in Chapter 8. In particular, a large colour MR jet area, increased transmitral inflow velocities, systolic flow reversal in the pulmonary veins and a strong continuous-wave (CW) MR signal are all useful signs for detecting significant MR (Fig. 6.12). Quantitative methods such as calculation of the effective regurgitant orifice area (EROA) and the regurgitant volume and regurgitant fraction can also be performed.

As for MR, tricuspid regurgitation (TR) is found in almost all patients with DCM; TR occurs secondary to tricuspid annular dilatation. The degree of TR is variable; ranging from mild to severe. The severity of TR is evaluated via the traditional methods which are described in detail in Chapter 9. The peak velocity of the TR signal can also be used in the estimation of the right ventricular systolic pressure (RVSP).

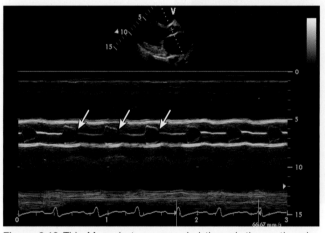

Figure 6.10 This M-mode trace recorded through the aortic valve and left atrium shows a tapered or gradual closure of the aortic valve throughout systole (*arrows*). Also observe that there is minimal anterior motion of the aortic root during systole. Both of these findings are consistent with a reduced cardiac output and poor left ventricular systolic function.

Table 6.8 Grading of Diastolic Function and Associated Left Ventricular Filling Pressures (LVFP)

Stage of LV Diastolic Dysfunction	Grade	LVFP
Impaired relaxation	Grade 1a	Normal
	Grade 1b	Elevated LVEDP *
Pseudonormalisation	Grade 2	Moderate increase in left atrial pressure (LAP)
Reversible restrictive filling#	Grade 3a	Marked increase in LAP
Irreversible restrictive filling#	Grade 3b	Marked increase in LAP

* An elevated left ventricular end-diastolic pressure (LVEDP) should be suspected when the AR_{dur}-A_{dur} ≥ 30 ms and/or the AR velocity > 35 cm/s.
# Reversible restrictive filling can be differentiated from an irreversible restrictive filling by asking the patient to perform the Valsalva manoeuvre. If the transmitral flow profile reverts to either a pseudonormal filling profile or an impaired relaxation profile, this is consistent with reversible restrictive filling; if the transmitral flow profile does not change then this is consistent with irreversible restrictive filling.

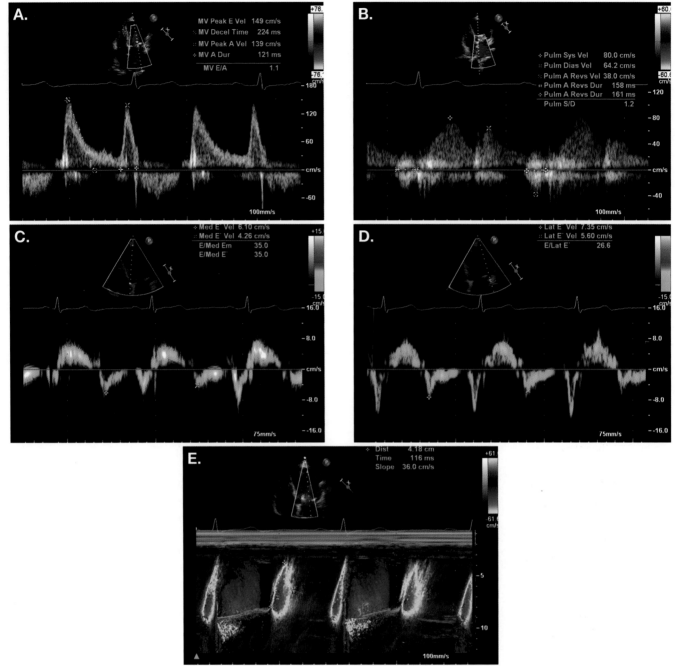

Figure 6.11 Left ventricular (LV) diastolic function in a patient with a dilated cardiomyopathy is assessed via the transmitral inflow profile (A), pulmonary venous profile (B), septal annular Doppler tissue imaging (DTI) (C), lateral annular DTI (D), and the flow propagation velocity (E). The transmitral inflow shows a 'normal' flow profile. However, the pulmonary venous A reversal velocity is elevated at 38 cm/s and the difference between the pulmonary venous A reversal duration (159 ms) and the mitral A duration (121 ms) is 38 ms; these findings are consistent with increased left ventricular end-diastolic pressure (LVEDP). In addition, the E/e' ratio derived from the septal and lateral annular DTI are both markedly increased (35 and 26.6, respectively); this is consistent with increased left atrial pressure (LAP). The flow propagation slope is also slow (36 cm/s); this is consistent with impaired LV relaxation. Based on the evidence of an increased LVEDP, an increased LAP and underlying impaired LV relaxation, this is grade II diastolic dysfunction (pseudonormalisation).

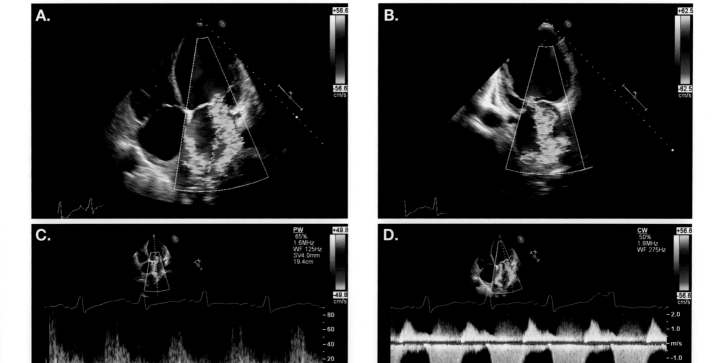

Figure 6.12 The colour flow Doppler images recorded from the apical 4-chamber view (A) and apical 2-chamber view (B) show severe mitral regurgitation (MR); observe the large MR jet filling the dilated left atrium. The pulmonary venous pulsed-wave Doppler trace (C) shows systolic flow reversal into the right upper pulmonary vein (*arrows*); this is also consistent with severe MR. The continuous-wave Doppler trace (D) reveals a strong MR signal and increased transmitral inflow velocities; these features are again consistent with severe MR.

Technical Tips

- **Diastolic dysfunction precedes systolic dysfunction**

  All patients with a DCM will have diastolic dysfunction. Consequently, patients with a DCM and "normal" transmitral profile will have grade II diastolic dysfunction (that is, pseudonormalisation).

- **Variation in Profiles**

  Patients with DCM can move between an abnormal relaxation pattern, pseudonormalisation and a restrictive filling profile as the disease progresses. Likewise, patients may revert from a restrictive filling profile to pseudonormalisation or an abnormal relaxation pattern with successful medical management.

- **Restrictive Physiology versus Restrictive Cardiomyopathy**

  Restrictive physiology does not mean that the patient has a restrictive cardiomyopathy. Similarly, patients with a restrictive cardiomyopathy do not always have a restrictive filling profile.

- **Transmitral Inflow Direction**

  In normal individuals, transmitral inflow is directed approximately 20 degrees laterally to the cardiac apex; flow then continues down the lateral wall, around the apex and up to the LV outflow tract (*curved arrow, below left*). In patients with DCM, LV enlargement alters the normal relationship between the mitral valve apparatus and the interventricular septum. As a result, the mitral orifice is oriented more towards the lateral wall of the LV. Therefore, transmitral inflow is directed progressively more laterally such that optimal transducer position for alignment with transmitral inflow may be 40 degrees

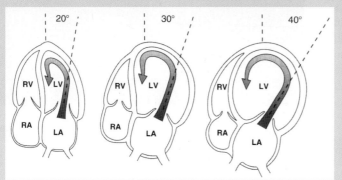

or more from the standard apical imaging position (*curved arrow, below middle and right*). This means that the sonographer may have to readjust the apical view to a more lateral position to ensure that the flow is aligned parallel to the ultrasound beam. Colour flow Doppler will also assist in the determining the direction of blood flow.

Adapted from Appleton CP, Jensen JL, Hatle LK, Oh JK. Doppler evaluation of left and right ventricular diastolic function: a technical guide for obtaining optimal flow velocity recordings. *J Am Soc Echocardiogr.* Vol. 10(3), page 272, © 1997, with permission from Elsevier.

Exclusion of LV and/or RV thrombus

Thrombus occurs due to stasis of blood flow. The recognition of LV thrombus in patients with DCM is especially important as LV thrombus is a potential source for systemic embolisation. The 2D echocardiographic features of thrombus include the appearance of echo-dense material within the chamber cavity; the echogenicity of thrombus is usually distinct from underlying endocardium (Fig. 6.13). Importantly, 2D image optimisation is fundamental for the detection of LV thrombus. Therefore, the sonographer should:

- Use the highest possible transducer frequency (to improve spatial resolution),
- Use harmonic imaging (to improve contrast resolution),
- Use a shallow field of view (thrombus usually at the apex),
- Reposition the focal zone (to improve lateral resolution),
- Slowly and carefully pan through the ventricle (anterior to posterior) from all possible imaging planes,
- Confirm the presence of thrombus in more than one imaging plane.

It is also important to be aware that poor image quality may mask LV thrombus (especially at the apex) while normal anatomic structures and imaging artefacts may mimic LV thrombus. Anatomic structures mimicking LV thrombus include: (1) aberrant fibrous cords or accessory bands, (2) ruptured papillary muscle and/or cords, and (3) prominent LV trabeculations. Colour flow Doppler imaging or the injection of intravenous contrast agents may be very useful in the determining the presence or absence of thrombus in these situations (see Fig. 5.26 and 5.27).

Role of Echocardiography in Cardiac Resynchronization Therapy (CRT)

LV dilatation and impaired systolic function can result in desynchronised ventricular contraction which effectively reduces the LVEF and increases the severity of MR. Cardiac resynchronization therapy (CRT) aims to resynchronize ventricular contractility thereby improving the LVEF and reducing MR severity. This is achieved by biventricular pacing whereby the RV is paced in the traditional manner and the lateral wall of the LV is paced by placing a pacing wire down the coronary sinus and into a coronary vein on that LV wall.

A positive response to CRT includes a decrease in NYHA class by one class, an increase in exercise capacity, improved quality of life, less hospital admissions, evidence of reversed LV remodelling, improved systolic function, and a decrease in MR severity. However, in approximately 20-30% of patients receiving CRT there is no apparent clinical improvement; these patients are referred to as non-responders. Various echocardiographic techniques have been investigated in an attempt to distinguish between CRT responders and non-responders. Echocardiography can also be utilised to determine the degree of LV reverse remodelling and the reduction in MR severity, and to optimise atrioventricular and interventricular intervals following CRT.

Echocardiographic Measures of Dyssynchrony

Dyssynchrony can be classified as interventricular dyssynchrony and/or intraventricular dyssynchrony. Interventricular dyssynchrony refers to dyssynchronous contraction between the LV and RV while intraventricular dyssynchrony refers to dyssynchronous contraction within the LV. Comparisons of selected measures of dyssynchrony including methods, normal values, cut-off values for identifying dyssynchrony, advantages and limitations are summarized in Table 6.9.

Interventricular dyssynchrony

Interventricular dyssynchrony or interventricular mechanical delay (IVMD) can be measured using PW Doppler as well as DTI. A normal interventricular conduction time is < 20 ms; a delay ≥ 40 ms is an indicator of interventricular dyssynchrony. Using PW Doppler, IVMD is derived from two measurements: (1) the RV pre-ejection period (RVPEP) and (2) the LV pre-ejection period (LVPEP) (Fig. 6.14). The IVMD is then derived as the difference between the LVPEP and the RVPEP.

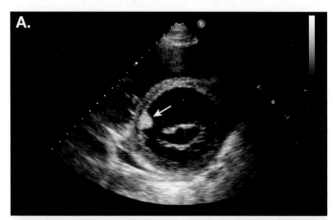

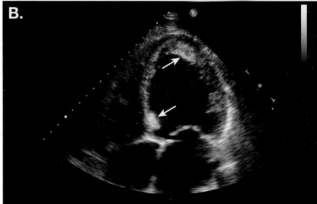

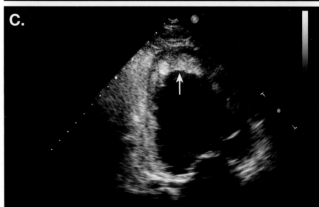

Figure 6.13 These images were recorded from a patient with a dilated cardiomyopathy and left ventricular (LV) thrombus. Observe that there are two prominent echogenic masses within the LV (*arrows*). An echogenic mass on the inferior septum is seen in the parasternal short axis view (A) and in the apical 4-chamber view (B); an echogenic mass at the LV apex is seen in the apical 4-chamber view and in the apical 2-chamber view (C). The appearance of these masses is consistent with a laminar thrombus.

Using DTI, IVMD is derived from two measurements: (1) the time to systolic peak from the RV lateral annulus (Ts [RV]) and (2) the time to systolic peak from the LV lateral annulus (Ts [LV]) (Fig. 6.15). The IVMD is then derived as the difference between the Ts [LV] and the Ts [RV].

Intraventricular dyssynchrony

Several methods have been described for measuring intraventricular dyssynchrony. They include the septal to posterior wall delay (SPWD), the opposing wall delay (OWD), and by calculating the standard deviation of the time-to-peak systolic velocity from 12 sites (Yu index).

The SPWD is a measure of radial intraventricular dyssynchrony. This measurement can be derived from two M-mode measurements: (1) the time to the first posterior peak of the IVS after the QRS (interval A) and (2) the time to the first anterior peak of the posterior wall following the QRS (interval B) (Fig. 6.16). The SPWD is then derived as the difference between interval B and interval A. Alternatively, the SPWD can be measured as the interval between the peak posterior deflection of the IVS and the peak anterior deflection of the PW. The normal SPWD is < 50 ms; a SPWD ≥ 130 ms is an indicator of intraventricular radial dyssynchrony.

The OWD is a measure of longitudinal intraventricular dyssynchrony. This measurement can be derived from pulsed and colour DTI from either an apical 4-chamber view or apical long axis view. For example, from the apical 4-chamber view, two measurements are required: (1) the time to systolic peak from the septal mitral annulus (Ts [S]) and (2) the time to systolic peak from the lateral mitral annulus (Ts [L]) (Fig. 6.17). In this instance, the opposing wall delay corresponds to the septal to lateral delay (SLD) which is derived as the difference between (Ts [S]) and (Ts [L]). The normal SLD is < 50 ms; a SLD ≥ 65 ms is an indicator of intraventricular longitudinal dyssynchrony.

The Yu index is also a measure of longitudinal intraventricular dyssynchrony. This index is derived from colour DTI by measuring the time to systolic peak (Ts) from 12 sites of the LV myocardium: Ts is measured from the basal and mid segments of the apical 4-chamber view, the apical 2-chamber view, and the apical long axis view. The Yu index is then calculated as the standard deviation (SD) of these 12 Ts measurements. The normal Yu index is < 30 ms; a SD ≥ 33 ms is an indicator of intraventricular longitudinal dyssynchrony.

> This section on CRT provides a brief overview of the role of transthoracic echocardiography in this therapy. It should be noted that advanced techniques such as strain, speckle tracking and 3D echocardiography have also been used in guiding CRT (see the Further Reading section of this Chapter for selected articles on this topic).

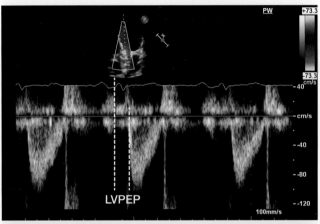

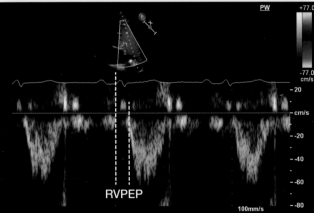

Figure 6.14 Interventricular mechanical delay (IVMD) via pulsed-wave (PW) Doppler is derived from the left ventricular pre-ejection period (LVPEP) and the right ventricular pre-ejection period (RVPEP). From the PW Doppler signal recorded from the left ventricular outflow tract, the LVPEP is measured from the onset of the QRS complex of the ECG to the onset of systolic flow (*top*). From the PW Doppler signal recorded from the right ventricular outflow tract, the RVPEP is measured from the onset of the QRS complex of the ECG to the onset of systolic flow (*bottom*). The IVMD is calculated as the difference between the LVPEP and the RVPEP: IVMD = LVPEP – RVPEP.

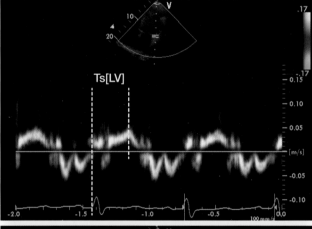

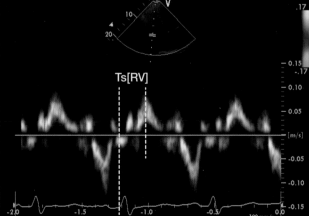

Figure 6.15 Interventricular mechanical delay (IVMD) via Doppler tissue imaging (DTI) is derived from the onset of the QRS complex of the ECG to the systolic myocardial peak (s') at the left ventricular lateral annulus (Ts [LV]) (*top*) and at the right ventricular lateral annulus (Ts [RV]) (*bottom*). The IVMD is calculated as the difference between the Ts [LV] and Ts [RV]: IVMD = Ts [LV] – Ts [RV].

Echocardiographic Optimisation of CRT

Optimisation of the atrioventricular (AV) interval and interventricular or ventricular-to-ventricular (VV) interval may also improve the response to CRT and echocardiography may be utilised to assist with optimisation of these intervals.

AV Optimisation

AV optimisation adjusts the AV intervals to improve LV diastolic filling. For example, if the AV interval is too short, the atrial component of LA contractility may be absent or interrupted by the premature ventricular contraction and early closure of the mitral valve; if the AV interval is too long then early diastolic filling may be abbreviated.

The transmitral inflow profile can be used to identify when AV optimisation might be necessary and to assist in the optimisation of the AV interval. In particular, an optimal AV interval is based on adequate separation of the E and A waves with an identifiable A wave that terminates before the QRS complex, or when the mitral valve closure click aligns with the end of the A wave and the QRS complex.

VV Optimisation

VV optimisation adjusts the sequence and timing of LV and RV pacing to improve SV and the LVEF. Measurement of the SPWD and the LV outflow tract (LVOT) velocity time integral (VTI) can be utilised to determine an optimal VV interval. In particular, the shortest SPWD with the highest LVOT VTI indicates an optimal VV interval.

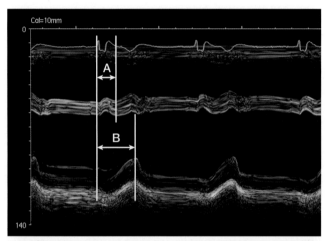

Figure 6.16 The septal to posterior wall delay (SPWD) can be derived via M-mode and is measured from the onset of the QRS complex of the ECG to the first posterior peak of the interventricular septum after the QRS (Interval A) and from the onset of the QRS complex of the ECG to the first anterior peak of the posterior wall following the QRS (Interval B). The SPWD is derived as the difference between interval B and interval A: SPWD = Interval B − Interval A.

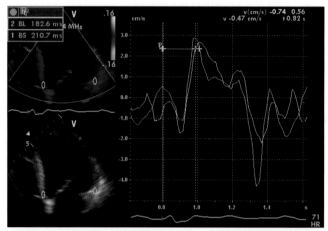

Figure 6.17 Longitudinal intraventricular mechanical delay via colour Doppler tissue imaging (DTI) is derived from the time to the systolic peak from the basal septal mitral annulus (BS) and the time to the systolic peak from the basal lateral mitral annulus (BL). The time to systolic peak is measured from the onset of the QRS complex of the ECG to the peak systolic myocardial velocity (s'). The septal to lateral delay (SLD) is derived as the difference between the BS and BL; in this example, the SLD is 28 ms.

Table 6.9 Selected M-Mode and Doppler Indices for Dyssynchrony

Parameter	Method	Normal	Cut-off	Advantages	Disadvantages
Interventricular dyssynchrony					
Interventricular Mechanical Delay (IVMD)	Routine pulsed-wave Doppler (RVOT and LVOT)	< 20 ms	≥ 40 ms	Widely available; no advanced technical requirements; highly reproducible	Nonspecific; affected by LV and RV function
Intraventricular dyssynchrony					
Septal to Posterior Wall Delay (SPWD)	M-mode (parasternal mid-LV view)	< 50 ms	≥ 130 ms	Widely available; rapidly applied; no advanced technical requirements	Largely affected by passive motion or tethering; difficulties with segmental akinesis
Opposing Wall Delay (OWD)	Colour tissue Doppler peak velocity (apical 4-chamber or long-axis views)	< 50 ms	≥ 65 ms	Rapidly applied; offline analysis is possible	Requires colour TD equipment; affected by passive motion tethering
Yu Index	Colour tissue Doppler, 12-segment SD (apical 4-chamber, 2-chamber, & long-axis views)	< 30 ms	≥ 33 ms	More complete detection of longitudinal dyssynchrony; offline analysis is possible	Requires colour TD equipment; more time-consuming; affected by passive motion tethering

LV = left ventricle; LVOT = left ventricular outflow tract; RV = right ventricle; RVOT = right ventricular outflow tract; SD = standard deviation; TD = tissue Doppler
Adapted from Gorcsan J 3rd, Abraham T, Agler DA, Bax JJ, Derumeaux G, Grimm RA, Martin R, Steinberg JS, Sutton MS, Yu CM; American Society of Echocardiography Dyssynchrony Writing Group. Echocardiography for cardiac resynchronization therapy: recommendations for performance and reporting--a report from the American Society of Echocardiography Dyssynchrony Writing Group endorsed by the Heart Rhythm Society. *J Am Soc Echocardiogr.* Vol. 21(3), page 205, © 2008 reproduced with permission from Elsevier

Hypertrophic Cardiomyopathy

Hypertrophic cardiomyopathy (HCM) refers to hypertrophy of the LV that occurs in the absence of an obvious underlying cause such as hypertension or severe aortic stenosis. Hypertrophy in HCM is often asymmetric rather than concentric. Most commonly the interventricular septum (IVS) is hypertrophied to a greater degree than the rest of the LV; however, there are a number of variants of HCM (Fig. 6.18).

HCM can also be subdivided into two groups based on the presence or absence of dynamic LV outflow tract (LVOT) obstruction. Non-obstructive HCM refers to the absence of a dynamic LVOT gradient while hypertrophic obstructive cardiomyopathy (HOCM) refers to the presence of a dynamic LVOT gradient. Numerous terms have been used to describe HCM/HOCM; these terms are listed in Table 6.10.

Aetiology of HCM

HCM is a genetic disease that is inherited in an autosomal dominant pattern. HCM is caused by specific gene mutations resulting in alterations of the contractile elements of the cardiac sarcomere which secondarily leads to myocardial hypertrophy and fibrosis.

As stated above, the pattern of ventricular hypertrophy is variable; most commonly there is asymmetric septal hypertrophy (ASH). Apical HCM, characterised by primary hypertrophy of the LV apex, is a variant of HCM that is seen in approximately 25% of Japanese patients with HCM and is rarely seen in non-Japanese populations.

Pathophysiology of HCM

The characteristic pathologic features of HCM are ventricular hypertrophy and myocardial disarray (Fig. 6.19). The pathophysiological responses in HCM are dependent upon the site and extent of hypertrophy. In particular, pathophysiological abnormalities that are commonly seen include diastolic dysfunction, myocardial ischaemia, LVOT obstruction, MR (secondary to mitral valve and subvalvular apparatus abnormalities), and cardiac arrhythmias.

Typically, the ventricular chambers are small with normal or hyperdynamic systolic function. Diastolic dysfunction is invariably present and is characterised by abnormal stiffness of the LV with resultant impaired ventricular filling which in turn leads to increased LV filling pressures.

Myocardial ischaemia may occur secondary to: (1) increased LV muscle mass which increases myocardial oxygen demand, (2) decreased capillary network which decreases myocardial oxygen supply, (3) elevated intracavity LV pressures which compress the intramyocardial coronary arteries, and (4) elevated LV filling pressures which lower the diastolic aorta-to-LV pressure gradient and, therefore, the coronary artery perfusion pressure.

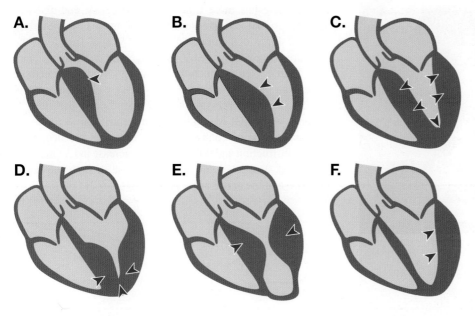

Figure 6.18 These drawings illustrate the various types of hypertrophic cardiomyopathy (HCM); the areas of hypertrophy are indicated by the arrowheads.
A = asymmetric (septal) HCM with left ventricular outflow tract (LVOT) obstruction;
B = asymmetric (septal) HCM without LVOT obstruction;
C = concentric hypertrophy;
D = apical HCM;
E = midventricular HCM with an apical aneurysm;
F = posterior wall hypertrophy with no septal involvement.

Table 6.10 Various Terminologies for HCM/HOCM

• Apical hypertrophic cardiomyopathy	• Idiopathic hypertrophic cardiomyopathy
• Asymmetric septal hypertrophy	• Idiopathic hypertrophic subaortic stenosis (IHSS)
• Brock's disease	• Idiopathic muscular hypertrophic subaortic stenosis
• Diffuse muscular subaortic stenosis	• Left ventricular muscular stenosis
• Diffuse subvalvular aortic stenosis	• Mid-ventricular hypertrophic cardiomyopathy
• Familial hypertrophic subaortic stenosis	• Mid-ventricular hypertrophic obstructive cardiomyopathy
• Functional obstructive cardiomyopathy	• Muscular aortic stenosis of the left ventricle
• Functional obstruction of the left ventricle	• Muscular subaortic stenosis
• Functional subaortic stenosis	• Non-obstructive hypertrophic cardiomyopathy
• Hypertrophic cardiomyopathy	• Subaortic hypertrophic obstructive cardiomyopathy
• Hypertrophic obstructive cardiomyopathy	• Subaortic hypertrophic stenosis
• Hypertrophic subaortic stenosis	• Subaortic muscular stenosis
	• Teare's disease

Approximately 25-40% of patients with HCM have a dynamic LVOT obstruction or HOCM. HOCM can be further subdivided into: (1) obstruction at rest (persistent), (2) mild obstruction at rest with significant obstruction occurring following provocation (provocable), or (3) no obstruction at rest with significant obstruction apparent following provocation (latent).

Mechanism of LVOT Obstruction

The mechanism for dynamic LVOT obstruction in HOCM relates to ASH and systolic anterior motion (SAM) of the mitral valve. SAM of the mitral valve refers to the marked and abnormal forward movement of the anterior or both mitral leaflets toward the LVOT during systole. A number of causes for mitral SAM have been proposed including: (1) the Venturi effect, (2) malposition of the papillary muscles, and (3) displacement of the valve apparatus.

The Venturi effect is a suction effect caused by ASH which narrows the LVOT during the systolic ejection period; this produces a pressure drop in the LVOT which effectively "sucks" the anterior mitral leaflet upward and toward the hypertrophied IVS. Furthermore, central displacement of the valve apparatus and anterior displacement of the papillary muscles may decrease the tension of the tendinous cords of

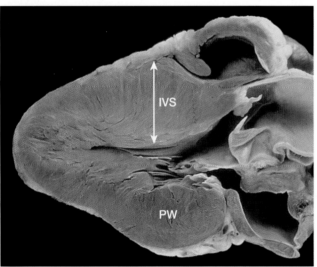

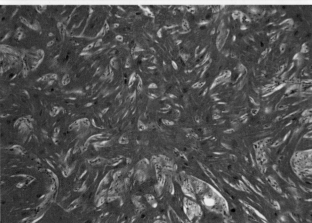

Figure 6.19 Gross and histological specimens show the characteristic features of hypertrophic cardiomyopathy. The gross cardiac specimen shows marked hypertrophy of the interventricular septum (IVS). In particular the IVS is much thicker than the posterior wall (PW); this is consistent with asymmetric septal hypertrophy. The histological example of cardiac muscle displays myocyte disarray.
By permission of Mayo Foundation for Medical Education and Research. All rights reserved. Courtesy of William D. Edwards, MD.

the anterior mitral leaflet predisposing the valve to be drawn anteriorly by Venturi effects (Fig. 6.20).

SAM of the anterior mitral leaflet also causes incomplete coaptation of the mitral leaflets and/or distortion of the mitral valve apparatus during systole which leads to MR.

Provocation of LVOT Obstruction

As stated above, some patients with HOCM do not exhibit dynamic LVOT obstruction at rest or have only mild LVOT obstruction at rest. In this subset of patients, dynamic LVOT obstruction may be produced by provocation. In particular, dynamic LVOT obstruction occurs when the outflow tract is narrowed by an increased force of LV contraction. The force of LV contraction can be induced by decreasing preload, decreasing afterload, or a combination of these.

For example, vasodilators such as amyl nitrate and glyceryl trinitrate (GTN) and/or the Valsalva manoeuvre may increase the force of LV contraction and induce dynamic LVOT obstruction by decreasing both arterial pressure (afterload) and ventricular volume (preload). An increased force of LV contraction also occurs during exercise or following a ventricular ectopic beat. Dynamic LVOT obstruction following a ventricular ectopic beat is also referred to as the Brockenbrough–Braunwald–Morrow sign. In particular, this sign can be used to differentiate between fixed obstruction (as seen with a subaortic membrane or aortic stenosis) and dynamic LVOT obstruction. Following a ventricular ectopic, the ventricle has more time to fill so the LV end-diastolic volume (preload) is increased and based on the Frank–Starling law, the force of contraction of the LV and, therefore, the pressure generated by the LV will be greater on the subsequent beat. With a fixed obstruction, following a ventricular ectopic there is an increase in the LV pressure as well as an increase in both the aortic pressure and the aortic pulse pressure. In patients with HOCM, following a ventricular ectopic the increased force of contraction also increases the degree of LVOT obstruction and this leads to an increase in LV pressure, a reduced stroke volume and a decrease in both the aortic pressure and the aortic pulse pressure (Fig. 6.21).

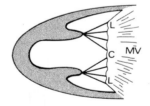 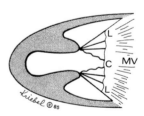

Figure 6.20 This schematic of cordal geometry illustrates the effects of papillary muscle malposition on distribution of tension to the mitral valve (MV). Compare the normal papillary muscle position and normal cordal tensions (*left*) to that of hypertrophic cardiomyopathy (HCM) with systolic anterior motion (*right*). In HCM the papillary muscle tips are displaced toward one another and this geometry can produce relative cordal 'slackness' in the central leaflet portions as indicated by the wavy lines. Resultant decreased cordal tension on the midportion of the leaflet predisposes the valve to be drawn anteriorly during systole. L = lateral edge of the mitral valve; C = central portion of the mitral valve.
Reprinted from Jiang L, Levine RA, King ME, Weyman AE, An integrated mechanism for systolic anterior motion of the mitral valve in hypertrophic cardiomyopathy based on echocardiographic observations, *American Heart Journal*, Vol. 113(3), page 640, © 1987 with permission from Elsevier.

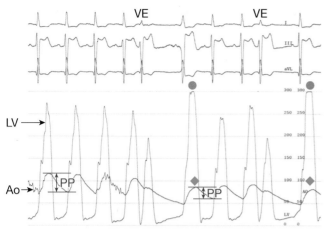

Figure 6.21 Simultaneous pressure recordings of the left ventricle (LV) and the aorta (Ao) demonstrate the pressure gradient between the LV and the aorta in a patient with hypertrophic obstructive cardiomyopathy. The aortic pulse pressure (PP) which is the difference between the systolic and diastolic pressures is also highlighted. Observe that following a ventricular ectopic (VE), the LV pressure rises (*pink dots*) while the aortic pressure (*green diamonds*) and the aortic pulse pressure (PP) both decrease. There is also a significant increase in the degree of LV outflow tract obstruction following the ectopic beats. This effect is known as the Brockenbrough-Braunwald-Morrow sign.

Clinical Manifestations of HCM

The majority of patients with HCM are asymptomatic or only mildly symptomatic with the most common symptom being exertional dyspnoea. Other clinical manifestations associated with HCM include dizziness, syncope and presyncope, chest pain, palpitations, orthopnoea, paroxysmal nocturnal dyspnoea, atrial fibrillation and other symptoms associated with heart failure. Progressive heart failure may develop with preserved systolic function with or without outflow obstruction; this may occasionally evolve to systolic dysfunction (end-stage HCM). Sudden cardiac death (SCD) may also occur in asymptomatic or mildly symptomatic patients and SCD is often the first clinical manifestation of HCM, occurring without warning signs or symptoms [6.1].

Role of Echocardiography in HCM

The aims and objectives of echocardiography in the assessment of patients with HCM/HOCM include:
- Determining the presence and distribution of hypertrophy,
- Assessment of LV systolic function,
- Evaluation of LV diastolic function,
- Determining the presence, location and magnitude of dynamic LVOT obstruction (including the response of the LVOT gradient to provocative manoeuvres),
- Assessment of the mechanism and degree of MR,
- Guidance during, and assessment following, septal reduction procedures.

Presence and Distribution of Hypertrophy

The echocardiographic criterion for HCM is the presence of LV hypertrophy greater than 1.5 cm in the absence of an identifiable cause for hypertrophy. The most common morphological variant of HCM is ASH which is defined as an IVS-to-posterior wall thickness ratio greater than 1.3:1; this is best appreciated from the parasternal long axis view (Fig. 6.22).

As stated above, there are many other variants of HCM; for example, hypertrophy can be concentric or isolated to the LV free wall or the LV apex. The parasternal short axis views of the LV are very useful in determining the distribution and extent of hypertrophy while the apical views can be used to identify apical HCM or midventricular HCM with an apical aneurysm (Fig. 6.23). In particular, the recognition of apical HCM is based on the characteristic 'Ace of Spades' appearance of the LV cavity when viewed from the apical views during diastole. Myocardial contrast may be required to identify apical HCM and midventricular HCM with an apical aneurysm (Fig. 6.24). Careful assessment of the RV wall thickness is also warranted in patients with HCM as approximately one-third of patients with HCM also have RV involvement.

Assessment of LV Systolic Function

Systolic function of the LV is assessed in the traditional manner as detailed in Chapter 2. In particular, LV systolic function is usually normal or hyperdynamic in patients with HCM. However, LV systolic dysfunction can be seen in patients with so-called "burnt-out" or "end-stage" HCM. Burnt-out or end-stage HCM is also typically associated with LV dilatation and a regression of ventricular hypertrophy.

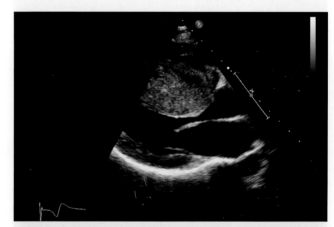

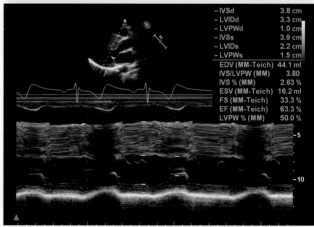

Figure 6.22 The 2D image shows the characteristic features of asymmetric septal hypertrophy (ASH) which is the most common variant of hypertrophic cardiomyopathy (*top*). The M-mode trace also demonstrates ASH (*bottom*). The IVS at end-diastole (IVSd) measures 3.8 cm and the posterior wall at end-diastole (LVPWd) measures 1.0 cm; the IVS to posterior wall thickness ratio (IVS/LVPW) is 3.80.

[6.1] Maron BJ, Maron MS. Hypertrophic cardiomyopathy. *Lancet*. 2013. Jan 19;381(9862):242-55.

Assessment of LV Diastolic Function

Diastolic dysfunction in HCM occurs due to increased LV stiffness which leads to impaired ventricular filling and increased LV filling pressures. The grade of LV diastolic dysfunction and the presence of elevated LV filling pressures is based on the comprehensive assessment of all diastolic parameters. The detailed approach for the assessment of LV diastolic function is described in Chapter 3.

Importantly, asynchronous relaxation of the LV may lead to isovolumetric relaxation flow (IVRF). Normally, no flow occurs during the isovolumic relaxation (IVR) period. However, in HCM there may be asynchronous relaxation of the LV. For example, if the LV apex relaxes earlier than normal, an intraventricular pressure gradient between the base of the LV and the LV apex is created during IVR; this results in antegrade flow from the base of the LV to the LV apex (Fig. 6.25). Recognition of IVRF is important as it may be confused with the transmitral E velocity. Differentiation between IVRF and the transmitral E velocity is based on the timing of flow compared with the ECG.

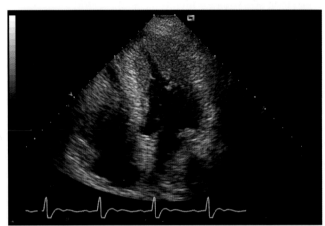

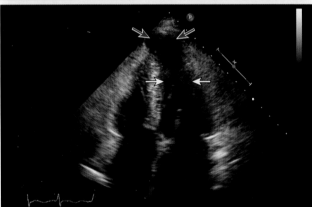

Figure 6.23 These apical 4-chamber images show two of the variants of hypertrophic cardiomyopathy (HCM). The apical variant of HCM is characterised by an 'Ace of Spades' appearance of the LV cavity during diastole (*top*). The midventricular HCM with an apical aneurysm is characterised by midventricular hypertrophy (*white arrows*) with an aneurysm at the left ventricular apex (*red arrows*) (*bottom*).

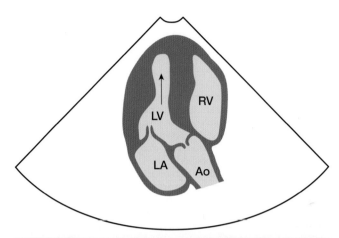

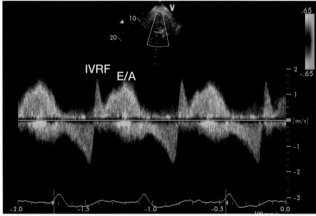

Figure 6.25 Isovolumic relaxation flow (IVRF) occurs when there is asynchronous left ventricular (LV) relaxation. When the LV apex relaxes earlier than normal an intraventricular pressure gradient between the base of the LV and the LV apex is created during isovolumic relaxation (*arrow, top*). On the transmitral inflow trace, this flow appears as antegrade flow prior to diastole (*bottom*). Observe that on this transmitral trace, there is fusion of the early diastolic velocity and the velocity with atrial contraction (E/A).

Ao = aorta; LA = left atrium; LV = left ventricle; RV = right ventricle.

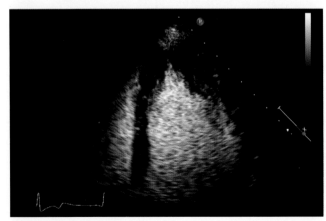

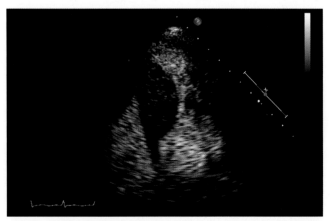

Figure 6.24 These images show the use of a myocardial contrast agent in a patient with apical hypertrophic cardiomyopathy (HCM) (*left*) and a patient with mid cavity HCM with an apical aneurysm (*right*). Note that the blood pool appears 'white' while the myocardium appears 'black'.

Presence, Location and Magnitude of Dynamic LVOT Obstruction

As stated above, the most common variant of HCM is ASH. ASH in conjunction with mitral SAM leads to dynamic LVOT obstruction or HOCM. Mitral SAM can be identified on 2D echocardiography and on the M-mode trace (Fig. 6.26). In particular, SAM is best appreciated via M-mode due to its superior temporal resolution. In addition, M-mode can be used to determine the severity of SAM and this can be used to indirectly predict the magnitude of LVOT obstruction. For example, mild SAM is identified

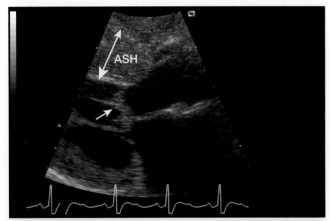

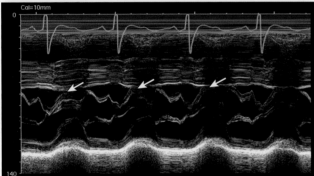

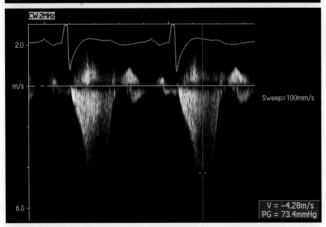

Figure 6.26 The 2D image (*top*) recorded from a zoomed parasternal long axis view demonstrates marked systolic anterior motion (SAM) of the anterior mitral valve leaflet (*arrow*). Also observe the marked asymmetric septal hypertrophy (ASH). The M-mode trace (*middle*) recorded from the same patient also shows ASH and SAM of the mitral valve (*arrows*); also observe on this trace that the anterior mitral leaflet has prolonged contact with the interventricular septum during systole; this suggests the presence of a significant left ventricular outflow tract (LVOT) gradient. The continuous-wave (CW) Doppler trace (*bottom*) confirms the presence of a significant LVOT gradient; the peak velocity is measured at 4.3 m/s yielding a peak pressure gradient of 73 mm Hg. Also observe that the LVOT signal is late peaking or 'dagger-shaped' which is consistent with dynamic LVOT obstruction.

when the mitral leaflet comes within less than 10 mm of the IVS; moderate SAM is identified when the mitral leaflet makes brief contact with the septum, and severe SAM is identified when the mitral leaflet has prolonged contact with the septum. The magnitude of LVOT obstruction is dependent upon: (1) the closeness of the anterior mitral leaflet to the IVS, (2) the onset of SAM to the onset of SAM-septal contact, and (3) the duration of SAM-septal contact (Fig. 6.27). For example, low pressure gradients across the LVOT can be predicted when SAM-septal contact occurs late in systole and is of short duration while high pressure gradients may be expected when the SAM-septal contact occurs early in systole and when the duration of contact is long.

CW Doppler is used to estimate the degree of LVOT obstruction by measuring the peak velocity across the LVOT (Fig. 6.26). The CW Doppler signal can also be used to differentiate a dynamic LVOT gradient from fixed LVOT obstructions such as discrete subaortic stenosis or subaortic membranes. In particular, with dynamic LVOT obstruction the LVOT signal peaks in mid-late systole and has a 'dagger' shape while the CW Doppler signal in fixed LVOT obstruction peaks in early systole similar to that seen with aortic stenosis.

PW Doppler can also be used to determine the precise anatomic location of the LV cavity obstruction; this is performed by interrogating the various levels of the LV cavity from the LV apex to the LVOT. Likewise, colour flow Doppler can also be utilised to identify the level of LV obstruction (Fig. 6.28). One of the limitations of PW Doppler in assessing HOCM is that the peak velocities may not be resolved; for example, when the

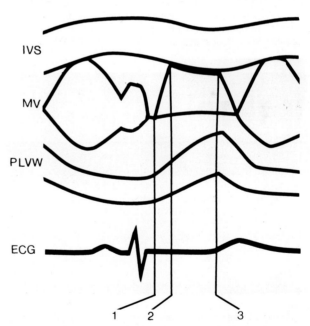

Figure 6.27 This schematic illustrates the variables that affect the degree of left ventricular outflow tract obstruction in hypertrophic obstructive cardiomyopathy. The numbers refer to points of measurement: 1 = onset of mitral systolic anterior motion (SAM); 2 = onset of SAM-septal contact; 3 = end of SAM-septal contact. The duration of SAM-septal contact is measured from point 2 to point 3. The period of onset of SAM to the onset of SAM-septal contact is measured from point 1 to point 2.

ECG = electrocardiogram; IVS = interventricular septum; MV = mitral valve; PLVW = posterior left ventricular wall.

Reproduced from Pollick C, Rakowski H, Wigle ED. Muscular subaortic stenosis: the quantitative relationship between systolic anterior motion and the pressure gradient. *Circulation*, 69(1): page 44; © 1984 Lippincott, Williams & Wilkins with permission.

Doppler shift exceeds the Nyquist limit the signal aliases and the peak velocity cannot be determined.

Another clue to the presence of significant LVOT obstruction is mid-systolic notching of the aortic valve. Mid-systolic notching (also known as mid-systolic closure) occurs when the LVOT gradient peaks in mid-late systole. At this time, LVOT obstruction is maximal and the pressure gradient between the LV and the aorta declines. As a result, aortic flow is interrupted and the aortic valve begins to move towards a closed position. The aortic valve frequently re-opens for the second half of systole and then closes normally at end-systole. Mid-systolic notching is best appreciated via M-mode due to its superior temporal resolution (Fig. 6.29).

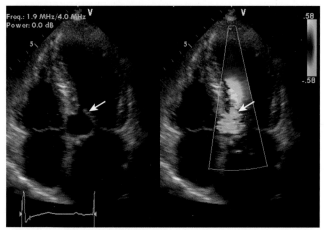

Figure 6.28 This image is recorded from the apical 4-chamber view. Observe on the 2D image that there is systolic anterior motion (SAM) of the mitral valve leaflet (*arrow*) which narrows the left ventricular outflow tract (LVOT). The colour flow Doppler image shows aliasing of the colour signal within the LVOT just downstream from the mitral SAM (*arrow*).

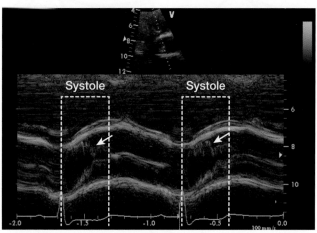

Figure 6.29 This M-mode trace recorded from a zoomed parasternal long axis view of the aortic valve demonstrates mid-systolic notching of the aortic valve (*arrows*). This sign is a characteristic feature of left ventricular outflow tract obstruction.

Mitral SAM and mid-systolic aortic valve notching are not pathognomonic of HOCM. Mitral SAM may also occur whenever there is a small left ventricular (LV) cavity with hyperdynamic systolic function while mid-systolic closure of the aortic valve may be seen when there is discrete subaortic stenosis or a subaortic membrane. Likewise, the absence of SAM and mid-systolic aortic valve notching does not exclude the diagnosis of HOCM as the LV outflow tract gradient may be absent at rest.

Response of the LVOT Gradient to Provocative Manoeuvres
HOCM is characterised by a dynamic pressure gradient across the LVOT. This means that the pressure gradient is dependent upon loading conditions and the contractile force of the myocardium. As previously stated, some patients with HOCM do not exhibit dynamic LVOT obstruction at rest or have only mild LVOT obstruction at rest. In these patients, dynamic LVOT obstruction may be provoked by certain medications, exercise, or the Valsalva manoeuvre. For example, in patients with latent LVOT obstruction, the LVOT velocities will increase with exercise or approximately 4 - 5 beats after the onset of strain in the Valsalva manoeuvre (Fig. 6.30). A marked increase in the LVOT gradient may also be noted following a ventricular ectopic which is consistent with the Brockenbrough–Braunwald–Morrow sign (Fig. 6.31).

Assessment of the Mechanism and Degree of MR
As previously stated, MR is often caused by mitral SAM due to incomplete coaptation of the mitral leaflets and/or distortion of the mitral valve apparatus during systole. The mechanism for MR in HOCM is referred to as "eject => obstruct => leak"; that is, when the LV ejects, LVOT obstruction follows and MR occurs as a consequence. MR secondary to SAM typically occurs in mid to late systole and the MR jet is usually posteriorly directed (Fig. 6.32). In particular, the timing and MR jet direction aids in differentiating MR due to SAM from MR due to primary mitral valve pathology.

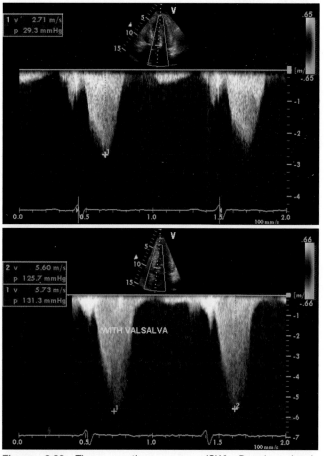

Figure 6.30 These continuous-wave (CW) Doppler signals were recorded from a patient with hypertrophic obstructive cardiomyopathy. At rest, the peak velocity across the left ventricular outflow tract (LVOT) was 2.7 m/s, yielding a peak pressure gradient of 29 mm Hg (*top*). Following the Valsalva manoeuvre, the peak velocity significantly increased to 5.6-5.7 m/s, yielding a peak pressure gradient of 126-131 mm Hg (*bottom*).

In the presence of MR, the LVOT gradient can be cross-checked using the peak MR velocity. Recall that the MR signal reflects the pressure gradient between the LV and LA during systole:

Equation 6.1

$$4V_{MR}^2 = LVSP - LAP$$

where V_{MR} = peak mitral regurgitant velocity (m/s)
 LVSP = left ventricular systolic pressure (mm Hg)
 LAP = left atrial pressure (mm Hg)

By measuring the MR velocity and by estimating the LA pressure, this equation can be rearranged to calculate the LV systolic pressure (LVSP):

Equation 6.2

$$LVSP = 4V_{MR}^2 + LAP$$

Then from the estimated LVSP and the aortic systolic pressure (which is assumed to be equal to the systolic blood pressure), the LVOT pressure gradient can be derived:

Equation 6.3

$$\Delta P_{LVOT} = LVSP - SBP$$

where ΔP_{LVOT} = left ventricular outflow tract pressure
         gradient (mm Hg)
 LVSP = left ventricular systolic pressure (mm Hg)
 SBP = systolic blood pressure (mm Hg)

MR and HOCM
Not all mitral regurgitation (MR) in hypertrophic obstructive cardiomyopathy (HOCM) occurs due to systolic anterior motion (SAM) of the mitral valve; MR may also occur due to primary valve pathology. In particular, recognition of coexistent primary mitral valve pathology is very important as patients undergoing surgical repair of HOCM may also require additional mitral valve surgery.

As for left ventricular outflow (LVOT) obstruction, MR is dynamic so the MR severity is dependent upon the loading conditions and LV contractile force. For example, any increase in LVOT obstruction will increase the degree of MR while a decrease in LVOT obstruction will decrease the MR. Furthermore, LVOT obstruction increases when there is a decrease in afterload and preload and decreases when there is an increase in the afterload and preload. Therefore, it follows that "HOCM MR" will also increase with a decrease in afterload and preload, and decrease with an increase in the afterload and preload. Note that this response is opposite to that which occurs in other mechanisms of MR.

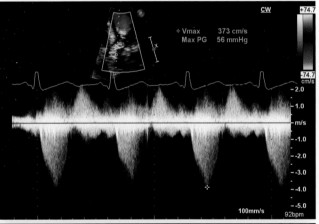

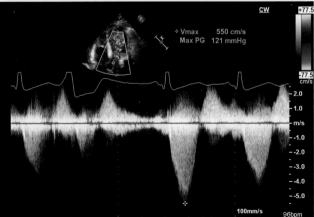

Figure 6.31 These continuous-wave (CW) Doppler signals were recorded from a patient with hypertrophic obstructive cardiomyopathy. During sinus rhythm, the peak velocity across the left ventricular outflow tract (LVOT) was 3.7 m/s, yielding a peak pressure gradient of 56 mm Hg (*top*). Following a ventricular ectopic beat, the peak velocity increased to 5.5 m/s, yielding a peak pressure gradient of 121 mm Hg (*bottom*).

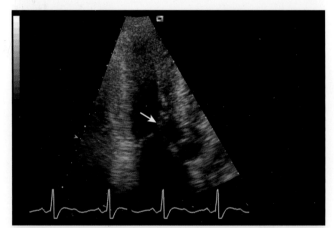

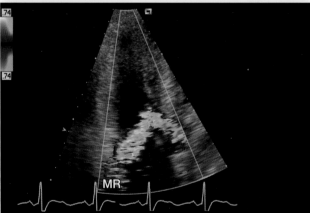

Figure 6.32 These images were recorded from the apical long axis view. The 2D image (*top*) demonstrates narrowing of the left ventricular outflow tract (LVOT) due to asymmetric septal hypertrophy (ASH) and systolic anterior motion (SAM) of the mitral valve (*arrow*). The corresponding colour flow Doppler image (*bottom*) shows turbulent flow within the LVOT consistent with dynamic LVOT obstruction; an eccentric jet of posteriorly directed mitral regurgitation (MR) is also shown. MR is most likely the result of mitral SAM and incomplete coaptation of the mitral leaflets during systole.

Guidance During, and Assessment Following Septal Reduction Procedures

Septal reduction procedures such as surgical septal myectomy and alcohol septal ablation aim to relieve or abolish LVOT obstruction in HOCM.

Surgical Septal Myectomy

Surgical septal myectomy is performed via an aortotomy and involves the resection or debulking of the basal IVS. This procedure effectively widens the LVOT, thus, eliminating mitral SAM and abolishes the LVOT obstruction.

Potential complications of this procedure include an iatrogenic ventricular septal defect (VSD) and aortic regurgitation (AR). An iatrogenic VSD may result if too much myocardium is resected while AR may occur due to either direct injury to the aortic valve via the aortotomy or resection of the myocardium too close to the aortic annulus resulting in destablisation of the right coronary cusp.

Following surgical septal myectomy, echocardiography has an important role in determining the resultant LVOT gradient, excluding an iatrogenic VSD, and assessing the presence and degree of AR.

Alcohol Septal Ablation

Alcohol septal ablation or transcoronary alcohol septal ablation for hypertrophy (TASH) is a percutaneous procedure whereby a small volume of alcohol is injected into a major septal

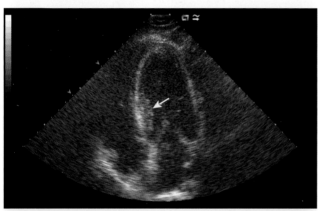

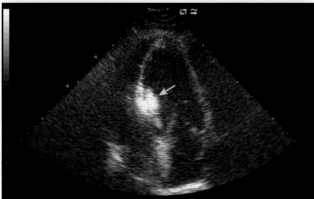

Figure 6.33 These images were recorded before (*top*) and following (*bottom*) alcohol septal ablation. On the baseline 2D image, asymmetric septal hypertrophy is apparent (*white arrow*). Following the injection of myocardial contrast (Levovist) into the septal perforator of the left anterior descending coronary artery, the site of perfusion is identified by an intense echo bright region in the basal interventricular septum (*yellow arrow*).

perforator branch of the left anterior descending coronary artery. This causes a localised myocardial infarction of the basal IVS. As a result the basal IVS becomes akinetic and over time the IVS becomes scarred and thinned; this effectively widens the LVOT, resolves or decreases mitral SAM and abolishes or reduces the LVOT obstruction.

Echocardiography can be used to guide TASH as well as evaluate the success of this procedure. In particular, myocardial contrast echocardiography can be used to facilitate selection of the optimal septal perforator branch (Fig. 6.33). By injecting a myocardial contrast agent into the septal perforator, the precise perfusion site of the selected septal perforator can be identified to ensure that the perfusion area corresponds to the basal IVS. Following the procedure, echocardiography is utilised to determine the resultant LVOT gradient and to assess the degree of LV remodelling of the basal IVS (Fig. 6.34).

Mimics of HCM

As stated above, HCM may be concentric and as there are a number of conditions that can cause a concentric increase in LV wall thickness these conditions may be confused with HCM. Examples causing concentric LV hypertrophy (LVH) include systemic hypertension, severe aortic stenosis, coarctation of the aorta, chronic renal disease and glycogen storage diseases. Infiltrative diseases such as amyloidosis may also produce increased LV wall thickness. These diseases can be differentiated from HCM based on various tests and observations (Table 6.11).

"Athlete's heart" is another condition that can mimic HCM. Cardiac remodelling may develop in some highly trained athletes who participate in endurance sports such as rowing, canoeing, swimming, cycling, cross-country skiing and ultra-endurance running. This remodelling includes an increase in LV, RV and LA chamber dimensions as well as an increase in the absolute LV wall thickness. These morphologic changes are thought to be related to physiologic adaptations to intense training as well as a number of demographic factors including age, gender, ethnicity, body size, and the type of endurance sport. The physiological upper limit for LV wall thickness in a highly trained athlete is 16 mm; therefore, LV wall thickness >16 mm should be considered pathological [6.2]. However, when the LV wall thickness is increased but <16 mm, other 'routine' echocardiographic measurements and findings can be used to distinguish between "athlete's heart" and HCM (Table 6.12).

"Athlete's heart" can also be differentiated from HCM based on gender. For example, the LV wall thickness does not usually exceed 12 mm in female athletes so an increased LV wall thickness >12 mm in a female athlete may be indicative of HCM. In addition, regression of ventricular hypertrophy following a short period of complete deconditioning can also be used to differentiate "athlete's heart" from HCM. For example, after suspending training for a 2-3 month period, the LV wall thickness decreases by approximately 2-3 mm in an "athlete's heart" while the LV wall thickness will remain unchanged in HCM. Importantly, evidence of changes in wall thickness with deconditioning is best identified via high-quality serial imaging such as cardiac magnetic resonance imaging, rather than echocardiography.

[6.2] Rawlins J, Bhan A, Sharma S. Left ventricular hypertrophy in athletes. *Eur J Echocardiogr.* 2009 May;10(3):350-6.

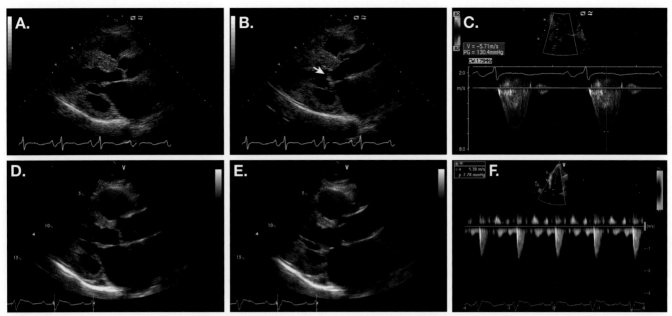

Figure 6.34 These images were recorded before (*top*) and 18 months following alcohol septal ablation (*bottom*). Observe that prior to the procedure, the 2D images show asymmetric septal hypertrophy (ASH) (A), systolic anterior motion (SAM) of the mitral valve (*arrow*) (B), and a peak pressure gradient across the left ventricular outflow tract (LVOT) of 130 mm Hg (C). 18 months after the procedure, a marked decrease in the interventricular septal thickness is apparent (D); in addition, mitral SAM is no longer evident (E) and the pressure gradient across the LVOT is now only 8 mm Hg (F).

Table 6.11 Mimics of Hypertrophic Cardiomyopathy (HCM)

Mimics of HCM	Differentiation from HCM
Aortic stenosis (AS)	Echocardiographic features consistent with AS (see Chapter 7)
Chronic renal failure	Clinical history
Coarctation of the Aorta (CoAo)	Echocardiographic features consistent with CoAo (see Chapter 15)
Fabry's disease	Evidence of α-galactosidase deficiency (see Chapter 14)
Friedreich's ataxia	Clinical findings; genetic testing (see Chapter 14)
Hypertension	History of chronic elevation in blood pressure
Infiltrative disease (e.g. Amyloidosis)	Low voltages on the ECG; endomyocardial biopsy (see Chapter 14)

Table 6.12 Echocardiographic Parameters distinguishing Athlete's Heart from Hypertrophic Cardiomyopathy (HCM)

Parameter	Athlete's Heart	HCM
Left ventricular (LV) wall thickness	< 16 mm	Usually > 16 mm
Pattern of LV Hypertrophy	Symmetric thickening (difference 2 mm or less between all portions of the LV)	Typically asymmetric (ASH most common)
LV cavity size	Enlarged (EDD ≥ 55 mm)	Normal or reduced (EDD ≤ 50 mm) May be increased in 'end stage' or 'burnt-out' HCM
LV cavity shape	Ellipsoid shape	Abnormal or distorted
Left ventricular outflow tract (LVOT)	Normal or enlarged LVOT obstruction not inducible; mitral SAM absent	Narrowed LVOT obstruction inducible in about 2/3 of cases due to mitral SAM
Left atrium (LA) and LV size	Enlarged LA and LV	Enlarged LA with normal LV size
Diastolic function	Normal or supranormal	Always abnormal (evidence of impaired LV relaxation)
Doppler tissue imaging (DTI)	Systolic and early diastolic velocities preserved	Systolic and early diastolic velocities decreased

ASH = asymmetric septal hypertrophy; EDD = end-diastolic dimension; SAM = systolic anterior motion
Based on data from: [1] Pelliccia A, Maron MS, Maron BJ. Assessment of left ventricular hypertrophy in a trained athlete: differential diagnosis of physiologic athlete's heart from pathologic hypertrophy. *Prog Cardiovasc Dis.* 2012; 54(5):387-96 and [2] Rawlins J, Bhan A, Sharma S. Left ventricular hypertrophy in athletes. *Eur J Echocardiogr.* 2009 May;10(3):350-6.

Restrictive Cardiomyopathy

Restrictive cardiomyopathy (RCM) refers to any heart muscle disease that results in impaired ventricular filling with normal or reduced diastolic volumes of either or both ventricles with normal or near-normal systolic function and wall thickness.

Aetiology of RCM

The cause of RCM may be idiopathic or it may occur secondary to other local and systemic disorders (Table 6.13). In particular, infiltrative and storage disorders cause RCM via infiltration or deposition of pathologic substances within or between myocardial cells resulting in increased ventricular wall thickness and stiffness. In noninfiltrative disorders, the abnormal myocardium also leads to increased myocardial stiffness causing a RCM. Endomyocardial disorders cause RCM by myocardial and/or endocardial fibrosis or scarring of the endomyocardial surface.

The most common specific cause of RCM in developed countries is cardiac amyloidosis while endomyocardial fibrosis is the most common specific cause of RCM in underdeveloped countries. Details regarding many of the specific, systemic causes of RCM listed in Table 6.13 are discussed in Chapter 14.

Table 6.13 Classification of Types of Restrictive Cardiomyopathy According to Cause

Cause	Example
Myocardial	
- Noninfiltrative	Idiopathic cardiomyopathy* Familial cardiomyopathy Hypertrophic cardiomyopathy Scleroderma Pseudoxanthoma elasticum Diabetic cardiomyopathy
- Infiltrative	Amyloidosis* Sarcoidosis* Gaucher disease Hurler disease Fatty infiltration
- Storage Disease	Haemochromatosis Fabry disease Glycogen storage disease
Endomyocardial	Endomyocardial fibrosis* Hypereosinophilic syndrome Carcinoid heart disease Metastatic cancers Radiation* Toxic effects of anthracycline* Drugs causing fibrous endocarditis (serotonin, methysergide, ergotamine, mercurial agents, busulfan)

*These conditions are more likely to be encountered in clinical practice. Reproduced from Kushwaha SS, Fallon JT, Fuster V. Restrictive cardiomyopathy. *N Engl J Med.* Jan 23;336(4), page 269, © 1997 with permission from the Massachusetts Medical Society.

Pathophysiology of RCM

The hallmark of RCM is abnormal diastolic function which occurs due to increased myocardial stiffness and poor chamber compliance. Recall that ventricular filling and the resultant ventricular pressures and volumes are determined by the compliance or the stiffness of the ventricle (see Chapter 2). In particular, when there is a stiff, non-compliant ventricle diastolic filling of the ventricle is restricted. Therefore, in early diastole there is rapid filling of the ventricles as per normal, however, due to the stiff, non-compliant myocardium for a small increase in diastolic volume there is a simultaneous and relatively larger increase in diastolic ventricular pressure; this results in premature termination of early diastolic filling. On the haemodynamic pressure trace, this appears as a characteristic 'dip-and-plateau' or 'square root' sign (Fig 6.35).

Ventricular systolic function in the early stages of the disease is typically normal (but this may deteriorate as the disease progresses). Additionally, the marked elevation in atrial pressures leads to marked atrial enlargement. Therefore, the classic anatomic features of a RCM include marked atrial dilatation with normal sized ventricles (Fig. 6.36).

Clinical Manifestations of RCM

The clinical manifestations associated with RCM are related to biventricular heart failure; these symptoms include dyspnoea, peripheral oedema, fatigue and weakness, decreased exercise tolerance, an increased jugular venous pressure and ascites.

Role of Echocardiography in RCM

The primary aims and objectives of echocardiography in the assessment of patients with RCM include:
- Establishing the diagnosis of RCM,
- Assessment of ventricular size and systolic function,
- Evaluation of LV diastolic function.

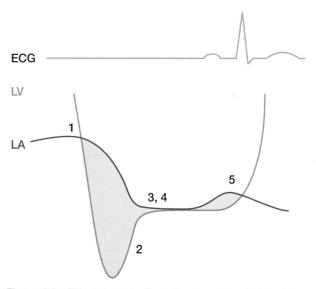

Figure 6.35 This schematic illustrates the characteristic "dip and plateau" pattern seen on the left ventricular (LV) pressure trace with restrictive filling. When there is poor LV compliance, there is (1) a marked increase in left atrial (LA) pressure, (2) a rapid rise in LV pressure with early diastolic filling, (3) a rapid equalization of LV and LA pressures, and (4) an abrupt termination of early diastolic filling which occurs when the fixed volume of the ventricles is reached. In addition, as the ventricle has reached its fixed volume in early diastole, there is minimal filling with atrial contraction (5).

Establishing the Diagnosis of RCM

The characteristic echocardiographic features of RCM include marked biatrial dilatation with normal sized ventricles and normal or near-normal systolic function (Fig. 6.37). A small circumferential pericardial effusion is also commonly seen.

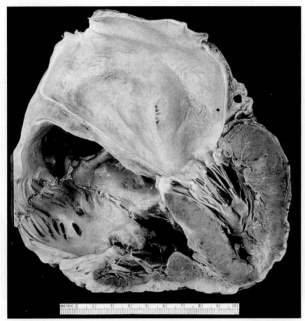

Figure 6.36 This gross cardiac specimen shows the characteristic features of restrictive cardiomyopathy which includes marked biatrial enlargement with normal-sized ventricles.
By permission of Mayo Foundation for Medical Education and Research. All rights reserved. Courtesy of William D. Edwards, MD.

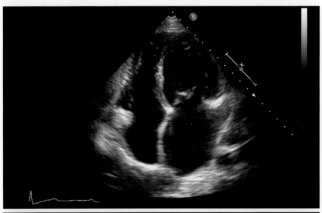

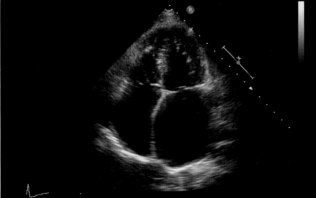

Figure 6.37 These apical 4-chamber images were recorded at end-diastole (*top*) and end-systole (*bottom*) in a patient with idiopathic restrictive cardiomyopathy. Observe the markedly dilated atria with normal-sized ventricles; the ejection fraction is also normal at 62% (calculated by the biplane Simpson's method).

Specific systemic diseases that cause RCM such as amyloidosis, sarcoidosis, hypereosinophilic syndrome, and carcinoid heart disease have characteristic echocardiographic features; these features are described in Chapter 14.

Assessment of Ventricular Size and Systolic Function

The assessment of LV and RV systolic function is assessed in the traditional manner as detailed in Chapter 2. In particular, in the early stages of the disease ventricular size and systolic function are usually normal. However, as the disease progresses systolic function may deteriorate.

Evaluation of LV Diastolic Function

The hallmark of RCM is diastolic dysfunction which is related to increased myocardial stiffness and poor ventricular compliance. RCM may be associated with a classic restrictive diastolic filling profile (Fig. 6.38). Importantly, however, not

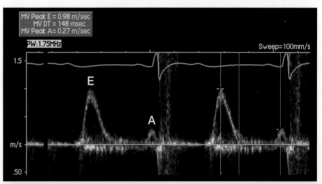

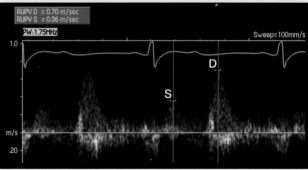

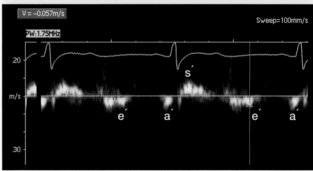

Figure 6.38 Left ventricular (LV) diastolic function in a patient with a restrictive cardiomyopathy was assessed via the transmitral inflow profile (*top*), pulmonary venous profile (*middle*), and lateral annular Doppler tissue imaging (DTI) (*bottom*). The transmitral inflow shows a classic restrictive filling profile with an E/A ratio ≥ 2 and a deceleration time less than 160 ms. The pulmonary venous trace is also consistent with a restrictive filling profile; observe that the diastolic velocity (D) is increased and there is a marked reduction in the pulmonary systolic velocity (S). In addition, the E/e' ratio derived from the transmitral E velocity and DTI early diastolic velocity (e') of 5 cm/s is increased at 18; this is consistent with increased left atrial pressure.
E = early diastolic velocity; A = velocity with atrial contraction; a' = myocardial velocity with atrial contraction; s' = systolic myocardial velocity.

all cases of RCM produce restrictive haemodynamics. In particular, a patient with RCM may exhibit any grade of diastolic dysfunction. The grades of diastolic dysfunction are summarized in Table 6.8. The detailed approach for the assessment of LV diastolic function is described in Chapter 3.

RCM versus Constrictive Pericarditis

The characteristic clinical and physiological presentation of patients with RCM may be identical to that seen in patients with constrictive pericarditis (CP). Importantly, CP is a treatable cause of diastolic heart failure and, therefore, identification of this disorder is crucial as most symptoms can be reversed by surgical pericardiectomy. Echocardiography in the assessment of CP as well as the role of echocardiography in differentiation between RCM and CP are discussed in Chapter 12.

> ### RCM versus Restrictive Physiology
> Patients with a restrictive cardiomyopathy (RCM) do not always have a restrictive filling profile; in particular, diastolic dysfunction can vary in severity from an abnormal relaxation pattern, to pseudonormalisation, to restrictive filling. Likewise, a restrictive filling pattern does not mean that the patient has a RCM. Restrictive physiology may occur in any condition where there is poor left ventricular compliance and increased left atrial pressures.

Arrhythmogenic Right Ventricular Cardiomyopathy

Arrhythmogenic right ventricular dysplasia or cardiomyopathy (ARVD/C) is an uncommon inherited disorder characterised clinically by ventricular arrhythmias, heart failure and sudden death and structurally by progressive fibrofatty replacement of the RV myocardium.

Aetiology of ARVD/C

ARVC/D is a predominantly genetic disorder of autosomal dominant inheritance characterised by fibrofatty replacement of the RV myocardium (Fig.6.39). The diagnosis of ARVD/C is based on the presence of major and minor criteria that include structural, histological, ECG, arrhythmic, and genetic factors (Table 6.14). On the basis of this classification, a definitive diagnosis of ARVD/C is fulfilled in the presence of 2 major criteria, or 1 major and 2 minor criteria, or 4 minor criteria from different categories. A borderline diagnosis is suspected in the presence of 1 major and 1 minor criteria, or 3 minor criteria from different categories; and a possible diagnosis is suspected in the presence of 1 major criterion, or 2 minor criteria from different categories.

Pathophysiology of ARVD/C

Fibrofatty replacement leads to RV thinning and aneurysmal dilatation. RV aneurysms most commonly affect the inflow, apical, and outflow portions of the RV; this pattern of aneurysmal formation is referred to as the "triangle of dysplasia" (Fig. 6.40). While the LV is spared in the majority of cases, fibrofatty replacement of the LV myocardium may also occur in the later stages of the disease progression.

The replacement of the RV myocardium by fibrofatty tissue has been related to three basic mechanisms: (1) apoptosis or programmed cell death, (2) inflammatory heart disease with a spectrum of clinical presentations ranging from acute myocarditis to fibrous healing, and (3) myocardial dystrophy independent of myocarditis possibly reflecting genetically determined atrophy [6.3].

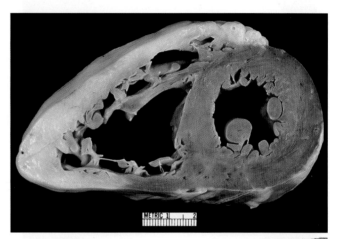

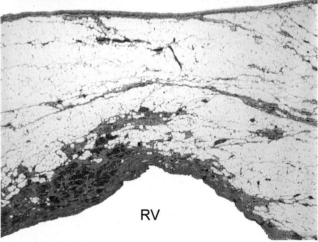

RV

Figure 6.39 Gross and histological specimens of arrhythmogenic right ventricular dysplasia/cardiomyopathy (ARVD/C) are shown. In the gross specimen observe that the majority of the right ventricular (RV) myocardium has been replaced by yellow fat. The histological example of the RV shows massive myocardial replacement with fibrous tissue (blue stained) and the adipose tissue (white 'bubbles'); only a small amount of RV myocardium remains (red stained).
By permission of Mayo Foundation for Medical Education and Research. All rights reserved. Courtesy of William D. Edwards, MD.

> "Exercise induced right ventricular dysplasia/cardiomyopathy" (EIRVD/C) is thought to be an acquired form of ARVD/C seen in athletes who participate in extreme endurance sports. A possible mechanism of EIRVD/C includes cumulative and progressive RV myocardial damage caused by repeated bouts of intense, ultra-endurance exercise leading to myocardial inflammation and fibrosis, potential arrhythmogenesis, and RV myocardial dysfunction.

[6.3] Corrado D, Fontaine G, Marcus FI, McKenna WJ, Nava A, Thiene G, Wichter T. Arrhythmogenic right ventricular dysplasia/cardiomyopathy: need for an international registry. Study Group on Arrhythmogenic Right Ventricular Dysplasia/Cardiomyopathy of the Working Groups on Myocardial and Pericardial Disease and Arrhythmias of the European Society of Cardiology and of the Scientific Council on Cardiomyopathies of the World Heart Federation. *Circulation*. 2000 Mar 21;101(11):E101-6.

Table 6.14 Diagnostic Criteria for Arrhythmogenic Right Ventricular Dysplasia/Cardiomyopathy (ARVD/C)

Features	Major Diagnostic Criteria	Minor Diagnostic Criteria
Global or regional dysfunction and structural alterations	**By 2D echo:** Regional RV akinesia, dyskinesia, or aneurysm *and* 1 of the following: • PLAX RVOT $\geq$ 32 mm (or PLAX/BSA $\geq$ 19 mm/m^2) • PSAX RVOT $\geq$ 36 mm (or PSAX/BSA $\geq$ 21 mm/m^2) • *or* fractional area change $\leq$ 33% **By MRI:** Regional RV akinesia or dyskinesia or dyssynchronous RV contraction *and* 1 of the following: • Ratio of RVEDV to BSA $\geq$110 mL/m^2 (male) or $\geq$100 mL/m^2 (female) • *or* RV ejection fraction $\leq$ 40% **By RV angiography:** Regional RV akinesia, dyskinesia, or aneurysm	**By 2D echo:** Regional RV akinesia or dyskinesia *and* 1 of the following: • PLAX RVOT $\geq$ 29 to <32 mm (or PLAX/BSA $\geq$16 to <19 mm/m^2) • PSAX RVOT $\geq$ 32 to <36 mm (or PSAX/BSA $\geq$18 to <21 mm/m^2) • *or* fractional area change >33% to $\leq$ 40% **By MRI:** Regional RV akinesia or dyskinesia or dyssynchronous RV contraction *and* 1 of the following: • Ratio of RVEDV to BSA $\geq$ 100 to <110 mL/m^2 (male) or $\geq$ 90 to <100 mL/m^2 (female) • *or* RV ejection fraction >40% to $\leq$ 45%
Tissue characterization of walls	Residual myocytes <60% by morphometric analysis (or <50% if estimated), with fibrous replacement of RV free wall myocardium in $\geq$1 sample, with or without fatty replacement of tissue on endomyocardial biopsy	Residual myocytes 60% to 75% by morphometric analysis (or 50% to 65% if estimated), with fibrous replacement of RV free wall myocardium in $\geq$ 1 sample, with or without fatty replacement of tissue on endomyocardial biopsy
ECG Repolarization abnormalities	Inverted T waves in right precordial leads (V1, V2, and V3) or beyond in individuals >14 years of age (in the absence of complete RBBB block QRS $\geq$120 ms)	Inverted T waves in leads V1 and V2 in individuals >14 years of age (in the absence of complete RBBB) or in V4, V5, or V6 Inverted T waves in leads V1, V2, V3, and V4 in individuals >14 years of age in the presence of complete RBBB
ECG Depolarization/ conduction abnormalities	Epsilon wave (reproducible low-amplitude signals between the end of the QRS complex to onset of the T wave) in the right precordial leads (V1 to V3)	Late potentials by SAECG in $\geq$1 of 3 parameters in the absence of a QRS duration of $\geq$110 ms on the standard ECG Filtered QRS duration (fQRS) $\geq$114 ms Duration of terminal QRS <40 μV (low-amplitude signal duration) $\geq$ 38 ms Root-mean-square voltage of terminal 40 ms $\leq$ 20 μV Terminal activation duration of QRS $\geq$ 55 ms measured from the nadir of the S wave to the end of the QRS, including R', in V1, V2, or V3, in the absence of complete RBBB
Arrhythmias	Nonsustained or sustained VT of LBBB morphology with superior axis (negative or indeterminate QRS in leads II, III, and aVF and positive in lead aVL)	Nonsustained or sustained VT of RV outflow configuration, LBBB morphology with inferior axis (positive QRS in leads II, III, and aVF and negative in lead aVL) or of unknown axis > 500 ventricular extrasystoles per 24 hours (Holter)
Family history	ARVD/C confirmed in a 1st-degree relative who meets current Task Force criteria ARVD/C confirmed pathologically at autopsy or surgery in a 1st-degree relative Identification of a pathogenic mutation* categorized as associated or probably associated with ARVD/C in the patient under evaluation	History of ARVD/C in a 1st-degree relative in whom it is not possible or practical to determine whether the family member meets current Task Force criteria Premature sudden death (<35 years of age) due to suspected ARVD/C in a 1st-degree relative ARVD/C confirmed pathologically or by current Task Force criteria in 2nd-degree relative

BSA = body surface area; LBBB = left bundle branch block; LV = left ventricle; MRI = magnetic resonance imaging; PLAX = parasternal long axis; PSAX = parasternal short axis; RBBB = right bundle branch block; RV = right ventricle; RVEDV = right ventricular end-diastolic volume; RVOT = right ventricular outflow tract; SAECG = signal averaged ECG; VT = ventricular tachycardia.

Diagnostic terminology: Definite diagnosis: 2 major criteria, or 1 major and 2 minor criteria, or 4 minor criteria from different categories; Borderline diagnosis: 1 major and 1 minor criteria, or 3 minor criteria from different categories; Possible diagnosis: 1 major criterion, or 2 minor criteria from different categories.

* A pathogenic mutation is a DNA alteration associated with ARVD/C that (1) alters or is expected to alter the encoded protein, (2) is unobserved or rare in a large non-ARVD/C control population, and (3) either alters or is predicted to alter the structure or function of the protein or has demonstrated linkage to the disease phenotype in a conclusive pedigree.

Adapted from Marcus FI, McKenna WJ, Sherrill D, Basso C, Bauce B, Bluemke DA, Calkins H, Corrado D, Cox MG, Daubert JP, Fontaine G, Gear K, Hauer R, Nava A, Picard MH, Protonotarios N, Saffitz JE, Sanborn DM, Steinberg JS, Tandri H, Thiene G, Towbin JA, Tsatsopoulou A, Wichter T, Zareba W. Diagnosis of arrhythmogenic right ventricular cardiomyopathy/dysplasia: proposed modification of the Task Force Criteria. *Eur Heart J.* Apr;31(7), pages 808-809, © 2010, with permission of Oxford University Press.

Clinical Manifestations of ARVD/C

The clinical presentation of ARVD/C usually consists of arrhythmias ranging from isolated ventricular ectopics to sustained ventricular tachycardia (VT), or ventricular fibrillation (VF) leading to sudden cardiac death. Patients typically present between the second and fourth decades. However, young adolescent patients can also present following an episode of sudden cardiac death.

Role of Echocardiography in ARVD/C

The primary aims and objectives of echocardiography in the assessment of patients with ARVD/C include:
• Establishing the diagnosis of ARVD/C,
• Assessment of RV systolic function,
• Assessment of LV systolic function,
• Evaluation of TR severity including estimation of the RVSP.

Establishing the Diagnosis of ARVD/C

As indicated in Table 6.14, 2D echocardiography has an important role in the diagnosis of ARVD/C. In particular, echocardiography can be used to identify major and minor criteria based on global or regional RV dysfunction and RV structural alterations. For example, regional RV akinesia, dyskinesia, or aneurysm and dilatation of the RV outflow tract (RVOT) are major criteria of ARVD/C (Fig. 6.41, A-C). It is important to note, however, that there is a wide spectrum of RV involvement including discrete RV aneurysms, segmental RV thinning with akinesis/dyskinesis, global RV thinning with akinesis/dyskinesis/aneurysms, and marked RV dilatation with poor systolic function. Other clues to the presence of ARVD/C include a hyper-reflective moderator band and an abnormal trabecular pattern or trabecular derangement (Fig. 6.41, D-E). Importantly, a careful evaluation of the RV from all possible echocardiographic views is required; these views include: (1) the parasternal long axis of the RV inflow, (2) the parasternal long axis of the RVOT, (3) the parasternal short axis views, (4) the apical 4-chamber; (5) the RV focused apical 4-chamber, and (6) the subcostal views.

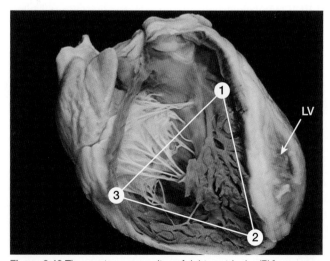

Figure 6.40 The most common sites of right ventricular (RV) aneurysm formation are at: (1) the anterior infundibulum (RV outflow), (2) the RV apex, and (3) the inferior or diaphragmatic aspect of the RV (RV inflow). These 3 regions constitute the "triangle of dysplasia". LV = left ventricle. Pathology photo from Anderson RH and Becker AE. 1980, Cardiac Anatomy. An Integrated Text and Color Atlas, Gower Medical Publishing Ltd, pp 3.12, with permission from Robert H. Anderson, M.D., FRCPath. University College London.

Assessment of RV Systolic Function

RV systolic function is assessed in the usual manner as described in detail in Chapter 2. For example, measurements of RV systolic function include the DTI systolic velocity, TAPSE, FAC and/or the RV MPI. Importantly, more than one measure of RV function should be used to distinguish between normal and abnormal RV systolic function.

Assessment of LV Systolic Function

Although the LV is not usually affected by ARVD/C, fibrofatty replacement of the LV myocardium may occur in the later stages of the disease. Therefore, in patients with advanced ARVD/C, a careful evaluation of regional and global LV systolic function is also important. Global LV systolic function is assessed in the traditional manner as detailed in Chapter 2; the assessment of regional LV systolic function is described in Chapter 5.

Evaluation of TR Severity

Most patients with ARVD/C will have some degree of functional TR. In these patients, TR occurs secondary to tricuspid annular dilatation. The degree of TR is variable and can range from mild to severe. The severity of TR is evaluated via the traditional methods which are described in detail in Chapter 9. In particular, a large colour TR jet area, increased forward flow velocities across the tricuspid valve, systolic flow reversal in the hepatic veins, and a strong TR CW Doppler signal are all useful signs for detecting significant TR.

Importantly, in advanced ARVD/C there may be 'free' or 'wide-open' TR. In these patients, the tricuspid regurgitant

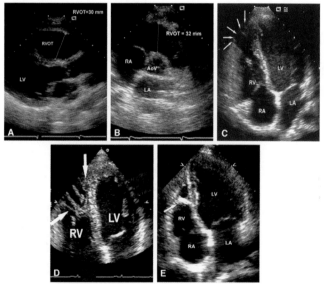

Figure 6.41 These images show the echocardiographic features associated with arrhythmogenic right ventricular dysplasia/cardiomyopathy (ARVD/C). The parasternal long axis view and short axis view show right ventricular outflow tract (RVOT) enlargement (A and B, respectively). The apical 4-chamber views show a focal RV apical aneurysm (C, *arrows*), excessive trabeculations (D, *arrows*), and a hyper-reflective moderator band (E, *arrow*). AoV = aortic valve; LA = left atrium; LV = left ventricle; RA = right atrium; RV = right ventricle.
Reproduced from Yoerger DM, Marcus F, Sherrill D, Calkins H, Towbin JA, Zareba W, Picard MH; Multidisciplinary Study of Right Ventricular Dysplasia Investigators. Echocardiographic findings in patients meeting task force criteria for arrhythmogenic right ventricular dysplasia: new insights from the multidisciplinary study of right ventricular dysplasia, *J Am Coll Cardiol,* Vol 45(6), page 862, © 2005, with permission from Elsevier.

orifice is very large; therefore, in the absence of pulmonary hypertension, the pressure differential between the RA and RV is very small. As a result, there is little or no aliasing of the TR jet so TR may be significantly underestimated on the colour Doppler examination.

From the peak TR velocity, the RVSP can be estimated in the standard manner. However, if there is 'free' or 'wide-open' TR, the TR velocity is usually very low as stated above. In this situation, the RVSP cannot be accurately estimated from the peak TR velocity. This is because while the TR velocity will still reflect the pressure difference between the RV and RA in systole, the RAP is unknown and it may be as high as 40 mm Hg.

Left Ventricular Non-Compaction

Left ventricular non-compaction (LVNC) is an abnormality of the LV myocardium characterised by numerous prominent LV trabeculations and deep intertrabecular recesses that communicate with the LV cavity. LVNC is a well-known abnormality that is associated with a number of congenital heart diseases. LVNC without other associated morphologic cardiac abnormalities is referred to as "isolated" LV non-compaction (ILVNC). LVNC is included in the unclassified cardiomyopathy category.

Aetiology of LVNC

LVNC is a rare congenital abnormality. Several pathogenetic concepts have been proposed to explain the occurrence of this condition. The most popular of these theories is that LVNC occurs due to the failure of normal trabecular resorption or compaction during embryonic development resulting in a bilayered LV myocardium.

In early embryonic development of the ventricular myocardium, prominent myocardial trabeculations form. The intertrabecular spaces and deep intertrabecular recesses serve to supply the myocardium with blood in the absence of a yet established coronary circulation. As development continues, compaction of these trabeculations occurs so that the intertrabecular spaces are transformed into capillaries, trabeculations become flattened or disappear, and the formation of coronary vessels establishes the coronary circulation. Compaction of the ventricular myocardium normally progresses from epicardium to endocardium and from the base of the heart toward the apex. An abnormal arrest in this process is thought to produce the characteristic bilayered ventricular appearance associated with ILVNC (Fig. 6.42).

Pathophysiology of LVNC

LV systolic dysfunction is frequently associated with ILVNC. In particular, non-compacted myocardial segments have reduced contractile potential compared with compacted myocardium. Therefore, the degree of LV systolic dysfunction is determined by the extent of myocardial non-compaction and the severity of the disease.

Clinical Manifestations of LVNC

A number of clinical manifestations of ILVNC have been described; these include a high incidence of heart failure, atrial and ventricular arrhythmias, and endocardial clot with systemic embolisation. Incidences of sudden cardiac death in patients with ILVNC have also been reported.

Echocardiographic Features of LVNC

Several echocardiographic criteria for the diagnosis of ILVNC have been described; these include the absence of coexisting cardiac abnormalities plus:

- the appearance of more than three trabeculations protruding from the LV wall, apically to the papillary muscles, visible in a single image plane (trabeculations are defined as localised protrusions of the ventricular wall with the same echogenicity as the myocardium and moving synchronously with ventricular contractions) (Fig. 6.43);
- the appearance of blood flow from the LV cavity into the intertrabecular recesses as visualised by colour Doppler imaging (Fig. 6.43);
- a two-layered or bilayered myocardium, with a thin outer compacted layer (epicardial) and a thickened inner non-compacted layer (endocardial) (Fig. 6.44).

In particular, two ratios have been described to confirm the diagnosis of ILVNC. The X/Y ratio is derived from: (1) the distance between the epicardial surface and trough of a trabecular recess (X), and (2) the distance between the epicardial surface and peak of the trabeculation (Y). For the

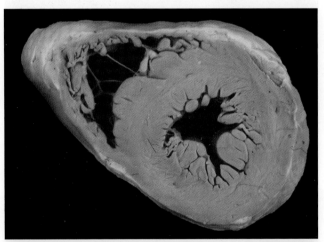
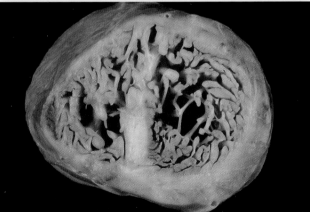

Figure 6.42 Gross specimens of a normal heart (*top*) and a heart with left ventricular non-compaction (*bottom*) are shown in short axis cuts. Observe the bilayered appearance of the ventricular myocardium in the non-compacted heart compared with the normal heart; the non-compacted layer consists of numerous prominent ventricular trabeculations and deep intertrabecular recesses. These deep intertrabecular recesses communicate with the ventricular cavity.
By permission of Mayo Foundation for Medical Education and Research. All rights reserved. Courtesy of William D. Edwards, MD.

X/Y ratio, measurements are performed from the parasternal short axis and apical views at end-diastole. An X/Y ratio ≤ 0.5 is consistent with ILVNC [6.4]. The NC/C ratio is determined from: (1) the non-compacted layer thickness (NC), and (2) the compacted layer thickness (C). Measurements are performed from the parasternal short axis view at end-systole (Fig. 6.44). A ratio greater than 2 is consistent with ILVNC [6.5, 6.6].

It should also be noted that the degree of myocardial involvement of the LV is typically segmental, with the apex being nearly always involved and the mid LV lateral wall segments being involved in the majority of cases; involvement of the basal LV wall segments is rare (Fig. 6.45).

In patients where conventional echocardiographic images are suboptimal or the diagnosis is uncertain, contrast echocardiography can be used to identify LV trabeculations and to confirm communication between the deep intertrabecular recesses and the LV cavity (Fig. 6.46).

Due to the predominately apical involvement of ILVNC, misdiagnosis of this abnormality for the apical form of hypertrophic cardiomyopathy, endomyocardial fibrosis, or an apical LV mass may occur. Awareness of this abnormality as well as the echocardiographic features of ILVNC should avoid misdiagnosis.

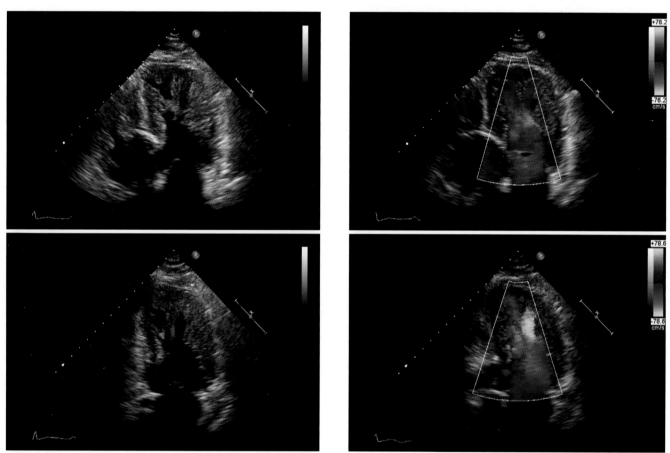

Figure 6.43 These images were recorded from a patient with isolated left ventricular non-compaction (ILVNC). The upper images are apical 4-chamber images and the lower images are apical 2-chamber images. On the 2D images, the non-compacted layer consists of the numerous trabeculations with deep intertrabecular recesses that appear to communicate with the left ventricular (LV) cavity. The colour flow Doppler images nicely demonstrate the deep intertrabecular recesses confirming that these recesses are in continuity with the LV cavity.

[6.4] Chin TK, Perloff JK, Williams RG, Jue K, Mohrmann R. Isolated noncompaction of left ventricular myocardium. A study of eight cases. *Circulation.* 1990 Aug;82(2):507-13.

[6.5] Jenni R, Oechslin E, Schneider J, Attenhofer Jost C, Kaufmann PA. Echocardiographic and pathoanatomical characteristics of isolated left ventricular non-compaction: a step towards classification as a distinct cardiomyopathy. *Heart.* 2001 Dec;86(6):666-71.

[6.5] Paterick TE, Umland MM, Jan MF, Ammar KA, Kramer C, Khandheria BK, Seward JB, Tajik AJ. Left ventricular noncompaction: a 25-year odyssey. *J Am Soc Echocardiogr.* 2012 Apr;25(4):363-75.

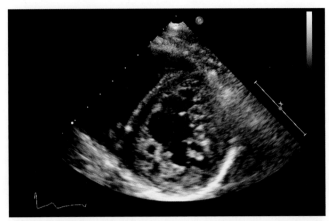 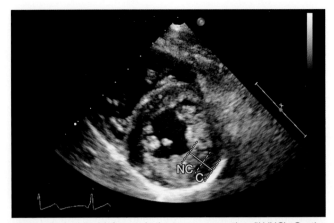

Figure 6.44 These parasternal short axis images were recorded from a patient with isolated left ventricular non-compaction (ILVNC). On the end-diastolic frame, there are multiple trabeculations protruding from the left ventricle (LV) (*left*). On the end-systolic frame, an obvious two-layered effect is seen with a thin outer compacted layer (C) and a thickened inner non-compacted layer (NC) (*right*). The ratio of non-compacted to compacted layers can be derived by measuring the compacted layer (C) and the non-compacted layer (NC); the ratio is then derived as NC divided by C. A ratio > 2 is consistent with ILVNC.

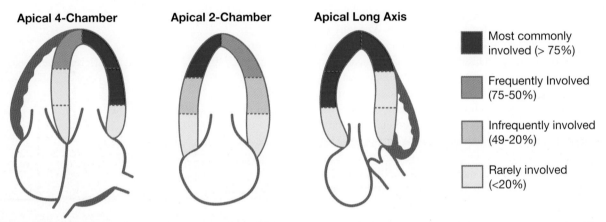

Figure 6.45 These schematics illustrate the distribution of prominent trabeculations seen in isolated left ventricular non-compaction. The most frequently involved segments include the LV apex and the mid-lateral segments.

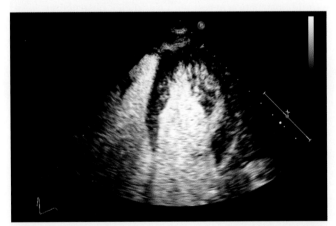

Figure 6.46 This image recorded from the apical 4-chamber view shows the use of a myocardial contrast agent in a patient with isolated left ventricular non-compaction (ILVNC). Numerous left ventricular (LV) trabeculations are noted; the deep intertrabecular recesses and their continuity with the LV cavity are also nicely demonstrated.

Key Points

Dilated Cardiomyopathy (DCM): Basic Concepts
- *Aetiology*: familial and genetic factors, viral myocarditis and other cytotoxic insults, and immunological abnormalities
- *Pathophysiology*: all 4 cardiac chambers usually dilated; LV dilatation occurs in an attempt to maintain a normal cardiac output, however, increased LV size also increases wall stress ultimately resulting in reduced stroke volume and contractility; LA dilatation occurs secondary to elevated LV filling pressures +/- MR; dilatation of right heart chambers occurs due to the myopathic process or secondary to elevated pulmonary pressures
- *Clinical manifestations*: relate to heart failure; symptoms include dyspnoea, peripheral oedema, fatigue and weakness, and decreased exercise tolerance

Role of Echo in DCM
- Assessment of chamber size
- Assessment of LV systolic function:
  - Contrast echo may be required to enhance endocardial border definition and improve accuracy of LV volume measurements
- Evaluation of LV diastolic function
- Assessment of RV systolic function
- Evaluation of the degree of valvular regurgitation
- Exclusion of LV and/or RV thrombus:
  - Contrast echo may be required to determine the presence or absence of LV thrombus

Role of Echo in Cardiac Resynchronization Therapy (CRT)
- Identify interventricular dyssynchrony and intraventricular dyssynchrony:
  - Interventricular dyssynchrony (dyssynchronous contraction between the LV and RV) is derived as difference between:
    ○ LVPEP and RVPEP (measured via PW Doppler)
    ○ Time to peak from LV and RV lateral annulus (measured via DTI)
  - Intraventricular dyssynchrony (dyssynchronous contraction within the LV) is derived from the:
    ○ Septal to posterior wall delay (derived via M-mode)
    ○ Opposing wall delay (derived via PW or colour DTI)
    ○ Yu index (standard deviation (SD) of time to systolic peak measured from 12 LV segments)
- Determine the degree of LV reverse remodelling and the reduction in MR severity
- Optimisation of atrioventricular and interventricular intervals following CRT

Hypertrophic Cardiomyopathy (HCM): Basic Concepts
- *Aetiology*: genetic disease inherited in an autosomal dominant pattern
- *Pathophysiology*: characterised by ventricular hypertrophy and myocardial disarray which leads to diastolic dysfunction +/- myocardial ischaemia; approximately 25-40% patients have dynamic LVOT obstruction or HOCM:
  - HOCM classified as persistent (obstruction at rest), provocable (mild obstruction at rest with significant obstruction occurring following provocation), or latent (no obstruction at rest with significant obstruction apparent following provocation)
  - Mechanism for HOCM relates to ASH and mitral SAM
- *Clinical manifestations*: majority of patients are asymptomatic or only mildly symptomatic; most common symptom is exertional dyspnoea; other clinical manifestations include dizziness, syncope and presyncope, angina, palpitations, orthopnoea, paroxysmal nocturnal dyspnoea, and sudden cardiac death

Role of Echo in HCM
- Determine the presence and distribution of hypertrophy:
  - Contrast echo may be required to make the diagnosis of apical HCM and midventricular HCM with an apical aneurysm
- Assessment of LV systolic function
- Evaluation of LV diastolic function
- Determine the presence, location and magnitude of dynamic LVOT obstruction (including the response of the LVOT gradient to provocative manoeuvres)
- Assessment of the mechanism and degree of MR
- Guidance during, and assessment following, septal reduction procedures:
  - Contrast echo is used to facilitate selection of the optimal septal perforator branch in alcohol septal ablation
- Differentiation between HCM and mimics of HCM:
  - Mimics of HCM include systemic hypertension, severe AS, coarctation of the aorta, chronic renal disease, glycogen storage diseases, infiltrative diseases, and "Athlete's heart"
  - Distinction based on clinical features and characteristic echocardiographic findings

(continued over...)

Key Points (continued)

Restrictive Cardiomyopathy (RCM): Basic Concepts
- *Aetiology*: idiopathic or secondary to other local and systemic disorders
- *Pathophysiology*: characterised by diastolic dysfunction due to myocardial stiffness and poor chamber compliance; systolic ventricular function is usually normal (early stages of disease); marked elevation in atrial pressures results in marked biatrial dilatation
- *Clinical manifestations*: related to biventricular heart failure; includes dyspnoea, peripheral oedema, fatigue and weakness, decreased exercise tolerance, an increased jugular venous pressure and ascites

Role of Echo in RCM
- Establish the diagnosis of RCM
- Assessment of ventricular size and systolic function
- Evaluation of left ventricular diastolic function:
  - may show classic restrictive diastolic filling profile or may vary from an abnormal relaxation pattern to pseudonormalisation to restrictive filling
  - restrictive filling profile does not mean patient has RCM (restrictive physiology may occur in any condition where there is poor LV compliance and increased LA pressures)
- Differentiation between RCM and constrictive pericarditis

Arrhythmogenic Right Ventricular Dysplasia/Cardiomyopathy (ARVD/C): Basic Concepts
- *Aetiology*: inherited autosomal dominant disease; diagnosis based on structural, histological, ECG, arrhythmic, and genetic factors
- *Pathophysiology*: characterised by fibrofatty replacement of the RV myocardium resulting in RV thinning and aneurysmal dilatation; RV aneurysms most commonly affect the RV inflow, RV apex, and RV outflow ("triangle of dysplasia")
- *Clinical manifestations*: arrhythmias ranging from isolated ventricular ectopics to sustained ventricular tachycardia (VT), or ventricular fibrillation (VF) leading to sudden cardiac death

Role of Echo in ARVD/C
- Establish the diagnosis of ARVD/C
- Assessment of RV systolic function
- Assessment of LV systolic function
- Evaluation of TR severity including the estimation of RVSP

Isolated Left Ventricular Non-Compaction (ILVNC): Basic Concepts
- *Aetiology*: rare congenital abnormality; thought to occur due to failure of normal trabecular resorption or compaction during embryonic development resulting in a bilayered LV myocardium
- *Pathophysiology*: LV systolic dysfunction frequently present; degree of LV systolic dysfunction is determined by the extent of myocardial non-compaction and disease severity
- *Clinical manifestations*: include high incidences of heart failure, atrial and ventricular arrhythmias, and endocardial clot with systemic embolisation; incidences of sudden cardiac death have also been reported

Echo features of ILVNC
- Absence of coexisting cardiac abnormalities plus:
  - > 3 trabeculations protruding from LV wall, apically to the papillary muscles and visible in a single image plane,
  - Evidence of blood flow from LV cavity into intertrabecular recesses,
  - 2-layered myocardium: thin outer compacted (C) layer and thickened inner non-compacted (NC) layer; NC/C ratio > 2 is diagnostic
- Degree of LV involvement is typically segmental:
  - the apex is nearly always involved
  - the mid LV lateral wall segments are involved in the majority of cases
  - involvement of the basal LV wall segments is rare
- Contrast echo may be required to make the diagnosis when image quality is suboptimal

Further Reading (listed in alphabetical order)

General

Elliott P, Andersson B, Arbustini E, Bilinska Z, Cecchi F, Charron P, Dubourg O, Kühl U, Maisch B, McKenna WJ, Monserrat L, Pankuweit S, Rapezzi C, Seferovic P, Tavazzi L, Keren A. Classification of the cardiomyopathies: a position statement from the European Society Of Cardiology Working Group on Myocardial and Pericardial Diseases. *Eur Heart J.* 2008 Jan;29(2):270-6.

Maisch B, Noutsias M, Ruppert V, Richter A, Pankuweit S. Cardiomyopathies: classification, diagnosis, and treatment. *Heart Fail Clin.* 2012 Jan;8(1):53-78.

Maron BJ, Towbin JA, Thiene G, Antzelevitch C, Corrado D, Arnett D, Moss AJ, Seidman CE, Young JB; American Heart Association; Council on Clinical Cardiology, Heart Failure and Transplantation Committee; Quality of Care and Outcomes Research and Functional Genomics and Translational Biology Interdisciplinary Working Groups; Council on Epidemiology and Prevention. Contemporary definitions and classification of the cardiomyopathies: an American Heart Association Scientific Statement from the Council on Clinical Cardiology, Heart Failure and Transplantation Committee; Quality of Care and Outcomes Research and Functional Genomics and Translational Biology Interdisciplinary Working Groups; and Council on Epidemiology and Prevention. *Circulation.* 2006 Apr 11;113(14):1807-16.

Dilated Cardiomyopathy

Thomas DE, Wheeler R, Yousef ZR, Masani ND. The role of echocardiography in guiding management in dilated cardiomyopathy. *Eur J Echocardiogr.* 2009 Dec;10(8):iii15-21.

CRT

Gorcsan J 3rd, Abraham T, Agler DA, Bax JJ, Derumeaux G, Grimm RA, Martin R, Steinberg JS, Sutton MS, Yu CM; American Society of Echocardiography Dyssynchrony Writing Group. Echocardiography for cardiac resynchronization therapy: recommendations for performance and reporting--a report from the American Society of Echocardiography Dyssynchrony Writing Group endorsed by the Heart Rhythm Society. *J Am Soc Echocardiogr.* 2008 Mar;21(3):191-213.

Kapetanakis S, Bhan A, Murgatroyd F, Kearney MT, Gall N, Zhang Q, Yu CM, Monaghan MJ. Real-time 3D echo in patient selection for cardiac resynchronization therapy. *JACC Cardiovasc Imaging.* 2011 Jan;4(1):16-26.

Tavazzi L. Ventricular pacing: a promising new therapeutic strategy in heart failure. For whom? *Eur Heart J.* 2000 Aug;21(15):1211-4.

Wang CL, Powell BD, Redfield MM, Miyazaki C, Fine NM, Olson LJ, Cha YM, Espinosa RE, Hayes DL, Hodge DO, Lin G, Friedman PA, Oh JK. Left ventricular discoordination index measured by speckle tracking strain rate imaging predicts reverse remodelling and survival after cardiac resynchronization therapy. *Eur J Heart Fail.* 2012 May;14(5):517-25.

Hypertrophic Cardiomyopathy

Butz T, van Buuren F, Mellwig KP, Langer C, Plehn G, Meissner A, Trappe HJ, Horstkotte D, Faber L. Two-dimensional strain analysis of the global and regional myocardial function for the differentiation of pathologic and physiologic left ventricular hypertrophy: a study in athletes and in patients with hypertrophic cardiomyopathy. Int J Cardiovasc Imaging. 2011 Jan;27(1):91-100.

Maron BJ, Maron MS. Hypertrophic cardiomyopathy. *Lancet.* 2013. Jan 19;381(9862):242-55.

Nagueh SF, Bierig SM, Budoff MJ, Desai M, Dilsizian V, Eidem B, Goldstein SA, Hung J, Maron MS, Ommen SR, Woo A; American Society of Echocardiography; American Society of Nuclear Cardiology; Society for Cardiovascular Magnetic Resonance; Society of Cardiovascular Computed Tomography. American Society of Echocardiography clinical recommendations for multimodality cardiovascular imaging of patients with hypertrophic cardiomyopathy: Endorsed by the American Society of Nuclear Cardiology, Society for Cardiovascular Magnetic Resonance, and Society of Cardiovascular Computed Tomography. *J Am Soc Echocardiogr.* 2011 May;24(5):473-98.

Palka P, Lange A, Fleming AD, Donnelly JE, Dutka DP, Starkey IR, Shaw TR, Sutherland GR, Fox KA. Differences in myocardial velocity gradient measured throughout the cardiac cycle in patients with hypertrophic cardiomyopathy, athletes and patients with left ventricular hypertrophy due to hypertension. J Am Coll Cardiol. 1997 Sep;30(3):760-8

Pelliccia A, Maron MS, Maron BJ. Assessment of left ventricular hypertrophy in a trained athlete: differential diagnosis of physiologic athlete's heart from pathologic hypertrophy. *Prog Cardiovasc Dis.* 2012; 54(5):387-96

Rawlins J, Bhan A, Sharma S. Left ventricular hypertrophy in athletes. *Eur J Echocardiogr.* 2009 May;10(3):350-6

Williams LK, Frenneaux MP, Steeds RP. Echocardiography in hypertrophic cardiomyopathy diagnosis, prognosis, and role in management. *Eur J Echocardiogr.* 2009 Dec;10(8):iii9-14.

Restrictive Cardiomyopathy

Kushwaha SS, Fallon JT, Fuster V. Restrictive cardiomyopathy. *N Engl J Med.* 1997 Jan 23;336(4):267-76.

Nihoyannopoulos P, Dawson D. Restrictive cardiomyopathies. *Eur J Echocardiogr.* 2009 Dec;10(8):iii23-33.

Arrhythmogenic Right Ventricular Dysplasia/Cardiomyopathy

Harper RW, Mottram PM. Exercise-induced right ventricular dysplasia/cardiomyopathy--an emerging condition distinct from arrhythmogenic right ventricular dysplasia/cardiomyopathy. *Heart Lung Circ.* 2009 Jun;18(3):233-5.

La Gerche A, Burns AT, Mooney DJ, Inder WJ, Taylor AJ, Bogaert J, Macisaac AI, Heidbüchel H, Prior DL. Exercise-induced right ventricular dysfunction and structural remodelling in endurance athletes. *Eur Heart J.* 2012 Apr;33(8):998-1006.

Marcus FI, McKenna WJ, Sherrill D, Basso C, Bauce B, Bluemke DA, Calkins H, Corrado D, Cox MG, Daubert JP, Fontaine G, Gear K, Hauer R, Nava A, Picard MH, Protonotarios N, Saffitz JE, Sanborn DM, Steinberg JS, Tandri H, Thiene G, Towbin JA, Tsatsopoulou A, Wichter T, Zareba W. Diagnosis of arrhythmogenic right ventricular cardiomyopathy/dysplasia: proposed modification of the Task Force Criteria. *Eur Heart J.* 2010 Apr;31(7):806-14.

Muthappan P, Calkins H. Arrhythmogenic right ventricular dysplasia. *Prog Cardiovasc Dis.* 2008 Jul-Aug;51(1):31-43.

Yoerger DM, Marcus F, Sherrill D, Calkins H, Towbin JA, Zareba W, Picard MH; Multidisciplinary Study of Right Ventricular Dysplasia Investigators. Echocardiographic findings in patients meeting task force criteria for arrhythmogenic right ventricular dysplasia: new insights from the multidisciplinary study of right ventricular dysplasia. *J Am Coll Cardiol.* 2005 Mar 15;45(6):860-5.

Left Ventricular Non-Compaction

Chin TK, Perloff JK, Williams RG, Jue K, Mohrmann R. Isolated noncompaction of left ventricular myocardium. A study of eight cases. *Circulation.* 1990 Aug;82(2):507-13.

Jenni R, Oechslin E, Schneider J, Attenhofer Jost C, Kaufmann PA. Echocardiographic and pathoanatomical characteristics of isolated left ventricular non-compaction: a step towards classification as a distinct cardiomyopathy. *Heart.* 2001 Dec;86(6):666-71.

Kohli SK, Pantazis AA, Shah JS, Adeyemi B, Jackson G, McKenna WJ, Sharma S, Elliott PM. Diagnosis of left-ventricular non-compaction in patients with left-ventricular systolic dysfunction: time for a reappraisal of diagnostic criteria? *Eur Heart J.* 2008 Jan;29(1):89-95.

Niemann M, Liu D, Hu K, Cikes M, Beer M, Herrmann S, Gaudron PD, Hillenbrand H, Voelker W, Ertl G, Weidemann F. Echocardiographic quantification of regional deformation helps to distinguish isolated left ventricular non-compaction from dilated cardiomyopathy. *Eur J Heart Fail.* 2012 Feb;14(2):155-61.

Oechslin E, Jenni R. Left ventricular non-compaction revisited: a distinct phenotype with genetic heterogeneity? *Eur Heart J.* 2011 Jun;32(12):1446-56.

Paterick TE, Umland MM, Jan MF, Ammar KA, Kramer C, Khandheria BK, Seward JB, Tajik AJ. Left ventricular noncompaction: a 25-year odyssey. *J Am Soc Echocardiogr.* 2012 Apr;25(4):363-75.

Stöllberger C, Finsterer J. Left ventricular hypertrabeculation/noncompaction. *J Am Soc Echocardiogr.* 2004 Jan;17(1):91-100.

Aortic Valve Disease

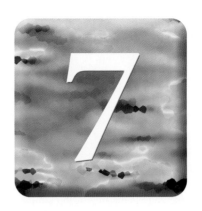

Anatomy of the Aortic Valve and Aortic Root

The aortic valve is one of four cardiac valves in the heart. It is composed of endocardium and connective tissue reinforced by fibres which prevent the valve from turning inside out. Because of its half moon shape, it is also described as a semilunar valve.

With respect to surface anatomy, the aortic valve is the cardiac 'centrepiece' and lies to the left of the sternum opposite the third intercostal space (Fig. 7.1). Internally, the aortic valve is located between the left ventricular outflow tract (LVOT) and the ascending aorta in the centre of the heart; it is in close proximity to the other cardiac valves (Fig. 7.2). The primary function of the aortic valve is to prevent the backflow of blood into the left ventricle (LV) during ventricular diastole.

The aortic valve anatomy can be described in terms of its four principal components: (1) the annulus, (2) the cusps, (3) the commissures, and (4) the interleaflet triangles.

Aortic Annulus

The aortic annulus provides a structural support to the semilunar aortic cusps. Importantly, the aortic annulus is not a simple ring. It is demarcated by the hinges of the leaflets to the aortic wall and as a result forms a crown-like structure. There are three circular anatomic rings associated with the crown-like aortic annulus (Fig. 7.3). The base of the crown is formed by the basal attachment points of the aortic leaflets within the LV; this forms the virtual ring. The top of the crown relates to the peripheral attachment of the aortic leaflets with the aortic wall. At this site there is an anatomical ridge or ring known as the sinotubular (ST) ridge or ST junction. The third circular ring is the anatomical junction in the middle of the aortic root referred to as the ventriculoarterial junction; this junction marks the transition from ventricular to arterial walls and is crossed by the hinge-lines of the aortic valve cusps.

Aortic Cusps

There are three almost equal-sized aortic valve leaflets or cusps which have a half-moon or semilunar shape (Fig. 7.4). Three expanded outward pouches of the aortic root are associated with each cusp; these are the sinuses of Valsalva. These sinuses are confined proximally by the attachments of the valve

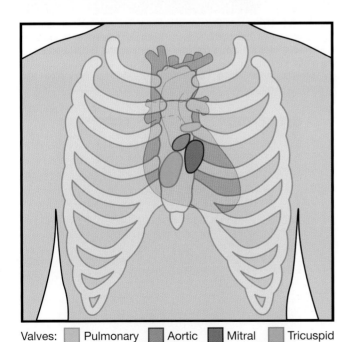

Valves: ☐ Pulmonary ☐ Aortic ☐ Mitral ☐ Tricuspid

Figure 7.1 This schematic illustrates the location of the heart valves with respect to the anterior chest wall. The aortic valve (*red circle*) lies to the left of the sternum opposite the 3rd intercostal space; the mitral valve (*purple circle*) lies to the left of the sternum opposite the 4th costal cartilage; the pulmonary valve (*blue circle*) lies behind the medial end of the 3rd costal cartilage; the tricuspid valve (*green circle*) lies towards the right of the sternum opposite the 4th intercostal space.

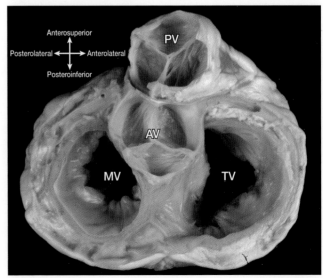

Figure 7.2 This specimen shows the anatomic relationship between the cardiac valves as viewed from the posterolateral oblique aspect. AV = aortic valve; MV = mitral valve; PV = pulmonary valve; TV = tricuspid valve. By permission of Mayo Foundation for Medical Education and Research. All rights reserved. Courtesy of William D. Edwards, MD.

leaflets and distally by the ST junction. The sinus is defined as the space between the edge of the leaflets and the aorta. The sinuses are named according to the coronary arteries arising from them: the right coronary sinus, the left coronary sinus, and the non-coronary sinus. Likewise, the three aortic valve cusps are named based on the sinuses that they overlie; therefore, the aortic cusps are referred to as the right coronary cusp (RCC), the left coronary cusp (LCC) and the non-coronary cusp (NCC). The RCC and the LCC are of a similar size and the NCC is usually slightly larger than the other two cusps. Each cusp has two free edges which it shares with its adjacent cusps. Below the free edge is an area of thickening that corresponds

to the closing edge of the valve.

At the centre of each cusp is a fibrous tissue node; these nodes are referred to as the nodules of Arantius. These nodes are located at the contact site of valve cusp closure. Lambl's excrescences may also be present. These excrescences are filiform fronds that occur on the ventricular side of the aortic valve at the site of valve closure (Fig. 7.5).

Aortic Commissures

During valve closure, adjacent aortic cusps contact one another along the surfaces between the free and closing edges. The entire zone of apposition of the aortic closure is referred to as the commissure. Hence, in the closed position, the commissure of the aortic valve extends from the peripheral attachment at the ST junction to the centre of the valve orifice (Fig. 7.6).

> In echocardiography, the term commissure refers to only the peripheral points of attachment of the valve at the aortic wall. With reference to Figure 7.6 the 'echo' commissure is located at the position of the stars.

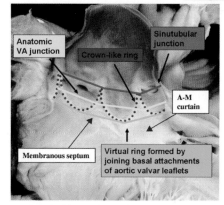

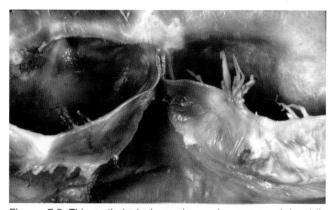

Figure 7.5 This pathological specimen shows several Lambl's excrescences of the aortic valve. These excrescences appear as filamentous strands along the free edges and the closing edges of the aortic valve.

By permission of Mayo Foundation for Medical Education and Research. All rights reserved. Courtesy of William D. Edwards, MD.

Figure 7.3 A, Three dimensional arrangement of the aortic root shows 3 circular "rings," the aortic annulus is a crown-like ring from which the aortic leaflets are suspended. **B,** The aortic leaflets have been removed from this specimen of the aortic root, showing the location of the 3 rings relative to the crown-like hinges of the leaflets. **VA** = ventriculoarterial; **A-M** =aortic-mitral.

Reproduced from Piazza N, de Jaegere P, Schultz C, Becker AE, Serruys PW, Anderson RH. Anatomy of the aortic valvar complex and its implications for transcatheter implantation of the aortic valve. *Circ Cardiovasc Interv.* © 2008 Aug;1(1):74-81, with permission.

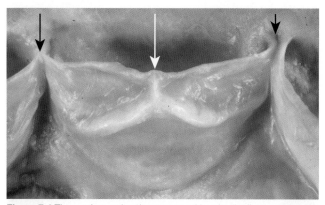

Figure 7.4 The aortic root has been opened longitudinally to expose the aortic valve; the non-coronary (posterior) cusp is shown. Observe that the aortic leaflet appears as a delicate, half-moon or semilunar cusp with its commissures extending to the level of the sinotubular junction (*black arrows*). The nodule of Arantius can be seen at the centre of the cusp (*white arrow*); the pouch behind the cusp is the aortic sinus of Valsalva.

By permission of Mayo Foundation for Medical Education and Research. All rights reserved. Courtesy of William D. Edwards, MD.

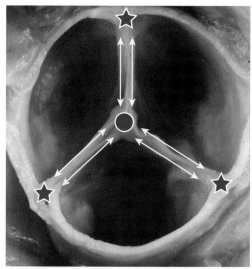

Figure 7.6 In the closed position the free edges of the aortic valve cusps (*white arrows*) extend from the commissures at the sinotubular junction (*stars*) to the centre of the valve orifice (*circle*).

By permission of Mayo Foundation for Medical Education and Research. All rights reserved. Courtesy of William D. Edwards, MD.

Interleaflet Triangles

Below the three commissures lie three areas called the interleaflet triangles which are considered as extensions of the LVOT (Fig. 7.7). Each triangle extends distally to the level of the ST junction. The triangle between the LCC and NCC, also referred to as the aortomitral curtain, is continuous with the anterior leaflet of the mitral valve. The triangle between the LCC and RCC is the potential space between the aorta and the right ventricular outflow tract (RVOT). The triangle between the RCC and NCC is in direct continuity with the membranous ventricular septum; this triangle is also in close proximity to the bundle of His.

Aortic Root Anatomy

The aortic root is the section of the aorta between the LVOT and the ascending aorta; it is bounded by the basal attachment of the aortic cusps to the virtual ring proximally and the peripheral attachment of the aortic cusps to the ST junction distally (Fig. 7.8). Therefore, the length of the aortic root is defined by the 'length' or 'height' of the aortic cusps. Encompassed within the aortic root are the aortic valve leaflets, the sinuses of Valsalva, the commissures, and the interleaflet triangles.

Aortic Stenosis

Aetiology of Aortic Stenosis

Aortic stenosis (AS) refers to the obstruction of blood flow across the aortic valve. Valvular AS can be caused by a congenital malformation of the valve or from an acquired deformation of the valve.

Congenital Aortic Stenosis

Congenitally abnormal aortic valves which may present as AS in the adult patient include: (1) unicuspid aortic valves and (2) bicuspid aortic valves.

Unicuspid Aortic Valves

The incidence of a unicuspid aortic valve (UAV) is very rare. A UAV occurs when there is fusion between two of the three developing aortic valve leaflets or fusion of all three developing leaflets resulting in an abnormal valve with a solitary opening. There are two types of UAV: acommissural and unicommissural (Fig. 7.9). In a unicuspid acommissural aortic valve there is a single membrane-like leaflet with a central orifice and no apparent commissural attachment to the aortic root (Fig. 7.9, left). The unicommissural type is more common than the acommissural type and it has an eccentric orifice with one commissural attachment to the aorta; the free edge of this type arises from a single aortic attachment which continues to encircle the entire orifice and returns to the aortic wall near its original attachment (Fig. 7.9, right). Due to its eccentric opening this type of unicuspid valve is described as having a "key-hole" or "tear-drop" appearance.

UAVs are usually stenotic at birth (a UAV is the most common type of aortic valve structure in infants and young children with congenital AS). UAVs are associated with dilatation of the aorta, aortic dissection, and dystrophic calcification.

Bicuspid Aortic Valves

A bicuspid aortic valve (BAV) occurs in approximately 1-2% of the general population. There is male to female ratio of about 3:1 and a familial reoccurrence of about 9%. Stenosis of a BAV is the most common cause of isolated AS in patients under 50 years.

Essentially there are two types of bicuspid aortic valves: those with a raphe (or seam) and those without (Fig. 7.10). In the BAV with a raphe the most common site of cuspal fusion is between the RCC and LCC (about 85% of cases) followed by fusion between the RCC and NCC (about 15% of cases); LCC and NCC fusion is rarely seen.

A BAV without a raphe or a 'true' BAV is less commonly seen accounting for only 10% of BAVs. Typically a true BAV usually has near-equal size cusps. The orientation of these cusps is variable: commissures may be located anteriorly and posteriorly or medially and laterally.

Importantly, BAV is associated with aortopathies such as aortic root dilatation, aortic aneurysm and aortic dissection as well as a number of congenital heart lesions including coarctation of the aorta, supravalvular aortic stenosis and ventricular septal defects (see Chapter 15, Congenital Aortic Stenosis).

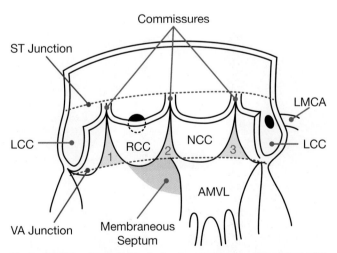

Figure 7.7 This schematic illustrates the relationship of the interleaflet triangles with the commissures and aortic valve leaflets (see text for further details). **1** = right/left coronary interleaflet triangle; **2** = right/non-coronary interleaflet triangle; **3** = non-/left coronary interleaflet triangle; **AMVL** = anterior mitral valve leaflet; **LCC** = left coronary cusp; **LMCA** = left main coronary artery; **NCC** = non-coronary cusp; **RCC** = right coronary cusp; **ST** = sinotubular; **VA** = ventriculoarterial.

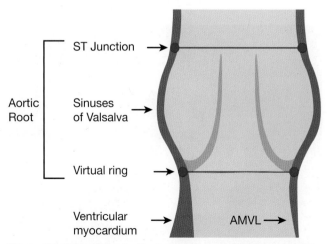

Figure 7.8 This schematic illustrates the aortic root anatomy. The aortic root extends from the basal attachment of the aortic cusps at the virtual ring to the sinotubular (ST) junction. The sinuses of Valsalva are the expanded portions or outward pouches of the aortic root. These sinuses extend from the proximal attachments of the aortic valve leaflets at the virtual ring (aortic annulus) to the distal attachment of the valve leaflets at the ST junction. **AMVL** = anterior mitral valve leaflet.

Acquired Aortic Stenosis

Acquired aortic valve diseases which may cause AS include: (1) senile calcification of the aortic valve and (2) rheumatic valve disease.

Senile Calcification of the Aortic Valve

Senile degeneration of previously normal trileaflet aortic valves results from calcification of the valve leaflets. This is the most common cause of AS typically occurring in the 8th and 9th decades of life. The cusps are immobilised by a deposit of calcium along their flexion lines that begins at their bases and progresses toward the free edge (Fig. 7.11, left). These calcium deposits prevent the cusps from opening normally in systole. Commissural fusion with calcific AS is usually absent.

Degenerative "wear and tear", as a result of the normal mechanical stress on the aortic valve, is a proposed mechanism for this type of AS. Senile AS is commonly accompanied by mitral annular calcification and calcification of the coronary arteries.

Rheumatic Valve Disease

Rheumatic valve disease occurs secondarily to an episode or recurrent episodes of acute rheumatic fever (ARF). ARF occurs due to a group A beta-haemolytic Streptococcus infection and is most commonly encountered in developing nations and disadvantaged communities where there is overcrowding and malnutrition. ARF typically develops in children and adolescents between the ages of 5–14 years, however cases do occur in adults; the disease is rare in children under three years of age.

Valvular disease due to ARF occurs several years after the initial episode of ARF. An autoimmune response leads to chronic inflammation, commissural fusion, thickening, and calcification of cardiac valves. In rheumatic AS, this inflammatory process ultimately leads to retraction and stiffening of the free borders of the aortic cusps reducing the aortic orifice to a round or triangular opening (Fig. 7.11, right). Fusion usually affects all commissures equally but it may also be limited to only a single commissure; in this instance, the aortic valve becomes functionally bicuspid. Associated valvular calcification may or may not be present. The severity of the stenosis depends on the number of commissures that are adherent and the extent of commissural fusion. Importantly, rheumatic AS rarely occurs in isolation and is usually associated with mitral valve stenosis.

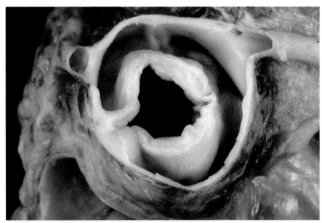
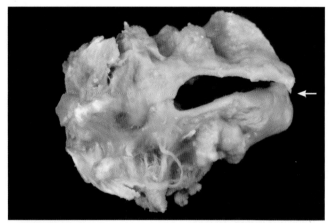

Figure 7.9 Pathological examples of unicuspid unicommissural aortic valves are shown. Observe that the unicommissural type of unicuspid valve has an eccentric opening ('keyhole" or "tear-drop" appearance) with a single commissural attachment to the aortic root (*arrow*). The non-calcified valve (*left*) had only mild stenosis, whereas the heavily calcified valve (*right*) was severely stenotic. Figure 9.40A shows an example of a unicuspid acommissural valve.
By permission of Mayo Foundation for Medical Education and Research. All rights reserved. Courtesy of William D. Edwards, MD.

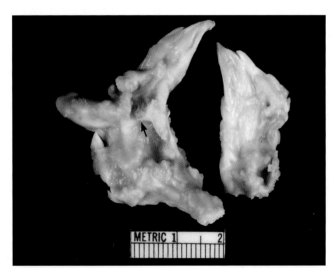
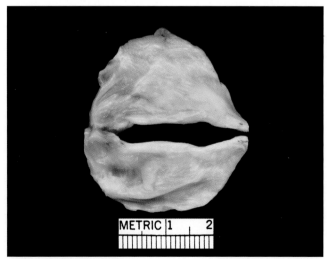

Figure 7.10 Pathological examples are shown of congenitally bicuspid aortic valves. Note that the bicuspid valve with a raphe (*left*) has one larger cusp to its left and one smaller cusp to the right; the raphe is seen in the centre of the larger cusp (*arrow*). Observe that the bicuspid valve without a raphe (*right*) has equal-size cusps.
By permission of Mayo Foundation for Medical Education and Research. All rights reserved. Courtesy of William D. Edwards, MD.

> **Rheumatic Valve Disease**
> The valve most commonly affected by rheumatic heart disease is the mitral valve (65-70%) followed by the aortic valve (25%). The tricuspid valve is deformed in about 10% of patients; rheumatic tricuspid valve disease is almost always associated with mitral and aortic valve disease. The pulmonary valve is rarely affected.

Other Causes of LVOT Obstruction

Congenital obstruction to the outflow of blood from the LV to the aorta can also occur at the subvalvular and supravalvular levels. These lesions are discussed in further detail in Chapter 15.

Subvalvular LVOT obstruction may also occur due to dynamic obstruction. Dynamic obstruction may result from asymmetric septal hypertrophy which causes systolic anterior motion (SAM) of the anterior mitral valve into the LVOT; this is a feature of hypertrophic obstructive cardiomyopathy (see Chapter 6). Dynamic obstruction may also occur in elderly patients with concentric left ventricular hypertrophy (LVH) due to chronic hypertension; in these patients the aorta shifts to the right creating a basal interventricular septal bulge. This septal bulge can cause SAM of the anterior mitral valve into the LVOT resulting in dynamic LVOT obstruction.

Pathophysiology of Aortic Stenosis

Calcification, fibrosis and/or commissural fusion can hinder cusp mobility, cause thickening of the cusps or prevent complete valvular opening; all of which result in a decreased valve area and obstruction to LV emptying during ventricular systole.

In the adult patient, AS is a chronic lesion whereby the degree of LVOT obstruction gradually increases over time. Initially the LV end diastolic volume and systolic function remain normal and LV output is maintained by the development of LVH. LVH allows the LV to sustain large pressure gradients across the stenotic valve for many years without a reduction in the cardiac output, LV dilatation or the development of symptoms. However, as the LV becomes less compliant the LV end-diastolic pressure (LVEDP) increases and the LV dilates in order to maintain a normal cardiac output (see the Frank-Starling mechanism in Chapter 2). In addition, increased end-systolic wall stress due to the increased afterload placed on the LV ultimately results in a reduction in the LV stroke volume and contractility (see Laplace's law in Chapter 2).

Clinical Manifestations of Aortic Stenosis

The clinical manifestations of AS relate to the pathophysiological responses to chronic, severe AS. The primary manifestations of severe AS include angina pectoris, syncope, and congestive heart failure.

Angina Pectoris

Many patients with AS also have coexistent coronary artery disease (CAD). Therefore, these patients may also suffer angina. Furthermore, angina may be exacerbated by LVH. The mechanisms of myocardial ischaemia and subsequent angina in severe AS (unrelated to CAD) include:

• compression of the intramyocardial coronary arteries due to elevated intracavity LV pressures, prolonged contraction and impaired myocardial relaxation,
• increased myocardial oxygen demand of the hypertrophied LV due to elevated LV systolic pressure and prolongation of the LV ejection time,
• impaired coronary blood flow due to elevation of LVEDP which lowers the diastolic aorta-to-LV pressure gradient and, therefore, the coronary artery perfusion pressure;
• decreased coronary perfusion time due to a decrease in the diastolic filling period,
• reduced coronary flow reserve.

Syncope or Presyncope

Patients with severe AS may experience syncope with exertion or rarely at rest. With exertion, syncope is caused by decreased cerebral perfusion due to peripheral vasodilatation and the inability of the heart to increase cardiac output across a fixed stenotic valve orifice. Syncope may also occur due to baroreceptor dysfunction and a vasodepressor response to increased LV systolic pressures during exercise. Syncope or presyncope may also be due to exercise-induced vasodilation which results in hypotension.

Congestive Heart Failure

Congestive heart failure (CHF) or congestive cardiac failure (CCF) refers to the inability of the heart to supply sufficient blood flow to meet the needs of the body. CHF can result from a number of cardiac causes including AS. The common symptoms of CHF include dyspnoea, peripheral oedema and decreased exercise tolerance.

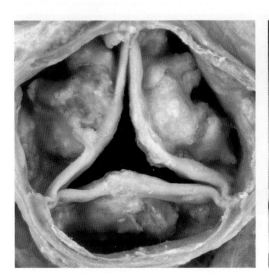
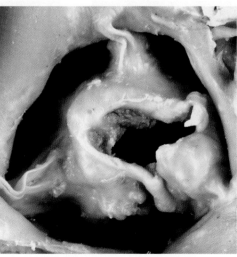

Figure 7.11 Pathological examples are shown of calcific aortic valve disease associated with severe stenosis.
The valve with degenerative disease (left) shows arch-like calcification of the cusps with no commissural fusion. In contrast, the valve with rheumatic disease shows marked commissural fusion, as well as further deformity by fibrosis and calcification.
By permission of Mayo Foundation for Medical Education and Research. All rights reserved. Courtesy of William D. Edwards, MD.

Role of Echocardiography in Aortic Stenosis

The aims and objectives of echocardiography in the assessment of AS are to:

- Determine the aetiology of the lesion (e.g. congenital, degenerative, rheumatic),
- Exclude other causes of LVOT obstruction,
- Assess LV size and systolic and diastolic function,
- Assess the degree of LVH,
- Measure aortic dimensions,
- Estimate the severity of the stenosis,
- Identify associated valve lesions.

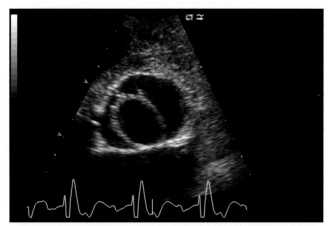

Figure 7.12 An example of a unicommissural unicuspid aortic valve as seen from the parasternal short axis view. Note that in this systolic still frame there is only one commissure extending to the aortic periphery (at 6 o'clock position) and the orifice of the valve appears elliptical in shape.

Aetiology of Aortic Stenosis

As stated above valvular AS may be due to a congenital malformation of the valve (unicuspid or bicuspid) or it may occur due to 'acquired' deformation of the valve (rheumatic or degenerative).

Unicuspid Aortic Valve

The diagnosis of a UAV is made from the parasternal short axis (PSAX) view. The key to the diagnosis of a UAV is based on identifying the commissural attachments to the aortic root during systole. As previously mentioned, UAVs may be acommissural or unicommissural. In an acommissural UAV there is no commissural attachment to the aortic root; the appearance of this type of UAV is described as having a 'volcano' appearance. In a unicommissural UAV there is only one commissural attachment to the aortic root; as a result the 2D appearance of this type of UAV displays a characteristic eccentric orifice opening during systole (Fig. 7.12).

Bicuspid Aortic Valve

As stated previously, BAVs vary based on the presence or absence of a raphe and on the orientation of the cusps.

As for the diagnosis of a UAV, a BAV is also identified from the PSAX view during systole based on identifying the commissural attachments to the aortic root. A BAV is, therefore, diagnosed when only two cusps are seen and when there are only two commissural attachments to the aortic root (Fig. 7.13). BAVs are further discussed in Chapter 15.

─────────────────── **Panel A** ───────────────────

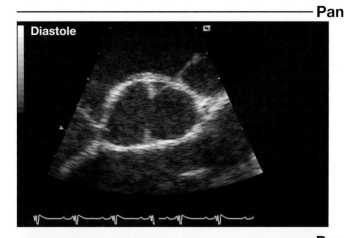
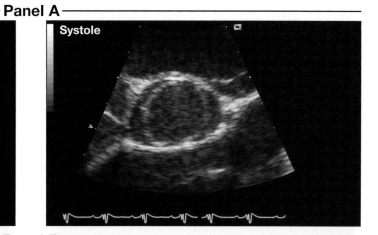

─────────────────── **Panel B** ───────────────────

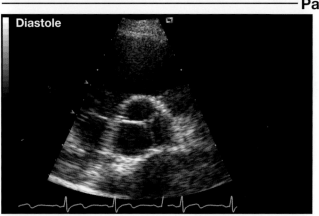
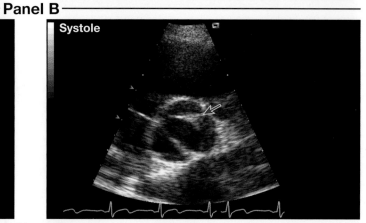

Figure 7.13 Examples of different types of bicuspid aortic valves (BAV) are shown; images were recorded from the parasternal short axis view. **Panel A:** Diastolic and systolic frames of a true BAV with no raphe are shown; cusps are termed medial and lateral. **Panel B:** Diastolic and systolic frames of a BAV with a raphe are shown; observe that the valve appears to be trileaflet in the diastolic frame but is clearly bicuspid in systole with only two commissures opening out to the aortic root; a raphe between the right and left cusps is evident (*arrow*).

Rheumatic Aortic Stenosis

Rheumatic valve disease almost always involves the mitral valve. Therefore, identification of rheumatic AS usually occurs when rheumatic mitral valve disease is also seen. Rheumatic AS is characterized by fusion of the aortic commissures and thickening of the aortic leaflet edges (Fig. 7.14). Typically, there is focal thickening that is limited to the free edges of the leaflets which appears as 'brighter' echoes compared to the rest of the leaflet. With advancing age, calcification is usually superimposed on the deformed valve and leaflet motion becomes further restricted.

Calcific Aortic Stenosis

The calcified valve associated with senile degenerative AS is characterised by increased reflectivity from the thickened, deformed valve cusps (Fig. 7.15)

Subvalvular Aortic Stenosis

Subvalvular AS can occur due to a fixed congenital lesion within the LVOT or dynamic obstruction to LV outflow proximal to the aortic valve. An example of dynamic obstruction secondary to SAM of the anterior mitral valve is shown in figure 7.16.

Assessment of Left Ventricular Size, Wall Thickness and Systolic and Diastolic Function

Left ventricular size, wall thickness and systolic function can be assessed by both M-mode and 2D echocardiography in the traditional manner (see Chapter 2).

As mentioned previously, LVH is a compensatory response that occurs due to chronic pressure overload. Therefore, the degree of LVH may offer an indirect clue as to the severity of AS; that is, the greater the LVH, the more significant the stenosis. However, it is important to remember that LVH can occur due to chronic systemic hypertension also. Furthermore, it has been

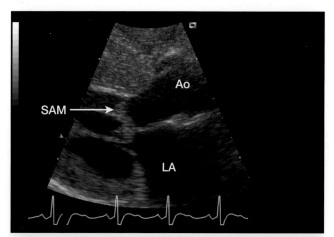

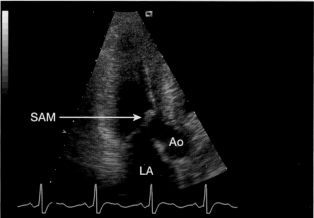

Figure 7.16 This zoomed parasternal long axis view (*top*) and zoomed apical long view (*bottom*) were recorded from a patient with hypertrophic obstructive cardiomyopathy. Systolic anterior motion (*SAM*) of the mitral valve results in dynamic left ventricular outflow tract obstruction (*arrows*). **Ao** = aorta; **LA** = left atrium.

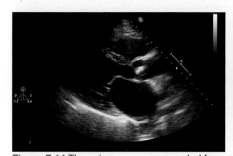
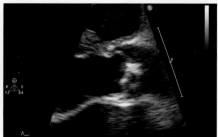
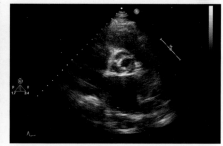

Figure 7.14 These images were recorded from a patient with rheumatic valve disease. From the parasternal long axis both rheumatic mitral valve stenosis and rheumatic aortic valve stenosis are shown in diastole (*left*); observe the diastolic doming of the mitral valve as well as the thickened aortic cusps. From the zoomed parasternal long axis view, systolic doming of the aortic valve and leaflet thickening is apparent (*middle*). From a systolic frame recorded from the parasternal short axis at the aortic valve level, thickening of the aortic cusps, reduced systolic opening and commissural fusion between the right coronary and non-coronary cusps is evident (*right*).

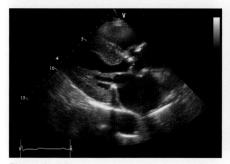
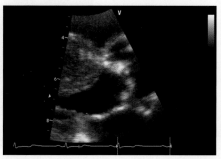
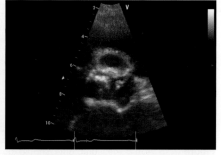

Figure 7.15 These images were recorded from a patient with calcific aortic stenosis. The parasternal long axis view (*left*), zoomed parasternal long axis view (*middle*) and the parasternal short axis view (*right*) all show extensive calcification of the aortic valve (bright areas). Reduced systolic opening of the valve is also apparent on the middle and right images. Note that calcification of the mitral annulus is also present (*left image*).

noted that patients can have haemodynamically significant AS without significant LVH. LV wall thickness can be measured from the 2D image or M-mode trace recorded from the parasternal long and short axis views (Fig. 7.17). In addition, the calculation of LV mass is also useful in determining the degree of LVH. The reference limits and various partition values of LV wall thickness and LV mass can be found in Chapter 4 (Table 4.8).

LV diastolic function should also be evaluated in the usual manner. The methods for assessing LV diastolic function and LV filling pressures are described in detail in Chapter 3.

Measurements of the Aorta

In patients with AS, there may be associated post-stenotic dilatation of the aortic root. This is more commonly seen in congenital aortic stenosis but may also be present in patients with acquired AS.

Measurements of the aorta that should be routinely performed include the trans-sinus diameter at the sinuses of Valsalva, the ST junction, and the ascending aorta (Fig. 7.18). These measurements are performed from a high parasternal long axis view at end-diastole using the leading edge to leading edge technique. The normal values for these measurements can be found in Chapter 11 (Table 11.1).

In addition, the LVOT diameter is measured. The LVOT diameter is measured from a zoomed parasternal long axis view at mid-systole using the inner edge to inner edge technique (Fig. 7.19). This important measurement is required for the calculation of the aortic valve area (AVA) by the continuity equation. Therefore, accurate measurements are crucial. For this reason measurements should be averaged over at least 2 consecutive cardiac cycles; if these two measurements vary by 2 mm or more, additional measurements should be performed until a consistent and reproducible value is obtained.

When evaluating patients for suitability for transcatheter aortic valve implantation (TAVI), the sinus height should also be measured. The sinus height is measured as the distance from the aortic annulus to the ST junction, perpendicular to the annular plane (Fig. 7.20).

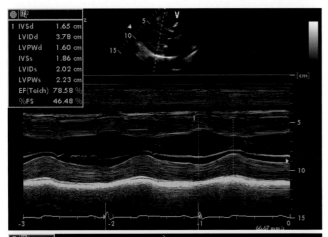

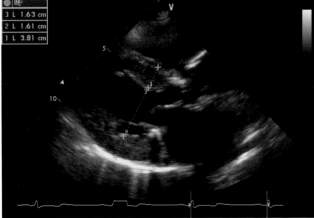

Figure 7.17 M-mode measurements (*top*) and 2D measurements (*bottom*) of left ventricular wall thickness and cavity size recorded in a patient with severe aortic stenosis are shown. These measurements are consistent with severe concentric left ventricular hypertrophy; the M-mode trace also confirms the presence of normal systolic function.

> The LVOT diameter can be measured at the aortic annulus (virtual aortic ring) or at an arbitrary region 0.5-1.0 cm proximal to the aortic valve. Theoretically, for stroke volume (SV) calculations, the diameter should be measured at the same location as the velocity time integral measurement. Therefore, for the LVOT SV, the LVOT diameter should be measured 0.5-1.0 cm proximal to the aortic valve. However, the aortic annulus has distinctive anatomical landmarks which can be clearly defined; these anatomical reference points allow for a more accurate and reproducible measurement across serial studies. For this reason, measurements of the LVOT diameter at our institution are measured at the annulus.

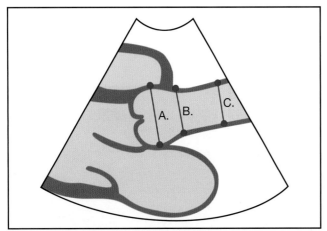

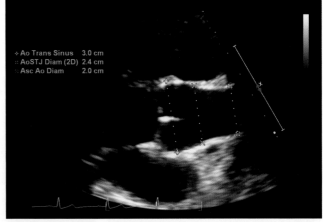

Figure 7.18 Aortic measurements should be routinely performed in all patients with aortic stenosis. The schematic to the left illustrates various measurements of the aorta: **A** = trans-sinus diameter at the sinuses of Valsalva; **B** = sinotubular junction; **C** = ascending aorta. The image to the right shows actual measurements at the trans-sinus level **(1)**, at the sinotubular junction **(2)** and at the ascending aorta **(3)**. All measurements are performed at end-diastole from a high parasternal long axis view using the leading edge to leading edge technique.

Estimation of Severity

The severity of AS is most commonly based on haemodynamic parameters such as:
- peak velocity,
- mean pressure gradient,
- aortic valve area (AVA),
- indexed aortic valve area,
- dimensionless severity index (velocity ratio).

The criteria for defining the various grades of AS based on these measurements are listed in Table 7.1.
Other less frequently used methods for assessing the severity of AS include:
- maximal aortic cusp separation (MAC),
- 2D planimetry of the AVA.

Velocities and Pressure Gradients

Transaortic valve velocities are recorded via continuous-wave (CW) Doppler. From the Doppler velocity trace the transvalvular pressure gradients are estimated by application of the simplified Bernoulli equation (see Chapter 1). The maximum instantaneous pressure gradient is measured from

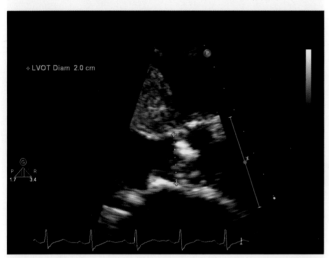

Figure 7.19 The left ventricular outflow tract diameter (LVOT Diam) is measured from a zoomed parasternal long axis view at mid-systole. Using the inner edge to inner edge technique, callipers are placed at the interface of the septal endocardium to the anterior mitral leaflet, parallel to the aortic annulus. Measurements should be averaged over at least 2 consecutive cardiac cycles.

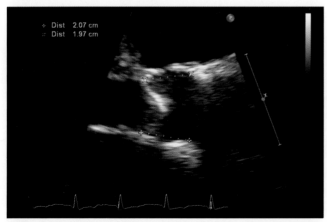

Figure 7.20 Measurements of the sinus height are shown on this image. The sinus height is measured from a zoomed parasternal long axis view at end-diastole as the distance between the aortic annulus and the sinotubular junction, perpendicular to the annular plane.

the peak Doppler velocity while the mean pressure gradient is calculated by tracing the Doppler signal over the systolic flow period (Fig. 7.21).
The limitations of pressure gradient estimations are discussed in detail in Chapter 1. With respect to AS, the most common pitfalls encountered include the underestimation of AS velocity and pressure gradients due to suboptimal alignment of the ultrasound beam with the AS jet. Overestimation of the AS pressure gradient can occur when there is a coexistent increase in LVOT velocities and when the mitral regurgitation (MR) signal is misinterpreted for the AS signal.

Parallel Alignment with the AS Jet

The accuracy of Doppler velocities is highly dependent on the angle of intercept between the Doppler beam and flow direction. In particular, the highest Doppler velocities are recorded when flow is aligned parallel with the Doppler beam. Because the AS jet direction can be significantly 'distorted' by the stenotic valve, AS velocities must be interrogated from multiple windows. These windows include the apical position, the suprasternal notch, the right supraclavicular fossa and the right parasternal window (Table 7.2). Rarely, signals may also be recorded from the subcostal window when the AS jet is especially eccentric.
The AS signal which displays the highest velocity is used to measure the peak velocity, maximum and mean pressure gradients, and for calculation of the AVA; AS signals of lower values recorded from other views are ignored and are not reported (Fig. 7.22). In addition, the acoustic window that provides the highest AS velocity should be stated within the report; this information is useful for serial studies as the window that reveals the highest velocity usually remains the same.
Importantly, while 2D guided CW Doppler is able to reliably record AS signals, AS signals are best recorded with the non-imaging CW transducer. The three advantages of this dedicated CW probe include:
1. this probe has a higher signal-to-noise ratio; the higher the ratio, the less obtrusive the background noise so a superior signal quality is obtained;
2. this probe allows better access to small intercostal spaces which enables optimal positioning and angulation of the transducer, and

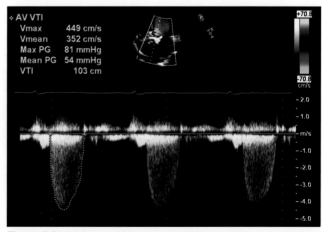

Figure 7.21 On this continuous-wave (CW) Doppler trace recorded across the aortic valve, the peak velocity is measured at 4.5 m/s. Using the simplified Bernoulli equation this translates to a maximum pressure gradient of 81 mm Hg. The mean pressure gradient is derived by tracing the aortic CW Doppler signal; the mean pressure gradient in this example is 54 mm Hg.

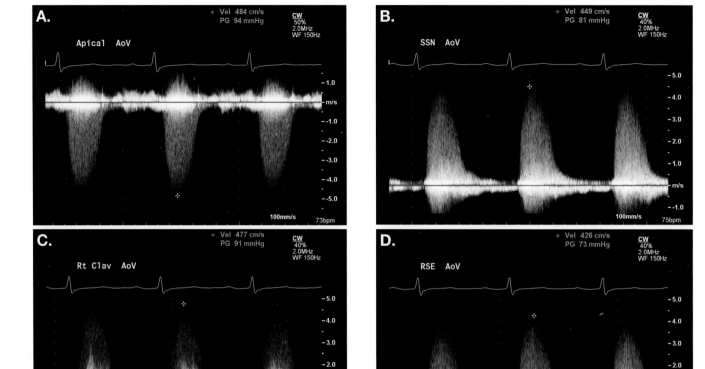

Figure 7.22 Aortic signals are recorded from the apical window **(A)**, the suprasternal notch (SSN) **(B)**, the right supraclavicular fossa (Rt Clav) **(C)**, and the right sternal edge (RSE) **(D)**. The highest velocity is recorded from the apical window, therefore this signal should be used to measure the peak velocity, maximum and mean pressure gradients, and to calculate the aortic valve area.

Table 7.1 Recommendations for Classification of Aortic Stenosis (AS) Severity

	Aortic Sclerosis	Mild AS	Moderate AS	Severe AS
Aortic jet velocity (m/s)	≤ 2.5	2.6 - 2.9	3.0 - 4.0	> 4.0
Mean gradient (mm Hg)	-	< 20[b] (<30[a])	20 – 40[b] (30-50[a])	> 40[b] (>50[a])
AVA (cm²)	-	> 1.5	1.0 - 1.5	< 1.0
Indexed AVA (cm²/m²)	-	> 0.85	0.60 - 85	< 0.6
DSI (Velocity Ratio)	-	> 0.50	0.25 - 0.50	< 0.25

[a] European Society of Cardiology Guidelines.
[b] American Heart Association/American College of Cardiology Guidelines.
AVA = aortic valve area; **DSI** = dimensionless severity index.
Pressure gradients for severity only relevant in the setting of normal LV systolic function.
Reproduced from Baumgartner H, Hung J, Bermejo J, Chambers JB, Evangelista A, Griffin BP, Iung B, Otto CM, Pellikka PA, Quiñones M; American Society of Echocardiography; European Association of Echocardiography. Echocardiographic assessment of valve stenosis: EAE/ASE recommendations for clinical practice. *J Am Soc Echocardiogr*, Vol. 22(1), page 10, © 2009 with permission from Elsevier.

Table 7.2 Windows for Interrogation of Aortic Stenotic (AS) Signals

Acoustic Window	Transducer Position	Patient Position	AS Jet Direction
Apical	5th intercostal space	Left lateral decubitus	Below zero baseline
Right sternal edge	2nd or 3rd intercostal space*	Steep right lateral decubitus	Above zero baseline
Suprasternal notch	Suprasternal notch, steep inferior tilting	Supine with hyperextension of neck	Above zero baseline
Right supraclavicular fossa	Right supraclavicular fossa, steep medial angulation	Supine, head turned towards patient's left	Above zero baseline

* The signal is usually located an intercostal space higher than the window used to record the left parasternal images.

3. because the dedicated probe is 'blind', the operator is not biased to a particular location; that is, the operator must depend upon the audio quality and the spectral quality of the signal to determine if the stenotic jet has been located.

Corrected Pressure Gradients

Most commonly, the maximum pressure gradient is derived from the simplified Bernoulli equation:

Equation 7.1

$$\Delta P = 4\ V^2$$

where ΔP = the pressure difference between 2 points (mm Hg)
     V = peak velocity between 2 points (m/s)

The use of this simplified equation assumes that the velocity proximal to a narrowing is insignificant. If the velocity within the LVOT is elevated (≥ 1.2 m/s), the maximum and mean pressure gradients derived from the simplified Bernoulli equation will be overestimated (see Chapter 1). Therefore, when the LVOT ≥ 1.2 m/s, the maximum and mean pressure gradients must be corrected:

Equation 7.2

$$\Delta P_C = \Delta P_{AV} - \Delta P_{LVOT}$$

where ΔP_C = corrected maximum or mean pressure gradient (mm Hg)

ΔP_{AV} = maximum or mean pressure gradient across the aortic valve (mm Hg)

ΔP_{LVOT} = maximum or mean pressure gradient at the LVOT (mm Hg)

Aortic Stenosis versus Mitral Regurgitation

One of the limitations of the dedicated non-imaging CW transducer is that it is blind; this means that a MR signal may be confused for an AS signal. Confusion between these two signals occurs because both the AS and MR signals occur during systole, both signals are orientated in the same direction, and when AS is severe both signals are relatively high in velocity. Differentiation between AS and MR signals is based on: (1) the shape of the signal, (2) the duration of the signal, (3) diastolic signals, and (4) the velocity of the signals (Table 7.3).

The shape of the MR signal reflects the pressure difference between the LV and left atrium (LA) during systole (Fig. 7.23, left). Normally, the LA pressure is relatively low throughout the systolic period. As a result the pressure difference between the LV and LA is usually high through the entire systolic period; the pressure gradient peaks at mid to late systole. Therefore, the MR signal is parabolic in shape (Figure 7.23, right). In AS, the AS jet reflects the pressure difference between the LV and the aorta during systole (Fig. 7.24, left). The pressure difference between the LV and aorta is greatest in early systole and this pressure difference gradually declines as the aortic pressure increases over the systolic period. As a result the AS signal peaks in early systole and is more V-shaped (Fig. 7.24, right).

However, in patients with acute severe MR, the MR signal may peak in early systole and it may have a V-shaped appearance (Fig. 7.25). This appearance reflects a marked elevation in the LA pressure in mid-late systole which reduces the LV-LA pressure gradient in mid-late systole. Furthermore, in patients with critical AS, the AS jet may appear rounded; this occurs due to 'flattening' of the aortic pressure waveform (Fig. 7.26).

Table 7.3 Differentiation between Aortic Stenosis and Mitral Regurgitant Spectral Doppler Signals

	Aortic Stenosis (AS)	Mitral Regurgitation (MR)
Shape	Early systolic peak resulting in a V-shaped signal (exception: critical AS)	Mid-late systolic peak resulting in a parabolic-shaped signal (exception: acute, severe MR)
Duration	AS is shorter than MR (no flow during isovolumic periods)	MR is longer than AS (includes isovolumic periods)
Diastolic Signals	Mitral inflow is not continuous with AS signal	Mitral inflow is continuous with MR signal
Velocity	AS velocity is always lower than the MR velocity	MR velocity is always higher than AS velocity

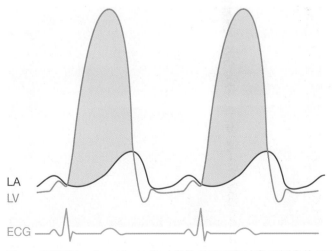
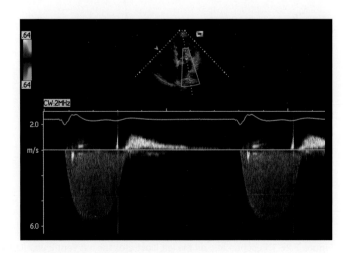

Figure 7.23 The schematic on the left illustrates the left atrial (LA) and left ventricular (LV) pressure traces. Mitral regurgitation (MR) reflects the pressure difference between the LV and LA during systole (*shaded area*). The image on the right is a continuous-wave Doppler trace of MR; observe that the MR signal has a parabolic shape with the peak velocity occurring in mid systole.

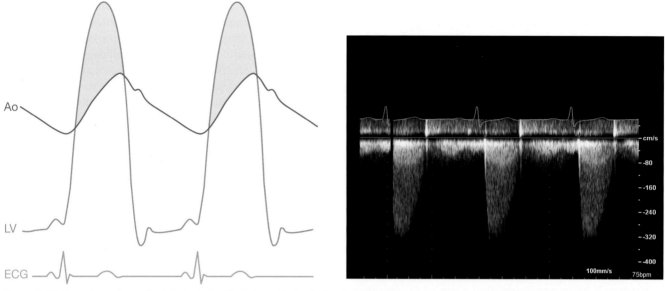

Figure 7.24 The schematic on the left illustrates the left ventricular (LV) and aortic (Ao) pressure traces. Aortic stenosis (AS) reflects the pressure difference between the LV and aorta during systole (*shaded area*). The image on the right is a continuous-wave Doppler trace of AS; observe that the AS signal has a V-shape with the peak velocity occurring in early systole.

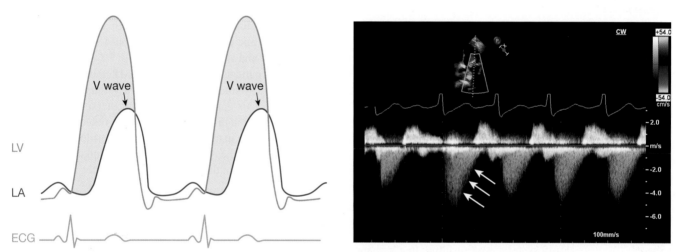

Figure 7.25 The schematic on the left illustrates the left atrial (LA) and left ventricular (LV) pressure traces as seen with acute, severe mitral regurgitation. The shaded area reflects the LV-LA pressure gradient. Observe the marked elevation in the LA pressure at mid-late systole (*V wave*) results in a decreased LV-LA pressure gradient. The image on the right is a continuous-wave Doppler trace of acute, severe MR; observe that the MR signal appears V-shaped with an early systolic peak. This is referred to as the V cut-off sign.

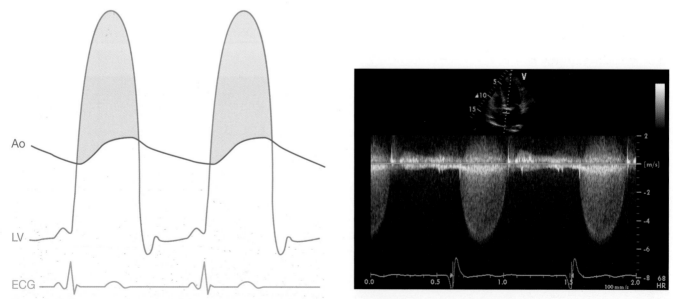

Figure 7.26 The schematic on the left illustrates the left ventricular (LV) and aortic (Ao) pressure traces as seen with critical aortic stenosis (AS). The shaded area reflects the pressure difference between the LV and aorta during systole. Observe that the flattening of the aortic pressure wave. The image on the right is a continuous-wave Doppler trace of critical AS; observe that the AS signal has a parabolic shape with the peak velocity occurring in mid-systole.

When AS and MR are coexistent, the duration of each signal is helpful in distinguishing between the two signals. The AS signal commences from the time of aortic valve opening to the closure of the aortic valve while the MR signal commences from the time of mitral valve closure to the next opening of the mitral valve. The MR duration incorporates both isovolumic contraction time (IVCT) and the isovolumic relaxation time (IVRT); therefore the duration of the MR signal is longer than the AS signal (Fig. 7.27).

In addition, identification of continuity between the diastolic and systolic signals is also valuable in differentiating AS from MR. The AS signal will display a 'gap' between the end of the mitral inflow signal and the start of the systolic signal (the IVCT) and a 'gap' between the end of the systolic signal and the beginning of the mitral inflow signal (the IVRT) (Fig. 7.28, left). The MR signal will show continuity between the mitral inflow signal and the systolic signal (Fig. 7.28, right).

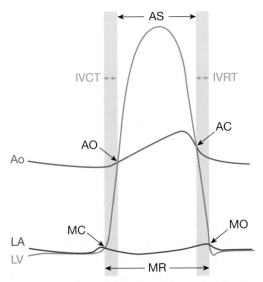

Figure 7.27 This schematic illustrates the difference in durations between the mitral regurgitant (MR) and aortic stenosis (AS) signals. The MR signal is longer than the AS signal because it incorporates the isovolumic contraction time (IVCT) as well as the isovolumic relaxation time (IVRT). The IVCT is the time interval between mitral valve closure (MC) and aortic valve opening (AO) while the IVRT is the time interval between aortic valve closure (AC) and mitral valve opening (MO). **Ao** = aortic pressure trace; **LA** = left atrial pressure trace; **LV** = left ventricular pressure trace.

When AS and MR are coexistent, the velocity of the MR jet will always be higher than the AS velocity (Fig. 7.29). In fact, the MR velocity can be used to cross-check the transaortic pressure gradient. Recall that the MR signal reflects the pressure gradient between the LV and LA during systole:

Equation 7.3

$$4V_{MR}^2 = LVSP - LAP$$

where $4V_{MR}$ = peak mitral regurgitant velocity (m/s)
LVSP = left ventricular systolic pressure (mm Hg)
LAP = left atrial pressure (mm Hg)

By measuring the MR velocity and by estimating the LA pressure, this equation can be rearranged to calculate the LV systolic pressure (LVSP):

Equation 7.4

$$LVSP = 4V_{MR}^2 + LAP$$

The LV-to-aortic pressure gradient can then be derived as the difference between the LVSP and the aortic systolic pressure. By assuming that the systolic arm blood pressure is equal to the aortic systolic pressure, the LV-to-aortic pressure gradient can be derived:

Equation 7.5

$$\Delta P_{LV-Ao} = LVSP - SBP$$

where ΔP_{LV-Ao} = left ventricular-to-aortic pressure gradient (mm Hg)
LVSP = left ventricular systolic pressure (mm Hg)
SBP = systolic blood pressure (mm Hg)

Importantly, it should be noted that when estimating the LV-to-aortic pressure gradient via this method, it is the peak-to-peak gradient that is being estimated (see Figure 1.7). This pressure gradient should correlate with the catheter-derived pressure gradient which measures the gradient between the peak LVSP and the peak aortic pressure. Note, however, that this peak-to-peak pressure gradient is different to the Doppler-derived pressure gradient which measures the maximum instantaneous pressure gradient between the LV and the aorta at the same instant in the cardiac cycle.

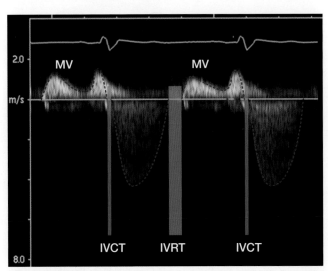 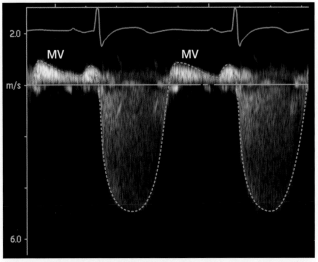

Figure 7.28 The aortic stenosis trace *(left)* shows a 'gap' between the end of the mitral inflow (MV) signal and the start of the systolic signal (IVCT) as well as a 'gap' between the end of the systolic signal and the beginning of the mitral inflow signal (IVRT). The mitral regurgitation trace *(right)* shows continuity between the mitral inflow signal and the systolic signal. **IVCT** = isovolumic contraction time; **IVRT** = isovolumic relaxation time.

Discordance between Doppler- and Catheter-derived Gradients
As discussed in Chapter 1, there may also be an apparent overestimation of Doppler-derived pressure gradients in patients with mild-moderate aortic valve stenosis (see Fig. 1.7) due to a phenomenon called "rapid pressure recovery" (see Fig. 1.8). In particular, overestimation of pressure gradients due to rapid pressure recovery is relevant when the ascending aorta is small (< 30 mm); when the ascending aorta is greater than 30 mm this phenomenon can be disregarded as a cause for overestimation of pressure gradients.

Flow Dependency
Another limitation of pressure gradients for the assessment of AS is that these gradients are flow dependent. For example, in high output states such as anaemia, or in patients with significant coexistent aortic regurgitation (AR), the transaortic velocities may be increased in the absence of severe AS; conversely, a low stroke volume as seen with severe LV systolic dysfunction may result in low transaortic pressure gradients in the presence of severe AS (see Discrepancies between AVA and Pressure Gradients below).

Aortic Valve Area
The transaortic pressure gradients are useful in assessing the severity of AS and for following its progression over time. However, as stated above, pressure gradients are dependent on the stroke volume (SV) across the valve. Therefore to 'compensate' for the changes in the SV, calculation of the AVA should be performed. The AVA, rather than the pressure gradients, is especially valuable in the serial assessment of AS.

> The normal aortic valve area in a normal sized adult is between 3.0 and 4.0 cm².

Calculation of the AVA is based upon the continuity equation (see Chapter 1). Recall that this principle is based on the assumption that the SV proximal to a narrowing is equal to the SV across the narrowing. In the estimation of the AVA via this principle, it is assumed that the SV across the LVOT will be identical to the SV across the stenotic aortic valve (Fig. 7.30). The SV is derived as the product of the cross-

sectional area (CSA) and the velocity time integral (VTI). For the LVOT, the CSA is derived from the LVOT diameter:

Equation 7.6

$$CSA = 0.785 \times D^2$$

where CSA = cross-sectional area (cm²)
  D = diameter (cm)

If the LVOT diameter can be measured to derive the CSA of the LVOT, and if the VTI across the LVOT and across the aortic valve can be measured, then the AVA can be derived (Fig. 7.31):

Equation 7.7

$$AVA = (CSA_{LVOT} \times VTI_{LVOT}) \div VTI_{AV}$$

where AVA   = aortic valve area (cm²)
  CSA_{LVOT} = cross-sectional area of the LVOT (cm²)
  VTI_{LVOT} = velocity time integral of the LVOT (cm)
  VTI_{AV} = velocity time integral across the stenotic aortic valve (cm)

This equation can be simplified by assuming that the flow duration across the LVOT and across the stenotic aortic valve are the same. Therefore, the VTI across the LVOT and across the stenotic aortic valve can be substituted with peak velocity at LVOT and the peak AS velocity:

Equation 7.8

$$AVA = (CSA_{LVOT} \times V_{LVOT}) \div V_{AV}$$

where AVA   = aortic valve area (cm²)
  CSA_{LVOT} = cross-sectional area of the LVOT (cm²)
  V_{LVOT} = peak velocity at the LVOT (m/s)
  V_{AV} = peak velocity across the stenotic aortic valve (m/s)

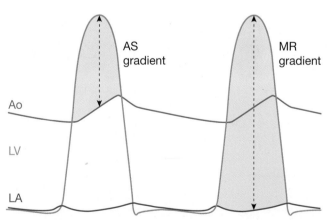

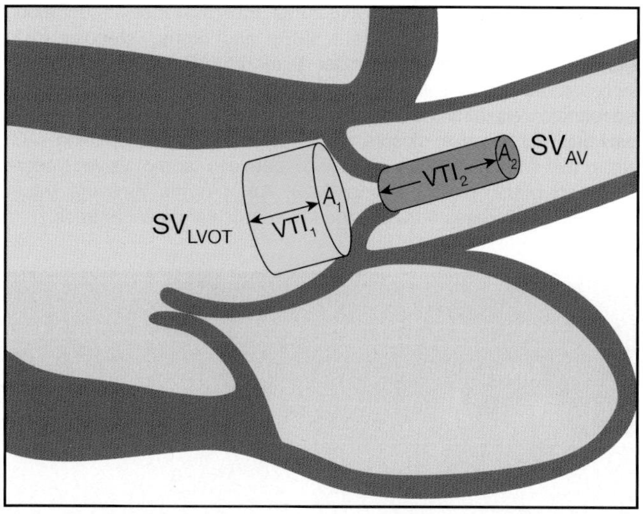

Figure 7.30 Stroke volume (SV) is derived as a product of the cross-sectional area (CSA) and the velocity time integral (VTI). As VTI is measured as a distance or 'height' it can be postulated that flow through the LVOT and across the aortic valve is cylindrical (the volume of a cylinder is derived from the CSA and the height of the cylinder). Hence, the SV across the left ventricular outflow tract (SV_LVOT) is the product of the CSA of the LVOT (A₁) and the height of the cylinder or the VTI of the LVOT (VTI₁); the SV across the aortic valve (SV_AV) is the product of the aortic valve area (A₂) and the height of the cylinder or the VTI across the aortic valve (VTI₂). Based on the continuity principle the SV_LVOT is equal to the SV_AV. Therefore, as the aortic valve area (A₂) decreases, the height of the cylinder or the VTI (VTI₂) must increase to maintain continuity of flow.

Figure 7.29 This schematic illustrates why the mitral regurgitant (MR) pressure gradient, between the left ventricle (LV) and left atrium (LA), will always exceed the aortic stenosis (AS) pressure gradient, between the aorta (Ao) and left ventricle (LV). Therefore, as the Doppler velocity reflects the pressure gradient, the MR velocity will always be higher than the AS velocity.

Indexed Aortic Valve Area

The AVA can be indexed to the body surface area (BSA) by simply dividing the AVA by the BSA:

Equation 7.9

$$IAVA = AVA \div BSA$$

where IAVA = indexed aortic valve area (cm²/m²)
AVA = aortic valve area (cm²)
BSA = body surface area (m²)

Indexing the AVA to BSA is important in two particular groups of patients: (1) the very large (but not obese) patient and (2) the very small adult patient. In the very small adult patient the AVA may fall into the severe range for AS severity by AVA but this might be functionally mild for this sized patient. For example, an AVA of 0.9 cm² in a patient who is 135 cm and only 40 kg may be only mildly stenotic for this patient.

In a patient of tall stature who has high transaortic pressure gradients the actual AVA may not fall into the severe range. For example, in a patient who is 210 cm tall weighing 110 kg an AVA of 1.3 cm² may in fact be functionally severe for this patient. Importantly, indexing the AVA for obese patients is not useful as the AVA does not increase with increasing body weight. Therefore, indexing of AVA is only useful in large but not obese patients.

The limitations of the continuity principle for valve area calculations are discussed in detail in Chapter 1 while the limitations of SV calculations using the LVOT are discussed in Chapter 2. With respect to the AVA, the most common pitfalls encountered include: (1) underestimation of the AS velocity and VTI due to suboptimal alignment of the ultrasound beam with blood flow direction, (2) underestimation of the LVOT velocity and VTI due to improper placement of the pulsed-wave (PW) Doppler sample volume within the LVOT and (3) errors in the LVOT diameter measurement (refer to Fig. 2.29). Another important limitation in calculating the AVA occurs when there is coexistent LVOT obstruction or when the LVOT flow is not laminar. This situation is often encountered in patients with a small LV cavity and basal hypertrophy of the interventricular septum. In these situations calculation of the AVA can be achieved by substituting the right ventricular outflow tract (RVOT) SV for the LVOT SV so long as there is no intracardiac shunt and no significant regurgitation across the aortic or pulmonary valves; that is, the SV across both the RVOT and the aortic valve are the same (Fig. 7.32).

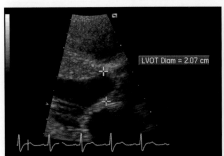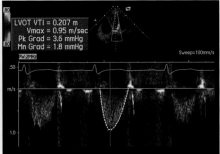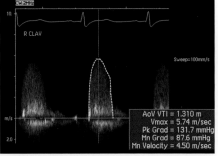

Figure 7.31 The aortic valve area (AVA) is calculated from the left ventricular outflow tract (LVOT) diameter, the LVOT velocity time integral (VTI) and the transaortic VTI. The LVOT diameter is measured from a zoomed parasternal long axis view of the LVOT (*left*). At mid-systole callipers are placed from the inner edge of the junction between the anterior aortic wall and the interventricular septum to the inner edge of the junction between the posterior aortic wall and the anterior leaflet of the mitral valve, perpendicular to the aortic root. From an apical 5-chamber view (*middle*), the LVOT VTI is traced from the pulsed-wave Doppler signal with a 2-4 mm sample volume placed 0.5 cm proximal to the aortic valve. The transaortic VTI is traced from the continuous-wave Doppler signal recorded from the window that provides the highest velocity across the stenotic aortic valve; this was the right supraclavicular window (R CLAV) in this case (*right*). The AVA via the VTI method in this example is calculated as:

$$
\begin{aligned}
AVA &= (CSA_{LVOT} \times VTI_{LVOT}) \div VTI_{AV} \\
&= (0.785 \times 2.07^2 \times 20.7) \div 131 \\
&= 0.5 \ cm^2
\end{aligned}
$$

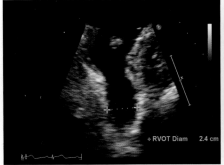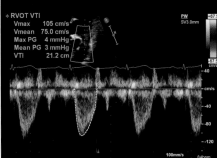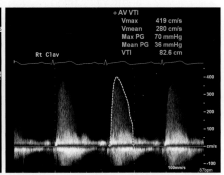

Figure 7.32 The aortic valve area (AVA) is calculated from the right ventricular outflow tract (RVOT) diameter, the RVOT velocity time integral (VTI) and the transaortic VTI. In this example, the RVOT diameter is measured from a zoomed subcostal 4-chamber view with anterior tilting (*left*). The diameter is measured at mid-systole via the inner edge to inner edge method. From the same zoomed view of the RVOT, the RVOT VTI is traced from the pulsed-wave Doppler signal with a 2-4 mm sample volume placed 0.5 cm proximal to the pulmonary valve (*middle*). The transaortic VTI is traced from the continuous-wave Doppler signal recorded from the window that provides the highest velocity across the stenotic aortic valve; this was the right supraclavicular window (Rt Clav) in this case (*right*). The AVA in this example is calculated as:

$$
\begin{aligned}
AVA &= (CSA_{RVOT} \times VTI_{RVOT}) \div VTI_{AV} \\
&= (0.785 \times 2.4^2 \times 21.2) \div 82.6 \\
&= 1.12 \ cm^2
\end{aligned}
$$

As previously mentioned, an important concept that results in a discrepancy between Doppler and invasive measurements of transaortic pressure gradients is the pressure recovery phenomenon. In particular, when there is rapid pressure recovery, the AVA derived by Doppler will be smaller than the AVA derived invasively. This is because the highest velocity (and largest pressure drop) detected by Doppler occurs at the vena contracta while the invasive method records the pressure drop between the LV and aortic root (see Fig. 1.8). To counter this discrepancy, an equation to calculate the pressure recovery adjusted effective valve area has been described; this is referred to as the energy loss index (ELI). This index is derived from the AVA, the aortic area at the level of the ST junction (Aa) and the BSA. The Aa is derived from the ST junction diameter using Equation 7.6.

Equation 7.10

$$ELI = [(AVA \times Aa) \div (Aa - AVA)] \div BSA$$

where ELI = energy loss index (cm^2/m^2)
      AVA = aortic valve area (cm^2)
      Aa   = aortic area at the sinotubular junction (cm^2)
      BSA = body surface area (m^2)

The significance of the ELI is based on the same criteria as the AVAi; that is, severe AS is defined as an ELI < 0.6 cm^2/m^2. In particular, calculation of this index is especially important in patients with small aortic roots (< 30 mm) where rapid pressure recovery is more often present. This index can also be used to confirm the presence of severe AS in asymptomatic patients; for example, asymptomatic AS patients may be misclassified as severe AS if pressure recovery is not taken into account.

Dimensionless Severity Index
The dimensionless severity index (DSI) or the velocity ratio is simply the ratio of the LVOT peak velocity (or VTI) divided by the transaortic peak velocity (or VTI):

Equation 7.11

$$DSI = V_{LVOT} \div V_{AV}$$

where DSI   = dimensionless severity index (unitless)
      V_{LVOT} = peak velocity (or VTI) at the LVOT (m/s)
      V_{AV} = peak velocity (or VTI) across the stenotic aortic valve (m/s)

The value of the DSI is that this index provides a useful clue as to the severity of stenosis based on two Doppler variables only. This parameter is especially valuable in situations where the LVOT diameter cannot be accurately measured due to suboptimal parasternal images.

Discrepancies between AVA and Pressure Gradients
Discrepancies between the AVA and pressure gradients in defining the severity of AS are commonly encountered. For example, the AVA may be consistent with severe AS (AVA ≤ 1.0 cm^2) yet the peak velocity may not fall within the severe range (velocity ≤ 4.0 m/s). Conversely, the peak velocity might be consistent with severe AS (velocity > 4.0 m/s) but the AVA may not meet the criteria for severe AS (AVA > 1.0 cm^2).

Severe AS by Velocity (> 4.0 m/s) but not by AVA (> 1.0 cm²)
Possible causes for severe AS based on the velocity but not

by AVA include measurement error, large body size, and high transaortic flow (Fig. 7.33, left).
Measurement errors can lead to an overestimation of the AVA due to overestimation of the LVOT diameter and/or LVOT VTI (refer to Fig. 2.29). In particular, overestimation of the LVOT VTI occurs when the PW Doppler sample volume is placed too close to the aortic valve.
In patients of a large stature, the AVA may not accurately reflect the severity of the AS. In these patients the AVA should be indexed to the BSA.
In addition, high velocities in the absence of severe AS may occur when there is a high flow rate across the aortic valve. This may occur with high output states such as anaemia, fever, tachycardia, sepsis and/or pregnancy. High flow rates across the aortic valve also occur when there is significant AR. In patients with moderate-severe AR, the LVOT SV is increased as this includes the normal forward SV plus the regurgitant AR volume. As a result higher transaortic velocities may be seen despite the absence of severe AS.

Severe AS by AVA (≤ 1.0 cm²) but not Peak Velocity (≤ 4.0 m/s)
Possible causes for severe AS based on the AVA but not by peak velocities include measurement error, small body size, and low transaortic flow (Fig. 7.33, right).
Measurement errors can lead to an underestimation of the AVA due to underestimation of the LVOT diameter and/or the LVOT VTI (refer to Fig. 2.29). Therefore, these measurements should be rechecked. In particular, underestimation of the LVOT VTI occurs when the PW Doppler sample volume is placed too far into the LVOT.
In patients of a small stature, the AVA may not accurately reflect the severity of the AS. In these patients, the AVA should be indexed to the BSA.
In addition, low velocities in the presence of severe AS may occur when there is low flow in the setting of a normal LV ejection fraction (LVEF) or when there is low flow in the setting of a reduced LVEF. Low flow in the setting of a normal LVEF can be seen in patients with marked LV concentric remodelling and a small LV cavity size (so-called 'paradoxical' low flow severe AS) or in patients with coexistent significant MR. In patients with moderate-severe MR, the LVOT SV is decreased because blood is being 'ejected' into the LA during systole. As a result, lower transaortic velocities may be seen despite the presence of severe AS. 'Paradoxical' low flow severe AS with preserved LVEF can be encountered in patients with a small and severely hypertrophied LV whereby there is a reduction in the overall SV. This condition can be identified when the indexed stroke volume (SVi) is < 35 mL/m^2, the LVEF is > 50%, and the indexed AVA is < 0.6 cm^2/m^2. The most common cause for low flow AS is LV systolic dysfunction. In this situation, there is either "true" severe AS that causes LV systolic dysfunction or "pseudo-severe" AS where there is really only moderate AS with another cause of LV systolic dysfunction. Distinction between these two conditions can be made via dobutamine stress echocardiography (see Role of Stress Echocardiography in Aortic Stenosis below). In addition, considering the degree of calcification of the aortic valve can be useful. For example, it would be expected that patients with true severe AS will have heavily calcified valves showing extensive thickening and calcification of all cusps; the absence of heavily calcified cusps would be suggestive of pseudo-AS.

Maximal Aortic Cusp Separation

The severity of AS can be indirectly evaluated by observation of restricted leaflet motion and measurement of the maximal aortic cusp separation (MACS). The MACS is the vertical distance between the RCC and the NCC measured at the onset of ventricular systole (Fig. 7.34). In patients with severe AS, restricted valve opening leads to a reduction in the MACS. However, there are several limitations of this measurement in the evaluation of AS. Firstly, this measurement is one dimensional (1D) and assumes that the MACS occurs perpendicular to the ultrasound beam which may not be the case. Secondly, it is also assumed that this 1D measurement reflects the overall geometry of the valve area but it does not account for asymmetric involvement of the leaflets, eccentric orifices, or severe distortion of the valve. Thirdly, extensive calcification or

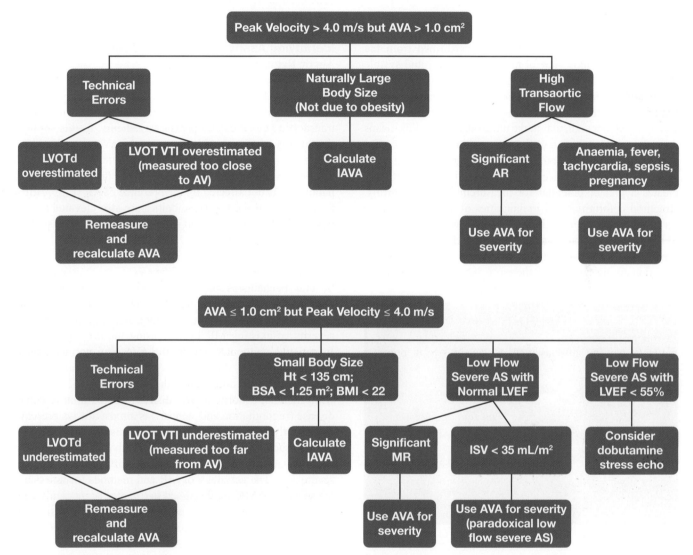

Figure 7.33 These flow charts illustrate the possible causes for discrepancies between the aortic valve area (AVA) and peak velocities and how the severity of aortic stenosis may be determined in these situations. See text for further details.
AR = aortic regurgitation; **AV** = aortic valve; **IAVA** = indexed aortic valve area; **BMI** = body mass index; **BSA** = body surface area; **Ht** = height; **LVEF** = left ventricular ejection fraction; **LVOTd** = left ventricular outflow tract diameter; **MR** = mitral regurgitation; **ISV** = indexed stroke volume.

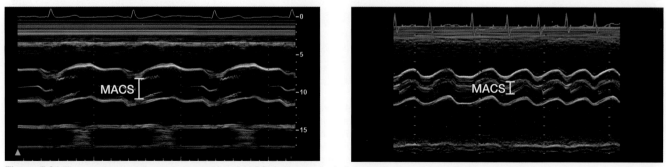

Figure 7.34 The maximal aortic cusp separation (MACS) is the vertical distance between the anterior and posterior cusps of the aortic valve measured at the onset of ventricular systole. The M-mode trace on the left displays normal aortic valve motion. Observe that during systole, the aortic leaflets snap open and lie parallel to the aortic root walls throughout systole resulting in a 'wide' MACS. At the end of ejection the leaflets abruptly close and coapt in the centre of the aortic root. The M-mode trace on the right was obtained through a stenotic aortic valve. Observe that the MACS is 'narrowed' indicating restricted aortic valve opening.

thickening of the valve leaflets typically results in the display of multiple echoes which significantly limits the feasibility and accuracy of this measurement. Fourthly, this measurement assumes that the cusps are maximally distended which may not be true when there is LV systolic dysfunction or low cardiac output states. Finally, the MACS is measured with the M-mode cursor placed at the trans-sinus level; however, in congenital AS the site of maximal obstruction occurs at the leaflet tips, not at the trans-sinus level.

Direct 2D Planimetry of the AVA

Direct planimetry of the AVA can be performed from the parasternal short axis view of the aortic valve at mid-systole (Fig. 7.35). While direct planimetry of the AVA is possible by 2D imaging there are several limitations to this measurement. Firstly, it is rare that all three aortic valve leaflets are sufficiently well imaged perpendicular to the ultrasound beam; this means that adequate delineation of the entire perimeter of the orifice area in systole is often not possible. Secondly, the triangular shape of the aortic orifice and the eccentricity of this valve creates a greater potential for measurement error. Thirdly, structural deformities and irregularities of the stenotic valve further exacerbate errors in orifice traces while calcification of the cusps often causes shadow and reverberation artefacts. Finally, the aortic valve moves rapidly in a superior-inferior direction during systole and, therefore, the valve orifice passes

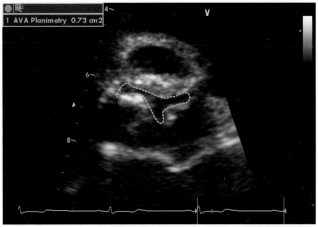

Figure 7.35 This is an example of 2D planimetry of the aortic valve area (AVA) in a severely stenotic aortic valve. The AVA is traced in mid-systole along the inner edge of the orifice.

rapidly through the scan plane making the localisation of the true aortic valve orifice more difficult.

In addition, while direct planimetry of the anatomical valve area provides the most precise evaluation of the true valve area, it is the effective orifice area (EOA) that is the primary predictor of clinical outcome [7.1]. Importantly, the EOA derived by haemodynamic calculation of the AVA is smaller than the true anatomical area. This is because the EOA is calculated downstream from the anatomical valve area at the vena contracta (see Fig. 1.21).

Identifying Associated Valve Lesions
Aortic Regurgitation

Some degree of AR is commonly associated with AS. The severity of AR is described later in this chapter. In particular, as mentioned above, significant AR can result in increased transaortic velocities and pressure gradients. In this setting, the severity of AS should be based on the AVA rather than the transaortic peak velocity and pressure gradients. Importantly, the accuracy of the AVA, which is a flow independent parameter, is not affected by the presence of AR (Fig. 7.36). Furthermore, if the LVOT velocities are also elevated (≥ 1.2 m/s), both the maximum and mean pressure gradients should be corrected using Equation 7.2 as previously stated.

Mitral Regurgitation

Several mechanisms may be responsible for MR in patients with severe AS. For example, MR may simply occur due to the increased LVSP. Furthermore, AS may increase the severity of existing MR by increasing the driving pressure from the LV to the LA. MR may also result from incomplete leaflet coaptation due to: (1) coexistent mitral annular calcification or (2) dilatation of the mitral annulus. In patients with rheumatic aortic valve disease, mixed mitral valve disease (regurgitation and stenosis) is almost always present. Importantly, identification of the mechanism and severity of MR is crucial as concomitant mitral valve surgery may be necessary in patients undergoing aortic valve replacement for severe AS. The aetiology of MR and methods for assessing the severity of MR are discussed in Chapter 8.

As mentioned previously, significant MR can result in decreased transaortic velocities and pressure gradients. In this situation, the severity of AS should be based on the AVA rather than the peak velocity and pressure gradients.

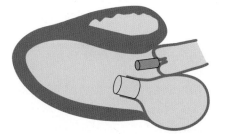 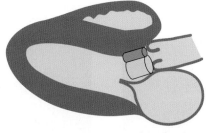 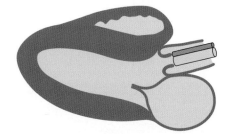

Figure 7.36 This schematic explains how the accuracy of the aortic valve area (AVA) calculation is not compromised by the presence of coexistent aortic regurgitation (AR). During diastole (*left*) the left ventricle accepts the forward stroke volume (SV) across the mitral valve [blue cylinder] and the aortic regurgitant volume (RV) [pink cylinder]. During systole the SV across the LVOT (*middle*) will include both the forward SV and the aortic RV. Likewise, during systole the SV across the aortic valve (*right*) will also include both the forward SV and the aortic RV. Therefore, the SV across the LVOT and across the aortic valve are the same despite the presence of AR; therefore, the calculation of the AVA based on this principle is still accurate.

[7.1] Baumgartner H, Hung J, Bermejo J, Chambers JB, Evangelista A, Griffin BP, Iung B, Otto CM, Pellikka PA, Quiñones M; American Society of Echocardiography; European Association of Echocardiography. Echocardiographic assessment of valve stenosis: EAE/ASE recommendations for clinical practice. *J Am Soc Echocardiogr.* 2009 Jan;22(1):page 8

Role of Stress Echocardiography in Aortic Stenosis

Essentially stress echocardiography can be used in two groups of patients: (1) patients with asymptomatic severe AS at rest and (2) patients with low flow, low gradient (LFLG) AS with associated LV systolic dysfunction.

In patients with asymptomatic severe AS at rest, exercise echocardiography (treadmill, or upright or semi-supine bicycle) may be utilized to: (1) determine if the patient has exercise-induced symptoms, (2) assess the compliance of the aortic valve, (3) assess haemodynamic severity of the stenosis, (4) assess LV contractile reserve and diastolic function, and (5) identify haemodynamic variables such as MR and pulmonary pressures (Table 7.4).

As previously mentioned, LFLG AS with associated LV systolic dysfunction may occur due to "true" severe AS or "pseudo-severe" AS. In both settings, the low flow state caused by LV systolic dysfunction is responsible for a calculated AVA consistent with severe AS. Distinction between these two clinical scenarios is important with respect to whom will benefit from an aortic valve replacement (AVR). To differentiate true severe AS from pseudo-severe AS dobutamine stress echocardiography may be used (Fig. 7.37). In patients with true AS, severe AS is responsible for LV systolic dysfunction. LV systolic dysfunction leads to a reduced SV which accounts for the reduced transvalvular gradients and an AVA in the severe range. In those patients with true AS plus LV contractile reserve, dobutamine will increase the cardiac output (SV ≥ 20%) as well as the transaortic gradient. As a result there is no change in the AVA; that is, the AVA remains consistent with severe AS. These patients have fixed AS with contractile reserve and usually benefit from an AVR (that is, improvements in symptomatic status and LVEF are observed). In patients with pseudo-severe AS, LV systolic dysfunction is unrelated to AS. That is, LV systolic dysfunction is due to another primary cause such as ischaemic heart disease, or cardiomyopathy. As for the true AS patients, LV systolic dysfunction also causes a reduced SV and a reduction in transvalvular gradients resulting in a calculated AVA in the severe range. In these patients dobutamine will increase the

cardiac output (SV ≥ 20%) but there will be no change or only a slight increase in the transaortic gradient and, therefore, the AVA actually increases. These patients have moderate AS and will not benefit from an AVR (that is, the LVEF does not significantly improve following an AVR).

A third scenario may also be seen where there is low gradient AS with no contractile reserve. In these patients, following dobutamine there is no change to the cardiac output, transaortic gradient or AVA. Thus, the severity of AS in these patients is indeterminate and the operative risk in these patients is high.

> This section provides a brief overview of the role of stress echocardiography in patients with low flow, low gradient AS. For a more comprehensive understanding of the role of stress echocardiography in these patients, including recommended protocols, readers are advised to review other sources as listed in the Further Reading section of this Chapter.

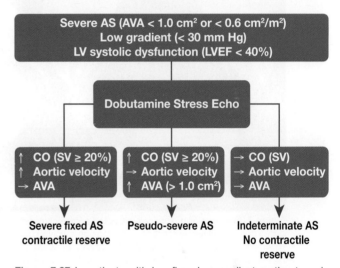

Figure 7.37 In patients with low flow, low gradient aortic stenosis (AS) dobutamine stress echocardiography can be used to distinguish between 3 groups: (1) true AS with contractile reserve, (2) pseudo-AS, and (3) indeterminate AS with no contractile reserve. See text for details. ↑ = increased; → = no change; **AVA** = aortic valve area; **CO** = cardiac output; **SV** = stroke volume.

Table 7.4 Abnormal Stress Echocardiographic Measurements in Asymptomatic Aortic Stenosis

Component	Findings
Valvular components	
Aortic valve area	Increased: compliant valve
	Stable: fixed and non-compliant valve
Mean gradient	Increased: fixed and non-compliant valve or presence of contractile reserve (should be correlated to ejection fraction)
	Decreased or no change: no contractile reserve
Left ventricular components	
Systolic function ejection fraction	Increased: presence of contractile reserve
	Stable or decreased: absence of contractile reserve
Strain imaging by TDI or speckle tracking	Decreased: absence of contractile reserve
Diastolic function E/e'	Increased: elevated filling pressure
Other components	
Mitral regurgitation	Worsening or occurrence: elevated global afterload
Transtricuspid gradient	Increased > 50 mm Hg: elevated pulmonary pressure

Reprinted from *Archives of Cardiovascular Disease*, Vol. 103 (4), O'Connor K, Lancellotti P, Donal E, Piérard LA, Exercise echocardiography in severe asymptomatic aortic stenosis, Page 264, © 2010, with permission from Elsevier.

Aortic Regurgitation

Aetiology of Aortic Regurgitation

Aortic regurgitation (AR) refers to the backward flow of blood flow from the aorta to the LV during diastole. AR may result from disorders of the aortic valve, the aortic root or a combination of both. Essentially the mechanisms of AR can be categorised into four groups: (1) cuspal abnormalities, (2) aortic root dilatation, (3) aortic root distortion, and (4) loss of commissural support (Table 7.5).

Cuspal Abnormalities

Cuspal abnormalities causing AR include congenital aortic valve abnormalities, rheumatic aortic valve disease, aortic

valve prolapse and infective endocarditis.

Congenital AR is usually related to abnormalities of leaflet morphology and cusp number; for example, BAV (Fig. 7.38, middle) or quadricuspid aortic valves. BAVs are discussed above (see Aetiology of Aortic Stenosis).

Quadricuspid aortic valves (QAV) are very, very rare. The most common haemodynamic abnormality associated with these types of valves is AR. In addition, anomalies of the coronary arteries which may include displacement of the right or left coronary ostium, a single coronary orifice or the presence of an accessory artery are also commonly associated with QAV. As for BAV, the anatomy of the QAV is variable; in particular, seven variations have been described (Fig. 7.39 and 7.40).

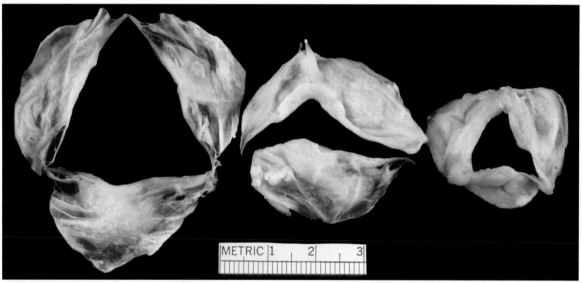

Figure 7.38 Examples of surgically resected aortic valves which caused aortic regurgitation are shown. *Left:* stretched and thinned cusps due to a dilated aortic root. *Middle:* a non-calcified bicuspid aortic valve (raphe on the 'top' cusp) with mild annular dilatation. *Right:* a rheumatic aortic valve with fibrotic and retracted aortic cusps and only minimal commissural fusion in this example.
By permission of Mayo Foundation for Medical Education and Research. All rights reserved. Courtesy of William D. Edwards, MD.

Table 7.5 Aetiology of Aortic Regurgitation

Structural Abnormality causing AR	Examples
Annular or aortic root dilatation	Aortic dissection Annuloaortic ectasia Bicuspid aortic valve Connective tissue disorders (e.g. Marfan syndrome, Ehlers-Danlos syndrome) Idiopathic aortic root dilatation Sinus of Valsalva aneurysm Systemic hypertension
Annular or aortic root distortion	Autoimmune diseases (e.g. ankylosing spondylitis, systemic lupus erythematosus) Aortitis (e.g. autoimmune disease, rheumatoid arthritis, syphilis, Takayasu arteritis)
Cusp abnormalities	Aortic valve prolapse Congenitally abnormal aortic valve (e.g. bicuspid aortic valve) Cusp rupture Degenerative calcific aortic valve Infective endocarditis Myxomatous aortic valve Rheumatic aortic valve disease Rheumatoid arthritis
Loss of commissural support	Aortic dissection Membranous ventricular septal defect (VSD) Trauma VSD associated with tetralogy of Fallot

Rheumatic aortic valve disease is discussed above (see Aetiology of Aortic Stenosis). In the rheumatic aortic valve, the cusps become infiltrated with fibrous tissue and retraction of the leaflets prevents cuspal apposition during diastole leading to AR (Fig. 7.38, right). "Isolated" AR is rare in patients with rheumatic aortic valve disease; AR is usually associated with some degree of aortic stenosis. Furthermore, as mentioned above, rheumatic aortic valve disease is usually associated with rheumatic mitral valve disease.

Aortic valve prolapse (AVP) is defined as downward displacement of aortic cusps below the points of attachment of the aortic valve leaflets (that is, displacement of the aortic cusps below the virtual ring). AVP may occur due to myxomatous degeneration of the valve or due to post-inflammatory changes associated with rheumatic valve disease. AVP may also occur secondary to aortic root dilatation, when there is a membranous ventricular septal defect, or following trauma.

AR secondary to infective endocarditis occurs when an aortic valve vegetation interferes with proper coaptation of the cusps, when the valve cusp is destroyed, or when there is perforation of the leaflet (Fig. 7.41).

Aortic Root Dilatation

Aortic root dilatation prevents normal leaflet coaption during diastole which leads to AR (see Fig. 7.42). Causes of aortic root dilatation include: (1) systemic hypertension, (2) atherosclerosis, (3) connective tissue disorders, (4) BAV, and (5) sinus of Valsalva aneurysms (Table 7.6). In some cases of aortic root dilatation no definite cause can be determined; this is referred to as idiopathic aortic root dilatation. Sinus of Valsalva aneurysms (SVA) and connective tissue disorders are discussed in more detail in Chapters 11 and 14, respectively.

Aortic Root Distortion

Aortic root distortion can occur due to aortitis which is associated with inflammatory processes such as ankylosing spondylitis, Takayasu arteritis and rheumatoid arthritis. In these conditions the aortic root becomes distorted and the aortic cusps may also be affected, becoming scarred; AR occurs as a consequence.

Loss of Commissural Support

Loss of commissural support leading to AR may occur with: (1) ventricular septal defects (VSD), (2) aortic dissections or

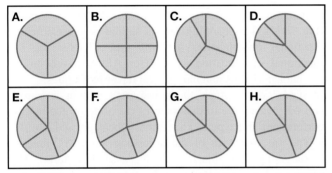

Figure 7.39 Various orientations of quadricuspid aortic valves (QAV) compared with a normal trileaflet valve are illustrated: **A** = Normal trileaflet aortic valve; **B** = QAV with 4 equal-sized cusps (most common); **C** = QAV with 3 equal-sized cusps and 1 smaller cusp; **D** = QAV with 2 equal-sized larger cusps and 2 equal-sized smaller cusps; **E** = QAV with 1 larger cusp, 2 intermediate-sized cusps and 1 smaller cusp; **F** = QAV with 3 equal-sized cusps and 1 larger cusp; **G** = QAV with 2 larger cusps and 2 unequal smaller cusps; **H** = QAV with 4 unequal-sized cusps.

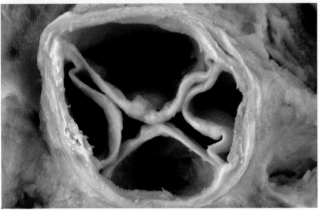
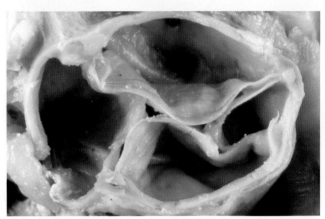

Figure 7.40 Pathological examples of a quadricuspid aortic valve (QAV) with 4 equal-sized cusps (*left*) and a QAV with 3 equal-sized cusps and 1 smaller (supernumerary) cusp (*right*) are shown.
By permission of Mayo Foundation for Medical Education and Research. All rights reserved. Courtesy of William D. Edwards, MD.

Table 7.6 Causes and Mechanisms of Aortic Root Dilatation

Cause	Mechanism of Aortic Root Dilatation
Systemic Hypertension	Elevation in aortic wall stress caused by chronic, severe elevation in blood pressure
Atherosclerotic Plaques	Destruction of underlying tunica media and subsequent weakening of the aortic wall
Connective Tissue Disorders	Medial degeneration causing weakening of aortic wall due to loss of normal collagenous and elastic framework and appearance of cystic spaces filled with mucoid material
Bicuspid Aortic Valve	Two main theories: (1) genetic theory: aortic wall fragility is a consequence of a developmental defect (i.e. medial degeneration) or (2) haemodynamic theory: abnormal stress on the aortic wall induced by eccentric turbulent flow through bicuspid valve
Sinus of Valsalva Aneurysms	Localised weakening of wall of sinus of Valsalva leading to focal bulging of associated coronary sinus and subsequent asymmetric aortic root dilatation

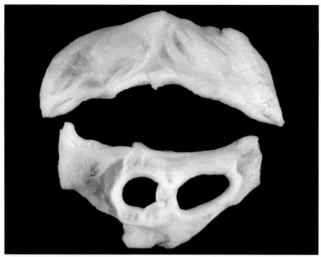

Figure 7.41 This pathological specimen resected at surgery shows a bicuspid aortic valve with two old perforations of the 'bottom' cusp caused by infective endocarditis.

By permission of Mayo Foundation for Medical Education and Research. All rights reserved. Courtesy of William D. Edwards, MD.

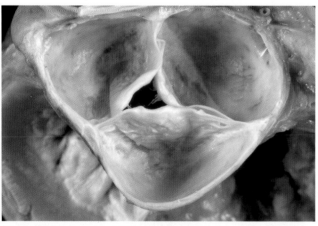

Figure 7.42 This gross pathological specimen shows dilatation of the aortic annulus. This condition prevents the aortic cusps from coapting normally during diastole which leads to central aortic regurgitation.

By permission of Mayo Foundation for Medical Education and Research. All rights reserved. Courtesy of William D. Edwards, MD.

(3) aortic trauma. For example, membranous VSDs or VSDs associated with tetralogy of Fallot may result in distortion or incomplete support of the valve cusps or annulus (Fig. 7.43). Trauma resulting from tearing of the ascending aorta and loss of commissural support can cause prolapse of a cusp. Tears of the aortic cusps may also be seen in cases of trauma where the patient has suffered a non-penetrating injury caused by a motor vehicle accident, a fall from a height, or by a blow to the chest wall. Type A aortic dissections can also cause AR due to loss of commissural support. This condition is discussed in more detail in Chapter 11.

Functional Classification of Aortic Regurgitation

A functional classification for AR has also been proposed (Fig. 7.44). This classification is similar to the Carpentier functional classification for MR (see Chapter 8). The functional classification system for AR is based on the mechanisms of AR and the surgical repair techniques.

In type I dysfunction, the aortic cusp motion is normal and AR occurs due to dilatation of the aorta or due to cusp perforation. This type can be further subcategorised into:
- Type Ia: aneurysm of the ascending aorta (ST junction enlargement and dilatation of the ascending aorta). This type is often associated with degenerative and aneurysmal changes of the aortic arch,
- Type Ib: aneurysm of the aortic root (dilatation of the sinuses of Valsalva and the ST junction). This type is typically associated with connective tissue disorders where there is degenerative disease of the media,
- Type Ic: isolated dilatation of the ventriculoarterial junction,
- Type Id: AR results from cusp perforation without a primary functional aortic annular lesion and annular dilatation. This type is usually associated with traumatic aortic injury or infective endocarditis.

Type II dysfunction refers to leaflet prolapse as a result of excessive cusp tissue or commissural disruption. Type III refers to leaflet restriction, which may occur in bicuspid, degenerative, or rheumatic valvular disease and as a result of calcification, thickening, and fibrosis of the aortic leaflets.

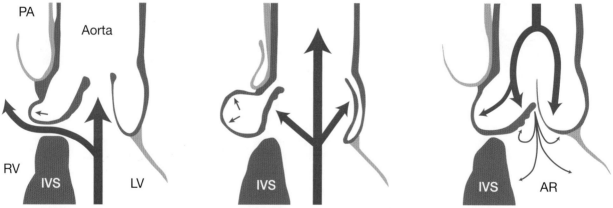

Figure 7.43 This schematic illustrates the proposed mechanism of aortic regurgitation (AR) associated with a ventricular septal defect (VSD). In early systole ejected blood from the left ventricle (LV) will be shunted through the VSD (left). The anatomically unsupported cusp and aortic sinus are then drawn or 'sucked' into the right ventricle (RV) (middle); this is known as the Venturi effect. In diastole (right), the intra-aortic pressure forces the aortic valve leaflet to close, but the unsupported cusp is pushed down into the left ventricular outflow tract away from the opposed coronary cusp, resulting in AR. **IVS** = interventricular septum; **PA** = pulmonary artery.
From Tatsuno K, Konno S, Ando M, Sakakibara S. Pathogenetic mechanisms of prolapsing aortic valve and aortic regurgitation associated with ventricular septal defect. Anatomical, angiographic, and surgical considerations. *Circulation*, Nov;48(5): page 1030, © 1973, Lippincott, Williams & Wilkins, Redrawn in colour with permission.

Importantly, patients may have either single or multiple lesions contributing to their AR. For example, patients with isolated type Ib AR due to aneurysmal aortic root dilatation would be expected to have a central AR jet. The presence of an aneurysmal aortic root dilatation with an eccentric AR jet suggests concomitant leaflet prolapse (type II) or restriction (type III).

Pathophysiology of Aortic Regurgitation

The pathophysiology of AR can be discussed in terms of acute, severe and chronic, severe AR.

Acute, severe AR typically occurs due to infective endocarditis, type A aortic dissection or cardiac trauma. In the acute situation, the aortic regurgitant volume (RV) fills a normal sized LV (the LV has not had time to compensate for an increased diastolic volume by dilating). This means that the LV cannot accommodate the combined large RV as well as the normal inflow of blood from the LA. As a result there is a marked elevation in the left ventricular end-diastolic pressure (LVEDP). In particular, if the LVEDP exceeds the LA pressure, there will be a pressure gradient between the LV and LA during diastole when the mitral valve is open; this leads to diastolic MR. Further increases in the LVEDP may lead to premature closure of the mitral valve. Rarely, the LVEDP may exceed the aortic diastolic pressure; in this instance, premature opening of the aortic valve occurs.

In the chronic situation, a significant aortic RV leads to gradual LV dilatation. As LV end-diastolic volume (LVEDV) increases, LV compliance also increases. An increase in LV compliance means that the LV is able to accept a larger volume of blood without a significant increase in the diastolic pressure (see Fig. 3.4). Therefore, in chronic, severe AR LVEDP can remain near normal for an extended period. This increase in the LVEDV also allows for an increase in the forward SV (see the Frank-Starling principle in Chapter 2). Therefore, initially, LV systolic function is normal and there is a normal LVEF. However, continued chronic, severe AR leads to an eventual decline in the LVEF and forward SV.

LV wall thickness is usually normal or mildly increased in chronic, severe AR. However, eccentric hypertrophy is usually present due to an increase in LV mass secondary to chamber dilatation rather than increased wall thickness (see Chapter 4).

Clinical Manifestations of Aortic Regurgitation

In chronic, severe AR, the clinical manifestations relate to the pathophysiological responses that occur due to the increased mass of the dilated LV. For example, patients may develop symptoms of congestive heart failure (see Clinical Manifestations of Aortic Stenosis above).

Myocardial ischaemia and angina are relatively uncommon in pure AR. However, in chronic, severe AR increased LV mass and LV dilatation result in increased myocardial oxygen demand and this can lead to myocardial ischaemia and chest pain. In addition, reduced diastolic perfusion pressure of the coronary arteries may lead to inadequate coronary blood flow which can also result in myocardial ischaemia and chest pain.

Role of Echocardiography in Aortic Regurgitation

The aims and objectives of echocardiography in the assessment of AR are to:
- Determine the aetiology of the lesion (e.g. congenital, degenerative, or rheumatic)
- Assess LV size and systolic function
- Measure the aortic dimensions
- Estimate the severity of the regurgitation (semiquantitative and/or quantitative methods).

'Physiological' or mild degrees of mitral, tricuspid and pulmonary regurgitation are quite common in the normal population; however, 'physiological' or mild degrees AR are not normally seen. Therefore, whenever AR is detected, close inspection of the aortic valve and aortic root are warranted.

Functional Type	Type I				Type II	Type III
	Ia	Ib	Ic	Id		
Cusp Motion	Normal	Normal	Normal	Normal	Excessive	Restricted
Cause of AR	Dilatation of STJ & AscAo	Dilatation of SV & STJ	Isolated dilatation of VAJ	Cusp perforation	Cusp prolapse	Calcification, thickening, &/or fibrosis of cusps
Illustrative example	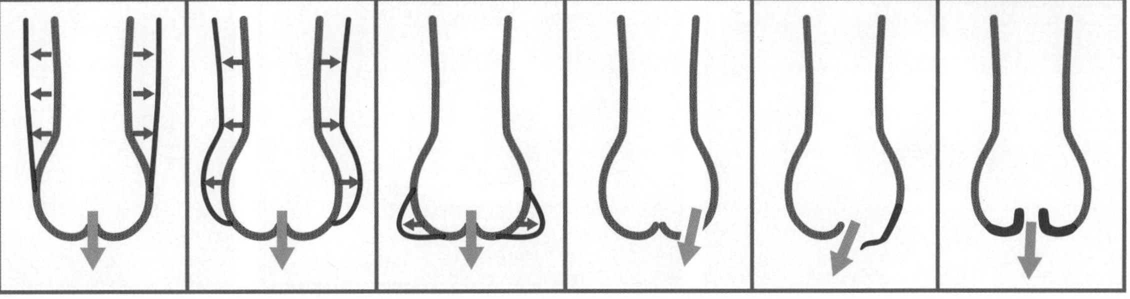					

Figure 7.44 This figure illustrates the functional classification of aortic regurgitation (AR). See text for further details.
AscAo = ascending aorta; **STJ** = sinotubular junction; **SVA** = sinuses of Valsalva; **VAJ** = ventriculoarterial junction.
Adapted from Boodhwani M, de Kerchove L, Glineur D, Poncelet A, Rubay J, Astarci P, Verhelst R, Noirhomme P, El Khoury G. Repair-oriented classification of aortic insufficiency: impact on surgical techniques and clinical outcomes, *J Thorac Cardiovasc Surg*, Feb;137(2), page 287, © 2009, with permission from Elsevier.

Aetiology of Aortic Regurgitation

As stated above AR may be due to cuspal abnormalities of the aortic valve or due to aortic root dilatation. In particular, many valvular causes of AS also result in some degree of AR. The echocardiographic appearance of BAVs, rheumatic aortic valves and calcific aortic valves has been described above under Aortic Stenosis.

Quadricuspid Aortic Valve

The diagnosis of a QAV is made from the PSAX view (Fig. 7.45). The key to the diagnosis of a QAV is based on identifying four aortic cusps during diastole. The characteristic appearance of a QAV with four equal-sized cusps is an "X" or a "+" configuration which is formed by the commissural lines of the closed valve during diastole.

Aortic Valve Endocarditis

Infective endocarditis (IE) of the aortic valve is one of the most common causes of acute, severe AR. The classic appearance of an aortic valve vegetation is a hypermobile mass or masses attached to the ventricular surface of the aortic valve which shows different tissue characteristics compared to underlying tissue (Fig. 7.46). On real-time imaging, these vegetations demonstrate independent, high frequency motion. The use of echocardiography in the assessment of IE is discussed in more detail in Chapter 13.

Ventricular Septal Defect

As stated above, a membranous VSD or a VSD associated with tetralogy of Fallot may result in AR due to prolapse of the aortic valve (Fig. 7.47). The mechanism of AR due to a VSD is a result of functional and haemodynamic factors. The functional factor is the lack of adequate anatomical support of the valve while the haemodynamic factor can be explained by the Venturi effect (see Fig. 7.43).

> Cuspal perforation secondary to IE should be suspected whenever the AR jet appears to arise from the base of the cusp rather than at the site of cusp coaptation.

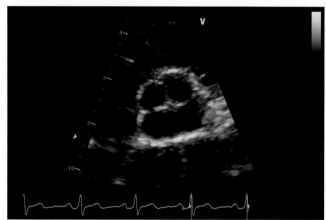
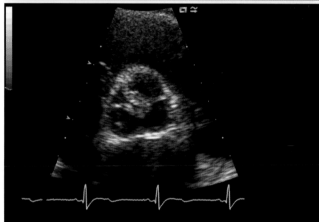

Figure 7.45 A QAV with 4 equal-sized cusps *(top)* and a QAV with 3 equal-sized cusps and 1 smaller cusp *(bottom)* are shown. These diastolic frames were recorded from a zoomed parasternal short axis view of the aortic valve.

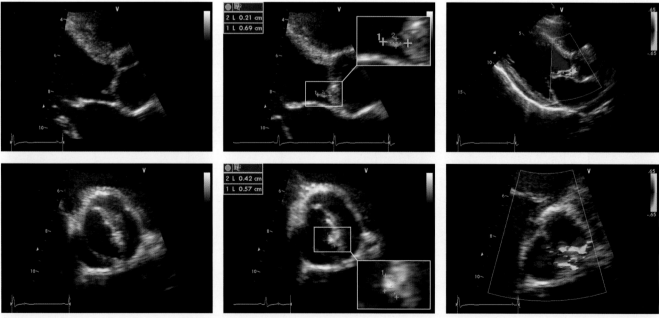

Figure 7.46 This is an example of a bicuspid aortic valve (BAV). The zoomed parasternal long axis images *(top left and middle)* show a small mass attached to the 'posterior' leaflet measuring 7 mm x 2 mm; associated aortic regurgitation (AR) is also noted *(top right)*. Also observe the eccentric closure of the aortic valve on these diastolic frames; this appearance is characteristic of a BAV. The zoomed parasternal short axis images *(bottom)* confirm the presence of a BAV with commissures seen at 11 and 5 o'clock. Again a small mass attached to the anterolateral leaflet posteriorly measuring 6 mm x 4 mm is seen with associated AR.

Aortic Root Dilatation

As mentioned above there are a number of conditions that cause dilatation of the aortic root which can lead to AR. An example of aortic root dilatation with a coaptation defect is shown in figure 7.48 (also refer to Chapter 11).

Aortic Dissection

An aortic dissection occurs when there is a tear in the intima resulting in blood entering the medial layer to create a false, blood-filled channel. Aortic dissections are classified according to the Stanford or DeBakey classifications (see Fig. 11.19). A type A aortic dissection is an important cause of AR. Several mechanisms for AR in Type A aortic dissections have been described (Fig. 7.49). These mechanisms include: (1) incomplete closure of a normal aortic valve due to ST junction dilatation; (2) AVP due to extension of the dissection into the aortic root which disrupts normal leaflet attachments to the aortic wall; (3) prolapse of the dissection flap through normal aortic valve leaflets that disrupts leaflet coaptation; (4) asymmetrical dissection where pressure from the dissecting haematoma may depress one leaflet below the line of closure of the other two leaflets; and (5) loss of annular support or tearing of the leaflets themselves may render the valve incompetent.

On the 2D echocardiographic examination an aortic dissection can be identified by observing an intimal flap within the aortic root. On real-time echocardiography, this flap appears as a thin, undulating structure within the aortic lumen. Aortic dissections are discussed in further detail in Chapter 11.

Assessment of Left Ventricular Size, Wall Thickness and Systolic Function

LV size, wall thickness and systolic function can be assessed by both M-mode and 2D echocardiography in the traditional manner (see Chapter 2). As previously mentioned, chronic volume overload of the LV secondary to chronic and significant AR leads to progressive LV dilatation. As a result, the LV tends to adopt a more spherical shape (Fig. 7.50).

In the early stages of AR, LV systolic function remains normal. However, with chronic, severe AR the LV function will eventually decline.

LV measurements are critical for the serial follow-up of patients with AR. In particular, the LV end-diastolic dimension (LVEDD), the LV end-systolic dimension (LVESD) and the LVEF are important parameters used in the determination of the patient management and in aiding the timing of surgery in chronic severe, AR. For this reason, it is crucial that these measurements are accurately performed.

Measurements of the Aorta

In patients with AR, the aorta is often dilated. Measurements of the aorta that should be routinely performed include trans-sinus diameter at the sinuses of Valsalva, the ST junction, and the ascending aorta. In addition, the LVOT diameter is also measured. The measurement technique for each of these dimensions is described above under Aortic Stenosis (see Fig 7.18 and 7.19).

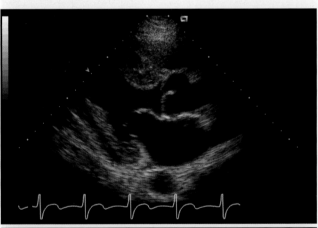

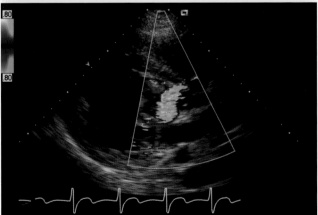

Figure 7.47 This is an example of a membranous ventricular septal defect (VSD) causing aortic regurgitation (AR). These diastolic frames were recorded from the parasternal long axis view. The 2D image shows that the right coronary cusp (RCC) is being 'sucked' into the VSD (*top*). The colour Doppler image shows AR due to prolapse of the RCC into the VSD (*bottom*).

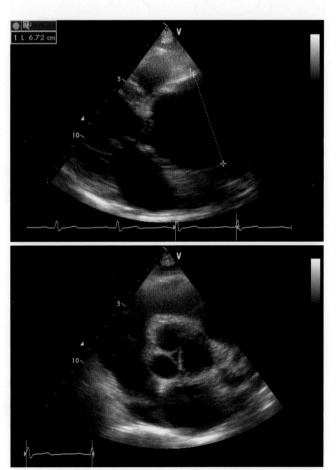

Figure 7.48 The parasternal long axis view shows marked dilatation of the aortic root, sinotubular junction and ascending aorta which measures 6.7 cm (*top*). From the parasternal short axis view a coaptation defect or 'hole' between the aortic cusps at end diastole is evident (*bottom*).

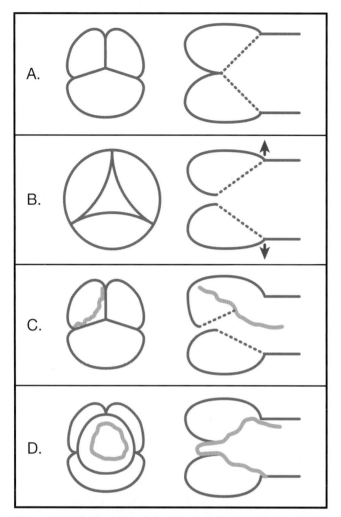

Figure 7.49 Mechanisms of functional aortic regurgitation (AR) in type A aortic dissection: **Panel A** is a schematic of normal aortic valve anatomy in the short-axis view (*left*) and long-axis view (*right*). The dotted lines represent the attachment of the leaflet tips to the sinotubular (ST) junction. Note that the leaflet tips coapt fully in diastole (*short-axis view*) and that the diameter of the ST junction is similar to that at the base of the annulus. **Panel B** shows incomplete leaflet closure which occurs when the ST junction dilates (*arrows*) relative to the aortic annulus; this leads to leaflet tethering and a persistent diastolic orifice which is best visualized in the short-axis view. **Panel C** shows aortic leaflet prolapse that occurs when the dissection extends into the aortic root and disrupts normal leaflet attachments to the aortic wall, thereby resulting in abnormal leaflet coaptation and eccentric AR. This is usually best visualized in the long-axis view where one or more leaflets are seen prolapsing into the left ventricular outflow tract in diastole. **Panel D** shows dissection flap prolapse that occurs when a redundant dissection flap prolapses through intrinsically normal aortic leaflets resulting in AR.

Reproduced from *J Am Coll Cardiol*, Vol. 36(3), Movsowitz HD, Levine RA, Hilgenberg AD, Isselbacher EM. Transesophageal echocardiographic description of the mechanisms of aortic regurgitation in acute type A aortic dissection: implications for aortic valve repair, page 885, © 2000 with permission from Elsevier.

Estimation of Severity

An accurate assessment of AR severity requires a comprehensive evaluation of indirect signs of AR severity on colour and spectral Doppler +/- the performance of quantitative calculations.

Indirect Signs for Assessing AR Severity: Colour Doppler Imaging

Colour Doppler flow imaging (CFI) provides a quick and easy method for identifying the presence of AR. CFI also provides indirect clues to the severity of AR. In particular, assessment of: (1) the colour jet height compared with the LVOT height, (2) the colour jet area compared with the LVOT area, and (3) the vena contracta width are very useful in determining the severity of AR. These methods are discussed in detail below; the criteria for defining the various grades of AR based on these methods are summarised in Table 7.7.

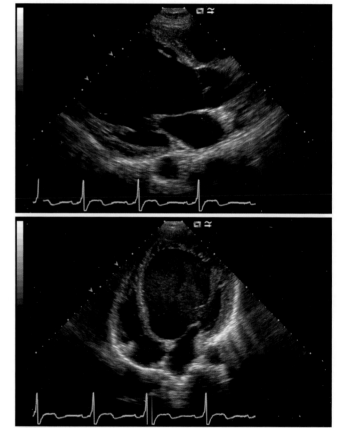

Figure 7.50 In this patient with chronic severe aortic regurgitation (AR), marked left ventricular (LV) dilatation is apparent from the parasternal long axis view (*top*) and the apical 4-chamber view (*bottom*). Observe that the LV is not only dilated but has also assumed a more spherical shape. LV dilatation occurs as a result of volume overloading of the ventricle due to AR; in particular, the diastolic volume LV is a combination of the forward stroke volume from the MV plus the AR regurgitant volume.

Table 7.7 Qualitative Colour Doppler Parameters for Grading Aortic Regurgitation Severity

Parameter	Mild	Moderate		Severe
Jet Height Ratio (%)	< 25	25-45	46-64	≥ 65
Jet Area Ratio (%)	<5	5-20	21-59	≥ 60
Vena Contracta Width (cm)	< 0.3	0.3-0.6		> 0.6

Using a Nyquist limit of 50–60 cm/s moderate regurgitation can be classified into mild-to-moderate and moderate-to-severe regurgitation as shown.
Reference: Zoghbi WA, Enriquez-Sarano M, Foster E, Grayburn PA, Kraft CD, Levine RA, Nihoyannopoulos P, Otto CM, Quinones MA, Rakowski H, Stewart WJ, Waggoner A, Weissman NJ; American Society of Echocardiography. Recommendations for evaluation of the severity of native valvular regurgitation with two-dimensional and Doppler echocardiography. *J Am Soc Echocardiogr*. 2003 Jul;16(7):777-802.

Colour Jet Height and Colour Jet Height Ratio

The maximal AR colour jet height (JH) is determined from the parasternal long axis view via colour Doppler imaging or a colour Doppler M-mode trace. In particular, comparison of the AR jet height to the LVOT height, the jet height ratio, provides a better estimation of AR severity (Fig. 7.51 and 7.52). Most commonly, an 'eyeball' evaluation, rather than direct measurements of the JH and/or jet height ratio is performed.

Colour Jet Area and Colour Jet Area Ratio

The AR colour jet area is determined from the colour Doppler image recorded from the parasternal short axis view at the level of the LVOT (Fig. 7.53). This colour jet area provides an estimation of the regurgitant orifice size. Comparison of the AR jet area to LVOT area, the jet area ratio, may also be performed from this view. As for the jet height ratio, most commonly, an 'eyeball' evaluation, rather than direct measurement of the jet area or jet area ratio is performed.

Vena Contracta Width

The vena contracta (VC) is defined as the narrowest part of the jet downstream from the narrowed orifice (see Fig. 1.21). With respect to regurgitant jets, the VC is the narrowest region of the regurgitant jet which occurs between the proximal flow convergence zone and the actual regurgitant jet. The vena contracta width (VC-W) of a regurgitant jet provides an estimate of the effective regurgitant orifice size.

VC-W is best measured when it appears perpendicular to the ultrasound beam. Therefore, for AR this measurement is best performed from the parasternal long axis view (Fig. 7.54). Measurement of the VC-W requires all three components of the regurgitant flow to be seen; this includes: (1) the flow convergence dome, (2) the VC and (3) the regurgitant jet.

> The VC-W is not the same as the AR jet height. The AR jet height is measured about 0.5-1.0 cm proximal to the aortic valve, while the VC-W is measured at the narrowest neck of the jet.

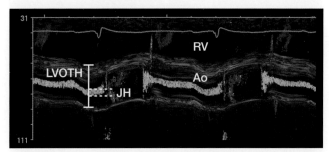

Figure 7.52 This M-mode trace was recorded from the parasternal long axis view. The M-mode cursor was placed through the left ventricular outflow tract. The aortic regurgitant (AR) jet appears as a mosaic line within the lumen of the aorta. The AR jet height (JH) is measured as the maximal anteroposterior diameter of the AR jet and the left ventricular outflow tract height (LVOTH) is measured using the leading edge to leading edge technique; both measurements are performed at end-diastole. Ao = aorta; RV = right ventricle.

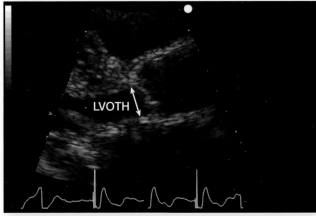

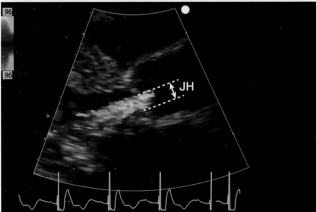

Figure 7.51 These images were recorded from a zoomed parasternal long axis view at end-diastole. The left ventricular outflow tract height (LVOTH) is measured at end-diastole at the hinge points of the valve (*top*). The colour Doppler image was recorded from the same view and shows an aortic regurgitant (AR) jet (*bottom*). The AR jet height (JH) is measured as the maximal height of the AR jet at the same level as the LVOTH. The regurgitant jet height-to-LVOT height ratio (JH/LVOTH) is simply calculated by dividing the AR jet height (JH) by the LVOT height.

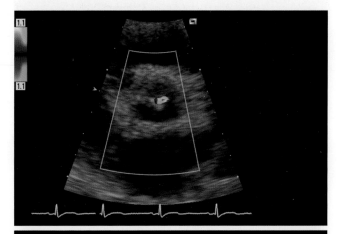

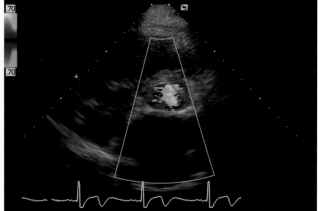

Figure 7.53 These diastolic still frame images were recorded from a parasternal short axis view at the level of the left ventricular outflow tract (LVOT). In the example of mild aortic regurgitation (AR), the AR jet area occupies only a small area of the LVOT (*top*). In the example of severe AR, the AR jet area fills the entire LVOT (*bottom*).

Limitations of CFI Indirect Signs

There are numerous technical and physiological factors that can affect the colour Doppler image which are unrelated to the severity of AR (Table 7.8).

In particular, recall that Doppler techniques detect the motion of moving red blood cells (RBC). As such any RBC in motion will create a Doppler shift and this Doppler shift is detected by the ultrasound machine. Therefore, RBCs displaced by the regurgitant jet will be incorporated into the 'colour regurgitant volume'. As a result, the RV will be overestimated on the colour Doppler display.

Another important technical factor to consider is the angle of interrogation between the ultrasound beam and the regurgitant jet. Like the heart, regurgitant jets are also 3-dimensional. Therefore, the sonographer must carefully angle through the valve to ensure that the regurgitant jet is clearly delineated.

A limitation of the VC-W in the assessment of regurgitation severity is the assumption that the regurgitant orifice is almost circular. However, the regurgitant orifice is often elliptic or irregular in shape. In these circumstances, the VC-W will vary depending on the imaging view. In addition, the VC-W value is a relatively small number so small measurement errors may lead to underestimation or overestimation of the AR severity. Furthermore, the VC-W cannot be used in the presence of multiple jets as the respective widths are not additive.

While not strictly a limitation, it is worthwhile mentioning that the maximal length of the AR jet into the LV cavity correlates poorly with the severity of AR (Fig. 7.55). Studies have indicated that the length of the regurgitant jet more closely relates to the driving pressure across the regurgitant orifice rather than to the regurgitant orifice size.

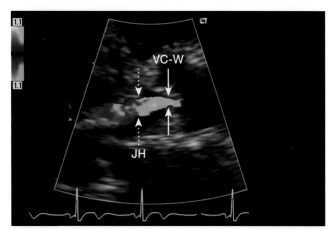

Figure 7.54 This colour flow Doppler image showing aortic regurgitation (AR) was recorded from a zoomed parasternal long axis view. The vena contracta width (VC-W) is measured at the narrowest neck of the AR flow region at the junction of flow convergence zone and the regurgitant jet. Note that the VC-W is performed at a different level to the AR jet height (JH) which is measured further into the LVOT.

Indirect Signs for Assessing AR Severity: Spectral Doppler

Indirect signs of AR severity can also be provided by PW and CW spectral Doppler signals. PW Doppler methods include the presence and/or the duration of diastolic flow reversal in the descending and abdominal aorta. CW Doppler methods include the intensity of the AR signal and the pressure half-time of the AR signal. The criteria for defining the various grades of AR via these methods are summarised in Table 7.9.

Intensity of AR CW Signal

In theory, the density or intensity of the spectral Doppler signal of a regurgitant jet is proportional to the number of RBCs travelling within the regurgitant jet. Therefore, the greater the regurgitation, the denser the regurgitant CW signal. For example, a weak AR Doppler signal is suggestive of relatively mild AR whereas a strong signal is suggestive of more significant AR (Fig. 7.56).

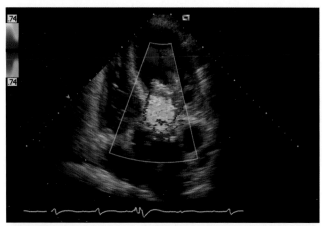

Figure 7.55 This image was recorded from an apical 5-chamber view. Aortic regurgitation (AR) is clearly severe based on the AR jet filling the entire left ventricular outflow tract. Despite this, the length of this jet is very short. The width of the AR jet at its origin rather than the AR jet length is important in determining the severity of AR.

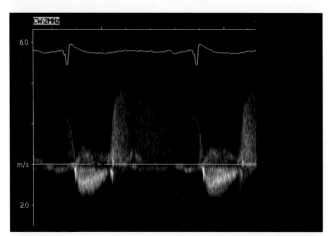

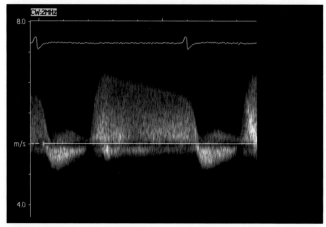

Figure 7.56 These continuous-wave spectral Doppler signals were recorded from two different patients. The weak aortic regurgitant (AR) signal *(left)* suggests that the severity of AR is not very significant. The stronger AR signal *(right)* suggests that the severity of AR is more significant in this patient compared with the patient on the left.

Flow Reversals

Pan-diastolic flow reversal in the descending aorta and/or abdominal aorta can be demonstrated by PW Doppler.

Interrogation of the descending aorta is performed from the suprasternal window. A PW sample volume is positioned approximately 1 cm distal to the origin of the left subclavian artery. Normally, flow within the descending aorta is predominantly systolic, although a small amount of retrograde, early diastolic flow can be recorded occasionally; when present this retrograde flow is less than 60 cm/s and occurs during the first 1/3 of diastole only (Fig. 7.57, left). When there is moderate or more AR, diastolic flow reversal is pan-diastolic (Fig. 7.57, right).

Investigation of the abdominal aorta is performed from the subcostal window. A PW sample volume is positioned within the abdominal aorta. Normally, from this view, only antegrade systolic flow towards the transducer (above the zero baseline) is observed (Fig. 7.58, left). When there is severe AR, pan-diastolic flow reversal may be detected (Fig. 7.58, right). In particular, the presence of pan-diastolic flow reversal in the abdominal aorta is a very specific sign of severe AR.

CFI and colour Doppler M-mode can also be used to identify diastolic flow reversal in the descending and abdominal aorta (Fig. 7.59).

AR Pressure Half-Time

The AR Doppler signal reflects the pressure gradient between the aorta and the LV during diastole. Therefore, the slope of this velocity spectrum reflects the rate of decline in the pressure gradient between the aorta and the LV over the diastolic period. The highest AR velocity occurs shortly after the aortic valve closes, when the pressure gradient between the LV and aorta is at its maximum. The AR velocity then gradually declines throughout diastole due to: (1) a fall in the aortic diastolic pressure due to forward run-off to the periphery as well as regurgitation back into the LV, and (2) the rise in LV diastolic pressure due to normal mitral inflow into the LV as well as the aortic RV back into the LV.

Table 7.8 Physiological and Technical Factors affecting CFI in the Assessment of Valvular Regurgitation

Physiological Factors	Technical Factors
Driving pressure	Angle of intercept
Eccentric jets	Attenuation
Influence of coexistent jets or flow streams	Colour Doppler gain and filter settings
Receiving chamber size and compliance	Colour velocity scale
Regurgitant volume	Frame rate
Size and shape of regurgitant orifice	Pulse repetition frequency
Wall impingement	Transducer frequency

Table 7.9 Qualitative Spectral Doppler Parameters for Grading Aortic Regurgitation Severity

Parameter [Ref.]	Mild	Moderate	Severe
Flow reversal – Descending aorta (PW) [1,2]	Brief, early diastolic	Intermediate	Pan-diastolic
Flow reversal – Abdominal aorta (PW) [3]	-	-	Pan-diastolic
Intensity of AR signal (CW) [1,2]	Incomplete or faint	Dense	Dense
AR pressure half-time (CW) (ms) [1,2] ^	> 500	500 – 200	< 200

CW = contunous-wave Doppler; PW = pulsed-wave Doppler.
^ dependent upon LV compliance: e.g. may be lengthened in chronic adaptation to severe AR, may be shortened with other causes of elevated LV diastolic pressures in absence of severe AR.
Reference: [1] Zoghbi WA, Enriquez-Sarano M, Foster E, Grayburn PA, Kraft CD, Levine RA, Nihoyannopoulos P, Otto CM, Quinones MA, Rakowski H, Stewart WJ, Waggoner A, Weissman NJ; American Society of Echocardiography. Recommendations for evaluation of the severity of native valvular regurgitation with two-dimensional and Doppler echocardiography. *J Am Soc Echocardiogr.* 2003 Jul;16(7):777-802; **[2]** Lancellotti P, Tribouilloy C, Hagendorff A, Moura L, Popescu BA, Agricola E, Monin JL, Pierard LA, Badano L, Zamorano JL; European Association of Echocardiography. European Association of Echocardiography recommendations for the assessment of valvular regurgitation. Part 1: aortic and pulmonary regurgitation (native valve disease). *Eur J Echocardiogr.* 2010 Apr;11(3):223-44; **[3]** Takenaka K, Dabestani A, Gardin JM, Russell D, Clark S, Allfie A, Henry WL. A simple Doppler echocardiographic method for estimating severity of aortic regurgitation. *Am J Cardiol.* 1986 Jun 1;57(15):1340-3.

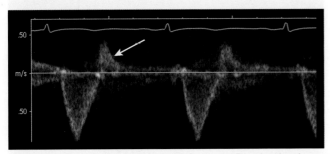 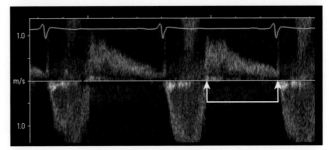

Figure 7.57 These two pulsed-wave (PW) spectral Doppler signals were recorded from the suprasternal window with the PW sample volume placed approximately 1 cm distal to the origin of the left subclavian artery. In the normal patient with no aortic regurgitation (AR) (*left*), there is a short period of low velocity, early diastolic flow reversal; this flow lasts less than one-third of diastole and the peak early diastolic velocity is < 60 cm/s (*arrow*). In the patient with severe AR (*right*), pan-diastolic flow reversal is present (*between the arrows*); that is, flow reversal occurs throughout the diastolic period.

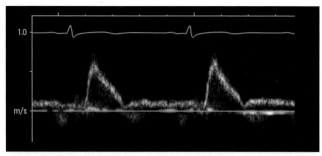 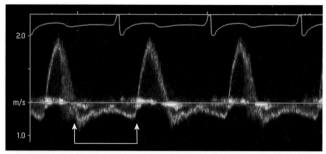

Figure 7.58 These pulsed-wave (PW) spectral Doppler signals were recorded from the subcostal window with the PW sample volume placed within the abdominal aorta. In the normal patient (*left*), flow is antegrade only (above the zero baseline) and no flow reversal is noted during diastole. In the patient with severe AR (*right*), pan-diastolic flow reversal is present (*between the arrows*); this appears as flow below the zero baseline.

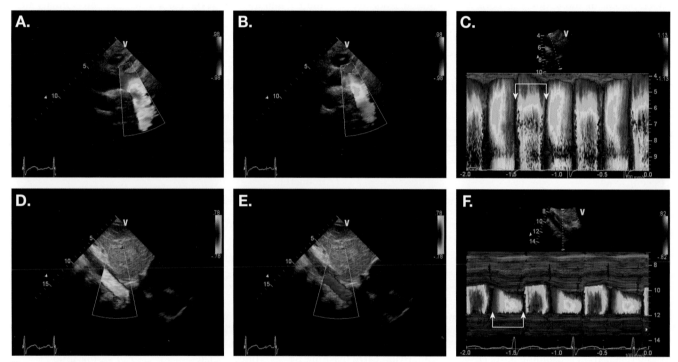

Figure 7.59 Colour flow Doppler images (CFI) and colour Doppler M-mode traces from a patient with severe aortic regurgitation (AR) are shown. The top images were recorded from the suprasternal view of the aorta while the bottom images were recorded from the subcostal view of the abdominal aorta. CFI of the descending aorta during systole **(A)** shows aliased flow away from the transducer; aliased flow occurs due to the increased stroke volume being ejected from the left ventricle. CFI of the descending aorta during diastole **(B)** shows red flow towards the transducer; this flow is very abnormal and is consistent with significant AR. The colour Doppler M-mode trace **(C)** was recorded with the M-mode cursor placed along the descending aorta. Observe that during the entire diastolic period colour is seen filling the aortic lumen (*arrows*); this represents pan-diastolic flow reversal in the descending aorta. CFI of the abdominal aorta during systole **(D)** shows aliased flow toward the transducer. CFI of the abdominal aorta during diastole **(E)** shows blue flow away from the transducer; this flow is very abnormal and is consistent with severe AR. The colour Doppler M-mode trace **(F)** was recorded with the M-mode cursor transecting the abdominal aorta. Observe that during the entire diastolic period colour is seen filling the aortic lumen (*arrows*); this represents pan-diastolic flow reversal in the abdominal aorta.

The rate of decline of the AR velocity spectrum can be measured using the slope and pressure half-time (P½t). The slope is measured as the rate of decline of the aortic velocities from their initial peak while the P½t represents the time taken for the pressure to fall to half of its initial value (Fig. 7.60).

With mild AR, the initial early diastolic pressure gradient between the aorta and LV is high and this gradient gradually decreases throughout diastole due to a gradual decline in aortic diastolic pressure and a gradual rise in the LVEDP (Fig. 7.61, left). In the presence of acute severe AR, the aortic pressure declines rapidly and the LVEDP rises rapidly. As a result the P½t of the AR signal shortens significantly (Fig. 7.61, right).

Limitations of Spectral Doppler Indirect Signs

The intensity of the AR signal can be affected by a number of factors. For example, Doppler gain affects the overall

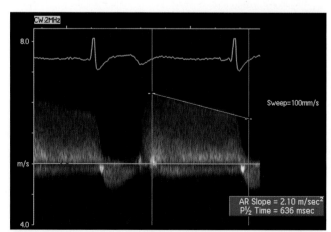

Figure 7.60 The aortic regurgitant (AR) Doppler velocity spectrum reflects the rate of decline in the pressure gradient between the aorta and the LV during diastole. From this spectrum the slope of the AR signal (AR Slope) and the pressure half-time (P½ Time) can be derived.

intensity of the regurgitant jet; if the gain is set too low then the signal intensity will also be decreased. In addition, poor alignment of the AR jet with the Doppler beam will result in a suboptimal AR signal; this is especially a problem with eccentric jets.

The presence of pan-diastolic flow reversal in the descending and abdominal aorta strongly supports the diagnosis of severe AR. Because diastolic velocities are low it is crucial that the velocity scale and wall filters are appropriately set to optimally display these low velocity signals. In particular, if the wall filters are set too high, pan-diastolic flow may be totally missed. Pan-diastolic flow reversal within the descending and abdominal aorta in the *absence* of severe AR may also be encountered. For example, reduced aortic compliance as seen with advancing age may increase the velocity and prolong the duration of diastolic reversal in the absence of significant AR. Pan-diastolic flow reversal in the absence of severe AR may also occur when there is another low pressure 'outlet' from the aorta; that is, when there is flow from the aorta into another low pressure chamber or vessel. Examples include significant left-to-right shunts through a patent ductus arteriosus, an aorto-pulmonary window, or an aorta-pulmonary artery fistula, and in an aortic dissection where flow from the aorta enters the low pressure false lumen.

Importantly, the AR P½t simply reflects the pressure gradient between the aorta and LV over diastole. Therefore, this gradient is not only dependent on the severity of AR, it is also dependent on systemic vascular resistance (SVR) and LV compliance. For example, the P½t can be short in the *absence* of severe AR when there is poor LV compliance. In this case, there is a

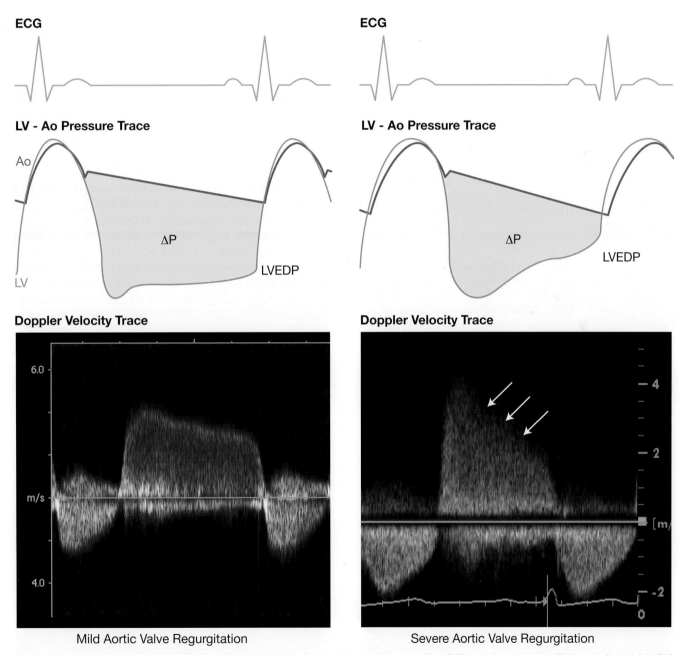

Mild Aortic Valve Regurgitation

Severe Aortic Valve Regurgitation

Figure 7.61 The aortic regurgitant (AR) Doppler signal is a function of the pressure gradient (ΔP) between the aorta (Ao) and left ventricle (LV) during diastole. The top schematic illustrates the pressure tracings of the aorta and the LV while the Doppler velocity spectra corresponding to these schematics are displayed below. With mild AR (*left*), the ΔP between the aorta and the LV in early diastole is high. This gradient then gradually decreases throughout diastole due to a gradual decline in the aortic diastolic pressure and only a small increase in the LV end-diastolic pressure (LVEDP). The resultant Doppler spectrum depicts a reasonably 'flat' (prolonged) deceleration slope. With acute, severe AR (*right*), the aortic pressure drops rapidly during diastole and the LVEDP also rises rapidly. This results in a rapid decline (shortening) of the diastolic slope of the regurgitant Doppler velocity curve (*triple arrows*).

rapid rise in LV diastolic pressure due to myocardial causes; this leads to an elevation in the LVEDP and a subsequent shortening of the P½t. Conversely, in chronic, severe AR, the AR P½t may be prolonged when there is a compliant LV; that is, the LV is able to accept a large volume of blood without a significant increase in the LVEDP. Furthermore, the AR P½t may be lengthened when the SVR is increased or when there is a dilated and compliant aorta.

Quantitative Methods for AR Severity
Quantitative calculations for the assessment of AR severity include the:
• Regurgitant volume,
• Regurgitant fraction,
• Effective regurgitant orifice area.
The criteria for defining the various grades of AR based on these methods are listed in Table 7.10.

Regurgitant Volume
Regurgitant volume (RV) is defined as the volume of blood that leaks (regurgitates) through an incompetent valve. RV can be calculated using the SV method or the proximal isovelocity surface area (PISA) method.

Estimation of LVEDP from the AR Doppler Signal
Recall that the AR velocity reflects the pressure difference between the aorta and the LV. Therefore, the AR velocity at end-diastole reflects the pressure difference between the aortic diastolic pressure and the LVEDP:

Equation 7.12

$$4V_{AR\text{-}ED}^2 = AoDP - LVEDP$$

where $V_{AR\text{-}ED}^2$ = peak AR velocity at end-diastole (m/s)
LVEDP = left ventricular end-diastolic pressure (mm Hg)
AoDP = aortic diastolic pressure (mm Hg)

By measuring the peak AR velocity at end-diastole and the aortic diastolic blood pressure (DBP), the above equation can be rearranged to calculate the LVEDP:

Equation 7.13

$$LVEDP = DBP - 4V_{AR\text{-}ED}^2$$

where LVEDP = left ventricular end-diastolic pressure (mm Hg)
DBP = diastolic blood pressure (mm Hg)
$V_{AR\text{-}ED}^2$ = peak AR velocity at end-diastole (m/s)

Caveat: The important limitation of this calculation is that two relatively large pressures (aortic diastolic blood pressure and the aorta-LV pressure gradient) are used to estimate a relatively low pressure (LVEDP).

A. Stroke Volume Method
The basic concepts of SV calculations and how these calculations can be used to estimate the RV are described in Chapter 1. Recall that the calculation of RV is based on the estimations of the SV across the leaking valve and the SV across a competent (non-leaking) valve. In the case of AR, the RV can be calculated from the LVOT SV and, providing that there is no MR, the SV across the mitral annulus:

Equation 7.14

$$RV_{AR} = SV_{LVOT} - SV_{MA}$$

where RV_{AR} = aortic regurgitant volume (mL)
SV_{LVOT} = stroke volume across left ventricular outflow tract (mL)
SV_{MA} = stroke volume across mitral annulus (mL)

Recall that the SV is a product of the CSA and the VTI. Therefore, to perform this calculation four sets of measurements are required (Fig. 7.62):
1. LVOT diameter (used to calculate the LVOT CSA)
2. LVOT VTI
3. mitral annular diameter (used to calculate the mitral annular CSA)
4. mitral annular VTI

In the event that MR is present, the aortic RV can still be calculated by substituting the RVOT SV for the mitral annular SV, providing that there is no intracardiac shunt and no significant regurgitation across the pulmonary valve.
The limitations of RV calculations via this method are the same as those limitations described for SV calculations (see Chapter 2). In particular, common errors in mitral annular measurements include: (1) not measuring the annulus at the correct phase of the cardiac cycle, and (2) not measuring the annulus at the same site as the VTI signal. Importantly, any error in the annular measurement is magnified because the diameter is squared to derive the CSA. Common VTI measurements errors include: (1) non-parallel alignment between the Doppler beam and blood flow, (2) incorrect placement of the PW Doppler sample volume (especially at the mitral annulus), (3) failure to optimise the Doppler trace, and (4) not tracing the modal velocity.

B. PISA Method
The RV via PISA method is based on first estimating the effective regurgitant orifice area (EROA) via the PISA technique (discussed below) and then by tracing the VTI of the regurgitant jet. Calculation of the RV via this technique is based on the standard SV equation. Recall that the SV is a product of the CSA and VTI. Based on this relationship between SV, CSA and VTI, the RV is simply derived by substituting the RV for SV, EROA for CSA and

---

Table 7.10 **Quantitative Methods for Grading Aortic Regurgitation Severity**

Parameter	Mild	Moderate		Severe
Regurgitant Volume (mL)	< 30	30-44	45-59	≥ 60
Regurgitant Fraction (%)	<30	30-39	40-49	≥ 50
Effective Regurgitant Orifice Area (cm²)	< 0.10	0.10-0.19	0.20-0.29	≥ 0.30

Moderate regurgitation can be classified into mild-to-moderate and moderate-to-severe regurgitation as shown.
Reference: Zoghbi WA, Enriquez-Sarano M, Foster E, Grayburn PA, Kraft CD, Levine RA, Nihoyannopoulos P, Otto CM, Quinones MA, Rakowski H, Stewart WJ, Waggoner A, Weissman NJ; American Society of Echocardiography. Recommendations for evaluation of the severity of native valvular regurgitation with two-dimensional and Doppler echocardiography. *J Am Soc Echocardiogr.* 2003 Jul;16(7):777-802.

RV using 2D LV Volumes

In theory, it is possible to calculate the aortic RV using the SV derived from the LV end-diastolic and end-systolic volumes (SV_{2D}) and the mitral annular SV (SV_{MA}). The SV_{2D} reflects the amount of blood being ejected from the LV across the LVOT; therefore, the SV_{2D} can be used as a surrogate for the LVOT SV (SV_{LVOT}). Therefore, to calculate the aortic RV, the SV_{MA} is subtracted from the SV_{2D} ($RV_{AR} = SV_{2D} - SV_{MA}$).

This method, however, is not advised for the calculation of RV as: (1) 2D echocardiography has a known tendency to significantly underestimate LV volumes and, therefore, the SV_{2D} will also be underestimated, and (2) calculation of the SV_{MA} in itself has significant limitations (typically the largest source of error in the RV calculation is the SV_{MA} rather than the SV_{LVOT}).

VTI of the regurgitant jet (VTI_{RJ}) for the VTI:

Equation 7.15

$$RV = EROA \times VTI_{RJ}$$

where RV = regurgitant volume (mL)

EROA = effective regurgitant orifice area (cm^2)

VTI_{RJ} = velocity time integral of regurgitant jet (cm)

Therefore, to perform this calculation for AR the following are required (see Fig. 7.63):

1. EROA for AR
2. VTI of the AR jet

The limitations of RV calculations via this method are the same as those limitations described for the calculation of the EROA via the PISA technique (see Chapter 2 and below).

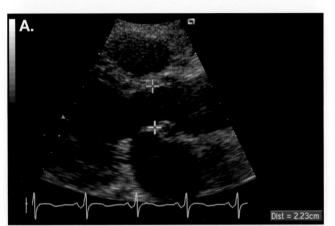

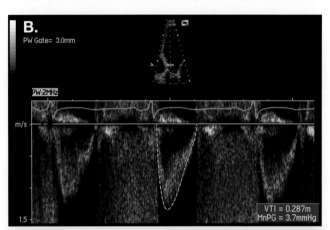

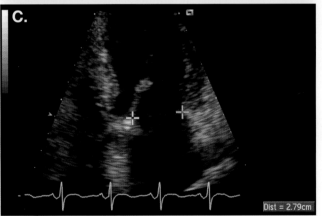

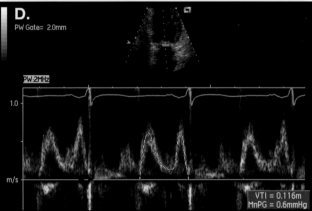

Figure 7.62 The regurgitant volume (RV) for aortic regurgitation (AR) is calculated from the stroke volume across the left ventricular outflow tract (SV_{LVOT}) and the SV across the mitral annulus (SV_{MA}). SV_{LVOT} is derived from the LVOT diameter and velocity time integral (VTI). The LVOT diameter is measured from a zoomed parasternal long axis view of the LVOT **(A)**. At mid-systole callipers are placed from the inner edge of the junction between the anterior aortic wall and the interventricular septum to the inner edge of the junction between the posterior aortic wall and the anterior leaflet of the mitral valve, perpendicular to the aortic root. From an apical 5-chamber view, the LVOT VTI is recorded via a pulsed-wave (PW) Doppler signal with a 2-4 mm sample volume placed 0.5 cm proximal to the aortic valve **(B)**.

SV_{MA} is derived from the mitral annular diameter and VTI at the mitral annulus. The mitral annular diameter is measured from a zoomed apical 4-chamber view of the mitral valve at early diastole (2-3 frames after end-systole); callipers are placed from where the leaflets insert into the ventricular myocardium using the inner edge to inner edge technique **(C)**. From the same apical 4-chamber view the mitral annular VTI is recorded via a PW Doppler signal with a 1-2 mm sample volume placed at the level of the mitral annulus; the VTI is traced along the modal velocity **(D)**. The aortic RV in this example is calculated as:

RV_{AR} = SV_{LVOT} - SV_{MA}
= ($CSA_{LVOT} \times VTI_{LVOT}$) - ($CSA_{MA} \times VTI_{MA}$)
= ($0.785 \times 2.23^2 \times 28.7$) - ($0.785 \times 2.79^2 \times 11.6$)
= 112 - 71
= 41 mL

The aortic RF in this example is calculated as:
RF_{AR} = ($RV \div SV_{LVOT}$) × 100
= (41 ÷ 112) × 100
= 37%

Regurgitant Fraction

The regurgitant fraction (RF) is defined as the regurgitant volume expressed as a percentage of the total SV across the incompetent valve. Therefore, in the case of AR, the aortic RF is simply derived from the aortic RV and the SV across the LVOT (Fig. 7.62):

Equation 7.16

$$RF_{AR} = (RV_{AR} \div SV_{LVOT}) \times 100$$

where RF_{AR} = aortic regurgitant fraction (%)

RV_{AR} = aortic regurgitant volume (mL)

SV_{LVOT} = stroke volume across left ventricular outflow tract (mL)

The limitations of this calculation include those limitations described for RV calculations via the SV method (see above).

Technical Tip for RV and RF calculations via SV method

The RV and RF calculations via the SV method are calculated from the SV derived from the LVOT and the mitral annulus. Knowledge of the normal values for the VTI and annular diameters at these sites is helpful when undertaking these measurements. For example, in a patient with AR, the mitral annular parameters would be expected to be close to the normal range; therefore, if the mitral annular VTI measures are well outside the normal range, this would be a clue that this measurement has not been performed correctly.

The normal VTI and annular measurements for the LVOT and mitral annulus are tabled below.

Measurement	Normal values
Mitral annular diameter	3.0 - 3.5 cm
Mitral annular VTI	10 - 13 cm
LVOT diameter	1.8 - 2.2 cm
LVOT VTI	18 - 22 cm

Effective Regurgitant Orifice Area

The effective regurgitant orifice area (EROA) is the size of the 'hole' in the incompetent valve. The EROA can be calculated using the SV method or the PISA method.

A. Stroke Volume Method

The SV method for calculating the EROA is based on the relationship between SV, CSA and VTI as described by Equation 7.15 above. Therefore, if the RV and the VTI of the regurgitant signal are measured, this equation can be rearranged to calculate the EROA:

Equation 7.17

$$EROA = RV \div VTI_{RJ}$$

where EROA = effective regurgitant orifice area (cm²)

RV = regurgitant volume (mL)

VTI_{RJ} = velocity time integral of regurgitant jet (cm)

B. PISA Method for EROA

The basic concepts of the PISA principle in the calculation of the effective orifice area are described in Chapter 1. Recall that this calculation is based on the continuity principle which states that flow proximal to a narrowed orifice must equal flow through the narrowed orifice.

In the case of AR, the EROA can be calculated from the radius of the proximal flow convergence dome, the velocity at the radius and the peak velocity of the AR jet (Fig. 7.63):

Equation 7.18

$$EROA = (2\pi\, r^2 \times V_N) \div V_{AR}$$

where EROA = effective regurgitant orifice area (cm²)

$2\pi r^2$ = surface area of the hemispheric shell derived from the flow convergence radius [r] proximal to the stenotic valve (cm²)

V_N = colour Nyquist limit at the radial distance of the hemispheric shell (cm/s)

V_{AR} = peak velocity of the aortic regurgitant jet (cm/s)

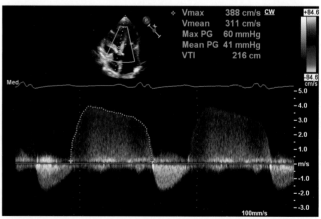

Figure 7.63 The effective regurgitant orifice area (EROA) for aortic regurgitation (AR) is calculated via the proximal isovelocity surface area (PISA) method. From a zoomed apical 5-chamber view of the aortic valve (*left*), the proximal flow convergence radius is measured on the aortic side in early diastole; callipers are placed between the aortic leaflets and the first aliased velocity. The colour Nyquist limit at this radius is the velocity at the top of the colour bar as flow is towards the transducer so the velocity at which flow aliases is the velocity at the top of the colour bar. From the continuous-wave Doppler trace (*right*), the peak early diastolic velocity (Vmax) is measured. The aortic EROA in this example is calculated as:

EROA = $(2\pi r^2 \times V_N) \div V_{AR}$

= $(6.28 \times 0.6^2 \times 44.7) \div 388$

= 0.26 cm²

From the EROA and the VTI of the AR signal, the RV can also be calculated as:

RV = EROA × VTI_{AR}

= 0.26 × 216

= 56 mL

PISA Tips for calculating the Aortic EROA and RV

- Zoom on the aortic valve (AV) from the view that best displays the AR jet (e.g. left parasternal long axis view, right parasternal long view or any apical view).
- Only attempt this measurement when a hemispheric PISA dome is seen on the aortic side of the AV.
- Shift the colour baseline in the direction of flow to increase the PISA dome (baseline is shifted downwards from the parasternal views and upwards from the apical views).
- Simply decreasing the colour velocity scale rather than baseline shift will also increase the size of the PISA dome.
- From an early diastolic frame, measure the PISA radius from the AV to the first aliased velocity (at the red-blue interface).
- When measuring the peak AR velocity, ensure that the ultrasound beam is aligned parallel with flow; remember that this might be a left parasternal view or a right parasternal view.
- Because the EROA is a measure of the regurgitant orifice area in early diastole, the VTI of the AR jet should be traced to calculate the aortic RV as this reflects the severity of AR over the entire diastolic period (see Equation 7.15).

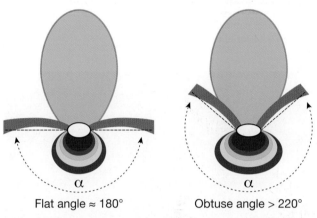

Flat angle ≈ 180°   Obtuse angle > 220°

Figure 7.64 Calculation of the effective regurgitant orifice area (EROA) via the proximal isovelocity surface area (PISA) method assumes that the flow convergence zone proximal to the regurgitant orifice is flat with a flow convergence angle (α) of 180 degrees (*left*). However, when there is an ascending aortic aneurysm, the flow convergence zone may be obtuse with the flow convergence angle (α) often exceeding 220° (*right*). This leads to 'flattening' of the flow convergence zone; in this situation, the EROA calculated via equation 7.18 will be underestimated. Therefore, when the flow convergence zone proximal to the regurgitant orifice is > 220°, the corrected EROA should be calculated by multiplying the EROA by α/180. The angle α is either estimated or measured off-line.

The limitations of EROA calculations are the same as those limitations described for the PISA method (see Chapter 2). In particular, for AR the feasibility of this technique is limited by aortic valve calcifications. In addition, it should be remembered that this method estimates the EROA at early diastole and this EROA may not be maintained over the entire diastolic period. Therefore, the aortic RV via PISA should also be estimated to provide an assessment of AR severity over the diastolic period. In the presence of ascending aortic aneurysms, the valvular plane may be deformed with the flow convergence angle often exceeding 220 degrees. In this situation, calculation of the EROA without angle correction will underestimate the EROA (Fig. 7.64). Therefore, angle correction is required to account for the non-planar flow convergence zone; calculation of the corrected EROA is derived by multiplying the EROA by α/180.

Other Signs of Severe AR

As discussed, there are a number of limitations associated with indirect signs and quantitative methods for assessing the severity of AR. Therefore, it is important to be aware of other clues that are indicative of severe AR. These signs along with the mechanism for each sign are summarised in Table 7.11 and illustrated in figures 7.65-7.67.

Table 7.11 Additional Echocardiographic Signs of Severe Aortic Regurgitation

Signs of Severe AR	Mechanism
Pulsatile aortic arch on 2D imaging from suprasternal window	Marked increase in stroke volume (SV) of the left ventricle (LV) and a hyperdynamic circulation.
Hyperdynamic motion of interventricular septum on M-mode (Fig. 7.65, A)	Occurs as a result of LV volume overload and an unequal SV of the LV compared with the right ventricle.
Diastolic mitral regurgitation via PW Doppler, CFI and/or colour Doppler M-mode (Fig. 7.66, A)	Consistent with a significant elevation in left ventricular end-diastolic pressure (LVEDP); following atrial contraction there is a transient increase in LVEDP above LA pressure while the mitral valve is still open.
Premature mitral valve closure on M-mode (Fig. 7.67)	Consistent with a marked elevation in LVEDP (usually only seen with acute, severe AR); when LVEDP exceeds LA pressure, the mitral valve closes prematurely.
Premature aortic valve opening on M-mode (Fig. 7.65, B)	Consistent with a marked elevation in LVEDP (usually only seen with acute, severe AR); when LVEDP exceeds aortic diastolic pressure the aortic valve opens prematurely.
Increased LVOT velocities via PW Doppler (Fig. 7.65, C)	Increased SV across the left ventricular outflow tract due to the combination of forward SV across the mitral valve plus the aortic RV.
Short transmitral deceleration time (Fig. 7.66, A)	With severe AR, there may be a rapid and sharp rise in the LV diastolic pressure. This causes a marked reduction in the transmitral deceleration time which mimics a restrictive filling pattern.
'A-dip' on AR CW Doppler (Fig. 7.66, B)	Consistent with a significant elevation in LVEDP in association with increased LA pressure and low diastolic aortic pressure. Following atrial contraction, there is an increase in the LV diastolic pressure which reduces the aorta-LV pressure gradient at this point in time.

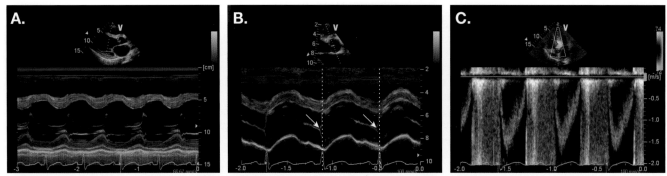

Figure 7.65 In this patient with severe aortic regurgitation (AR), three classic signs of severe AR are shown. On the M-mode trace of the left ventricle, hyperdynamic motion of the interventricular septum is evident **(A)**. On the M-mode trace recorded through the aortic valve, premature opening of the aortic valve (*arrows*) prior to the onset of systole (*vertical dashed lines*) is seen **(B)**. Also observe on this M-mode trace the marked 'thickening' of the anterior aortic wall. This patient also had an anterior aortic root abscess associated with infective endocarditis; this area of thickening was considered to be consistent with phlegmon (pus). Increased left ventricular outflow tract (LVOT) velocities are seen on the pulsed-wave Doppler trace recorded with the sample volume within the LVOT **(C)**. See Table 7.11 for further details.

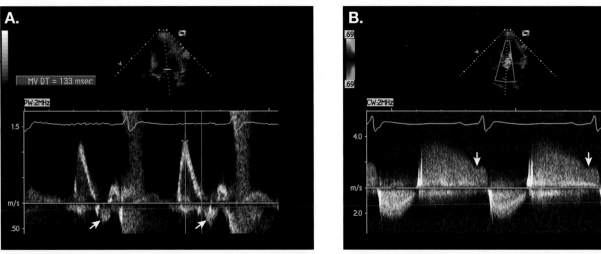

Figure 7.66 In this patient with severe aortic regurgitation (AR) three classic signs of an elevated left ventricular end-diastolic pressure are shown. On the pulsed-wave Doppler transmitral inflow trace, a "restrictive filling pattern" is shown (E velocity = 1.2 m/s, A velocity = 0.3 m/s, E:A ratio 4, DT = 133 ms) as well as diastolic mitral regurgitation (*arrows*) **(A)**. On the continuous-wave Doppler trace, an 'a-dip' is seen interrupting the AR jet (*arrows*) **(B)**; the AR pressure half-time was measured at 206 ms. See Table 7.11 for further details.

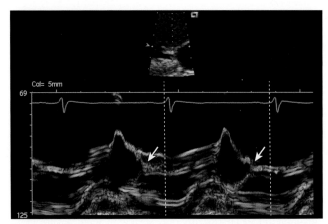

Figure 7.67 On this M-mode trace recorded through the mitral valve leaflets, premature closure of the mitral valve (*arrows*) prior to the end of diastole (*vertical dashed lines*) is seen. Also note the appearance of fine diastolic flutter of the mitral valve which is seen when the aortic regurgitation jet slams into the open mitral leaflets. See Table 7.11 for further details.

Key Points

Anatomy of the Aortic Valve
- The aortic valve is the cardiac 'centrepiece'; it consists of three almost equal-sized, semilunar leaflets that are named based on the origin of the coronary arteries: right coronary cusp, left coronary cusp and non-coronary cusp.
- Aortic cusps are supported by a crown-like annulus which can be defined by three rings: the virtual ring, the ST ridge and the ventriculoarterial junction.
- The aortic root is defined by the length of the aortic leaflets and is bounded by the virtual ring and the ST junction.
- Three expanded pouches of the aortic root form the sinuses of Valsalva.

Aortic Stenosis: Basic Concepts
- *Aetiology:* congenital (e.g. unicuspid or bicuspid valve) or acquired (e.g. senile calcification or rheumatic); other causes of LVOT obstruction include fixed congenital lesions above and below the valve (supravalvular or subvalvular AS) and dynamic LVOT obstruction.
- *Pathophysiology:* in early stages of AS, LV size is normal with normal systolic function; LVH develops to maintain cardiac output; in advanced stages of the AS, LV dilates and systolic function declines.
- *Clinical manifestations:* angina, syncope or presyncope and congestive cardiac failure (CCF).

Role of Echo in Aortic Stenosis
- Determine the aetiology of the lesion (e.g. congenital, degenerative, rheumatic)
- Exclude other causes of LVOT obstruction
- Assess LV size and systolic and diastolic function
- Assess the degree of LVH
- Measure aortic dimensions
- Estimate the severity of stenosis via:
  - Peak velocity
  - Mean gradient
  - AVA and indexed AVA
  - Dimensionless severity index (velocity ratio)
- Identify associated valve lesions

Stress Echo in Aortic Stenosis
- Role in patients with asymptomatic severe AS at rest:
  - determine if the patient has exercise-induced symptoms,
  - to assess the compliance of the aortic valve, the haemodynamic severity of the stenosis, LV contractile reserve and diastolic function, and other components such as MR and pulmonary pressures.
- Role in patients with low flow, low gradient AS with associated LV systolic dysfunction:
  - Differentiate true AS from pseudo-AS
  - *True AS:* AVA unchanged with increasing cardiac output
  - *Pseudo-AS:* AVA increases with increasing cardiac output

Aortic Regurgitation: Basic Concepts
- *Aetiology:* annular or aortic root dilatation, annular or aortic root distortion, cuspal abnormalities, loss of commissural support
- *Functional classification:* based on the mechanisms of AR and the surgical repair techniques:
  - Type I: aortic cusp motion is normal and AR occurs due to the enlargement or dilatation of the aorta or due to cuspal perforation; subcategorised in types Ia, Ib, Ic and Id,
  - Type II: leaflet prolapse as a result of excessive cusp tissue or commissural disruption,
  - Type III: leaflet restriction as a result of calcification, thickening, and fibrosis of the aortic valve leaflets.
- *Pathophysiology:* dependent on whether acute or chronic AR:
  - Acute severe AR: associated with a normal LV size and a marked elevation in LVEDP,
  - Chronic severe AR: LV dilatation, eccentric hypertrophy, LVEDP usually normal, LV systolic function may be normal but gradually declines.
- *Clinical manifestations:* CCF, myocardial ischaemia and chest pain may occur due to increased myocardial oxygen demand caused by significant LV dilatation and increased LV mass.

Role of Echo in Aortic Regurgitation
- Determine the aetiology of the lesion (e.g. congenital, degenerative, or rheumatic)
- Assess LV size and systolic function
- Measure aortic dimensions
- Estimate the severity of regurgitation via:
  - Indirect signs by colour Doppler imaging (e.g. jet height, jet area, VC-W)
  - Indirect signs by spectral Doppler (e.g. intensity of AR jet, diastolic flow reversal in descending and abdominal aorta, P½t)
  - Quantification by calculation of aortic RV, RF and/or EROA

Further Reading (listed in alphabetical order)

Aortic Valve Anatomy

Anderson RH. Clinical anatomy of the aortic root. *Heart*. 2000 Dec;84(6):670-3.

Ho SY. Structure and anatomy of the aortic root. *Eur J Echocardiogr*. 2009 Jan;10(1):i3-10.

Piazza N, de Jaegere P, Schultz C, Becker AE, Serruys PW, Anderson RH. Anatomy of the aortic valvar complex and its implications for transcatheter implantation of the aortic valve. *Circ Cardiovasc Interv*. 2008 Aug;1(1):74-81.

Aortic Stenosis

Bahlmann E, Cramariuc D, Gerdts E, Gohlke-Baerwolf C, Nienaber CA, Eriksen E, Wachtell K, Chambers J, Kuck KH, Ray S. Impact of pressure recovery on echocardiographic assessment of asymptomatic aortic stenosis: a SEAS substudy. *JACC Cardiovasc Imaging*. 2010 Jun;3(6):555-62.

Baumgartner H, Hung J, Bermejo J, Chambers JB, Evangelista A, Griffin BP, Iung B, Otto CM, Pellikka PA, Quiñones M; American Society of Echocardiography; European Association of Echocardiography. Echocardiographic assessment of valve stenosis: EAE/ASE recommendations for clinical practice. *J Am Soc Echocardiogr*. 2009 Jan;22(1):1-23

Chambers JB. Aortic stenosis. *Eur J Echocardiogr*. 2009 Jan;10(1):i11-9.

Chambers J. Low "gradient", low flow aortic stenosis. *Heart*. 2006 Apr;92(4):554-8.

Dumesnil JG, Pibarot P, Carabello B. Paradoxical low flow and/or low gradient severe aortic stenosis despite preserved left ventricular ejection fraction: implications for diagnosis and treatment. *Eur Heart J*. 2010 Feb;31(3):281-9.

Stress Echo in Aortic Stenosis

Ennezat PV, Maréchaux S, Iung B, Chauvel C, LeJemtel TH, Pibarot P. Exercise testing and exercise stress echocardiography in asymptomatic aortic valve stenosis. *Heart*. 2009 Jun;95(11):877-84.

Grayburn PA, Eichhorn EJ. Dobutamine challenge for low-gradient aortic stenosis. *Circulation*. 2002 Aug 13;106(7):763-5.

O'Connor K, Lancellotti P, Donal E, Piérard LA. Exercise echocardiography in severe asymptomatic aortic stenosis. *Arch Cardiovasc Dis*. 2010 Apr;103(4):262-9.

Aortic Regurgitation

El Khoury G, Glineur D, Rubay J, Verhelst R, d'Acoz Y, Poncelet A, Astarci P, Noirhomme P, van Dyck M. Functional classification of aortic root/valve abnormalities and their correlation with etiologies and surgical procedures. *Curr Opin Cardiol*. 2005 Mar;20(2):115-21.

Lancellotti P, Tribouilloy C, Hagendorff A, Moura L, Popescu BA, Agricola E, Monin JL, Pierard LA, Badano L, Zamorano JL; European Association of Echocardiography. European Association of Echocardiography recommendations for the assessment of valvular regurgitation. Part 1: aortic and pulmonary regurgitation (native valve disease). *Eur J Echocardiogr*. 2010 Apr;11(3):223-44.

le Polain de Waroux JB, Pouleur AC, Goffinet C, Vancraeynest D, Van Dyck M, Robert A, Gerber BL, Pasquet A, El Khoury G, Vanoverschelde JL. Functional anatomy of aortic regurgitation: accuracy, prediction of surgical repairability, and outcome implications of transesophageal echocardiography. *Circulation*. 2007 Sep 11;116(11 Suppl):I264-9.

Zoghbi WA, Enriquez-Sarano M, Foster E, Grayburn PA, Kraft CD, Levine RA, Nihoyannopoulos P, Otto CM, Quinones MA, Rakowski H, Stewart WJ, Waggoner A, Weissman NJ; American Society of Echocardiography. Recommendations for evaluation of the severity of native valvular regurgitation with two-dimensional and Doppler echocardiography. *J Am Soc Echocardiogr*. 2003 Jul;16(7):777-802.

Mitral Valve Disease

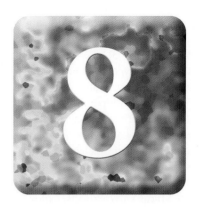

Anatomy of the Mitral Valve

The mitral valve is one of four cardiac valves in the heart. It is composed of endocardium and connective tissue. With respect to surface anatomy, the mitral valve lies to the left of the sternum behind the fourth intercostal space (see Fig. 7.1). Internally, the mitral valve is located slightly posterior and lateral to the aortic valve; it is in close proximity to the other cardiac valves (see Fig. 7.2). The primary function of the mitral valve is to prevent the backflow of blood into the left atrium (LA) during ventricular systole.

The mitral valve is considered in terms of the mitral valve "complex". This complex is composed of several individual components which all need to function in unison to ensure competency of the valve. The five principal anatomical components that form the mitral valve complex include (Fig. 8.1): (1) the valve annulus, (2) the valve leaflets, (3) the commissures, (4) the tendinous cords, and (5) the papillary muscles and left ventricular (LV) myocardium. The mitral valve derives its name from the anatomical resemblance of the valve 'complex' to a bishop's mitre.

Mitral Annulus

The mitral annulus depicts the anatomical junction between the LA and the LV and it provides a structural support to the mitral leaflets. From an 'en face' 2D perspective, the mitral annulus is D-shaped (Fig. 8.1,D). The straight border of the anterior annulus is closely aligned with the aortic valve; the region between the straight border of the anterior annulus and the aortic valve is the aortomitral curtain (Fig. 8.1,C). This curtain depicts the region of fibrous continuity between the anterior mitral leaflet and the aortic valve. At each end of the aortomitral curtain are the right and left fibrous trigones which anchor the annulus to the LV walls. The right fibrous trigone is continuous with the membranous interventricular septum, mitral annulus, tricuspid annulus, and non-coronary cusp of the aortic annulus; the atrioventricular (AV) conduction bundle passes through this trigone. The left fibrous trigone is beneath the left coronary cusp of the aortic annulus and attaches to the adjacent LV wall.

The posterior mitral annulus is less developed and is more flexible than the anterior mitral annulus as it is not connected to

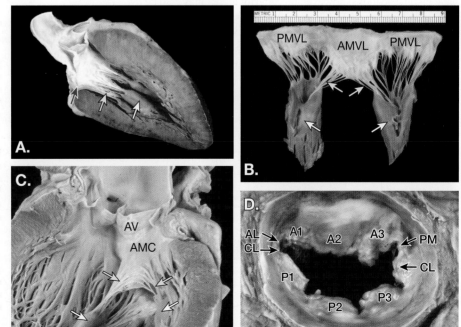

Figure 8.1 These gross pathological specimens show the normal anatomy of the mitral valve complex. **Photo A** shows a long axis of the mitral valve complex. **Photo B** shows the mitral valve opened out (cut open along the middle scallop of the posterior mitral leaflet). **Photo C** shows the mitral valve complex with the left ventricular outflow tract opened from the front. **Photo D** shows a short axis of the mitral valve from the left atrial aspect.

The annulus supports the mitral leaflets (*red arrow in A*) and appears D-shaped from the left atrial aspect (D). The anterior mitral valve leaflet (AMVL) has twice the height and half the annular length of the posterior mitral valve leaflet (PMVL) (B). Between the aortic valve (AV) and AMVL is an area of fibrous continuity, the aortomitral curtain (AMC) (C). In short axis, the three distinct scallops of the PMVL (P1, P2 and P3) and the corresponding opposing regions of the AMVL (A1, A2 and A3) can be seen (D); in addition, the commissural leaflets (CL) extending between the ends of the closure line and the mitral annulus can also be seen. The posteromedial (PM) and anterolateral (AL) commissures which separate the anterior and posterior leaflets are also depicted. The connections of the tendinous cords (*yellow arrows*) between the papillary muscles (*white arrows*) and the mitral leaflets are also shown (A-C); observe that each papillary muscle supplies cords to both mitral leaflets (B). See text for further details.

By permission of Mayo Foundation for Medical Education and Research. All rights reserved. Courtesy of William D. Edwards, MD.

any rigid structure. For this reason, dilatation and calcification most commonly occur at the posterior mitral annulus.

When viewed from a 3D perspective during systole, the mitral annulus has a hyperbolic paraboloid shape or "saddle" shape (Fig. 8.2). In particular, the annulus has two high points or peaks at the midpoint of the anterior and posterior leaflets with the anterior point peaking above the posterior point. There are also two low points or troughs located posteromedially and anterolaterally near the commissures. This saddle-shaped configuration of the mitral annulus and mitral leaflets is important in the assessment of mitral valve prolapse (see Mitral Valve Prolapse below).

Mitral Leaflets

There are two mitral valve leaflets. The anterior leaflet, also known as the aortic leaflet, has a semi-circular shape and attaches to approximately one-third of the mitral annular circumference. As stated above, there is fibrous continuity between the anterior mitral leaflet and the aortic valve; this is the aortomitral curtain.

The posterior leaflet, also known as the mural leaflet, has a quadrangular shape and attaches to approximately two-thirds of the mitral annular circumference. Although the posterior leaflet occupies two-thirds of the mitral annulus, the base-to-tip diameter or "height" of the posterior leaflet is less than the anterior leaflet. Therefore, the anterior and posterior leaflets are almost equal in area (Fig. 8.1,B & D).

The posterior leaflet usually has well defined indentations or clefts which divides the leaflet into scallops. While the number of scallops in the posterior leaflet varies markedly from individual to individual, three distinct, asymmetrical scallops can be identified in most individuals (Fig. 8.1,D). These scallops are identified as lateral, middle and medial; the middle scallop is most commonly the largest. For simplification, these scallops are also referred to as P1 (lateral scallop), P2 (middle scallop), and P3 (medial scallop); this is the so-called Carpentier anatomic classification. The anterior leaflet does not have distinct scallops; however, the anterior leaflet may also be subdivided into the A1, A2, and A3 regions corresponding to the opposing posterior leaflet scallops (Fig. 8.1,D).

On the atrial surface of the valve there are two zones in the anterior leaflet and three zones in the posterior leaflet (Fig. 8.3). The zone near the free margin (tips) of both leaflets is the rough zone. This thick zone, which extends for several millimetres, depicts the coaptation surface where the two leaflets meet during ventricular systole; this zone is the main region for cordal attachments. The clear zone is also present in both leaflets; this zone is thin and almost translucent and receives no cordal attachments. The basal zone, which is only present on the posterior leaflet, is located closest to the mitral annulus and also receives cordal attachments. The clear zone of the anterior leaflet and the basal and clear zones of the mitral leaflets are also referred to as the smooth zones.

At the microscopic level, the mitral valve is composed of three layers (Fig. 8.4). The fibrosa is found at the base of the free edge of the valve and is composed of dense collagen with occasional elastin fibres; this layer forms the basic mechanical support of the mitral valve. The spongiosa is the 'middle' layer and this layer contains loosely arranged connective tissue, proteoglycans and a small amount of elastic fibres and is most prominent in the free edge of the valve. The atrialis covers the atrial aspect of the spongiosa and is continuous with the LA endocardium; this layer is composed of thin endothelium-covered collagen and elastic tissue.

Mitral Commissures

When closed, the anterior and posterior leaflets meet to form a curved closure line or zone of apposition which when viewed from the LA resembles a smile. At each end of the closure line is a commissure (Fig. 8.1,D). The commissures are named anterolateral and posteromedial based on their anatomical location. These commissures divide the leaflets into anterior and posterior. Because the closure does not extend to the annulus, there is a portion of the mitral leaflet tissue which is distinct from the leaflets, between the ends of the closure line and the mitral annulus; the tissue in these areas is referred to as the "commissural" leaflets.

Tendinous Cords

The tendinous cords, or chordae tendinae, are string-like fibres that attach the mitral leaflets to either the papillary muscles or directly to the ventricular myocardium (Fig. 8.1, A-C). These cords are primarily responsible for anchoring the valve, maintaining ventricular geometry, and preventing prolapse of the mitral leaflets into the LA during systole. There are some 120 cords which are classified into various groups according to their origin and site of attachment to the mitral leaflets. Detailed cordal anatomy is beyond the scope of this text; however, cords can generally be described as primary, secondary or basal cords. Primary cords, or cords of the first order, insert into the free edge of the leaflets; these cords are also commonly referred to as free edge cords or rough

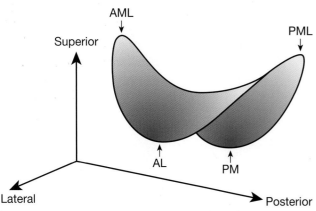

Figure 8.2 This schematic illustrates the 3D saddle-shape of the mitral annulus. The midpoints of the anterior mitral leaflet (AML) and posterior mitral leaflet (PML) form two high points and the posteromedial (PM) and anterolateral (AL) commissures form two low points of the mitral annulus.

> There are no cordal attachments between the mitral valve and the interventricular septum (IVS). Fibrous or fibromuscular strands extending between the IVS and the papillary muscles or the ventricular wall are false tendons. Unlike true tendinous cords, false tendons do not attach to the mitral leaflets. False tendons are common anatomic variants of the normal left ventricle and should not be mistaken for pathologies such as ruptured cords, vegetations or subaortic membranes. False tendons are also known as anomalous cords, false cords, ventricular bands, pseudotendons, aberrant tendons or 'heart strings'.

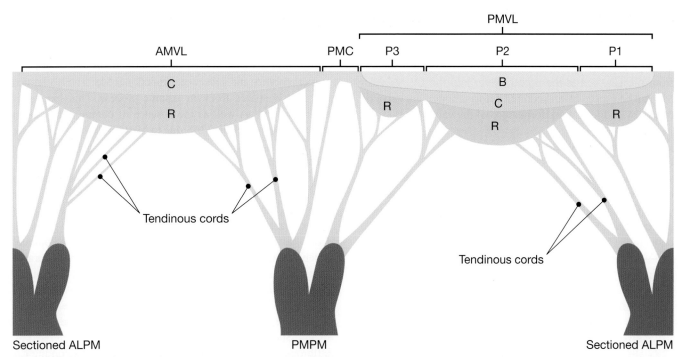

Figure 8.3 This schematic illustrates the various zones of the mitral leaflets. The anterior mitral valve leaflet (AMVL) has a clear zone (C) and a rough zone (R) while the posterior mitral valve leaflet (PMVL) has a clear zone (C), a rough zone (R) and a basal zone (B). The clear and basal zones are also referred to as the smooth zone. The rough zone depicts the region of leaflet coaptation. The basal and rough zones have cordal insertions while there are no cordal insertions to the clear zone. See text for further details. ALPM = anterolateral papillary muscle; PMC = posteromedial commissure; PMPM = posteromedial papillary muscle; P1 = medial scallop; P2 = middle scallop; P3 = lateral scallop.

edge cords. Commissural cords, which support the free edge of the commissural leaflets, are also primary cords. Secondary cords, or cords of the second order, insert beyond the free margin, typically inserting at the junction of the rough and clear zones on the ventricular surface of the leaflets; these cords are commonly referred to as strut cords. Free edge, commissural and strut cords characteristically branch in fan-like fashion. Basal cords, or cords of the third order, originate from the LV wall or small ventricular trabeculations and attach to the basal zone on the ventricular surface of the posterior leaflet.

Papillary Muscles and Left Ventricular Myocardium

There are two prominent groups of papillary muscles arising from the LV walls between the apical and middle thirds of the ventricle (Fig. 8.1,B). Contraction of the papillary muscles pulls the two mitral leaflets toward one another thereby promoting valve closure during systole. The papillary muscle groups are named based on their position in relation to the anterolateral and posteromedial mitral commissures.

The anterolateral papillary muscle has a single body which bifurcates into two heads. The posteromedial papillary muscle usually has two bodies and trifurcates into three heads. Each papillary muscle provides cords to both leaflets.

The anterolateral papillary muscle is supplied by branches of the left anterior descending coronary artery and left circumflex artery while the posteromedial papillary muscle is supplied by the posterior descending coronary artery. For this reason, the posteromedial muscle, which has a single coronary artery supply, is more vulnerable to ischaemic episodes and complications of myocardial infarction.

The two papillary muscles in the LV are commonly referred to as anterolateral and posteromedial. This terminology is a consequence of anatomists taking the heart out of the body and sitting it on its apex when describing the orientation of the structures within it. However, the true orientation of the papillary muscles with respect to their position in the body is: (1) inferiorly and anteriorly, against the septum, and (2) superiorly and posteriorly, towards the posterior margin of the heart.

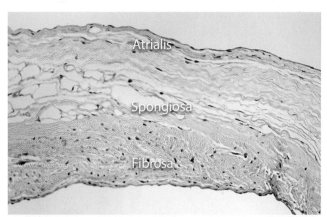

Figure 8.4 This histological specimen shows the three layers of the mitral valve (haematoxylin and eosin stain at x 400 objective). The fibrosa is found at the base of the free edge of the valve and is composed of dense collagen with occasional elastin fibres. The spongiosa is the 'middle' layer and contains loosely arranged connective tissue, proteoglycans and a small amount of elastic fibres. The atrialis covers the atrial aspect of the spongiosa in the basal and mid portion of the valve; this layer is composed of thin endothelium-covered collagen and elastic tissue.
Reproduced from www.e-heart.org with permission from E Rene Rodriguez, M.D., Professor of Pathology, Cleveland Clinic.

Mitral Stenosis

Aetiology of Mitral Stenosis

Mitral stenosis (MS) refers to the obstruction of blood flow from the LA, across the mitral valve, into the LV. Valvular MS can be caused by an acquired deformation of the valve or, rarely, by congenital malformations of the valve.

Congenital Mitral Stenosis

Congenital causes of MS are rare and are usually associated with other cardiac defects. Most commonly, congenital causes of MS will be detected in infancy or childhood. The anatomy of congenital MS is variable and may involve a number of components of the mitral valve complex. Examples of congenital MS include annular hypoplasia, commissural fusion, shortened cords, anomalous mitral arcade, anomalous position of the papillary muscles, and parachute mitral valves.

Acquired Mitral Stenosis

The most common causes of acquired MS include rheumatic valve disease and extensive mitral annular calcification.

Rheumatic Valve Disease

As discussed in Chapter 7, rheumatic valve disease occurs secondary to an episode or recurrent episodes of acute rheumatic fever (ARF) which occurs due to a group A beta-haemolytic Streptococcus infection. Rheumatic valvular disease occurs several years after the initial episode of ARF as an autoimmune response.

Rheumatic MS results from fusion of the mitral commissures, thickening and fibrosis of the mitral leaflets, leaflet calcification, and thickening, shortening and matting of the tendinous cords (Fig. 8.5, left). The resultant narrowing of the orifice forms a "fish mouth" appearance (Fig. 8.5, right). Calcification of the leaflets and commissures is also common.

Extensive Mitral Annular Calcification

Mitral annular calcification (MAC) is a degenerative process most commonly involving the posterior annulus of the mitral valve (Fig. 8.6). MAC frequently occurs in patients with mitral valve diseases such as fibroelastic deficiency of the mitral valve or Barlow's disease, in patients with systemic hypertension or metabolic diseases such as diabetes and hypercalcemia, in patients on renal dialysis, or in elderly

individuals (so-called degenerative calcific disease); MAC is also encountered in patients with Marfan syndrome.

Heavy or excessive MAC may extend into the body of the valve leaflets and subvalvular apparatus leading to reduced leaflet mobility and subsequent functional MS. The leaflet tips are usually spared from the calcific process. This sparing of the leaflet tips as well as the absence of commissural fusion differentiates functional MS due to MAC from rheumatic MS.

Other Causes of LV Inflow Obstruction

Congenital obstruction to LV inflow can also occur due to cor triatriatum or supravalvular stenosing ring; these rare congenital heart abnormalities are often associated with other congenital heart abnormalities.

Cor triatriatum occurs during embryological development when the common pulmonary vein fails to be incorporated into the LA. As a result there is a perforated interatrial, fibromuscular membrane that partitions the LA into a proximal accessory chamber that receives the pulmonary veins and a distal 'true' LA which contains the LA appendage and the fossa ovalis. Supravalvular stenosing mitral ring is characterised by a fibrous, shelf-like membrane of connective tissue on the LA side of a structurally normal mitral valve.

Obstruction to LV inflow can also occur due to mass lesions such as large mitral valve vegetations or left atrial myxomas which prolapse through the mitral valve in diastole.

Pathophysiology of Mitral Stenosis

Mitral stenosis decreases the mitral valve area and, therefore, obstructs LA emptying during diastole. In an attempt to maintain an adequate forward flow through the mitral valve, the LA pressure increases in order to increase the driving pressure across the stenotic mitral valve. This increase in LA pressure leads to dilatation of the LA. LA dilatation increases the risk for the development of atrial fibrillation (AF) and/or LA thrombus formation.

Furthermore, the passive backward transmission of elevated LA pressures to the pulmonary circulation leads to secondary pulmonary hypertension (PHTN). PHTN in patients with MS may also occur due to pulmonary arteriolar constriction caused by LA and pulmonary venous hypertension, organic obliterative changes in the pulmonary vascular bed, and/or pulmonary vasoconstriction.

In response to the increased pulmonary arterial pressures, the

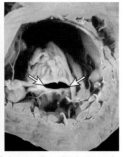

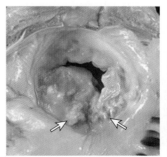

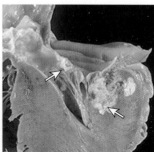

Figure 8.5 Gross pathological examples of rheumatic mitral stenosis are shown from two different patients in a long axis section (*left*) and a short axis section (*right*). The long axis section shows mitral leaflet and and cordal thickening, a large left atrial thrombus (*) is also present. The short axis section shows diffuse leaflet thickening; the fish-mouth appearance of the valve is caused by commissural fusion (*arrows*). By permission of Mayo Foundation for Medical Education and Research. All rights reserved. Courtesy of William D. Edwards, MD.

Figure 8.6 These gross pathological specimens show mitral annular calcification viewed from the left atrium (*left*) and via a cut section of myocardium (*right*). Calcific nodules appear at the base of the anterior mitral leaflet (*arrows*) and extend into the leaflet body; observe that the tips of the mitral leaflets are spared and commissural fusion is absent. Reproduced from Kumar et al: Robbins and Cotran Pathologic Basis of Disease, 8th Edition, Chapter 11, page 402, © 2009 Saunders, with permission from Elsevier.

right ventricle (RV) dilates. RV systolic function may be normal or impaired depending upon the degree and chronicity of PHTN. RV dilatation also leads to dilatation of the tricuspid annulus and varying degrees of tricuspid regurgitation (TR). Haemodynamically significant TR leads to an elevated jugular venous pressure, liver congestion, ascites, and pedal oedema.

Clinical Manifestations of Mitral Stenosis

The clinical manifestations of MS relate to the pathophysiological responses to chronic, severe MS. The common clinical manifestations of severe MS occur due to pulmonary venous congestion, a low cardiac output, AF or right heart failure. Common, atypical and rare symptoms of MS as well as their causes are summarised in Table 8.1.

Role of Echocardiography in Mitral Stenosis

The aims and objectives of echocardiography in the assessment of MS are to:
- Determine the aetiology of the lesion (e.g. rheumatic, congenital, other causes of LV inflow obstruction),
- Score the mitral valve (to determine suitability for balloon valvuloplasty),
- Assess the LA (LA size, presence or absence of thrombus),
- Assess LV size and systolic function,
- Estimate the severity of the stenosis (including an estimation of right ventricular systolic pressure),
- Identify associated valve lesions.

Aetiology of Mitral Stenosis

As stated above, the most common cause of acquired MS is rheumatic valve disease. Other causes of functional MS include extensive MAC and obstruction of LV inflow by large mass lesions. Congenital causes of MS include cor triatriatum, supravalvular stenosing ring and parachute mitral valves.

Rheumatic Mitral Stenosis

On the 2D echocardiographic examination, rheumatic MS is characterised by diastolic doming of the mitral valve leaflets. This occurs due to commissural fusion of the rheumatic mitral leaflets. Diastolic doming of the mitral leaflets is best seen from the parasternal long axis and apical views (Fig. 8.7). In particular, from the parasternal long axis view the anterior mitral leaflet demonstrates a characteristic "hockey stick" appearance. The posterior mitral leaflet, being 'shorter' than the anterior mitral leaflet, is often fixed with restricted motion. From the parasternal short axis view, commissural fusion with a significant reduction in the mitral valve orifice is observed (Fig. 8.8). Variable degrees of valvular calcification and subvalvular thickening may also be seen on the 2D images (Fig. 8.9).

> While diastolic doming of the anterior mitral leaflet is a 'hallmark' feature of MS, this may not be evident when the leaflets become extensively fibrosed or calcified. In this instance, the leaflets appear fixed and immobile.

Mitral Annular Calcification

As stated above, MAC of the posterior mitral annulus is also common amongst various patient populations. On the 2D echocardiographic examination, MAC appears as an area of increased echogenicity with acoustic shadowing distal to the MAC. Functional MS can occur when MAC extends into the anterior annulus and towards the base of the mitral leaflets; calcification may also extend down into the tendinous cords. On the 2D echocardiographic examination, extensive areas of increased echogenicity are noted (Fig. 8.10). On real-time imaging, the mitral leaflet tips appear mobile while the bases of the leaflets appear rigid. In particular, this acoustic shadowing artefact is very useful in differentiating calcification from mitral annular abscesses and tumours (Fig. 8.11).

Table 8.1 Clinical Symptoms of Mitral Stenosis

Clinical Symptoms	Cause
Common Symptoms	
Dyspnoea (most common symptom) occurs at rest or on exertion Paroxysmal nocturnal dyspnoea Orthopnoea	Pulmonary congestion due to elevated left atrial (LA) pressures and/or pulmonary hypertension (PHTN) Exacerbated by: • increase in blood flow across stenotic valve (e.g. exercise, pregnancy) or • reduction in diastolic filling time (e.g. atrial fibrillation, tachycardia)
Fatigue	Decreased cardiac output, especially with exercise Exacerbated by atrial fibrillation
Pulmonary oedema	Pulmonary congestion due to elevated LA pressures and/or PHTN
Right heart failure (e.g. hepatic congestion, ascites and/or peripheral oedema)	Secondary due to PHTN
Palpitations	Atrial fibrillation
Atypical or Rare Symptoms	
Chest pain (resembling angina)	Likely secondary due to PHTN
Haemoptysis (blood-stained sputum)	Increased pulmonary pressures and vascular congestion or ruptured bronchial veins
Persistent cough	Compression of bronchi by the enlarged LA
Hoarseness (Ortner's or cardiovocal syndrome)	Secondary to compression of the left recurrent laryngeal nerve against the pulmonary artery by a markedly dilated LA or left pulmonary artery (very rare)

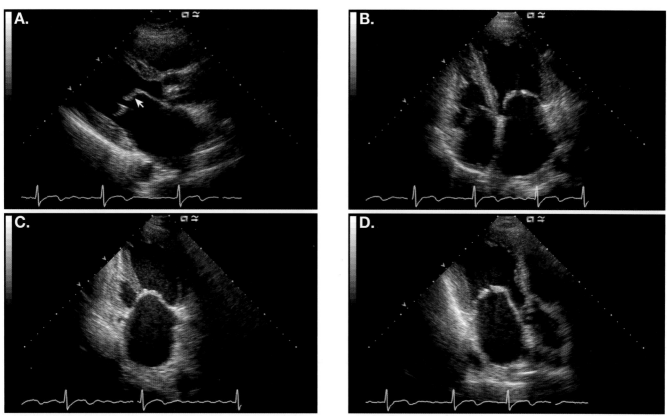

Figure 8.7 The characteristic appearances of rheumatic mitral stenosis are shown in the parasternal long axis view of the left ventricle (A), apical 4-chamber view (B), apical 2-chamber view (C) and apical long axis view (D). Observe the diastolic doming of the mitral valve leaflets which is most prominent in the anterior mitral leaflet (*arrow*); from the parasternal long axis view, diastolic doming of the anterior mitral valve leaflet exhibits characteristic "hockey-stick" appearance. Rheumatic aortic valve disease is also apparent from the parasternal long axis and apical long axis views.

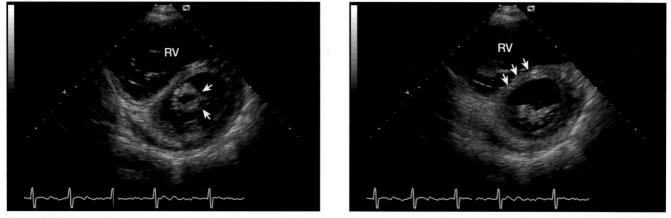

Figure 8.8 These two images were acquired from the parasternal short axis view at the tips of the mitral leaflets. The diastolic frame (*left*) shows narrowing of the mitral orifice and commissural fusion which is most extensive at the anterolateral commissure (*arrows*). The systolic frame (*right*) shows systolic flattening of the interventricular septum consistent with pulmonary hypertension (*arrows*). Right ventricular (RV) dilatation is also seen.

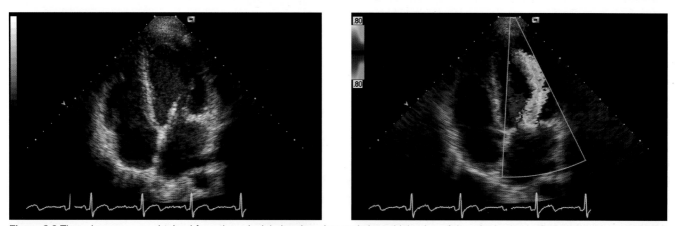

Figure 8.9 These images were obtained from the apical 4 chamber view and show thickening of the mitral valve leaflets which extends into the tendinous cords creating a subvalvular tunnel effect (*left*). Colour flow imaging highlights this subvalvular tunneling effect (*right*).

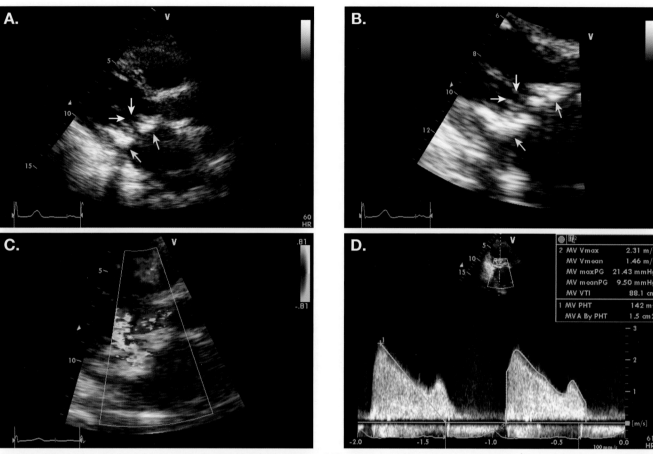

Figure 8.10 These images show an example of extensive mitral annular calcification causing functional mitral stenosis. Observe that in the parasternal long axis views there is extensive calcification of the anterior and posterior mitral annuli (*yellow arrows*) with sparing of the mitral leaflet tips (*white arrows*) (A & B). On the colour Doppler image, turbulent flow across the mitral valve is noted (C). Via continuous-wave Doppler, the mean pressure gradient (MV mean PG) across the mitral valve is 10 mm Hg and the pressure half-time (PHT) is 142 ms (D).

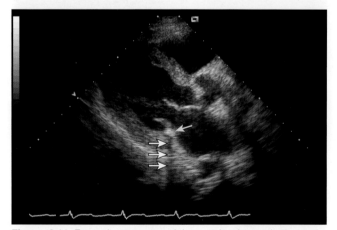

Figure 8.11 From the parasternal long axis view, mitral annular calcification is seen as a bright echogenic area in the posterior mitral annulus (*yellow arrow*) with acoustic shadowing distal to the calcified annulus (*white arrows*).

Cor Triatriatum and Supravalvular Stenosing Ring

Cor triatriatum and supravalvular stenosing ring are rare congenital heart abnormalities that result in the partial obstruction of the LV inflow. On the 2D echocardiographic examination, the diagnosis of cor triatriatum can be made by identifying the interatrial membrane transecting the LA cavity (Fig. 8.12). This membrane is best viewed when it is imaged perpendicular to the ultrasound beam; therefore, it is best seen from the apical views. In particular, because the membrane is relatively thin it can be easily missed from the parasternal long axis view when the membrane is aligned

parallel to the ultrasound beam. Location of the membrane orifice can be made by colour flow Doppler imaging; importantly, it should be noted that there can be more than one orifice within the membrane.

On the 2D echocardiographic examination, a supravalvular mitral ring can also be diagnosed by identification of an interatrial membrane transecting the LA cavity. The distinction between cor triatriatum and supravalvular mitral ring is based on the location of the membrane within the LA (Fig. 8.13). In cor triatriatum, the membrane is found superior to the ostium of the LA appendage while with a supravalvular mitral ring the membrane is located inferior to the ostium of the LA appendage and immediately superior to the mitral annulus.

Parachute Mitral Valve

A parachute mitral valve (PMV) is characterised by a single or fused papillary muscle which occurs due to abnormal LV myocardial compaction during embryological development. Therefore, all cord attachments to the mitral leaflets arise from this single papillary muscle; the cords are usually also underdeveloped. The single papillary muscle and abnormal cords restrict the motion of the mitral leaflets, effectively causing MS. A PMV often occurs as part of Shone's anomaly. On 2D echocardiography, a PMV can be diagnosed from the parasternal short axis view by the presence of a single papillary muscle or from the apical 4-chamber view by a characteristic diastolic, "pear-shaped" appearance of the LA and the funnel-shaped mitral valve leaflets (Fig. 8.14).

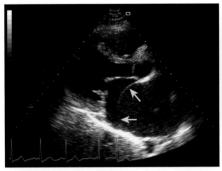 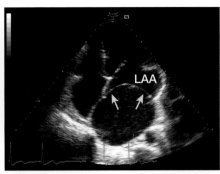 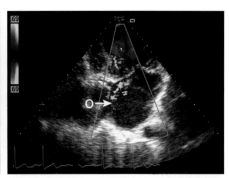

Figure 8.12 These images were recorded from a patient with cor triatriatum. From the parasternal long axis view (*left*) and from the apical 4-chamber view (*middle*), the interatrial membrane is seen transecting the left atrial cavity (*yellow arrows*). This membrane appears as a fine linear structure; on real-time imaging this membrane bows towards the mitral orifice during diastole. Observe that the membrane is superior to the left atrial appendage (LAA). On the colour Doppler image, the orifice in the membrane (O) is identified by the turbulent flow at the medial aspect of the membrane (*right*).

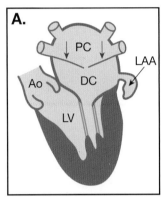 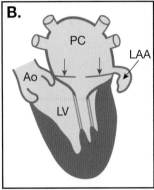

Figure 8.13 Panel A: This schematic illustrates the anatomy associated with cor triatriatum. Observe that the obstructing membrane (*red arrows*) transects the left atrium (LA) superior to the ostium of the left atrial appendage (LAA) dividing the LA into a proximal chamber (PC) which receives the pulmonary veins and a distal chamber (DC).
Panel B: This schematic illustrates the anatomy associated with a supravalvular mitral stenosing ring. Observe that the obstructing membrane dividing the LA is located inferior to the ostium of the LAA and immediately superior to the mitral annulus (*red arrows*). Ao = aorta; LV = left ventricle.

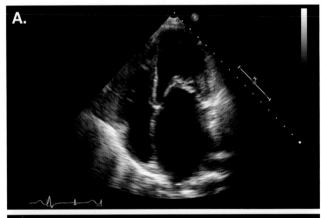 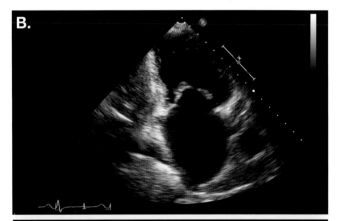

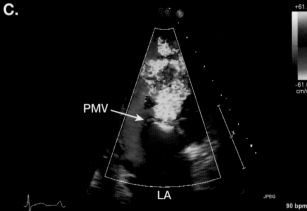 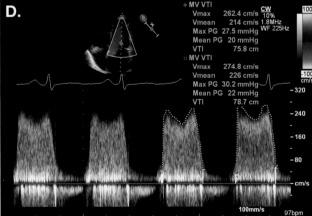

Figure 8.14 These diastolic frames, recorded from the apical 4-chamber view (A) and the apical 2-chamber view (B), show the characteristic pear-shaped appearance of the left atrium (LA) associated with a parachute mitral valve (PMV). The LA forms the base of the 'pear' and the funnel-shaped mitral valve leaflets form the top of the 'pear'. From the apical 4-chamber view, colour flow Doppler imaging confirms the presence of mitral stenosis across the PMV (C); the mean transmitral pressure gradient via continuous-wave Doppler was 21 mm Hg (D).

Shone's anomaly, also known as Shone's complex or Shone's syndrome, is a rare congenital heart condition characterised by four left-sided obstructive cardiac lesions. These defects include: (1) a supravalvular mitral ring or membrane, (2) a parachute mitral valve, (3) subaortic stenosis (membranous or muscular), and (4) aortic coarctation. A bicuspid aortic valve is also often included in this syndrome.

Left Atrial Myxoma

Myxomas are the most common primary tumours of the heart and are usually benign. Most commonly, these tumours occur within the LA and are attached to the fossa ovalis. On the 2D echocardiographic examination, myxomas have a globular, finely speckled appearance. When tumours are large they can prolapse through the mitral valve during diastole resulting in obstruction to LV inflow and, therefore, functional MS (Fig. 8.15). These tumours are discussed in further detail in Chapter 13.

Mitral Valve Score Index

In patients with valvular MS, it is important to determine whether or not the valve is suitable for a percutaneous balloon mitral valvuloplasty (PBMV). In particular, the outcome of the PBMV procedure can be predicted by scoring the anatomical appearance of the mitral valve by 2D echocardiography. For example, the mitral valve can be scored based on the criteria proposed by Wilkins et al and Padial et al.

The Wilkins criterion for scoring the mitral valve is based on the assessment of: (1) leaflet mobility, (2) subvalvular thickening, (3) leaflet thickness and (4) leaflet calcification. Each of these parameters is scored from 1 to 4 so a total score between 4 and 16 will be obtained (Table 8.2). A score of ≤ 8 recognises patients who will have a good result post valvuloplasty while a score greater than 8 identifies those patients who are less likely to have good result [8.1].

The Padial scoring system can be used to determine the degree of mitral regurgitation (MR) that is likely to occur following a PBMV. Scoring the mitral valve by the Padial criteria is based on the assessment of: (1) the thickening of each leaflet, (2)

commissure calcification, and (3) subvalvular disease. Each of these parameters is scored from 1 to 4 so a total score between 4 and 16 will be obtained (Table 8.3). A score of ≥ 10 identifies those patients likely to develop severe MR following a mitral balloon valvuloplasty via the Inoue technique [8.2]. The degree of commissural fusion is an additional important determinant of outcome following a PBMV.

Scoring of the mitral valve should be evaluated from multiple echocardiographic views. Also as the degree of subvalvular thickening is important in the scoring of the mitral valve, careful examination of the subvalvular apparatus is required. Therefore, from the parasternal long axis view, the transducer should be angled medially and laterally so that the tendinous cords and papillary muscles can be carefully inspected (Fig. 8.16). To examine the subvalvular thickening from the apical 4-chamber view, the transducer is tilted posteriorly into the left ventricle and from the apical 2-chamber view the transducer is angled medially and laterally.

Other factors that are considered in determining whether or not the patient is suitable for percutaneous balloon mitral valvuloplasty (PBMV) include: (1) the degree of mitral regurgitation (MR) and (2) the presence of left atrial (LA) thrombus.

PBMV results in the splitting of the mitral commissures, therefore, patients with more than mild MR are not suitable for this procedure as further splitting of the valve may lead to more significant MR. Furthermore, the technique for a PBMV involves trans-septal puncture of the interatrial septum so that the balloon catheter can be passed from the right atrium to the LA; the catheter is then manipulated through the LA, across the mitral valve, into the left ventricle. In the presence of LA thrombus, manipulation of the catheter in the LA may lead to systemic embolisation. Therefore, patients with LA thrombus are not suitable for this procedure. Due to the limitations of transthoracic echocardiography in detecting LA thrombus, transoesophageal echocardiography is recommended for all patients being considered for PBMV.

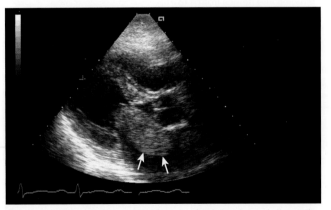
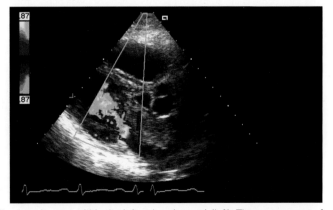

Figure 8.15 From the parasternal long axis view a large, echogenic mobile mass is seen within the left atrium (*arrows*) (*left*). The appearance of this mass is consistent with a myxoma. Observe that the myxoma is prolapsing through the mitral valve during diastole; turbulent flow on the colour Doppler image confirms that the tumour is obstructing left ventricular inflow and causing functional mitral stenosis (*right*).

[8.1] Wilkins GT, Weyman AE, Abascal VM, Block PC, Palacios IF. Percutaneous balloon dilatation of the mitral valve: an analysis of echocardiographic variables related to outcome and the mechanism of dilatation. *Br Heart J.* 1988 Oct;60(4):299-308.

[8.2] Padial LR, Abascal VM, Moreno PR, Weyman AE, Levine RA, Palacios IF. Echocardiography can predict the development of severe mitral regurgitation after percutaneous mitral valvuloplasty by the Inoue technique. *Am J Cardiol.* 1999 Apr 15;83(8):1210-3.

Assessment of the Left Atrium

As MS leads to dilatation of the LA, assessment of LA size is important. All measurements of LA size are performed at end-systole. The maximal anterior-posterior dimension of the LA can be measured from the parasternal long axis view via M-mode or 2D imaging while the LA area can be traced from the apical 4-chamber view. However, the preferred method for measuring LA size is the biplane area-length method (Fig. 8.17). Accuracy of this volume measurement relies on several variables which are discussed in Chapter 3 (see Table 3.2).

Patients with MS are prone to the development of AF. AF combined with a dilated LA results in stasis of blood flow which can lead to thrombus formation within the LA. Most commonly, thrombus forms within the LA appendage, though it may also occur in the body of the LA.

The echocardiographic appearance of thrombus is variable (Fig. 8.18-8.19). Thrombus may appear as an echogenic mass layered over the endocardial surface of the LA (laminated or mural thrombus), it may appear as a protruding echogenic mass within the LA cavity (pedunculated thrombus), or it may appear as a 'free' mobile echogenic mass within the LA cavity; furthermore, multiple thrombi may be present.

While it is possible to identify LA thrombus via transthoracic echocardiography, the sensitivity for detecting LA thrombus within the LA appendage is quite low due to the difficulty in adequately imaging this structure. Therefore, transoesophageal echocardiography is often required to exclude LA thrombus, especially if the patient is being considered for PBMV.

Thrombus may also be expected or anticipated in the presence of spontaneous echocardiographic contrast (SEC) within the LA cavity. On real-time echocardiographic imaging, SEC appears as a semi-organised pattern of swirling, 'smoke-like' echoes within the LA cavity or LA appendage; based on this appearance SEC is often referred to as 'smoke'. The presence of 'smoke' is considered a precursor of thrombus formation.

Assessment of LV Size and Systolic Function

LV size and systolic function are usually normal in patients with MS. These parameters can be assessed by both M-mode and 2D echocardiography in the traditional manner (see Chapter 2).

Estimation of Severity

Grading of the severity of MS is based on several haemodynamic parameters such as:
• mean pressure gradient,
• mitral valve area (MVA),
• estimation of right ventricular systolic pressure (RVSP).

The criteria for defining the various grades of MS based on these methods are listed in Table 8.4. Another 'out-dated' method for assessing the severity of MS is the mitral EF slope.

Table 8.2 Grading of Mitral Valve Characteristics by the Wilkins et al. Criteria

Grade	Mobility	Subvalvular Thickening	Leaflet Thickening	Calcification
1	Highly mobile valve with only leaflet tips restricted	Minimal thickening just below the mitral leaflets	Leaflets near normal in thickness (4-5 mm)	A single area of increased echo brightness
2	Leaflet mid and base portions have normal mobility	Thickening of chordal structures extending up to ⅓ of the chordal length	Mid-leaflets normal, considerable thickening of margins (5-8 mm)	Scattered areas of brightness confined to leaflet margins
3	Valve continues to move forward in diastole, mainly from the base	Thickening extending to the distal ⅓ of the chords	Thickening extending through the entire leaflet (5-8 mm)	Brightness extending into the mid-portion of the leaflets
4	No or minimal forward movement of the leaflets in diastole	Extensive thickening and shortening of all chordal structures extending down to the papillary muscles	Considerable thickening of all leaflet tissue (>8-10 mm)	Extensive brightness throughout much of the leaflet tissue

The total score is the sum of the score for each of these echocardiographic features and ranges from 4 to 16.
Reproduced from Wilkins GT, Weyman AE, Abascal VM, Block PC, Palacios IF. Percutaneous balloon dilatation of the mitral valve: an analysis of echocardiographic variables related to outcome and the mechanism of dilatation. *Br Heart J*, Oct;60(4), page 300, © 1988 with permission from BMJ Publishing Group Ltd.

Table 8.3 Echocardiographic Score for Severe Mitral Regurgitation Following Percutaneous Mitral Balloon Valvotomy by the Padial et al. Criteria

Grade	Leaflet Thickening (score each leaflet separately)	Commissure Calcification	Subvalvular Disease
1	Leaflet near normal (4-5 mm) or with only one thick segment	Fibrosis and/or calcium in only one commissure	Minimal thickening of chordal structures just below the valve
2	Leaflet fibrotic and/or calcified evenly; no thin areas	Both commissures mildly affected	Thickening of chordae extending up to ⅓ of chordal length
3	Leaflet fibrotic and/or calcified with uneven distribution; thinner segments are mildly thickened (5-8 mm)	Calcium in both commissures; one markedly affected	Thickening of the distal ⅓ of the chordae
4	Leaflet fibrotic and/or calcified with uneven distribution; thinner segments are near normal (4-5 mm)	Calcium in both commissures; both markedly affected	Extensive thickening and shortening of all chordae extending down to the papillary muscle

The total score is the sum of the score for each of these echocardiographic features and ranges from 4 to 16.
Reproduced from Padial LR, Abascal VM, Moreno PR, Weyman AE, Levine RA, Palacios IF. Echocardiography can predict the development of severe mitral regurgitation after percutaneous mitral valvuloplasty by the Inoue technique. *American Journal of Cardiology*, Vol. Apr 15;83(8), page 1211, © 1999 with permission from Elsevier.

Table 8.4 Recommendations for Classification of Mitral Stenosis Severity

	Mild MS	Moderate MS	Severe MS
Specific findings:			
MVA (cm²)	> 1.5	1.0 - 1.5	< 1.0
Supportive findings:			
Mean Gradient (mm Hg) [a]	< 5	5 – 10	> 10
RVSP (mm Hg)	< 30	30 - 50	> 50

[a] At heart rates between 60 and 80 bpm and in sinus rhythm.
Source: Baumgartner H, Hung J, Bermejo J, Chambers JB, Evangelista A, Griffin BP, Iung B, Otto CM, Pellikka PA, Quiñones M; American Society of Echocardiography; European Association of Echocardiography. Echocardiographic assessment of valve stenosis: EAE/ASE recommendations for clinical practice. *J Am Soc Echocardiogr*, Vol. 22(1), page 17, © 2009 with permission from Elsevier.

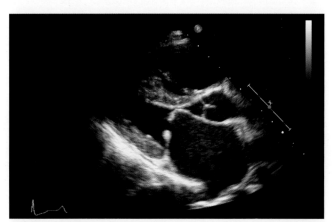 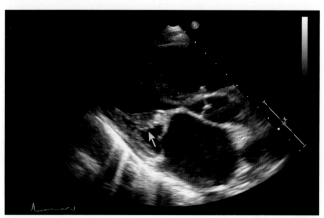

Figure 8.16 These two images were recorded from the parasternal long axis view in a patient with mitral stenosis. Observe that from the standard parasternal long axis view, there appears to be minimal or no subvalvular involvement (*left*). However, by angling medially through the valve, significant subvalvular thickening and cordal shortening can be appreciated (*arrow*) (*right*).

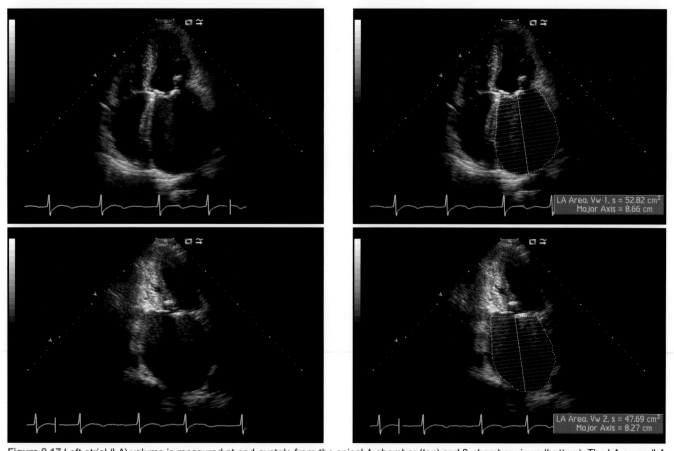

Figure 8.17 Left atrial (LA) volume is measured at end-systole from the apical 4-chamber (*top*) and 2-chamber views (*bottom*). The LA areas (LA Area Vw 1 and LA Area Vw 2) are measured by tracing around the blood-tissue interface. The major axis (length) of the atrium is measured from a line drawn perpendicularly from the centre of the mitral annulus to the superior aspect of the left atrium. The LA volume (LAV) in this example is:

LAV = *(0.85 × LA Area Vw 1 × LA Area Vw 2) ÷ major axis (shortest)*
= *(0.85 × 52.82 × 47.69) ÷ 8.27*
= *259 mL*

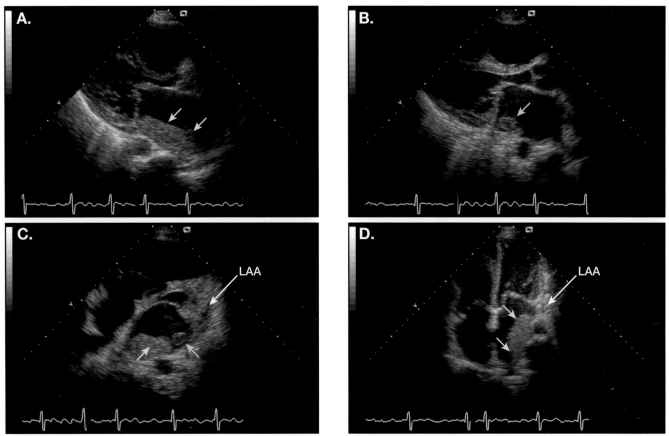

Figure 8.18 These transthoracic images show multiple echogenic masses within the left atrial (LA) cavity in a patient with severe mitral stenosis and atrial fibrillation. Images are recorded from the parasternal long axis view (A), the parasternal long axis view with slight medial tilting (B), the parasternal short axis view (C), and the apical 4-chamber view (D). In this clinical setting, the appearance of these masses is consistent with LA thrombus. Observe the large thrombus which extends posteriorly and laterally along the LA wall (*yellow arrows*). A smaller pedunculated thrombus is also noted (*blue arrows*); thrombus within the LA appendage (LAA) is present as well (*white arrow*).

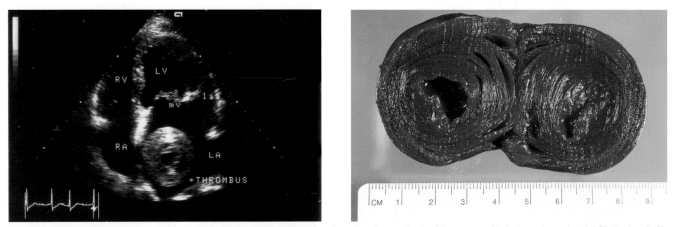

Figure 8.19 The 2D image shown was recorded from the apical 4-chamber view in a patient with severe mitral stenosis and atrial fibrillation (*left*). There is a large, ball-like, echogenic mass with an echolucent centre within the left atrial cavity (LA). On real-time imaging, this mass was freely mobile and 'bounced' around the LA cavity over the cardiac cycle, intermittently occluding the mitral orifice during diastole. At cardiac surgery, this mass was removed; the cut section of the mass reveals laminated thrombus and an area of central cavitation (*right*).
laa = left atrial appendage; LV = left ventricle; RA = right atrium; RV = right ventricle; mv = mitral valve.

Mean Pressure Gradients

Transmitral valve velocities are recorded via continuous-wave (CW) Doppler. From the CW Doppler velocity trace the transvalvular pressure gradients are estimated by application of the simplified Bernoulli equation (see Chapter 1).

In MS, the mean pressure gradient rather than the maximum instantaneous pressure gradient is important. This is because the diastolic pressure gradient varies over the diastolic period and the period of diastole is much longer than the period of systole. The mean pressure gradient is calculated by tracing the Doppler signal over the diastolic flow period (see Fig. 8.10 and 8.14). Importantly, the heart rate at which mean pressure gradients are measured should always be reported. In patients with AF, the mean pressure gradient should be averaged over five cycles, with the R-R intervals exhibiting minimal variation, and at heart rates that are close to normal. The limitations of pressure gradient estimations are discussed in detail in Chapter 1.

Mitral Valve Area

While the transmitral mean pressure gradients are useful in assessing the severity of MS, pressure gradients are dependent on the stroke volume (SV) across the valve. Therefore, to 'compensate' for the changes to the SV, calculation of the mitral valve area (MVA) should be performed. The MVA rather than the mean pressure gradient is especially valuable in the serial assessment of MS.

Caveats of Mean Pressure Gradients

CW Doppler versus PW Doppler
When assessing patients with mitral stenosis, continuous-wave (CW) Doppler rather than pulsed-wave (PW) Doppler is recommended. This is because the aim of the spectral Doppler assessment is to record the highest velocity and, therefore, the highest pressure gradient across the stenotic valve. Therefore, to achieve this goal with PW Doppler, the sample volume must be placed at the narrowest region of flow. If the sample volume is incorrectly positioned, then the highest velocity may be missed. As CW Doppler continuously 'samples' along the entire length of the ultrasound beam, the highest velocity will not be missed provided that the ultrasound beam is aligned parallel with flow.

Increased Pressure Gradients in the Absence of MS
Increased diastolic velocities and mean pressure gradients across the mitral valve in the absence of mitral stenosis (MS) may occur when there is tachycardia and/or significant mitral regurgitation (MR). In the case of MR, increased pressure gradients occur because the total stroke volume (SV) across the mitral valve is a combination of forward flow returning from the lungs plus the regurgitant volume that leaked through the mitral valve during systole. Increased velocities due to MR or tachycardia can be differentiated from increased velocities due to MS by the deceleration slope of the early diastolic velocity. For example, in MS, the deceleration slope is prolonged as a longer time is taken for the blood to pass across the narrowed mitral orifice.

Value of Colour Flow Doppler
MS jets may be eccentric. Therefore, colour flow Doppler is very useful in identifying eccentric MS jets and in ensuring that the Doppler beam is aligned parallel with the MS jet.

> The normal mitral valve area in the average sized adult is approximately 4.0 to 5.0 cm².

Four methods can be used to calculate the MVA; these include:
1. 2D planimetry of the MVA,
2. Pressure half-time method,
3. Stroke volume method,
4. PISA method.

1. Direct 2D Planimetry of the MVA
Direct 2D planimetry of the MVA measures the anatomical area of the stenotic valve. This method does not rely on hypothetical assumptions regarding flow dynamics; therefore, direct planimetry of the MVA is regarded as the most accurate non-invasive method for determining the anatomical MVA in patients with MS.

The MVA is traced from a zoomed parasternal short axis view acquired at the tips of the stenotic valve. The MVA is traced along the inner margins of the valve orifice, at the blood-tissue interface, in mid-diastole (Fig. 8.20).

The reliability and accuracy of direct 2D planimetry of the MVA is dependent upon the ability to clearly delineate the mitral valve orifice, tracing of the orifice area at the correct level, gain settings, and the skill and experience of the operator. In particular, image optimisation is crucial to the accuracy of this measurement. Therefore, the highest possible transducer frequency should be selected to maximise the spatial resolution and the 2D gain settings should be optimised to minimise 'blooming' of the valve and to avoid areas of 'drop-out'. In particular, increased gain settings ('over-gaining') may produce a 'blooming' effect which can lead to an underestimation of the MVA. Furthermore, spatial resolution is poorer at lower transducer frequencies so lower transducer frequencies may lead to the 'drop-out' of echoes in the lateral margins of the mitral orifice leading to an overestimation of the MVA.

Another factor that affects the accuracy of direct planimetry of the MVA is the ability of the operator to identify the true valve orifice. In MS, there is fusion and tethering of the leaflet tips of the valve resulting in a funnel-shaped orifice. Therefore, it is crucial that the valve orifice is measured at the leaflet tips. If the MVA is measured at the base of the valve or obliquely through the valve, the MVA will be overestimated (Fig. 8.21).

Other factors which may limit clear delineation of the true mitral valve orifice include dense fibrosis or calcification along the margins of the leaflets. In particular, calcification distorts the valve orifice and the intense, bright echoes generated from calcification may cause the leaflets to appear thicker and the orifice to appear smaller leading to an underestimation of the MVA.

2. MVA via the Pressure-Half Time
The slope of the Doppler velocity spectrum across the mitral valve reflects the pressure difference between the LA and LV over diastole. In the normal mitral valve, diastolic blood flow from the LA to the LV is unimpeded and as the majority of LV filling occurs during early diastole, the early diastolic pressure gradient between the two chambers rapidly declines (Fig. 8.22, top). In MS, the rate of LA emptying is 'slowed' due to the narrowed mitral orifice and this prolongs the decline of the early diastolic pressure gradient between the LA and LV (Fig. 8.22, bottom).

In particular, measurement of the time taken for the early diastolic pressure gradient to fall to half its original value, or the pressure half-time (P½t), is inversely proportional to the MVA. The P½t can be measured from the Doppler velocity spectrum recorded across the mitral valve (Fig. 8.23).

It has been observed that patients with a MVA of 1.0 cm² have

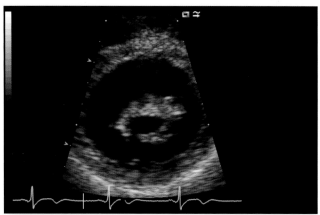

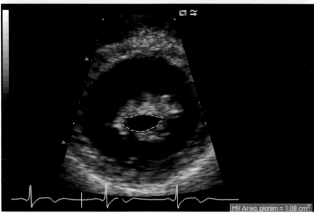

Figure 8.20 Planimetry of the mitral orifice is performed from a zoomed parasternal short axis view at the tips of the stenotic mitral valve (*top*). The mitral valve area is traced along the inner margin of the mitral orifice in mid-diastole (*bottom*).

Tips for Accurate Tracing of the MVA
1. Zoom on the mitral valve from the parasternal short axis view
2. From the papillary muscle level, slowly angle and tilt the transducer slightly medially and superiorly until the entire orifice of the stenotic mitral valve is just visible; this should correspond to the MVA at the leaflet tips
3. Optimise the 2D image by:
   • using the highest possible transducer frequency
   • adjusting the 2D gain and dynamic range so the mitral orifice is clearly delineated
   • setting the focal zone at the level of the mitral orifice
4. Using the cine-loop function, scroll to a mid-diastolic frame
5. Trace the MVA along the inner margins of the leaflets at the blood-tissue interface
6. Average at least 3 measurements when the patient is in sinus rhythm and 3-5 measurements when the patient is in AF. Measurements should be performed on consecutive beats if possible and post-ectopic beats should be avoided.

---

a P½t of approximately 220 ms[8.3]. Therefore, the MVA can be derived by dividing 220 by the P½t:

Equation 8.1

$$MVA = 220 \div P\tfrac{1}{2}t$$

where MVA = mitral valve area (cm²)
220   = empirical constant
P½t = pressure half-time (ms)

The P½t is also related to the deceleration time (DT) which is measured as the time taken for the peak early diastolic velocity to fall to zero (Fig. 8.24). The relationship between the P½t and the DT is that the P½t is equal to 29% of the DT and, therefore, the P½t can be derived from the DT as:

Equation 8.2

$$P\tfrac{1}{2}t = 0.29 \times DT$$

where P½t = pressure half-time (ms)
DT   = deceleration time (ms)

Furthermore, by combining Equations 8.1 and 8.2, the MVA can also be directly derived from the DT:

Equation 8.3

$$MVA = 759 \div DT$$

where MVA = mitral valve area (cm²)
759   = 220 ÷ 0.29
DT   = deceleration time (ms)

The limitations of the MVA derived by the P½t include arrhythmias, non-linear or curvilinear diastolic slopes, significant aortic regurgitation, acute changes in LA compliance, LV diastolic dysfunction, and the presence of an atrial shunt.

Arrhythmias

Many patients with MS are in AF. With AF, there are variations in the length of diastole and the P½t may vary accordingly. For this reason, measurements should be averaged over 3-5 cardiac cycles.

In patients with sinus tachycardia, the increased heart rate often results in fusion of the early diastolic velocity (E wave) and the velocity that follows atrial contraction (A wave). Therefore, when there is E/A fusion, accurate measurement of the P½t is not possible.

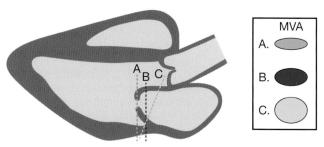

Figure 8.21 This schematic illustrates the effect of measuring the mitral valve area (MVA) at various levels through the valve. With rheumatic mitral stenosis, there is tethering at the leaflet tips with doming of the anterior leaflet during diastole. The correct level for planimetry of the MVA is at position A. Observe that if the MVA is traced through the body of the leaflets (B), the MVA will be overestimated. The MVA is also overestimated when the valve is transected obliquely (C).

[8.3] The 220 empirical constant is derived from the observation that patients with a P½t of approximately 220 ms had a functional MVA of 1.0 cm². Hatle L and Angelsen B. Doppler Ultrasound in Cardiology. Physical Principles and Clinical Applications. U.S.A. Lea and Febiger, pages 118-122, 1985.

Normal

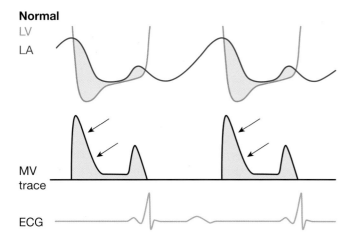

Mitral Stenosis

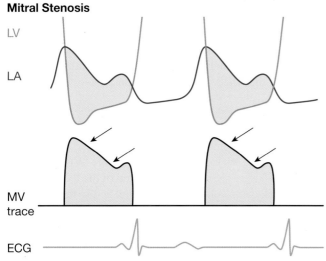

Figure 8.22 These schematic illustrates the relationship between the left ventricular (LV) and left atrial (LA) pressure traces and the transmitral inflow profile in the normal situation (*top*) and with mitral stenosis (*bottom*). In the normal situation, diastolic blood flow from the LA into the LV is unimpeded and as the majority of LV filling occurs during early diastole, the early diastolic pressure gradient between the two chambers rapidly declines. This effect is reflected in the transmitral inflow trace as a rapid deceleration of the early diastolic slope (*arrows*). In the case of mitral stenosis, the LA pressure is elevated and the rate of LA emptying is 'slowed' due to the narrowed mitral orifice. This effectively prolongs the decline of the early diastolic pressure gradient between the LA and LV. This effect is reflected in the transmitral inflow trace as prolongation of the deceleration slope (*arrows*).

Non-linear (Curvilinear) Diastolic Slope

In the majority of cases, the early diastolic velocity slope is linear and this allows the accurate measurement of the P½t and the subsequent MVA. However, curvilinear diastolic slopes ('ski-slopes') can lead to erroneous calculations of the MVA. The section of the curvilinear slope that is measured is dependent upon the end-diastolic pressure gradient. For example, when the end-diastolic velocity is elevated, the P½T is measured from the end-diastolic velocity back along the diastolic velocity curve (Fig. 8.25).

Significant Aortic Regurgitation

Severe aortic regurgitation (AR) may result in the overestimation of the MVA derived by the P½t. In this instance, the P½t is shortened due to a marked and rapid increase in the left ventricular end-diastolic pressure (LVEDP) which effectively reduces the pressure gradient between the LA and the LV at the end of diastole (Fig. 8.26). Furthermore, mistaking the AR signal for the MS signal is also possible. These signals can be easily differentiated based on their durations. For example, the AR signal commences at the closure of the aortic valve and continues until the next opening of the aortic valve. Therefore, the AR signal includes: (1) the time interval between aortic valve closure and mitral

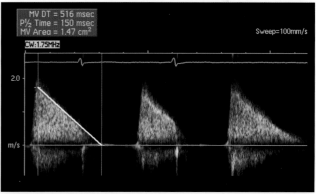

Figure 8.24 The transmitral deceleration time (DT) is derived by measuring along the early diastolic slope of the transmitral Doppler signal. In this example, the DT is 516 ms. The pressure half-time (P½ Time) can be derived from the DT as:

P½t = 0.29 × DT
     = 0.29 × 516
     = 150 ms

The mitral valve area (MVA) can then be calculated from the DT and the P½ time:

MVA = 220 ÷ P½ time   MVA = 759 ÷ DT
     = 220 ÷ 150   = 759 ÷ 516
     = 1.5 cm²   = 1.5 cm²

Figure 8.23 This figure illustrates how the pressure half-time (P½t) is measured from the transmitral Doppler velocity spectrum. Recall that simplified Bernoulli equation states that the relationship between pressure gradients (ΔP) and velocity (V) is $\Delta P = 4V^2$. Therefore, as the P½t is the time required for the pressure to decay to half its original value, using the Doppler velocity spectrum, the P½t is equal to the time taken for the peak velocity (Vmax) to fall to a value equivalent to Vmax ÷ √2. In the example shown, Vmax is 1.97 m/s and Vmax ÷ √2 is 1.39 m/s. Hence, the P½t is the time taken for the maximum velocity to fall from 1.97 m/s to 1.39 m/s; in this case, the P½t was 181 ms. The mitral valve area (MVA) can then be calculated from the P½t:

MVA = 220 ÷ P½t
     = 220 ÷ 181
     = 1.22 cm²

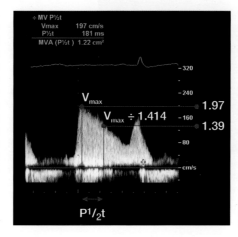

Peak pressure
$\Delta P = 4Vmax^2$

Half pressure
$\dfrac{\Delta P}{2} = 4V\frac{1}{2}^2$

and so...
$\dfrac{4Vmax^2}{2} = 4V\frac{1}{2}^2$

Rearranging this...
$4V\frac{1}{2}^2 = \dfrac{4Vmax^2}{2}$
$V\frac{1}{2} = \dfrac{Vmax}{\sqrt{2}} = \dfrac{Vmax}{1.414}$

valve opening, (2) the isovolumic relaxation period, and (3) the time interval between mitral valve closure and aortic valve opening, the isovolumic contraction period. Conversely, the transmitral inflow begins following the isovolumic relaxation period and terminates at the onset of the isovolumic contraction period. Therefore, the duration of the AR signal is always longer than the duration of the MS signal.

Acute Changes in LA Compliance

The P½t is not only inversely related to the MVA but it is also directly proportional to other factors such as the peak transmitral gradient and chamber compliance. In the normal situation, LA and LV compliance counteract one another. However, with acute changes in LA compliance, as occurs immediately following PBMV, the relationship between the P½t and the MVA is altered and the accuracy of the MVA calculated by the P½t declines. This adverse effect on the P½t is short-term such that calculation of the MVA by the P½t can be accurately performed 24 to 48 hours after PBMV.

Left Ventricular Diastolic Dysfunction

As described in Chapter 3, the DT is prolonged when LV relaxation is impaired and the DT is significantly shortened when there is a marked decrease in LV compliance. Therefore, in elderly patients with delayed LV relaxation, the MVA via the P½t method can be underestimated while an increase in LV stiffness will result in an overestimation of the MVA via the P½t method.

Atrial Septal Defect

In patients with MS and an atrial septal defect (ASD), the increased LA pressure due to MS increases left-to-right shunting across the ASD and this decreases the pressure gradient across the mitral valve during diastole. As a result, the MVA estimated via the P½t method will be overestimated.

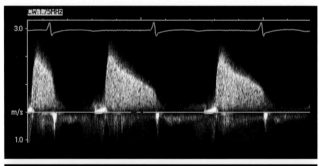

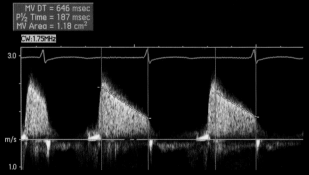

Figure 8.25 Observe the curvilinear diastolic slope on this transmitral Doppler trace (top). As the end-diastolic velocity is elevated, the pressure half-time (P½ Time) is measured from the peak end-diastolic velocity back along the diastolic slope (bottom).

The presence of mitral stenosis with an associated left-to-right shunt at the atrial level is referred to as Lutembacher Syndrome. Defects in the atrial septum usually occur due to stretching of a patent foramen ovale; however, congenital or acquired atrial septal defects may also be present.

3. MVA via the SV Continuity Method

The basic principles of the valve area calculations based on the SV continuity method are discussed in Chapter 1. Recall that this principle is based on the assumption that the SV proximal to a narrowing is equal to the SV across the narrowing. To estimate the MVA via this principle, it is assumed that the SV across the mitral valve will be identical to the SV across the left ventricular outflow tract (LVOT) (Fig. 8.27). The SV is derived as the product of the cross-sectional area (CSA) and the velocity time integral (VTI). Therefore, if the LVOT diameter can be measured to derive the CSA of the LVOT and if the VTI across the LVOT and across the mitral valve can be measured, then the MVA can be estimated (Fig. 8.28):

Equation 8.4

$$MVA = (CSA_{LVOT} \times VTI_{LVOT}) \div VTI_{MV}$$

where MVA = mitral valve area (cm²)
   CSA_{LVOT} = cross-sectional area of the LVOT (cm²)
   VTI_{LVOT} = velocity time integral of the LVOT (cm)
   VTI_{MV} = velocity time integral across the MV (cm)

The limitations of the continuity principle for valve area calculations are discussed in detail in Chapter 1 while limitations to SV calculations using the LVOT are discussed in Chapter 2. With respect to the MVA, the most common pitfalls encountered include: (1) underestimation of mitral VTI due to suboptimal alignment of the CW Doppler beam with blood flow direction, (2) underestimation of the LVOT velocity and VTI due to improper placement of the pulsed-wave (PW) Doppler sample volume in the LVOT, and (3) errors in the LVOT diameter measurement (refer to Fig. 2.29).

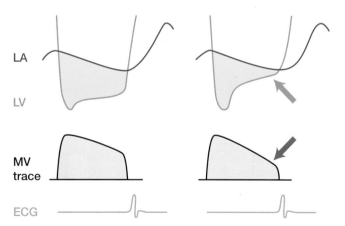

Figure 8.26 These schematic illustrations display the pressure difference between the left atrium (LA) and the left ventricle (LV). In severe mitral stenosis, the diastolic pressure gradient remains high throughout the diastolic period (left). When there is coexistent severe aortic regurgitation (AR), there is an increase in the LV volume which may result in a significant increase in the LVEDP (orange arrow). Therefore, even though the LA pressure remains high, the elevated LVEDP effectively decreases the pressure gradient between the LA and LV at end-diastole and this is reflected on the transmitral profile (blue arrow). Therefore, the resultant P½t is decreased and the MVA will be overestimated.

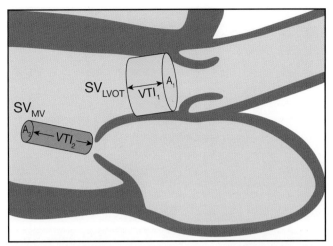

Figure 8.27 Stroke volume (SV) is derived as a product of the cross-sectional area (CSA) and the velocity time integral (VTI). As VTI is measured as a distance or 'height' it can be postulated that flow through the LVOT and across the mitral valve is cylindrical (the volume of a cylinder is derived as the product of the CSA and the height of the cylinder). Hence, the SV across the left ventricular outflow tract (SV_{LVOT}) is the product of the CSA of the LVOT (A_1) and the height of the cylinder or the VTI of the LVOT (VTI_1) and the SV across the mitral valve (SV_{AV}) is the product of the mitral valve area (A_2) and the height of the cylinder or the VTI across the mitral valve (VTI_2). Based on the continuity principle the SV_{LVOT} is equal to the SV_{MV}.

Another important limitation in calculating the MVA via the SV method occurs when there is coexistent AR and/or coexistent MR. In these circumstances, the SV across the mitral valve and across the LVOT are no longer equal. When there is MR, the SV across the mitral valve is increased because this SV includes the mitral regurgitant volume that leaked back through the mitral valve in systole plus the normal forward SV returning from the lungs; in this instance, the calculated MVA will be underestimated. When there is AR, the SV across the LVOT is increased because this SV includes the aortic regurgitant volume that leaked back across the aortic valve in diastole as well as the forward SV from the mitral valve; calculation of the MVA in this instance will be overestimated.

In the presence of AR or in situations when the LVOT parameters cannot be accurately estimated, the MVA can be calculated by substituting the right ventricular outflow tract (RVOT) SV for the SV of the LVOT. This method assumes that the SV across the mitral valve is equal to the SV across the RVOT. Therefore, there cannot be any significant mitral or pulmonary regurgitation or an intracardiac shunt or the measurement will be inaccurate. The SV of the RVOT is calculated from the RVOT diameter, which is used to derive the CSA of the RVOT, and the VTI across the RVOT.

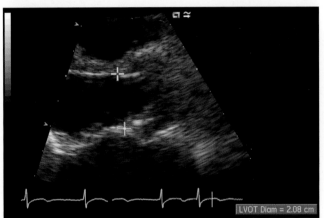

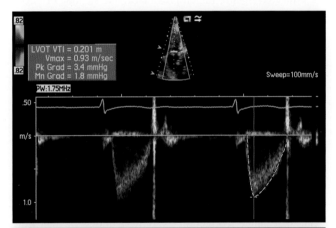

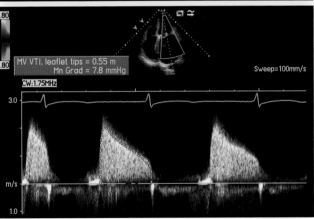

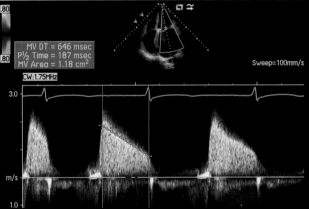

Figure 8.28 The mitral valve area (MVA) is calculated from the left ventricular outflow tract (LVOT) diameter, the LVOT velocity time integral (VTI) and the transmitral VTI. The LVOT diameter is measured from the zoomed parasternal long axis view of the LVOT (*top left*). At mid-systole callipers are placed from the inner edge of the junction between the anterior aortic wall and the interventricular septum to the inner edge of the junction between the posterior aortic wall and the anterior leaflet of the mitral valve, perpendicular to the aortic root. From an apical 5-chamber view, the LVOT VTI is traced from the pulsed-wave Doppler signal with a 2-4 mm sample volume placed 0.5 cm proximal to the aortic valve (*top right*). The transmitral VTI is traced from the continuous-wave Doppler signal recorded from the apical 4-chamber view (*bottom left*). The pressure half-time (P½ Time) is also measured (*bottom right*). The MVA via the stroke volume continuity method and via the pressure half-time method based on these measurements is calculated as:

$MVA = 220 \div P\frac{1}{2}\ time$ $MVA = (CSA_{LVOT} \times VTI_{LVOT}) \div VTI_{MV}$
$\quad\quad\ = 220 \div 187$ $\quad\quad\ = (0.785 \times 2.08^2 \times 20.1) \div 55$
$\quad\quad\ = 1.2\ cm^2$ $\quad\quad\ = 1.2\ cm^2$

Note: As the patient is in atrial fibrillation, all measurements should be averaged over 3-5 cardiac cycles.

4. MVA via the PISA Continuity Method

The basic concepts of the PISA principle in the calculation of the effective orifice area (EOA) are described in Chapter 1. Recall that this calculation is based on the continuity principle which states that flow proximal to a narrowed orifice must equal flow through the narrowed orifice.

In the case of MS, the EOA or MVA can be calculated from the radius of the proximal flow convergence dome, the velocity at the radius, and the peak early diastolic velocity of the MS jet:

Equation 8.5

$$EOA = (2\pi \, r^2 \times V_N) \div V_{max}$$

where EOA = effective orifice area or MVA (cm²)

$2\pi \, r^2$ = surface area of the hemispheric shell derived from the flow convergence radius [r] proximal to the stenotic valve (cm²)

V_N = colour Nyquist limit at the radial distance of the hemispheric shell (cm/s)

V_{max} = peak early diastolic velocity of the mitral stenotic jet (cm/s)

Importantly, the PISA principle is based on flow approaching a narrowed orifice that conforms to a flat planar surface. In MS however, the mitral leaflets usually form a funnel so that the flow convergence region proximal to the stenotic orifice is more funnel-shaped. Therefore, to account for the altered shape of the flow profile, the angle (α) of flow convergence must be measured and an angle correction factor of α/180 must be applied. Therefore, accounting for the angle correction factor, the MVA can be derived from the following equation (Fig. 8.29):

Equation 8.6

$$EOAc = EOA \times [\alpha \div 180]$$

where EOAc = corrected effective orifice area or MVA (cm²)

EOA = effective orifice area or MVA (cm²) calculated using Equation 8.6

α = angle of the mitral funnel

Note that angle correction is only required if the flow convergence zone is not flat. In some cases of MS, the valvular plane in diastole is flat or almost at 180 degrees; in these situations the EOA or MVA via PISA can be calculated without angle correction (Fig. 8.30).

Tips for calculating the MVA via PISA

• Zoom on the mitral valve from the apical 4-chamber view.
• Shift the colour baseline in the direction of flow to increase the PISA dome (from the apical views diastolic blood flow is towards the transducer so the baseline is shifted upwards). Note that simply decreasing the colour velocity scale rather than baseline shift will also increase the size of the PISA dome.
• From an early diastolic frame, measure the PISA radius from the valve tips to the first aliased velocity identified at the red-blue interface.
• Angle correction is required when the flow convergence zone is not flat. The mitral angle can be directly measured on some ultrasound machines but is more commonly estimated.
• Measure the peak E velocity via CW Doppler ensuring parallel alignment with blood flow direction.
• Convert all units to cm or cm/s when calculating the MVA.

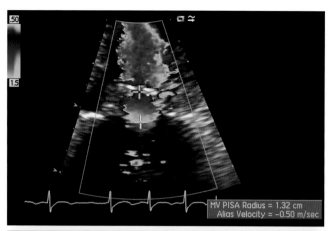

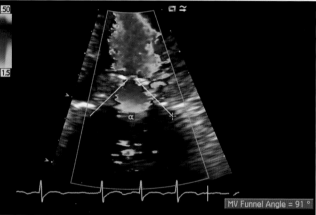

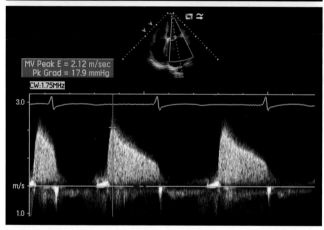

Figure 8.29 The effective orifice area (EOA) or the mitral valve area (MVA) is calculated via the proximal isovelocity surface area (PISA) method. From a zoomed apical 4-chamber view of the mitral valve, the PISA radius is measured on the left atrial side of the mitral valve in early diastole; callipers are placed between the mitral leaflets to the first aliased velocity (*top*). The colour Nyquist limit at this radius is 0.50 m/s or 50 cm/s; this value is noted at the top of the colour bar as flow is towards the transducer. The angle of the mitral valve funnel (α) is measured proximal to the stenotic orifice in the flow convergence region (*middle*). From the continuous-wave Doppler trace, the peak early diastolic velocity is measured at 2.12 m/s or 212 cm/s (*bottom*). The EOA in this example is calculated as:

$$
\begin{aligned}
EOAc &= EOA \times [\alpha \div 180] \\
&= [(2\pi \, r^2 \times V_N) \div V_{max}] \times [\alpha \div 180] \\
&= [(6.28 \times 1.32^2 \times 50) \div 212] \times [91 \div 180] \\
&= 2.58 \times 0.51 \\
&= 1.3 \; cm^2
\end{aligned}
$$

Note: As the patient is in atrial fibrillation, all measurements should be averaged over 3-5 cardiac cycles. In performing this calculation, it is important to convert all units to cm or cm/s.

The limitations of PISA calculations are the same as those limitations described in Chapter 2. In particular, for MS, it is not possible to perform the measurement of angle α on-line on many ultrasound systems and, therefore, this measurement must be either estimated or performed off-line using a protractor. Furthermore, the angle formed by the stenotic mitral valve leaflets is three dimensional. Therefore, the correction for angle α, which is performed in one imaging plane, may not be representative of the true leaflet geometry.

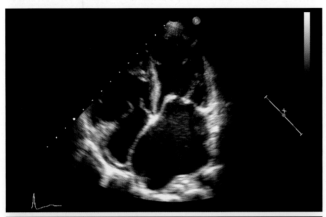

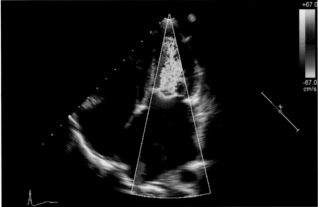

Figure 8.30 As shown in these two images, the mitral valvular plane is approximately 180 degrees (*top*). Therefore, the flow convergence zone proximal to the stenotic mitral orifice is flat (*bottom*). In this instance, the effective orifice area (EOA) or the mitral valve area (MVA) can be calculated via the PISA method without angle correction.

Which MVA Method and When?

In considering which MVA to perform in patients with MS, it is important to consider the advantages and limitations of each technique as well as the factors that affect the MVA calculation. Because 2D planimetry of the MVA provides a direct measurement of the anatomical valve area, this is the method of choice for estimation of the MVA. However, when 2D planimetry is not feasible, then the MVA can be calculated by the haemodynamic methods such as the P½t and the continuity methods (SV and PISA). Importantly, calculation of the MVA via haemodynamic methods provides an estimation of the EOA and this will be smaller than the true anatomical area (see Fig. 1.23). In addition, these haemodynamic estimates of the MVA are influenced by flow dynamics, intracardiac pressures, and chamber compliance. Figure 8.31 provides a flow chart for identifying which haemodynamic estimate of the MVA is best under varying conditions.

Pulmonary Hypertension

Pulmonary hypertension (PHTN) is commonly associated with MS. PHTN occurs secondary to elevated LA pressures which leads to a passive backward increase in the pulmonary venous pressures. In particular, the RVSP can be used as a supportive finding to MS severity (see Table 8.4).

The RVSP is estimated from the TR velocity in the standard manner. Other evidence of PHTN includes dilatation of the RV, RV hypertrophy, abnormal displacement or paradoxical systolic motion of the interventricular septum with a D-shaped LV (see Chapter 4).

Mitral EF Slope

Another (albeit outdated) method for assessing the severity of MS is the measurement of the M-mode mitral EF slope. The mitral EF slope is a measure of the slope of the anterior mitral leaflet during early diastole. This slope is a function of the rate of LA emptying and LV filling. In MS, the early diastolic closing motion of the leaflets occurs at a much slower rate than usual due to restriction of LA emptying and a persistent pressure gradient between LA and LV which holds the leaflets open for longer; this results in prolongation of the EF slope (Fig. 8.32).

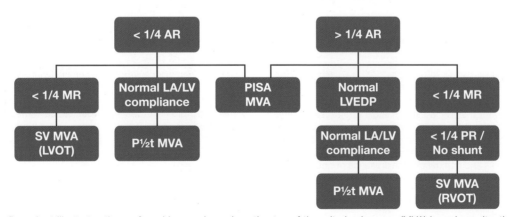

Figure 8.31 This flow chart illustrates the preferred haemodynamic estimates of the mitral valve area (MVA) in various situations based on the presence or absence of significant aortic regurgitation (AR). When there is grade 1/4 or less AR **and** less than grade 1/4 mitral regurgitation (MR), then the MVA can be calculated via the stroke volume (SV) continuity principle using the left ventricular outflow tract (LVOT) SV. When there is grade 1/4 or less AR **and** normal left atrial (LA) and left ventricular (LV) compliance, the MVA can also be calculated by the pressure half-time (P½t) method. When there is more than grade 1/4 AR **and** a normal left ventricular end-diastolic pressure (LVEDP) and normal LA and LV compliance, then the MVA can be calculated via the P½t method. When there is more than grade 1/4 AR **but** less than grade 1/4 MR and less than grade 1/4 pulmonary regurgitation (PR) **and** no intracardiac shunt, the MVA can be calculated via the SV continuity principle using the right ventricular outflow tract (RVOT) SV. Calculation of the MVA by the PISA technique is not affected by the degree of AR so this method can be used irrespective of the AR severity.

Although M-mode assessment for semi-quantifying the severity of MS has been superseded by Doppler techniques, the M-mode pattern of the mitral valve provides other clues to the presence of MS. These clues include: (1) thickening of the anterior and posterior mitral leaflets, (2) anterior motion of the posterior leaflet due to tethering of the leaflets and commissural fusion, and (3) absent or reduced mid-diastolic closure of the valve (Fig. 8.32). In particular, reduced or absent mid-diastolic closure occurs due to persistently high diastolic LA pressures which prevent the mitral valve moving towards a closed position following the early filling phase of diastole.

Identifying Associated Valve Lesions

Some degree of MR is commonly associated with MS. The severity of MR is described later in this chapter. In particular, when there is coexistent MR, the MVA via the SV continuity equation is not valid so the MVA should be calculated by 2D planimetry of the valve area or via the P½t or PISA methods. When PHTN is present, the RV is frequently dilated. Therefore, TR may occur secondary to annular dilatation. Methods for assessing the severity of TR are discussed in Chapter 9.

Furthermore, in cases of rheumatic MS, rheumatic involvement of the aortic valve +/- the tricuspid valve is quite common so a comprehensive assessment of the anatomy and function of these valves is also important.

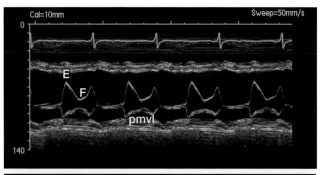

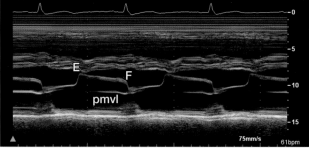

Figure 8.32 On the M-mode trace of a normal mitral valve, there is a rapid decline of the EF slope in early diastole (*top*). Also observe that the posterior mitral valve leaflet (pmvl) moves posteriorly over diastole. In mitral stenosis, there is prolongation of the EF slope (*bottom*). Also observe the posterior mitral valve leaflet (pmvl) moves anteriorly over diastole and that despite the presence of sinus rhythm, mid-diastolic closure is absent (see text for details).

> The following section provides a brief overview of the role of stress echocardiography in patients with MS. For a more comprehensive understanding of the role of stress echocardiography in these patients including recommended protocols readers are advised to review other sources as listed in the Further Reading section of this Chapter.

Role of Stress Echocardiography in Mitral Stenosis

Essentially stress echocardiography can be used in two groups of patients with MS: (1) patients with asymptomatic severe MS at rest, and (2) symptomatic patients with apparently mild MS.

In patients with asymptomatic severe MS at rest, defined as a mean transmitral pressure gradient > 10 mm Hg and MVA < 1.0 cm², stress echocardiography may be utilised to determine if the patient has exercise-induced symptoms.

In symptomatic patients with apparently mild MS, defined as a mean transmitral pressure gradient < 5 mm Hg and a MVA ≥ 1.5 cm², stress echocardiography may be employed to determine if there is a significant increase in the mean transmitral pressure gradient and/or RVSP during or immediately following stress. In particular, in those patients with 'true' mild MS, a stable or only mild increase in mean pressure gradient and only a mild increase in the RVSP will be demonstrated while in those patients with 'pseudo-mild' MS, the mean transmitral pressure gradient increases significantly or there is a marked increase in RVSP (Fig. 8.33). In particular, an increase in the mean transmitral gradient > 15 mm Hg and an increase in the RVSP > 60 mm Hg with exercise echocardiography may be an indication for PBMV if the mitral valve morphology is suitable for such a procedure [8.4]. With dobutamine stress echocardiography, an increased mean transmitral gradient ≥ 18 mm Hg has been shown to predict clinical deterioration or indicate the need for intervention [8.5].

> In symptomatic patients with apparent mild MS, the discordance between the patient's symptoms and haemodynamic data can be explained by the relationship between the heart rate and cardiac output, and transmitral flow and the diastolic filling time. For example, at rest or at low heart rates, transmitral flow is lowest and the diastolic filling time is longest, and therefore, the mean transmitral pressure gradient is only mildly increased. However, when the patient becomes 'active' or exercises, the cardiac output and heart rate increase and the diastolic filling period decreases. This leads to an increase in the LA and pulmonary capillary pressures which results in symptoms of dyspnoea on exertion.

[8.4] Bonow RO, Carabello BA, Chatterjee K, de Leon AC Jr, Faxon DP, Freed MD, Gaasch WH, Lytle BW, Nishimura RA, O'Gara PT, O'Rourke RA, Otto CM, Shah PM, Shanewise JS. 2008 focused update incorporated into the ACC/AHA 2006 guidelines for the management of patients with valvular heart disease: a report of the American College of Cardiology/American Heart Association Task Force on Practice Guidelines (Writing Committee to revise the 1998 guidelines for the management of patients with valvular heart disease). Endorsed by the Society of Cardiovascular Anesthesiologists, Society for Cardiovascular Angiography and Interventions, and Society of Thoracic Surgeons. *J Am Coll Cardiol.* 2008 Sep 23;52(13):e41.

[8.5] Reis G, Motta MS, Barbosa MM, Esteves WA, Souza SF, Bocchi EA. Dobutamine stress echocardiography for noninvasive assessment and risk stratification of patients with rheumatic mitral stenosis. *J Am Coll Cardiol.* 2004 Feb 4;43(3):393-401.

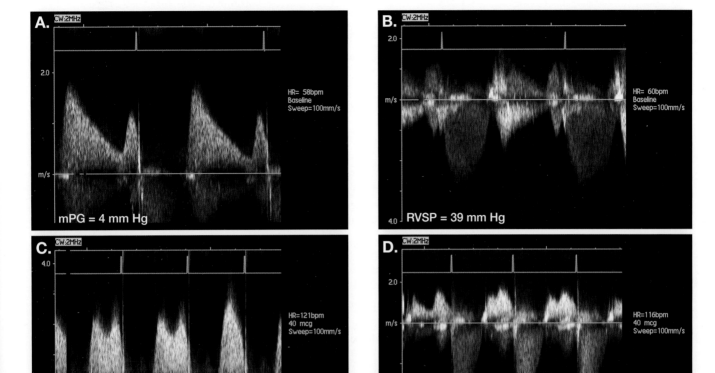

Figure 8.33 These spectral Doppler traces were recorded from a symptomatic patient with apparently mild mitral stenosis (MS). The mean transmitral pressure gradient (MPG) recorded at baseline (rest) was 4 mm Hg (A) and the estimated RVSP derived from the tricuspid regurgitant (TR) velocity was 39 mm Hg (B). At peak dobutamine infusion (40 mcg), the mean transmitral pressure gradient increased to 17 mm Hg (C) and the RVSP derived from the TR velocity increased to 94 mm Hg (D). This patient was, therefore, deemed to have severe, not mild, MS.

Mitral Regurgitation

Aetiology of Mitral Regurgitation

Mitral regurgitation (MR) refers to the backward flow of blood from the LV to the LA during systole. MR may result from a number of disorders of the mitral valve complex; accordingly, the mechanisms of MR can be categorised based on the structural abnormalities of the mitral valve complex (Table 8.5).

Leaflet Abnormalities

As listed in Table 8.5, there are numerous leaflet abnormalities that result in MR. The most common causes of MR include rheumatic valve disease and degenerative mitral valve disease (mitral valve prolapse). MR can also occur secondary to destruction of the mitral valve leaflets as a consequence of penetrating and non-penetrating trauma and/or endocarditis, congenital malformations such as a cleft anterior mitral valve associated with atrioventricular canal defect, or systolic anterior motion (SAM) of the anterior mitral leaflet secondary to hypertrophic obstructive cardiomyopathy (see Chapter 6, Hypertrophic Cardiomyopathy).

Rheumatic mitral valve disease is discussed above (see Aetiology of Mitral Stenosis). In the rheumatic mitral valve, MR occurs as a consequence of shortening, rigidity, deformity and retraction of one or both leaflets of the valve as well as shortening and fusion of the tendinous cords and papillary muscles.

Degenerative Mitral Valve Regurgitation

Degenerative mitral valve regurgitation (DMVR) refers to a spectrum of conditions in which infiltrative or dysplastic tissue changes cause elongation or rupture of the mitral valve cords resulting in leaflet prolapse (Fig. 8.34 and 8.35). Mitral valve prolapse (MVP), defined as the systolic billowing of the mitral leaflets into the LA, occurs as a consequence of DMVR whereby morphologic changes in the connective tissue of the valve cause structural lesions that prevent normal mitral complex function. These degenerative changes include cordal elongation, cordal rupture, leaflet tissue expansion and annular dilatation. There are three primary conditions responsible for DMVR: (1) Barlow's disease, (2) fibroelastic deficiency (FED), and (3) Marfan syndrome. The key differences between Barlow's disease and FED are listed in Table 8.6 and illustrated in Figure 8.34. Marfan syndrome is discussed in Chapter 14.

Mitral Annular Dilatation and Calcification

The normal mitral annulus is approximately 10 cm in circumference. During systole, contraction of the surrounding LV muscle causes the annulus to constrict and this constriction contributes to normal valve closure.

Dilatation of the LV leads to dilatation of the mitral annulus. As the mitral leaflets are of a fixed length, when there is dilatation of the annulus the mitral leaflets are unable to effectively coapt during systole; this leads to secondary MR. MR secondary to MAC occurs when the calcification prevents normal coaptation of the leaflets during systole.

Table 8.5 **Aetiology of Mitral Regurgitation**

Structural Abnormality causing MR	Examples
Annular dilatation	Dilated cardiomyopathy Ischaemic heart disease
Annular calcification	Degenerative calcific disease Marfan syndrome Systemic hypertension
Leaflet abnormalities	Bacterial endocarditis Congenitally abnormal mitral valve (e.g. cleft mitral valve) Connective tissue disorders (e.g. Marfan syndrome) Degenerative mitral valve regurgitation (e.g. Barlow's disease, fibroelastic deficiency) Hypertrophic obstructive cardiomyopathy (due to systolic anterior motion of the anterior mitral leaflet) Post intervention (e.g. post mitral balloon valvuloplasty) Rheumatic mitral disease Systemic diseases (e.g. systemic lupus erythematosus, hypereosinophilic syndrome)
Tendinous cord elongation	Degenerative mitral valve regurgitation
Tendinous cord maldevelopment	Parachute mitral valve Atrioventricular canal defects
Tendinous cord rupture	Bacterial endocarditis Degenerative mitral valve regurgitation Ischaemic heart disease Trauma
Papillary muscle and left ventricular dysfunction	Ischaemic heart disease
Papillary muscle malalignment	Dilated cardiomyopathy Hypertrophic obstructive cardiomyopathy Ischaemic heart disease
Papillary muscle rupture	Complication of myocardial infarction Trauma Bacterial endocarditis

Table 8.6 **Key Differences between Barlow's Disease and Fibroelastic Deficiency**

	Barlow's Disease	Fibroelastic Deficiency
Aetiology	Unknown	Unknown (may be ageing process)
Typical age	Young (< 60 years)	Older (≥ 60 years)
Microscopic appearance	Defective extracellular matrix resulting in a thickened spongiosa that impinges on the fibrosa	Connective tissue deficiency
Gross appearance • Annulus	Always dilated; calcification common	Variably dilated (less pronounced than Barlow's)
• Leaflets	Bulky, billowing leaflets Cul-de-sac at base of posterior leaflet	Thin leaflets
• Prolapsed segments	Multisegment prolapse Bileaflet prolapse is common	Prolapse of single segment (most commonly P2) May appear bulky
• Non-prolapsed segments	Billowing of body of both leaflets including non-prolapsing segments	No billowing of non-prolapsing segments
• Cordal rupture	Uncommon (elongation more common than rupture)	Common

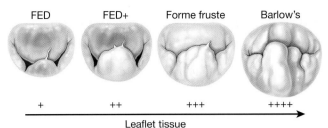

FED   FED+   Forme fruste   Barlow's

+   ++   +++   ++++

Leaflet tissue

Figure 8.34 This schematic illustrates the spectrum of degenerative mitral disease ranging from fibroelastic deficiency (FED) to Barlow's disease. In isolated FED there is a deficiency of collagen, with thin transparent leaflets and typically a ruptured thin cord. In longstanding prolapse, secondary myxomatous pathologic changes may occur in the prolapsing segment, resulting in leaflet thickening and expansion (FED+). Forme fruste designates degenerative disease with excess tissue with myxomatous changes in usually more than one leaflet segment, but usually does not involve a large valve size, distinguishing it from Barlow's disease. In the latter, the hallmarks are large valve size, with diffuse myxomatous changes and excess leaflet tissue, with thickened, elongated, and often ruptured cords.
Reproduced from Adams DH, Rosenhek R, Falk V. Degenerative mitral valve regurgitation: best practice revolution. *Eur Heart J.* © 2010 Aug;31(16):1959, with permission of Oxford University Press.

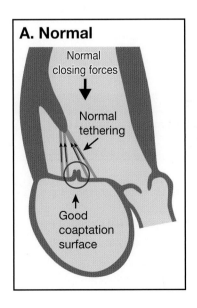

Figure 8.35 This pathological specimen shows marked prolapse of the posterior mitral leaflet (*yellow arrow*) with associated cordal rupture (*white arrow*). By permission of Mayo Foundation for Medical Education and Research. All rights reserved. Courtesy of William D. Edwards, MD.

Abnormalities of Tendinous Cords

The tendinous cords are an important component of the mitral valve complex. One of the primary functions of these cords is to prevent prolapse of the mitral leaflets into the LA during systole. MR can occur when there is elongation, rupture or maldevelopment of the cords.

Cordal rupture may occur as a consequence of bacterial endocarditis, trauma, rheumatic fever, or myxomatous proliferation. Cordal elongation may occur due to dysfunction of the papillary muscles which causes stretching and ultimately rupture of the cords; cordal elongation is also associated with DMVR. Congenital maldevelopment of the cords results in thickened or poorly defined cords as may occur with a parachute mitral valve or atrioventricular canal defects.

Abnormalities of Papillary Muscles and LV Wall

As for the tendinous cords, the papillary muscles and the LV wall to which they are attached are important components of the mitral valve complex. Contraction of the papillary muscles and LV wall pulls the two mitral leaflets toward one another and promotes valve closure during systole.

Papillary muscle rupture (PMR) is usually the consequence of an acute myocardial infarction (AMI) of the underlying LV wall. PMR is typically associated with acute, severe MR (see Chapter 5, Complications of Myocardial Infarction).

Malalignment of the papillary muscles may occur with LV dilatation or SAM of the anterior mitral valve leaflet secondary to hypertrophic obstructive cardiomyopathy (see Chapter 6, Hypertrophic Cardiomyopathy).

Ischaemic Mitral Regurgitation

Ischaemic mitral regurgitation (IMR) is generally defined as MR caused by segmental LV wall motion abnormalities which occur more than two weeks following an AMI. IMR can also occur in the presence of significant coronary artery disease in a territory supplying the papillary muscles and underlying LV myocardium. Importantly, in IMR the mitral valve leaflets and tendinous cords are structurally normal.

The mechanisms for IMR are complex with more than one mechanism contributing to MR. The principal mechanisms for IMR are listed in Table 8.7 and illustrated in Figure 8.36.

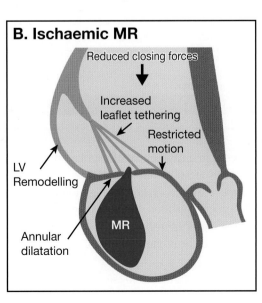

A. Normal

Normal closing forces

Normal tethering

Good coaptation surface

B. Ischaemic MR

Reduced closing forces

Increased leaflet tethering

Restricted motion

LV Remodelling

Annular dilatation

MR

Figure 8.36 Panel A: This schematic shows normal leaflet tethering with normal closing forces and a good leaflet coaptation surface between the anterior and posterior mitral leaflets.
Panel B: This schematic illustrates the mechanisms of ischaemic mitral regurgitation (IMR). Left ventricular (LV) remodelling due to ischaemia causes LV dilatation, mitral annular dilatation and papillary muscle displacement. The net effect of these changes is increased leaflet tethering or tenting, restricted systolic leaflet motion and reduced closing forces which prevent effective valve closure during systole; mitral regurgitation (MR) occurs as a consequence of these mechanisms.

Functional Classification of Mitral Regurgitation

A functional classification for MR has also been proposed. This classification was originally described by Carpentier as a functional rather than aetiological classification based on the surgical aim of mitral valve reconstruction which is to restore normal valve function rather than normal valve anatomy[8.6]. This functional classification is categorised by the opening and closing motions of the mitral leaflets such that type I refers to normal leaflet motion, type II refers to increased leaflet motion and type III refers to diminished or restricted leaflet motion (Fig. 8.37).

In the type I classification there is normal leaflet motion and MR occurs when there is a annular dilatation; leaflet perforation and cleft leaflets also fall into this classification. Type II refers to MR that occurs due to increased leaflet motion; this type therefore includes MVP, cordal elongation or rupture, and/or papillary muscle elongation or rupture.

Type III refers to MR that occurs due to restricted leaflet motion. This type can be further subcategorised into:

- type IIIa: restricted mitral leaflet motion during both diastole and systole that is caused by leaflet thickening and/or retraction, cordal thickening and/or shortening, and/or commissural fusion. This classification of MR is most often associated with rheumatic mitral valve disease.
- Type IIIb: restricted leaflet motion during systole only. The most common causes for this type of MR include LV dilatation with apical papillary muscle displacement as seen in ischaemic heart disease.

Importantly, it should be noted that more than one Carpentier type may coexist in any given individual. Furthermore, the Carpentier classification does not describe all mechanisms of MR. For example, MR due to SAM of the anterior mitral leaflet as seen with hypertrophic obstructive cardiomyopathy is not included in this classification.

Functional Type	Type I	Type II	Type III	
			IIIa	IIIb
Cusp Motion	Normal	Increased	Restricted during systole & diastole	Restricted during systole only
Example lesion	• Annular dilatation • Leaflet perforation • Cleft valve	• Prolapse • Cordal elongation • Cordal rupture • Papillary muscle elongation • Papillary muscle rupture	• Leaflet thickening and/or retraction • Cordal thickening and/or shortening • Commissural fusion	• Papillary muscle displacement and/or leaflet tethering
Illustrative example	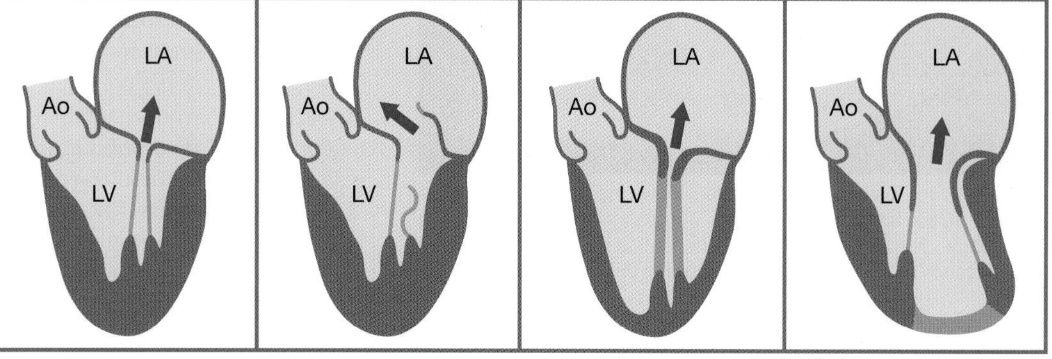			

Figure 8.37 This figure illustrates the functional classification for mitral regurgitation (MR). See text for further details. Ao = aorta; LA = left atrium; LV = left ventricle.

Table 8.7 **Principal Mechanisms of Ischaemic Mitral Regurgitation**

Mechanism	Cause of Mitral Regurgitation
Left ventricular (LV) remodelling	Decreased closing forces due to LV global or regional dysfunction and LV geometric distortion (LV dilatation) can lead to MR. LV geometrical changes result in displacement of papillary muscles which pulls the leaflets away from each other preventing adequate systolic leaflet coaptation.
Increased systolic tethering of the mitral leaflets	Papillary muscle displacement restricts systolic leaflet motion resulting in valve tenting or tethering which prevents complete leaflet coaptation during systole. Leaflet tethering may be symmetric (global LV remodelling) or asymmetric (regional LV remodelling).
Reduced leaflet closing forces	LV systolic dysfunction prevents the production of sufficient ventricular closing forces to adequately close the valve.
Annular dilatation	Annular dilatation pulls the leaflets further from one another preventing them from coapting during systole.

[8.6] Carpentier A. Cardiac valve surgery--the "French correction". *J Thorac Cardiovasc Surg.* 1983 Sep;86(3):323-37.

Pathophysiology of Mitral Regurgitation

The pathophysiology of MR can be discussed in terms of acute and chronic MR.

Acute, severe MR may occur due to PMR following an AMI or acute cardiac trauma. In the acute situation, the mitral regurgitant volume (RV) fills a normal sized LA as the LA has not had time to compensate for increased systolic volume by dilating. This results in a marked elevation in the LA pressure. In addition, as the pulmonary capillaries are not 'protected' by a dilated LA and are subjected to the markedly elevated LA pressure, the pulmonary capillary pressures also rise markedly and acute pulmonary oedema and PHTN ensue. Furthermore, the LV end-diastolic volume (LVEDV) is increased because the LV receives the mitral RV along with the normal forward flow returning from the lungs. At the same time, LV afterload is reduced because the LV is essentially ejecting into the LA. As a result, the LV is able to eject more completely so the LV end-systolic volume (LVESV) is decreased. Therefore, as the LVEDV is increased and the LVESV is decreased, the LV ejection fraction (LVEF) is usually greater than normal or "supernormal". However, because the majority of the SV is being ejected into the LA, the total forward SV to the body is significantly decreased resulting in a low cardiac output.

In the case of chronic 'compensated' MR, the heart has had time to develop compensatory mechanisms. In particular, chronically increased LA pressure results in LA dilatation and when the LA is dilated and still compliant, it can accommodate the mitral RV at a lower pressure, so that LA pressure is only mildly elevated. Over time, the increased LV volume causes increasing LV dilatation and hypertrophy. This allows for a larger increase in total SV so that forward SV is normal (see the Frank-Starling principle in Chapter 2). The LVEF also remains increased. However, as the severity of MR increases over time, the ability of the LV to augment its systolic function reaches its limit and LV systolic function then decreases. This is referred to as chronic 'decompensated' MR. In this situation, LV contractile function is reduced due to muscle damage caused by prolonged and severe LV volume overload. As a result, the weakened LV can no longer shorten adequately so the LVESV increases. This leads to a decrease in total and forward SV with a subsequent increase in LA and LV filling pressures. In addition, there is a further increase in LVEDV, without a concomitant decrease in LVESV; therefore, both the total and forward SV are decreased. The LVEF also declines but often remains within the "normal" range but this LVEF does not reflect the true contractile function of the ventricle. Furthermore, in chronic MR pulmonary hypertension is also common due to the backwards transmission of increased LA pressures to the pulmonary capillary bed.

Clinical Manifestations of Mitral Regurgitation

The clinical signs of MR are caused by backward flow of blood across the mitral valve, leading to increased LA pressures. The clinical manifestations of MR depend on the severity of MR as well as whether MR is acute or chronic.

Patients with acute MR typically present with frank pulmonary oedema, hypotension, and signs and symptoms of cardiogenic shock.

Patients with chronic MR may be relatively asymptomatic if the LV systolic function remains normal. In patients with chronic, symptomatic MR, the most common symptoms include generalised weakness, fatigue, and exercise intolerance. In more severe cases of chronic MR, signs of congestive heart failure, evidence of pulmonary congestion and pulmonary oedema may be present.

Role of Echocardiography in Mitral Regurgitation

The aims and objectives of echocardiography in the assessment of MR are to:
• Determine the aetiology of the lesion,
• Assess LA size,
• Assess LV size and systolic function,
• Estimate the severity of the regurgitation,
• Estimate RVSP.

Aetiology of Mitral Regurgitation

As discussed previously, the anatomy of the mitral valve complex consists of many components and disorders of any of these components can result in MR (see Table 8.5). Two important conditions that warrant special consideration are DMVR (MVP) and MR due to ischaemia.

> 'Physiological' or a mild degree of MR is commonly encountered in the normal population with the incidence of MR increasing with advancing age. MR may also be described in terms of functional or organic regurgitation. Organic or primary regurgitation refers to diseases that involve the leaflets and their supporting apparatus; that is, MR occurs due to intrinsic valvular disease. Functional or secondary regurgitation refers to diseases that affect the LV and LA resulting in altered ventricular geometry; so MR occurs due to annular dilatation of an otherwise normal mitral complex.

Mitral Valve Prolapse

As stated above, DMVR refers to a spectrum of conditions that ultimately result in MVP. MVP may be defined as the slipping of one or more mitral leaflets and/or scallops beyond the mitral annulus during systole.

In considering the echocardiographic appearance of MVP, it is important to be aware of a number of factors. Firstly, the orientation of the echocardiographic short axis view of the mitral scallops varies compared to the surgical or pathological short axis view of the scallops. For example, the surgical or pathological inspection of the mitral valve is typically viewed from above; that is, from the LA aspect of the valve. From the 2D parasternal short axis view of the mitral valve, the valve is viewed from below; that is, the valve is viewed from the LV aspect of the valve. As a result, from the 2D short axis view the lateral aspect of the valve appears to the right of the image while the medial aspect appears to the left of the image. Therefore, on 2D echocardiography, the mitral scallops are seen as a mirror image of the surgical or pathological view of the scallops (Fig. 8.38).

Secondly, while there may be prolapse of the whole leaflet, prolapse may be isolated to one or more mitral scallops. Therefore, an awareness of the various mitral scallops with respect to the various echocardiographic views is also required (Fig. 8.39).

Thirdly, the diagnosis of MVP via 2D echocardiography should not be made solely based on the appearance of the valve from the apical 4-chamber view. This is because the mitral annulus at end-systole is saddle-shaped; as a result the valve may appear to prolapse in the apical 4-chamber view simply due to the manner in which the valve is transected through the saddle-shaped annulus (Fig. 8.40).

The 2D diagnostic criterion for MVP is the bowing of one or both leaflets 2 mm or more above the mitral annulus in the parasternal long axis view (Fig. 8.41). M-mode can also be useful in confirming the presence of MVP. On the M-mode examination, MVP appears as "hammocking" of the mitral valve leaflets (Fig. 8.42).

The 2D appearance of the mitral valve can also be used to differentiate MVP due to Barlow's disease from FED (Fig. 8.43). Barlow's disease typically displays billowing of the body of both mitral leaflets; the leaflets also appear large, bulky (myxomatous), elongated and distended. Multi-segment prolapse is usually present and bileaflet prolapse is common. In addition, the cords appear thickened and mesh-like. Conversely, the mitral leaflets associated with FED appear thin and do not have a billowing or redundant appearance;

however, the prolapsing segment may appear thickened and bulky but this appearance is limited to the prolapsing segment only. In FED there is usually a single, prolapsing segment which is most commonly the middle scallop of the posterior leaflet (P2); bileaflet prolapse is uncommon.

Colour flow Doppler imaging is also very useful in determining whether prolapse relates to the anterior leaflet or the posterior leaflet. In particular, the MR jet is usually directed away from the prolapsing leaflet; that is, with posterior MVP the MR jet is directed or baffled anteriorly while with anterior MVP the MR jet is baffled posteriorly (Fig. 8.44 and 8.45). When there is bileaflet MVP the MR jet is usually central.

Flail leaflets versus Prolapse

Flail mitral valve leaflets can be differentiated from prolapsing mitral leaflets based on the direction of the tip of the leaflet. For example, in MVP the tip of the prolapsing leaflet points towards the LV cavity while in a flail mitral leaflet the tip of the flailed leaflet points towards the LA cavity.

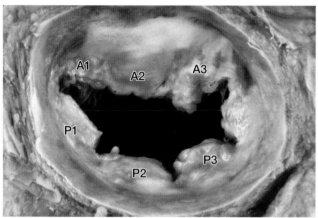
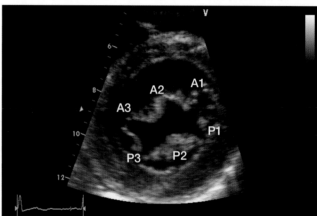

Figure 8.38 The pathological short axis view of the mitral scallops is viewed from the left atrial aspect (*left*). The posterior scallops are identified as P1, P2 and P3, and the opposing anterior scallops are identified as A1, A2 and A3. On the 2D parasternal short axis view of the mitral valve, the valve is viewed from the left ventricular aspect so the mitral scallops appear as a mirror image of the pathological scallops (*right*).
By permission of Mayo Foundation for Medical Education and Research. All rights reserved. Courtesy of William D. Edwards, MD.

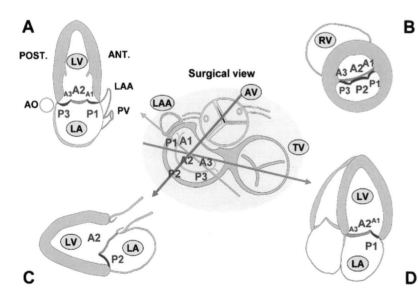

Figure 8.39 Four imaging planes used to assess the precise localisation of prolapsed or flail segments are illustrated. From the apical 2-chamber view, the most prominent scallops seen are P3, A2 and P1 (A). From the parasternal short-axis view, the anterior leaflet (A1, A2, and A3) and the three scallops of the posterior leaflet (P1, P2, and P3) are seen (B). From the parasternal long axis view, the middle segments of anterior (A2) and posterior (P2) leaflets are seen (C). From the apical 4-chamber view the anterior para commissural zone (between P1 and P2) is seen (D).
ANT. = anterior; AO = descending aorta; AV = aortic valve; LA = left atrium; LAA = left atrial appendage; LV = left ventricle; POST. = posterior; PV = pulmonary vein; RV = right ventricle; TV = tricuspid valve.
Reprinted from Monin JL, Dehant P, Roiron C, et al., Functional Assessment of Mitral Regurgitation by Transthoracic Echocardiography Using Standardized Imaging Planes, *J Am Coll Cardiol,* Vol 19, page 303, © 2005, with permission from Elsevier.

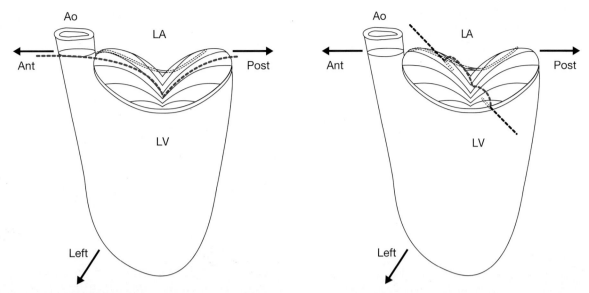

Figure 8.40 The mitral annulus is saddle-shaped, with two high points or peaks at the midpoint of the anterior and posterior leaflets and two low points or troughs located posteromedially and anterolaterally. These diagrams depict the 3D aspects of the mitral annulus with the dashed lines indicating the annular plane corresponding to the parasternal long axis view (*left*) and the apical 4 -chamber view (*right*). Observe that in the long axis plane, the leaflets appear to lie entirely below the intersections of the annulus while in the apical 4-chamber plane the leaflets appear to rise above the intersection of the annulus. As a result from the apical 4-chamber view the leaflets can appear to prolapse despite being normal. Ant = anterior; Ao = aorta; LA = left atrium; LV= left ventricle; Post = posterior; RA = right atrium.

Reproduced from Levine RA, Triulzi MO, Harrigan P, Weyman AE. The relationship of mitral annular shape to the diagnosis of mitral valve prolapse. *Circulation*, 75(4): page 761; © 1987 Lippincott, Williams & Wilkins with permission.

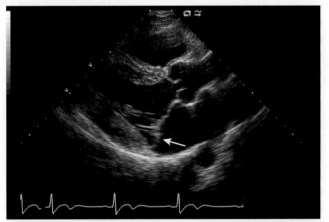
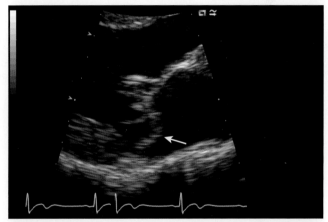

Figure 8.41 These systolic still frame images, recorded from the parasternal long axis view, demonstrate posterior mitral valve prolapse (*arrows*). Observe that when the mitral valve is closed in systole, the posterior leaflet bulges into the left atrium beyond the atrioventricular plane.

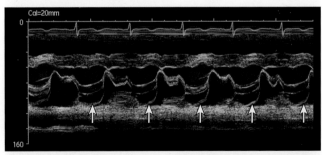

Figure 8.42 This M-mode trace through the mitral valve demonstrates "hammocking" of both the anterior and posterior mitral valve leaflets (*arrows*). This appearance is characteristic of mitral valve prolapse.

In patients with MVP, degeneration may involve the other cardiac valves; tricuspid valve prolapse is seen in about 40% of patients while pulmonary valve prolapse and aortic valve prolapse occur in about 10% and 2% of patients, respectively. Furthermore, about 20% of patients with a secundum atrial septal defect also have MVP.

Ischaemic Mitral Regurgitation

As stated above, IMR refers to MR resulting from segmental LV wall motion abnormalities following an AMI. Several clues to the presence of IMR can be appreciated on the 2D examination. These clues include: (1) segmental or regional wall motion abnormalities, (2) the presence of LV systolic dysfunction, (3) displacement of the papillary muscles, and (4) tethering or tenting of the mitral valve. In particular, systolic 'kinking' of the anterior mitral leaflet in its mid-belly, also known as the 'seagull' sign, is a characteristic feature associated with IMR (Fig. 8.46).

Various 2D parameters have also been described to predict the likelihood of persistent or recurrent MR following mitral valve repair in patients with IMR (Table 8.8). These parameters include the: (1) interpapillary muscle distance, (2) sphericity index, (3) tenting area, (4) coaptation depth, (5) posterior leaflet angle, and (6) anterior leaflet angle (Fig. 8.47-8.52). Consideration of these parameters may be important in selecting patients for mitral valve repair versus mitral valve replacement, or for new alternative procedures.

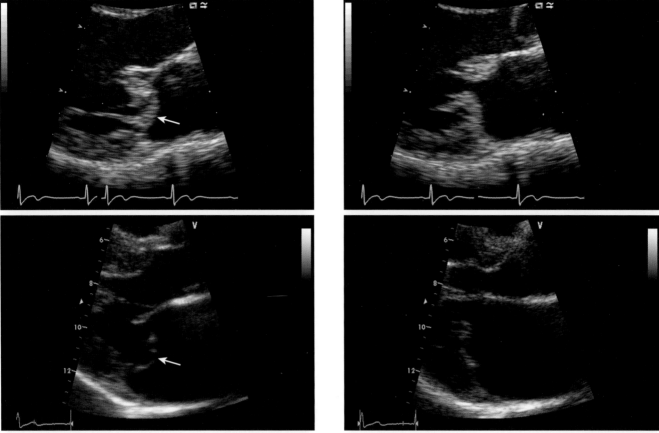

Figure 8.43 These zoomed views of the mitral valve were recorded from the parasternal long axis view. Systolic frames are shown to the left and diastolic frames are shown to the right. Mitral valve prolapse is indicated by the arrows. Observe that in a Barlow's valve, the leaflets appear thickened and bulky and prolapse involves multiple segments or scallops (*top*). With fibroelastic deficiency the leaflets appear thin and prolapse is typically isolated to one scallop; usually P2 as in this example (*bottom*).

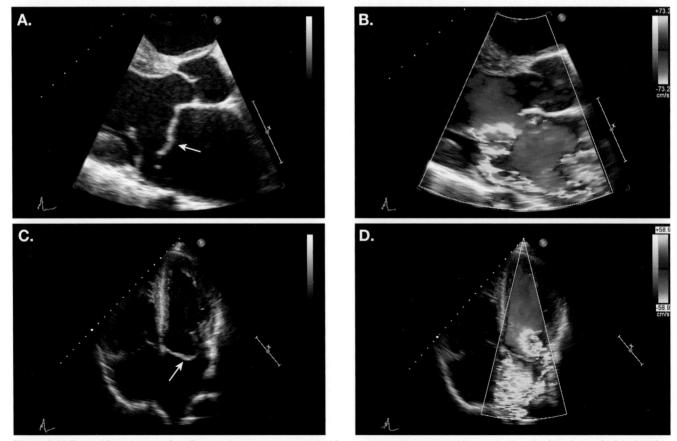

Figure 8.44 These 2D and colour flow Doppler images were recorded from a zoomed parasternal long axis view (*top*) and an apical 4-chamber view (*bottom*). Observe the flail anterior mitral valve leaflet on the 2D images (*arrows*). Observe on the colour Doppler images that the mitral regurgitant (MR) jet is baffled in a direction opposite to the flail leaflet. For example, from the parasternal long axis view, the MR jet is directed posteriorly (B) while from the apical 4-chamber view, the MR jet is baffled laterally (D).

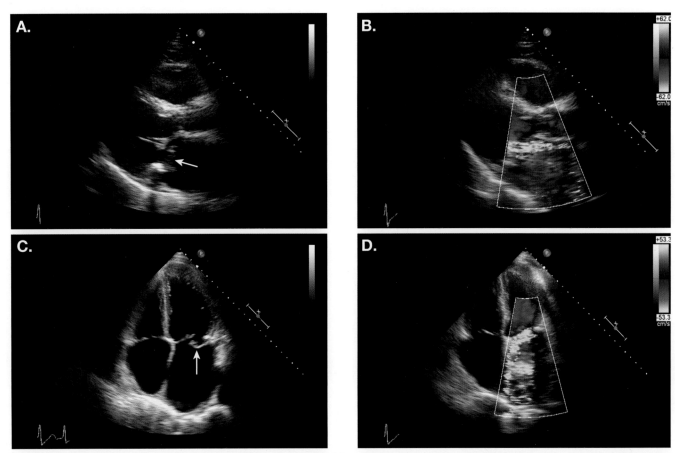

Figure 8.45 These 2D and colour flow Doppler images were recorded from the parasternal long axis view (*top*) and the apical 4-chamber view (*bottom*). Observe the marked prolapse of the posterior mitral valve leaflet on the 2D images (*arrows*). Observe on the colour Doppler images that the mitral regurgitant (MR) jet is baffled in a direction opposite to the prolapsing leaflet. For example, from the parasternal long axis view, the MR jet is directed anteriorly (B) while from the apical 4-chamber view, the MR jet is baffled medially (D).

Assessment of Left Atrial Size

Increased LA pressure leads to dilatation of the LA. As stated previously, the preferred method for measuring LA size is the biplane area-length method for LA volume. These measurements are performed in the manner described previously (under Mitral Stenosis). The accuracy of LA volume measurements relies on several variables which are detailed in Chapter 3 (see Table 3.2).

Assessment of Left Ventricular Size and Systolic Function

Left ventricular size, wall thickness and systolic function can be assessed by both M-mode and 2D echocardiography in the traditional manner (see Chapter 2). As previously mentioned, chronic volume overload of the LV secondary to chronic significant MR leads to progressive LV dilatation. As a result the LV tends to adopt a spherical shape.

In the early stages of MR, LV systolic function remains normal. However, with chronic severe MR, the LV function will eventually decline. Importantly, because the LVEF is load dependent, the LVEF is sensitive to changes in preload and afterload. Therefore, in MR, preload is increased and afterload is decreased so the LVEF may not accurately reflect the contractile function of the ventricle. That is, there may be significant underlying LV systolic dysfunction but the LVEF may remain normal. Therefore, in patients with MR, a greater lower limit for normal has been set. For example, in most cases the lower limit of normal for the LVEF is 55%, however, in patients with significant MR the lower limit of normal is 60%.

Furthermore, LV dimensions are critical for the serial follow-up of patients with MR. In particular, the LV end-diastolic dimension (LVEDD), the LV end-systolic dimension (LVESD) and the LVEF are used for determining the management of patients with chronic severe MR; for this reason, it is crucial that these measurements are accurately performed.

Estimation of Severity

An accurate assessment of the severity of MR requires a comprehensive evaluation of all possible Doppler variables. Therefore, the MR severity should be determined by looking for: (a) indirect signs of MR severity on colour and spectral Doppler and (b) by performing quantitative calculations.

Indirect Signs for Assessing MR Severity: Colour Doppler Flow Imaging

Colour Doppler flow imaging (CFI) provides a quick and easy method for identifying the presence of MR. CFI also provides indirect clues to MR severity. In particular, assessment of the colour jet area compared to the LA area, the flow convergence radius and the vena contracta width are very useful in determining the severity of MR. The criteria for defining the various grades of MR based on these methods are summarized in Table 8.9.

> MR jets can be quite complex, especially when there is MVP. Therefore, a thorough colour Doppler assessment of the MR jet is crucial. This includes slowly and carefully angling and tilting through the valve from multiple views; off-axis images and multiple clips may be required to show the full extent of the MR jet.

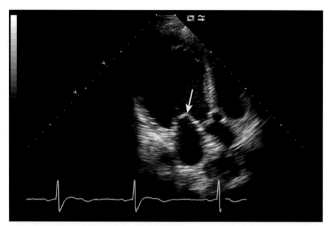

Figure 8.46 This image was recorded from the apical long axis view in mid systole. Observe the deformity of the anterior mitral valve which appears as a kinking of the leaflet in its mid-belly (*arrow*). This is also referred to as the 'seagull' sign; this appearance is caused by tethering of the anterior mitral valve leaflet by secondary tendinous cords.

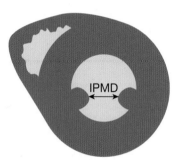

Figure 8.47 The interpapillary muscle distance (IPMD) is simply measured as the distance between the two papillary muscles at end-systole as viewed from the parasternal short axis view at the level of the papillary muscles.

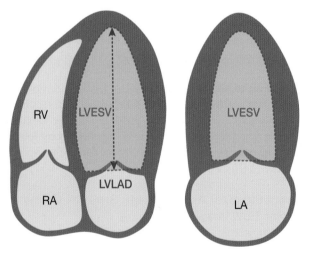

Figure 8.48 The sphericity index (SI) determines left ventricular geometry. This index is derived from the: (1) biplane LV volume end-systolic volume (LVESV) measured from the apical 4-chamber and apical 2-chamber views and (2) from the long-axis dimension of the left ventricle (LVLAD) measured in the apical 4-chamber view at end-systole. From the LVLAD measurement, the volume of a sphere (Vs) is calculated as π LVLAD^3 ÷ 6. The SI is then calculated as the LVESV divided by Vs.
LA = left atrium; RA = right atrium; RV = right ventricle.

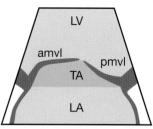

Figure 8.49 The tenting area (TA) is an index of mitral leaflet tethering and is defined as the smallest area between the mitral annulus and the two mitral leaflets. The TA is measured from a zoomed apical 4-chamber view of the mitral valve at mid-systole.
amvl = anterior mitral valve leaflet; LA = left atrium; LV = left ventricle; pmvl = posterior mitral valve leaflet.

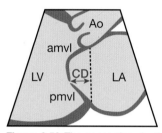
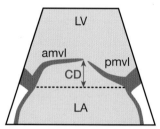

Figure 8.50 The coaptation depth (CD), also known as the tethering height, is defined as the shortest distance between leaflet coaptation and the mitral annulus plane during systole. The CD is measured from a zoomed view of the mitral valve recorded from either a parasternal long axis view (*left*) or apical 4-chamber view (*right*) at mid-systole.
Ao = aorta; amvl = anterior mitral valve leaflet; LA = left atrium; LV = left ventricle; pmvl = posterior mitral valve leaflet.

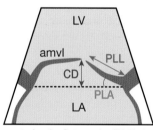

Figure 8.51 The posterior leaflet angle (PLA) is derived from two measurements performed from a zoomed apical 4-chamber view of the mitral valve, recorded at mid-systole. The coaptation distance (CD) is measured as the distance between the leaflet coaptation and the mitral annulus plane. The posterior leaflet length (PLL) is measured as the distance between the posterior annulus and the tip of the posterior leaflet. From these two measurements, the PLA is calculated as:

$$PLA = sin^{-1}\left[\frac{CD}{PLL}\right]$$

amvl = anterior mitral valve leaflet; LA = left atrium; LV = left ventricle.

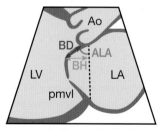

Figure 8.52 The anterior leaflet angle (ALA) is derived from two measurements performed from a zoomed parasternal long axis view of the mitral valve recorded at mid-systole. The bending height (BH) is measured between the annular line and the bending angle created by tethering in the body of the anterior leaflet. The bending distance (BD) is measured as the distance between the bending point and the anterior annulus. From these two measurements, the ALA is calculated as:

$$ALA = sin^{-1}\left[\frac{BH}{BD}\right]$$

Ao = aorta; amvl = anterior mitral valve leaflet; LA = left atrium; LV = left ventricle; pmvl = posterior mitral valve leaflet.

Table 8.8 Selected Pre-Operative 2D Echocardiographic Predictors of Post-Operative Persistent or Recurrent Mitral Regurgitation

Echo Parameter	Echo View	Cut-off Value	Sens. (%)	Spec. (%)	Ref.
Interpapillary Muscle Distance (iPMD)	PSAX	> 20 mm	96	97	1
Sphericity Index (systolic)	AP4-ch	≥ 0.7	100	100	2
Tenting Area (TA)	AP4-ch	≥ 2.5 cm^2	64	95	3
Coaptation Depth (CD)	AP4-ch	≥ 10 mm	64	90	3, 4
	PLAX	≥ 11 mm	81	84	
Posterior Leaflet Angle (PLA)	AP4-ch	$\geq 45^0$	100	95	3
Anterior Leaflet Angle (ALA)	PLAX	$\geq 39.5^0$	98	97	4

AP4-ch = apical 4-chamber view; PLAX = parasternal long axis view; PSAX = parasternal short axis view at the level of the papillary muscles; Ref. = reference; Sens. = sensitivity; Spec. = specificity.

References: [1] Roshanali F, Mandegar MH, Yousefnia MA, Rayatzadeh H, Alaeddini F. A prospective study of predicting factors in ischemic mitral regurgitation recurrence after ring annuloplasty. *Ann Thorac Surg.* 2007 Sept;84(3):745–9;
[2] Gelsomino S, Lorusso R, De Cicco G, Capecchi I, Rostagno C, Caciolli S, et al. Five-year echocardiographic results of combined undersized mitral ring annuloplasty and coronary artery bypass grafting for chronic ischaemic mitral regurgitation. *Eur Heart J.* 2008 Jan;29(2):231–40;
[3] Magne J, Pibarot P, Dagenais F, Hachicha Z, Dumesnil JG, Sénéchal M. Preoperative Posterior Leaflet Angle Accurately Predicts Outcome After Restrictive Mitral Valve Annuloplasty for Ischemic Mitral Regurgitation. *Circulation.* 2007 Feb 13;115(6):782–91;
[4] Gelsomino S, Lorusso R, Caciolli S, Capecchi I, Rostagno C, Chioccioli M, et al. Insights on left ventricular and valvular mechanisms of recurrent ischemic mitral regurgitation after restrictive annuloplasty and coronary artery bypass grafting. *J Thorac Cardiovasc Surg.* 2008 Aug;136(2):507–18.

Table 8.9 Qualitative Colour Doppler Parameters for Grading Mitral Regurgitation Severity

Parameter	Mild	Moderate	Severe
Jet area ratio (%)*	Small, central jet (< 4 cm^2 or < 20% of LA area)	Variable	Large central jet (usually >10 cm^2 or >40% of LA area) or variable size wall-impinging jet swirling in LA
Vena contracta width (cm)*	< 0.30	0.30-0.69	≥ 0.7
Flow convergence radius (cm)#	No or minimal flow convergence (< 0.4 central jet)	Variable	Large flow convergence (≥ 0.9 central jet)

* Using a Nyquist limit of 50–60 cm/s
# with a baseline shift at a Nyquist limit of 40 cm/s; cut-offs for eccentric jets are higher, and should be angle corrected.
Source: Zoghbi WA, Enriquez-Sarano M, Foster E, Grayburn PA, Kraft CD, Levine RA, Nihoyannopoulos P, Otto CM, Quinones MA, Rakowski H, Stewart WJ, Waggoner A, Weissman NJ; American Society of Echocardiography. Recommendations for evaluation of the severity of native valvular regurgitation with two-dimensional and Doppler echocardiography. *J Am Soc Echocardiogr.* 2003 Jul;16(7):777-802.

Colour Jet Area and Colour Jet Area Ratio

Comparing the size of the MR jet area to the LA area is a rapid way for semiquantitating the severity of MR. Because regurgitant jets are 3D, the MR jet area to LA area ratio must be evaluated by angling through the regurgitant jet (off-axis imaging may be required) and by using multiple orthogonal planes (Fig. 8.53). Most commonly, an 'eyeball' evaluation, rather than direct measurement, of the jet area ratio is performed.

Vena Contracta Width

The vena contracta (VC) is defined as the narrowest part of the jet downstream from the narrowed orifice (see Fig. 1.21). With respect to regurgitant jets, the VC is the narrowest region of the regurgitant jet which occurs between the proximal flow convergence zone and the actual regurgitant jet. The vena contracta width (VC-W) of a regurgitant jet provides an estimate of the effective regurgitant orifice size.

The VC-W is best measured when it appears perpendicular to the ultrasound beam. This is because this measurement is then performed along the axial plane and resolution along the axial plane is superior to resolution in the lateral plane. Accurate measurement of the VC-W requires all three components of the regurgitant flow to be seen. These three components are: (1) the flow convergence dome, (2) the VC, and (3) the regurgitant jet (Fig. 8.54).

Flow Convergence Radius

As the described in Chapter 1, as flow converges toward a narrowed orifice it accelerates in a laminar manner forming a flow convergence zone. This flow convergence zone is comprised of a series of concentric hemispheric shells of uniform velocity (isovelocities). As flow advances closer to the narrowed orifice, the area of each hemispheric shell decreases and the velocity of each shell increases. This assumption forms the basis of the PISA principle for the calculation of the EOA.

Typically, the PISA principle is used to calculate the effective regurgitant orifice area (EROA) (discussed later). However, measurement of the PISA radius or the flow convergence radius (FCR) proximal to a regurgitant orifice may provide an indirect clue as to the severity of valvular regurgitation; for example, the bigger the FCR the more significant the regurgitation. In the case of MR, the FCR is measured on the LV side of the mitral valve during systole at a colour Nyquist limit of approximately 40 cm/s (Fig. 8.55).

Limitations of CFI Indirect Signs

There are numerous technical and physiological factors that can affect the colour flow Doppler map unrelated to the severity of MR (see Table 7.8). In particular, recall that Doppler techniques detect the motion of moving red blood cells (RBC). As such any RBC in motion will create a Doppler shift and this Doppler shift is detected by the ultrasound machine. Therefore, RBCs in the receiving chamber that are displaced by the regurgitant jet will be incorporated into the 'colour regurgitant volume'. As a result, the RV will be overestimated on the colour Doppler display. The severity of regurgitation may also be underestimated when the regurgitant jet is eccentric. In these situations, the regurgitant jet is attracted to and 'hugs' the adjacent chamber

wall (Fig. 8.56). As a result the regurgitant jet area can appear significantly smaller than free jets due to jet distortion and loss of jet momentum. In this situation, the regurgitant jet area does not reflect the severity of regurgitation. The cause of this phenomenon is based on the Coandă effect. In these situations, alternate methods for assessing MR severity such as the FCR or other quantitative methods are required.

The principal limitation of the VC-W in the assessment of MR severity is the assumption that the regurgitant orifice is almost circular. However, the regurgitant orifice is often elliptic or irregular in shape rather than circular.

When there are multiple regurgitant jets, neither the VC-W nor the FCR can be used to qualitatively assess the severity of MR. This is because respective VC-Ws and FCRs are not additive.

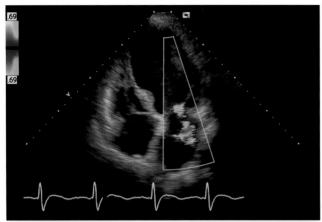

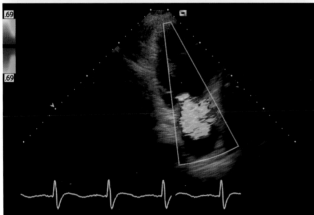

Figure 8.53 These two systolic colour flow Doppler still frame images were recorded from the same patient. These images highlight the importance of evaluating mitral regurgitation (MR) in multiple views. The apical 4-chamber image shows 'some' degree of MR (*top*). From this view alone, it is difficult to determine the degree of MR. From the apical 2-chamber image a greater degree of MR is evident (*bottom*). Based on this view the MR appears at least moderate.

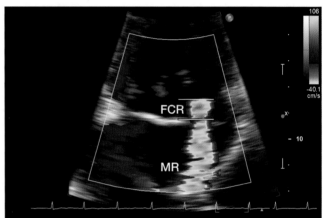

Figure 8.55 This zoomed image of the mitral valve was recorded from the apical 4-chamber view during systole. Colour flow imaging demonstrates mitral regurgitation (MR). The flow convergence zone proximal to the mitral valve is magnified by decreasing the colour Nyquist limit (V_N) to 40 cm/s; this is achieved by moving the colour baseline downwards in the direction of the MR jet. The flow convergence radius (FCR) is measured as the vertical distance from the mitral valve leaflets to the top of the flow convergence zone which is identified as the blue-red interface.

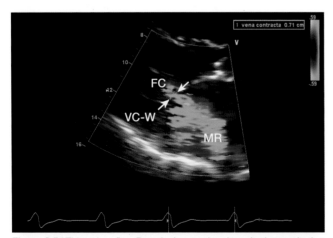

Figure 8.54 This colour flow Doppler image showing mitral regurgitation (MR) was recorded from a zoomed parasternal long axis view. The vena contracta width (VC-W) is measured at the narrowest neck of the MR flow region at the junction of the flow convergence zone (FC) and the regurgitant jet immediately below the flow convergence region.

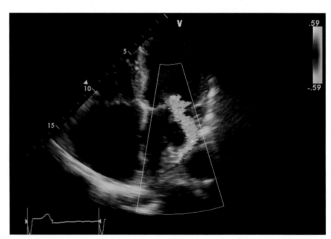

Figure 8.56 This colour Doppler image was recorded from the apical 4-chamber view in a patient with severe mitral regurgitation (MR). The Coandă effect is shown as the MR jet adheres to (hugs) the left atrial wall. Observe that the MR jet appears quite narrow despite the presence of a large flow convergence zone on the left ventricular side of the mitral valve. Consideration of the MR jet area alone will underestimate the MR severity in this case.

Indirect Signs for Assessing MR Severity: Spectral Doppler

Indirect signs of MR severity can also be provided by PW and CW spectral Doppler. PW Doppler methods include the transmitral inflow profile and the presence of systolic flow reversal in the pulmonary veins. CW Doppler methods include the intensity of the MR signal and the shape or contour of the MR signal. The criteria for defining the various grades of MR via these methods are summarized in Table 8.10.

Transmitral Inflow Velocities

The flow across the mitral valve in MR is the combination of the mitral RV and the normal SV returning from the lungs. Therefore, in patients with significant MR, the transmitral flow is often increased. This may be evident by an increased peak E velocity or a 'restrictive' filling pattern via PW Doppler or by increased mean transmitral pressure gradients as measured by CW Doppler. In particular, an A dominant velocity (E/A ratio < 1) essentially excludes the presence of severe MR.

Importantly, the value of the transmitral inflow pattern for semi-quantitating the severity of MR is more applicable to the older patient (greater than 50 yrs) or in conditions of impaired LV relaxation (for example, in hypertensive heart disease). This is because in these groups of patients, an abnormal relaxation pattern is expected so the presence of increased early diastolic transmitral inflow velocities indicates an increase in the LA pressure which can be attributed to the presence of significant MR.

Pulmonary Venous Flow Reversal

The presence of systolic flow reversal in the pulmonary veins demonstrated by PW Doppler is another clue to the presence of significant MR. Pulmonary venous flow is interrogated by PW Doppler from the apical 4-chamber view with a 3-5 mm sample volume placed at least 1 cm into the pulmonary vein. The normal pulmonary venous flow profile demonstrates predominant forward flow during systole and diastole with a small antegrade velocity occurring with atrial contraction (atrial flow reversal) (Fig. 8.57, top). With severe MR, systolic flow reversal may be present (Fig. 8.57, bottom). The presence of systolic flow reversal in the pulmonary veins is a very specific sign of severe MR; however, it is not very sensitive. That is, when present, pulmonary venous systolic flow reversal is a good indicator to the presence of significant MR; however, there can be significant MR without systolic flow reversal.

Intensity of MR CW Signal

In theory, the density or intensity of the spectral Doppler signal of a regurgitant jet is proportional to the number of RBC travelling within the regurgitant jet. Therefore, the greater the regurgitation, the denser the regurgitant CW signal. For example, a weak Doppler signal is suggestive of relatively mild valvular regurgitation whereas a strong signal is suggestive of more significant regurgitation.

Contour of MR CW Signal

The CW Doppler signal for MR reflects the pressure gradient between the LV and the LA during systole. Therefore, the contour of this velocity spectrum reflects the pressure gradient between the LV and the LA during systole. In particular, when there is mild MR, the LA pressure is usually normal; thus, the pressure difference between LV and LA is relatively high and remains consistently high throughout the entire systolic period; the resultant spectral Doppler signal shows a symmetrical or parabolic contour (Fig. 8.58, left). However, in the case of severe MR associated with an increased LA v-wave

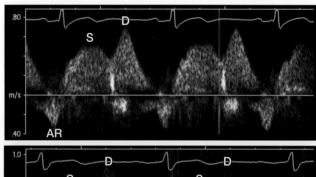
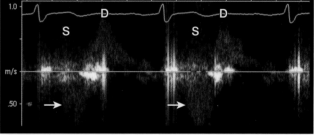

Figure 8.57 These pulsed-wave (PW) spectral Doppler signals were recorded from a patient with no mitral regurgitation (MR) (*top*) and a patient with severe MR (*bottom*). Both signals were recorded from the apical 4-chamber view with the PW sample volume placed approximately 1 cm into the right upper pulmonary vein. In the normal patient, three waveforms are seen: systolic forward flow (S), diastolic forward flow (D) and flow reversal with atrial contraction (AR). In the patient with severe MR, systolic flow reversal is present (*arrows*).

Table 8.10 Qualitative Spectral Doppler Parameters for Grading Mitral Regurgitation Severity

Parameter	Mild	Moderate	Severe
Transmitral inflow (PW)	A wave dominant #	Variable	E wave dominant (> 1.5 m/s)*
Pulmonary venous (PW)	Systolic dominance ^	Systolic blunting^	Systolic reversal
Intensity of MR signal (CW)	Incomplete or faint	Dense	Dense
MR Jet Contour (CW)	Parabolic	Usually parabolic	Early peaking or triangular

CW = continuous-wave Doppler; PW = pulsed-wave Doppler,
\# Usually after 50 years of age
* in the absence of other causes of elevated left atrial pressure and of mitral stenosis.
^ Unless other reasons for systolic blunting (e.g. atrial fibrillation, elevated LA pressure).

Sources: Zoghbi WA, Enriquez-Sarano M, Foster E, Grayburn PA, Kraft CD, Levine RA, Nihoyannopoulos P, Otto CM, Quinones MA, Rakowski H, Stewart WJ, Waggoner A, Weissman NJ; American Society of Echocardiography. Recommendations for evaluation of the severity of native valvular regurgitation with two-dimensional and Doppler echocardiography. *J Am Soc Echocardiogr.* 2003 Jul;16(7):777-802; Lancellotti P, Tribouilloy C, Hagendorff A, Moura L, Popescu BA, Agricola E, Monin JL, Pierard LA, Badano L, Zamorano JL; European Association of Echocardiography. European Association of Echocardiography recommendations for the assessment of valvular regurgitation. Part 2: mitral and tricuspid regurgitation (native valve disease). *Eur J Echocardiogr.* 2010 May;11(4):307-332.

pressure, the contour of the MR signal becomes triangular as the pressure difference between the LV and LA in mid-to-late systole decreases due to the marked elevation in the LA *v*-wave pressure (Fig. 8.58, right). The triangular appearance of the MR signal is also referred to as the 'V cut-off' sign.

Limitations of Spectral Doppler Indirect Signs

The intensity of the MR signal can be affected by a number of factors. For example, Doppler gain affects the overall intensity of the regurgitant jet; if the gain is set too low then the signal intensity will also be decreased. In addition, poor alignment of the MR jet with the Doppler beam will result in a suboptimal MR signal; this is especially a problem with eccentric jets.

The presence of systolic flow reversal in the pulmonary veins strongly supports the diagnosis of severe MR. However, systolic flow reversal within the pulmonary veins may be absent when the MR jet is eccentric. In addition, the systolic

ECG

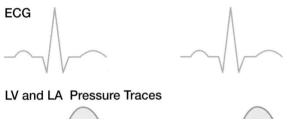

LV and LA Pressure Traces

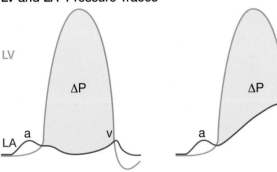

Doppler Velocity Curves

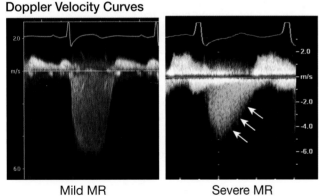

Mild MR   Severe MR

Figure 8.58 In mitral regurgitation (MR), the regurgitant Doppler velocity signal reflects the pressure difference (ΔP) between the left ventricle (LV) and the left atrium (LA) during systole. The top schematics illustrate the pressure tracings of the LV and the LA during systole while the Doppler velocity spectra corresponding to these traces are displayed below. The LA pressure trace consists of an *a*-wave which represents an increase in LA pressure with atrial contraction and a *v*-wave which represents an increase in LA pressure, caused by venous return into the LA, during ventricular systole. In mild MR (*left*), the ΔP between the LV and LA from early to late systole is relatively high; this results in a symmetrical, parabolic Doppler velocity curve. With severe MR (*right*), the ΔP between the LV and LA is high from early to mid systole as for mild MR. However, with an increased volume of blood entering the LA via the incompetent mitral valve, there is an increase in the *v*-wave of the LA pressure trace which leads to a decrease in the ΔP between the LV and LA toward the latter half of systole; this results in a rapid and asymmetric, V-shaped Doppler velocity curve (*triple arrows*).

velocity of the pulmonary venous flow profile is affected by LA pressure and AF. For example, systolic blunting is commonly encountered with AF due to the absence of effective LA relaxation. In addition, MR severity may be overestimated when the MR jet is aimed directly into the sampled vein.

An increased early diastolic velocity (E velocity) can be used to identify an increased forward SV across the mitral valve which is associated with significant MR; however, the peak E velocity is also affected by the heart rate, LA pressure, LV relaxation, and AF. For example, the E velocity may be increased in the absence of significant MR if the patient is tachycardic.

While the V cut-off sign is an indicator of a marked increase in the LA *v*-wave pressure, this is dependent on LA compliance. For example, this sign may be absent even when there is severe MR and when the LA compliance is high; that is, the LA is able to accept a large volume of blood without a significant increase in the LA pressure. Furthermore, this sign relies on the acquisition of a complete MR signal which is difficult to obtain in eccentric MR jets.

Estimation of LA Pressure from the MR Doppler Signal
The peak MR velocity reflects the pressure difference between the LV and the LA during systole:

Equation 8.7

$$4V_{MR}^2 = LVSP - LAP$$

where V_{MR} = peak MR velocity (m/s)
   LVSP = left ventricular systolic pressure (mm Hg)
   LAP = left atrial pressure (mm Hg)

In the absence of aortic stenosis or significant LVOT obstruction, the LVSP can be assumed to be the same as the systolic blood pressure (SBP). Therefore, by measuring the peak MR velocity and the SBP, the LAP can be estimated as:

Equation 8.8

$$LAP = SBP - 4V_{MR}^2$$

where LAP = left ventricular end-diastolic pressure (mm Hg)
   SBP = systolic blood pressure (mm Hg)
   V_{MR} = peak MR velocity (m/s)

Caveat: The important limitation of this calculation is that the difference between two relatively high pressures (SBP and the LV-LA pressure gradient) is used to estimate a relatively low pressure (LAP).

Quantitative Methods for MR Severity

Quantitative calculations for the assessment of MR severity include the:
• Regurgitant volume,
• Regurgitant fraction,
• Effective regurgitant orifice area.

The criteria for defining the various grades of MR based on these methods are listed in Table 8.11.

Regurgitant Volume

Regurgitant volume (RV) is defined as the volume of blood that leaks (regurgitates) through an incompetent valve. RV can be calculated using the SV method or the proximal isovelocity surface area (PISA) method.

A. Stroke volume method

The basic concepts of SV calculations and how these calculations can be used to estimate the RV are described in Chapter 1. Recall that the calculation of RV is based on the estimation of the SV across the leaking valve and the SV across a competent (non-leaking) valve. In the case of MR, the RV can be calculated from the mitral annular SV and, providing that there is no AR, the SV across the LVOT:

Equation 8.9

$$RV_{MR} = SV_{MA} - SV_{LVOT}$$

where RV_{MR} = mitral regurgitant volume (mL)
SV_{MA} = stroke volume across mitral annulus (mL)
SV_{LVOT} = stroke volume across left ventricular outflow tract (mL)

Recall that the SV is a product of the CSA and the VTI. Therefore, to perform this calculation four sets of measurements are required (Fig. 8.59):
1. LVOT diameter (used to calculate the LVOT CSA),
2. LVOT VTI,
3. mitral annular diameter (used to calculate the mitral annular CSA),
4. mitral annular VTI.

In the event that AR is present, the RV can still be calculated by substituting the SV derived from the RVOT for the LVOT SV, providing that there is no intracardiac shunt and no significant regurgitation across the pulmonary valve.

The limitations of RV calculations via this method are the same as those limitations described for SV calculations (see Chapter 2). In particular, common errors in mitral annular measurements include: (1) not measuring the annulus at the correct phase of the cardiac cycle, and (2) not measuring the annulus at the same site as the VTI signal. Importantly, any error in the annular measurement is magnified because

---

RV using 2D LV Volumes
In theory, it is possible to calculate the mitral RV (RV_{MR}) using the SV derived from 2D LV end-diastolic and end-systolic volumes (SV_{2D}) and the Doppler derived LVOT SV (SV_{LVOT}). The SV_{2D} reflects the amount of blood being ejected from the LV; therefore, this SV includes the SV_{LVOT} plus the RV_{MR}. So by subtracting the SV_{LVOT} from the SV_{2D}, the RV_{MR} can be estimated ($RV_{MR} = SV_{2D} - SV_{LVOT}$). This method however is **not** recommended for the calculation of the RV_{MR} as 2D echocardiography has a known tendency to significantly underestimate LV volumes; therefore, both the SV_{2D} and the RV_{MR} will also be underestimated.

---

the diameter is squared to derive the CSA. Common VTI measurement errors include: (1) non-parallel alignment between the Doppler beam and blood flow, (2) incorrect placement of the PW Doppler sample volume (that is, not placed at the mitral annulus), (3) failure to optimise the Doppler trace, and (4) not tracing the modal velocity.

B. PISA Method

The RV via the PISA method is based on first estimating the effective regurgitation orifice area (EROA) via the PISA technique (discussed below) and then by tracing the VTI of the regurgitant jet. Calculation of the RV via this technique is based on the standard SV equation whereby the SV is a product of the CSA and VTI. Based on this relationship between SV, CSA and VTI, the RV is simply derived by substituting the RV for SV, EROA for CSA, and VTI of the regurgitant jet (VTI_{RJ}) for the VTI:

Equation 8.10

$$RV = EROA \times VTI_{RJ}$$

where RV = regurgitant volume (mL)
EROA = effective regurgitant orifice area (cm^2)
VTI_{RJ} = velocity time integral of regurgitant jet (cm)

Therefore, to perform this calculation for MR two parameters are required (see Fig. 8.60):
1. EROA for MR,
2. VTI of the MR jet.

The limitations of RV calculations via this method are the same as those limitations described for the calculation of the EROA via the PISA technique (see Chapter 2 and below).

Regurgitant Fraction

Regurgitant fraction (RF) is defined as the percentage of the regurgitant volume compared with total SV across the incompetent valve. Therefore, in the case of MR calculation of the mitral RF is simply derived from the mitral RV and the SV across the mitral annulus (Fig. 8.59):

Equation 8.11

$$RF_{MR} = (RV_{MR} \div SV_{MA}) \times 100$$

where RF_{MR} = mitral regurgitant fraction (%)
RV_{MR} = mitral regurgitant volume (mL)
SV_{MA} = stroke volume across mitral annulus (mL)

The limitations of this calculation include those limitations described for RV calculations via the SV method (see above).

Table 8.11 Quantitative Methods for Grading Mitral Regurgitation Severity

Parameter	Mild	Moderate		Severe
Regurgitant Volume (mL)	< 30	30-44	45-59	≥ 60
Regurgitant Fraction (%)	<30	30-39	40-49	≥ 50
Effective Regurgitant Orifice Area (cm^2)	< 0.20	0.20-0.29	0.30-0.39	≥ 0.40

Moderate regurgitation can be classified into mild-to-moderate and moderate-to-severe regurgitation as shown.
Source: Zoghbi WA, Enriquez-Sarano M, Foster E, Grayburn PA, Kraft CD, Levine RA, Nihoyannopoulos P, Otto CM, Quinones MA, Rakowski H, Stewart WJ, Waggoner A, Weissman NJ; American Society of Echocardiography. Recommendations for evaluation of the severity of native valvular regurgitation with two-dimensional and Doppler echocardiography. *J Am Soc Echocardiogr.* 2003 Jul;16(7):777-802.

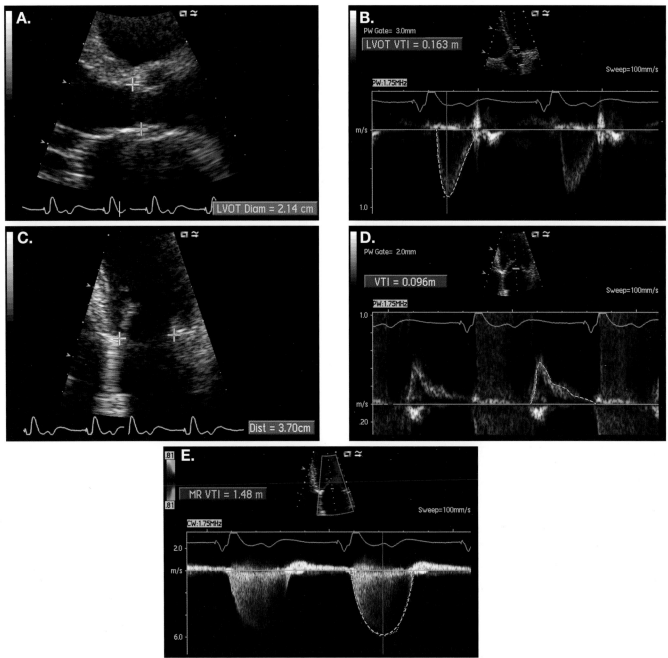

Figure 8.59 The regurgitant volume (RV) for mitral regurgitation (MR) is calculated from the SV across the mitral annulus (SV$_{MA}$) and the stroke volume across the left ventricular outflow tract (SV$_{LVOT}$). SV$_{LVOT}$ is derived from the LVOT diameter and velocity time integral (VTI). The LVOT diameter is measured from zoomed parasternal long axis view of the LVOT (A). At mid-systole callipers are placed from the inner junction between the anterior aortic wall and the interventricular septum to the inner junction between the posterior aortic wall and the anterior leaflet of the mitral valve, perpendicular to the aortic root. From an apical 5-chamber view the LVOT VTI is recorded via pulsed-wave (PW) Doppler signal with a 2-4 mm sample volume placed 0.5 cm proximal to the aortic valve (B). SV$_{MA}$ is derived from the mitral annular diameter and VTI at the mitral annulus. The mitral annular diameter is measured from a zoomed apical 4-chamber view of the mitral valve at early diastole (2-3 frames after end-systole); callipers are placed from where the leaflets insert into the ventricular myocardium using the inner edge to inner edge technique (C). From the same apical 4-chamber view the mitral annular VTI is recorded via PW Doppler signal with a 1-2 mm sample volume placed at the level of the mitral annulus; the VTI is traced along the modal velocity (D). The mitral RV in this example is calculated as:

$$RV_{MR} = SV_{MA} - SV_{LVOT}$$
$$= (CSA_{MA} \times VTI_{MA}) - (CSA_{LVOT} \times VTI_{LVOT})$$
$$= (0.785 \times 3.7^2 \times 9.6) - (0.785 \times 2.14^2 \times 16.3)$$
$$= 103 - 59$$
$$= 44 \text{ mL}$$

The mitral RF in this example is calculated as:

$$RF_{MR} = (RV_{MR} \div SV_{MA}) \times 100$$
$$= (44 \div 103) \times 100$$
$$= 43\%$$

By tracing the VTI of the MR signal (E), the effective regurgitant orifice area (EROA) can also be derived as:

$$EROA_{MR} = RV_{MR} \div VTI_{MR}$$
$$= 44 \div 148$$
$$= 0.30 \text{ cm}^2$$

Note: When performing these calculations, all units should be first converted to cm or cm/s and all measurements should be averaged over at least 2 consecutive cardiac cycles when there is sinus rhythm or over 3-5 cardiac cycles when there is atrial fibrillation.

Technical Tip for RV and RF calculations

RV and RF calculations via the SV method are calculated from the SV derived from the LVOT and the mitral annulus. Knowledge of the normal values for the VTI and annular diameters at these sites is helpful when undertaking these measurements. For example, in a patient with MR, the LVOT parameters would be expected to be close to the normal range; therefore, if the LVOT measurements are well outside the normal range, this would be a clue that this measurement has not been performed correctly.

The normal VTI and annular measurements for the LVOT and mitral annulus are tabled below.

Measurement	Normal values
Mitral annular diameter	3.0 - 3.5 cm
Mitral annular VTI	10 - 13 cm
LVOT diameter	1.8 - 2.2 cm
LVOT VTI	18 - 22 cm

Effective Regurgitant Orifice Area

The effective regurgitant orifice area (EROA) is the size of the 'hole' in the incompetent valve. The EROA can be calculated using the SV method or the PISA method.

A. Stroke Volume Method

The SV method for calculating the EROA is based on the relationship between SV, CSA and VTI as previously described. Therefore, if the RV and the VTI of the regurgitant signal are measured, then this equation can be arranged to calculate the EROA (Fig. 8.59):

Equation 8.12

$$EROA = RV \div VTI_{RJ}$$

where EROA = effective regurgitant orifice area (cm²)

RV   = regurgitant volume (mL)

VTI_{RJ} = velocity time integral of regurgitant jet (cm)

B. PISA Method for EROA

The basic concepts of the PISA principle in the calculation of the effective orifice area are described in Chapter 1. Recall that this calculation is based on the continuity principle which states that flow proximal to a narrowed orifice must equal flow through the narrowed orifice.

In the case of MR, the EROA can be calculated from the radius of the proximal flow convergence dome, the velocity at this radius, and the peak velocity of the MR jet (Fig. 8.60):

Equation 8.13

$$EROA_{MR} = (2\pi r^2 \times V_N) \div V_{MR}$$

where $EROA_{MR}$ = mitral effective regurgitant orifice area (cm²)

$2\pi r^2$ = surface area of the hemispheric shell derived from the flow convergence radius [r] proximal to the mitral valve (cm²)

V_N = colour Nyquist limit at the radial distance of the hemispheric shell (cm/s)

V_{MR} = peak velocity of mitral regurgitant jet (cm/s)

The limitations of EROA calculations are the same as those limitations described for the PISA method (see Chapter 2). In particular, in patients with MVP, calculation of the EROA via

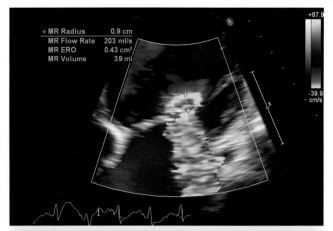

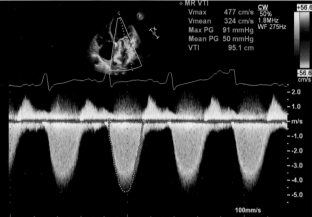

Figure 8.60 The effective regurgitant orifice area (EROA) for mitral regurgitation (MR) is calculated via the proximal isovelocity surface area (PISA) method. From a zoomed apical 4-chamber view of the mitral valve the proximal flow convergence radius (MR radius) is measured on the left ventricular side of the mitral valve in mid-late systole (*top*); callipers are placed between the mitral leaflets to the first aliased velocity. The colour Nyquist limit at this radius is noted at the bottom of the colour bar as flow is directed away from the transducer. From the continuous-wave Doppler trace, the peak MR velocity (Vmax) is measured (*bottom*). The mitral EROA in this example is calculated as:

$EROA_{MR} = (2\pi r^2 \times V_N) \div V_{MR}$
      $= (6.28 \times 0.9^2 \times 39.9) \div 477$
      $= 0.43 \ cm^2$

From the mitral EROA and the VTI of the MR signal, the mitral RV can also be calculated as:

RV_{MR} $= EROA \times VTI_{MR}$
      $= 0.43 \times 95.1$
      $= 41 \ mL$

PISA Tips for calculating the EROA and RV

- Zoom on the mitral valve from the view that best displays the MR jet (left parasternal long axis view, or any apical view).
- Only attempt this measurement when a hemispheric PISA dome is seen on the left ventricular side of the mitral valve.
- Shift the colour baseline in the direction of flow to increase the PISA dome (baseline is shifted downwards).
- Simply decreasing the colour velocity scale rather than baseline shift will also increase the size of the PISA dome.
- From a mid-late systolic frame, measure the radius from the valve tips to the first aliased velocity (identified at the red-blue interface).
- When measuring the peak MR velocity, ensure that the Doppler beam is aligned parallel with flow.

the PISA technique is difficult for a number of reasons. Firstly, the PISA radius may progressively increase over the systolic period (Fig. 8.61). To avoid underestimation or overestimation of the EROA in these instances, measurement of the PISA radius should be performed at the same time as the peak MR velocity; that is, the PISA radius should be measured in mid-late systole. Secondly, MVP prolapse often occurs in mid-late systole so the degree of MR may not be constant throughout systole; that is, significant MR is often confined to the latter

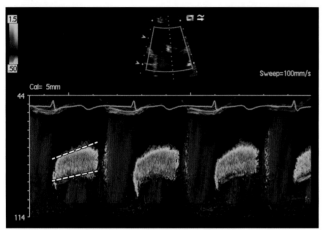

Figure 8.61 This colour Doppler M-mode trace of a mitral regurgitant (MR) jet was recorded from the apical 4-chamber view. Observe how the radius of the MR jet increases over the systolic period (distance between *dashed lines*).

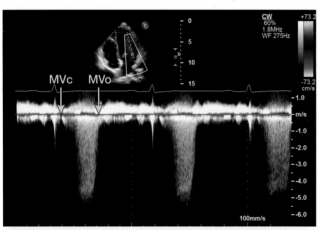

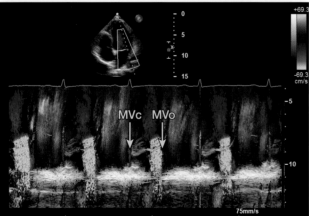

Figure 8.62 These traces were recorded from the apical 4-chamber view in a patient with mitral valve prolapse (MVP) and mitral regurgitation (MR). The continuous-wave Doppler trace of MR (*top*) and the colour Doppler M-mode trace (*bottom*) both demonstrate a short MR signal which occurs in mid-late systole. This is characteristically seen in MVP. MVc = mitral valve closure; MVo = mitral valve opening.

half of systole (Fig. 8.62). Therefore, determining the severity of MR based only on the EROA may overestimate the MR severity. In these cases the mitral RV should be calculated. Thirdly, with MVP, MR jets are often eccentric when the proximal flow convergence region encroaches on surrounding structures such as the LV walls; in this situation, flow constraint pushes the contours outwards from the regurgitant orifice and, therefore, the flow proximal to the mitral valve (PISA dome) is no longer hemispherical. As such measurement of the PISA radius in this case will overestimate the EROA. Therefore, in this situation, angle correction is required to account for non-planar flow convergence; calculation of the corrected EROA is derived by multiplying the EROA by $\alpha/180$ (Fig. 8.63). Fourthly, patients with MVP often have more than one jet. In this case, calculation of the EROA via the PISA method is not valid and the estimation of the RV and RF via the stroke volume method may be more useful in these patients.

> Calculation of the EROA by PISA requires measurement of the peak MR velocity. However, in some instances the peak MR velocity cannot be derived when the jet is eccentric and/or when there is suboptimal alignment between the Doppler beam and MR jet. In these situations, by assuming that the pressure gradient between the LV and LA is 100 mm Hg and by setting the colour Nyquist limit to 40 cm/s, the EROA can be estimated by simply measuring the radius of the first aliasing contour and multiplying the square of this radius by 0.5: EROA (cm^2) = 0.5 × r^2

Estimation of RVSP

In the presence of MR, it is crucial to attempt to obtain an estimation of the RVSP using the TR signal. Recall that in patients with significant MR and elevated LA pressures, an increase in the pulmonary venous and pulmonary capillary pressures can lead to PHTN and exertional dyspnoea. Therefore, the estimation of pulmonary artery pressures is extremely important in patients with MR. The RVSP is estimated from the TR velocity in the standard manner.

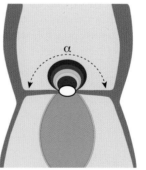

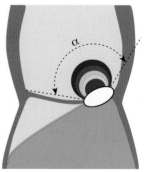

Flat angle ≈ 180°   Obtuse angle > 180°

Figure 8.63 Calculation of the effective regurgitant orifice area (EROA) via PISA assumes that the flow convergence zone proximal to the regurgitant orifice is flat with a flow convergence angle (α) of 180 degrees (*left*). However, when there is mitral valve prolapse the flow convergence angle (α) may be less than 180 degrees (*right*). This leads to 'funnelling' of the flow convergence zone due to flow constraint caused by the left ventricular wall. This flow constraint prohibits the formation of concentric hemispheres and pushes the contours outwards from the regurgitant orifice; calculation of the EROA in this situation will be overestimated. Therefore, in this situation the corrected EROA may be calculated by multiplying the EROA by $\alpha/180$. The angle α is either estimated or measured off-line.

Key Points

Anatomy of the Mitral Valve Complex
- The mitral valve "complex" is composed of several components including the valve annulus, the valve leaflets, the commissures, the tendinous cords, and the papillary muscles and LV myocardium.
- The D-shaped mitral annulus provides structural support to the mitral leaflets and is the anatomical junction between the LA and the LV.
- There are two mitral valve leaflets: anterior and posterior. The posterior mitral valve leaflet has well defined indentations or clefts referred to as scallops; these are defined as lateral, middle and medial or P1, P2, and P3, respectively.
- The mitral commissures, anterolateral and posteromedial, divide the anterior and posterior mitral leaflets; commissural leaflets refer to the mitral leaflet tissue between the end of the commissural closure line and the mitral annulus.
- Tendinous cords are string-like fibres that attach the leaflets to the papillary muscles or directly to the LV myocardium; they prevent prolapse of the leaflets into the LA during systole.
- Two papillary muscles, anterolateral and posteromedial, arise from the LV walls; contraction of these papillary muscles during systole promotes valve closure.

Mitral Stenosis: Basic Concepts
- *Aetiology:* most common acquired causes include rheumatic valve disease and extensive MAC; congenital causes are rare; other causes of LV inflow obstruction include congenital lesions such as cor triatriatum or supravalvular stenosing ring and mass lesions such as large mitral valve vegetations and left atrial myxomas.
- *Pathophysiology*: MS results in increased LA pressures and PHTN; RV dilatation and systolic dysfunction may occur due to PHTN.
- *Clinical manifestations:* include pulmonary venous congestion, a low cardiac output, AF or right heart failure.

Role of Echo in Mitral Stenosis
- Determine the aetiology of the lesion (e.g. rheumatic, congenital, other causes of LV inflow obstruction).
- Score the mitral valve (to determine suitability for balloon valvuloplasty).
- Assess LA (e.g. LA size and presence or absence of LA thrombus).
- Assess LV size and systolic function.
- Estimate the severity of the stenosis (including an estimation of RVSP).
- Identify associated valve lesions.

Stress Echo in Mitral Stenosis
- *Asymptomatic severe MS at rest:* determine if the patient has exercise-induced symptoms.
- *Symptomatic patients with apparently mild MS at rest:* determine if the mean transmitral pressure gradient and/or RVSP increase during or immediately following stress.

Mitral Regurgitation: Basic Concepts
- *Aetiology:* annular dilatation, annular calcification, leaflet abnormalities, cordal elongation, rupture or maldevelopment, papillary muscle and/or LV dysfunction, papillary muscle maldevelopment or rupture.
- *Functional classification:* based on functional mechanisms of MR:
  - Type I: normal leaflet motion with MR occurring due to annular dilatation, leaflet perforation or cleft leaflets
  - Type II: MR that occurs due to increased leaflet motion; e.g. MVP, cordal elongation or rupture, or papillary muscle elongation or rupture
  - Type III: MR occurring due to leaflet restriction; subcategorised as type IIIa (restricted leaflets during systole and diastole as seen with rheumatic disease) and type IIIb (restricted leaflets in systole only as seen with ischaemic heart disease).
- *Pathophysiology:* dependent on whether acute or chronic MR:
  - Acute severe MR: associated with a normal LV and LA size and a marked elevation in LA pressure resulting in acute pulmonary oedema and PHTN; LV systolic function usually hyperdynamic
  - Chronic severe MR: LV and LA dilatation, mild elevation in LA pressure; LV systolic function often normal but does not reflect true contractile LV function; PHTN often present.
- *Clinical manifestations:* dependent on severity and chronicity of MR; patients with acute MR typically present with frank pulmonary oedema, hypotension, and signs and symptoms of cardiogenic shock; patients with chronic MR may be relatively asymptomatic but in more severe cases congestive heart failure, pulmonary congestion and pulmonary oedema may be present.

Role of Echo in Mitral Regurgitation
- Determine the aetiology of the lesion.
- Assess LA size.
- Assess LV size and systolic function.
- Estimate the severity of the regurgitation via:
  - Indirect signs by colour Doppler imaging (e.g. jet area, VC-W, flow convergence radius)
  - Indirect signs by spectral Doppler (e.g. transmitral inflow velocities, systolic flow reversal in pulmonary veins, intensity and shape of MR jet)
  - Quantification by calculation of RV, RF and/or EROA.
- Estimate RVSP.

Further Reading (listed in alphabetical order)

Mitral Valve Anatomy

Anderson RH and Kanani M. Mitral valve repair: critical analysis of the anatomy discussed. Multimedia Manual of Cardiothoracic Surgery. 2007. doi:10.1510/mmcts.2006.002147.

Di Mauro M, Gallina S, D'Amico MA, Izzicupo P, Lanuti P, Bascelli A, Di Fonso A, Bartoloni G, Calafiore AM, Di Baldassarre A. Functional mitral regurgitation. From normal to pathological anatomy of mitral valve. *Int J Cardiol. 2011 Dec 20.* [Epub ahead of print]

Ho SY. Anatomy of the mitral valve. *Heart.* 2002 Nov;88 Suppl 4:iv5-10.

McCarthy KP, Ring L, Rana BS. Anatomy of the mitral valve: understanding the mitral valve complex in mitral regurgitation. *Eur J Echocardiogr.* 2010 Dec;11(10):i3-9.

Mitral Stenosis

Baumgartner H, Hung J, Bermejo J, Chambers JB, Evangelista A, Griffin BP, Iung B, Otto CM, Pellikka PA, Quiñones M; American Society of Echocardiography; European Association of Echocardiography. Echocardiographic assessment of valve stenosis: EAE/ASE recommendations for clinical practice. *J Am Soc Echocardiogr.* 2009 Jan;22(1):1-23

Das P, Prendergast B. Imaging in mitral stenosis: assessment before, during and after percutaneous balloon mitral valvuloplasty. *Expert Rev Cardiovasc Ther.* 2003 Nov;1(4):549-57.

González-Torrecilla E, García-Fernández MA, Pérez-David E, Bermejo J, Moreno M, Delcán JL. Predictors of left atrial spontaneous echo contrast and thrombi in patients with mitral stenosis and atrial fibrillation. *Am J Cardiol.* 2000 Sep 1;86(5):529-34.

Krishnamoorthy KM, Tharakan JA, Titus T, Ajithkumar VK, Bhat A, Harikrishnan SP, Padmakumar R. Usefulness of transthoracic echocardiography for identification of left atrial thrombus before balloon mitral valvuloplasty. *Am J Cardiol.* 2003 Nov 1;92(9):1132-4.

Padial LR, Abascal VM, Moreno PR, Weyman AE, Levine RA, Palacios IF. Echocardiography can predict the development of severe mitral regurgitation after percutaneous mitral valvuloplasty by the Inoue technique. *Am J Cardiol.* 1999 Apr 15;83(8):1210-3.

Séguéla PE, Houyel L, Acar P. Congenital malformations of the mitral valve. *Arch Cardiovasc Dis.* 2011 Aug;104(8-9):465-79.

Wilkins GT, Weyman AE, Abascal VM, Block PC, Palacios IF. Percutaneous balloon dilatation of the mitral valve: an analysis of echocardiographic variables related to outcome and the mechanism of dilatation. *Br Heart J.* 1988 Oct;60(4):299-308.

Stress Echo In MS

Picano E, Pibarot P, Lancellotti P, Monin JL, Bonow RO. The emerging role of exercise testing and stress echocardiography in valvular heart disease. *J Am Coll Cardiol.* 2009 Dec 8;54(24):2251-60.

Reis G, Motta MS, Barbosa MM, Esteves WA, Souza SF, Bocchi EA. Dobutamine stress echocardiography for noninvasive assessment and risk stratification of patients with rheumatic mitral stenosis. *J Am Coll Cardiol.* 2004 Feb 4;43(3):393-401.

Mitral Regurgitation

Adams DH, Rosenhek R, Falk V. Degenerative mitral valve regurgitation: best practice revolution. *Eur Heart J.* 2010 Aug;31(16):1958-66.

Anyanwu AC, Adams DH. Etiologic classification of degenerative mitral valve disease: Barlow's disease and fibroelastic deficiency. *Semin Thorac Cardiovasc Surg.* 2007 Summer;19(2):90-6.

Carpentier A. Cardiac valve surgery--the "French correction". *J Thorac Cardiovasc Surg.* 1983 Sep;86(3):323-37.

Hayek E, Gring CN, Griffin BP. Mitral valve prolapse. *Lancet.* 2005 Feb 5-11;365(9458):507-18.

Lancellotti P, Tribouilloy C, Hagendorff A, Moura L, Popescu BA, Agricola E, Monin JL, Pierard LA, Badano L, Zamorano JL; European Association of Echocardiography. European Association of Echocardiography recommendations for the assessment of valvular regurgitation. Part 2: mitral and tricuspid regurgitation (native valve disease). *Eur J Echocardiogr.* 2010 May;11(4):307-332.

Marwick TH, Lancellotti P, Pierard L. Ischaemic mitral regurgitation: mechanisms and diagnosis. *Heart.* 2009 Oct;95(20):1711-8.

Zoghbi WA, Enriquez-Sarano M, Foster E, Grayburn PA, Kraft CD, Levine RA, Nihoyannopoulos P, Otto CM, Quinones MA, Rakowski H, Stewart WJ, Waggoner A, Weissman NJ; American Society of Echocardiography. Recommendations for evaluation of the severity of native valvular regurgitation with two-dimensional and Doppler echocardiography. *J Am Soc Echocardiogr.* 2003 Jul;16(7):777-802

Tricuspid and Pulmonary Valve Disease

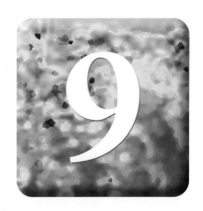

Anatomy of the Tricuspid Valve

The tricuspid valve is the largest of the four cardiac valves in the heart. It is composed of endocardium and connective tissue. With respect to surface anatomy, the tricuspid valve lies to the right of the sternum opposite the fourth intercostal space (see Fig. 7.1). Internally, the tricuspid valve is located slightly posterior and medial to the aortic valve and is in close proximity to the other cardiac valves (see Fig. 7.2). The primary function of the tricuspid valve is to prevent the backflow of blood into the right atrium (RA) during ventricular systole.

As for the mitral valve, the tricuspid valve is considered in terms of the tricuspid valve "complex". This complex is consists of: (1) a fibrous annulus, (2) three leaflets (anterior, posterior, and septal), (3) the tendinous cords, (4) two discrete papillary muscles and one rudimentary papillary muscle, and (5) the right ventricular (RV) myocardium. Valve competency depends upon the successful function of each of these components.

Tricuspid Annulus

The tricuspid annulus provides a structural support to the tricuspid leaflets and forms the anatomical junction between the RA and the RV. The tricuspid annulus is oval in shape and is approximately 20% larger than the mitral annulus.

As for the mitral annulus, the tricuspid annulus is a complex 3-dimensional structure. However, unlike the mitral annulus which has a more symmetric "saddle-shape" during systole, the tricuspid annulus has a nonplanar, elliptical-shape with two high points oriented superiorly towards the RA and two low points oriented inferiorly toward the RV (Fig. 9.1).

Tricuspid Leaflets

The tricuspid valve has three triangular-shaped, unequal-sized leaflets (Fig. 9.2). The anterior leaflet, also referred to as the infundibular or superior leaflet, is the largest tricuspid leaflet; it has a semicircular shape and attaches to the right atrioventricular junction. The septal leaflet, also referred to as the medial leaflet, is the smallest leaflet and is also semicircular in shape; this leaflet attaches from the posterior left ventricular (LV) wall across to the interventricular septum (IVS). Significantly, the insertion of the septal leaflet is more apical relative to the septal insertion of the anterior

mitral leaflet (Fig. 9.3). The posterior leaflet, also referred to as the marginal or inferior leaflet, has a trapezoidal shape and it has a mural attachment. As for the posterior mitral leaflet, the posterior tricuspid leaflet has several indentations or clefts which divide the leaflet into scallops. Mostly commonly, there are three scallops which are referred to as the anteroposterior scallop, posteroseptal scallop and middle scallop (Fig. 9.4).

Tricuspid Commissures

When closed, the tricuspid leaflets meet to form a Y-shaped closure line or zone of apposition (Fig. 9.2,C). At each end of the closure line is a commissure. The commissures are named anteroseptal, anteroposterior and posteroseptal based on their anatomical location. These commissures divide the leaflets into anterior, septal and posterior.

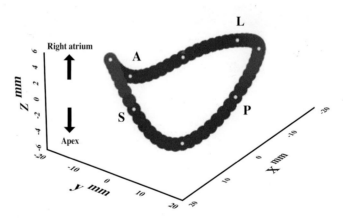

Figure 9.1 This schematic illustrates the 3D shape of the tricuspid annulus (TA). This reconstructed ring shape for tricuspid annuloplasty is based on the average results obtained in healthy subjects at the time of minimum TA area. The positive x-y-z axis indicates the respective directions toward the septum (S), the posterior (P) wall, and the right atrium. At the yellow dots, the average of each of the manually selected TA locations is shown. The reconstructed TA locations were colour coded by assigning shades of red to points located above the best-fit plane toward the atrium and shades of blue to points located below the best-fit plane toward the apex. A = anterior; L = lateral. Reproduced from Fukuda S, Saracino G, Matsumura Y, Daimon M, Tran H, Greenberg NL, Hozumi T, Yoshikawa J, Thomas JD, Shiota T.. Three-Dimensional Geometry of the Tricuspid Annulus in Healthy Subjects and in Patients with Functional Tricuspid Regurgitation: A Real-Time, 3-Dimensional Echocardiographic Study. *Circulation*, 114(1 Suppl): page I-497; © 2006 Wolters Kluwer Health with permission.

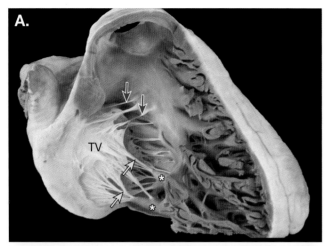

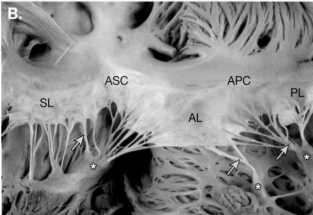

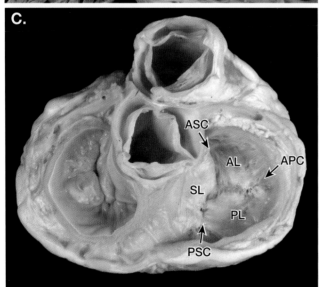

Figure 9.2 These gross pathological specimens show the normal anatomy of the tricuspid valve complex. **Photo A** shows the entire tricuspid valve complex, with the right ventricular free wall removed. **Photo B** shows the tricuspid valve opened out. **Photo C** shows a short axis of the tricuspid valve in its closed position as viewed from the right atrial aspect. The connections of the tendinous cords (*yellow arrows*) between the papillary muscles (*) and the tricuspid leaflets (TV) are also shown (A–B). Also observe the cordal attachments between the septal leaflet and the interventricular septum (*red arrows*) (A). The three leaflets of the tricuspid valve are the anterior leaflet (AL), posterior leaflet (PL) and septal leaflet (SL). The three commissures include the anteroseptal commissure (ASC), the anteroposterior commissure (APC) and the posteroseptal commissure (PSC). Note that the specimen shown in Photo C is simulated systole with opened semilunar valves and closed atrioventricular valves; Figure 7.2 shows the same specimen in simulated diastole with opened atrioventricular valves and closed semilunar valves.

By permission of Mayo Foundation for Medical Education and Research. All rights reserved. Courtesy of William D. Edwards, MD.

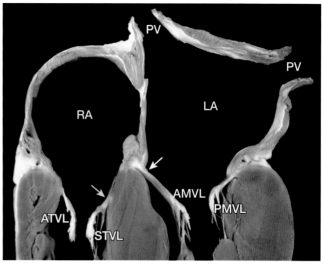

Figure 9.3 This gross pathological specimen illustrates the normal anatomical relationship between the anterior mitral valve leaflet (AMVL) and septal tricuspid valve leaflet (STVL). Observe that the insertion of the STVL (*yellow arrow*) is 'lower' than the insertion of the AMVL (*white arrow*). This normal apical displacement of the STVL distinguishes the tricuspid valve leaflet from the mitral valve. The myocardium between the insertion levels of two valves represents the atrioventricular septum, because it lies between the right atrium and the left ventricle. ATVL = anterior tricuspid valve leaflet; LA = left atrium; PMVL = posterior mitral valve leaflet; PV = pulmonary vein; RA = right atrium.

By permission of Mayo Foundation for Medical Education and Research. All rights reserved. Courtesy of William D. Edwards, MD.

Tendinous Cords

The tendinous cords, or chordae tendinae, are string-like fibres that attach the tricuspid leaflets to the papillary muscles (Fig. 9.4). Accessory cords that attach from the septal leaflet to the IVS, the moderator band or the RV free wall are also frequently found. In fact, a characteristic feature of the tricuspid valve is the presence of multiple cordal attachments from the septal leaflet to the IVS. There are more than 100 cords which can be classified into various groups according to their origin and site of attachment to the tricuspid leaflets. As for the mitral valve, these cords are primarily responsible for anchoring the valve and preventing prolapse of the tricuspid leaflets into the RA during systole.

Papillary Muscles

The number of papillary muscles within the RV is variable. Usually there are three groups of papillary muscles with each group being composed of up to three muscles. The anterior papillary muscle is the largest, the posterior papillary muscle often bifurcates into two heads (bifid) or trifurcates into three heads (trifid), and the septal papillary muscle is the smallest and is sometimes referred to as a rudimentary papillary muscle. Typically, each papillary muscle supplies cords to two adjacent tricuspid valve leaflets. For example, the anterior papillary muscle provides cords to the anterior and posterior tricuspid leaflets; the posterior papillary muscle provides cords to the posterior and septal tricuspid leaflets, and the septal papillary muscle supplies cords to the septal and anterior tricuspid leaflets (Fig. 9.4).

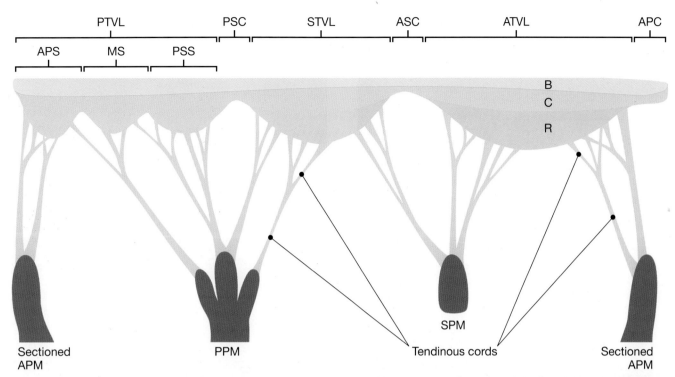

Figure 9.4 This schematic illustrates the various zones, commissures and cordal attachments of the tricuspid leaflets. All three leaflets have a clear zone (C), a rough zone (R) and a basal zone (B). The clear and basal zones are also referred to as the smooth zone. The rough zone depicts the region of leaflet coaptation. The basal and rough zones have cordal insertions while there are no cordal insertions to the clear zone. The posterior tricuspid valve leaflet (PTVL) is divided into three scallops. See text for further details.

ATVL = anterior tricuspid valve leaflet; APC = anteroposterior commissure; APS = anteroposterior scallop; APM = anterior papillary muscle; ASC = anteroseptal commissure; MS = middle scallop; PPM = posterior papillary muscle; PSC = posteroseptal commissure; PSS = posteroseptal scallop; SPM = septal papillary muscle; STVL =septal tricuspid valve leaflet.

Each ventricle is identified by its atrioventricular (AV) valve; that is, the tricuspid valve always leads to the morphological right ventricle (RV) and the mitral valve always leads to the morphological left ventricle (LV). Hence, identifying the AV valves will identify each ventricle. The tricuspid valve can be differentiated from the mitral valve by the apical (inferior) displacement of the septal tricuspid leaflet relative to the anterior mitral valve leaflet. Other clues that can be used to distinguish the tricuspid valve from the mitral valve are listed below.

	Tricuspid Valve	**Mitral Valve**
Number of leaflets	3	2 (exception, with a cleft anterior mitral leaflet may appear trileaflet)
Cordal attachment	Attachments between septal tricuspid leaflet directly to interventricular septum	Cordal insertions between the mitral valve and LV myocardium are never seen
Number of papillary muscles	Variability in number and arrangement	Regular arrangement of two groups of papillary muscles
Relationship to semilunar valve	Separated from the pulmonary valve by infundibulum	Fibrous continuity with the aortic valve

Recognition of the tricuspid valve and RV become especially important in the assessment of congenital heart disease.

Echo Imaging of the Tricuspid Valve

There are a number of transthoracic echocardiographic views that can be utilised to image the tricuspid valve. These views include the parasternal long axis of the RV inflow, the parasternal short axis at the aortic valve level, the apical 4-chamber view and the subcostal views (Fig. 9.5). Typically, only two of the three tricuspid valve leaflets are seen from any one imaging view; in addition, there may be some variation as to which two leaflets are seen depending upon the imaging plane cut. From the parasternal long axis of the RV inflow, the posterior and anterior leaflets are usually seen but the septal and anterior leaflets may also be seen from this view. From the parasternal short axis view at the level of the aortic valve, the anterior and septal leaflets are usually seen but the anterior and posterior leaflets may also be seen from this view. From the apical 4-chamber view, the septal and anterior leaflets are seen. Tricuspid leaflets seen from the subcostal views correspond to the same leaflets seen from the apical 4-chamber and parasternal short axis views.

When the RV is dilated, all three tricuspid leaflets may be seen from a parasternal short axis view (Fig. 9.6).

From the parasternal long axis view of right ventricular inflow, when a portion of the left ventricle is seen then the 'leftward' tricuspid leaflet is the septal leaflet and when only the right ventricle is seen then the 'leftward' tricuspid leaflet is the posterior leaflet.

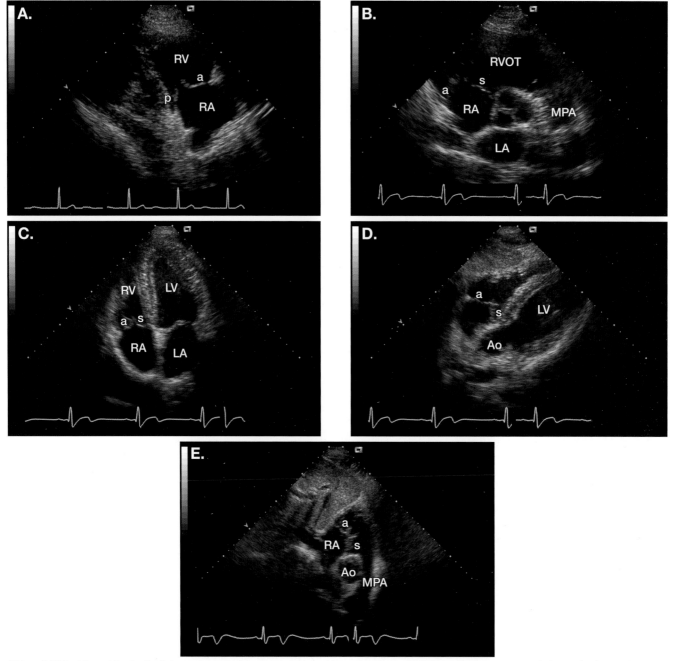

Figure 9.5 The tricuspid valve leaflets can be seen from the parasternal long axis view of RV inflow (A), the parasternal short axis view at the aortic valve level (B), the apical 4-chamber view (C), the subcostal 5-chamber view (D), and the subcostal short axis view (E). a = anterior tricuspid leaflet; LA = left atrium; LV = left ventricle; MPA = main pulmonary artery; p = posterior tricuspid leaflet; RA = right atrium; RV = right ventricle; RVOT = right ventricular outflow tract; s = septal tricuspid leaflet.

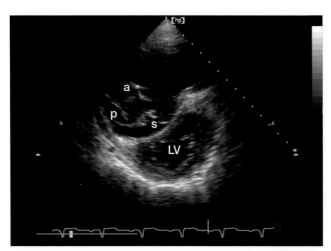

Figure 9.6 This parasternal short axis image at the papillary muscle level was recorded from a patient with pulmonary arterial hypertension. Observe that all three tricuspid valve leaflets can be seen. a = anterior tricuspid leaflet; LV = left ventricle; p = posterior tricuspid leaflet; s = septal tricuspid leaflet.

Tricuspid Stenosis

Aetiology of Tricuspid Stenosis

Tricuspid stenosis (TS) refers to the obstruction of blood flow from the RA, across the tricuspid valve, into the RV. Valvular TS can be caused by an acquired deformation of the valve or, rarely by congenital malformations of the valve.

Congenital Tricuspid Valve Disease

Congenital causes of TS are rare and are usually associated with other congenital cardiac defects. The anatomy of congenital TS is variable and may involve a number of components of the tricuspid valve complex. Examples of congenital TS include maldeveloped leaflets, shortened or malformed tendinous cords, annular hypoplasia, abnormalities of the papillary muscles, or any combination of these defects.

Acquired Tricuspid Valve Disease

Rheumatic valve disease is the most common cause of TS. As discussed in Chapters 7 and 8, rheumatic valve disease occurs secondary to an episode or recurrent episodes of acute rheumatic fever (ARF) which occurs due to a group A beta-haemolytic Streptococcus infection. Rheumatic valvular disease occurs several years after the initial episode of ARF as an autoimmune response. Rheumatic TS almost never occurs as an isolated lesion and is almost always associated with rheumatic mitral and aortic valve disease. The anatomical changes in rheumatic TS resemble those of rheumatic mitral stenosis (MS); that is, leaflets are thickened and fibrotic, commissures are fused, and the tendinous cords are thick, short and matted (Fig. 9.7).

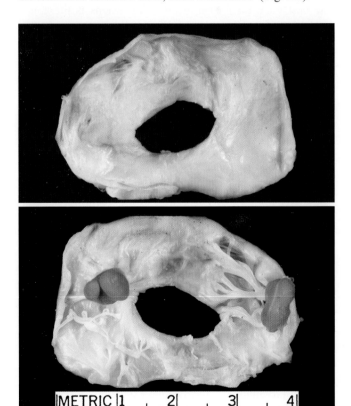

Figure 9.7 Gross pathological specimen with rheumatic tricuspid stenosis is shown as viewed from the right atrium (*top*) and from the right ventricle (*bottom*). Observe the marked fusion of all three commissures, with less prominent thickening of the tricuspid leaflets and tendinous cords.
By permission of Mayo Foundation for Medical Education and Research. All rights reserved. Courtesy of William D. Edwards, MD.

Another less commonly encountered cause of acquired TS is carcinoid heart disease. Carcinoid heart disease is caused by a rare, malignant neuroendrocrine tumour. These tumours secrete excessive amounts of the hormone serotonin which damages the tricuspid and pulmonic valves; in particular, increased circulating quantities of serotonin result in the formation of thick, pearly white plaque-like deposits on the endocardial surfaces of the tricuspid leaflets (Fig. 9.8). These plaques cause the valve to become thickened, retracted and rigid; therefore, the valve becomes both stenotic and regurgitant. Carcinoid heart disease is discussed in detail in Chapter 14 (Systemic Diseases with Cardiac Manifestations).

Other Causes of RV Inflow Obstruction

Congenital obstruction to RV inflow can also occur due to cor triatriatum dexter. Large mass lesions such as large tricuspid valve vegetations, right heart thrombus or right heart tumours may also obstruct tricuspid inflow.

Pathophysiology of Tricuspid Stenosis

TS effectively decreases the tricuspid valve area and results in the obstruction of RA emptying during diastole. In an attempt to maintain an adequate forward flow through the tricuspid valve, the RA pressure increases in order to increase the driving pressure across the stenotic valve. This increase in RA pressure leads to dilatation of the RA. In addition, increased RA pressure also hampers venous return into the RA and this leads to systemic venous congestion, jugular venous distension, ascites, and peripheral oedema.

Clinical Manifestations of Tricuspid Stenosis

The clinical manifestations of TS relate to the pathophysiological responses to chronic, severe TS. These manifestations include fatigue (due to a low cardiac output), abdominal discomfort and swelling (due to systemic venous congestion), and dyspnoea (due to concomitant mitral stenosis).

Importantly, as rheumatic TS usually occurs in association with rheumatic mitral valve disease, the clinical manifestations of severe MS are also seen; these manifestations include pulmonary venous congestion, a low cardiac output, atrial fibrillation and right heart failure.

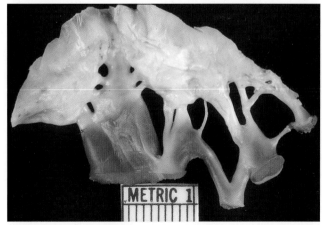

Figure 9.8 This is a gross pathological specimen of carcinoid tricuspid valve disease. Observe that the tricuspid leaflets are significantly thickened and the tendinous cords are markedly abnormal with thick, white plaques extending along the length of the cords and into the papillary muscles.
By permission of Mayo Foundation for Medical Education and Research. All rights reserved. Courtesy of William D. Edwards, MD.

Role of Echocardiography in Tricuspid Stenosis

The aims and objectives of echocardiography in the assessment of TS are to:

- Determine the aetiology of the lesion,
- Assess RA size,
- Assess RV size and systolic function,
- Estimate the severity of the stenosis,
- Estimate right ventricular systolic pressure,
- Identify associated valve lesions.

Aetiology of Tricuspid Stenosis

As stated above, the most common cause of TS is rheumatic valve disease. Other causes of TS include carcinoid heart disease, obstruction of RV inflow by large mass lesions and, rarely, congenital anomalies.

Rheumatic Tricuspid Stenosis

As for rheumatic MS, on the 2D echocardiographic examination, rheumatic TS is characterised by diastolic doming of the tricuspid valve leaflets. Diastolic tricuspid leaflet doming is best appreciated from the parasternal long axis view of the RV inflow or from the apical 4-chamber view (Fig. 9.9). On colour Doppler imaging, turbulent flow across the valve is also noted during diastole.

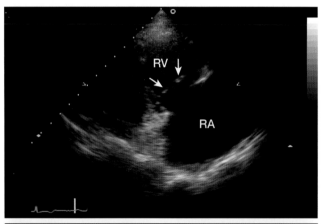

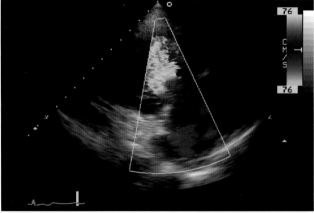

Figure 9.9 These images were recorded from the parasternal long axis view of the right ventricular inflow. Observe the diastolic doming of the tricuspid leaflets (*arrows*) which is characteristic of rheumatic tricuspid valve stenosis (*top*). Colour Doppler imaging confirms the presence of turbulent flow across the tricuspid valve (*bottom*). RA = right atrium; RV = right ventricle.

Carcinoid Tricuspid Valve Disease

The characteristic 2D echocardiographic appearance of carcinoid tricuspid valve disease is thickened and retracted leaflets with the valve remaining in a fixed semi-open position throughout the cardiac cycle (Fig. 9.10). As a result the valve is both stenotic and incompetent so on the colour Doppler examination, turbulent flow across the valve during diastole and significant tricuspid regurgitation (TR) during systole are also noted.

Differentiating Carcinoid from Rheumatic Tricuspid Valve Disease

While the carcinoid tricuspid valve may appear similar to that of rheumatic tricuspid valve disease, it is important to remember that TS due to rheumatic disease is almost always associated with mitral stenosis. Therefore, the absence of mitral stenosis or the presence of a normal mitral valve should alert the sonographer to other aetiologies of TS such as carcinoid heart disease.

Other Causes of Tricuspid Stenosis

Functional TS can also result from obstruction of RV inflow by large mass lesions such as right heart thrombus, right heart tumours, or large tricuspid valve vegetations. Examples of these lesions are shown in Figures 9.11-9.12.

Assessment of Right Atrial Size

A chronic elevation in RA pressure leads to RA dilatation. The best view for measuring RA dimensions is the apical 4-chamber view. From this view, the RA area is traced at end-systole along the blood-tissue interface from the lateral to the medial tricuspid annulus, being sure to exclude the vena cava, RA appendage and the tricuspid valve funnel (the area between the leaflets and the annulus) (Fig. 9.13, top).

Additional measurements of the RA size include the RA length (major or long axis) and the mid-RA diameter (minor or short axis) (Fig. 9.13, bottom). The RA length is measured from the centre of the tricuspid annulus to the centre of the superior RA wall, parallel to the interatrial septum. The mid-RA minor diameter is measured across the mid level of the RA from the RA free wall to the interatrial septum, perpendicular to the RA length.

The upper limits for normal for the RA area, RA length and RA diameter are 18 cm², 5.3 cm and 4.4 cm, respectively [9.1].

Assessment of Right Ventricular Size and Systolic Function

RV size and systolic function are assessed in the usual manner as described in detail in Chapter 2. For example, RV linear dimensions are measured from an RV-focused apical 4-chamber view at end-diastole. Measurements of RV systolic function include the Doppler tissue imaging systolic velocity, the tricuspid annular plane systolic excursion (TAPSE), the fractional area change and/or the RV myocardial performance index. Importantly, more than one measure of RV function should be used to distinguish between normal and abnormal RV systolic function.

[9.1] Rudski LG, Lai WW, Afilalo J, Hua L, Handschumacher MD, Chandrasekaran K, Solomon SD, Louie EK, Schiller NB. Guidelines for the echocardiographic assessment of the right heart in adults: a report from the American Society of Echocardiography endorsed by the European Association of Echocardiography, a registered branch of the European Society of Cardiology, and the Canadian Society of Echocardiography. *J Am Soc Echocardiogr.* 2010 Jul;23(7):691.

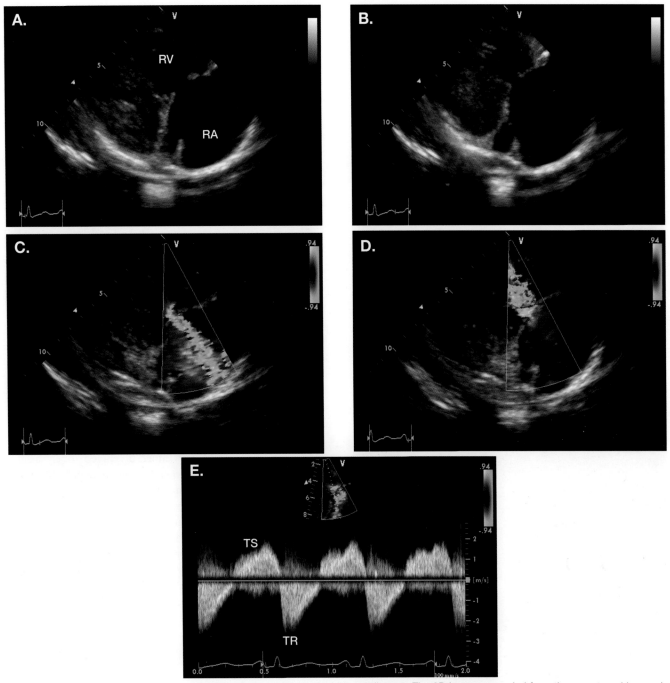

Figure 9.10 These images were recorded from a patient with carcinoid heart disease. The 2D images recorded from the parasternal long axis view of the right ventricular inflow show an end-diastolic frame (**A**) and an end-systolic frame (**B**); observe that the tricuspid valve remains in a partially open position during systole. On the colour Doppler images, turbulent flow is noted during systole (**C**) and diastole (**D**) confirming the presence of both tricuspid regurgitation (TR) and tricuspid stenosis (TS). The continuous-wave Doppler shows several characteristic features of significant TS and TR (**E**). The mean tricuspid gradient averaged over the respiratory cycle measured 4 mm Hg. The TR signal shows an early peaking systolic velocity with rapid deceleration indicating a high right atrial pressure.

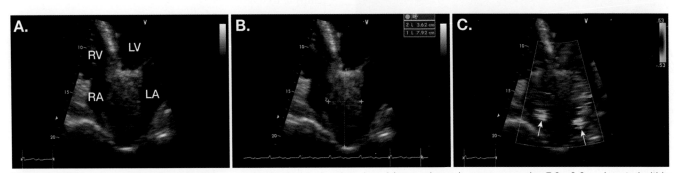

Figure 9.11 These images were recorded from a zoomed apical 4-chamber view. A large echogenic mass measuring 7.9 x 3.6 cm is noted within the right atrial (RA) cavity with apparent infiltration into the left atrium (LA) (**A & B**). Colour flow Doppler shows turbulence in the vicinity of RA and LA inflow (*arrows*) suggesting inflow obstruction (**C**). At cardiac magnetic resonance imaging this mass was diagnosed as an angiosarcoma.

Estimation of Severity

The severity of TS is based on haemodynamic parameters such as the:

* mean pressure gradient,
* tricuspid inflow velocity time integral,
* pressure half-time,
* tricuspid valve area (TVA).

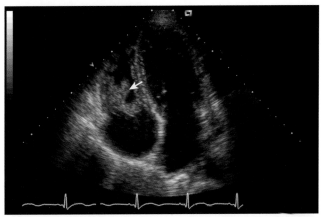

Figure 9.12 This image recorded from the apical 4-chamber view shows a very large tricuspid valve vegetation (*arrow*). Large mass lesions such as this can impede blood flow from the right atrium to the right ventricle effectively causing tricuspid stenosis.

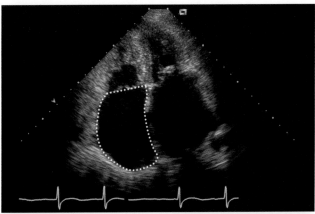

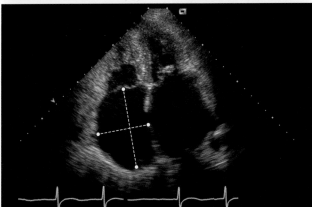

Figure 9.13 From the apical 4-chamber view at end-systole, the right atrial (RA) area is traced at the blood-tissue interface from the lateral to the medial tricuspid annulus (*top*). The RA length and RA diameter can also be measured (*bottom*). The RA length is measured from the centre of the tricuspid annulus to the superior RA wall, parallel with the interatrial septum and the RA diameter is measured at the mid level of the RA from the RA free wall to the interatrial septum, perpendicular to the RA length.

The criteria for identifying haemodynamically significant TS based on these parameters are listed in Table 9.1. Supportive signs of significant TS include evidence of increased RA pressures such as moderate or severe RA dilatation, and/or dilatation of the inferior vena cava (IVC).

Mean Pressure Gradients and Tricuspid Inflow Velocity Time Integral

Tricuspid inflow velocities are recorded via continuous-wave (CW) Doppler from a parasternal long axis view of the RV inflow, a parasternal short axis view or from the apical 4-chamber view. The view selected for these measurements is the one in which parallel alignment between the TS jet and the ultrasound beam is best achieved. By tracing the tricuspid inflow Doppler signal over the diastolic flow period, both the velocity time integral (VTI) and mean pressure gradient can be derived. The mean pressure gradient is estimated by application of the simplified Bernoulli equation (see Chapter 1). The VTI is simply a measure of the area under the Doppler curve; the VTI measurement may be considered as a surrogate of the mean pressure gradient. As for MS, the mean TS pressure gradient rather than the maximum instantaneous pressure gradient is important. This is because the diastolic pressure gradient varies over the diastolic period and the period of diastole is much longer than the period of systole.

Furthermore, due to augmentation of systemic venous return to the right heart during inspiration, tricuspid inflow velocities are typically increased with inspiration. Therefore, measurements should be either averaged over a full respiratory cycle (5-7 beats) or measured at end-expiratory apnoea [9.2] (Fig. 9.14). In addition, as tachycardia can increase transvalvular pressure gradients, measurements should be performed at heart rates that are close to normal. In the presence of atrial fibrillation, measurements should be averaged over two respiratory cycles.

The limitations of pressure gradient estimations are discussed in detail in Chapter 1.

Table 9.1 Findings Indicative of Haemodynamically Significant Tricuspid Stenosis

	Significant TS
Specific findings	
Mean gradient (mm Hg)	≥ 5
Inflow VTI (cm)	> 60
Pressure half-time (ms)	190
TVA (cm²)	≤ 1.0
Supportive findings:	
• Enlarged RA ($\geq$ moderate dilatation)	
• Dilated IVC	

IVC = inferior vena cava; RA = right atrium; TVA = tricuspid valve area; VTI = velocity time integral.
Source: Baumgartner H, Hung J, Bermejo J, Chambers JB, Evangelista A, Griffin BP, Iung B, Otto CM, Pellikka PA, Quinones M; American Society of Echocardiography; European Association of Echocardiography. Echocardiographic assessment of valve stenosis: EAE/ASE recommendations for clinical practice. *J Am Soc Echocardiogr,* Vol. 22(1), page 19, © 2009 with permission from Elsevier.

[9.2] Measurements of right heart Doppler parameters averaged over 5-7 consecutive beats is nearly identical to measurements obtained during apnoea. Zoghbi WA, Habib JB, Quiñones MA. Doppler assessment of right ventricular filling in a normal population: comparison with left ventricular filling dynamics. *Circulation.* 1990;82:1316-1324.

Pressure-Half Time

The basic principles of the pressure half-time (P½t) for TS are essentially the same as described for MS (see Fig. 8.22). In the case of the tricuspid valve, the diastolic slope of the Doppler velocity spectrum reflects the pressure difference between the RA and RV. In the normal tricuspid valve, diastolic blood flow from the RA to the RV is unimpeded and as the majority of RV filling occurs during early diastole, the pressure gradient following early diastole rapidly declines. In TS, the rate of RA emptying is 'slowed' due to the narrowed tricuspid orifice and this prolongs the decline of the early diastolic pressure gradient between the RA and RV.

The P½t of the TS signal is measured as the time taken for the early diastolic pressure gradient to fall to half its original value (Fig. 9.15). A P½t measured on an end-inspiratory beat greater than 190 ms is associated with severe TS. It has also been proposed that the tricuspid valve area (TVA) may be estimated by dividing a constant of 190 by the P½t; however, this method is not well validated.

The principal limitation of the P½t measurement occurs when there is tachycardia. In this instance, increased heart rates result in fusion of the early diastolic velocity (E wave) and the velocity that follows atrial contraction (A wave). Therefore, when there is E/A fusion, accurate measurement of the P½t is not possible.

Tricuspid Valve Area

While the mean tricuspid pressure gradient is a useful parameter in assessing the severity of TS, this pressure gradient is dependent upon the cardiac output. For example, in patients with mild stenosis, elevated mean gradients can be found when there is a high cardiac output such as occurs during exercise, pregnancy, in anxious patients, or when there is coexistent severe TR. Therefore, in these instances the transvalvular gradients may be elevated despite the presence of mild stenosis. Conversely, when the cardiac output is reduced, the amount of blood flowing through the stenotic valve is reduced and the gradient is also reduced; therefore, transvalvular gradients may be relatively low despite the presence of significant stenosis. Hence, to 'compensate' for variable flow conditions, calculation of the TVA can be performed. While the TVA can

be estimated by dividing a constant of 190 by the P½t, this method is not well validated. Calculation of the TVA can also be estimated based on the continuity principle. The basic continuity principle for valve area calculations is discussed in Chapter 1. Recall that this principle is based on the assumption that the stroke volume (SV) proximal to a narrowing is equal to the SV across the narrowing.

To estimate the TVA via this principle, it is assumed that the SV across the tricuspid valve will be identical to the SV across the left ventricular outflow tract (LVOT) (Fig. 9.16). The SV is derived as the product of the cross-sectional area (CSA) and the VTI. Therefore, if the LVOT diameter can be measured to derive the CSA of the LVOT and if the VTI across the LVOT and across the tricuspid valve can be measured, then the TVA can be derived:

Equation 9.1

$$TVA = (CSA_{LVOT} \times VTI_{LVOT}) \div VTI_{TV}$$

where TVA = tricuspid valve area (cm²)
CSA_{LVOT} = cross-sectional area of the LVOT (cm²)
VTI_{LVOT} = velocity time integral of the LVOT (cm)
VTI_{TV} = velocity time integral across the tricuspid valve (cm)

> The normal tricuspid valve area in a normal sized adult is approximately 6.0 to 7.0 cm².

The limitations of the continuity principle for valve area calculations are discussed in detail in Chapter 1 while limitations to SV calculations using the LVOT are discussed in Chapter 2. The most common pitfalls encountered for calculation of the TVA include: (1) underestimation of the tricuspid VTI due to suboptimal alignment of the ultrasound beam with blood flow direction, (2) underestimation of the LVOT VTI due to improper placement of the pulsed-wave (PW) Doppler sample volume in the LVOT, and (3) errors in the LVOT diameter measurement (refer to Fig. 2.29).

Another important limitation in calculating the TVA occurs when there is coexistent TR and/or coexistent aortic regurgitation (AR). In particular, as TS is almost always associated with TR, The TVA cannot be calculated. This is

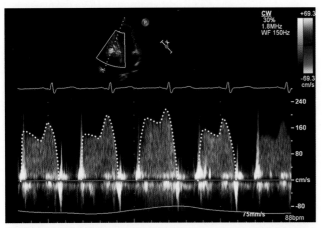

Figure 9.14 This continuous-wave Doppler trace was recorded through the tricuspid valve. The respiratory trace is the green line at the bottom of the image. The transtricuspid velocities fluctuate with respiration and therefore all measurements should be averaged over the respiratory cycle. In this example, the averaged peak early diastolic velocity was 1.8 m/s, the averaged diastolic velocity time integral was 60 cm, and the averaged mean pressure gradient was 8 mm Hg.

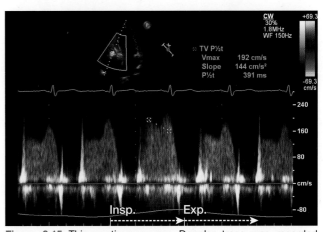

Figure 9.15 This continuous-wave Doppler trace was recorded through the tricuspid valve. The respiratory trace is the green line at the bottom of the image. The pressure half-time (P½t) is measured on the end-inspiratory beat. Insp. = inspiration; Exp. = expiration.

because the SV across the tricuspid valve is no longer the same as the SV across the LVOT. When there is TR, the SV across the tricuspid valve is increased because this SV includes the tricuspid regurgitant volume that leaked back through the tricuspid valve in systole plus the normal forward SV returning from the body; calculation of the TVA in this instance will be underestimated.

When there is coexistent AR, the SV across the LVOT is increased because this SV includes the aortic regurgitant volume as well as the forward SV across the mitral valve; therefore, calculation of the TVA in this instance will be overestimated. In the presence of AR or in situations when the LVOT parameters cannot be accurately estimated and providing that there is no significant tricuspid or pulmonary regurgitation, the TVA can be calculated using the right ventricular outflow tract (RVOT) SV.

> **TVA via Continuity**
> Calculation of the TVA via the continuity equation is usually not practicable in patients with tricuspid stenosis (TS). This is because TS is almost always associated with tricuspid regurgitation (TR). In this instance, the stroke volume across the tricuspid valve and across the 'reference' valve is no longer the same. The TVA via the continuity equation is more feasible in those patients who have a prosthetic tricuspid valve and no TR (see Chapter 10).

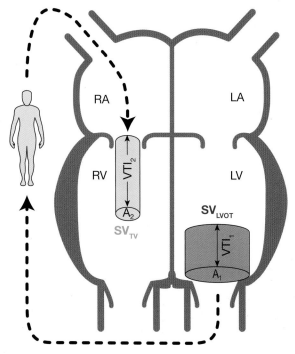

Figure 9.16 Stroke volume (SV) is derived as a product of the cross-sectional area (CSA) and the velocity time integral (VTI). As VTI is measured as a distance or 'height' it can be postulated that flow through the LVOT and across the tricuspid valve is cylindrical (the volume of a cylinder is derived as the product of the CSA and the height of the cylinder). Therefore, the SV across the left ventricular outflow tract (SV$_{LVOT}$) is the product of the CSA of the LVOT (A$_1$) and the height of the cylinder or the VTI of the LVOT (VTI$_1$) and the SV across the tricuspid valve (SV$_{TV}$) is the product of the tricuspid valve area (A$_2$) and the height of the cylinder or the VTI across the tricuspid valve (VTI$_2$). Based on the continuity principle the SV$_{LVOT}$ should be the same as the SV$_{TV}$; that is, all blood ejected across the LVOT will ultimately pass across the tricuspid valve so long as there is no aortic or tricuspid regurgitation, or an intracardiac shunt.

Identifying Associated Valve Lesions

As previously stated, the most common cause of TS is rheumatic valve disease and rheumatic TS rarely occurs in isolation. In particular, rheumatic TS is commonly associated with rheumatic involvement of the mitral and aortic valves; therefore, a comprehensive assessment of the anatomy and function of these valves is also important. Methods for assessing rheumatic aortic and mitral valve disease are discussed in Chapters 7 and 8, respectively.

TS is also commonly associated with TR. Methods for assessing the severity of TR are described later in this chapter. In particular, when there is coexistent TR, the TVA via the continuity principle is not valid so other parameters should be considered for determining the severity of TS (see Table 9.1).

Tricuspid Regurgitation
Aetiology of Tricuspid Regurgitation

Tricuspid regurgitation (TR) refers to the backward flow of blood from the RV to the RA during systole. As for mitral regurgitation (MR), TR may result from a number of disorders of the tricuspid valve complex. More commonly, the aetiology of TR is described in terms of functional or organic regurgitation (Table 9.2). Organic or primary regurgitation refers to diseases that involve the leaflets and the supporting apparatus; that is, TR occurs due to intrinsic valvular disease. Functional or secondary regurgitation refers to diseases that alter the annular geometry so TR occurs due to annular dilatation and subsequent poor leaflet coaptation of an otherwise normal tricuspid valve. Another unusual cause of TR is mechanical interference to valve closure caused by pacemaker wires and automatic implantable cardioverter defibrillator (AICD) leads.

Table 9.2 Aetiology of Tricuspid Regurgitation

Causes of TR	Examples
Functional causes (Annular dilatation)	• Atrial fibrillation (chronic) • Atrial septal defects • Dilated cardiomyopathy • Pulmonary hypertension • Pulmonary regurgitation • Right ventricular (RV) dysplasia • Right heart failure (2⁰ to left heart failure) • RV infarction
Organic causes (Disorders of tricuspid complex)	• Carcinoid tricuspid valve disease • Congenitally abnormal tricuspid valve (e.g. Ebstein's anomaly, atrioventricular canal defects) • Connective tissue disorders (e.g. Marfan syndrome) • Iatrogenic (e.g. post RV endomyocardial biopsy) • Infective endocarditis • Myxomatous disease (e.g. tricuspid valve prolapse) • Radiation injury • Rheumatic tricuspid disease • RV infarction • Trauma (e.g. motor vehicle accident, fall from a great height)

Rheumatic Tricuspid Valve Disease

As previously discussed, rheumatic valve disease occurs secondary to an episode or recurrent episodes of ARF. Rheumatic tricuspid valve disease almost never occurs as an isolated lesion and is almost always associated with rheumatic mitral and aortic valve disease. Structural changes to the tricuspid valve complex associated with rheumatic tricuspid disease result in TR as well as TS.

Carcinoid Tricuspid Valve Disease

As previously described, carcinoid heart disease is caused by a rare, malignant neuroendrocrine tumour that secretes excessive amounts of the hormone serotonin which damages the tricuspid valve. This leads to the formation of plaques which cause the valve to become thickened, retracted and rigid (see Fig. 9.8). As a result the valve becomes both stenotic and regurgitant. This systemic disease is discussed in detail in Chapter 14 (Systemic Diseases with Cardiac Manifestations).

Traumatic Tricuspid Valve Rupture

Violent external cardiac compression in conjunction with sudden pulmonary outflow obstruction applies great strain on the tendinous cords and papillary muscle attachments to the tricuspid valve. This may result in tearing and rupture of the tricuspid subvalvular apparatus. Late valve rupture may also occur when there is papillary muscle contusion and late necrosis. In blunt chest trauma, the anterior tricuspid valve leaflet is most often injured and may become flail due to cordal rupture and/or papillary muscle rupture.

Tricuspid Valve Prolapse

Tricuspid valve prolapse (TVP) is defined as the systolic billowing or displacement of one or more tricuspid leaflets, above the tricuspid annular plane, into the RA (Fig. 9.17). Isolated TVP may occur rarely, more commonly however, TVP is found together with mitral valve prolapse.

Ebstein's Anomaly

Ebstein's anomaly is a rare congenital malformation of the tricuspid valve. This anomaly is thought to occur due to the failure of the developing tricuspid leaflets to delaminate (split) from the inlet portion of the ventricle. This leads to the following characteristic features of this anomaly: (1) adhesion of the septal and posterior tricuspid leaflets to the underlying myocardium, (2) an exaggerated apical displacement of the functional tricuspid annulus including apical displacement of the septal tricuspid leaflet, (3) atrialisation and dilatation of a portion of the RV inflow tract, and (4) a small functional RV (Fig. 9.19). Importantly, it should be noted that this anomaly encompasses a wide spectrum of anatomic and functional abnormalities of the tricuspid valve and RV.

Other congenital heart lesions are frequently associated with this anomaly. The most commonly associated congenital heart malformation is an interatrial communication, either as a patent foramen ovale (PFO) or a secundum atrial septal defect (ASD). Ebstein's anomaly of the tricuspid valve is also commonly encountered in patients with congenitally corrected transposition of the great arteries and is also associated with ventricular septal defects. Other associated right heart anomalies include pulmonary valve lesions (atresia or stenosis) and a hypoplastic pulmonary artery; other associated left heart anomalies include bicuspid aortic valves, subaortic stenosis, coarctation of the aorta, mitral valve prolapse and LV morphological features resembling LV non-compaction. Ebstein's anomaly is also often associated with abnormal conduction pathways such as accessory AV pathways and Wolfe-Parkinson-White (WPW) syndrome.

Annular Dilatation

Annular dilatation is a functional cause of TR. In particular, despite the presence of structurally normal tricuspid leaflets, dilatation of the tricuspid annulus may result in incomplete or inadequate coaptation of the tricuspid leaflets during systole which leads to TR. Common conditions that lead to tricuspid annular dilatation include dilated cardiomyopathy, ASDs and pulmonary hypertension (Fig. 9.18).

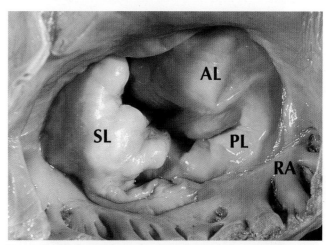

Figure 9.17 This gross pathological specimen shows prolapse of the anterior tricuspid leaflet (AL) and redundancy of the septal tricuspid leaflet (SL); the posterior tricuspid leaflet (PL) is normal.
RA = right atrium.
Reproduced from Virmani R, Burke AP, Farb A: Pathology of valvular heart disease. In Rahimtoola SH [ed]: Valvular Heart Disease. In Braunwald E [series ed]: Atlas of Heart Diseases. Vol 11. Philadelphia, Current Medicine, page 1.17, © 1997, with kind permission from Springer Science+Business Media B.V

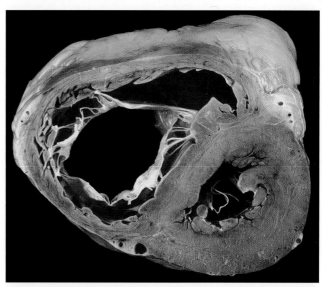

Figure 9.18 This gross pathological specimen from a patient with chronic pulmonary hypertension shows marked right ventricular (RV) dilatation and thickening of the RV walls. Severe tricuspid regurgitation was present as a consequence of marked tricuspid annular dilatation. Also observe the straightened ventricular septum and D-shaped appearance of the left ventricle which occurs due to RV dilatation and increased RV mass.
By permission of Mayo Foundation for Medical Education and Research. All rights reserved. Courtesy of William D. Edwards, MD.

Pathophysiology of Tricuspid Regurgitation

Tricuspid regurgitation is characterised by the backflow of blood from the RV into the RA during systole. When the RA is compliant, it is able to receive increased volumes without haemodynamic consequences. However, as RA compliance decreases, increases to the RA volume lead to an elevation of both RA and venous pressures which can lead to systemic venous congestion and signs and symptoms associated with right-sided congestive heart failure (CHF). In addition, diastolic volume overload of the RV causes RV dilatation which can lead to elevated RV end-diastolic pressures, which in turn, also leads to the development of right-sided CHF.

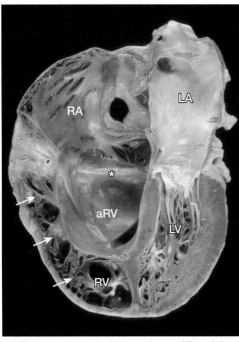

Figure 9.19 This gross pathological specimen of Ebstein's anomaly is cut in the 4-chamber plane. Observe that the anterior tricuspid leaflet is attached to the underlying ventricular myocardium at multiple points (*arrows*). There is also marked apical (downward) displacement of the functional tricuspid annulus. The atrialized portion of the right ventricle (aRV) lies between the true tricuspid annulus (*) and the tricuspid leaflets. The functional portion of the right ventricle (RV) is small and the RV free wall is very thin. LA = left atrium; LV = left ventricle; RA = right atrium.

By permission of Mayo Foundation for Medical Education and Research. All rights reserved. Courtesy of William D. Edwards, MD.

Clinical Manifestations of Tricuspid Regurgitation

The clinical manifestations of TR relate to a chronic elevation in RA and venous pressures and right-sided CHF. These manifestations include dyspnoea, orthopnoea, peripheral oedema, ascites, weight loss and cachexia, cyanosis, jaundice, and systolic pulsations of an enlarged, tender liver.

Role of Echocardiography in Tricuspid Regurgitation

The aims and objectives of echocardiography in the assessment of TR are to:
• Determine the aetiology of the lesion,
• Assess RA size,
• Assess RV size and systolic function,
• Estimate the severity of the regurgitation,
• Estimate right ventricular systolic pressure.

Aetiology of Tricuspid Regurgitation

As discussed previously, TR can result from intrinsic abnormalities of the tricuspid valve complex (organic TR) or secondary to annular dilatation (functional TR) (see Table 9.2). The characteristic echocardiographic features of various causes of TR are summarised below.

Rheumatic Tricuspid Stenosis

As previously described, rheumatic TS is characterised by the diastolic doming of the tricuspid valve leaflets. Rheumatic tricuspid valve disease results in thickening and retraction of the tricuspid leaflets and dilatation of the tricuspid annulus; the effect of these changes is incomplete leaflet coaptation during systole and TR (Fig. 9.20).

Carcinoid Tricuspid Valve Disease

As previously stated, the characteristic 2D echocardiographic feature of carcinoid tricuspid valve disease is thickened, retracted and immobile leaflets. Therefore, the valve remains in a fixed semi-open position throughout the cardiac cycle so there is coexistent stenosis and regurgitation (Fig. 9.21). Recall that while carcinoid tricuspid valve disease appears similar to rheumatic tricuspid valve disease, the absence of coexistent rheumatic mitral valve disease aids distinguishing carcinoid valve disease from rheumatic valve disease.

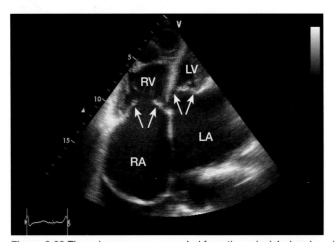
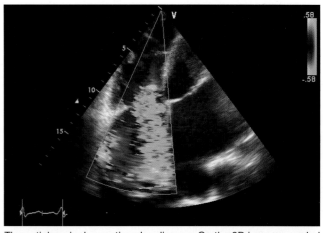

Figure 9.20 These images were recorded from the apical 4-chamber view. The aetiology is rheumatic valve disease. On the 2D image recorded during diastole, thickening and diastolic doming of both the tricuspid and mitral leaflets is evident (*arrows*); these features are characteristic of rheumatic valve disease (*left*). Marked biatrial and moderate right ventricular (RV) dilatation is also apparent. The colour Doppler image shows severe tricuspid regurgitation (*right*). LA = left atrium; LV = left ventricle; RA = right atrium.

Pulmonary Hypertension

Chronic, severe pulmonary hypertension is invariably associated with RV and, therefore, tricuspid annular dilatation. Tricuspid annular dilatation leads to incomplete or inadequate coaptation of the tricuspid leaflets during systole; in addition, apical descent of the papillary muscles further contributes to restricted systolic tricuspid leaflet motion. These changes result in functional TR (Fig. 9.22). Importantly, the peak TR velocity does not reflect the severity of TR; the TR velocity simply reflects the pressure difference between the RV and RA during systole. For example, there can be mild TR and very high TR velocities or there can be severe TR with low TR velocities.

> 'Physiological' or mild TR is often found in the normal population with incidence, but not severity, increasing with age.

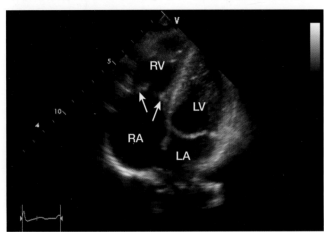
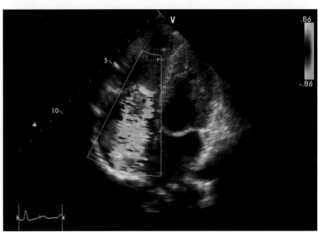

Figure 9.21 These images were recorded from an off-axis apical 4-chamber view. The aetiology is carcinoid tricuspid valve disease. On the 2D image recorded during systole, there is poor coaptation of the tricuspid valve leaflets with the leaflets remaining in a partially opened position (*arrows*). On the colour Doppler image, concomitant severe tricuspid regurgitation is apparent. LA = left atrium; LV = left ventricle; RA = right atrium; RV = right ventricle.

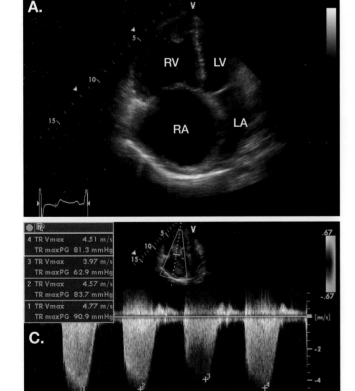
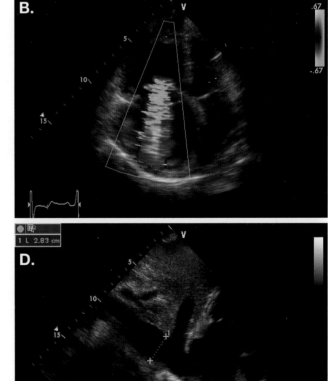

Figure 9.22 These images were recorded from a patient with idiopathic pulmonary arterial hypertension. The 2D image recorded from the apical 4-chamber view in systole shows marked dilatation of the right atrium (RA) and right ventricle (RV) (*top left*). The corresponding colour Doppler image shows significant tricuspid regurgitation (TR) secondary to dilatation of the tricuspid annulus (*top right*). The average TR velocity via continuous-wave Doppler was 4.45 m/s yielding an RV-to-RA pressure gradient of 80 mm Hg (*bottom left*). The inferior vena cava (IVC) was dilated with minimal collapse during respiration consistent with a RA pressure of 15 mm Hg (*bottom right*). Based on the TR velocity and the estimated RA pressure, the right ventricular systolic pressure was estimated at 95 mm Hg.

Tricuspid Valve Prolapse

As for mitral valve prolapse, the 2D diagnostic criterion for TVP is based on the systolic bowing of one or more tricuspid leaflets above the tricuspid annular plane. Other echocardiographic features of TVP include bulky (myxomatous) and elongated appearances of the tricuspid leaflets. As the tricuspid annulus has a complex 3D geometry similar to the mitral annulus, the tricuspid valve may mistakenly appear to prolapse when viewed in the apical 4-chamber view. For this reason, TVP is best diagnosed from the parasternal long axis view of the RV inflow or from the parasternal short axis view at the level of the aorta (Fig. 9.23).

Traumatic Tricuspid Valve Rupture

The characteristic 2D echocardiographic features of traumatic tricuspid valve rupture include a flail tricuspid leaflet and the presence of cordal rupture. A flail leaflet is identified when the tip of the leaflet points towards the RA during systole and ruptured cords appear as mobile, whip-like linear structures within the RA and RV (Fig. 9.24).

Ebstein's Anomaly

The characteristic 2D echocardiographic features of Ebstein's anomaly include the apical displacement of the tricuspid valve and the atrialisation of a portion of the RV inflow tract. This anomaly is best diagnosed from the apical 4-chamber view where the anatomic relationship between the insertion of the septal tricuspid leaflet and the anterior mitral leaflet is easily identified. The diagnostic criterion for this anomaly is based on the apical 4-chamber view and the apical displacement of the septal tricuspid leaflet insertion from the anterior mitral leaflet insertion greater than 8 mm/m^2 or more than 20 mm in adults (Fig. 9.25). In addition, the anterior tricuspid leaflet is often elongated and redundant. On real-time 2D imaging, the anterior leaflet displays a sail-like or whip-like motion. However, when the anterior leaflet is tethered to the RV free wall by accessory attachments, its motion may appear restricted rather than whip-like. Due to the gross abnormality of the tricuspid valve, TR is always present.

Displacement of the tricuspid valve results in dilatation of the RA which includes the morphological RA as well as an atrialized portion of the right ventricle (aRV) which lies between the true tricuspid annulus and the tricuspid leaflets (Fig. 9.26). By comparing the ratio of the combined area of the RA and aRV to the combined functional RV and left heart, the severity of Ebstein's anomaly can be graded (Fig. 9.27). This index, also known as the Celermajer index, also has prognostic value in newborns [9.3].

As a PFO or ASD are frequently associated with Ebstein's anomaly, careful interrogation of the interatrial septum is required. Importantly, shunting across the PFO or ASD is often right-to-left as the RA pressure often exceeds the LA pressure.

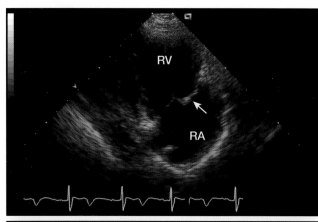

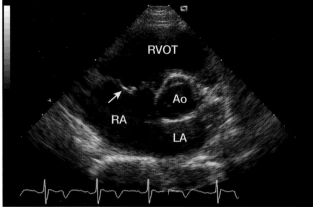

Figure 9.23 These systolic still frame images were recorded from the parasternal long axis view of the right ventricular inflow (*top*) and from the parasternal short axis view at the level of the aorta (*bottom*). Prolapse of the anterior tricuspid valve leaflet is evident on both images; observe that when the tricuspid valve is closed in systole, the anterior leaflet bows into the right atrium beyond the atrioventricular plane (*arrows*).
Ao = aorta; LA = left atrium; RA = right atrium; RV = right ventricle; RVOT = right ventricular outflow tract.

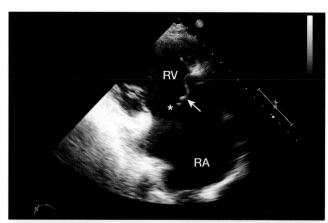

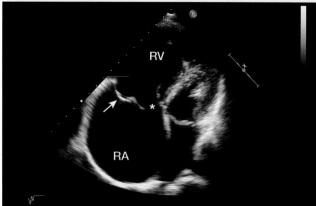

Figure 9.24 These systolic still frame images were recorded from the parasternal long axis view of the right ventricular inflow (*top*) and from the apical 4-chamber view (*bottom*). A flail anterior leaflet of the tricuspid valve is evident (*arrows*) and a very large coaptation defect is noted (*). The aetiology of this valve lesion was blunt chest trauma suffered 10 years prior to this presentation. RA = right atrium; RV = right ventricle.

[9.3] Celermajer DS, Cullen S, Sullivan ID, Spiegelhalter DJ, Wyse RK, Deanfield JE. Outcome in neonates with Ebstein's anomaly. *J Am Coll Cardiol.* 1992 Apr;19(5):1041-6.

Assessment of Right Atrial Size

Chronic RA volume overload due to chronic significant TR leads to RA dilatation. As stated above, the best view for measuring RA dimensions is the apical 4-chamber view. From this view, the RA area, the RA length (major or long axis) and the mid-RA diameter (minor or short axis) can be measured (see Fig. 9.13).

Assessment of Right Ventricular Size and Systolic Function

Chronic significant TR leads to chronic RV volume overload and progressive RV dilatation. Therefore, measurements of the RV size, performed from an RV-focused apical 4-chamber view at end-diastole, are important in the serial evaluation of patients with significant TR. Measurements of RV systolic function such as the Doppler tissue imaging systolic velocity, the TAPSE, the fractional area change and/or the RV myocardial performance index, are also an essential component of the echocardiographic examination in patients with TR. The methods for assessing RV size and systolic function are described in detail in Chapter 2.

Importantly, abnormal or paradoxical IVS motion is frequently seen when there is RV volume overload. RV volume overload results in increased RV diastolic filling pressures and when the RV diastolic pressure approaches or exceeds LV diastolic filling pressures, the IVS motion becomes paradoxical; that is, the IVS shifts leftwards towards the centre of the LV during diastole (see Fig. 2.40). Paradoxical IVS motion can be appreciated on the M-mode trace recorded through the

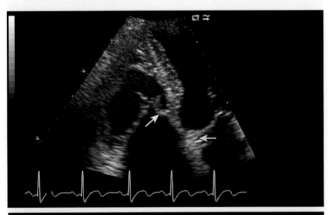

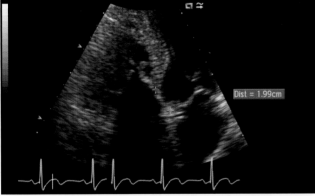

Figure 9.25 These images were recorded from a zoomed apical 4-chamber view. The patient has Ebstein's anomaly. Observe the apical displacement on the insertion of the septal leaflet of the tricuspid valve (*white arrow*) compared with the insertion of the anterior mitral valve (*yellow arrow*) (*top*). The distance between these two insertion points was measured at 20 mm and when indexed to the body surface area of 2.0 m², this distance was 10 mm/m² (*bottom*).

right and left ventricles and from 2D images recorded from the parasternal long axis and short axis views of the LV, and from the apical 4-chamber view.

Estimation of Severity

An accurate assessment of the severity of TR requires a comprehensive evaluation of all possible Doppler variables. Therefore, the TR severity should be determined by looking for indirect signs on the colour and spectral Doppler

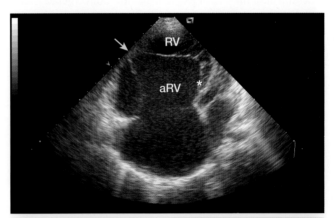

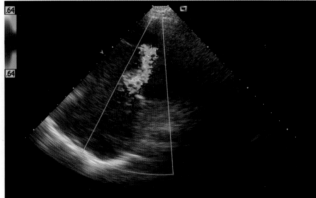

Figure 9.26 This is an extreme example of Ebstein's anomaly. Observe the marked apical displacement of the insertion of the septal tricuspid valve leaflet (*) and the sail-like appearance of the anterior tricuspid leaflet which is attached to the underlying ventricular myocardium (*yellow arrow*). A small functional right ventricle (RV) and a large atrialized portion of the right ventricle (aRV) is also apparent. The corresponding colour Doppler image shows tricuspid regurgitation. Colour Doppler is also very useful in identifying the apical displacement of the tricuspid orifice.

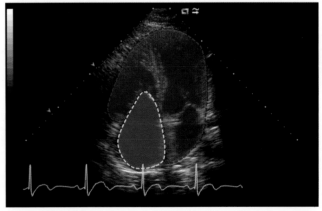

Figure 9.27 The Celermajer index is measured in an apical 4-chamber view at end-diastole and is calculated as the ratio of the combined area of the right atrium and atrialized right ventricle (*yellow area*) to the combined area of the functional right ventricle, left atrium, and left ventricle (*red area*).

examination. Quantitative calculations such as the regurgitant volume and the effective regurgitant orifice area are also theoretically possible.

Indirect Signs for Assessing TR Severity: Colour Doppler Imaging

Colour Doppler flow imaging (CFI) provides a quick and easy method for identifying the presence of TR. CFI also provides indirect clues to the severity of TR. In particular, assessment of the colour jet area, the flow convergence radius and the vena contracta width can be used to determine the TR severity. The criteria for defining the various grades of TR based on these methods are summarized in Table 9.3.

Colour Jet Area

Evaluation of the size of the TR jet area is a rapid way for semiquantitating the severity of TR. Because regurgitant jets are 3-dimensional, the TR jet area must be evaluated by carefully angling through the regurgitant jet and by using multiple orthogonal planes. Most commonly, an 'eyeball' evaluation rather than direct measurement of the jet area is used to estimate TR severity via this method (Fig. 9.28).

Vena Contracta Width

The vena contracta (VC) is defined as the narrowest part of a jet downstream from the narrowed orifice (see Fig. 1.21). With respect to regurgitant jets the VC is the narrowest region of the regurgitant jet which occurs between the proximal flow convergence zone and the actual regurgitant jet. The vena contracta width (VC-W) of a regurgitant jet provides an estimate of the effective regurgitant orifice size.

The VC-W for TR can be measured from the parasternal long axis of the RV inflow view or from the apical 4-chamber view. Accurate measurement of the VC-W requires all three components of the regurgitant flow to be seen; these three components are: (1) the flow convergence dome, (2) the VC and (3) the regurgitant jet (Fig. 9.29).

Flow Convergence Radius

As described in Chapter 1 as flow converges toward a narrowed orifice it accelerates in a laminar manner forming a flow convergence zone. This flow convergence zone is comprised of a series of concentric hemispheric shells of uniform velocity (isovelocities). As flow advances closer to the narrowed orifice, the area of each hemispheric shell decreases and the velocity of each shell increases. This assumption forms the basis of the proximal isovelocity surface area (PISA) principle for the calculation of the EOA. Typically, the PISA principle is used to calculate the effective regurgitant orifice area (EROA) (discussed later). However,

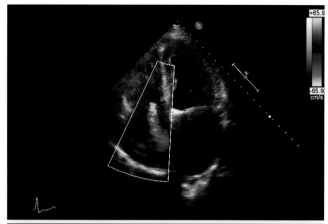

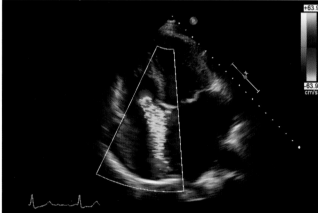

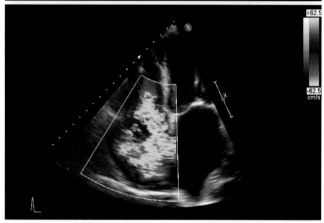

Figure 9.28 These three systolic colour flow Doppler still frame images were recorded from three different patients with varying degrees of tricuspid regurgitation (TR): mild TR (*top*), moderate TR (*middle*) and severe TR (*bottom*). The severity of TR is based on the TR colour jet area within the right atrium; the larger the colour jet area, the more severe the regurgitation.

Table 9.3 Qualitative Colour Doppler Parameters for Grading Tricuspid Regurgitation Severity

Parameter	Mild	Moderate	Severe
Jet area – central jets (cm²) *	< 5	5 – 10	> 10
Vena contracta width (cm) δ	Not defined	Not defined, but < 0.7	≥ 0.7
Flow convergence radius (cm) #	≤ 0.5	0.6 – 0.9	> 0.9

* Using a Nyquist limit of 50–60 cm/s; not valid in eccentric jets.
δ Using a Nyquist limit of 50–60 cm/s.
with a baseline shift at a Nyquist limit of 28 cm/s.
Source: Zoghbi WA, Enriquez-Sarano M, Foster E, Grayburn PA, Kraft CD, Levine RA, Nihoyannopoulos P, Otto CM, Quinones MA, Rakowski H, Stewart WJ, Waggoner A, Weissman NJ; American Society of Echocardiography. Recommendations for evaluation of the severity of native valvular regurgitation with two-dimensional and Doppler echocardiography. *J Am Soc Echocardiogr.* 2003 Jul;16(7):777-802.

measurement of the PISA radius or the flow convergence radius (FCR) proximal to a regurgitant orifice may provide an indirect clue as to the severity of valvular regurgitation; for example, the bigger the FCR the more significant the regurgitation.

In the case of TR, the FCR is measured on the RV side of the tricuspid valve during systole at a colour Nyquist limit of approximately 28 cm/s (Fig. 9.30).

Limitations of CFI Indirect Signs

There are numerous technical and physiological factors that can affect the colour flow Doppler map which are unrelated to the severity of TR (refer to Table 7.8).

In particular, recall that Doppler techniques detect the motion of moving red blood cells (RBCs). As such any RBCs in motion will create a Doppler shift and this Doppler shift is

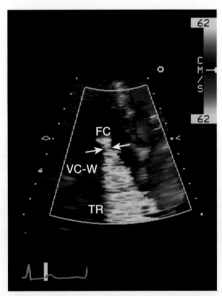

Figure 9.29 This colour flow Doppler image showing tricuspid regurgitation (TR) was recorded from a zoomed apical 4-chamber view. The vena contracta width (VC-W) is measured at the narrowest neck of the TR flow region at the junction of the flow convergence zone (FC) and the regurgitant jet immediately below the flow convergence region.

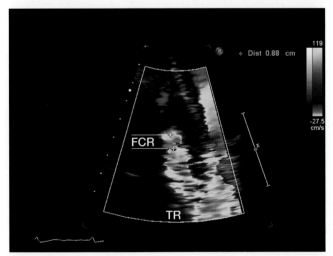

Figure 9.30 This zoomed image of the tricuspid valve was recorded from the apical 4-chamber view during systole. Colour flow imaging demonstrates tricuspid regurgitation (TR). The flow convergence zone proximal to the tricuspid valve was magnified by decreasing the colour Nyquist limit (V_N) to 27.5 cm/s; this is achieved by moving the colour baseline downwards in the direction of the TR jet. The flow convergence radius (FCR) is measured as the vertical distance from the tricuspid valve leaflets to the top of the flow convergence zone which is identified as the blue-red interface. In this example, the FCR is 0.88 cm.

detected by the ultrasound machine. Therefore, RBCs within the receiving chamber that are not within the regurgitant jet will be displaced by the regurgitant jet; therefore, the Doppler shifts created by these RBCs will be incorporated into the 'colour regurgitant volume'. As a result, the regurgitant volume will be overestimated on the colour Doppler display. The severity of regurgitation may also be underestimated when the regurgitant jet is eccentric. In these situations, the regurgitant jet is attracted to and 'hugs' the adjacent chamber wall; the cause of this phenomenon is based on the Coandă effect. In this instance, the regurgitant jet area can appear significantly smaller than free jets due to jet distortion and loss of jet momentum. Therefore, the regurgitant jet area does not reflect the severity of regurgitation. In these situations, alternate methods for assessing TR severity are required.

Another important limitation of CFI in the assessment of TR occurs when there is 'free' or 'wide-open' TR. In these patients, the tricuspid regurgitant orifice is very large; therefore, in the absence of pulmonary hypertension, the pressure differential between the RA and RV is very small and, therefore, little or no aliasing of the TR jet will occur. In fact, the TR velocity is often very low (< 2m/s) resulting in near equalisation of RV and RA pressures. As a result, this low turbulence, low velocity signal is visually unimpressive on CFI and may be overlooked or underestimated if colour flow Doppler alone is used to assess TR severity (Fig. 9.31).

As for MR, the principal limitation of the VC-W in the assessment of TR severity is the assumption that the regurgitant orifice is almost circular; however, the tricuspid regurgitant orifice is often elliptic or irregular in shape rather than circular. When there are multiple regurgitant jets, neither the VC-W nor the FCR can be used to qualitatively assess the severity of TR. This is because respective VC-Ws and FCRs are not additive. Furthermore, while a VC-W ≥ 0.7 cm is indicative of severe TR, values less than 0.7 cm are not accurate at distinguishing between mild and moderate TR.

Indirect Signs for Assessing TR Severity: Spectral Doppler

Indirect signs of TR severity can also be provided by PW and CW spectral Doppler. PW Doppler methods include the tricuspid inflow profile and the presence of systolic flow reversal in the hepatic veins. CW Doppler methods include the intensity of the TR signal and the shape or contour of the TR signal. The criteria for defining the various grades of TR via these methods are summarized in Table 9.4.

Tricuspid Inflow Velocities

When there is TR, the flow across the tricuspid valve is the combination of the tricuspid regurgitant volume and the normal SV returning from the body and coronary sinus. Therefore, in patients with significant TR, the tricuspid inflow velocities are often increased and this is reflected as an increased peak early diastolic (E) velocity via PW Doppler or by an increased mean trans-tricuspid pressure gradient as measured by CW Doppler. In particular, in the absence of TS, a peak E velocity ≥ 1.0 m/s is suggestive of severe TR.

Hepatic Venous Systolic Flow Reversal

The presence of systolic flow reversal in the hepatic veins demonstrated by PW Doppler is another clue to the presence of significant TR. Hepatic venous flow is interrogated by PW

Doppler from the subcostal window with a 3-5 mm sample volume placed at least 1 cm into one of the three hepatic veins (usually the middle hepatic vein).

The normal hepatic venous flow profile demonstrates predominant forward flow during systole and diastole with small antegrade velocities occurring with atrial contraction (atrial flow reversal) and ventricular contraction (ventricular flow reversal) (Fig. 9.32, top). With increasing degrees of TR, the hepatic vein systolic velocity becomes blunted or reduced; with severe TR, systolic flow reversal may be present (Fig. 9.32, bottom).

CFI and colour Doppler M-mode can also be used to identify systolic flow reversal in the hepatic veins. Colour Doppler M-mode, in particular, is very useful for displaying flow direction and for confirming the timing of flow over the cardiac cycle (Fig. 9.33).

While systolic flow reversal in the hepatic veins is a specific sign of severe TR, it is not very sensitive. That is, when present, hepatic venous systolic flow reversal is a good indicator to the presence of severe TR; however, there can be significant TR without systolic flow reversal.

Intensity of TR CW Signal

In theory, the density or intensity of the spectral Doppler signal of a regurgitant jet is proportional to the number of RBCs travelling within the regurgitant jet. Therefore, the greater the regurgitation, the denser the regurgitant CW signal. For example, a weak Doppler signal is suggestive of relatively mild valvular regurgitation whereas a strong signal is suggestive of more significant regurgitation.

Contour of TR CW Signal

The TR Doppler velocity signal reflects the pressure gradient between the RV and the RA during systole. Therefore, the contour of this velocity spectrum reflects the pressure difference between the RV and the RA during systole. In particular, when there is mild TR, the RA pressure is usually

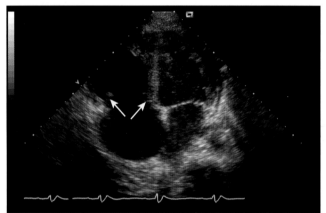

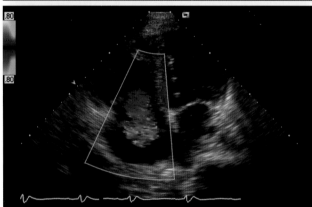

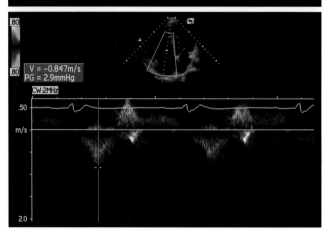

Figure 9.31 These images were recorded from a patient with 'free' or 'wide-open' tricuspid regurgitation (TR). The apical 4-chamber view during systole shows marked dilatation of the right heart chambers and poor coaptation of the tricuspid valve leaflets (*arrows*) (*top*). The corresponding colour flow Doppler of the TR jet appears essentially laminar with minimal turbulence and no aliasing (*middle*). This appearance occurs when the pressure difference between the RA and RV is minimal so the RA and RV are effectively operating as a single chamber. The continuous-wave Doppler signal of the TR jet confirms the presence of laminar, low velocity flow; the RV-to-RA pressure gradient is just 3 mm Hg (*bottom*).

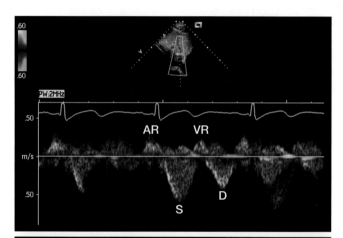

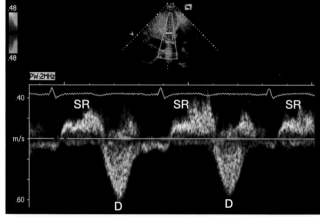

Figure 9.32 These pulsed-wave (PW) Doppler signals were recorded from a patient with no tricuspid regurgitation (TR) (*top*) and a patient with severe TR (*bottom*). Both signals were recorded from the subcostal window with the PW sample volume placed approximately 1 cm into the middle hepatic vein. In the patient with no TR, four waveforms are seen: systolic forward flow (S), diastolic forward flow (D), flow reversal with atrial contraction (AR) and flow reversal with ventricular contraction (VR). In the patient with severe TR, there is systolic flow reversal (SR) only and no systolic forward flow.

normal; thus, the pressure difference between the RV and RA is relatively high and remains consistently high throughout the entire systolic period; the resultant spectral Doppler signal shows a symmetrical or parabolic contour (Fig. 9.34, left). However, in the case of severe TR associated with an increased RA *v*-wave pressure, the contour of the TR signal becomes triangular as the pressure difference between the RV and RA in mid-to-late systole decreases due to the marked elevation in the RA *v*-wave pressure (Fig. 9.34, right). The triangular appearance of the TR signal is also referred to as the 'V cut-off' sign.

Limitations of Spectral Doppler Indirect Signs

When there is significant TR and an absence of co-existent TS, an increased E velocity across the tricuspid valve can be used to identify increased forward SV across the valve caused by significant TR. However, the peak E velocity is also affected by the heart rate, RA pressure, RV relaxation, and atrial fibrillation (AF). For example, tachycardia can lead to increased trans-tricuspid velocities in the absence of significant TR.

The presence of systolic flow reversal in the hepatic veins strongly supports the diagnosis of severe TR. However, systolic blunting may be encountered with AF, with increased RA pressures due to any cause, and in cases of RA and RV compliance abnormalities. Other limitations of hepatic venous Doppler relate to technical factors such as suboptimal

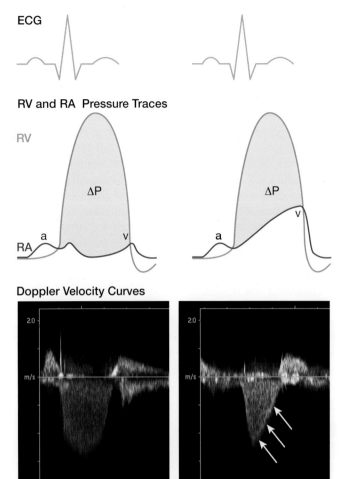

Figure 9.34 In tricuspid regurgitation (TR), the regurgitant Doppler velocity signal reflects the pressure difference (ΔP) between the right ventricle (RV) and the right atrium (RA) during systole. The top schematics illustrate the pressure tracings of the RV and the RA during systole while the Doppler velocity spectra corresponding to these traces are displayed below. The RA pressure trace consists of an *a* wave which represents an increase in RA pressure with atrial contraction and a *v* wave which represents an increase in RA pressure, caused by venous return into the RA, during ventricular systole. In mild TR (*left*), the ΔP between the RV and RA from early to late systole is relatively high. This results in a symmetrical, parabolic Doppler velocity curve. With severe TR (*right*), the ΔP between the RV and RA is high from early to mid systole as for mild TR. However, when there is severe TR, with an associated marked increase in the v wave of the RA pressure trace, there is a decrease in the ΔP between the RV and RA toward the latter half of systole. This results in a rapid and asymmetric, V-shaped Doppler velocity curve (*triple arrows*).

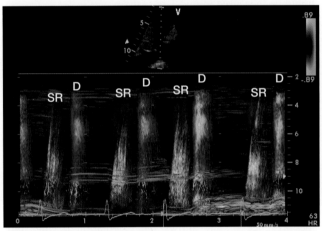

Figure 9.33 This colour Doppler M-mode trace was recorded from a patient with severe TR. This trace was recorded with the M-mode cursor placed within the middle hepatic vein. Systolic flow reversal (SR) into the hepatic vein is displayed; this appears as red flow towards the transducer during systole. Normal diastolic forward flow (D) is also noted; this appears as blue flow.

Table 9.4 Qualitative Spectral Doppler Parameters for Grading Tricuspid Regurgitation Severity

Parameter	Mild	Moderate	Severe
Tricuspid inflow (PW)	Normal	Normal	E wave dominant (≥ 1.0 m/s) *
Hepatic venous (PW)	Systolic dominance ^	Systolic blunting ^	Systolic reversal
Intensity of TR signal (CW)	Incomplete or faint	Dense	Dense
TR Jet Contour (CW)	Parabolic	Usually parabolic	Early peaking or triangular (peak < 2 m/s in massive TR)

CW = continuous-wave Doppler; PW = pulsed-wave Doppler
* in the absence of other causes of elevated right atrial pressure and of tricuspid stenosis.
^ Unless other reasons of systolic blunting (e.g. atrial fibrillation, elevated left atrial pressure).
Sources: Zoghbi WA, Enriquez-Sarano M, Foster E, Grayburn PA, Kraft CD, Levine RA, Nihoyannopoulos P, Otto CM, Quinones MA, Rakowski H, Stewart WJ, Waggoner A, Weissman NJ; American Society of Echocardiography. Recommendations for evaluation of the severity of native valvular regurgitation with two-dimensional and Doppler echocardiography. *J Am Soc Echocardiogr.* 2003 Jul;16(7):777-802; Lancellotti P, Tribouilloy C, Hagendorff A, Moura L, Popescu BA, Agricola E, Monin JL, Pierard LA, Badano L, Zamorano JL; European Association of Echocardiography. European Association of Echocardiography recommendations for the assessment of valvular regurgitation. Part 2: mitral and tricuspid regurgitation (native valve disease). *Eur J Echocardiogr.* 2010 May;11(4):307-332.

subcostal images and movement of the hepatic vein across the image display over the respiratory cycle.

The intensity of the TR signal can be affected by a number of factors. For example, Doppler gain affects the overall intensity of the regurgitant jet; if the gain is set too low then the signal intensity will also be decreased. In addition, poor alignment of the TR jet with the Doppler beam will result in a suboptimal TR signal; this is especially a problem with eccentric jets.

While the V cut-off sign is an indicator of a marked increase in the RA v-wave pressure, this is dependent on RA compliance. For example, this sign may be absent even when there is severe TR and when the RA compliance is high; that is, in this instance the RA is able to accept a large volume of blood without a significant increase in the RA pressure. Furthermore, the V cut-off sign relies on the acquisition of a complete TR signal which is difficult to achieve with eccentric TR jets.

Quantitative Methods for TR Severity

The severity of TR may be quantitatively assessed by calculating the regurgitant volume and the effective regurgitant orifice area via the PISA principle. The criteria for defining the various grades of TR based on these methods are listed in Table 9.5.

Effective Regurgitant Orifice Area

The effective regurgitant orifice area (EROA), which is a measure of the 'hole' size in the incompetent valve, can be calculated using the PISA method. The basic concepts of this principle in the calculation of the effective orifice area are described in Chapter 1. Recall that this calculation is based on the continuity principle which states that flow proximal to a narrowed orifice must equal flow through the narrowed orifice. In the case of TR, the EROA can be calculated from the radius of the proximal flow convergence dome, the velocity at the radius and the peak velocity of the TR jet (Fig. 9.35):

Equation 9.2

$$EROA_{TR} = (2\pi\ r^2 \times V_N) \div V_{TR}$$

where $EROA_{TR}$ = tricuspid effective regurgitant orifice area (cm²)

$2\pi\ r^2$ = surface area of the hemispheric shell derived from the flow convergence radius [r] proximal to the tricuspid valve (cm²)

V_N = colour Nyquist limit at the radial distance of the hemispheric shell (cm/s)

V_{TR} = peak velocity of the tricuspid regurgitant jet (cm/s)

Regurgitant Volume

Regurgitant volume (RV), defined as the volume of blood that leaks (regurgitates) through an incompetent valve, can

also be calculated based on the PISA principle. Calculation of the RV via this technique is based on the standard SV equation (Eq. 1.12). Recall that the SV is a product of the CSA and VTI. Based on this relationship between SV, CSA and VTI, the RV is simply derived by substituting the RV for SV, EROA for CSA and VTI of the regurgitant jet (VTI_{RJ}) for the VTI:

Equation 9.3

$$RV = EROA \times VTI_{RJ}$$

where RV = regurgitant volume (mL)

EROA = effective regurgitant orifice area (cm²)

VTI_{RJ} = velocity time integral of regurgitant jet (cm)

Therefore, to perform this calculation for TR two values are required (Fig. 9.35):
1. EROA for TR
2. VTI of the TR jet

The limitations of EROA and RV calculations are the same as those limitations described for the PISA method in Chapter 2. In particular, as described for MR, the PISA radius may progressively increase over the systolic period. Therefore, to avoid underestimation or overestimation of the EROA, measurement of the PISA radius should be performed at the same time as the peak TR velocity; that is, the PISA radius should be measured in mid-late systole.

Again, as for MR, the EROA may also be overestimated with eccentric TR jets when the proximal flow convergence region encroaches on surrounding structures such as the RV free wall. In this instance, flow constraint pushes the contours outwards from the regurgitant orifice; therefore, the flow proximal to the tricuspid valve (PISA dome) is no longer hemispherical.

Another limitation of the EROA via the PISA method is that this method is not valid when there are multiple regurgitant jets. Furthermore, while an EROA ≥ 0.40 cm² and a RV ≥ 45 mL are indicative of severe TR, values less than these are not accurate at distinguishing between mild and moderate TR.

Estimation of RVSP

The presence of TR allows the calculation of the right ventricular systolic pressure (RVSP). Recall that the peak systolic velocity of the TR signal reflects the pressure difference between the RV and RA in systole. Therefore, from the TR velocity and from an estimation of the RA pressure (RAP), it is possible to estimate the RVSP using the following equation:

Equation 9.4

$$RVSP = 4\ V_{TR}^2 + RAP$$

where RVSP = right ventricular systolic pressure (mm Hg)

V_{TR} = peak systolic TR velocity (m/s)

RAP = right atrial pressure (mm Hg)

Table 9.5 Quantitative Parameters for Grading Tricuspid Regurgitation Severity

Parameter	Mild	Moderate	Severe
Regurgitant Volume (mL)	Not defined	Not defined	≥ 45
Effective Regurgitant Orifice Area (cm²)	Not defined	Not defined	≥ 0.40

Sources: Lancellotti P, Tribouilloy C, Hagendorff A, Moura L, Popescu BA, Agricola E, Monin JL, Pierard LA, Badano L, Zamorano JL; European Association of Echocardiography. European Association of Echocardiography recommendations for the assessment of valvular regurgitation. Part 2: mitral and tricuspid regurgitation (native valve disease). *Eur J Echocardiogr.* 2010 May;11(4):307-332.

Estimation of the RAP can be determined using the inferior vena cava (IVC), hepatic venous (HV) Doppler parameters and/or Doppler tissue imaging (DTI) of the RV lateral annulus. These methods are described in detail in Chapter 4. Based on these measurements, the RAP can then be estimated (see Table 4.17).

Calculation of the RVSP with Free TR

When there is 'free' or 'wide-open' TR, the TR velocity is usually very low because the RA and RV are effectively functioning as a single chamber. In this situation, the RVSP cannot be accurately estimated from the peak TR velocity. This is because while the TR velocity will still reflect the pressure difference between the RV and RA in systole, the RAP is unknown and it may be as high as 40 mm Hg.

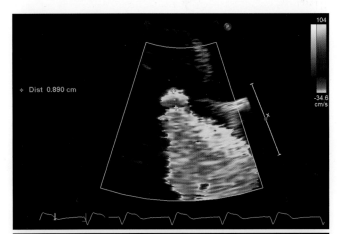

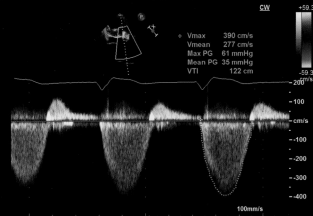

Figure 9.35 The effective regurgitant orifice area (EROA) for tricuspid regurgitation (TR) is calculated via the proximal isovelocity surface area (PISA) method. From a zoomed colour Doppler apical 4-chamber view of the tricuspid valve, the proximal flow convergence radius (Dist) is measured on the right ventricular side of the tricuspid valve in systole; callipers are placed between the tricuspid leaflets and the first aliased velocity (at the red-blue interface) (*top*). The colour Nyquist limit at this radius is noted at the bottom of the colour bar as flow is directed away from the transducer. From the continuous-wave Doppler trace, the peak TR velocity (Vmax) is measured (*bottom*). The tricuspid EROA in this example is calculated as:

$$EROA_{MR} = (2\pi\, r^2 \times V_N) \div V_{TR}$$
$$= (6.28 \times 0.89^2 \times 34.6) \div 390$$
$$= 0.44\ cm^2$$

From the tricuspid EROA and the VTI of the TR signal, the tricuspid RV can also be calculated as:

$$RV_{TR} = EROA \times VTI_{MR}$$
$$= 0.44 \times 122$$
$$= 54\ mL$$

Anatomy of the Pulmonary Valve and Pulmonary Root

The pulmonary valve is one of four cardiac valves in the heart. With respect to surface anatomy, the pulmonary valve is the most superiorly situated cardiac valve and lies behind the second and the third intercostal cartilages (see Fig. 7.1). Internally, the pulmonary valve is located between the RVOT and the main pulmonary artery (MPA); it is in close proximity the other cardiac valves (Fig. 9.36). The primary function of the pulmonary valve is to prevent backflow of blood into the RV during ventricular diastole.

Pulmonary Valve Anatomy

The structural anatomy of the pulmonary valve is very similar to that of the aortic valve in that it consists of four principal components: (1) the annulus, (2) the cusps, (3) the commissures, and (4) the interleaflet triangles. Like the aortic valve, the pulmonary valve is a semilunar valve with three half-moon shaped cusps. The cusps of the pulmonary valve are of approximately equal size; these cusps are named based on their anatomic location and/or their relationship with the aortic cusps; therefore, the pulmonary cusps are referred to as left or left-facing, right or right-facing and anterior or non-facing (Fig. 9.36). As for the aortic valve, at the centre of each pulmonary cusp is fibrous tissue node which is also known as the node of Arantii.

The principal differences between the pulmonary and aortic valves is that unlike the aortic valve which is in fibrous continuity with the mitral valve and the IVS, the pulmonary valve is separated from the tricuspid valve by a muscular fold and the pulmonary leaflets are not directly supported by the IVS.

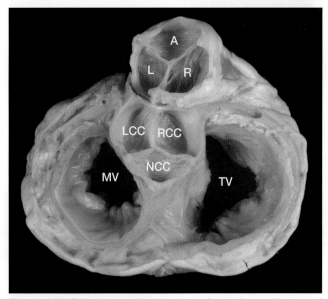

Figure 9.36 This gross pathological specimen shows the normal anatomy of the pulmonary valve; the valve is in its closed position and is viewed from above. The pulmonary valve has three cusps: (1) left-facing or left (L) which is adjacent to the left coronary cusp (LCC) of the aortic valve, (2) right facing or right (R) which is adjacent to the right coronary cusp (RCC) of the aortic valve, and (3) non-facing or anterior (A).

MV = mitral valve; NCC = non-coronary cusp; TV = tricuspid valve.

By permission of Mayo Foundation for Medical Education and Research. All rights reserved. Courtesy of William D. Edwards, MD.

Pulmonic Root Anatomy

The pulmonic root supports the pulmonary valve leaflets; it may be defined as the section of the pulmonary artery (PA) between the RVOT and the sinotubular (ST) junction of the PA. As for the aortic root, the ST junction of the PA relates to the peripheral attachment of the valve leaflets with the PA wall. The ST junction of the pulmonic root is not as pronounced as the ST junction of the aortic root.

Similar to the aortic root, there are 3 outward pouches or sinuses of the pulmonic root which are also referred to as sinuses of Valsalva. According to their relationship to the pulmonary valve leaflets, these sinuses are referred to as left or left-facing, right or right-facing, and anterior or non-facing. The MPA, which lies anterior to the aorta, bifurcates into the right and left pulmonary artery branches at approximately 4-5 cm from the RVOT. The right and left pulmonary arteries are of approximately equal size with the right pulmonary artery being slightly longer than the left.

Echo Imaging of the Pulmonary Valve

There are a number of transthoracic views that can be utilised to image the pulmonary valve; these views include the parasternal long axis of the RVOT, the parasternal short axis at the aortic valve or PA bifurcation levels, modified apical and subcostal 5-chamber views, and the subcostal short axis view (Fig. 9.37). As for the tricuspid valve, only two of the three leaflets of the pulmonary valve are usually seen from any one imaging view. Due to variations in the orientation of the pulmonary valve between individuals, it is difficult to accurately identify each pulmonary cusp. However, most commonly the two pulmonary cusps usually seen are the right

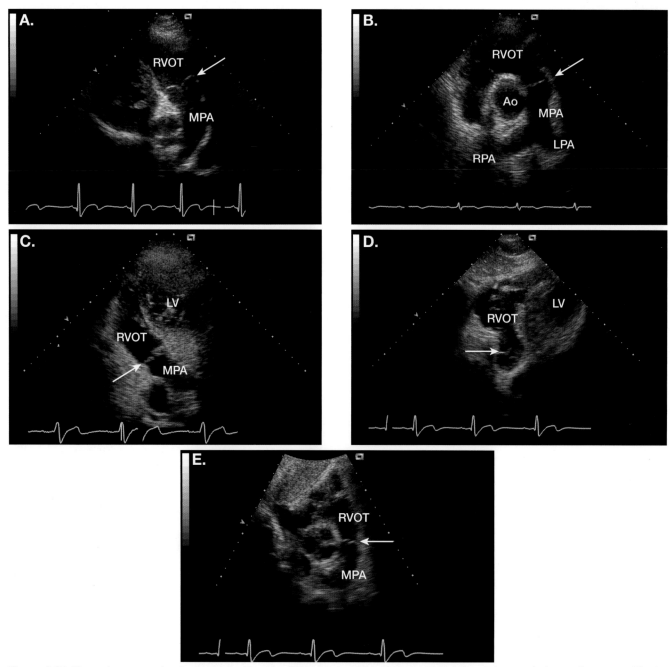

Figure 9.37 The pulmonary valve (*arrows*) can be seen from the parasternal long axis of the right ventricular outflow tract (**A**), the parasternal short axis at the pulmonary artery bifurcation level (**B**), a modified apical 5-chamber view with anterior tilt (**C**), a modified subcostal 5-chamber view with anterior tilt (**D**), and the subcostal short axis view (**E**). Ao = aorta; LPA = left pulmonary artery; LV = left ventricle; MPA = main pulmonary artery; RPA = right pulmonary artery; RVOT = right ventricular outflow tract.

and anterior cusps, with the right cusp being closest to the aorta. Infrequently, all three pulmonary valve leaflets may be seen from a parasternal short axis view (Fig. 9.38). In this situation, the three pulmonary cusps can be identified based on their relationship to the aortic valve cusps.

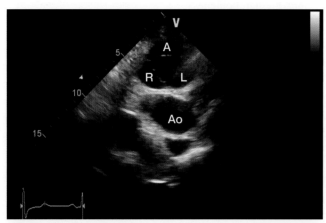

Figure 9.38 In this parasternal short axis image all three pulmonary valve leaflets can be seen. Identification of each pulmonary cusp is based on its anatomical relationship with the aortic cusps. A = anterior or non-facing cusp; Ao = aorta; L =left or left-facing cusp; R = right or right-facing cusp.

Pulmonary Stenosis

Aetiology of Pulmonary Stenosis

Pulmonary stenosis (PS) refers to the obstruction of blood flow from the RV, across the pulmonary valve, into the PA. By far, the most common cause of PS is congenital; acquired causes of PS are much less common.

Congenital Pulmonary Stenosis

Congenital causes of RVOT obstruction may occur at the valve level (valvular PS), below the pulmonary valve (subvalvular PS or infundibular stenosis), above the pulmonary valve (supravalvular PS), at the main pulmonary artery branches (branch stenosis) and/or in the peripheral pulmonary arteries (Fig. 9.39).

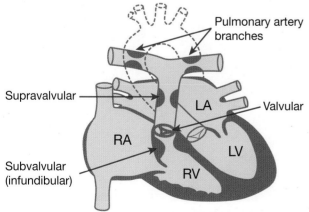

Figure 9.39 Sites for congenital right ventricular outflow tract obstruction may occur at multiple levels including: below the pulmonary valve (subpulmonary or infundibular stenosis), at the pulmonary valve (valvular stenosis), above the pulmonary valve (supravalvular stenosis) or within the main pulmonary artery branches (branch stenosis).
LA = left atrium; LV = left ventricle; RA = right atrium; RV = right ventricle.

Valvular PS

Three morphological types of congenital PS have been described: (1) the typical dome-shaped pulmonary valve, (2) the dysplastic pulmonary valve, and (3) the unicuspid or bicuspid pulmonary valve (Fig. 9.40).

The typical dome-shaped pulmonary valve is characterized by preserved valve mobility with a narrowed central opening caused by the presence of two to four rudimentary raphes; this is the most common type of congenital PS.

In the dysplastic pulmonary valve, the valve is trileaflet with severely thickened and deformed leaflets and, therefore, valve mobility is poor; this type of congenital PS is frequently associated with Noonan syndrome.

Unicuspid and bicuspid pulmonary valves form when there is fusion between the commissures of the pulmonary leaflets; unicuspid valves may be acommissural (central orifice and no apparent commissural attachment to the pulmonic root) or unicommissural (eccentric orifice with one commissural attachment to the pulmonic root). Bicuspid pulmonary valves are frequently found in patients with tetralogy of Fallot.

Subvalvular PS

Subvalvular PS is also often associated with tetralogy of Fallot (see Chapter 15) or it may be associated with other complex congenital heart lesions such as a double-chambered RV.

> A double-chambered right ventricle (DCRV) is characterised by the presence of aberrant hypertrophied muscle bundles that essentially divide or septate the RV cavity into a proximal high-pressure and a distal low-pressure chamber. This anomaly is frequently associated with other lesions such as a ventricular septal defect, pulmonary valve stenosis, and discrete subaortic stenosis.

Supravalvular PS

Supravalvular PS can occur as an isolated lesion or it may occur in association with tetralogy of Fallot or other syndromes such as Noonan's, William's or congenital rubella syndrome. Supravalvular PS may also occur secondary to residual scarring of the MPA following the removal of a PA band.

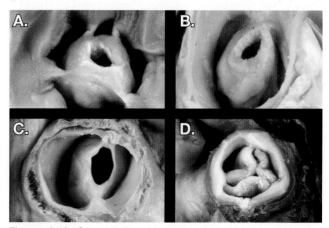

Figure 9.40 Congenitally abnormal pulmonary valves causing pulmonary stenosis include: unicuspid, acommissural valves (**A**), unicuspid, unicommissural valves (**B**), bicuspid valves (**C**), and dysplastic valves (**D**). See text for details.
By permission of Mayo Foundation for Medical Education and Research. All rights reserved. Courtesy of William D. Edwards, MD.

Pulmonary Artery Banding

Pulmonary artery banding (PAB) is a palliative procedure that is typically performed in patients with large left-to-right shunts. The PAB effectively reduces blood flow to the lungs to prevent the development of irreversible pulmonary hypertension. PAB is typically performed as part of a staged approach to a more definitive surgical repair of the shunt lesion. PAB may also be used in patients with more complex congenital heart lesions; for example, in cases where the left ventricle (LV) is the pulmonic ventricle and for when later anatomical corrective surgery is planned. In these patients, as the LV is the pulmonic ventricle it pumps at low pressures; so in order to prepare the LV to pump at systemic pressures, a PAB is applied to create pulmonary stenosis thereby subjecting the LV to higher pressures.

Branch Pulmonary Artery Stenosis

Branch PA stenosis may occur as a single lesion, at multiple sites, or diffusely throughout the PA tree. As for supravalvular PS, branch PA stenosis is often associated with other syndromes such as Noonan's, William's or congenital rubella syndrome. Branch PA stenosis may also coexist with valvular PS.

Acquired Pulmonary Stenosis

Acquired causes of PS are much less common than congenital causes. Rare, acquired causes of PS include rheumatic valve disease and carcinoid heart disease. Other lesions that can cause RVOT obstruction include extraneous tricuspid valve tissue, aneurysms of the aortic sinuses of Valsalva, aneurysms of the membranous IVS, hypertrophic cardiomyopathy, or mass lesions such as tumours, thrombus or vegetations. Acquired causes of supravalvular obstruction include mass lesions such as tumours, or narrowing at the anastomosis site following surgical procedures such as the Ross procedure or the arterial switch operation for complete transposition of the great arteries (see Chapters 10 and 15, respectively).

Pathophysiology of Pulmonary Stenosis

Pulmonary stenosis effectively obstructs RV emptying during ventricular systole. As a result and in an attempt to maintain flow across the stenotic valve, there is an increase in the RV pressure. Over time, a chronic increase in RV pressures leads to the development of RV hypertrophy (RVH) (Fig. 9.41). Furthermore, as the RV becomes less compliant the RV end-diastolic pressure (RVEDP) increases and the RV dilates in an attempt to maintain a normal cardiac output (see the Frank-Starling mechanism in Chapter 2). Increased end-systolic wall stress due to the increased afterload placed on the RV ultimately results in a reduction in the RV stroke volume and contractility (see Laplace's law in Chapter 2). This leads to the development of RV failure.

Clinical Manifestations of Pulmonary Stenosis

The clinical manifestations of PS relate to the severity of the obstruction. For example, patients with isolated mild to moderate PS may be asymptomatic while patients with severe PS may present with exertional fatigue, dyspnoea with exertion, or chest discomfort secondary to angina caused by marked RVH.

Role of Echocardiography in Pulmonary Stenosis

The aims and objectives of echocardiography in the assessment of PS are to:
• Determine the site of obstruction (e.g. valvular, subvalvular, supravalvular, branches),
• Assess valve morphology,
• Assess RV size and systolic function,
• Estimate the severity of the stenosis,
• Measure the pulmonary annulus (for pulmonary balloon valvuloplasty),
• Estimate pulmonary artery systolic pressures.

Site of Obstruction and Valve Morphology

As stated above, congenital RVOT obstruction may occur at multiple levels with the most common site of obstruction occurring at the valve level. The characteristic feature of valvular PS is systolic doming of the pulmonary valve leaflets; this systolic doming is best seen from the parasternal long axis view of the RVOT or from the parasternal short axis view of the RVOT (Fig. 9.42). Post stenotic dilatation of the MPA is commonly seen in cases of severe valvular PS.

Bicuspid or unicuspid pulmonary valves can only be diagnosed via 2D echocardiography when the valve is seen in its short axis. For example, in patients with transposition of the great arteries the PA is located in the aortic position (posterior displacement) so in the parasternal short axis view the pulmonary valve is seen in its short axis (Fig. 9.43). It is also feasible to determine the pulmonary valve morphology using 3D echocardiography with images acquired from either the parasternal long or short axis views [9.1].

Supravalvular PS may be identified by the appearance of narrowing above the pulmonary valve or on the PA side of the valve (Fig. 9.44); while subvalvular PS can be identified as thickening or narrowing below the pulmonary valve or on the RVOT side of the valve (Fig. 9.45). The use of colour flow Doppler imaging is also very useful in confirming the level of obstruction.

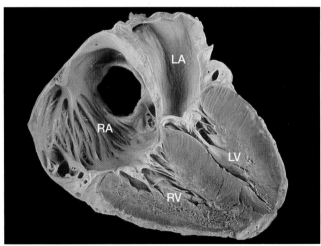

Figure 9.41 This gross pathological specimen is from a patient with chronic, severe pulmonary stenosis. Observe the marked dilatation of the right atrium (RA) and right ventricle (RV) as well as marked right ventricular hypertrophy. LA = left atrium; LV = left ventricle.
By permission of Mayo Foundation for Medical Education and Research. All rights reserved. Courtesy of William D. Edwards, MD.

[9.1] Kelly NF, Platts DG, Burstow DJ. Feasibility of pulmonary valve imaging using three-dimensional transthoracic echocardiography. *J Am Soc Echocardiogr.* 2010 Oct;23(10):1076-80.

Figure 9.42 These systolic still frame images were recorded from a patient with critical pulmonary stenosis. Observe that there is systolic doming of the pulmonary leaflets (*arrows*) on the unzoomed and zoomed 2D images recorded from the parasternal long axis view of the right ventricular outflow tract (*top images*). The colour Doppler image shows a narrow jet of blood being ejected through the 'pin-hole' pulmonary valve orifice (*bottom, left*). The peak velocity across the pulmonary valve recorded via continuous-wave Doppler was 6.2 m/s, yielding a pressure gradient of 155 mm Hg (*bottom, right*). MPA = main pulmonary artery; RVOT = right ventricular outflow tract.

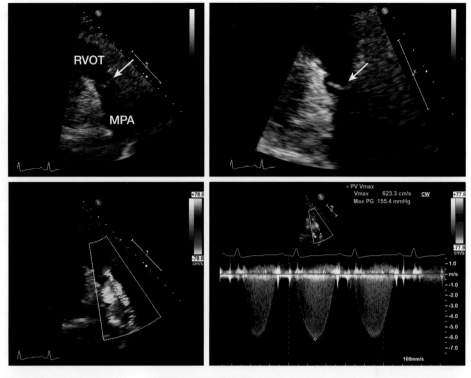

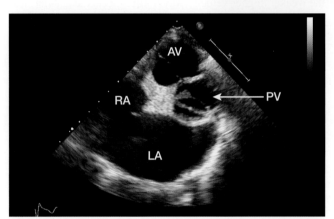

Figure 9.43 This image was recorded from a patient with complex congenital heart disease which included transposition of the great arteries. Because the aorta and pulmonary artery are transposed, from the parasternal short axis view the pulmonary valve can be seen in its short axis. Observe that the pulmonary valve (PV) is bicuspid. AV = aortic valve; LA = left atrium; RA = right atrium.

Stenosis of the aortic, mitral and tricuspid valves is easily recognised as the stenotic valves appear obviously thickened and calcified. However, in the congenitally dome-shaped, stenotic pulmonary valve the leaflet mobility is often preserved and the leaflets do not appear overly thickened; calcification is also uncommon. Therefore, pulmonary stenosis (PS) can easily be missed if 2D imaging only is used to assess the pulmonary valve.

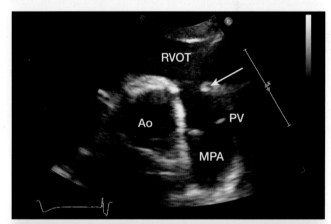

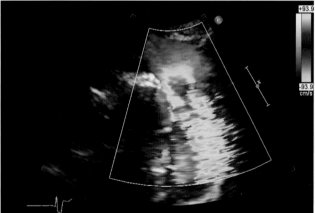

Figure 9.44 These images were recorded from a zoomed parasternal short axis view in a patient with a variant of tetralogy of Fallot. Observe the subvalvular muscular ridge below the pulmonary valve (PV) (*arrow*); systolic doming of the pulmonary valve is also apparent which is consistent with a degree of coexistent valvular stenosis (*top*). Colour flow Doppler imaging confirms the presence of turbulent flow below the pulmonary valve at the subvalvular level (*bottom*). Ao = aorta; MPA = main pulmonary artery; RVOT = right ventricular outflow tract.

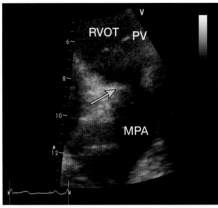 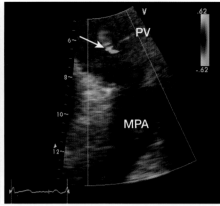 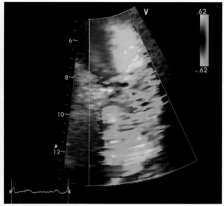

Figure 9.45 These images were recorded from a zoomed parasternal long axis view of the right ventricular outflow tract (RVOT) view. On the 2D image, supravalvular stenosis appears as a narrowing on the pulmonary arterial side of the valve (*arrow*) (*left*). Colour flow Doppler imaging serves to identify: (1) the pulmonary valve (PV) based on the origin of pulmonary regurgitation (PR) (*middle*) and (2) the level of obstruction based on the appearance of turbulent flow above the pulmonary valve (*right*).

Branch pulmonary artery (BPA) stenosis refers to obstruction at the right and/or left pulmonary artery branches. While 2D imaging may be able to identify narrowing of right and/or left pulmonary artery branches, BPA stenosis is best identified using colour flow Doppler imaging (Fig. 9.46, top). In particular, when assessing the PA via CFI it is important to ensure that the colour box length is adjusted to cover the PA bifurcation; BPA stenosis can easily be missed if the colour box does not cover the right and left pulmonary artery branches.

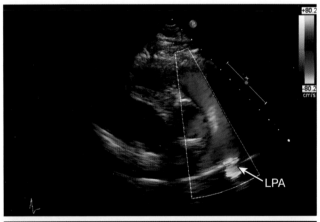

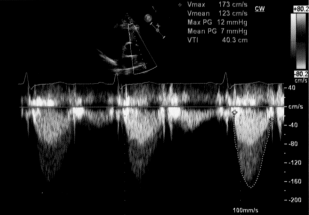

Figure 9.46 These images were recorded from a patient with branch pulmonary artery stenosis. The colour flow Doppler image recorded from the parasternal short axis view shows obvious turbulence at the origin of the left pulmonary artery (LPA) (*top*). The continuous-wave Doppler signal displays a 'layered' effect: the stronger, lower velocity waveform reflects blood flow across the pulmonary valve while the weaker, higher velocity waveform reflects the smaller flow stream across the branch stenosis (*bottom*). The peak velocity at the origin of the LPA was 1.73 m/s, yielding a peak pressure gradient of 12 mm Hg.

Another clue to the presence of BPA stenosis is based on the appearance of the CW Doppler signal recorded across the pulmonary valve; in the presence of BPA stenosis the CW signal has a 'layered' appearance consisting of two distinctly different waveforms of different velocities: the stronger, lower velocity waveform reflects blood flow across the pulmonary valve while the weaker, higher velocity waveform reflects the smaller flow stream across the branch stenosis (Fig. 9.46, bottom).

As mentioned above, while uncommon, there are a number of acquired causes of valvular PS, RVOT obstruction, and supravalvular obstruction. Echocardiographic examples of carcinoid pulmonary valve disease and RVOT obstruction due to an aortic sinus of Valsalva aneurysm are displayed in Figures 14.12 and 11.11, respectively; examples of RVOT obstruction due to thrombus and supravalvular obstruction due to a tumour mass are shown in Figures 9.47 and 9.48, respectively.

Assessment of RV Size and Systolic Function

The RV size and systolic function are assessed in the usual manner (see Chapter 2 and tricuspid valve disease above). In addition, as chronic pressure overload of the RV leads to the development of RVH, measurement of the RV wall thickness may also be attempted via M-mode or 2D imaging. RV wall thickness is measured at the peak of the R wave of the ECG (Fig. 9.49; also Fig. 4.32). A normal RV free wall thickness is 2-3 mm; a thickness of greater than 5 mm is considered abnormal.

While the RV wall thickness can be measured from the parasternal and apical views, it is best measured from the subcostal views as the epicardial border is usually easier to define from these views. From the parasternal views, the RV is in very close proximity to the chest wall so reverberation artefacts in the near field may obscure the epicardial border of the anterior RV wall. In addition, the echogenicity of the chest wall and the anterior RV wall are very similar so distinction between the epicardium of the anterior RV wall and the chest wall may be difficult from the parasternal views. From the apical views, RV wall thickness is measured across the width of the ultrasound beam in the lateral imaging plane; lateral resolution is generally poorer than the axial resolution so wherever possible relatively small dimensions should always be measured in the axial imaging plane (along the length of the ultrasound beam).

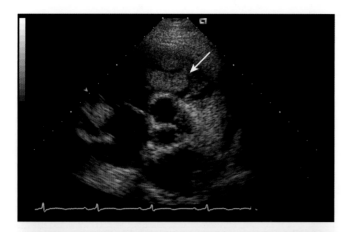

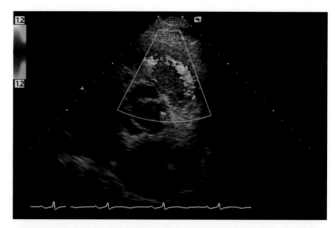

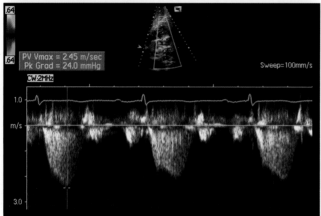

Figure 9.47 These images were recorded from the parasternal short axis view in a patient presenting with suspected acute pulmonary embolism. Observe the echogenic mass within the right ventricular outflow tract (RVOT) (*arrow*). Based on the appearance of this mass as well as the clinical presentation, this mass was most consistent with thrombus (*top left*). The systolic still frame colour flow Doppler image confirms that this thrombus is causing a degree of RVOT obstruction (*top right*); this is evident from the appearance of turbulent flow across the RVOT. Via continuous-wave Doppler the peak velocity across the RVOT was 2.45 m/s, yielding a peak pressure gradient of 24 mm Hg (*bottom left*).

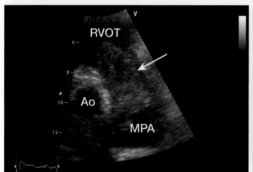

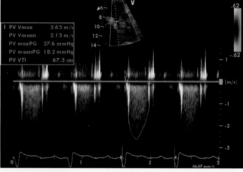

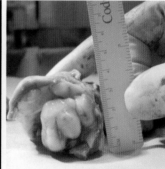

Figure 9.48 This image was recorded from a zoomed parasternal short axis view. Observe the large echogenic mass within the main pulmonary artery (MPA) (*arrow, left*); the appearance of this mass is consistent with either thrombus or a tumour. On the continuous-wave Doppler signal, the peak velocity across the MPA was 2.63 m/s, yielding a peak pressure gradient of 28 mm Hg (*middle*). This mass was surgically removed and, macroscopically the appearance of the mass was consistent with tumour (*right*). On the histological examination, the mass was diagnosed as angiosarcoma. Ao = aorta; RVOT = right ventricular outflow tract.

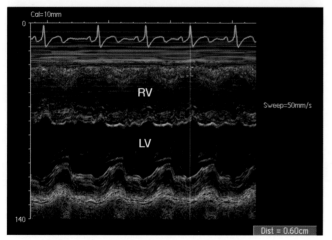

Figure 9.49 This M-mode trace was recorded from the parasternal long axis view in a patient with moderate pulmonary stenosis. The M-mode cursor is transecting the right and left ventricles. Right ventricular (RV) wall thickness is measured at the peak of the R wave of the ECG from the leading edge to the trailing edge of the anterior RV wall.
LV = left ventricle; RV = right ventricle.

Estimation of Severity

The severity of PS is assessed using the peak velocity and maximum pressure gradient across the pulmonary valve via CW Doppler (see Fig. 9.42). The criteria for defining the various grades of PS based on these values are listed in Table 9.6.

While the application of the continuity and PISA principles for the calculation of the pulmonary valve area (PVA) is theoretically feasible, these methods have not been validated for PS. In addition, the significance of the PVA for determining the various grades of severity of PS has not been described; therefore, calculation of the PVA is not useful in the assessment of PS severity.

The most common error in the estimation of pressure gradients relates to suboptimal alignment of the ultrasound beam with the PS jet. Another caveat is the presence of increased velocities and pressure gradients, secondary to increased flow across the pulmonary valve in the absence of PS. For example, increased velocities across the pulmonary valve may be encountered when there is an atrial septal defect, a ventricular septal defect or significant pulmonary regurgitation. In these cases, the transpulmonary velocities are increased secondary to an increased stroke volume across the valve; therefore, careful interrogation of the pulmonary valve leaflets and motion is required to determine if coexistent PS is also present.

Measurement of the Pulmonary Annulus

The procedure of choice for patients with severe or symptomatic congenital PS is balloon pulmonary valvuloplasty. In order to determine the optimal balloon size for successful dilatation of the valve, the size of the pulmonary annulus needs to be measured prior to the procedure. Measurement of the pulmonary annulus is best achieved from a zoomed parasternal long or short axis view of the RVOT (Fig. 9.50, top). Colour flow Doppler imaging may also be useful in delineating the lateral border of the RVOT (Fig. 9.50, bottom).

Estimation of Pulmonary Artery Systolic Pressure

In the absence of PS or RVOT obstruction, it is assumed that the RVSP is the same as the pulmonary artery systolic pressure (PASP). However, when there is RVOT obstruction or PS, the RVSP will be greater than the PASP as flow always travels from a higher pressure to a lower pressure area.

In particular, the RVSP will be equal to the sum of the PASP and the pressure gradient across the pulmonary valve (Fig. 9.51):

Equation 9.5

$$RVSP = PASP + \Delta P_{RV\text{-}PA}$$

where RVSP = right ventricular systolic pressure (mm Hg)
 PASP = pulmonary artery systolic pressure (mm Hg)
 $\Delta P_{RV\text{-}PA}$ = systolic pressure gradient between the RV and PA (mm Hg)

Therefore, by rearranging the above equation, the PASP can be derived:

Equation 9.6

$$PASP = RVSP - \Delta P_{RV\text{-}PA}$$

where PASP = pulmonary artery systolic pressure (mm Hg)
 RVSP = right ventricular systolic pressure (mm Hg)
 $\Delta P_{RV\text{-}PA}$ = systolic pressure gradient between the RV and PA (mm Hg)

Significant PS can be virtually excluded by the presence of a normal RVSP. When there is significant PS, the RVSP must be elevated as a higher RVSP is required to open the stenotic pulmonary valve. As such, the RVSP cannot be normal in patients with significant PS.

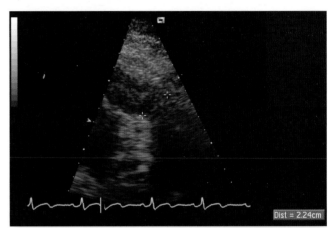

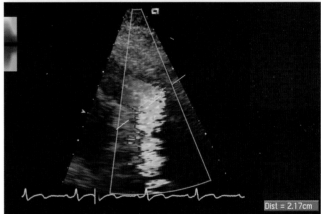

Figure 9.50 This zoomed view of the right ventricular outflow tract was recorded from the parasternal short axis view. The pulmonary annulus is measured during systole using the inner edge to inner edge technique (*top*). Using colour Doppler imaging, the borders of the pulmonary annulus may be enhanced to facilitate the measurement of the annulus (*bottom*).

Table 9.6 Recommendations for Classification of Pulmonary Stenosis Severity

	Mild PS	Moderate PS	Severe PS
Peak velocity (m/s)	< 3	3 – 4	> 4.0
Maximum Gradient (mm Hg)	< 36	36 - 64	> 64

Source: Baumgartner H, Hung J, Bermejo J, Chambers JB, Evangelista A, Griffin BP, Iung B, Otto CM, Pellikka PA, Quinones M; American Society of Echocardiography; European Association of Echocardiography. Echocardiographic assessment of valve stenosis: EAE/ASE recommendations for clinical practice. *J Am Soc Echocardiogr*, Vol. 22(1), page 20, © 2009 with permission from Elsevier.

As illustrated in Figure 9.51, the RVSP and the PASP do not peak at the same point in time and for this reason, the systolic pressure gradient between the RV and PA (ΔP_{RV-PA}) is referred to as the peak-to-peak pressure gradient. Therefore, the PASP is equal to the difference between the RVSP and the peak-to-peak pressure gradient across the pulmonary valve. Importantly, the peak-to-peak pressure gradient is different to the Doppler-derived pressure gradient which measures the maximum instantaneous pressure gradient between the RV and the PA at the same instant in the cardiac cycle. So in order to estimate the PASP via Doppler, the Doppler gradient that best correlates with the peak-to-peak pressure gradient is required; in most instances, this has been shown to be the mean pressure gradient [9.4]. Therefore, the PASP via Doppler can be estimated as:

Equation 9.7

$$PASP = RVSP - mPG_{PV}$$

where PASP = pulmonary artery systolic pressure (mm Hg)
     RVSP = right ventricular systolic pressure (mm Hg)
     mPG_{PV} = mean pressure gradient across the pulmonary valve (mm Hg)

However, in patients with very severe or critical PS, the Doppler maximum instantaneous pressure gradient and the peak-to-peak pressure gradient correlate extremely well. This is because in critical PS the pulmonary pressure waveform becomes quite 'flat', therefore the maximum instantaneous Doppler gradient and the peak-to-peak pressure gradient are very similar (Fig. 9.52). Therefore, in patients with critical PS, the PASP is estimated as the difference between the RVSP and the maximum instantaneous Doppler gradient across the valve:

Equation 9.8

$$PASP_C = RVSP - MIPG_{PV}$$

where $PASP_C$ = pulmonary artery systolic pressure in critical pulmonary stenosis (mm Hg)
     RVSP = right ventricular systolic pressure (mm Hg)
     $MIPG_{PV}$ = maximum instantaneous pressure gradient across the pulmonary valve (mm Hg)

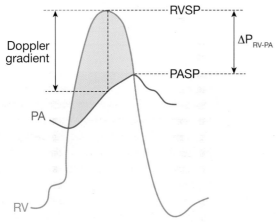

Figure 9.51 This schematic illustrates the right ventricular (RV) and pulmonary artery (PA) pressure traces in pulmonary stenosis. The pressure difference between the right ventricular systolic pressure (RVSP) and the pulmonary artery systolic pressure (PASP) is equivalent to the systolic pressure gradient between the RV and PA (ΔP_{RV-PA}). Observe that the RVSP peaks before the PASP; for this reason, the pressure gradient between the RV and PA is also referred to as the peak-to-peak pressure gradient.

Critical PS can be identified based on the shape of the Doppler profile (Fig. 9.53). In critical PS, the Doppler profile across the pulmonary valve appears rounded with the peak velocity occurring in mid systole.

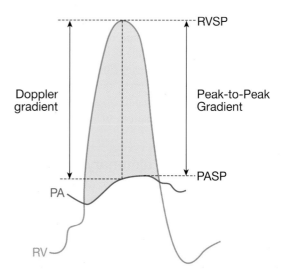

Figure 9.52 This schematic illustrates the right ventricular (RV) and pulmonary artery (PA) pressure traces in critical pulmonary stenosis. Observe that the Doppler-derived pressure gradient and the invasively-derived peak-to-peak pressure gradient are very similar due to damping and 'flattening' of the PA pressure trace.

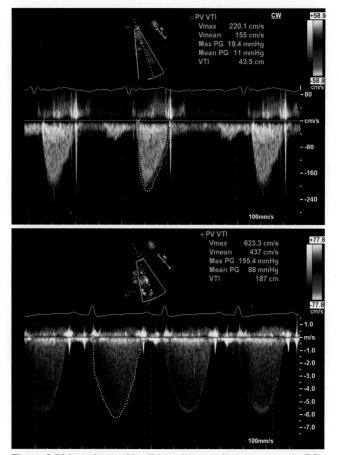

Figure 9.53 In patients with mild-moderate pulmonary stenosis (PS), the PS jet is V-shaped and the velocity peaks in early systole (*top*). In patients with critical PS, the PS jet appears rounded and the velocity peaks in mid systole (*bottom*); this occurs due to 'flattening' of the pulmonary pressure waveform as shown in Figure 9.52.

[9.4] Silvilairat S, Cabalka AK, Cetta F, Hagler DJ, O'Leary PW. Echocardiographic assessment of isolated pulmonary valve stenosis: which outpatient Doppler gradient has the most clinical validity? *J Am Soc Echocardiogr.* 2005 Nov;18(11):1137-42.

Pulmonary Regurgitation

Aetiology of Pulmonary Regurgitation

Pulmonary regurgitation (PR) refers to the backward flow of blood from the PA to the RV during diastole. As for TR, the aetiology of PR is described in terms of functional or organic regurgitation (Table 9.7). Organic or primary regurgitation refers to diseases that involve the leaflets; that is, PR occurs due to intrinsic valvular disease. Functional or secondary regurgitation refers to diseases that alter the annular geometry; therefore, PR occurs due to annular dilatation and subsequent poor leaflet coaptation of an otherwise normal pulmonary valve.

Pathophysiology of Pulmonary Regurgitation

As PR is characterised by the backflow of blood from the PA into the RV during diastole, this leads to RV, and eventually, RA dilatation. Secondary dilatation of the tricuspid annulus may also occur resulting in TR. Diastolic volume overload of the RV due to chronic, severe PR can also lead to an elevation in the RVEDP; in some cases, this may actually result in the equalisation of the PA and the RV pressures in diastole.

Clinical Manifestations of Pulmonary Regurgitation

The clinical manifestations of PR relate to the subsequent development of right-sided CHF. These manifestations include dyspnoea, peripheral oedema, and easy fatigability.

Role of Echocardiography in Pulmonary Regurgitation

The aims and objectives of echocardiography in the assessment of PR are to:
• Determine the aetiology of PR,
• Assess RV size and function,
• Estimate severity of regurgitation,
• Estimate PA pressures.

> 'Physiological' or a mild degree of PR is frequently encountered in the normal population with the incidence, but not the severity, of PR increasing with advancing age.

Aetiology of Pulmonary Regurgitation

Pulmonary regurgitation can result from intrinsic abnormalities of the pulmonary valve (organic PR) or more commonly secondary to annular dilatation (functional PR) (see Table 9.7). Echocardiographic examples of PR causes are illustrated in Figures 9.54-9.55; an example of carcinoid pulmonary valve disease can be seen in Figure 14.12.

Assessment of RV Size and Systolic Function

As stated above, chronic RV volume overload secondary to chronic significant PR leads to progressive RV dilatation. Therefore, measurements of the RV size, performed from an RV-focused apical 4-chamber view at end-diastole, are important in the serial evaluation of patients with significant PR. Assessment of RV systolic function is also important in the echocardiographic examination of patients with PR. The methods for assessing RV size and systolic function are described in detail in Chapter 2.

Importantly, as stated for TR, abnormal or paradoxical IVS motion is frequently seen when there is RV volume overload. In particular, RV volume overload results in increased RV diastolic filling pressures and when the RV diastolic pressure approaches or exceeds LV diastolic filling pressures, the IVS motion becomes paradoxical and shifts leftwards towards the LV during diastole (see Fig. 2.40).

Estimation of Severity

An accurate assessment of the PR severity requires a comprehensive evaluation of a number of echocardiographic parameters. In particular, PR severity should be determined by looking for indirect signs of significant PR based on the colour and spectral Doppler examination.

While quantitative calculations such as the regurgitant volume and the EROA are theoretically possible, these methods are rarely used. This is mainly because the significance of these quantitative values for determining the various grades of PR severity has not been described; therefore, quantitative calculations for PR are currently not advocated and are not described in this text.

Table 9.7 **Aetiology of Pulmonary Regurgitation**

Causes of PR	Examples
Functional causes (Annular dilatation)	• Coexistent congenital heart disease with right ventricular (RV) dilatation • Pulmonary artery dilatation; e.g. idiopathic, Marfan syndrome • Pulmonary hypertension • RV cardiomyopathy • RV infarction
Organic causes (Disorders of pulmonary valve)	• Carcinoid valve disease (rare) • Congenital lesions (e.g. isolated or associated with other congenital anomalies such as repaired tetralogy of Fallot) • Iatrogenic (e.g. post pulmonary valvuloplasty) • Infective endocarditis • Rheumatic valve disease (rare) • Trauma (rare)

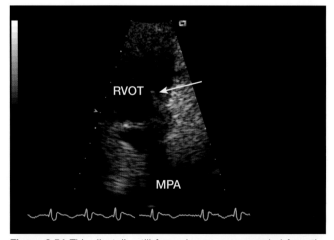

Figure 9.54 This diastolic still frame image was recorded from the parasternal long axis view of the right ventricular outflow in a patient with a previous pulmonary valvotomy for tetralogy of Fallot. A flail anterior leaflet of the pulmonary valve is evident (*arrow*).
MPA = main pulmonary artery; RVOT = right ventricular outflow tract.

Indirect Signs for Assessing PR Severity

Indirect signs for assessing PR severity include CFI and spectral Doppler variables. CFI provides a quick and easy method for identifying PR and the colour PR jet. The severity of PR can be determined from the PR jet width. CW Doppler indices that should be considered when assessing PR severity include the intensity of the PR signal, the deceleration slope of the PR signal, and the duration of the PR signal. Diastolic flow reversal into the branch pulmonary arteries provides another sign of significant PR; this sign can be appreciated via PW Doppler as well as via CFI. The criteria for defining the various grades of PR based on these methods are summarized in Table 9.8. In addition, the presence of pre-systolic forward flow across the pulmonary valve offers another clue to the presence of haemodynamically significant PR.

Colour Jet Width

The haemodynamic severity of PR can be readily evaluated based on the width of the PR jet; in particular, the wider the PR jet at its origin, the greater the severity of PR (Fig. 9.56). Similar to the colour jet height ratio used in AR, the ratio of the PR jet width to the RVOT (or pulmonary annular) diameter can also be used to semiquantitate PR severity. This ratio is measured from either the parasternal long axis or short axis views of the RVOT (Fig. 9.57). A PR jet-to-RVOT diameter ratio ≥ 50% is consistent with severe PR (Table 9.9). Although not currently listed as a method for assessing PR severity, VC-W can also be measured to assess the severity of PR. The VC-W for PR can be measured from the parasternal long or short axis views of the RVOT (Fig. 9.58).

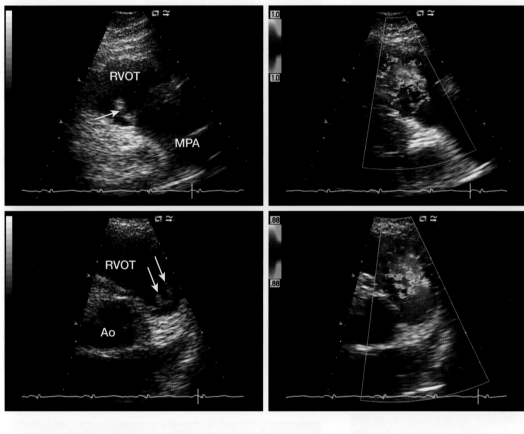

Figure 9.55 These images were acquired from the parasternal long axis and short axis views of the right ventricular outflow tract (RVOT) in a patient with clinically suspected infective endocarditis. The 2D images show multiple echo-dense masses attached to the pulmonary valve (*arrows*). On real-time imaging these masses appeared highly mobile prolapsing into the RVOT during diastole and into the main pulmonary artery (MPA) during systole. The colour flow Doppler images display severe pulmonary regurgitation. Based on the clinical presentation, the masses on the pulmonary valve were considered consistent with vegetations. Ao = aorta.

Table 9.8 Qualitative Doppler Parameters for Grading Pulmonary Regurgitation Severity

Parameter	Mild	Moderate	Severe
Jet width (mm) [1] * (CFI)	Small, usually <10 mm in length with a narrow origin	Intermediate	Large, with a wide origin; may be brief in duration
Flow reversal – BPA [2] (CFI or PW)	-	-	Diastolic flow reversal from BPA
Intensity of PR signal [1] (CW)	Faint	Dense	Dense
Deceleration of PR jet [1] † (CW)	Slow deceleration	Variable deceleration	Steep deceleration, early termination of diastolic flow

* Using a Nyquist limit of 50–60 cm/s; not valid in eccentric jets.

† Steep deceleration is not specific for severe PR

BPA = branch pulmonary arteries; CFI = colour flow imaging; CW = continuous-wave Doppler; PA = pulmonary artery; PR = pulmonary regurgitation; PW = pulsed-wave Doppler.

Sources: [1] Zoghbi WA, Enriquez-Sarano M, Foster E, Grayburn PA, Kraft CD, Levine RA, Nihoyannopoulos P, Otto CM, Quinones MA, Rakowski H, Stewart WJ, Waggoner A, Weissman NJ; American Society of Echocardiography. Recommendations for evaluation of the severity of native valvular regurgitation with two-dimensional and Doppler echocardiography. *J Am Soc Echocardiogr.* 2003 Jul;16(7):777-802. **[2]** Williams RV, Minich LL, Shaddy RE, Pagotto LT, Tani LY. Comparison of Doppler echocardiography with angiography for determining the severity of pulmonary regurgitation. *Am J Cardiol.* 2002 Jun 15;89(12):1438-41.

Limitations of CFI Indirect Signs

There are numerous technical and physiological factors that can affect the colour flow Doppler map which are unrelated to the severity of PR (refer to Table 7.8).

In particular, an important limitation of CFI in the assessment of PR occurs when there is severe and/or 'free' or 'wide-open' PR. In these patients, severe PR may be easily missed as the PR jet has a low velocity, PR flow appears laminar, and the duration of PR may be very brief. For instance, severe PR is often associated with a marked elevation in the RV diastolic pressures and when there is equalisation of the PA and the RV pressures there is no longer a driving pressure for PR so the PR jet terminates early (Fig. 9.59).

Furthermore, while measurement of the VC-W in the assessment of PR severity is possible, specific values for determining the various grades of PR severity based on this measurement have not been described. This measurement, however, might be useful in the serial evaluation of patients with PR.

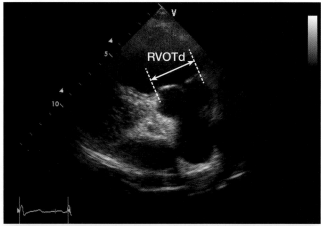

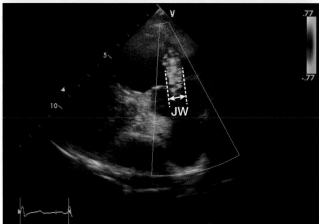

Figure 9.57 These diastolic images were recorded from a zoomed parasternal long axis view of the right ventricular outflow tract (RVOT). The RVOT diameter (RVOTd) is measured at the hinge points of the pulmonary valve leaflets (*top*). From the colour Doppler image recorded from the same view and at the same stage of diastole, the pulmonary regurgitant jet width (JW) is measured at the level of the RVOT (*bottom*). The ratio of the PR jet width to the RVOT diameter is simply calculated by dividing the PR jet width by the RVOT diameter.

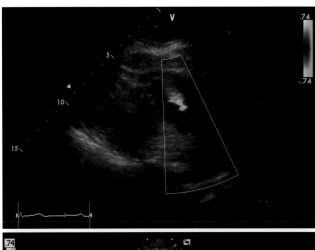

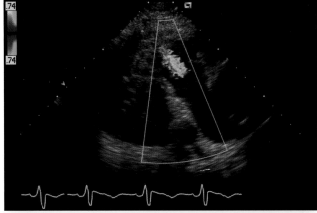

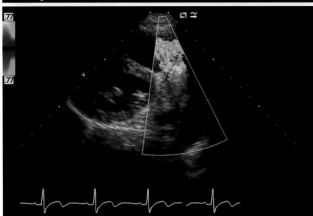

Figure 9.56 These three colour flow Doppler still frame images were recorded from three different patients with varying degrees of pulmonary regurgitation (PR): mild PR (*top*), moderate PR (*middle*) and severe PR (*bottom*). The PR severity is based on the width of the colour PR jet.

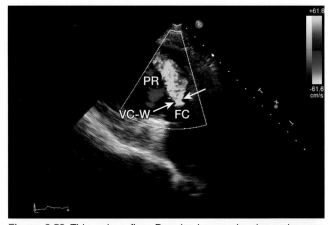

Figure 9.58 This colour flow Doppler image showing pulmonary regurgitation (PR) was recorded from the parasternal long axis of the right ventricular outflow tract. The vena contracta width (VC-W) is measured at the narrowest neck of the PR flow region at the junction of flow convergence zone (FC) and the regurgitant jet immediately below the flow convergence region.

Diastolic Flow Reversal in Pulmonary Branches

Another method for detecting severe PR is the detection of diastolic flow reversal in either the MPA or branch pulmonary arteries (Table 9.9). In particular, the presence of diastolic flow reversal in the PA branches is a very specific sign of severe PR. Diastolic flow reversal can be confirmed by CFI (Fig. 9.60);

however, diastolic flow reversal is best appreciated via PW Doppler. By PW Doppler, the presence of diastolic flow reversal in the branch pulmonary arteries is assessed from the parasternal long or short axis view with a 2-3 mm sample volume placed into the right and/or left pulmonary artery branch (Fig. 9.61).

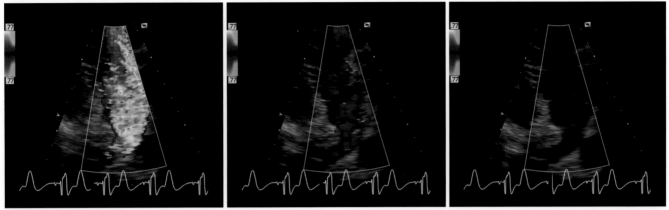

Figure 9.59 This series of colour Doppler images was recorded from a zoomed parasternal long axis view of the right ventricular outflow tract (RVOT) in a patient with 'free' or 'wide-open' pulmonary regurgitation (PR). In the early diastolic frame, severe PR is evident by the PR jet filling the RVOT (*left*). In mid diastole, the PR jet is less apparent (*middle*); this is because the pressure difference between the pulmonary artery (PA) and right ventricle (RV) has decreased due to an increase in the RV diastolic pressure. In late diastole, the PR jet is totally absent (*right*); early termination of the PR jet prior to the end of diastole occurs when there is equalisation between the PA and RV pressures.

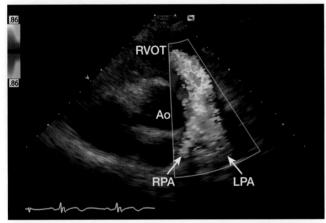

Figure 9.60 This diastolic still frame image was recorded from the parasternal short axis view. Diastolic flow reversal appears as red flow towards the transducer; this is observed within the main pulmonary artery and from the level of the right and left pulmonary artery branches. In particular, diastolic flow reversal at the pulmonary artery branches is a very sensitive and specific sign of severe PR.
Ao = aorta; LPA = left pulmonary artery; RPA = right pulmonary artery; RVOT = right ventricular outflow tract.

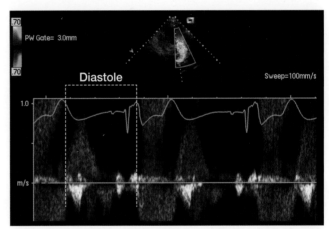

Figure 9.61 From the parasternal short axis view, a 2 mm sample volume is placed within the right pulmonary artery branch. On the spectral Doppler trace, diastolic flow reversal is identified as flow above the zero baseline during diastole. The detection of diastolic flow reversal at the pulmonary artery branches is a very sensitive and specific sign of severe PR.

Table 9.9 Sensitivity, Specificity and Predictive Valves of Doppler Echocardiographic Variables for Detecting Severe Pulmonary Regurgitation*

Parameter	Sens.	Spec.	PPV	NPV
MPA diastolic flow reversal	100%	39%	59%	100%
BPA diastolic flow reversal	87%	87%	87%	87%
PR jet/pulmonary annular diameter ratio ≥ 50%	94%	74%	76%	93%
P½t < 100 ms	90%	64%	78%	82%
PRi < 0.77	73%	47%	58%	64%

BPA = Branch pulmonary arteries; MPA = main pulmonary artery; NPV = negative predictive value; P½t = pressure half-time; PPV = positive predictive value; PR = pulmonary regurgitation; PRi = pulmonary regurgitant index; Sens. = sensitivity; Spec. = specificity.
* Severe PR defined as a PR fraction (PRF) > 40% by cardiac magnetic resonance imaging
Patient demographics: 36 patients (21 male, 15 female) with tetralogy of Fallot or pulmonary valve stenosis with prior pulmonary valvuloplasty or transannular or subannular patch repair; average age 33 ± 15 years.
Reproduced from Renella P, Aboulhosn J, Lohan DG, Jonnala P, Finn JP, Satou GM, Williams RJ, Child JS. Two-dimensional and Doppler echocardiography reliably predict severe pulmonary regurgitation as quantified by cardiac magnetic resonance. *J Am Soc Echocardiogr.* Vol. 23(8), page 884, © 2010 with permission from Elsevier.

Intensity of the PR CW Signal

In theory, the density or intensity of the spectral Doppler signal of a regurgitant jet is proportional to the number of RBCs travelling within the regurgitant jet. Therefore, the greater the regurgitation, the denser the regurgitant CW signal. For example, a weak Doppler signal is suggestive of relatively mild valvular regurgitation whereas a strong signal is suggestive of more significant regurgitation.

Deceleration of the PR Signal via CW Doppler

The PR velocity signal reflects the pressure gradient between the PA and the RV during diastole. The slope of this velocity curve, therefore, should reflect the rate of decline in the pressure gradient between the PA and the RV during diastole. The highest velocity occurs shortly after the pulmonary valve closes when the pressure gradient between PA and RV is at its maximum. The PR velocity then gradually declines throughout diastole as: (1) the PA pressure falls due to forward run-off to the lungs as well as regurgitation back into RV and

(2) the RV diastolic pressure rises due to normal tricuspid inflow into the RV as well as the pulmonary regurgitant volume back into the RV.

With mild PR, the initial early diastolic gradient between the PA and the RV is around 25 mm Hg (depending on the PA pressures). This gradient then declines slightly throughout diastole due to a gradual decline in PA diastolic pressure and a gradual rise in the RVEDP. As a result, the deceleration slope of the PR signal is quite prolonged (Fig. 9.62, left). In severe PR, the PA pressure falls rapidly due to a rapid run-off of the pulmonary regurgitant volume into the RV; at the same time, the RV diastolic pressure rapidly rises due to an increased volume into the RV. In addition, because the pressure difference between the PA and RV is relatively small, equalisation between the PA and RV pressures may occur before the end of diastole. In this instance, the deceleration slope of the PR signal appears very steep and short, and the PR signal terminates early (Fig. 9.62, right).

Therefore, when the PR signal ends prior to the end of diastole,

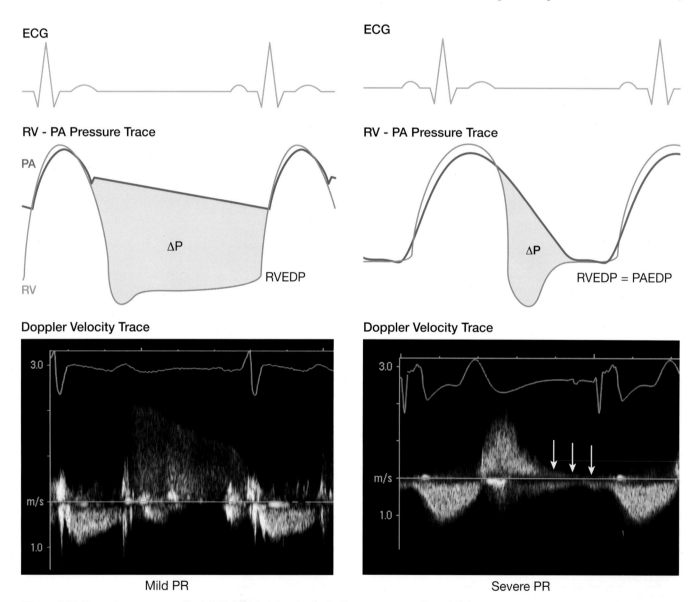

Figure 9.62 The pulmonary regurgitant (PR) Doppler signal reflects the pressure gradient (ΔP) between the pulmonary artery (PA) and right ventricle (RV) during diastole. The top schematic illustrates the pressure tracings of the PA and the RV while the Doppler velocity spectra corresponding to these schematics are displayed below. With mild PR (*left*), the ΔP between the PA and the RV in early diastole is around 25 mm Hg. This gradient then gradually decreases throughout diastole due to a gradual decline in the PA diastolic pressure and only a small increase in the RV end-diastolic pressure (RVEDP). The resultant Doppler spectrum depicts a reasonably 'flat' (prolonged) deceleration slope. With severe PR (*right*), the PA pressure drops rapidly during diastole and there is a marked increase in the RVEDP. Equalisation between the PA and RV pressures results in the early termination of the Doppler PR signal prior to the end of diastole (*triple arrows*).

this indicates equalisation between the PA and RV pressures. It can be postulated that the reason for this equalisation in diastolic pressures is due to the rapid rise in the RV diastolic pressure due to an increased volume of blood regurgitating into the RV which occurs when there is severe PR.

From the PR CW signal, the pressure half-time (P½t) and the PR index can be measured. The P½t of the PR signal, which represents the time taken for the pressure to fall to half of its initial value, is measured from the initial early diastolic PR velocity and along the deceleration slope (Fig. 9.63). A PR P½t less than 100 ms indicates the presence of severe PR (Table 9.9).

The PR index (PRi) is simply a measure of the ratio of the duration of the PR signal and the total diastolic duration (Fig. 9.64). A PRi less than 0.77 indicates severe PR (Table 9.9).

Pre-Systolic Flow across the Pulmonary Valve

The presence of forward flow across the pulmonary valve prior to the onset of systole is referred to as pre-systolic forward flow or late diastolic forward flow. The presence of this flow occurs when the RVEDP exceeds the pulmonary artery end-diastolic pressure (PAEDP).

In the setting of PR, pre-systolic forward flow provides another indicator of the presence of severe PR. The flow is best appreciated on the CW Doppler trace of the transpulmonary valve signal (Fig 9.64). It is important to note, however, that the RVEDP can also be increased secondary to poor RV compliance; for example, pre-systolic flow can be seen when there is a marked elevation in the RVEDP due to RV diastolic dysfunction. Thus, the presence of pre-systolic forward flow simply indicates that the RVEDP is elevated; in the setting of severe PR, it is assumed that the elevation in RVEDP is due to severe PR.

Limitations of Spectral Doppler Indirect Signs

The intensity of the PR signal can be affected by a number of factors. For example, Doppler gain affects the overall intensity of the regurgitant jet; if the gain is set too low then the signal intensity will also be decreased. In addition, poor alignment of the PR jet with the Doppler beam will result in a suboptimal PR signal.

The deceleration slope of the PR signal simply reflects the pressure gradient between the PA and RV over diastole. Therefore, this gradient is not only dependent on the severity of PR, it is also dependent on other factors such as RV compliance. In particular, a short PR P½t, early termination of the PR signal and pre-systolic forward flow are a result of a marked elevation in the RVEDP. The RVEDP can be elevated when there is severe PR but it can also be elevated when there is restrictive RV physiology.

Estimation of Pulmonary Artery Pressures

In the absence of PS or RVOT obstruction, it is assumed that the RVSP is the same as the pulmonary artery systolic pressure (PASP). The RVSP can be estimated as previously described. In addition, when there is PR, both the PAEDP and the mean pulmonary artery pressure (mPAP) can be estimated (Fig. 9.65).

Estimation of the PAEDP

As previously stated, the PR velocity reflects the pressure difference between the PA and the RV during diastole. Therefore, from the end-diastolic PR velocity and from an estimation of the RVEDP, it is possible to estimate the PAEDP:

Equation 9.9

$$PAEDP = 4\,V_{PR\text{-}ED}{}^2 + RVEDP$$

where PAEDP = pulmonary artery end-diastolic pressure (mm Hg)
$V_{PR\text{-}ED}$ = peak end-diastolic velocity of PR signal (m/s)
RVEDP = right ventricular end-diastolic pressure (mm Hg)

In the absence of tricuspid stenosis, it can be assumed that the RVEDP is equal to the RAP; therefore:

Equation 9.10

$$PAEDP = 4\,V_{PR\text{-}ED}{}^2 + RAP$$

where PAEDP = pulmonary artery end-diastolic pressure (mmHg)
$V_{PR\text{-}ED}$ = peak end-diastolic velocity of PR signal (m/s)
RAP = mean right atrial pressure (mmHg)

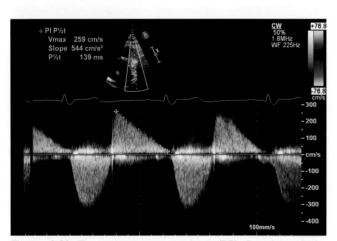

Figure 9.63 The pulmonary regurgitant (PR) Doppler velocity spectrum reflects the rate of decline in the pressure gradient between the pulmonary artery and the right ventricle during diastole. From this spectrum, the pressure half-time (P½t) is measured from the peak early diastolic PR signal along the deceleration slope. The P½t in this example is measured at 139 ms.

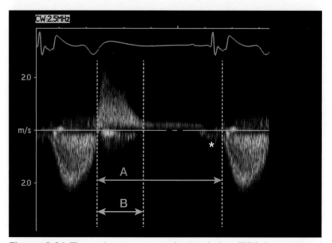

Figure 9.64 The pulmonary regurgitation index (PRi) is measured from the continuous-wave Doppler trace of the PR signal. The PR duration is measured from onset to end of the PR signal (B) and the total diastolic period is measured from end of the pulmonary forward flow signal to beginning of next forward flow signal (A). The PR index is then derived from the PR duration divided by the total diastolic period: PRi = B ÷ A. Also observe on this trace evidence of pre-systolic forward flow (*). See text for further details.

Estimation of the mPAP

Estimation of the mPAP from the PR signal is based on the assumption that the PR velocity at early diastole corresponds to the dicrotic notch on the PA pressure trace. The dicrotic notch, which reflects the closure of the pulmonary valve and the end of RV ejection, has been shown to be of a similar magnitude to mPAP [9.5]. Therefore, as the dicrotic notch reflects mPAP and as the peak PR pressure gradient corresponds to the pressure at the dicrotic notch (see Fig. 4.26), the mPAP can be estimated from the peak early diastolic PR velocity. Furthermore, adding the RAP to this derived pressure improves the correlation between the actual mPAP and the Doppler-estimated mPAP [9.6]:

Equation 9.11

$$mPAP = 4\,V_{PR\text{-}peak}{}^2 + RAP$$

where mPAP = mean pulmonary artery pressure (mm Hg)
$V_{PR\text{-}peak}$ = peak early diastolic PR velocity (m/s)
RAP = right atrial pressure (mm Hg)

Note that it is quite common to see a 'notch' or an 'a-dip' on the PR CW Doppler trace occurring just after the P wave of the ECG (arrows on opposite trace). This is seen in instances where the PA pressures are normal. Therefore, the diastolic pressure gradient between the PA and RV is quite small so following atrial contraction there is a transient drop in the PA-to-RV pressure gradient; that is, with atrial contraction there is a slight *increase* in the RV diastolic pressure which *decreases* the PA-to-RV pressure gradient. This is a normal finding and should not be confused with abnormal flow.

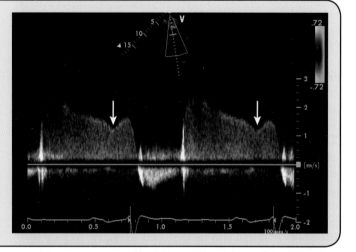

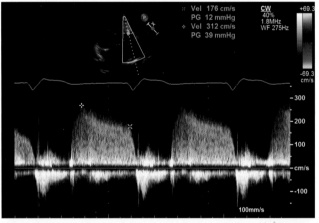

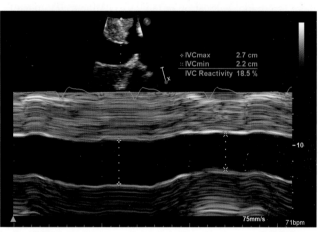

Figure 9.65 From the continuous-wave Doppler signal of pulmonary regurgitation (PR), the pulmonary artery end-diastole pressure (PAEDP) and the mean pulmonary artery pressures (mPAP) can be estimated (*left*). The PAEDP is derived from the peak end-diastolic PR velocity and the right atrial pressure (RAP) and the mPAP is derived from the peak early diastolic velocity and the RAP. In this case, the RAP is assumed to be 15 mm Hg as the IVC is dilated at 2.7 cm and only collapses 19% with inspiration (*right*).

$PAEDP = 4\,V_{PR\text{-}ED}{}^2 + RAP$
$\quad = 4\,(1.76)^2 + 15$
$\quad = 12 + 15$
$\quad = 27\ mm\ Hg$

$mPAP = 4\,V_{PR\text{-}peak}{}^2 + RAP$
$\quad = 4\,(3.12)^2 + 15$
$\quad = 39 + 15$
$\quad = 54\ mm\ Hg$

[9.5] Chemla D, Hébert JL, Coirault C, Salmeron S, Zamani K, Lecarpentier Y. Matching dicrotic notch and mean pulmonary artery pressures: implications for effective arterial elastance. *Am J Physiol.* 1996 Oct;271(4 Pt 2):H1287-95.

[9.6] Abbas AE, Fortuin FD, Schiller NB, Appleton CP, Moreno CA, Lester SJ. Echocardiographic determination of mean pulmonary artery pressure. *Am J Cardiol.* 2003 Dec 1;92(11):1373-6.

Key Points

Anatomy of the Tricuspid Valve Complex
- Tricuspid valve "complex" is composed of several components (valve annulus, valve leaflets, commissures, tendinous cords, and papillary muscles and RV myocardium).
- Three tricuspid valve leaflets are anterior, septal and posterior.
- Tendinous cords attach the leaflets with papillary muscles, RV myocardium or IVS (characteristic feature of the tricuspid valve is the presence of multiple cordal attachments from the septal leaflet to the IVS).
- Papillary muscles are variable; usually there are three distinct groups: anterior, posterior and septal.

Echo Imaging of the Tricuspid Valve
- Usually only two of the three tricuspid leaflets are seen from any one imaging plane:
  - Parasternal long axis of the RV inflow: posterior and anterior leaflets most commonly seen,
  - Parasternal short axis view: anterior and septal leaflets most commonly seen,
  - Apical 4-chamber view: septal and anterior leaflets,
  - Subcostal views: leaflets correspond to the leaflets seen from the apical 4-chamber and parasternal short axis views.

Tricuspid Stenosis: Basic Concepts
- *Aetiology*: the most common cause is rheumatic valve disease.
- *Pathophysiology*: TS results in increased RA pressures and RA dilatation; increased RA pressure hampers venous return into the RA leading to systemic venous congestion, jugular venous distension, ascites, and peripheral oedema.
- *Clinical manifestations:* relate to chronicity and severity of TS; includes fatigue, abdominal discomfort and swelling, and dyspnoea.

Role of Echo in Tricuspid Stenosis
- Determine the aetiology of the lesion,
- Assess RA size,
- Assess RV size and systolic function,
- Estimate the severity of the stenosis (via mean pressure gradient +/- TVA),
- Estimate RVSP,
- Identify associated valve lesions.

Tricuspid Regurgitation: Basic Concepts
- *Aetiology*: functional causes (2^0 to annular dilatation) and organic causes (disorders of tricuspid complex).
- *Pathophysiology*: Chronic severe TR leads to RA and RV dilatation, elevated RA and venous pressures, and elevated RVEDP.
- *Clinical manifestations*: relate to a chronic elevation in RA and venous pressures and right-sided CHF; include dyspnoea, orthopnoea, peripheral oedema, ascites, weight loss and cachexia, cyanosis, jaundice, and systolic pulsations of an enlarged, tender liver.

Role of Echo in Tricuspid Regurgitation
- Determine the aetiology of the lesion,
- Assess RA size,
- Assess RV size and systolic function,
- Estimate the severity of the regurgitation via:
  - Indirect signs by CFI (e.g. jet area, VC-W, flow convergence radius),
  - Indirect signs by spectral Doppler (e.g. inflow velocities, systolic reversal into hepatic veins, intensity and shape of TR jet),
  - Possible quantification of RV and EROA via PISA,
  - Estimate RVSP.

Anatomy of the Pulmonary Valve
- Pulmonary valve consists of three almost equal-sized, semilunar leaflets named based on their anatomic location and/or their relationship with the aortic cusps: right or right-facing, left or left-facing, and anterior or non-facing.
- Pulmonary valve is separated from tricuspid valve by a muscular fold, leaflets are not directly supported by the IVS.
- Pulmonic root is similar to the aortic root and includes 3 sinuses of Valsalva.
- MPA is anterior to the aorta and bifurcates at approximately 4-5 cm from the RVOT into right and left branches.

Echo Imaging of the Pulmonary Valve
- Pulmonary valve can be imaged from the parasternal long axis of the RVOT, the parasternal short axis, modified apical and subcostal 5-chamber views, and the subcostal short axis.
- Usually only two of the three pulmonary leaflets are seen from any one imaging plane: most commonly the right and anterior cusps are seen (the right cusp being closest to the aorta).

Pulmonary Stenosis: Basic Concepts
- *Aetiology*: most common cause is congenital valvular PS; RVOT obstruction may also occur below valve (subvalvular or infundibular), above valve (supravalvular), at the PA branches and/or in the peripheral pulmonary arteries.
- *Pathophysiology*: chronic elevation in RV pressures results in RVH; as RV becomes less compliant RVEDP increases and the RV dilates; increased end-systolic wall stress results in a reduction in the RV stroke volume and contractility.
- *Clinical manifestations*: asymptomatic (mild-moderate PS); exertional fatigue, dyspnoea with exertion, or chest discomfort secondary to angina caused by marked RVH (severe PS).

Key Points (continued)

Role of Echo in Pulmonary Stenosis
- Determine the site of obstruction,
- Assess valve morphology,
- Assess RV size and systolic and diastolic function,
- Estimate the severity of the stenosis (maximum pressure gradient),
- Measure the pulmonary annulus (for pulmonary balloon valvuloplasty),
- Estimate pulmonary artery systolic pressures (PASP = RVSP – MIPG or mPG depending on severity of PS).

Pulmonary Regurgitation: Basic Concepts
- *Aetiology*: classified according to functional causes (secondary to annular dilatation) and organic causes (disorders of pulmonary valve).
- *Pathophysiology*: chronic severe PR leads to RV and RA dilatation and an elevation in RVEDP.
- *Clinical manifestations:* relate to right-sided CHF; includes dyspnoea, peripheral oedema, and easy fatigability.

Role of Echo in Pulmonary Regurgitation
- Determine the aetiology of PR,
- Assess RV size and systolic function,
- Estimate the severity of the regurgitation via:
  - Indirect signs by CFI (e.g. jet width, VC-W),
  - Indirect signs by spectral Doppler (e.g. intensity of PR jet, deceleration of PR jet, early termination of PR signal, diastolic flow reversal in PA branches),
- Quantification not advocated due to lack of validated data.

Further Reading (listed in alphabetical order)

Tricuspid Valve Disease

Attenhofer Jost CH, Connolly HM, Dearani JA, Edwards WD, Danielson GK. Ebstein's anomaly. *Circulation.* 2007 Jan 16;115(2):277-85

Baumgartner H, Hung J, Bermejo J, Chambers JB, Evangelista A, Griffin BP, Iung B, Otto CM, Pellikka PA, Quiñones M; American Society of Echocardiography; European Association of Echocardiography. Echocardiographic assessment of valve stenosis: EAE/ASE recommendations for clinical practice. *J Am Soc Echocardiogr.* 2009 Jan;22(1):1-23

Celermajer DS, Cullen S, Sullivan ID, Spiegelhalter DJ, Wyse RK, Deanfield JE. Outcome in neonates with Ebstein's anomaly. *J Am Coll Cardiol.* 1992 Apr;19(5):1041-6.

Lancellotti P, Tribouilloy C, Hagendorff A, Moura L, Popescu BA, Agricola E, Monin JL, Pierard LA, Badano L, Zamorano JL; European Association of Echocardiography. European Association of Echocardiography recommendations for the assessment of valvular regurgitation. Part 2: mitral and tricuspid regurgitation (native valve disease). *Eur J Echocardiogr.* 2010 May;11(4):307-332.

Martinez RM, O'Leary PW, Anderson RH. Anatomy and echocardiography of the normal and abnormal tricuspid valve. *Cardiol Young.* 2006 Sep;16 Suppl 3:4-11.

Rogers JH, Bolling SF. The tricuspid valve: current perspective and evolving management of tricuspid regurgitation. *Circulation.* 2009 May 26;119(20):2718-25.

Shah PM. Tricuspid and pulmonary valve disease evaluation and management. *Rev Esp Cardiol.* 2010 Nov;63(11):1349-65.

Silver MD, Lam JH, Ranganathan N, Wigle ED. Morphology of the human tricuspid valve. *Circulation.* 1971 Mar;43(3):333-48.

Zoghbi WA, Enriquez-Sarano M, Foster E, Grayburn PA, Kraft CD, Levine RA, Nihoyannopoulos P, Otto CM, Quinones MA, Rakowski H, Stewart WJ, Waggoner A, Weissman NJ; American Society of Echocardiography. Recommendations for evaluation of the severity of native valvular regurgitation with two-dimensional and Doppler echocardiography. *J Am Soc Echocardiogr.* 2003 Jul;16(7):777-802.

Pulmonary Valve Disease

Abbas AE, Fortuin FD, Schiller NB, Appleton CP, Moreno CA, Lester SJ. Echocardiographic determination of mean pulmonary artery pressure. *Am J Cardiol.* 2003 Dec 1;92(11):1373-6.

Bashore TM. Adult congenital heart disease: right ventricular outflow tract lesions. *Circulation.* 2007 Apr 10;115(14):1933-47.

Baumgartner H, Hung J, Bermejo J, Chambers JB, Evangelista A, Griffin BP, Iung B, Otto CM, Pellikka PA, Quiñones M; American Society of Echocardiography; European Association of Echocardiography. Echocardiographic assessment of valve stenosis: EAE/ASE recommendations for clinical practice. *J Am Soc Echocardiogr.* 2009 Jan;22(1):1-23

Chemla D, Hébert JL, Coirault C, Salmeron S, Zamani K, Lecarpentier Y. Matching dicrotic notch and mean pulmonary artery pressures: implications for effective arterial elastance. *Am J Physiol.* 1996 Oct;271(4 Pt 2):H1287-95.

Martinez RM, Anderson RH. Echocardiographic features of the morphologically right ventriculo-arterial junction. *Cardiol Young.* 2005 Feb;15 Suppl 1:17-26.

Pierard LA, Badano L, Zamorano JL; European Association of Echocardiography. European Association of Echocardiography recommendations for the assessment of valvular regurgitation. Part 1: aortic and pulmonary regurgitation (native valve disease). *Eur J Echocardiogr.* 2010 Apr;11(3):223-44.

Rhodes JF, Hijazi ZM, Sommer RJ. Pathophysiology of congenital heart disease in the adult, part II. Simple obstructive lesions. *Circulation.* 2008 Mar 4;117(9):1228-37.

Shah PM. Tricuspid and pulmonary valve disease evaluation and management. *Rev Esp Cardiol.* 2010 Nov;63(11):1349-65.

Silvilairat S, Cabalka AK, Cetta F, Hagler DJ, O'Leary PW. Echocardiographic assessment of isolated pulmonary valve stenosis: which outpatient Doppler gradient has the most clinical validity? *J Am Soc Echocardiogr.* 2005 Nov;18(11):1137-42.

Silversides CK, Veldtman GR, Crossin J, Merchant N, Webb GD, McCrindle BW, Siu SC, Therrien J. Pressure half-time predicts hemodynamically significant pulmonary regurgitation in adult patients with repaired tetralogy of fallot. *J Am Soc Echocardiogr.* 2003 Oct;16(10):1057-62.

Stamm C, Anderson RH, Ho SY. Clinical anatomy of the normal pulmonary root compared with that in isolated pulmonary valvular stenosis. *J Am Coll Cardiol.* 1998 May;31(6):1420-5.

Williams RV, Minich LL, Shaddy RE, Pagotto LT, Tani LY. Comparison of Doppler echocardiography with angiography for determining the severity of pulmonary regurgitation. *Am J Cardiol.* 2002 Jun 15;89(12):1438-41.

Zoghbi WA, Enriquez-Sarano M, Foster E, Grayburn PA, Kraft CD, Levine RA, Nihoyannopoulos P, Otto CM, Quinones MA, Rakowski H, Stewart WJ, Waggoner A, Weissman NJ; American Society of Echocardiography. Recommendations for evaluation of the severity of native valvular regurgitation with two-dimensional and Doppler echocardiography. *J Am Soc Echocardiogr.* 2003 Jul;16(7):777-802.

Prosthetic Valves

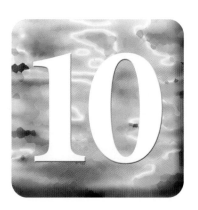

Basic Concepts

Prosthetic Valve Replacements

Prosthetic valve replacement for valvular heart disease was first introduced in the early 1960's. Since this time, many prosthetic heart valves have been designed and implanted with new and improved prosthetic valves being constantly developed. Prosthetic heart valves can be simply classified as either biological (tissue) valves or mechanical valves. Biological valves include human valves (allografts or homografts) and valves constructed from animal tissue (xenografts or heterografts). Included in the biological valves are the newer percutaneous valves which can be implanted in the aortic or pulmonary positions. Allograft valves are inserted into either the aortic or pulmonary position as a valve only replacement or as a valved conduit. Xenograft valves are typically composed of porcine or bovine tissue. These valves may be mounted on a metal support (stented bioprosthesis) or without a metal support (stentless bioprosthesis); stentless valves are only used in the aortic position.

Mechanical valves are made from non-biological materials such as pyrolytic carbon, polymeric silicone or titanium. Mechanical valves are further classified according to their occluder/leaflet structure. For example, the bileaflet tilting disc valve has two equal sized semicircular discs which form two large lateral orifices and one smaller central orifice when in the open position, the single tilting disc design has a single hinged disc which forms major and minor orifices when in the open position, and the ball-cage valves contain a ball occluder (poppet) within a wire cage.

Because each prosthetic heart valve is different, it is crucial that the sonographer is aware of the various types and designs of prosthetic valves. In particular, the echocardiographic appearances of mechanical prosthetic valves vary depending upon its basic structure, occluder mechanism and motion, and haemodynamic flow patterns. Tables 10.1-10.3 provide examples of prosthetic valves that may be commonly encountered. Importantly, these tables are not all-inclusive and only selected examples are described.

Table 10.1 Biological Homograft (Tissue) Valves

Valve Type		Description	Flow Characteristics
Allograft (Homograft)		• Aortic valve from human donor • Used only in aortic position • Stentless • Typically harvested as a block of tissue including aortic valve and ascending aorta	• Similar flow characteristics as native valve • Central flow • Trivial or no regurgitation • Low stenosis rate • Low thrombosis rate • Failure secondary to increasing regurgitation
Autograft (Ross Procedure)		• Native pulmonary valve resected and sewn into aortic position (autograft) • Allograft then placed in pulmonary position • Coronary arteries reimplanted to autograft	• Native valve flow characteristics for both valves • Central flow • Trivial or no regurgitation • Failure due to: (1) dilatation of autograft root leading to progression of aortic regurgitation, and/or (2) pulmonary allograft degeneration

Allograft photograph courtesy of Dr Darryl Burstow. Autograft Illustration courtesy of Tau Boga ©

Table 10.2 Biological Xenograft (Tissue) Valves

Stented Valves			
Description • Stented bioprosthetic valves consist of porcine aortic valves or valves created from pericardium which are mounted on a metallic stent • Porcine valve may be an entire valve from a single pig or a composite from 2 or 3 individual pigs • Pericardial valves (Perimount valves) are usually bovine in origin but may be porcine or equine **Flow Characteristics** • Central flow dynamics • Relatively stenotic in smaller sizes • Trivial or no regurgitation • Failure due to leaflet degeneration such as leaflet thickening, calcification and tearing resulting in stenosis and regurgitation	Mitroflow® Aortic Pericardial Valve (Sorin Group) 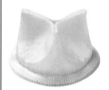	Carpentier-Edwards Mitral Porcine Bioprosthesis (Edwards Lifesciences) 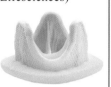	Medtronic Mosaic® Bioprosthesis heart valve (Medtronic Inc.)

Stentless Valves			
Description • Stentless valves are placed in the aortic position only • Stentless xenograft valves usually consist of a portion of porcine aorta • Aortic segment may be relatively long or may be sculpted to fit under the coronary arteries **Flow Characteristics** • Central flow • Improved flow characteristics compared to stented valves (larger valve area for given annulus size) • Trivial or no regurgitation	Cryolife O'Brien (CLOB) Valve® (Cryolife International, Inc.) 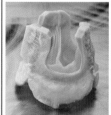	Freestyle® Stentless Porcine Valve (Medtronic Inc.) 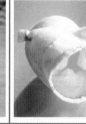	Toronto SPV® (St. Jude Medical, Inc.) 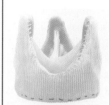

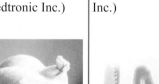

Percutaneous Valves			
Description • Tissue valves composed from bovine or porcine tissue and mounted on a balloon-expandable or self-expandable stent • Percutaneous aortic valves are placed in patients with severe calcific aortic stenosis considered to be high-risk or non-operable for conventional valve replacement surgery • Percutaneous pulmonary valves are placed in patients with repaired congenital heart lesions plus pulmonary valve stenosis and/or regurgitation in a right ventricle-to-pulmonary artery conduit. Percutaneous intervention is performed in these patients to avoid multiple open heart operations **Flow Characteristics** • Central flow • Small central regurgitant jets are common • Perivalvular regurgitation is common (but not normal) in the aortic valves • Long term durability uncertain at this stage	CoreValve® (Aortic) (Medtronic Inc.) Self-expandable 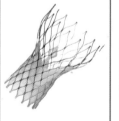	Edwards SAPIEN transcatheter heart valve (Edwards Lifesciences) Balloon-expandable 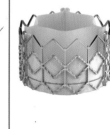	Melody® Valve (Pulmonary) (Medtronic Inc.) Balloon-expandable 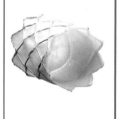

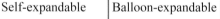
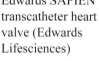
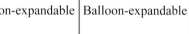

Mitroflow® Aortic Pericardial Valve reproduced from Piazza N, Bleiziffer S, Brockmann G, Hendrick R, Deutsch MA, Opitz A, Mazzitelli D, Tassani-Prell P, Schreiber C, Lange R. Transcatheter aortic valve implantation for failing surgical aortic bioprosthetic valve: from concept to clinical application and evaluation (part 1). *JACC Cardiovasc Interv.* Vol. 4(7), page 723 © 2011, with permission from Elsevier.

Images of Carpentier-Edwards Mitral Porcine Bioprosthesis and Edwards SAPIEN transcatheter heart valve courtesy of Edwards Lifesciences LLC, Irvine, CA. Carpentier-Edwards and Edwards SAPIEN are trademarks of Edwards Lifesciences Corporation.

Medtronic Mosaic® Bioprosthesis heart valve, CoreValve® (Aortic) and Melody® Valve (Pulmonary) reproduced with permission from Medtronic Inc.

Images of Cryo-Life, Freestyle and Toronto valves reproduced from Westaby S, Huysmans HA, David TE. Stentless aortic bioprostheses: compelling data from the Second International Symposium. *Ann Thorac Surg.* Vol. (1), pages 236 & 239, © 1998, with permission from Elsevier.

Table 10.3 **Mechanical Prosthetic Valves**

Bileaflet Tilting Disc Valves

Description
- 2 equal-sized semicircular discs attached to central hinge
- Open valve consists of 3 orifices: 1 small, slit-like central orifice between open discs and 2 larger semicircular lateral orifices
- Designs differ in composition and purity of pyrolytic carbon, shape and opening angle of the leaflets, design of the pivots, size and shape of the housing, and design of the sewing ring
- Opening angle ranges from 75-90°; closing angle ranges from 25-40°

Flow Characteristics
- Complex flow dynamics with 2 large lateral orifices and 1 smaller central orifice
- Higher velocities in central orifice have been reported
- Normal leakage volume regurgitation common: appears as 3 jets - 2 peripheral jets where closed leaflets meet housing, and 1 central jet where closed discs meet each other

ATS Bileaflet Valve (ATS Medical)	St. Jude Medical Bileaflet Valve (St. Jude Medical)	On-X® Prosthetic Heart Valve (On-X Life Technologies, Inc.)
Opening angle 85°; closing angle 25°	Opening angle 85°; closing angle 25-30°	Opening angle 90°; closing angle 40°
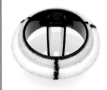	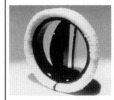	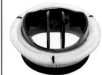

Single Tilting Disc Valves

Description
- Single hinged circular disc within rigid annulus
- Open valve consists of 2 distinct orifices of different sizes
- Variable opening angle of disc (ranges from 60° to 80°)

Flow Characteristics
- Flow through a major and a minor orifice (semi-central flow)
- Leakage and closing volume regurgitation common around central strut and between disc and sewing ring (peripheral jets)

Bjork-Shiley (Pfizer, Inc.)	Medtronic-Hall (Medtronic Inc.)	Lillehei-Kaster (Medical Inc.)
Opening angle 60°	Opening angle 75° (aortic); 70° (mitral)	Opening angle 80°
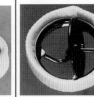	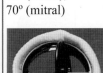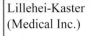	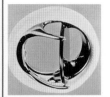

Ball-Cage Valves

Description
- Silastic ball (poppet) housed within a stellite alloy cage composed of three or four U-shaped, monocast struts joining at the apex
- Rarely implanted these days

Flow Characteristics
- Non-central flow dynamics with lateral flow diverging around ball occluder
- 'Stenotic' especially in small sized valves
- Closing volume regurgitation common; true valvular (leakage) regurgitation uncommon

Starr-Edwards heart valve (Edwards Lifesciences)

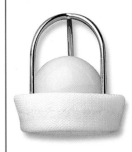

ATS Bileaflet Valve reproduced with permission from Medtronic Inc.
Images of St. Jude Medical, Bjork-Shiley, Medtronic-Hall and Lillehei-Kaster valves reproduced from Gott VL, Alejo DE, Cameron DE. Mechanical heart valves: 50 years of evolution. *Ann Thorac Surg.* Vol. 76(6), page S2235, © 2003, with permission from Elsevier.
On-X® Prosthetic Heart Valve image reproduced with permission from On-X Life Technologies, Inc.
Starr-Edwards heart valve image courtesy of Edwards Lifesciences LLC, Irvine, CA. Starr-Edwards is a trademark of Edwards Lifesciences Corporation.

With the exception of the allograft and stentless valves, all prosthetic valves are inherently stenotic and have a trivial or mild degree of transprosthetic regurgitation. The degree of obstruction varies according to the type and size of the valve while the appearance of 'physiologic' regurgitation also varies with the type and design of the prosthetic valve. In particular, 'physiologic' regurgitation is commonly seen with mechanical valves and may appear as 'closing volume' or 'leakage volume'. Closing volume occurs due to the displacement of blood when the occluder shuts (closes). Leakage volume refers to built-in transprosthetic regurgitation which aims to prevent thrombus formation at potential points of stasis by a "washing out" mechanism; these 'washing jets' appear as transprosthetic regurgitation at the hinge points of the occluder.

Surgical Valve Repair

When possible, valve repair is preferred to valve replacement. This is because prosthetic valves do not last forever and there is a potential for complications to occur with these valves; furthermore, mechanical prosthetic valves require lifelong anticoagulation. In fact, valve repair for mitral and tricuspid regurgitation is considered the surgical treatment of choice.

Several techniques have been described for mitral and tricuspid valve repair. These techniques include the use of neocords, cordal transfer, triangular and quadrangular resection as well as the insertion of annuloplasty rings (Fig. 10.1-10.3). It is important to note that surgical valve repair techniques will vary between institutions and according to the expertise of the cardiac surgeon.

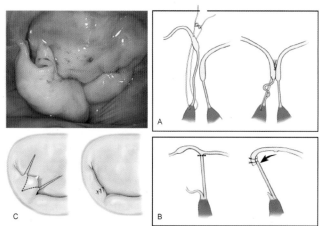

Figure 10.1 An intra-operative photograph of fibroelastic deficiency (FED) of the mitral valve is shown (*top left*). The drawings illustrate the various surgical techniques that can be performed for these leaflets without excess tissue and with single segment prolapse, which may or may not be thickened. A: The neocordal technique involves the attachment of artificial cords from the head of the papillary muscle to the free edge of the unsupported prolapsing leaflet. B: Cordal transfer involves the transfer of normal cords from another part of the valve to the unsupported free edge of the prolapsing leaflet. C: Triangular resection involves the resection of a triangular section of the prolapsing segment followed by the leaflet edges being sewn together.
Reproduced from Chikwe J, Adams DH, State of the art: degenerative mitral valve disease. *Heart Lung Circ.* Vol. 18(5), page 321, © 2009, with permission from Elsevier.

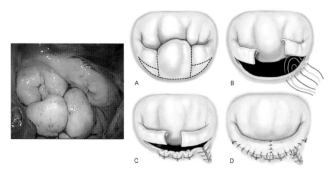

Figure 10.2 An intra-operative photograph of a Barlow's mitral valve is shown (*left*). The drawings illustrate quadrangular resection of the posterior leaflet with a sliding-plasty. This surgical technique is commonly used to repair these thickened mitral leaflets with excess tissue and multisegment mitral valve prolapse. A: The resection line for quadrangular resection and leaflet sliding-plasty is identified and a quadrangular resection is performed. B: Sutures are then placed to vertically plicate (compress) the posterior annulus. C: Leaflet sliding plasty is then performed. D: The procedure is concluded by completed suture lines.
Reproduced from Chikwe J, Adams DH, State of the art: degenerative mitral valve disease. *Heart Lung Circ.* Vol. 18(5), page 321, © 2009, with permission from Elsevier.

Percutaneous Mitral Valve Repair

Several approaches have been proposed for the percutaneous repair of degenerative and functional mitral regurgitation (MR). These approaches include direct leaflet repair, direct or indirect annular remodelling, and ventricular remodelling. An example of one such approach for percutaneous mitral valve repair is the MitraClip® device. This device is an edge-to-edge repair that effectively 'clamps' together the anterior and posterior mitral leaflets to create a double orifice mitral valve (Fig. 10.4).

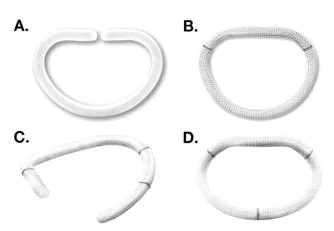

Figure 10.3 Selected examples of annuloplasty rings are shown. A: Carpentier-Edwards Classic Annuloplasty Ring (Edwards Lifesciences); B: Carpentier-Edwards Physio Annuloplasty Ring (Edwards Lifesciences); C: Contour 3D® annuloplasty ring (Medtronic); D: Medtronic Profile 3D® annuloplasty ring (Medtronic. Inc.). The principal goal of these 3D rigid or flexible annuloplasty rings is to remodel the valve annulus whilst preserving the annular motion.
Images A and B courtesy of Edwards Lifesciences LLC, Irvine, CA. Carpentier-Edwards, Carpentier-Edwards Classic and Carpentier-Edwards Physio, are trademarks of Edwards Lifesciences Corporation. Images C and D reproduced with permission from Medtronic Inc.

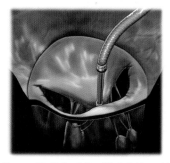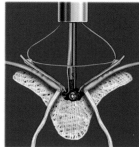

Figure 10.4 The MitraClip® (Abbott Vascular, Menlo Park, California) is implanted in the A2-P2 region of the mitral valve. The partially opened clip demonstrates tissue penetration into the clip (*left*). Once proper leaflet grasping is confirmed, the clip is closed to enhance coaptation. The free edges of the leaflets are then engaged between the clip arms and the grippers (*right*). Figure illustration by Craig Skaggs.
Reproduced from Maisano F, La Canna G, Colombo A, Alfieri O. The evolution from surgery to percutaneous mitral valve interventions: the role of the edge-to-edge technique. *J Am Coll Cardiol.* Vol. 58(21), page 2175, © 2011, with permission from Elsevier.

Role of Echocardiography

Echocardiography has a vital role in the pre-operative, peri-operative and post-operative assessment of prosthetic valves. Most commonly, the peri-operative assessment of prosthetic valves is performed by transoesophageal echocardiography (TOE). In particular, TOE has a very important role in guiding valve placement during transcatheter aortic valve implantation (TAVI), also known as transcatheter aortic valve replacement (TAVR), and in guiding clip placement for percutaneous mitral valve repair. The peri-operative assessment of prosthetic valves will not be discussed further as this is a very specialised technique which is most commonly performed by the echocardiologist.

Pre-operative Assessment

An obvious and crucial pre-operative role of echocardiography in patients undergoing 'conventional' prosthetic valve surgery is to confirm that the patient does, in fact, have severe valve disease. Importantly, when there is severe valvular regurgitation it is essential that the precise mechanism of regurgitation is identified. For example, valve replacement may not be required in patients with severe MR secondary to systolic anterior motion of the mitral valve; this is because MR in these patients is due to dynamic left ventricular outflow tract (LVOT) obstruction rather than a primary problem with the mitral valve complex.

Pre-Allograft Replacement

An accurate measurement of the LVOT diameter is required for all patients having an allograft aortic valve replacement (AVR). This is because the allograft valves are stored frozen in a tissue bank and, therefore, need to be thawed prior to the operation. The size of allograft valve selected for the operation is based on the LVOT diameter; therefore, an accurate measurement of this diameter is crucial to ensure that an appropriately sized valve is chosen.

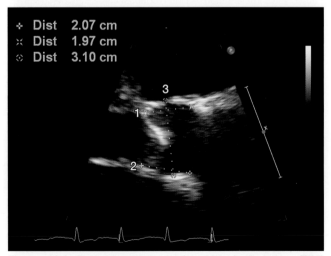

Figure 10.5 Pre-transcatheter aortic valve implantation (TAVI) measurements of the trans-sinus diameter (sinus of Valsalva width) and the sinus height are shown. These measurements are performed from a zoomed parasternal long axis view at end-diastole. The anterior and posterior sinus heights are measured as the distance between the aortic annulus to the sinotubular junction, perpendicular to the annular plane (1 and 2). The trans-sinus diameter is measured using the leading edge to leading edge technique, parallel to the annular plane (3). The aortic annulus or left ventricular outflow tract diameter is measured between the insertion points of the right coronary cusp (1) and the non-coronary cusp (2).

Pre-Ross Procedure

For the Ross procedure, the native pulmonary valve is resected and placed into aortic position (autograft) and an allograft is placed in pulmonary position (see Table 10.1). This procedure is typically performed in young adults and children because in these patients failure of allograft aortic valves is commonly encountered due to a vigorous immune response. In addition, with this procedure there is no requirement for anticoagulation which is especially important in young women of child-bearing age. Other advantages of this operation include the superior longevity of the pulmonary autograft and the pulmonary allograft. In particular, the pulmonary allograft tends to last longer due to lower pressures through this right-sided valve and as the pulmonary autograft is living tissue, it has the potential to grow with the patient.

The role of echocardiography prior to this operation includes determining that the pulmonary valve is anatomically and functionally normal (as this valve will become the aortic valve) and to confirm that the pulmonary and aortic annuli are of a similar size. 3D echocardiography may be especially useful in determining that the pulmonary valve is trileaflet.

Pre-TAVI Procedure

The pre-operative role of echocardiography in TAVI includes confirming that the patient has severe aortic stenosis (AS), identifying patient suitability for the procedure and determining the prosthesis size.

Severe AS is defined as an aortic valve area (AVA) < 1 cm^2 (or < 0.6 cm^2/m^2) and a mean pressure gradient of > 40 mm Hg (or transaortic peak systolic velocity of > 4 m/s). The severity of AS is determined in the traditional manner (see Chapter 7). Patient suitability is based on both anatomical and clinical criteria. Clinical criteria include patients with a high or prohibitive surgical risk which is quantified using the logistic European System for Cardiac Operative Risk Evaluation (EuroSCORE) or the Society of Thoracic Surgeons (STS) Predicted Risk of Mortality score. In particular, patients with a EuroSCORE of ≥ 15- 20% or an STS score ≥ 10% are considered candidates for the TAVI procedure.

Anatomic criteria include an extensive list of parameters that are assessed by echocardiography, computer tomography (CT) or cardiac magnetic resonance imaging (CMRI), and angiography. The specific echocardiographic selection inclusion and exclusion criteria for the CoreValve are listed in Tables 10.4-10.5; similar criteria are used for the Edwards SAPIEN valve.

Importantly, the size of the prosthesis is selected based on the diameter of the aortic annulus (Table 10.5); therefore, an accurate measurement of this diameter is crucial to ensure that an appropriately sized valve is selected. In addition, aortic dimensions such as the LVOT diameter at the aortic annulus, the LVOT diameter 5 mm from the aortic annulus, the trans-sinus diameter (sinus of Valsalva width) and the sinus height should also be measured (Fig. 10.5). A thorough assessment of aortic valve morphology is also required as patients with unicuspid and bicuspid aortic valves are not optimal candidates for TAVI because the valvular orifice is elliptical and may predispose the prosthetic valve to perivalvular aortic regurgitation (AR).

Table 10.4A **Medtronic CoreValve® Patient Evaluation Criteria**

Diagnostic Findings by Echo	Selection Criteria	
	Recommended	Not Recommended
Atrial or Ventricular Thrombus	Not Present	Present
Sub Aortic Stenosis	Not Present	Present
LV Ejection Fraction	≥ 20%	< 20% without contractile reserve
Mitral Regurgitation	≤ Grade 2	> Grade 2 (organic reason)

Table 10.4B **General Medical Guidance for Use of CoreValve***

Diagnostic Findings by Echo	Selection Criteria	
	Recommended	Moderate-High Risk
LV Hypertrophy	Normal to Moderate 0.6 - 1.6 cm	Severe ≥ 1.7 cm
Anatomic Considerations for 26 mm CoreValve Device		
Sinus of Valsalva Width	≥ 27 mm	< 27 mm
Sinus of Valsalva Height	≥ 15 mm	< 15 mm
Anatomic Considerations for 29 mm CoreValve Device		
Sinus of Valsalva Width	≥ 29 mm	< 29 mm
Sinus of Valsalva Height	≥ 15 mm	< 15 mm
Anatomic Considerations for 31 mm CoreValve Device		
Sinus of Valsalva Width	≥ 29 mm	< 29 mm
Sinus of Valsalva Height	≥ 15 mm	< 15 mm

* General medical guidance reflects the experience to date with the product, but final judgment remains with the implanting physician(s). Based on Medtronic data (Medtronic, Inc. PDF (UC201106402 EE) 2011)

Table 10.5 **Selection of Transcatheter Aortic Valve Size**

CoreValve Device		Edwards-SAPIEN XT Valve	
CoreValve Size	Aortic Annulus Size	SAPIEN XT Size	Aortic Annulus Size
23 mm	17–20 mm	20 mm	16–19 mm
26 mm	20-23 mm	23 mm	18-21 mm
29 mm	24-27 mm	26 mm	22-25 mm
31 mm	26-29 mm	29 mm	25-27 mm

Source: Mylotte D, Martucci G, Piazza N. Patient selection for transcatheter aortic valve implantation: An interventional cardiology perspective. *Ann Cardiothorac Surg.* 2012;1(2):206-215.

Pre-MitraClip Procedure

The role of echocardiography prior to the MitraClip procedure includes confirming that the patient has severe MR and determining anatomic suitability for the procedure. MR severity is assessed in the traditional manner using semiquantitative and quantitative techniques (see Chapter 8). Patient suitability is based on both clinical and anatomical criteria (Table 10.6 and Fig. 10.6). Importantly, the sonographer should be aware of the anatomical variables when assessing patients considered for the MitraClip procedure.

Post-operative Assessment: General Considerations

For all prosthetic valves, the comprehensive echocardiographic examination includes:

• measurements of cardiac chamber dimensions (including the ascending aorta when an AVR is in-situ),
• evaluation of ventricular systolic function,
• assessment of coexistent native valve lesions,
• estimation of right ventricular systolic pressure (RVSP).

Measurements of Cardiac Chamber Dimensions

The degree of chamber dilatation and ventricular wall thickness is dependent on the type and chronicity of valve disease present prior to surgery. For example, in patients with chronic severe MR prior to surgery, marked dilatation of the left atrium (LA) and LV would be expected; if coexistent pulmonary hypertension was also present pre-operatively then dilatation of the right heart chambers and increased right ventricular (RV) wall thickness would also be expected. In patients with chronic severe AS prior to surgery, a concentric increase in LV wall thickness is usually present.

In the post-operative patient, echocardiography can be used to assess and monitor the regression of chamber dilatation and ventricular wall thickness. These measurements are performed in the standard manner (see Chapter 2). In addition, progressive dilatation of the ascending aorta may occur following an AVR; therefore, careful assessment of the ascending aorta is required in these patients. Aortic measurements are performed from a high parasternal window and/or from the right sternal edge (Fig. 10.7).

Evaluation of Ventricular Systolic Function

Echocardiography is also important in the assessment of ventricular systolic function. In particular, echocardiography is used to monitor the recovery of LV systolic function in patients where there was a pre-operative reduction in function. The assessment of left and right ventricular systolic function is carried out in the tradition manner (see Chapter 2).

Table 10.6 Anatomical Selection Criteria for the MitraClip Device

Recommended anatomical criteria (from EVEREST trial)
MR originates from the A2-P2 area
Coaptation length ≥ 2 mm
Coaptation depth < 11 mm
Flail gap < 10 mm
Flail width < 15 mm
Mitral valve orifice area > 4 cm²
Additional criteria for caution
Short posterior leaflet (< 8 mm)
Restricted posterior leaflet prolapse/flail width >15 mm
Calcification in the grasping area
Cleft or subcommissures in the area of the jet

EVEREST = Endovascular Valve Edge-to-edge REpair STudy; MR = mitral regurgitation.
Reproduced from Maisano F, La Canna G, Colombo A, Alfieri O. The evolution from surgery to percutaneous mitral valve interventions: the role of the edge-to-edge technique.
J Am Coll Cardiol. Vol. 58(21), page 2179, © 2011, with permission from Elsevier.

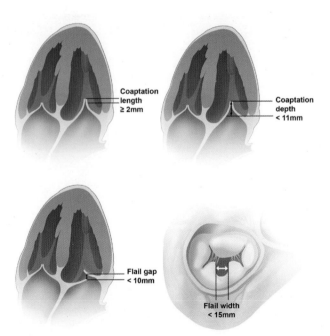

Figure 10.6 Key anatomic eligibility criteria for the MitraClip are illustrated. Measurements are best performed via transoesophageal echocardiography using a 4-chamber view. For patients with functional mitral regurgitation (MR), the coaptation length must be at least 2 mm and the coaptation depth must be < 11 mm (*top*). For patients with degenerative MR and a flail leaflet, the flail gap must be < 10 mm, and the flail width must be < 15 mm (*bottom*). These anatomic characteristics are necessary for sufficient leaflet tissue for mechanical coaptation when the MitraClip device is used.
Reproduced from Feldman T, Kar S, Rinaldi M, Fail P, Hermiller J, Smalling R et al. Percutaneous mitral repair with the MitraClip system: safety and midterm durability in the initial EVEREST (Endovascular Valve Edge-to-edge REpair STudy) cohort. *J Am Coll Cardiol*, Vol. 54(8), page 639, © 2009, with permission from Elsevier.

Following open heart surgery, abnormal or paradoxical motion of the interventricular septum is commonly encountered. This abnormal motion may recover or may persist. Possible mechanisms for this abnormal motion include: (1) ischaemia to the septum during cardiopulmonary bypass, (2) total displacement of heart anteriorly during systole secondary to adhesions between sternum and heart, or (3) changes in cardiac motion secondary to the pericardiotomy.

Assessment of Coexistent Native Valve Lesions

One of the most common causes for severe valve disease is rheumatic heart disease. Rheumatic heart disease often affects more than one cardiac valve but only one valve lesion may be severe enough to require replacement or repair. Hence, coexistent native valve disease may still be present post-operatively. The echocardiographic assessment of these valvular lesions is carried out in the usual manner (see Chapters 7-9).

Estimation of RVSP

Right ventricular systolic pressure (RVSP) is another important parameter that should be assessed in patients following valve replacement or repair. This is particularly important in patients following mitral valve replacement (MVR) who had secondary pulmonary hypertension prior to surgery. Furthermore, an elevation in the RVSP may be an indirect sign of the presence of significant regurgitation in a MVR. RVSP is estimated from the tricuspid regurgitant (TR) velocity in the usual manner.

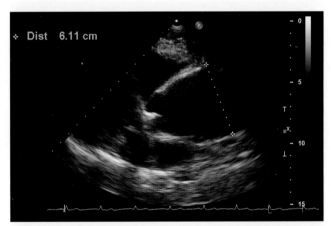

Figure 10.7 The ascending aorta is measured from a high parasternal long axis view. Measurements are performed at end-diastole using the leading edge to leading edge technique, parallel with the aortic annulus. Observe that the ascending aorta in this patient with an allograft aortic valve replacement is markedly dilated at 6.1 cm.

Post-operative Assessment: Prosthetic Valve

A comprehensive assessment of the prosthetic valve itself is also important in the post-operative patient. This assessment includes:

- a baseline assessment of the prosthetic valve (early post-operative assessment),
- 2D assessment of the prosthetic valve (morphology, seating and mobility),
- haemodynamic assessment of prosthetic valve parameters (discussed in a separate section below),
- evaluation of the degree and type of prosthetic valve regurgitation.

Baseline Study

The baseline study should be performed within the first two months following surgery and, ideally, after the patient has been discharged from hospital. The primary aim of the early, post-operative baseline study is to acquire haemodynamic data at a time when the prosthetic valve is functioning normally. The baseline study also provides a reference point for that particular prosthetic valve which can be compared to future studies; that is, the baseline study serves as a 'normal reference' for the individual patient so the patient serves as his/her own 'control'. Other advantages of the baseline study include the recognition of prosthesis-patient mismatch (PPM), facilitating the detection of prosthetic valve dysfunction, and identifying suspected infective endocarditis. PPM occurs when the effective orifice area (EOA) of a normally functioning prosthetic valve is too small in relation to the patient's body size, leading to abnormally high transprosthetic gradients. PPM may be difficult to differentiate from 'acquired' valvular stenosis if only a single study is performed at a time when prosthesis obstruction is suspected. Furthermore, following the progression of prosthetic valve stenosis and regurgitation is difficult if only a single study is performed at a time when an 'abnormal' prosthesis is suspected. In these cases, the baseline study can be compared with subsequent studies to track changes in valvular haemodynamics over time. Likewise, in the clinical setting of suspected infective endocarditis, the baseline study can be helpful by comparing valve appearance 'then' to valve appearance 'now'; this is especially valuable in the assessment of MVRs as redundant cords may be easily mistaken for vegetations.

The baseline study also allows the monitoring of: (1) the regression of ventricular hypertrophy (pre-operative stenotic valve lesions), (2) the regression of chamber dilatation (pre-operative regurgitant valve lesions), (3) the recovery of LV systolic function (if reduced pre-operatively), and (4) the reduction in pulmonary artery systolic pressures (pre-operative pulmonary hypertension).

> Ideally, the baseline study should be performed after the patient has been discharged from hospital. Studies performed too early in the post-operative period are often technically challenging and can result in an incomplete and/or inadequate assessment of prosthetic valve haemodynamics which essentially defeats the aim of the baseline echo study. Reasons for a suboptimal study in the very early post-operative period include: (1) chest tenderness, (2) reduced patient mobility, and (3) the presence of bandages, chest drains and temporary pacing wires which limit access to suitable acoustic windows.

2D Assessment of Prosthetic Valves

2D imaging of prosthetic valves, especially mechanical valves, is challenging due to the acoustic properties of the prosthetic materials which cause increased echogenicity and imaging artefacts distal to the prosthesis. These acoustic factors typically impede visualisation of the prosthetic valve structures

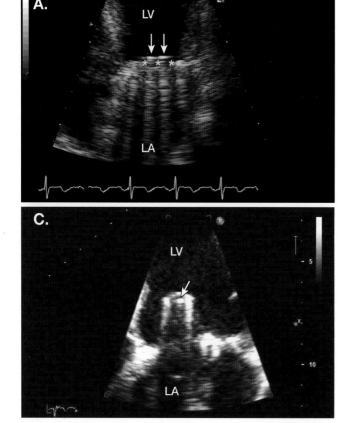
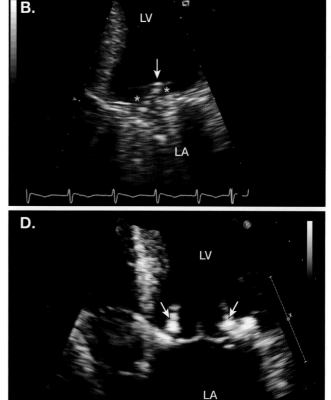

Figure 10.8 Echocardiographic examples of various mitral prosthetic valves are shown. All images are recorded from a zoomed apical 4-chamber view of the mitral prosthesis A: Bileaflet tilting disc (St Jude): observe how the two discs open in parallel (*arrows*). As a result, there are two large lateral orifices (*yellow* *) and one smaller central orifice (blue *). Reverberation artefacts are also seen within the left atrium arising from the sewing ring and the two discs. B: Single leaflet tilting disc valve (Lillehei-Kaster): this single disc valve opens to an angle of approximately 80⁰ (*arrow*). Two distinct orifices of different sizes are seen: one major (*yellow* *) and one minor (blue *). C: Caged-ball valve (Starr-Edwards): the ball (poppet) is seen within the metal cage (*arrow*). Flow through this valve diverges laterally around ball occluder. D: Stented xenograft valve (Mosaic): the stent posts of this valve project into the left ventricle (*arrows*). The leaflets are seen between the struts and appear thin similar to a native valve. LA = left atrium; LV = left ventricle.

and surrounding cardiac anatomy. Therefore, it is important to assess the prosthesis from multiple on-axis and off-axis imaging views.

Prior to commencing the examination, the type and size of the prosthetic valve should be established. Knowledge of these characteristics is important as the 2D appearance of the valve is dependent on the type of prosthesis; for example, a single tilting disc valve will look different to a bileaflet tilting disc valve. Furthermore, it is not always possible to differentiate between the various types of prosthetic valves by 2D imaging alone; for example, all stented bioprosthetic valves look alike while bileaflet tilting disc valves also appear very similar. Echocardiographic examples of various types of prosthetic valves are shown in Figures 10.8-10.9. Awareness of the prosthetic valve size is also essential for the haemodynamic assessment of the valve (discussed below).

The 2D examination of the prosthetic valve should include an evaluation of the valve appearance, the seating of the valve within the native annulus, and the opening and closing motion of the leaflets/occluders. In particular, for mechanical valves, it is also important to consider the opening angle of the discs compared to the normal known opening angles (see Table 10.3). The most common causes for reduced opening angles include valvular thrombosis and pannus formation (see Prosthetic Valve Complications below).

The valve bed and the appearance of the sewing ring should also be assessed to ensure that the sewing ring is stable and the valve is well-seated. For example, a "rocking" motion of the valve is a characteristic feature of prosthetic valve dehiscence (see Prosthetic Valve Complications below).

Any extraneous echoes should also be noted; for example, leaflet calcification or abnormal echo densities attached to the sewing ring, occluder, leaflets, stents, or cage should be reported. Importantly, remnant mitral subvalvular apparatus following a MVR with cordal preservation may mimic vegetations; therefore, it is important to note whether or not a cordal preservation procedure was performed.

Another commonly encountered phenomenon observed with mechanical prosthetic valves is microbubbles within the cardiac chambers (Fig. 10.10). These microbubbles appear as very small, echogenic bubbles downstream from the valve which last for several seconds; this appearance is especially prominent with harmonic imaging and occurs due to carbon dioxide degassing. This normal phenomenon should not be confused with spontaneous echo contrast which is considered a precursor for thrombus formation.

Occluder motion for mechanical AVRs is often best appreciated from zoomed apical 5-chamber and apical long axis views where the open occluder is orientated parallel to the ultrasound beam and, therefore, shielding of these structures by the valve stent can be avoided.

The leaflet excursion for MVRs is often well seen from a low parasternal short axis view of the mitral prosthesis.

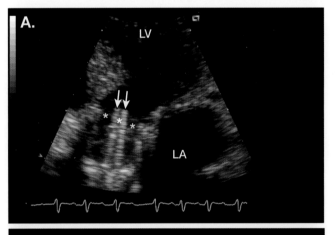

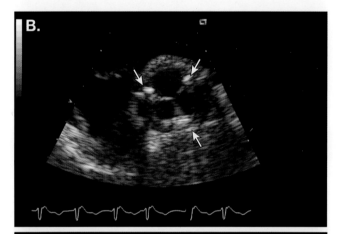

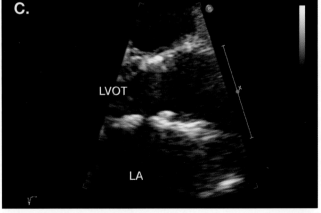

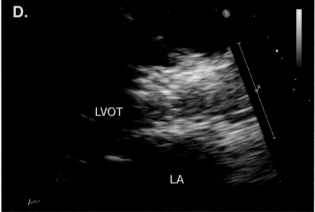

Figure 10.9 Echocardiographic examples of various aortic prosthetic valves are shown. All images are zoomed views. A: Bileaflet tilting disc (ATS): from the apical 5-chamber view in systole the two discs are seen to open in parallel (*arrows*). As a result, there are two large lateral orifices (*yellow **) and one smaller central orifice (*white **). B: Stented xenograft (Carpentier-Edwards): from the parasternal short axis view in diastole, all three struts of this valve are clearly seen (*arrows*). These stents are located in positions similar to the native valve commissures. C: Stentless xenograft valve (Cryo-Life O'Brien): from the parasternal long axis view, this valve appears similar to a native aortic valve. D: Percutaneous valve (CoreValve): from this parasternal long axis view, the valve leaflets cannot be seen; however, this image nicely illustrates the wire frame of this valve. LA = left atrium; LV = left ventricle; LVOT = left ventricular outflow tract.

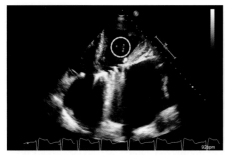 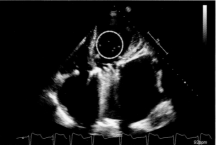 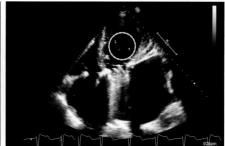

Figure 10.10 This series of images shows microbubbles within the left ventricle (*circled*). These microbubbles are created by the degassing phenomenon which occurs as carbon dioxide separates from blood as blood flows through this 31 mm St Jude mitral valve replacement (see text for details). Images are recorded from an apical 4-chamber view.

Degree and Type of Prosthetic Valve Regurgitation

As indicated in Tables 10.1-10.3, 'physiological' transprosthetic regurgitation is frequently present in all types of mechanical valves and is also common in many biological valves. The appearance of regurgitation is related to the flow profiles through each valve. For example, with the bileaflet tilting disc valves two small leakage jets are often seen at the periphery of the valve (Fig. 10.11). Importantly, this normal prosthetic valve regurgitation should be distinguished from pathological regurgitation (see Complications of Prosthetic Valves below).

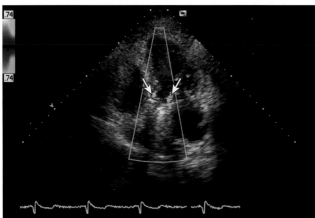

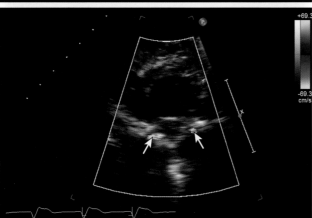

Figure 10.11 Normal leakage volume regurgitation through bileaflet tilting disc valves in the aortic and mitral position are shown; images were acquired from two different patients. The image of the aortic prosthesis was recorded from the apical 5-chamber view (*top*). The image of the mitral prosthesis was recorded from the parasternal short axis view (*bottom*). Observe that these normal jets appear at the periphery of the valve where the closed discs meet the housing (*arrows*). The jets appear short and narrow in the case of the aortic prosthesis and small in area in the case of the mitral prosthesis.

Haemodynamic Assessment of Prosthetic Valves

The haemodynamic assessment of prosthetic valves includes measurement of the transprosthetic velocities and the maximum and/or mean pressure gradients, estimation of the EOA, and the calculation of the Doppler velocity index (DVI). For mitral and tricuspid prosthetic valves, the pressure half-time is also measured.

As previously stated, prior to performing an echocardiogram in a patient with a prosthetic valve, it is crucial that the type and size of prosthetic valve is known. This is because the normal haemodynamic values for prosthetic valves are based on the valve type and size as well as on the position of the valve. The normal Doppler haemodynamic values for various prosthetic valves are listed in Appendices 1-4.

All haemodynamic measurements should be averaged over at least two consecutive cardiac cycles when the patient is in sinus rhythm. In patients with atrial fibrillation (AF), measurements should be averaged over five cycles, on beats that exhibit minimal variation in the R-R intervals, and at a heart rate that is close to normal.

Transprosthetic Velocities and Pressure Gradients

The peak velocities and pressure gradients are measured via continuous-wave (CW) Doppler from the view which best aligns flow parallel with the ultrasound beam. Parallel alignment of the Doppler beam with transprosthetic flow can be assisted by using colour flow imaging (CFI); this is especially useful in the Starr-Edwards valve where flow diverges laterally around the ball occluder (Fig. 10.12). CFI is also useful in distinguishing laminar from turbulent flow (Fig. 10.13).

From the spectral Doppler trace, transprosthetic pressure gradients are estimated by application of the simplified Bernoulli equation (see Chapter 1). The maximum instantaneous pressure gradient is measured from the peak Doppler velocity while the mean pressure gradient is calculated by tracing the Doppler signal over the flow period. For prosthetic mitral and tricuspid valves, the mean pressure gradient rather than the maximum pressure gradient is important as the transprosthetic pressure gradient varies over the diastolic period. In addition, for mitral and tricuspid prosthetic valves, the heart rate at which mean pressure gradients are measured should also be reported; this is especially important at rapid heart rates where the mean gradients tend to be increased.

AVR Caveats

Importantly, mechanical AVRs must be assessed using the non-imaging CW Doppler probe from multiple acoustic windows in a manner as described for native AS. This is because the transprosthetic jet direction may be quite eccentric. In normal biological valves, especially allograft, autograft and stentless bioprostheses, flow characteristics are very similar to the native aortic valve so the CW Doppler assessment is usually adequate from the apical window. However, when the valve leaflets are thickened, these valves must be interrogated from multiple acoustic windows as the

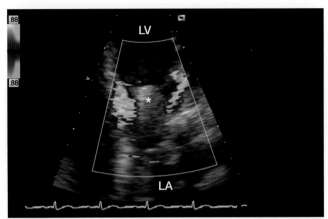

Figure 10.12 This zoomed apical 4-chamber view was recorded from a patient with a Starr-Edwards mitral valve replacement. Observe that transprosthetic flow diverges laterally around ball occluder (*).

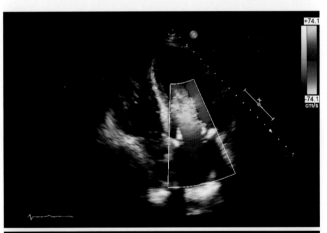

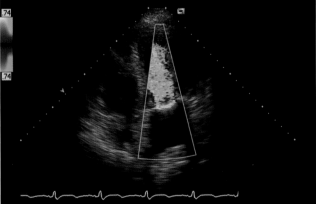

Figure 10.13 These two images were recorded from two different patients with a stented Xenograft mitral valve replacement (MVR). Images are from the apical 4-chamber view during diastole. Diastolic flow through the MVR on the top image appears laminar; this is consistent with normal transprosthetic flow. Diastolic flow through the MVR on the bottom image appears turbulent; this is consistent with an obstructed MVR.

stenotic jet direction is often eccentric.

Calculation of pressure gradients via the simplified Bernoulli equation assumes that the velocity proximal to a narrowing is insignificant (< 1.0 m/s). If the velocity within the LVOT is elevated (≥ 1.2 m/s), the maximum and mean pressure gradients derived from the simplified Bernoulli equation will be overestimated (see Chapter 1). Therefore, when the LVOT velocity is ≥ 1.2 m/s, corrected maximum and mean pressure gradients should be derived by using the 'expanded' Bernoulli equation:

Equation 10.1

$$\Delta P_C = \Delta P_{AVR} - \Delta P_{LVOT}$$

where ΔP_C = corrected maximum or mean pressure gradient (mm Hg)

ΔP_{AVR} = maximum or mean pressure gradient across the AVR (mm Hg)

ΔP_{LVOT} = maximum or mean pressure gradient at the LVOT (mm Hg)

The CW Doppler interrogation of mechanical AVRs must be performed from multiple transducer positions, even in haemodynamically normal valves. This is because these valves are inherently stenotic and the structure of mechanical valves often leads to eccentric transprosthetic jets. Therefore, in order to ensure accurate velocities are recorded it is imperative to interrogate these valves from the apex, suprasternal notch, right supraclavicular fossa and the right sternal edge. The window from which the maximal velocity is obtained should also be recorded in the report for future reference; this information is useful for serial studies as the window that reveals the highest velocity usually remains the same. However, if the valve becomes stenotic the window providing the highest velocity may vary.

Effective Orifice Area

Pressure gradients are dependent upon the stroke volume (SV) across the valve as well as the prosthetic valve characteristics. Calculation of the EOA accounts for the volumetric flow at the time of the study and therefore 'compensates' for SV changes. For this reason, the EOA rather than pressure gradients are especially valuable in the serial assessment of prosthetic valves. Estimation of the EOA is based upon the continuity principle (see Chapter 1). In particular, assuming that the SV across the LVOT is the same as the SV across the prosthetic valve, the prosthetic EOA can be calculated from the LVOT SV (derived from the LVOT diameter and velocity time integral [VTI]) and the prosthetic valve VTI (Fig. 10.14-10.15):

Equation 10.2

$$EOA_{VTI} = (CSA_{LVOT} \times VTI_{LVOT}) \div VTI_{PrV}$$

where EOA_{VTI} = effective orifice area [VTI method] (cm²)

CSA_{LVOT} = cross-sectional area of the LVOT (cm²)

VTI_{LVOT} = velocity time integral of the LVOT (cm)

VTI_{PrV} = velocity time integral across the prosthetic valve (cm)

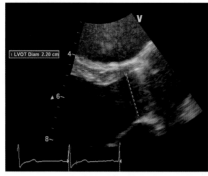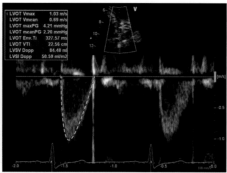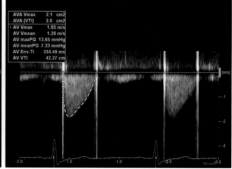

Figure 10.14 A 22 mm ATS-AP aortic valve replacement (AVR) is in-situ. The effective orifice area (EOA) is calculated from the: (1) left ventricular outflow tract (LVOT) diameter, (2) LVOT velocity time integral (VTI), and (3) VTI across the AVR. The LVOT diameter is measured from zoomed parasternal long axis view of the LVOT (*left*). At mid-systole, the LVOT diameter is measured, perpendicular to the aortic root, using the inner edge to inner edge technique. From an apical 5-chamber view (*middle*), the LVOT VTI is traced from the pulsed-wave Doppler signal with a 2-4 mm sample volume placed 5 mm proximal to the prosthetic aortic valve. The transaortic VTI is traced from the continuous-wave Doppler signal recorded from the window that provides the highest velocity across the AVR; this was the apical window in this case (*right*). The EOA via the VTI and Vmax methods in this example are calculated below.

$$EOA_{VTI} = (CSA_{LVOT} \times VTI_{LVOT}) \div VTI_{AVR}$$
$$= (0.785 \times 2.2^2 \times 22.56) \div 42.27$$
$$= 2.0 \ cm^2$$

$$EOA_{Vmax} = (CSA_{LVOT} \times V_{LVOT}) \div V_{AVR}$$
$$= (0.785 \times 2.2^2 \times 1.03) \div 1.85$$
$$= 2.1 \ cm^2$$

The Doppler velocity index (DVI) can also be derived as the ratio of the LVOT VTI and the AVR VTI or peak velocities through the LVOT and the AVR:

$$DVI_{VTI} = VTI_{LVOT} \div VTI_{AVR}$$
$$= 22.56 \div 42.27$$
$$= 0.53$$

$$DVI_{Vmax} = V_{LVOT} \div V_{AVR}$$
$$= 1.03 \div 1.85$$
$$= 0.56$$

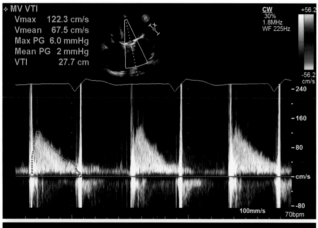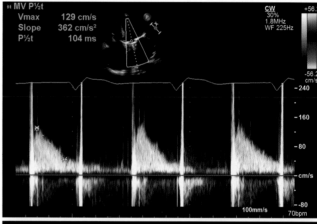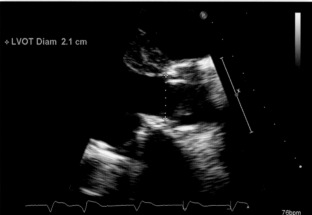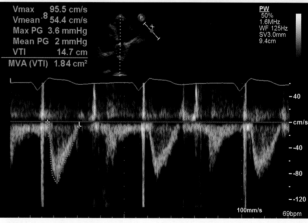

Figure 10.15 A 33 mm St Jude mitral valve replacement (MVR) is in-situ. Haemodynamic measurements include the pressure half-time, the mean MVR pressure gradient, the effective orifice area (EOA), and the Doppler velocity index (DVI). From the continuous-wave Doppler signal recorded from the apical 4-chamber view, the MVR signal is traced to derive the velocity time integral (VTI) and the mean pressure gradient (*top, left*). The P½t is measured along the peak early diastolic slope (*top, right*). The EOA is calculated from the: (1) left ventricular outflow tract (LVOT) diameter, (2) LVOT VTI, and (3) VTI across the MVR. The LVOT diameter is measured from zoomed parasternal long axis view of the LVOT (*bottom, left*). At mid-systole, callipers are placed from the inner edge of the junction between the anterior aortic wall and the interventricular septum to the inner edge of the junction between the posterior aortic wall and the anterior aspect of the MVR, perpendicular to the aortic root. From an apical 5-chamber view (*bottom, right*), the LVOT VTI is traced from the pulsed-wave Doppler signal with a 2-4 mm sample volume placed 5 mm proximal to the aortic valve. The EOA in this example is calculated as:

$$EOA = (CSA_{LVOT} \times VTI_{LVOT}) \div VTI_{MVR}$$
$$= (0.785 \times 2.1^2 \times 14.7) \div 27.7$$
$$= 1.8 \ cm^2$$

The DVI is derived as the ratio of the MVR VTI and the LVOT VTI:

$$DVI = VTI_{MVR} \div VTI_{LVOT}$$
$$= 27.7 \div 14.7$$
$$= 1.9$$

Note: As the patient is in atrial fibrillation, all measurements should be averaged over 3-5 cardiac cycles.

Indexed Effective Orifice Area

The EOA can also be indexed to the body surface area (BSA) by simply dividing the EOA by the BSA:

Equation 10.3

$$IEOA = EOA \div BSA$$

where IEOA = indexed effective orifice area (cm^2/m^2)

EOA = effective orifice area (cm^2)

BSA = body surface area (m^2)

Indexing the EOA to BSA is very useful in identifying patients with PPM (see Complications of Prosthetic Valves below).

Non-Laminar LVOT Flow

In patients with small LV cavities and basal hypertrophy of the interventricular septum, coexistent obstruction or non-laminar flow within the LVOT may occur. In this situation, the LVOT stroke volume (SV) cannot be used to calculate the EOA. Instead the EOA can be estimated by substituting the right ventricular outflow tract (RVOT) SV for the LVOT SV providing that there is no intracardiac shunt and no significant prosthetic or pulmonary valve regurgitation; that is, the SV across the RVOT and across the prosthetic valve are the same.

Coexistent Aortic Regurgitation

When there is coexistent aortic regurgitation (AR), the SV across the LVOT and across the AVR will still be the same so the EOA can still be accurately calculated using the LVOT SV. However, the LVOT SV cannot be used to calculate the EOA in prosthetic mitral, tricuspid and/or pulmonary valves when there is AR. In this situation, the EOA can be estimated by substituting the RVOT SV for the LVOT SV providing that there is no intracardiac shunt and no significant prosthetic or pulmonary valve regurgitation; that is, the SV across the RVOT and across the prosthetic valve is the same.

AVR Caveats

In the presence of an AVR and assuming that the flow duration across the LVOT and the AVR are the same, Equation 10.2 can be simplified by substituting the VTI across the LVOT and AVR with the peak velocities across the LVOT and AVR. This is referred to as the Vmax method:

Equation 10.3

$$EOA_{Vmax} = (CSA_{LVOT} \times V_{LVOT}) \div V_{AVR}$$

where EOA_{Vmax} = effective orifice area [Vmax method] (cm^2)

CSA_{LVOT} = cross-sectional area of the LVOT (cm^2)

V_{LVOT} = peak velocity at the LVOT (m/s)

V_{AVR} = peak velocity across the AVR (m/s)

The most common errors encountered in the calculation of the EOA in an AVR include underestimation of the LVOT VTI, substituting of the LVOT diameter with the prosthesis size, and measurement of the internal prosthetic valve dimension instead of the LVOT diameter (Fig. 10.16). In particular, when the prosthetic valve is implanted in the supra-annular position, the substitution of the LVOT diameter with the prosthesis size leads to an overestimation of the EOA. As a general rule, the LVOT diameter should be within ± 2 mm of the surgically implanted AVR size if the valve is placed at the level of the aortic annulus (intra-annulus). In cases where the LVOT diameter is difficult to measure, the surgically implanted AVR size may be used as a substitute; this substitution should be noted in the report and this diameter should be used in subsequent serial studies.

EOA in TAVI

Typically, measurements of the LVOT diameter and VTI are performed just proximal to the prosthetic valve stent or sewing ring. However, in the transcatheter valves, the proximal portion of the valve extends deeper into the LVOT. For example, in the self-expandable CoreValve, the stent is much longer and it may be quite low in the LVOT; while with the balloon-expandable Edwards SAPIEN valve the apical border of the stent is just below the native aortic valve annulus. Therefore, measurements of the LVOT diameter and VTI vary according to the type of transcatheter valve in-situ (Fig. 10.17 -10.18).

Importantly, the LVOT VTI should be measured proximal to the flow acceleration zone and the LVOT diameter should then be measured at the same anatomic location. In particular, for the percutaneous valves, measurements should be performed immediately proximal to the stent (pre-stent region) rather than at the base of the prosthetic valve leaflets (in-stent precusp region). The rationale for using pre-stent measurements in

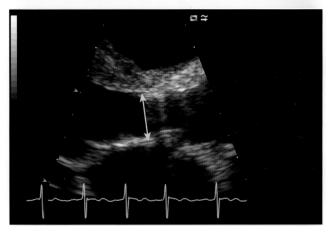

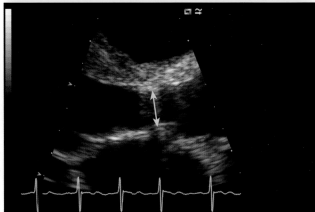

Figure 10.16 Two possible measurements of the left ventricular outflow tract (LVOT) diameter with an aortic valve replacement (AVR) are shown: the correct method (*top*) and the incorrect method (*bottom*). The correct method for measuring the LVOT diameter is approximately 5 mm from the aortic annulus, perpendicular to the aortic root, using the inner edge to inner edge technique (*top*). Incorrectly measuring the internal prosthesis dimension as the LVOT diameter will significantly underestimate the LVOT diameter and the resultant effective orifice area (*bottom*).

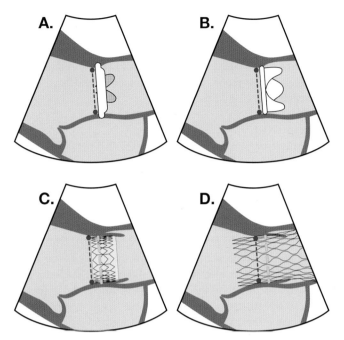

Figure 10.17 Measurements for the left ventricular outflow tract (LVOT) diameter in surgically placed and transcatheter aortic valves are illustrated. The red dashed line represents the LVOT diameter and the blue dashed line represents the level of the valve cusps in the transcatheter aortic valves. A & B: For surgically placed valves, the LVOT diameter is measured just proximal to the prosthetic valve. C: For the percutaneous valves, the LVOT diameter is measured at the apical end of the stent (pre-stent). D: For the self-expandable CoreValve where the stent sits low in the LVOT, the LVOT diameter is measured within the stent (in-stent) and just proximal to the valve cusps.

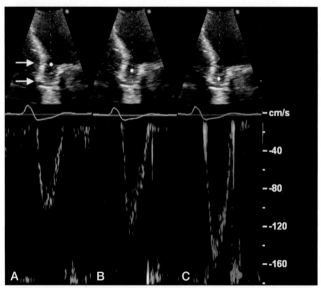

Figure 10.18 This figure demonstrates three discrete pulsed-wave Doppler spectra and sampling positions acquired from the apical 5-chamber view in an Edwards SAPIEN valve: A = pre-stent, B = in-stent precusp, and C = in-stent postcusp. There is flow acceleration in the stent proximal to the cusps (B) as well as additional flow acceleration distal to the cusps (C). The stent is identifiable as two parallel bright lines, the ends of which are indicated by the white arrows. The red arrow points to the position of the cusps. For calculating the effective orifice area and the Doppler velocity index, the sample volume should be placed in the pre-stent position (A). Reproduced from Shames S, Koczo A, Hahn R, Jin Z, Picard MH, Gillam LD. Flow characteristics of the SAPIEN aortic valve: the importance of recognizing in-stent flow acceleration for the echocardiographic assessment of valve function. *J Am Soc Echocardiogr.* Vol. 25(6), page 605, © 2012, with permission from Elsevier.

these valves is two-fold. Firstly, flow acceleration in the LVOT occurs at the in-stent position; therefore, the pulsed-wave Doppler sample volume should be placed in the pre-stent position and not at the in-stent precusp position. Secondly, the LVOT diameter should be measured at the same location as the VTI. The additional advantages of measuring the LVOT diameter pre-stent include: (1) the apical border of the stent provides more precise and reproducible anatomic landmarks for the LVOT diameter measurement, and (2) the pre-stent region avoids reverberation and acoustic shadowing artefacts over the cusps which occur due to fibrocalcific remodelling around the prosthesis. Importantly, if the CoreValve sits low into the LVOT then the LVOT diameter should be measured in-stent just proximal to the valve cusps (Fig. 10.17D).

Doppler Velocity Index

Doppler velocity index (DVI) is simply a dimensionless ratio that is derived from the LVOT VTI and the transprosthetic VTI. This ratio provides a quick and easy method for identifying prosthetic valve dysfunction (Table 10.7). Furthermore, as this index is not dependent on valve size, in an individual patient where the LVOT diameter can be assumed to remain constant, the DVI measured at an early post-operative study can serve as the patient's control value and, therefore, acts as a "finger-print" for that patient.

Calculation of this ratio differs according to the site of the prosthetic valve. For an AVR, the DVI is calculated as the ratio of the LVOT VTI (or peak velocity) and the AVR VTI (or peak velocity) (see Fig. 10.14):

Equation 10.5

$$DVI_{AVR} = V_{LVOT} \ (or \ VTI_{LVOT}) \div V_{AVR} \ (or \ VTI_{AVR})$$

where DVI_{AVR} = Doppler velocity index for aortic valve replacement (unitless)
V_{LVOT} = peak velocity at the LVOT (m/s)
VTI_{LVOT} = velocity time integral at the LVOT (cm)
V_{AVR} = peak velocity across the aortic valve replacement (m/s)
VTI_{AVR} = velocity time integral across the aortic valve replacement (cm)

For a MVR and a tricuspid valve replacement (TVR), the DVI is calculated as the ratio of the transprosthetic VTI and the LVOT VTI (Fig. 10.15):

Equation 10.6

$$DVI_{MVR} = VTI_{MVR} \div VTI_{LVOT}$$

where DVI_{MVR} = Doppler velocity index for mitral valve replacement (unitless)
VTI_{MVR} = velocity time integral across the mitral valve replacement (cm)
VTI_{LVOT} = velocity time integral at the LVOT (cm)

Equation 10.7

$$DVI_{TVR} = VTI_{TVR} \div VTI_{LVOT}$$

where DVI_{TVR} = Doppler velocity index for tricuspid valve replacement (unitless)
VTI_{TVR} = velocity time integral across the tricuspid valve replacement (cm)
VTI_{LVOT} = velocity time integral at the LVOT (cm)

Pressure Half-time

The diastolic slope of the Doppler velocity spectrum across the MVR reflects the pressure difference between the LA and LV over the diastolic period. Likewise, the diastolic slope of the Doppler velocity spectrum across a TVR reflects the pressure difference between the right atrium (RA) and the RV over the diastolic period. From these diastolic slopes, the pressure half-time (P½t) is measured as the time taken for the early diastolic pressure gradient to fall to half its original value (see Fig. 10.15).

Importantly, the P½t cannot be used to determine the EOA in a MVR or a TVR. This is because the constants used to estimate the EOA in native mitral and tricuspid stenosis have not been validated in prosthetic valves. In particular, estimation of the EOA for MVR using the P½t method tends to grossly overestimate the EOA [10.1-2]. However, while the P½t cannot be used to estimate the EOA, it still provides important information regarding the normality of prosthetic valve haemodynamics. For example, as for native stenosis, prolongation of the P½t is expected when there is MVR/TVR obstruction or stenosis. Furthermore, in MVRs, consideration of the P½t in combination with the peak E velocity and DVI can be used to distinguish between normal, obstructed, and regurgitant valves (see Table 10.7 and Fig. 10.19).

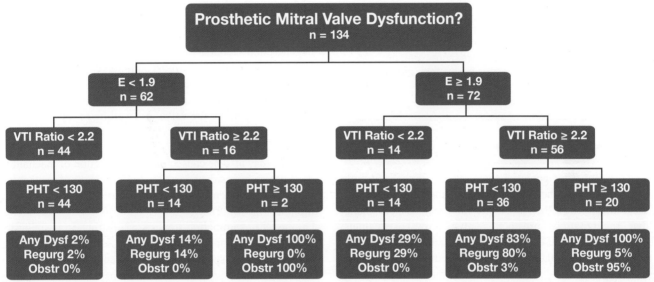

Figure 10.19 This flow chart shows the outcome of the 134 patients according to the various Doppler variables associated with prosthetic mitral valve dysfunction: peak early velocity (E) of mitral inflow (m/s), the VTI ratio (VTI$_{MVR}$/VTI$_{LVOT}$) and pressure half-time (PHT) (ms). The end of each branch of the tree depicts the conditional probability for the presence of significant prosthetic mitral valve dysfunction (regurgitation or stenosis). In 4 patients, VTI$_{LVOT}$ could not be determined and the PHT could also not be determined in 1 of these patients. Based on this flow chart, the likelihood of prosthetic dysfunction can be predicted. Dysf = dysfunction; Obstr = obstruction; Regurg = regurgitation.
Reproduced from Fernandes V, Olmos L, Nagueh SF, Quiñones MA, Zoghbi WA. Peak early diastolic velocity rather than pressure half-time is the best index of mechanical prosthetic mitral valve function. *Am J Cardiol.* Vol. 89(6), page 708, © 2002, with permission from Elsevier.

Table 10.7 Normal and Abnormal Doppler Velocity Indices (DVI)

Prosthetic Valve	Normal DVI	Abnormal DVI	Ref.
Aortic Valve	≥ 0.3	< 0.3 *	1
Mitral Valve	< 2.2 ψ	≥ 2.2 #	2
Tricuspid Valve	< 3.3 §	≥ 3.3 ^	3

* < 0.25 highly suggestive of significant valve obstruction

ψ Combination of transmitral E velocity < 1.9 m/s, DVI < 2.2, and pressure half-time (P½t) < 130 ms highly predictive of normal mechanical mitral valve prosthesis function

\# Higher values indicate possible prosthetic valve dysfunction (obstruction or regurgitation); combination of transmitral E velocity ≥ 1.9 m/s, DVI ≥ 2.2, and P½t < 130 ms suggests significant prosthetic and/or periprosthetic regurgitation for mechanical mitral valve prostheses; combination of transmitral E velocity ≥ 1.9 m/s, DVI ≥ 2.2, and P½t ≥ 130 ms suggests significant prosthetic obstruction for mechanical mitral valve prostheses

§ combination of transtricuspid E velocity < 2.1 m/s, DVI < 3.3, and P½t < 200 ms likely to be highly predictive of normal prosthetic tricuspid valve function

^ Higher values indicate possible prosthetic valve dysfunction (obstruction or regurgitation); combination of transtricuspid E velocity ≥ 2.1 m/s, DVI ≥ 3.3, and P½t < 200 ms suggests significant prosthetic and/or periprosthetic regurgitation

References (Ref.): [1] Zoghbi WA, Chambers JB, Dumesnil JG, et al. Recommendations for evaluation of prosthetic valves with echocardiography and Doppler ultrasound: a report From the American Society of Echocardiography's Guidelines and Standards Committee and the Task Force on Prosthetic Valves. *J Am Soc Echocardiogr.* 2009 Sep;22(9):975-1014. **[2]** Fernandes V, Olmos L, Nagueh SF, Quiñones MA, Zoghbi WA. Peak early diastolic velocity rather than pressure half-time is the best index of mechanical prosthetic mitral valve function. *Am J Cardiol.* 2002 Mar 15;89(6):704-10. **[3]** Blauwet LA, Danielson GK, Burkhart HM, Dearani JA, Malouf JF, Connolly HM, Hodge DO, Herges RM, Miller FA Jr. Comprehensive Echocardiographic Assessment of the Hemodynamic Parameters of 285 Tricuspid Valve Bioprostheses Early after Implantation. *J Am Soc Echocardiogr.* 2010 Oct;23(10):1045-1059.

[10.1] Dumesnil JG, Honos GN, Lemieux M, Beauchemin J. Validation and applications of mitral prosthetic valvular areas calculated by Doppler echocardiography. *Am J Cardiol.* 1990;65:1443–1448.
[10.2] Malouf JF, Ballo M, Connolly HM, Hodge DO, Herges RM, Mullany CJ, Miller FA. Doppler echocardiography of 119 normal-functioning St. Jude Medical mitral valve prostheses: a comprehensive assessment including time-velocity integral ratio and prosthesis performance index. *J Am Soc Echocardiogr* 2005; 18:252-256.

Mitral Valve Repairs

Mitral valve repairs should be assessed in the same manner as prosthetic mitral valves. In particular, haemodynamic parameters measured for mitral valve repairs include: (1) the peak transmitral velocities, (2) the mean pressure gradient, (3) the pressure half-time, and (4) the effective orifice area (EOA). Importantly, the EOA via the continuity equation is based on the assumption that the stroke volume across the mitral valve and through the LVOT is the same; therefore, the EOA can only be estimated when MR and AR is graded as 1/4 or less. In addition, as for a prosthetic MVR, the pressure half-time cannot be used to estimate the EOA.

Tricuspid Valve Repairs

The haemodynamic parameters measured for tricuspid valve repairs include: (1) the peak transtricuspid velocities, and (2) the mean pressure gradient. As transtricuspid velocities vary over the respiratory period, measurements should be averaged over a full respiratory cycle.

Complications of Prosthetic Valves

There are numerous potential complications associated with prosthetic valves; these complications include prosthesis-patient mismatch (PPM), prosthetic valve stenosis, prosthetic valve regurgitation, prosthetic valve thrombosis/pannus formation, prosthetic valve dehiscence, and prosthetic valve endocarditis (Fig. 10.20). Pericardial haematoma following cardiac surgery and haematoma around the aorta following AVR are other potential complications which may occur in the early post-operative period.

Prosthesis-Patient Mismatch

PPM occurs when a normally functioning prosthetic valve is too small in relation to the patient's body size; this leads to abnormally high transprosthetic gradients compared with the normal range for the valve subtype and size. Recognition of PPM is important as this condition is associated with suboptimal haemodynamic stasis, reduced exercise tolerance, more adverse cardiac events and lower survival. The best method of identifying PPM is based on the EOA indexed to the BSA (IEOA). IEOA values used to identify and to quantify PPM in the aortic, mitral and tricuspid positions are listed in Table 10.8. Other clues to the presence of PPM include elevated transprosthetic gradients in the setting of normal prosthetic leaflet/disc motion with no significant change in the EOA or DVI compared with the baseline or serial studies.

Importantly, as PPM leads to abnormally high transprosthetic gradients it may be confused with prosthetic valve stenosis; these two conditions can be differentiated by considering a number of variables (see Prosthetic Valve Stenosis below).

> PPM is more commonly encountered in aortic prostheses. However, PPM associated with mitral and/or tricuspid prostheses may be seen in individuals in whom a small prosthesis was inserted in early childhood.

Prosthetic Valve Stenosis/Obstruction

The aetiology of prosthetic valve stenosis or obstruction is dependent on the valve type. In the bioprosthetic valves, stenosis is typically caused by leaflet thickening and degeneration secondary to fibrocalcific changes (Fig. 10.21). In mechanical valves, the most common cause of obstruction is thrombosis and/or pannus formation. Mechanical valve obstruction may also occur due to a faulty disc design, acute dehiscence of the valve, or swelling of the poppet in a ball-caged valve (so-called poppet-cage variance). In patients who have a MVR with cordal preservation, functional MVR stenosis may also be caused by the obstruction of mechanical disc motion by residual cordal tissue. Evidence of mechanical valve obstruction may be seen as restricted mechanical disc motion (Fig. 10.22).

On the CFI examination stenosis or obstruction is suggested by the presence of turbulent flow across the valve (see Fig. 10.13). On the spectral Doppler examination stenosis or obstruction is suggested by high transprosthetic velocities and pressure gradients, a decrease in the EOA, a decrease in the DVI for AVRs, and an increase in the DVI and prolongation of the P½t in MVRs and/or TVRs. Tables 10.9 and 10.10 summarise the Doppler echocardiographic criteria for detection and quantification of prosthetic valve stenosis.

> With mechanical valves, the mobility of the occluder is often difficult to visualise due to reverberation and acoustic shadowing artefacts. However, reverberation artefacts can be very useful. For example, in a normal bileaflet tilting disc valve, symmetrical reverberation artefacts during opening and closing of the valve are expected; the presence of a fixed reverberation artefact suggests that the disc remains in a fixed closed position over the cardiac cycle (see Fig. 10.22). Likewise an absent reverberation artefact suggests that the disc remains in a fixed open position over the cardiac cycle.

Table 10.8 Threshold Values of Indexed Effective Orifice Area (IEOA) for the Identification and Quantification of PPM in Aortic, Mitral and Tricuspid Prostheses

	Mild or not clinically significant PPM	Moderate PPM	Severe PPM	Ref.
IEOA (AVR) (cm²/m²)	> 0.85	0.85 – 0.66	≤ 0.65	1
IEOA (MVR) (cm²/m²)	> 1.2	1.2 – 1.0	≤ 0.9	1
IEOA (TVR) (cm²/m²)	-	-	≤ 0.9	2

AVR = aortic valve replacement; MVR = mitral valve replacement; TVR = tricuspid valve replacement

References (Ref.): [1] Pibarot P, Dumesnil JG. Prosthetic heart valves: selection of the optimal prosthesis and long-term management. *Circulation*. 2009 Feb 24;119(7):1034-48. **[2]** Blauwet LA, Burkhart HM, Dearani JA, Malouf JF, Connolly HM, Hodge DO, Herges RM, Miller FA Jr. Comprehensive echocardiographic assessment of mechanical tricuspid valve prostheses based on early post-implantation echocardiographic studies. *J Am Soc Echocardiogr*. 2011 Apr;24(4):414-24.

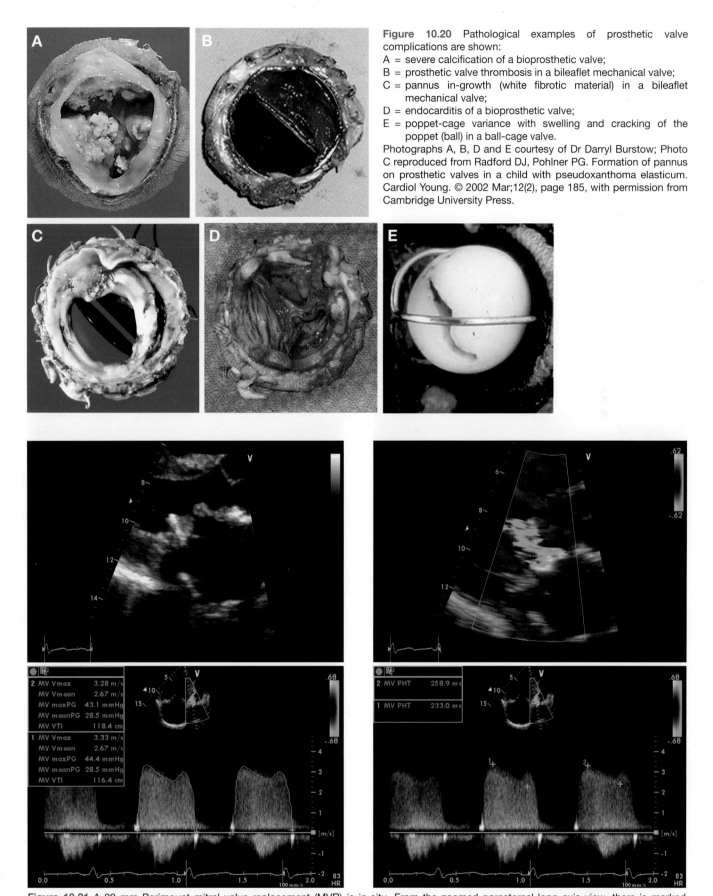

Figure 10.20 Pathological examples of prosthetic valve complications are shown:

A = severe calcification of a bioprosthetic valve;

B = prosthetic valve thrombosis in a bileaflet mechanical valve;

C = pannus in-growth (white fibrotic material) in a bileaflet mechanical valve;

D = endocarditis of a bioprosthetic valve;

E = poppet-cage variance with swelling and cracking of the poppet (ball) in a ball-cage valve.

Photographs A, B, D and E courtesy of Dr Darryl Burstow; Photo C reproduced from Radford DJ, Pohlner PG. Formation of pannus on prosthetic valves in a child with pseudoxanthoma elasticum. Cardiol Young. © 2002 Mar;12(2), page 185, with permission from Cambridge University Press.

Figure 10.21 A 29 mm Perimount mitral valve replacement (MVR) is in-situ. From the zoomed parasternal long axis view, there is marked thickening of the bioprosthetic mitral valve leaflets (*top, left*). The corresponding colour flow Doppler image confirms the presence of turbulent flow across the valve which is consistent with prosthetic valve stenosis (*top, right*). On the spectral Doppler traces recorded across the MVR, the peak early diastolic velocity (MV Vmax) and the mean pressure gradient (MV meanPG) are markedly elevated at 3.3 m/s and 29 mm Hg, respectively (*bottom, left*); the pressure half-time (MV PHT) is also prolonged at 233-259 ms (*bottom, right*).

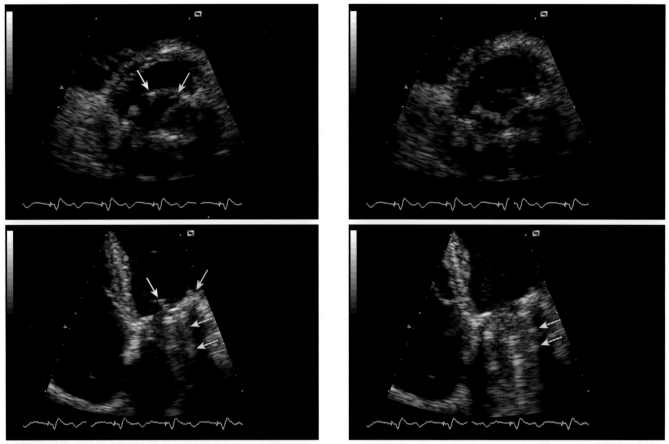

Figure 10.22 A 29 mm ATS mitral valve replacement is in-situ. Images are recorded from a zoomed parasternal short axis view (*top*) and an apical 4-chamber view (*bottom*); the images on the left are diastolic frames and the images on the right are systolic frames. Observe that during diastole only the medial disc is opening (*white arrow*) and the lateral disc is struck closed (*yellow arrow*). Also observe that in the apical 4-chamber view the reverberation artefacts arising from the struck lateral disc do not vary between the diastolic and systolic frames (*blue arrows*); this is a clue to the presence of a stuck prosthetic valve disc.

Table 10.9 **Doppler Echocardiographic Criteria for Detection and Quantification of Prosthetic Aortic and/or Mitral Stenosis/Obstruction**

Aortic Valves *	Normal	Possible stenosis	Suggests severe stenosis
Peak velocity (m/s) †	< 3	3 - 4	> 4
Mean gradient (mm Hg) †	< 20	20 - 35	> 35
DVI	≥ 0.30	0.29 - 0.25	< 0.25
EOA (cm²)	> 1.2	1.2 - 0.8	< 0.8
Contour of AVR jet ††	Triangular, early peaking	Triangular to intermediate	Rounded, symmetrical
Acceleration time (ms) ††	< 80	80 - 100	> 100
Mitral Valves	**Normal ****	**Possible stenosis δ**	**Suggests severe stenosis**δ**
Peak velocity (m/s) # §	< 1.9	1.9 – 2.5	≥ 2.5
Mean gradient (mm Hg) # §	≤ 5	6 - 10	> 10
DVI # §	< 2.2	2.2 – 2.5	> 2.5
EOA (cm²)	≥ 2.0	1.0 – 2.0	< 1.0
P½t (ms)	< 130	130 – 200	> 200

DVI = Doppler velocity index; EOA = effective orifice area; P½t = pressure half-time.
* In conditions of normal or near normal stroke volume (50-70 mL) through the aortic valve.
† These parameters are more affected by flow, including low cardiac output and concomitant prosthetic valve regurgitation.
†† These parameters are highly influenced by left ventricular chronotropy and function.
** Best specificity for normality or abnormality is seen if the majority of the parameters listed are normal or abnormal, respectively.
δ Values of the parameters should prompt a closer evaluation of valve function and/or other considerations such as increased flow, increased heart rate, or prosthesis-patient mismatch.
Slightly higher cut-off values than shown may be seen in some bioprosthetic valves.
§ These parameters are also abnormal in the presence of significant prosthetic mitral valve regurgitation.
Adapted from Zoghbi WA, Chambers JB, Dumesnil JG, et al. Recommendations for evaluation of prosthetic valves with echocardiography and Doppler ultrasound: a report From the American Society of Echocardiography's Guidelines and Standards Committee and the Task Force on Prosthetic Valves. *J Am Soc Echocardiogr.* 2009 Sep;22(9):975-1014.

Importantly, elevated gradients across prosthetic valves are not only caused by prosthetic valve stenosis or obstruction; elevated gradients may also occur secondary to PPM (discussed above), high flow conditions (high output states), prosthetic valve regurgitation, or rapid pressure recovery (RPR). For example, recall that RPR can result in localised high transvalvular velocities (see Chapter 1). RPR may be encountered in the small-sized bileaflet mechanical valves where the velocity at the smaller central orifice is higher than the velocities at the larger lateral orifices. Therefore, measuring velocities through the central orifice leads to overestimation of pressure gradients and an underestimation of EOA. While this phenomenon is usually only problematic in the small-sized bileaflet AVR (19–21 mm), it has also been observed in ball-cage prostheses.

Table 10.10 Doppler Echocardiographic Criteria for Detection of Prosthetic Tricuspid Stenosis

	Consider stenosis*
Peak velocity (m/s) †	> 1.7
Mean gradient (mm Hg) †	≥ 6
P½t (ms)	≥ 230

P½t = pressure half-time.
* Because of respiratory variation, average ≥ 5 cycles.
† May be increased also with concomitant prosthetic valve regurgitation.
Source: Zoghbi WA, Chambers JB, Dumesnil JG, et al. Recommendations for evaluation of prosthetic valves with echocardiography and Doppler ultrasound: a report From the American Society of Echocardiography's Guidelines and Standards Committee and the Task Force on Prosthetic Valves. *J Am Soc Echocardiogr.* 2009 Sep;22(9):1001.

In addition, if the aorta is of a small diameter, RPR within the aorta immediately distal to an AVR may also occur further exaggerating this phenomenon.

Algorithms for interpreting the cause of elevated transprosthetic pressure gradients after aortic or mitral valve replacement are illustrated in Figures 10.23-10.24.

Stress Echocardiography in Prosthetic Valves

As for native aortic and mitral valve disease, stress echocardiography can be useful in patients with prosthetic valves. Essentially stress echocardiography may be useful in two groups of patients with suspected prosthetic valve obstruction or PPM: (1) symptomatic patients with discordant resting transprosthetic haemodynamics, and (2) patients with a reduced transprosthetic EOA and low transprosthetic gradients in the setting of low flow states.

In symptomatic patients with discordant resting transprosthetic haemodynamics, the presence of significant prosthetic valve obstruction or PPM is expected when there is a rise in the mean AVR pressure gradient > 15mm Hg with stress or if the mean MVR pressure gradient rises above 18 mm Hg with stress [10.3].

Patients with a reduced transprosthetic EOA and low transprosthetic gradients in the setting of low flow states may have "true" prosthetic valve stenosis or PPM, or "pseudo" prosthetic valve stenosis or PPM. In both settings, the low flow state caused by LV systolic dysfunction is responsible for a reduced prosthetic EOA. As in low flow, low gradient AS, dobutamine stress echo can be used to differentiate between true stenosis/PPM and pseudo stenosis/PPM (Fig. 10.25). Importantly, Dobutamine stress echocardiography does not

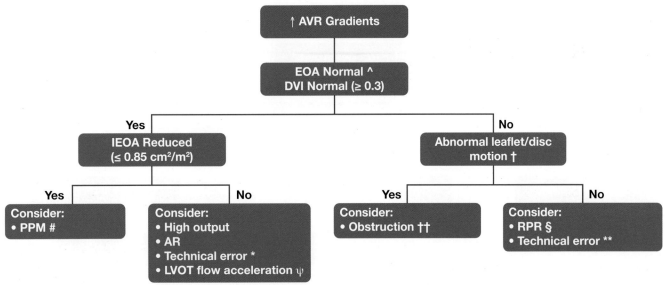

Figure 10.23 Algorithm for interpreting elevated transprosthetic pressure gradients after aortic valve replacement (AVR).
DVI = Doppler velocity index; EOA = effective orifice area; IEOA = indexed effective orifice area; LVOT = left ventricular outflow tract; PPM = Prosthesis-patient mismatch; RPR = rapid pressure recovery.
^ Normal values compared with normal range for valve subtype and size
#IEOA and DVI unchanged compared with baseline study
* Consider overestimation of LVOT diameter and/or LVOT velocity time integral (sample volume placed too close to AVR)
† If leaflet/disc motion unclear by transthoracic echocardiography, consider cinefluoroscopy
†† Consider significant prosthetic valve obstruction when AVR signal has a rounded velocity contour or AVR signal that peaks in mid-systole, when acceleration time (AT) is prolonged (> 100 ms) and when the AT to left ventricular ejection time ratio is > 0.37
§ Bileaflet valves only, small AVR size (19-21 mm)
ψ Recalculate EOA using RVOT stroke volume (only in absence of significant aortic or pulmonary regurgitation, RVOT obstruction, or intracardiac shunt)
** Consider underestimation of LVOT diameter and/or LVOT velocity time integral (sample volume placed too far from AVR)

[10.3] Zoghbi WA, Chambers JB, Dumesnil JG, et al. Recommendations for evaluation of prosthetic valves with echocardiography and Doppler ultrasound: a report From the American Society of Echocardiography's Guidelines and Standards Committee and the Task Force on Prosthetic Valves. *J Am Soc Echocardiogr.* 2009 Sep;22(9):975-1014.

distinguish between prosthetic valve stenosis and PPM. For this purpose, the EOA after normalisation of the cardiac output following stress echocardiography should be considered (see Figures 10.23-10.24).

Prosthesis Valve Regurgitation

As previously stated, most mechanical prostheses have mild physiological closing and leakage volume regurgitation and this normal in-built regurgitation should be recognised and differentiated from pathological leaks.

On CFI, physiological regurgitant jets are usually short, narrow and non-turbulent. The size and number of these normal regurgitant jets depends upon the valve design. For example, in the bileaflet valves there are one to two central jets and two peripheral jets while in the ball-caged valves there is usually one central closing volume jet.

Pathological regurgitation may be transvalvular and/or paravalvular. As for prosthetic valve stenosis/obstruction, the aetiology of pathological prosthetic valve regurgitation

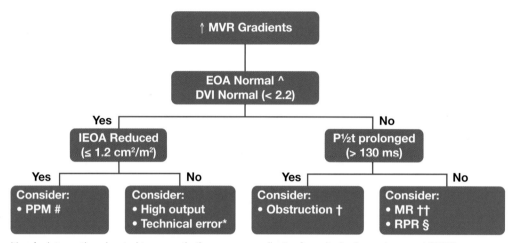

Figure 10.24 Algorithm for interpreting elevated transprosthetic pressure gradients after mitral valve replacement (MVR).
DVI = Doppler velocity index; EOA = effective orifice area; IEOA = indexed effective orifice area; MR = mitral regurgitation; P½t = pressure half-time; PPM = Prosthesis-patient mismatch; RPR = rapid pressure recovery.
^ Normal values compared with normal range for valve subtype and size
\#IEOA and DVI unchanged compared with baseline study
† Consider transoesophageal echocardiography and/or cinefluoroscopy to confirm
† † Consider transoesophageal echocardiography to confirm
§ Rarely encountered in MVR, consider when small-sized bileaflet MVR in-situ
* Consider overestimation of LVOT diameter and/or LVOT velocity time integral (sample volume placed too close to aortic valve)

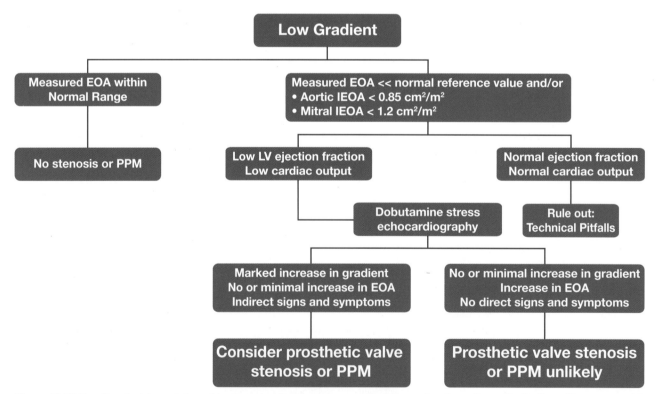

Figure 10.25 Algorithm for interpretation of low transprosthetic pressure gradients in conjunction with small effective orifice areas and low left ventricular (LV) ejection fraction.
EOA = effective orifice area; IEOA = indexed effective orifice area; PPM = Prosthesis-patient mismatch.
Reproduced from Pibarot P, Dumesil JG and Magne J. Chapter 20 Prosthetic Valve Dysfunction, page 456. In: Valvular Heart Disease, Edited by: Wang A and Bashore TM, © 2009 Humana Press; with kind permission from Springer Science+Business Media B.V.

is dependent on the valve type. In the bioprosthetic valves, transvalvular regurgitation is typically caused by leaflet degeneration. In mechanical valves, the most common cause of transvalvular regurgitation is thrombosis and/or pannus formation which prevents complete closure of the discs.

Paravalvular regurgitation can occur due to prosthetic valve dehiscence and other associated abnormalities of the valve bed such as vegetations or fibrosis, and calcification of the native annulus. In the TAVI valves, paravalvular AR may occur due to incomplete prosthesis apposition to the native annulus due to ridges of calcium, implantation of the valve too low or too deep leading to paravalvular leakage through uncovered portions of the prosthesis, or implantation of a prosthesis too small for the valve annulus.

The Doppler assessment of prosthetic valve regurgitation is assessed by the standard qualitative and quantitative parameters used for native valve regurgitation (Table 10.11). Each of these parameters is discussed in detail within the relevant chapters for each native valve. Importantly, CFI is especially useful in distinguishing between transvalvular and paravalvular regurgitation; transvalvular regurgitation occurs within the sewing ring while paravalvular regurgitation arises outside the sewing ring, between the sewing ring and the valve annulus (Fig. 10.26).

As for the CFI assessment of native valve regurgitation, the evaluation of prosthetic valve regurgitation should be performed in multiple views and at multiple imaging planes including off-axis imaging. In particular, for AVRs the best plane for assessing paravalvular AR is generally just below the annulus while the best plane for assessing transvalvular AR is just below the prosthetic valve cusps. The severity of paravalvular AR can be estimated by the percentage of the sewing ring circumference that is occupied by the regurgitant jet (Fig. 10.27).

In patients with a mechanical MVR, assessment of prosthetic valve regurgitation by transthoracic echocardiography (TTE) is especially difficult. This is due to imaging artefacts distal to the MVR which obscure the LA so the MR jet area is difficult to image. A clue to the presence of significant prosthetic valve MR is the presence of systolic flow convergence on the LV side of the MVR (Fig. 10.28). Other indirect spectral Doppler clues of significant MR include: (1) the presence of a strong MR CW Doppler signal, (2) increased transmitral flow velocities (and mean pressure gradients) in the absence of prosthetic stenosis, PPM or high output states, (3) an increased DVI, and/or (4) an increased RVSP. In particular, a DVI $\geq$ 2.2 in combination with a peak transprosthetic E velocity $\geq$ 1.9 m/s and a P½t < 130 ms are suggestive of significant prosthetic MVR regurgitation (see Fig. 10.19).

As for native valve regurgitation, the assessment of chamber size, ventricular systolic function, and pulmonary pressures is also important.

> Paravalvular regurgitation is always abnormal. An important clinical sign suggestive of paravalvular regurgitation is the presence of haemolysis. Haemolysis, or the release of haemoglobin from red blood cells (RBC), occurs secondary to RBC destruction as RBC are "squeezed" through the rigid, small paravalvular orifice.

Prosthetic Valve Thrombosis/Pannus Formation

Prosthetic valve thrombus (PVT) refers to the formation of a blood clot around the prosthetic valve. PVT frequently interferes with prosthetic valve function; in particular, the valve may be stuck closed resulting in significant obstruction, or stuck open resulting in significant regurgitation. PVT may occur in both mechanical and bioprosthetic valves but is more commonly seen in mechanical valves where there is inadequate antithrombotic therapy (international normalized ratio [INR] $\leq$ 2.5).

Pannus refers to a slow in-growth of fibrous tissue over the prosthetic valve sewing ring. This is a healing response whereby excessive scarring or keloid formation occurs. Pannus formation has been observed in both mechanical and bioprosthetic valves but is more commonly encountered with mechanical valves. This abnormal over-exuberant

Table 10.11 Qualitative and Quantitative Doppler Parameters for Grading Prosthetic Valve Regurgitation Severity

Prosthetic Valve	Qualitative CFI Parameters	Qualitative Spectral Doppler Parameters	Quantitative Parameters
Aortic position	• Jet height ratio • Jet area ratio • Vena contracta width	• Intensity of AR CW jet • AR P½t • Diastolic flow reversal (desc. & abdo. aorta)	• Regurgitant volume • Regurgitant fraction
Mitral position	• Jet area ratio • Vena contracta width • Flow convergence radius	• Pulmonary venous PW • Intensity of MR CW jet • MR jet contour	• Regurgitant volume • Regurgitant fraction • Effective regurgitant orifice area
Tricuspid position	• Jet area • Vena contracta width • Flow convergence radius	• Hepatic venous PW • Intensity of TR CW jet • TR jet contour	-
Pulmonary position	• Jet width	• Diastolic flow reversal (branch PA) • Intensity of PR CW jet • Deceleration of PR	-

abdo. = abdominal; AR = aortic regurgitation; CFI = colour flow imaging; CW = continuous wave Doppler; desc. = descending; MR = mitral regurgitation; P½t = pressure half-time; PA = pulmonary arteries; PR = pulmonary regurgitation; PW = pulsed wave Doppler; TR = tricuspid regurgitation.

Panel A

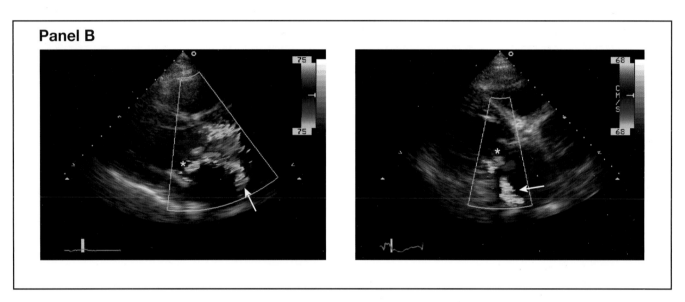

Panel B

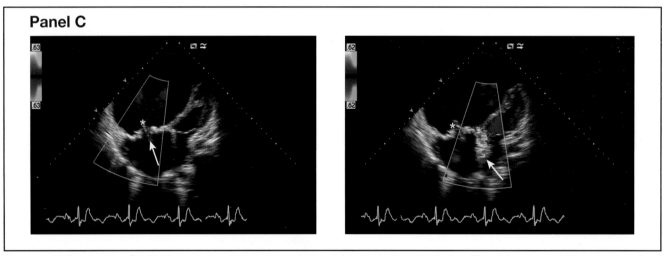

Panel C

Figure 10.26 These colour Doppler images demonstrate transvalvular and paravalvular regurgitation. The white arrows indicate the regurgitant jet(s) and yellow stars indicate the centre of the region between the prosthetic valve sewing ring.

Panel A: Zoomed parasternal long axis views from two different patients: mild transvalvular aortic regurgitation (AR) in an allograft AVR (*left*) and moderate paravalvular AR in a percutaneous valve (*right*) are shown.

Panel B: Parasternal long axis views from two different patients with a stented bioprosthetic mitral valve. Anteriorly directed transvalvular mitral regurgitation (MR) (*left*) and posteriorly directed moderate paravalvular MR (*right*) are shown. Observe that off-axis imaging was required to demonstrate the paravalvular MR.

Panel C: Apical 4-chamber views from the same patient with a stented bioprosthetic tricuspid valve replacement: trace transvalvular tricuspid regurgitation (TR) (*left*) and moderate paravalvular TR (*right*) are shown. Observe that transvalvular regurgitation occurs within the sewing ring while paravalvular regurgitation arises outside the sewing ring, between the sewing ring and the valve annulus.

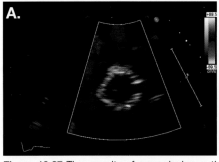 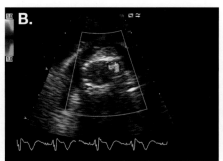 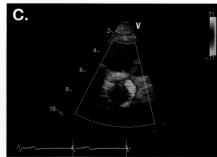

Figure 10.27 The severity of paravalvular aortic regurgitation (PAR) can be estimated by assessing the circumferential extent of the paravalvular regurgitant jet. PAR is graded as mild when the jet(s) occupies <10%of the sewing ring (A), moderate when the jet(s) occupy 10% to 20% of the sewing ring (B), and severe when the jet(s) occupy >20% of the sewing ring (C). Alternatively, considering that there are 60 minutes around a clock face, then mild PAR is < 6 minutes of the clock face, moderate PAR is 6-12 minutes of the clock face and severe PAR is > 12 minutes of the clock face.

fibrous reaction, which usually develops over many years, may interfere with occluder/leaflet motion and may narrow the orifice of the prosthesis resulting in significant obstruction. Secondary thrombus formation can also occur.

As stated above, both thrombus and pannus may lead to prosthetic valve obstruction. Initial echocardiographic clues to the presence of thrombus/pannus include: (1) an increase in transprosthetic pressure gradients compared with the baseline study or compared with established normal values, (2) a reduced EOA compared with the baseline study or compared with established normal values, (3) reduced or absent prosthetic leaflets/disc mobility, and/or (4) the visualisation of the echogenic material around the prosthetic valve.

The distinction between thrombus and pannus is important as the management strategies for each is different. For example, PVT may be treatable with thrombolytic therapy while thrombolysis is ineffective in pannus. Severe prosthetic valve obstruction due to pannus formation or PVT which does not resolve with thrombolytic therapy may require a repeat valve replacement. Echocardiographic and clinical parameters that are useful in differentiating between PVT and pannus formation are listed in Table 10.12 and are illustrated in Figure 10.29.

In patients with PVT, serial Doppler studies have an important role in guiding the duration and the efficacy of

thrombolytic therapy. A successful haemodynamic response to thrombolytic therapy is the normalisation of transprosthetic pressure gradients and prosthetic disc/occluder motion.

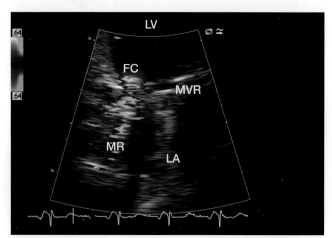

Figure 10.28 This systolic still frame image was recorded from a zoomed apical 4-chamber view; a 31 mm bileaflet mitral valve replacement (MVR) is in-situ. Observe that there is a dome of systolic flow convergence (FC) on the left ventricular (LV) side of the MVR. This is a clue to the presence of significant transprosthetic mitral regurgitation (MR). As the FC arises outside the sewing ring, paravalvular MR is most likely.
LA = left atrium.

Table 10.12 **Parameters for Differentiating Prosthetic Valve Thrombus from Pannus Formation**

Parameters	Thrombus	Pannus
Clinical	• Time from valve surgery to valve malfunction shorter (≈ 2 months) • Symptom duration before reoperation shorter (< 1 month) • Inadequate anticoagulation *	• Time from valve surgery to valve malfunction longer (> 12 months) • Symptom duration before reoperation longer (≈ 10 months) • Adequate anticoagulation*
Echocardiography	• Larger • Soft tissue appearance (similar to myocardium) • Mobile • Extension of mass beyond limits of prosthetic valve ring to adjacent cardiac structures • More common in MVR than AVR	• Smaller • Echo dense appearance • Firmly fixed • Annular location (along valvular plane) • More common in AVR than MVR

* Adequate anticoagulation defined as International Normalized Ratio (INR) ≥ 2.5 at the time of diagnosis
AVR = aortic valve replacement; MVR = mitral valve replacement
Source: Barbetseas J, Nagueh SF, Pitsavos C, Toutouzas PK, Quiñones MA, Zoghbi WA. Differentiating thrombus from pannus formation in obstructed mechanical prosthetic valves: an evaluation of clinical, transthoracic and transesophageal echocardiographic parameters. *J Am Coll Cardiol.* 1998 Nov;32(5):1410-7.

Prosthetic Valve Dehiscence

Prosthetic valve dehiscence (PVD) refers to partial separation of the prosthetic sewing ring from the native valve annulus. This is a serious prosthetic valve complication as it can result in significant obstruction to forward flow as well as significant paravalvular regurgitation. The aetiology of prosthetic valve dehiscence includes "unraveling" of the sutures or the pulling away of the prosthetic valve from the native valve annulus secondary to infective endocarditis.

The characteristic 2D echo appearance of prosthetic valve dehiscence is "rocking" of the prosthetic valve at an angle far in excess of its normal excursion (Fig. 10.30). Evidence of an echo-free space between the prosthetic valve and native valve annulus with associated paravalvular regurgitation is also another clue to PVD (Fig. 10.31).

PVD can also occur following a modified Bentall procedure whereby a bioprosthetic valved conduit is inserted within the native aortic root. PVD following this procedure may result in the compression of, and therefore significant obstruction to, the prosthetic valve as blood flow enters the space between the native aortic root and the conduit (Fig. 10.32).

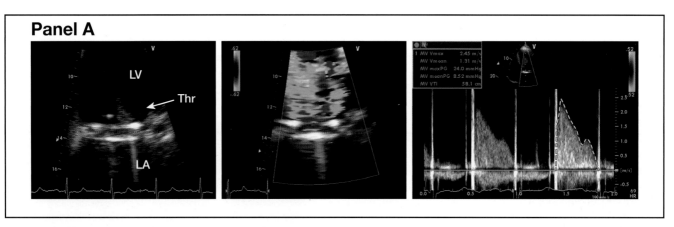

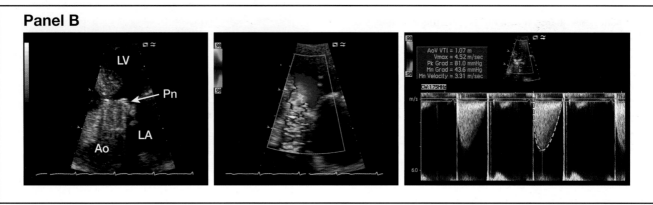

Figure 10.29 Panel A: Echocardiographic images of a bileaflet mitral valve replacement (MVR) recorded from zoomed apical 4-chamber are shown. Thrombus (Thr) appears as a soft tissue mass on the left ventricular (LV) side of the MVR (*left*). Obstruction of the valve is confirmed by colour flow imaging (*middle*). The mean pressure gradient across the MVR is 9 mm Hg (*right*). **Panel B:** Echocardiographic images of a bileaflet aortic valve replacement (AVR) recorded from zoomed apical 5-chamber are shown. Pannus (Pn) appears as a dense echogenic mass at the lateral aspect of the AVR (*left*). Obstruction to the valve is confirmed by colour flow imaging (*middle*). The maximum pressure gradient across the AVR is 81 mm Hg with a mean pressure gradient of 44 mm Hg (*right*).
Ao = aorta; LA = left atrium.

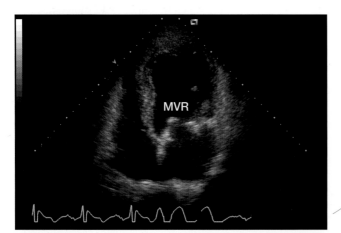 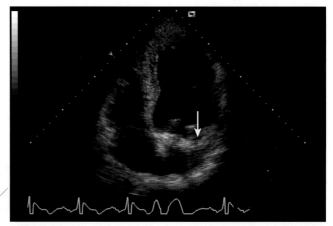

Figure 10.30 These two images of a bioprosthetic mitral valve replacement (MVR) are recorded from the apical 4 chamber view. Observe the marked displacement of the lateral aspect of the MVR (*arrow*) on the systolic frame (*right*) compared with the diastolic frame (*left*). On real-time imaging excessive "rocking" of the MVR was observed. This appearance is characteristic of acute prosthetic valve dehiscence.

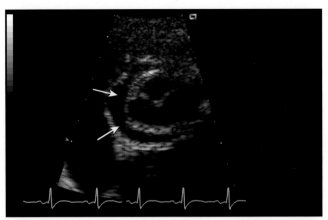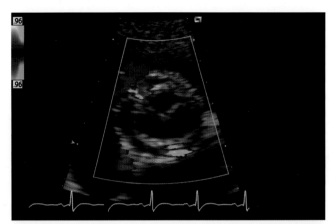

Figure 10.31 These images of a 25 mm stentless aortic valve replacement (AVR) were recorded from a zoomed parasternal short axis of the AVR. Observe the separation of the AVR from the aortic annulus (*left, arrows*); this appearance is characteristic of partial prosthetic valve dehiscence. The colour flow Doppler image also reveals the presence of paravalvular aortic regurgitation between the sewing ring and the AVR (*right*).

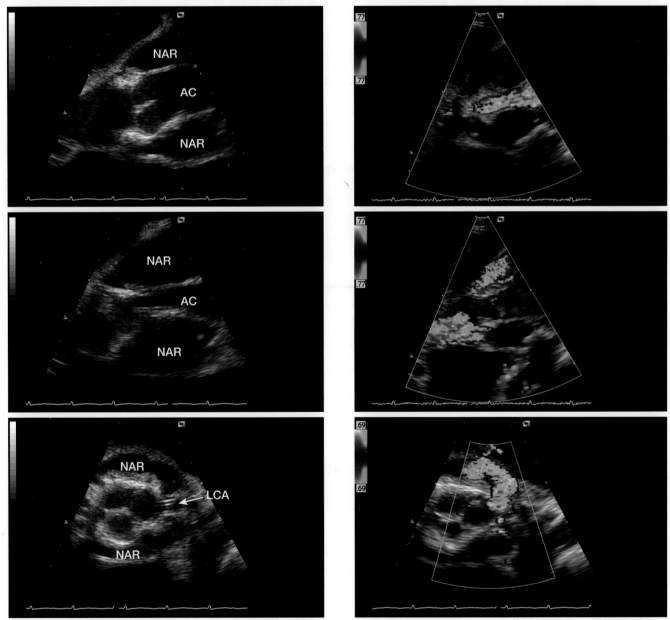

Figure 10.32 These images were recorded from a patient who had an Allograft conduit (AC) inserted within the native aortic root (NAR). From a zoomed parasternal long axis view, diastolic and systolic frames are shown (*top & middle, respectively*). Dehiscence of the proximal anastomosis site is evident by the separation between the NAR and the AC. During systole, blood flow into this space results in compression of the Allograft causing severe obstruction to outflow; observe the turbulent flow within the conduit on the colour Doppler image (*top, right*). During diastole, significant valvular and paravalvular aortic regurgitation (AR) is also evident (*middle, right*). From a zoomed parasternal short axis view (*bottom, left*), the likely origin of dehiscence appears to be at the reimplantation site of the left coronary artery (LCA) into the conduit; the colour Doppler image also pinpoints the origin of dehiscence at this site (*bottom, right*).

Prosthetic Valve Endocarditis

Prosthetic valve endocarditis (PVE) is another serious complication which occurs due to an infection of the prosthetic valve leaflets (bioprosthetic valves) or between the sewing ring and the native valve annulus (bioprosthetic and mechanical valves).

The characteristic echocardiographic features of vegetations include an independently hypermobile mass which has a different echo appearance to underlying tissue; vegetations may also intermittently or persistently impair valve closure and valve opening resulting in varying degrees of prosthetic valve regurgitation and/or stenosis (Fig. 10.33-10.36).

Endocarditis can be further complicated by leaflet perforation (bioprosthetic valves) valve bed abnormalities, such as paravalvular abscesses, dehiscence and paravalvular regurgitation, fistula, or pseudoaneurysms (Fig. 10.37).

The detection of PVE is very challenging by TTE due to imaging artefacts produced by and occurring around the prosthetic valve. TOE has a higher sensitivity and specificity for the detection of PVE due to its superior spatial and temporal resolution; therefore, when the TTE findings are inconclusive and the clinical suspicion for PVE is high, TOE is required. TOE is also valuable for the early detection of valve bed complications associated with PVE.

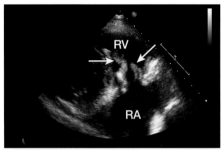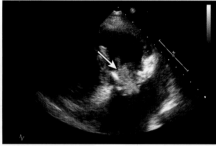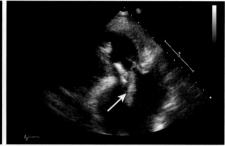

Figure 10.33 This series of images, recorded from the parasternal long axis of right ventricular (RV) inflow, was acquired in a patient with a bioprosthetic tricuspid valve replacement who presented with suspected infective endocarditis. Observe the very large, echogenic mass attached to the tricuspid valve (*arrows*). The mobility of the mass can be appreciated over the cardiac cycle: diastole (*left*), mid systole (*middle*) and late systole (*right*). RA = right atrium.

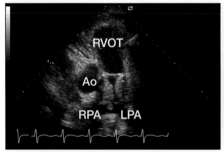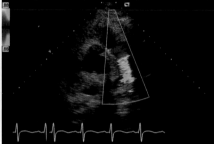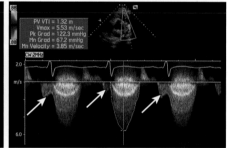

Figure 10.34 This series of images was acquired from a patient with a pulmonary valve conduit who presented with a staphylococcal sepsis. Observe on the 2D images, recorded from a parasternal short axis view, that there is diffuse narrowing of the pulmonary conduit secondary to marked soft tissue thickening of the conduit walls (*left*). A large mass attached to the distal end of the conduit, immediately proximal to the pulmonary artery bifurcation, is also seen; on real-time imaging this mass was independently mobile. Colour flow imaging reveals turbulent flow through the conduit (*middle*). The continuous-wave Doppler examination confirms the presence of significant obstruction with a peak pressure gradient of 122 mm Hg and a mean pressure gradient of 67 mm Hg (*right*). Pre-systolic flow across the pulmonary valve is also observed (*arrows*); this indicates that there is marked increase in the right ventricular diastolic pressure which exceeds the pulmonary artery diastolic pressure resulting in premature opening of the pulmonary valve.
Ao = aorta; LPA = left pulmonary artery; RPA = right pulmonary artery; RVOT = right ventricular outflow tract.

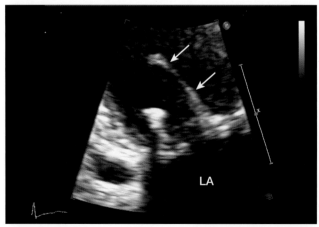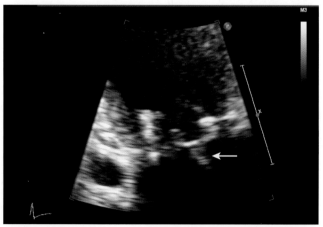

Figure 10.35 These zoomed apical 2-chamber view images were recorded from a patient with a 29mm Mosaic mitral valve replacement and infective endocarditis. In diastole (*left*), a large, elongated echodense mass attached to the anterior leaflet is seen (*arrow*); in systole (*right*), this mass can be seen to prolapse into the left atrium (LA) (*arrow*).

Furthermore, TOE allows improved visualisation of the LA surface of the MVR which is virtually always obscured by artefactual echoes on TTE.

Infective endocarditis is also discussed in greater detail in Chapter 13.

> Differentiation between vegetations and other echogenic masses, such as pannus, thrombus, sutures, torn cusps, or residual cordal tissue, is very difficult. However, consideration of the clinical presentation as well as comparison of the current study with the baseline study is very useful in determining the nature of these masses.

Haematoma

Another complication of cardiac surgery is loculated pericardial haematoma. In particular, loculated pericardial haematomas can form around the right atrium (RA) in the region where the venous cannulas are inserted for

cardiopulmonary bypass. Importantly, these haematomas can compress the RA resulting in significant haemodynamic compromise which may require re-operation to remove the clot. On 2D imaging loculated pericardial haematomas appear as a heterogeneous or homogeneous mass anterior and lateral to the RA (Figure 10.38).

Peri-aortic haematoma can also occur following an AVR and the Bentall procedure. In these cases, the accumulation of blood around the aortic root occurs as a consequence of a small leak from the suture line. On 2D imaging peri-aortic haematoma appears as a heterogeneous or homogeneous mass surrounding the aorta (Figure 10.39). Peri-aortic haematomas usually spontaneously resolve over 3 to 6 months.

Note that the appearance of the haematoma depends on the extent of clot formation. For example, when blood is completely clotted within the haematoma the mass will appear homogeneous; if there is a combination of clotted and unclotted blood within the haematoma the mass will appear heterogeneous.

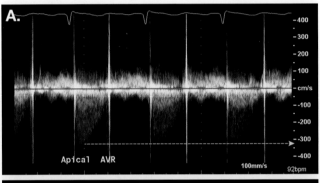

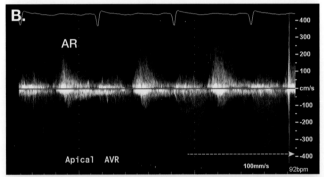

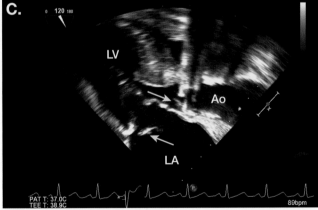

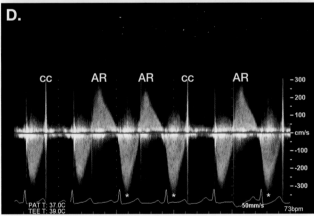

Figure 10.36 These images were recorded from a patient with a bileaflet aortic valve replacement (AVR) and infective endocarditis of the native mitral valve. On the transthoracic echocardiographic examination, two continuous-wave (CW) Doppler traces were acquired. One trace showed normal AVR signals with normal opening and closing clicks (A). A second trace showed evidence of severe aortic regurgitation (AR) (B). Observe on this trace that the AR pressure half-time is very short and that valve clicks are absent; systolic forward flow velocities are also elevated compared to trace A. The subsequent transoesophageal echocardiogram demonstrated echogenic masses, consistent with vegetations, attached to the left atrial (LA) surface of the posterior mitral valve leaflet (*yellow arrow*) and attached to the AVR (*blue arrow*) (C). On real-time imaging, the AVR vegetation became intermittently trapped within the AVR discs resulting in the valve sticking in an open position, thus, causing intermittent, severe AR. The CW Doppler signal also demonstrated intermittent, severe AR (D). This was evident by: (1) the presence of an AR signal with a very short pressure half-time, (2) the absence of closing clicks (cc) on the second, third and fifth beats indicating the absence of valve closure at the end of systole, and (3) increased systolic velocities following each AR signal consistent with an increased total stroke volume across the AVR (*).
Ao = aorta; LV = left ventricle.

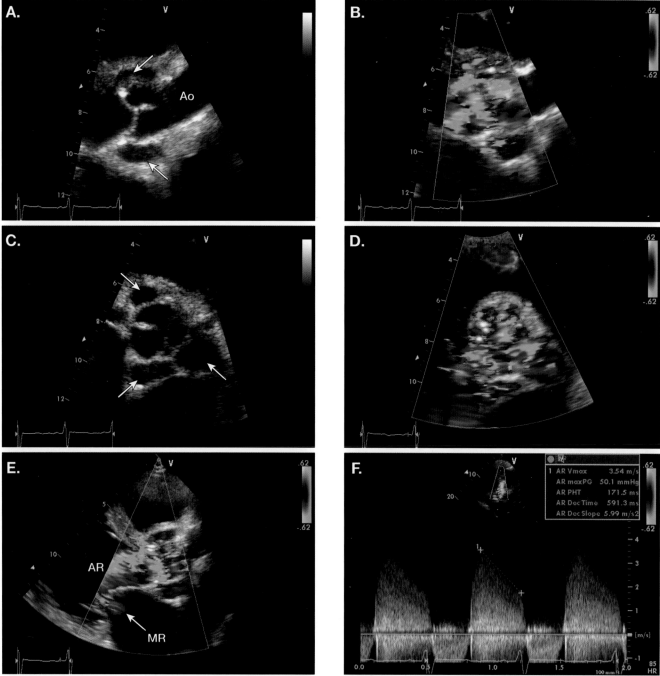

Figure 10.37 These images were recorded from a patient with an Allograft aortic valve replacement and recurrent staphylococcal sepsis. 2D images recorded from zoomed parasternal long axis (A) and short axis (C) views show partial dehiscence of the prosthetic valve and multiple para-aortic cavities (*arrows*). On the colour flow images recorded during systole, communication between the aorta and these para-aortic cavities is noted (B and D). Severe aortic regurgitation (AR) is also evident on the colour Doppler image acquired from the parasternal long axis view during diastole (E); direct communication between the para-aortic cavities and the left ventricle is also observed. Continuous-wave Doppler signal revealed a very short AR pressure half-time (AR PHT) of 172 ms (F); this reflects a marked elevation in the left ventricular end-diastolic pressure (LVEDP). The marked increase in LVEDP has also resulted in diastolic mitral regurgitation (MR) (E). Diastolic MR occurs when the LVEDP exceeds left atrial (LA) pressure resulting in retrograde flow from the LV, across the open mitral valve, into the LA.
Ao = aorta.

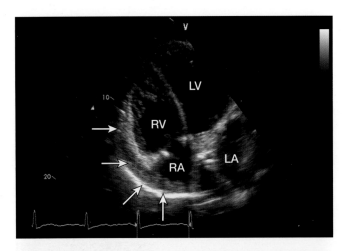

Figure 10.38 This image was recorded from the apical 4-chamber view on day 4 post aortic and mitral valve replacement. Observe the homogenous thickening of the pericardium adjacent to the right heart (*arrows*). This appearance is consistent with a pericardial haematoma. LA = left atrium; LV = left ventricle; RA = right atrium; RV = right ventricle.

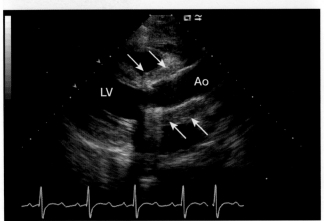 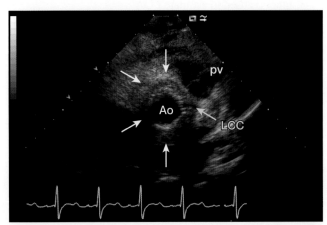

Figure 10.39 These images were recorded from the parasternal long axis view (*left*) and the parasternal short axis view (*right*) following a Bentall procedure with a St Jude aortic valve replacement (day 5 post-op). Observe the large homogenous mass surrounding the aorta (Ao) (*white arrows*). This appearance is characteristic of clotted blood and is consistent with peri-aortic haematoma. The left coronary artery (LCC) can also be seen in the parasternal short axis image tracking through the haematoma (*yellow arrow*). LV = left ventricle; pv = pulmonary valve.

Key Points

General Points
- Prosthetic valves can be classified as biological (tissue) or mechanical
- The echocardiographic appearance of prosthetic valves varies according to type
- Mechanical valve appearances vary depending upon the basic structure, occluder mechanism and motion, and haemodynamic flow patterns across the valve
- All prosthetic valves, with the exception of the allograft and stentless valves, are inherently stenotic
- Most prosthetic valves have trivial or mild degrees of transprosthetic regurgitation such as:
  - Closing volume: displacement of blood when the occluder shuts
  - Leakage volume (or washing jets): built-in transprosthetic regurgitation associated with mechanical valves
- Where possible, valve repair (especially of mitral and tricuspid valves) is preferable to valve replacement

Role of Echo in Prosthetic Valves: General
- Pre-operative: confirm presence of severe valve disease; determine suitability for percutaneous procedures
- Peri-operative: usually via TOE; especially important in guiding valve placement during TAVI and in guiding clip placement for percutaneous mitral valve repair
- Post-operative:
  - measurements of cardiac chamber dimensions (and ascending aorta for AVR)
  - evaluation of ventricular systolic function
  - assessment of coexistent native valve lesions
  - estimation of RVSP
- Baseline post-operative assessment is crucial:
  - Acquire baseline haemodynamics (comparison for future studies)
  - Recognition of PPM
  - Facilitates detection of dysfunction
  - Suspected endocarditis ('then' versus 'now' appearance)
  - Regression of hypertrophy and chamber dilatation, recovery of LV systolic function, reduction in RVSP

(continued over...)

Key Points (continued)

Haemodynamic Assessment
- Transprosthetic velocities and pressure gradients:
  - Corrected gradients for AVR when LVOT velocity $\geq$ 1.2 m/s
- Effective orifice area (EOA):
  - Assuming flow through LVOT is laminar and that LVOT stroke volume (LVOT SV) and prosthetic valve (PrV) stroke volume are the same: then EOA = LVOT SV $\div$ PrV VTI
  - Indexed EOA (IEOA) useful in identifying PPM
  - TAVI: for Edwards SAPIEN valves, LVOT diameter and VTI measured immediately proximal to the stent (pre-stent position)
- Doppler velocity Index (DVI):
  - Derived from LVOT VTI and PrV VTI
  - Quick method for identifying normal and abnormal PrV function
- Pressure Half-time (P½t):
  - For MVR and TVR
  - Cannot be used to estimate EOA

Prosthetic Valve Complications
- Prosthesis-Patient Mismatch (PPM):
  - normally functioning prosthetic valve is too small in relation to the patient's body size
  - results in abnormally high transprosthetic gradients compared with normal values
  - recognised based on IEOA
- Prosthesis Valve Stenosis/Obstruction:
  - Bioprosthetic valves: most common cause is leaflet degeneration
  - Mechanical valves: most common cause is thrombus and/or pannus
  - Stress echo useful in patients with:
    - Symptoms and discordant resting transprosthetic haemodynamics
    - Reduced transprosthetic EOA and low transprosthetic gradients in the setting of low flow states
- Prosthesis Valve Regurgitation:
  - Physiological jets are usually short, narrow and non-turbulent
  - Pathological regurgitation may be transvalvular and/or paravalvular
  - Transvalvular:
    - Most commonly caused by leaflet degeneration (bioprosthetic valves) or thrombosis and/or pannus formation (mechanical valves)
    - On CFI: regurgitation occurs within the sewing ring
  - Paravalvular:
    - Can occur due to prosthetic valve dehiscence and other abnormalities of the valve bed
    - TAVI valves: paravalvular AR may occur due to incomplete prosthesis apposition with native annulus, implantation of prosthesis too small for valve annulus, or implantation of valve too low
    - On CFI: regurgitation arises outside the sewing ring, between the sewing ring and the valve annulus
- Prosthetic Valve Thrombosis/Pannus Formation:
  - Can result in significant PrV obstruction and/or regurgitation
  - Distinction between thrombus and pannus is important because each has different management strategies
  - Thrombus and pannus can be differentiated based on clinical and echocardiographic parameters
- Prosthetic Valve Dehiscence (PVD):
  - Defined as partial separation of prosthetic sewing ring from native valve annulus
  - Characteristic 2D echo feature of PVD: 'rocking' of the PrV
- Prosthetic Valve Endocarditis (PVE):
  - infection of PrV leaflets (bioprosthetic valves) or between sewing ring and native valve annulus (bioprosthetic and mechanical valves)
  - Characteristic 2D echo feature of vegetations: independent, hypermobile mass with a different echo appearance to underlying tissue
  - Vegetations may intermittently or persistently impair valve closure and valve opening resulting PrV in regurgitation and/or stenosis
  - PVE can be further complicated by leaflet perforation (bioprosthetic valves), other valve bed abnormalities (abscesses, dehiscence and paravalvular regurgitation, fistula, or pseudoaneurysms)
  - TOE often required (higher sensitivity and specificity for detection of PVE due to its superior spatial and temporal resolution)
- Haematoma:
  - Loculated pericardial haematomas can form anterior and lateral to the RA
  - Compromise of the RA by loculated pericardial haematomas can result in significant haemodynamic compromise
  - Peri-aortic haematomas can form following an AVR or the Bentall procedure; these haematomas tend to spontaneously resolve over 3-6 months

Further Reading (listed in alphabetical order)

General

Chikwe J, Adams DH. State of the art: degenerative mitral valve disease. *Heart Lung Circ.* 2009 Oct;18(5):319-29.

Pibarot P, Dumesnil JG. Prosthetic heart valves: selection of the optimal prosthesis and long-term management. *Circulation.* 2009 Feb 24;119(7):1034-48.

Pibarot P, Dumesnil JG. Doppler echocardiographic evaluation of prosthetic valve function. *Heart.* 2012 Jan;98(1):69-78.

Zabalgoitia M. Echocardiographic assessment of prosthetic heart valves. *Curr Probl Cardiol.* 2000 Mar;25(3):157-218.

Zoghbi WA, Chambers JB, Dumesnil JG, Foster E, Gottdiener JS, Grayburn PA, Khandheria BK, Levine RA, Marx GR, Miller FA Jr, Nakatani S, Quiñones MA, Rakowski H, Rodriguez LL, Swaminathan M, Waggoner AD, Weissman NJ, Zabalgoitia M. Recommendations for evaluation of prosthetic valves with echocardiography and Doppler ultrasound: a report From the American Society of Echocardiography's Guidelines and Standards Committee and the Task Force on Prosthetic Valves, developed in conjunction with the American College of Cardiology Cardiovascular Imaging Committee, Cardiac Imaging Committee of the American Heart Association, the European Association of Echocardiography, a registered branch of the European Society of Cardiology, the Japanese Society of Echocardiography and the Canadian Society of Echocardiography. *J Am Soc Echocardiogr.* 2009 Sep;22(9):975-1014.

Percutaneous Valves

Bloomfield GS, Gillam LD, Hahn RT, Kapadia S, Leipsic J, Lerakis S, Tuzcu M, Douglas PS. A practical guide to multimodality imaging of transcatheter aortic valve replacement. JACC *Cardiovasc Imaging.* 2012 Apr;5(4):441-55.

Cavalcante JL, Rodriguez LL, Kapadia S, Tuzcu EM, Stewart WJ. Role of echocardiography in percutaneous mitral valve interventions. JACC *Cardiovasc Imaging.* 2012 Jul;5(7):733-46.

Clavel MA, Rodés-Cabau J, Dumont É, Bagur R, Bergeron S, De Larochellière R, Doyle D, Larose E, Dumesnil JG, Pibarot P. Validation and characterization of transcatheter aortic valve effective orifice area measured by Doppler echocardiography. JACC *Cardiovasc Imaging.* 2011 Oct;4(10):1053-62.

Feldman T, Kar S, Rinaldi M, Fail P, Hermiller J, Smalling R, Whitlow PL, Gray W, Low R, Herrmann HC, Lim S, Foster E, Glower D; EVEREST Investigators. Percutaneous mitral repair with the MitraClip system: safety and midterm durability in the initial EVEREST (Endovascular Valve Edge-to-Edge REpair Study) cohort. *J Am Coll Cardiol.* 2009 Aug 18;54(8):686-94.

Maisano F, La Canna G, Colombo A, Alfieri O. The evolution from surgery to percutaneous mitral valve interventions: the role of the edge-to-edge technique. *J Am Coll Cardiol.* 2011 Nov 15;58(21):2174-82.

Shames S, Koczo A, Hahn R, Jin Z, Picard MH, Gillam LD. Flow characteristics of the SAPIEN aortic valve: the importance of recognizing in-stent flow acceleration for the echocardiographic assessment of valve function. *J Am Soc Echocardiogr.* 2012 Jun;25(6):603-9.

Zamorano JL, Badano LP, Bruce C, Chan KL, Gonçalves A, Hahn RT, Keane MG, La Canna G, Monaghan MJ, Nihoyannopoulos P, Silvestry FE, Vanoverschelde JL, Gillam LD. EAE/ASE recommendations for the use of echocardiography in new transcatheter interventions for valvular heart disease. *J Am Soc Echocardiogr.* 2011 Sep;24(9):937-65

Complications

Bach DS. Echo/Doppler evaluation of hemodynamics after aortic valve replacement: principles of interrogation and evaluation of high gradients. JACC *Cardiovasc Imaging.* 2010 Mar;3(3):296-304.

Barbetseas J, Nagueh SF, Pitsavos C, Toutouzas PK, Quiñones MA, Zoghbi WA. Differentiating thrombus from pannus formation in obstructed mechanical prosthetic valves: an evaluation of clinical, transthoracic and transesophageal echocardiographic parameters. *J Am Coll Cardiol.* 1998 Nov;32(5):1410-7.

Fernandes V, Olmos L, Nagueh SF, Quiñones MA, Zoghbi WA. Peak early diastolic velocity rather than pressure half-time is the best index of mechanical prosthetic mitral valve function. *Am J Cardiol.* 2002 Mar 15;89(6):704-10.

Pibarot P, Dumesnil JG. Doppler echocardiographic evaluation of prosthetic valve function. *Heart.* 2012 Jan;98(1):69-78.

Pibarot P, Dumesnil JG. Prosthesis-patient mismatch: definition, clinical impact, and prevention. *Heart.* 2006 Aug;92(8):1022-9.

Rahimtoola SH. The problem of valve prosthesis-patient mismatch. *Circulation.* 1978 Jul;58(1):20-4.

Normal Values

Blauwet LA, Burkhart HM, Dearani JA, Malouf JF, Connolly HM, Hodge DO, Herges RM, Miller FA Jr. Comprehensive echocardiographic assessment of mechanical tricuspid valve prostheses based on early post-implantation echocardiographic studies. *J Am Soc Echocardiogr.* 2011 Apr;24(4):414-24.

Blauwet LA, Danielson GK, Burkhart HM, Dearani JA, Malouf JF, Connolly HM, Hodge DO, Herges RM, Miller FA Jr. Comprehensive echocardiographic assessment of the hemodynamic parameters of 285 tricuspid valve bioprostheses early after implantation. *J Am Soc Echocardiogr.* 2010 Oct;23(10):1045-1059, 1059.e1-2.

Blauwet LA, Malouf JF, Connolly HM, Hodge DO, Evans KN, Herges RM, Sundt TM 3rd, Miller FA Jr. Comprehensive echocardiographic assessment of normal mitral Medtronic Hancock II, Medtronic Mosaic, and Carpentier-Edwards Perimount bioprostheses early after implantation. *J Am Soc Echocardiogr.* 2010 Jun;23(6):656-66.

Bleiziffer S, Eichinger WB, Hettich IM, Ruzicka D, Badiu CC, Guenzinger R, Bauernschmitt R, Lange R. Hemodynamic characterization of the Sorin Mitroflow pericardial bioprosthesis at rest and exercise. *J Heart Valve Dis.* 2009 Jan;18(1):95-100.

Novaro GM, Connolly HM, Miller FA. Doppler hemodynamics of 51 clinically and echocardiographically normal pulmonary valve prostheses. *Mayo Clin Proc.* 2001 Feb;76(2):155-60.

Rajani R, Mukherjee D, Chambers JB. Doppler echocardiography in normally functioning replacement aortic valves: a review of 129 studies. *J Heart Valve Dis.* 2007 Sep;16(5):519-35.

Rosenhek R, Binder T, Maurer G, Baumgartner H. Normal values for Doppler echocardiographic assessment of heart valve prostheses. *J Am Soc Echocardiogr.* 2003 Nov;16(11):1116-27.

Ruzicka DJ, Hettich I, Hutter A, Bleiziffer S, Badiu CC, Bauernschmitt R, Lange R, Eichinger WB. The complete supraannular concept: in vivo hemodynamics of bovine and porcine aortic bioprostheses. *Circulation.* 2009 Sep 15;120(11 Suppl):S139-45.

Sadeghpour A, Saadatifar H, Kiavar M, Esmaeilzadeh M, Maleki M, Ojaghi Z, Noohi F, Samiei N, Mohebbi A. Doppler echocardiographic assessment of pulmonary prostheses: a comprehensive assessment including velocity time integral ratio and prosthesis effective orifice area. *Congenit Heart Dis.* 2008 Nov-Dec;3(6):415-21.

Spethmann S, Dreger H, Schattke S, Baldenhofer G, Saghabalyan D, Stangl V, Laule M, Baumann G, Stangl K, Knebel F. Doppler haemodynamics and effective orifice areas of Edwards SAPIEN and CoreValve transcatheter aortic valves. *Eur Heart J Cardiovasc Imaging.* 2012 Aug;13(8):690-6.

Diseases of the Aorta

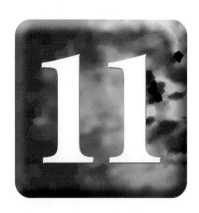

Anatomy and Structure of the Aorta

Basic Structure of Aortic Walls

The aorta, as for all blood vessels except for capillaries and venules, consists of three distinct layers: (1) the tunica intima, (2) the tunica media and (3) the tunica adventitia (Fig. 11.1).

The tunica intima is the innermost layer and is comprised of an endothelial lining and connective tissue. Beneath the connective tissue is the internal elastic lamina, which separates this inner layer from the tunica media. The tunica media is the middle layer and is composed of smooth muscle tissue, elastic fibres and connective tissue. A second layer of elastic fibres, the external elastic lamina, separates the tunica media from the tunica adventitia. The tunica adventitia is the outermost layer and is composed mostly of connective tissue. The adventitia links the vessels to the surrounding tissues.

The strength of the aorta lies in the media, which is composed of laminated and intertwining sheets of elastic tissue arranged in a spiral manner. The aorta is also supplied by a network of small vessels, the vasa vasorum; these vessels are located within the adventitia.

Segments of the Aorta

The aorta consists of the thoracic and abdominal portions. The thoracic aorta is the section of aorta that lies above the diaphragm while the abdominal aorta is the section of aorta that lies below the diaphragm (Fig. 11.2).

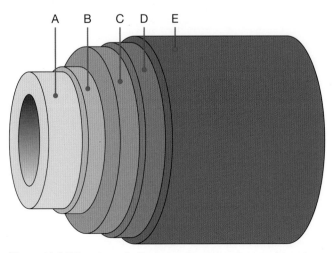

Figure 11.1 This schematic illustrates the various layers of an artery: A = tunica intima; B = internal elastic lamina; C = tunica media; D = external elastic lamina; E = tunica adventitia.

The thoracic aorta consists of five segments:

1. The aortic root is the section of the aorta between the left ventricular outflow tract (LVOT) and the ascending aorta; it is bounded by the basal attachment of the aortic cusps to the virtual ring proximally and the peripheral attachment of the aortic cusps to the sinotubular (ST) junction distally.

2. The ascending aorta which is approximately 5 cm in length extends from the ST junction and terminates at the origin of the brachiocephalic artery.

3. The aortic arch gives rise to the three major head and neck vessels and is located entirely within the superior mediastinum. This segment of the aorta is approximately 4 cm in length and extends from the origin of the brachiocephalic artery to the ligamentum arteriosum which lies directly opposite the left subclavian artery.

4. The aortic isthmus is a very small segment of the aorta that is located at the site of the ligamentum arteriosum. The aorta is especially vulnerable to trauma at the aortic isthmus because it is here that the ascending aorta and arch are relatively fixed to the thoracic cage by the pleural reflections, the intercostal arteries, and the left subclavian artery.

5. The descending thoracic aorta extends from the aortic isthmus to the diaphragm and is located in the posterior mediastinum.

The abdominal aorta consists of two segments:

1. The suprarenal segment extends from the diaphragm to the origin of the renal arteries.

2. The infrarenal segment extends from below the origin of the renal arteries to the bifurcation of the aorta into the common iliac arteries.

2D Imaging and Measurements of the Aorta

2D Imaging of the Aorta

The various long axis segments of the aorta can be viewed from multiple acoustic windows (Fig. 11.3).

From the standard left parasternal view, the aortic valve, aortic root, and proximal ascending aorta can be imaged (Fig. 11.4,A). In addition, the descending aorta in its short axis can also be visualised posterior to the left atrium (LA). From an intercostal space higher, a longer portion of the ascending aorta is often seen (Fig. 11.4,B).

From the parasternal short axis at the level of the aorta, a short axis of the descending aorta can be seen posterior to the LA (Fig. 11.4,C). From this imaging plane it is often possible

The brachiocephalic artery is also often referred to as the brachiocephalic trunk or innominate artery. This artery bifurcates into the right subclavian and right common carotid arteries.

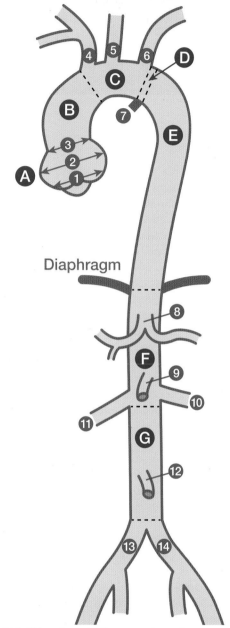

Figure 11.2 This schematic illustrates the various segments of the thoracic and abdominal aorta. The thoracic aorta consists of the aortic root **(A)**, the ascending aorta **(B)**, the aortic arch **(C)**, the aortic isthmus **(D)** and the descending thoracic aorta **(E)**. The aortic root extends from the basal attachment of the aortic cusps at the virtual ring **(1)** to the sinotubular (ST) junction **(3)**; the aortic sinuses **(2)** are incorporated within the aortic root. The ascending aorta extends from the ST junction **(3)** to the origin of the brachiocephalic artery **(4)**. The aortic arch is the section of aorta from the origin of the brachiocephalic artery **(4)** to the ligamentum arteriosum **(7)**. All head and neck vessels arise from the aortic arch; these vessels include the brachiocephalic artery **(4)**, the left common carotid artery **(5)** and the left subclavian artery **(6)**. The aortic isthmus is the portion of aorta at the ligamentum arteriosum **(7)**. The descending thoracic aorta extends from the aortic isthmus to the diaphragm. The abdominal aorta consists of the suprarenal segment **(F)** and the infrarenal segment **(G)**. The suprarenal segment extends from diaphragm to the origin of the renal arteries **(10** and **11)**; the coeliac artery **(8)** and the superior mesenteric artery **(9)** are included in this section of the abdominal aorta. The infrarenal segment extends from below the origin of the renal arteries to the bifurcation into the common iliac arteries **(13** and **14)**; the inferior mesenteric artery **(12)** is included in this section. This figure is not drawn to scale.

to open the descending aorta into its long axis by rotating the transducer anti-clockwise 90 degrees (Fig. 11.4,D).

From the apical 4-chamber view, the short axis of the descending aorta can be seen lateral to the LA (Fig. 11.4,E). The long axis of the descending aorta can also been imaged from the apical 2-chamber view (Fig. 11.4,F).

From the apical 5-chamber and apical long axis views, the proximal aortic root can be seen; however, the parasternal views are better for imaging this segment of the aorta as the aorta is closer to the transducer from the parasternal window. From the subcostal view, the long axis of the abdominal aorta can be visualised (Fig. 11.4,G). From the subcostal 5-chamber view the proximal aortic root can be seen.

From the suprasternal view, the aortic arch and the descending aorta are imaged (Fig. 11.4,H). When image quality is exceptionally good the ascending aorta may also be imaged from this window.

As the aorta dilates, the aortic root and ascending aorta move towards the right of the sternum. As a result the ascending aorta can also be imaged from the right parasternal transducer position (Fig. 11.5).

In the presence of a left pleural effusion an additional ultrasonic window for visualisation of the descending aorta is provided (Fig. 11.6).

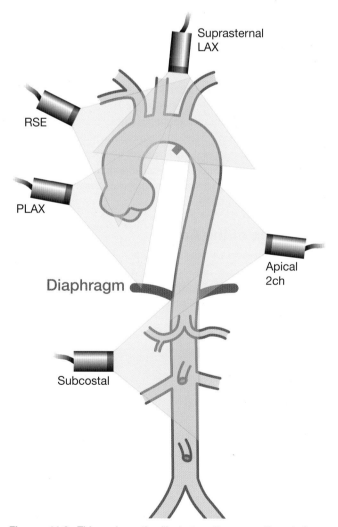

Figure 11.3 This schematic illustrates the acoustic windows that can be utilised to image the various segments of the aorta. 2ch = 2-chamber view; LAX = long axis; PLAX = parasternal long axis; RSE = right sternal edge.

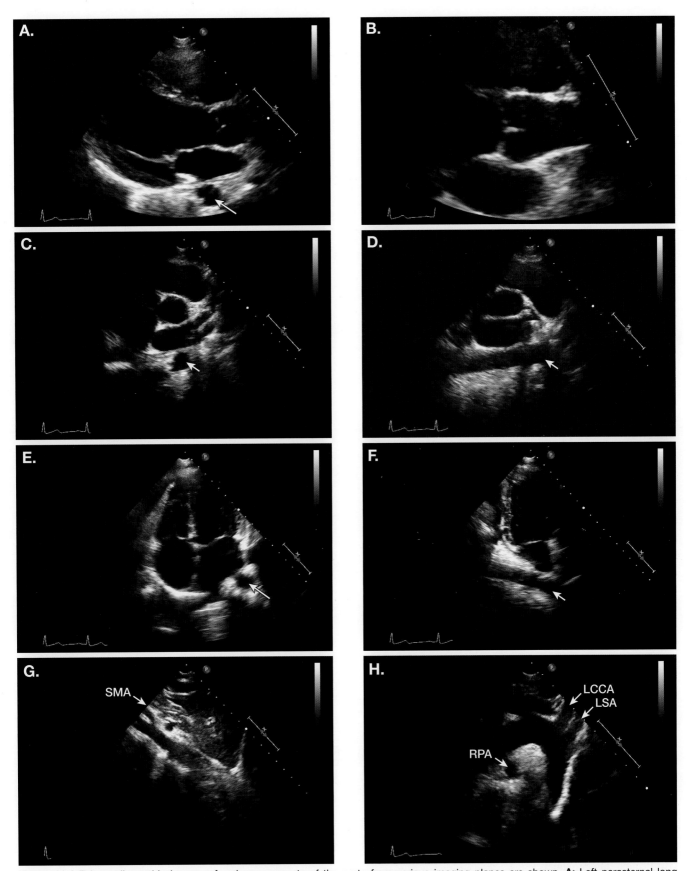

Figure 11.4 Echocardiographic images of various segments of the aorta from various imaging planes are shown. **A:** Left parasternal long axis view of the aortic root and ascending aorta; the short axis of the descending aorta is also seen (*arrow*); **B:** High left parasternal long axis view of the aortic root and ascending aorta; **C:** Standard parasternal short axis view showing the descending aorta in its short axis (*arrow*); **D:** Parasternal short axis view rotated slightly anti-clockwise to show the long axis of the descending aorta (*arrow*); **E:** Apical 4-chamber view showing the short axis of the descending aorta lateral to the left atrium (*arrow*); **F:** Apical 2-chamber view rotated anti-clockwise and tilted inferiorly to show the long axis of the descending aorta (*arrow*); **G:** Subcostal view orientated to show the long axis of the proximal (suprarenal) abdominal aorta; **H:** Suprasternal long axis view showing the aortic arch and descending thoracic aorta. LCCA = left common carotid artery; LSA = left subclavian artery; RPA = right pulmonary artery; SMA = superior mesenteric artery

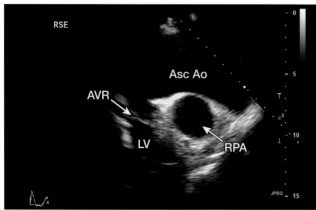

Figure 11.5 This image of the ascending aorta (AscAo) was recorded from the right parasternal edge (RSE). To acquire this view the transducer is placed in the first, second or third intercostal space at the right sternal border; the transducer is perpendicular to the chest wall and is rotated so that the image index marker is at the 1 o'clock position. AVR = aortic valve replacement; LV = left ventricle; RPA = right pulmonary artery.

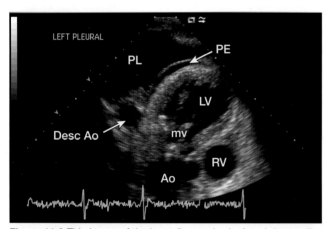

Figure 11.6 This image of the heart (long axis view) and descending thoracic aorta (in its short axis) was recorded from the posterior view using the left pleural effusion as an acoustic window. To acquire this image the patient is in a sitting position or is rolled into the right lateral decubitus position. The transducer is placed near the patient's left scapula perpendicular to the posterior thoracic wall. The transducer is then orientated to show heart and descending thoracic aorta; observe that a small pericardial effusion (PE) is also present. Ao = aortic root; Desc Ao= descending aorta; LV = left ventricle; mv = mitral valve; PL = pleural effusion; RV = right ventricle.

Measurements of the Aorta

From the above mentioned views, various measurements of the aorta can be performed. From the parasternal long axis views routine measurements of the aorta include the LVOT diameter, trans-sinus diameter at the sinuses of Valsalva, the ST junction, and the ascending aorta (Fig. 11.7,A&B). These measurements, except for the LVOT diameter, are performed at end-diastole via the leading edge to leading edge technique. The LVOT diameter is measured via the inner edge to inner edge technique at mid-systole. The LVOT diameter is measured at the level of the aortic annulus from the cuspal insertion of the right coronary cusp into the ventricular septum to where the non-coronary cusp 'meets' the anterior mitral leaflet. It has also be suggested that the LVOT diameter should be measured 0.5-1.0 cm proximal to the aortic valve when this value is used to calculate the LVOT stroke volume (both the LVOT diameter and LVOT velocity time integral are measured at the same anatomic location).

From the suprasternal long axis views, measurements of the aortic arch and descending aorta can be performed (Fig. 11.7,C). These measurements are performed at end-diastole. The aortic arch is measured via the leading edge to leading edge technique. As the descending aorta is parallel with the ultrasound beam, it is measured via the inner edge to inner edge technique (leading edges are only encountered when the ultrasound beam is perpendicular to an interface).

The absolute and indexed normal values of the various aortic segments are listed in Table 11.1.

> **Technical Tip**
> From the subcostal window the abdominal aorta may be confused with the inferior vena cava (IVC). Differentiation of the aorta from the IVC can be made by recognition of the systolic pulsations of the aorta and the more vertical course of the aorta. The IVC can be identified based on its variation in size with respiration; it also has a more horizontal course compared to the aorta. In addition, the hepatic veins can usually be seen draining into the IVC and the IVC can be followed to confirm its drainage into the right atrium.

Table 11.1 Absolute and Indexed Normal Values of Aortic Segments

Aortic Level	Women		Men	
	Absolute Values (cm)	Indexed Values (cm/m²)	Absolute Values (cm)	Indexed Values (cm/m²)
LVOT diameter [1]	2.3 ± 0.2	1.3 ± 0.1	2.6 ± 0.3	1.3 ± 0.1
Sinus of Valsalva [1]	3.0 ± 0.3	1.8 ± 0.2	3.4 ± 0.3	1.7 ± 0.2
Sinotubular junction [1]	2.6 ± 0.3	1.5 ± 0.2	2.9 ± 0.3	1.5 ± 0.2
Ascending aorta [1]	2.7 ± 0.4	1.6 ± 0.3	3.0 ± 0.4	1.5 ± 0.3
Aortic arch (just proximal to brachiocephalic artery) [2]	2.2 - 3.6 (range)		2.2 - 3.6 (range)	
Descending aorta (opposite ligamentum arteriosum) [2]	2.0 - 3.0 (range)		2.0 - 3.0 (range)	

LVOT = Left ventricular outflow tract or aortic annulus.
Source: [1] Roman MJ, Devereux RB, Kramer-Fox R, O'Loughlin J. Two-dimensional echocardiographic aortic root dimensions in normal children and adults. *Am J Cardiol*. 1989 Sep 1;64(8):507-12. **[2]** Evangelista A, Flachskampf FA, Erbel R, Antonini-Canterin F, Vlachopoulos C, Rocchi G, Sicari R, Nihoyannopoulos P, Zamorano J; European Association of Echocardiography; Document Reviewers:, Pepi M, Breithardt OA, Plonska-Gosciniak E. Echocardiography in aortic diseases: EAE recommendations for clinical practice. *Eur J Echocardiogr*. 2011 Aug;12(8):642 (Corrigendum).

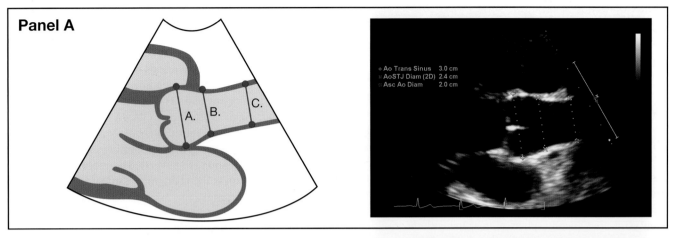

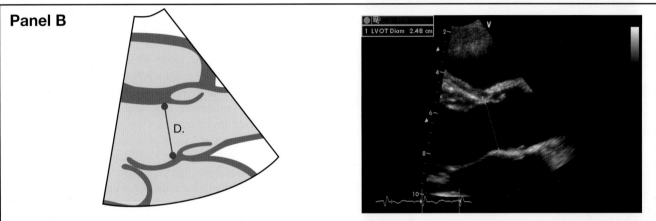

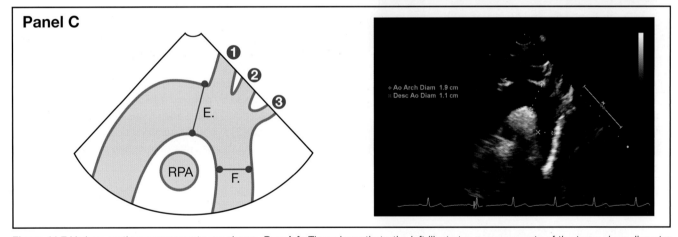

Figure 11.7 Various aortic measurements are shown. **Panel A:** The schematic to the left illustrates measurements of the trans-sinus diameter **(A)**, the sinotubular junction (STJ) **(B)** and the ascending aorta **(C)** performed from the parasternal long axis view. The image to the right shows actual measurements of the aorta at these levels. All measurements are performed at end-diastole via the leading edge to leading edge technique. **Panel B:** The schematic to the left illustrates the measurement of the left ventricular outflow tract (LVOT) diameter **(D)**. The image to the right shows actual measurements of the LVOT diameter. This measurement is performed at mid-systole via the inner edge to inner edge method. **Panel C:** The schematic to the left illustrates the measurement of the aortic arch diameter **(E)** and the descending aorta **(F)** from the suprasternal long axis view. The image to the right shows actual measurements of the aorta at these levels. Note that all three head and neck vessels are not usually seen in the suprasternal long axis view as these vessels arise from the aorta in slightly different planes. Measurements are performed at end-diastole; the arch is measured via the leading edge to leading edge technique and the descending aorta is measured via the inner edge to inner edge method. 1 = brachiocephalic artery; 2 = left common carotid artery; 3 = left subclavian artery; RPA = right pulmonary artery.

Aortic Measurement Technique
The recommended method for measuring the thoracic aorta is via the leading edge to leading edge technique at end-diastole. However, some institutions prefer the inner edge to inner edge technique to increase reproducibility and match the methods used by other imaging technologies such as magnetic resonance imaging (MRI) and computed tomography (CT) scanning. Furthermore, at times the aortic walls are better delineated during systole so measurements may be more accurate at this phase of the cardiac cycle. Importantly, if measuring the thoracic aorta via the inner edge to inner edge technique or at end-systole rather than at end-diastole, the normal values as per Table 11.1 cannot be applied as these normative data were obtained using the leading edge technique at end-diastole.

Aortic Aneurysms

Definition

An aortic aneurysm is defined as a dilatation involving all layers of the aorta 1.5 times greater than the normal arterial diameter.

Types of Aneurysms

There are three main types of aortic aneurysms: (1) saccular, (2) fusiform, and (3) a false aneurysm or pseudoaneurysm (Fig. 11.8).

A saccular aneurysm occurs when there is weakening in the vessel wall at one point or one side of the vessel; this leads to an expansion or "outpouching" of the vessel wall. These aneurysms are typically spherical in shape with the mouth of the aneurysm being smaller than the body of the aneurysm. A fusiform aneurysm occurs when there is a uniform and symmetrical dilatation of the entire circumference of the vessel. These aneurysms are typically 'spindle-shaped'. Both saccular and fusiform aneurysms are true aneurysms; that is the wall of the aneurysm involves all three arterial layers.

A pseudoaneurysm or false aneurysm represents a contained rupture of the arterial wall; that is, there is a collection of blood outside the vessel wall which is confined by the tunica adventitia. Recognition of a pseudoaneurysm is important as there a significant risk of full rupture.

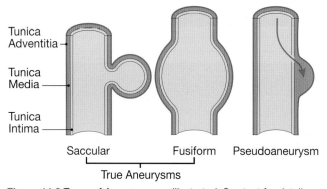

Figure 11.8 Types of Aneurysms as illustrated. See text for details.

Location of Aortic Aneurysms

Aortic aneurysms are divided into thoracic aortic aneurysms, thoracoabdominal aortic aneurysms, and abdominal aortic aneurysms. Thoracic aortic aneurysms (TAA) can be further subcategorised into: (1) ascending aortic aneurysms, (2) aortic arch aneurysms and (3) descending aortic aneurysms. Thoracoabdominal aneurysms (TAAA) refer to thoracic aneurysms that extend into the abdomen. These aneurysms are divided into five groups according to the modified Crawford classification (Fig. 11.9). The most common type of aortic aneurysm is the abdominal aortic aneurysm (AAA) below the renal arteries.

Aetiology of Aortic Aneurysms

Aortic aneurysms usually occur in a weakened area of the aortic wall which has been damaged by the destruction of the medial elastic elements. The risk factors for aortic aneurysm formation are listed in Table 11.2. In particular, smoking markedly increases the risk for AAA.

Destruction of the tunica media can occur due to several causes. The aetiology, examples, type and location of aneurysms are summarised in Table 11.3. The most common cause of ascending aortic aneurysms is annuloaortic ectasia and medial degeneration. Medial degeneration is characterized by disruption and loss of elastic fibres, increased deposition of proteoglycans and loss of smooth muscle cells within the media.

Atherosclerosis is the second most common cause of ascending aortic aneurysms and the most common cause of AAA. Atherosclerosis is a focal disease of muscular arteries in which the intima becomes thickened by fibrofatty plaques. The development of invasive atheromas leads to extensive destruction of elastic fibres and muscle cells in the medial layer which then weakens the aorta and predisposes this segment of the aorta to aneurysmal formation.

Aneurysms caused by primary infections of the aorta are rare. Types of infectious aortic aneurysms include: (1) mycotic aneurysms and (2) syphilitic aneurysms. Mycotic aneurysms (bacterial or fungal) arise due to infection of the aortic walls.

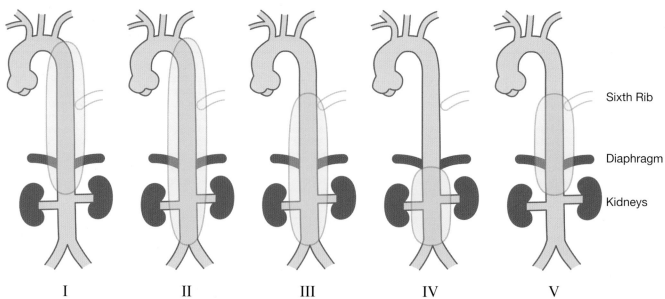

Figure 11.9 Modified Crawford classification of thoracoabdominal aortic aneurysms. **Type I:** involves the descending thoracic aorta from the left subclavian artery down to the abdominal aorta above the renal arteries. **Type II:** extends distal to the left subclavian artery to the aortic bifurcation. **Type III:** extends from the sixth intercostal space to the aortic bifurcation. **Type IV:** extends from the diaphragm to the aortic bifurcation (entire abdominal aorta). **Type V:** extends from the sixth intercostal space to above the renal arteries.

Infection of the aorta can occur due to:
1. seeding of the vasa vasorum during haematogenous spread,
2. direct invasion of the wall from the aortic lumen,
3. septic emboli (usually from infective endocarditis),
4. spread of infection from neighbouring structures,
5. traumatic aortic injury with subsequent infection.

Syphilis was once a common cause of ascending aortic aneurysms. With this disease, the muscular and elastic medial elements are destroyed by infective and inflammatory responses. This leads to weakening of the aortic wall and aneurysmal dilatation. Syphilitic aneurysms most commonly involve the ascending aorta and aortic arch. Less commonly syphilitic aneurysms occur in the proximal descending aorta and they rarely occur in the abdominal aorta.

Table 11.2 **Risk factors for Aortic Aneurysms**

Risk factors for Aortic Aneurysms
Advanced age
Bicuspid or unicuspid aortic valves
Chronic obstructive lung disease
Cigarette smoking
Coronary artery disease
Dyslipidemia
Family history
Genetic disorders
Hypertension
Male gender

Complications of Aortic Aneurysms

One of the most important complications of aortic aneurysms is aortic aneurysm rupture; in particular, the larger the aneurysm the greater the likelihood of rupture. Another life-threatening complication of aortic aneurysms is acute aortic dissection.

Other complications of aneurysms include thrombus formation due to stasis of blood flow, embolism of formed thrombus, and vascular obstruction.

In patients with aortic root and ascending aorta aneurysms, aortic regurgitation (AR) commonly occurs secondary to annular dilatation.

Echocardiography in Thoracic Aortic Aneurysms

The role of echocardiography in the assessment of aortic aneurysms includes:
• Identifying the presence and site of an aortic aneurysm,
• Measuring the size of aortic aneurysm,
• Assessing the severity of associated AR.

Identifying the Presence and Site of an Aortic Aneurysm

In most patients, 2D echocardiography is able to visualise the aortic root, the aortic arch, the descending aorta as well as the abdominal aorta. When aortic aneurysms are expected or known then the aorta should be viewed and measured from all possible imaging planes. The aorta should also be thoroughly interrogated in patient populations predisposed to aneurysms.

Table 11.3 **Aortic Aneurysms: Aetiology, Examples, Location and Type**

Aetiology	Examples	Location	Type
Annuloaortic ectasia and medial degeneration	Isolated condition Marfan syndrome Bicuspid aortic valve Advanced age	Aortic root Ascending aorta Aortic arch	Fusiform
Aortic Arteritis (inflammation)	Takayasu's arteritis Giant-cell arteritis	Variable	Fusiform
Aortic dissection (weakening of false lumen)	Type A or Type B	Variable	Pseudoaneurysm
Atherosclerosis (weakening of vessel walls)	Atherosclerotic plaques	Ascending aorta Descending aorta Abdominal aorta	Fusiform (or saccular in ascending, descending & abdominal aorta)
Defective collagen & medial degeneration	Ehlers-Danlos syndrome (Type IV)	Variable	Fusiform
Infection (medial degeneration [MD] or inflammatory changes)	Bacterial or mycotic (inflammatory) Syphilitic (MD)	Aortic root (syphilis) Variable (Mycotic)	Fusiform, saccular or pseudoaneurysm (saccular most common)
Post surgical (weakening of anastomotic walls)	Aortic valve replacement	Anastomosis site	Fusiform
Post-stenotic dilatation (haemodynamic insult)	Aortic stenosis (AS) Coarctation (CoAo)	Ascending aorta (AS) Descending aorta (CoAo)	Fusiform
Pseudoaneurysms	Trauma Infection Surgical procedures	Variable	Pseudoaneurysm
Trauma (damaged vessel wall)	Motor vehicle accident Fall from height	Aortic isthmus Proximal descending aorta	Pseudoaneurysm

Patient populations predisposed to aortic aneurysms include patients with Marfan syndrome, bicuspid aortic valves, aortic stenosis, prosthetic aortic valves and systemic hypertension (see Table 11.3). Regular serial echocardiograms are also recommended in patients with Marfan syndrome and other diseases with a known predisposition for aortic aneurysms as well as in patients with dilated aortas due to any cause. Examples of aortic aneurysms are displayed in Figure 11.10.

> ### Abdominal Aortic Aneurysms
> On the routine transthoracic examination (TTE), the suprarenal (proximal) abdominal aorta is often imaged from the subcostal window. However, as more than 90% of AAA's are infrarenal, a normal-sized suprarenal aorta does not exclude an AAA. Typically the investigation for AAA is performed in the general ultrasound laboratory; although some echocardiographic laboratories also routinely interrogate the infrarenal abdominal aorta. Measurements of the infrarenal abdominal aorta are performed at the site of the maximum diameter below the renal arteries in the longitudinal and transverse planes; callipers are placed from outer wall to the outer wall.

Measuring the Size of the Aortic Aneurysm
When images are optimal, accurate measurement of the aortic dimensions is possible. Measurement at all levels of the thoracic aorta should be attempted including measurements at the LVOT, trans-sinus dimension, ST junction, ascending aorta, aortic arch, and descending aorta. The measurement technique for aortic dimensions is described above and demonstrated in Figure 11.7. Importantly, accurate aortic measurements are crucial as elective intervention in patients with aortic aneurysms is based on the size of the aneurysm, the rate of growth of the aneurysm as well as the underlying aetiology and symptoms (Table 11.4). Elective intervention in these patients is indicated due to the high risk of rupture or aortic dissection when aortic sizes are larger than the criteria listed. In addition, concomitant repair of the aortic root or replacement of the ascending aorta may be considered in patients undergoing aortic valve repair or replacement who have an ascending aorta or aortic root of greater than 4.5 cm.

Severity of Aortic Regurgitation
Aortic aneurysms of the aortic root and ascending aorta are often associated with AR. In these cases, AR is most commonly due to annular dilatation (see Fig. 7.44). The severity of AR is assessed in the usual manner (see Chapter 7).

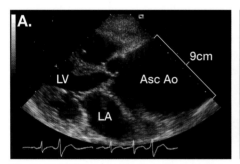 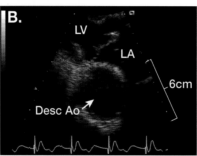 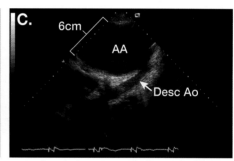

Figure 11.10 These images show three aortic aneurysm sites from three different patients. **A:** From the parasternal long axis view an aneurysm of the ascending aorta (Asc Ao) is shown; observe that the ascending aorta is approximately 9 cm wide with effacement of the sinotubular junction. **B:** From this zoomed and slightly off-axis parasternal long axis view an aneurysm of the descending aorta (Desc Ao) is shown; the maximum diameter of this aneurysm was measured at 5.6 cm. **C:** From the suprasternal view an aneurysm of the aortic arch (AA) is shown; observe that the maximum arch diameter is more than 6 cm. LA = left atrium; LV = left ventricle.

Table 11.4 Thresholds for Elective Intervention for Aortic Aneurysms based on Aortic Dimensions

Site of Aneurysm	Patient Population	Criteria
Ascending aorta	Patients with degenerative thoracic aneurysm, chronic aortic dissection, intramural hematoma, penetrating atherosclerotic ulcer, mycotic aneurysm, or pseudoaneurysm	≥ 5.5 cm
	Marfan syndrome or other genetically mediated disorders#	4.0 – 5.0 cm
	Any patient population	Growth rate > 0.5 cm/year in aorta < 5.5 cm in diameter
	Patients undergoing aortic valve repair or replacement with dilated aortic root or ascending aorta	Consider concomitant aortic root or ascending replacement if > 4.5 cm
	Marfan syndrome, other genetic diseases or bicuspid aortic valves	Ratio of maximal ascending or aortic root area (cm²) divided by the patient's height (m) > 10
Descending thoracic aorta	General population	> 6.0 cm*
		> 5.5 cm ^

\# includes Ehlers Danlos syndrome, Turner Syndrome, bicuspid aortic valve or familial thoracic aortic aneurysms.
* repaired via open surgical technique; ^ repaired with endovascular technique or Marfan patients.
Source: Hiratzka LF, Bakris GL, Beckman JA, et al. 2010 ACCF/AHA/AATS/ACR/ASA/SCA/SCAI/SIR/STS/SVM guidelines for the diagnosis and management of patients with thoracic aortic disease: a report of the American College of Cardiology Foundation/American Heart Association Task Force on Practice Guidelines, American Association for Thoracic Surgery, American College of Radiology, American Stroke Association, Society of Cardiovascular Anesthesiologists, Society for Cardiovascular Angiography and Interventions, Society of Interventional Radiology, Society of Thoracic Surgeons, and Society for Vascular Medicine. *J Am Coll Cardiol.* 2010 Apr 6;55(14):e27-e129.

Sinus of Valsalva Aneurysms

Anatomy of the Sinus of Valsalva

Recall that the aortic root is the segment of the aorta between the LVOT and the ascending aorta; it is bounded by the basal attachment of the aortic cusps to the virtual ring proximally and the peripheral attachment of the aortic cusps to the ST junction distally (see Fig. 7.8). There are three sinuses of Valsalva which form distinct out-pouchings of the aortic wall. The sinuses originate at the aortic annulus and end at the ST junction. The sinuses are named according to the coronary arteries arising from within them; that is, the right coronary sinus, the left coronary sinus, and the non-coronary sinus.

Definition of Sinus of Valsalva Aneurysms

A sinus of Valsalva aneurysm (SVA) is a rare congenital anomaly where there is dilatation of a single sinus of Valsalva which is a result of congenital weakening or absence of the media in one of the aortic sinuses. Under the continued strain of aortic pressure, the weakened sinus gradually dilates and eventually forms an aneurysm.

Types and Associated Lesions

The most common site of a SVA is the right sinus (65% - 85%) followed by the non-coronary sinus (10% - 30%). SVA of the left sinus is very rare (< 5%). There are a number of congenital anomalies associated with a congenital SVA. For example, SVAs are commonly associated with a bicuspid aortic valve and a ventricular septal defect (VSD) is commonly associated with a right SVA. Less commonly pulmonary stenosis, coarctation, and atrial septal defect are associated with a SVA.

Complications of SVA

Rupture of a SVA results in a fistulous communication between the aorta and another site. The site of rupture and the resultant fistulous communication is dependent upon the origin of the SVA. A right SVA protrudes towards the right ventricle (RV) and/or the right ventricular outflow tract (RVOT). Therefore, rupture of a right SVA usually results in a fistulous communication between the aorta and the RV or RVOT. Less commonly a ruptured right SVA results in a fistulous communication between the aorta and the right atrium (RA).

A non-coronary SVA protrudes towards the RA. Therefore, rupture of a non-coronary SVA usually results in a fistulous communication between the aorta and the RA, and less commonly between the aorta and the RV.

A left SVA typically protrudes towards the LA but it may also protrude into the pulmonary artery, the left ventricle (LV), the myocardium, or the pericardial space beneath the left coronary artery. Rupture of the left SVA is rare; however, isolated cases of left SVA rupture into the LA, LV and pericardium have been reported. Rupture into the pericardium is almost always fatal due to the development of cardiac tamponade.

As mentioned, an associated VSD is most frequently seen with a right SVA. In particular, deformation of the right sinus of Valsalva in association with a VSD can lead to aortic valve prolapse and subsequent AR (see Fig. 7.43).

Other complications associated with an unruptured SVA have also been reported. These complications include obstruction of the RVOT, conduction abnormalities due to the compression of the bundle of His and proximal portions of the right bundle and left bundle branches, and myocardial ischaemia or infarction due to compression or obstruction of the coronary ostia by the SVA.

Echocardiography in SVA

Echocardiography is able to identify the presence of a SVA, determine the type or location of the SVA, establish the size of the SVA, and identify associated lesions and complications.

SVAs are best seen from the parasternal short axis view at the level of the aortic valve. Aneurysms appear as 'ballooning' of the coronary sinus into the adjacent chamber or chambers (Fig. 11.11).

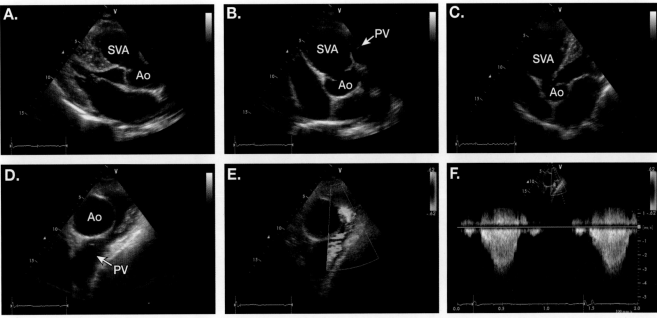

Figure 11.11 A large right sinus of Valsalva aneurysm (SVA) is shown. Images are recorded from the parasternal long axis view **(A)**, the parasternal short axis view **(B)**, the apical 5-chamber view **(C)** and a high parasternal short axis view **(D)**. Right ventricular outflow tract (RVOT) obstruction due to the significant protrusion of this aneurysm into the RVOT is also apparent **(D)**. Colour Doppler imaging **(E)** confirms the presence of turbulent flow across the RVOT. The peak velocity across the RVOT was approximately 3 m/s, yielding a pressure gradient of 36 mm Hg **(F)**. Ao = aorta; PV = pulmonary valve.

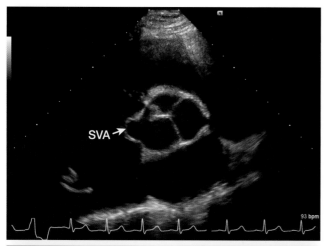

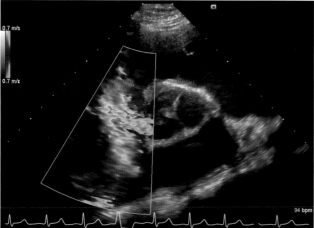

Figure 11.12 A ruptured non-coronary sinus of Valsalva aneurysm (SVA) is displayed in the parasternal short axis view. The SVA has a typical windsock appearance (*top*). Colour flow imaging confirms the communication between the aorta and the right atrium (*bottom*).

SVA may also be an acquired lesion occurring secondary to other disease processes involving the aortic root and sinuses. These diseases include medial degeneration, atherosclerosis, endocarditis, and trauma. In most instances, more than one sinus of Valsalva is affected in which case there is an aneurysm of the aortic root rather a SVA.

Ruptured SVAs have a typical 'wind-sock' appearance on 2D echocardiography. On spectral and colour Doppler imaging abnormal continuous flow from the aorta to the respective chamber is seen (Fig. 11.12). As ruptures usually occur between the aorta and the RV, RA or LA, the velocity of the spectral Doppler signal will be high throughout the cardiac cycle as this signal reflects the pressure difference between the aorta and these lower pressured chambers.

Acute Aortic Syndromes
Definition
Acute aortic syndromes (AAS) refer to the spectrum of life-threatening aortic emergencies caused by non-traumatic acute aortic injury. These conditions include aortic dissection, intramural haematoma (IMH) and penetrating atherosclerotic ulcer (PAU) (Fig. 11.13).

IMH and PAU are briefly discussed below. Aortic dissection is discussed in detail in the following section.

Intramural Haematoma
IMH refers to the presence of blood or haemorrhage within the media of the aortic wall but there is no intimal tear (see Fig. 11.13, top right). This condition is therefore also referred to as "dissection without intimal tear". The lack of an intimal tear distinguishes IMH from classical aortic dissection and PAU. The likely cause of IMH is rupture of the vasa vasorum within the aortic wall which results in haemorrhaging into the media that extends into the adventitia (Fig. 11.14). This condition can account for up to 10-30% of patients presenting with AAS.

Propagation of the haematoma along the medial aortic layer weakens the aorta. This may then progress to outward rupture of the aortic wall with resultant haemorrhage extending into the mediastinum, pericardium or pleura, or to inward disruption of the intima leading to an aortic dissection, a penetrating ulcer or a pseudoaneurysm.

The characteristic echocardiographic feature of IMH is a circular or crescentic hypoechoic area of the aortic wall more than 5 mm in thickness (Fig. 11.15). While IMH can be seen on TTE it is better appreciated on TOE due to its superior spatial resolution and its ability to more completely image the distal ascending aorta and aortic arch.

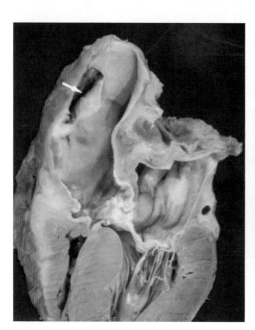

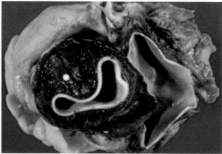

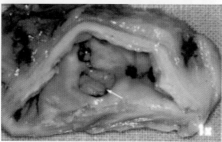

Figure 11.13 These pathological specimens show examples of acute aortic syndromes.
Left: A type A aortic dissection with an entrance tear in the ascending aorta (*arrow*).
Top Right: A cross section of the ascending aorta showing an intramural aortic haematoma (*asterisk*).
Bottom Right: A cross section of the descending thoracic aorta with a penetrating atherosclerotic aortic ulcer (*arrow*).
Reproduced from Vilacosta I, Román JA. Acute aortic syndrome, *Heart*, Apr;85(4), pages 366 and 367, © 2001 with permission from BMJ Publishing Group Ltd.

Penetrating Atherosclerotic Ulcer

PAU refers to an ulcerating atherosclerotic lesion that 'blisters' and erodes through the elastic lamina of the aortic wall and into the intima (see Fig. 11.13, bottom right). This ulcer then penetrates into the media to form a haematoma (Fig. 11.16). This is an uncommon condition accounting for less than 5% of patients presenting with AAS.

PAU may occur as a complication of IMH and it may also

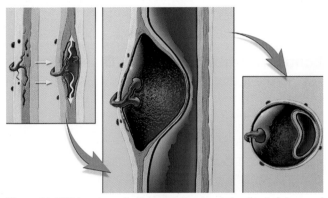

Figure 11.14 This schematic illustrates the events leading to intramural haematoma, from rupture of vasa vasorum feeding the aortic media to creation of intramedial haematoma with an intact intimal layer.
Reproduced from Macura KJ, Corl FM, Fishman EK, Bluemke DA. Pathogenesis in acute aortic syndromes: aortic dissection, intramural hematoma, and penetrating atherosclerotic aortic ulcer. *AJR Am J Roentgenol.* © 2003 Aug;181(2), page 312, with permission from the American Journal of Roentgenology.

lead to an aortic dissection. Erosion through the adventitia may lead to the formation of a pseudoaneurysm.

These lesions are best diagnosed by contrast-enhanced CT or MRI. On TOE, PAU may appear in areas of extensive aortic atheromas as a crater-like 'pocket' with irregular edges within the aortic intima (Fig. 11.17).

Aortic Dissections

Definition and Classification

Aortic dissection is the most common cause of AAS accounting for approximately 80%-90% of all cases.

An aortic dissection occurs when there is a tear in the intima resulting in blood entering the medial layer to create a false, blood-filled channel that is separated from the true lumen by an intimal flap (Fig. 11.18). Aortic dissections are classified according to the Stanford or DeBakey classifications (Fig. 11.19). Via the DeBakey classification, a Type I aortic dissection involves both the ascending aorta and aortic arch, Type II is confined to the ascending aorta, while Type III begins in the descending aorta. Type III may be further subdivided into Type IIIa where the dissection is confined to the descending thoracic aorta and Type IIIb where the dissection extends into the abdominal aorta and iliac arteries. The Stanford classification is based solely on whether or not the ascending aorta is involved irrespective of the entry site or the distal extent of the dissection. Therefore, a Type A dissection includes all dissections involving the ascending

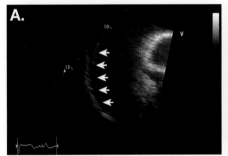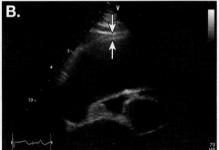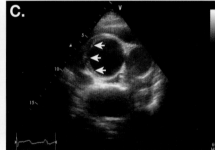

Figure 11.15 These images were recorded from the suprasternal window. Observe the intramural haematoma within the ascending aorta **(A)** and aortic arch **(B)** as indicated by the arrows; haematoma appears as a soft tissue, hypoechoic echodensity. In the short axis plane **(C)** the characteristic crescentic shape of the intramural haematoma is evident (*arrows*).

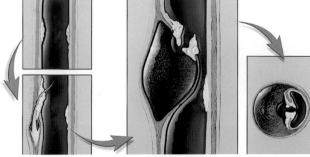

Figure 11.16 This schematic illustrates the events leading to penetrating aortic ulcer from the formation of extensive aortic atheroma confined to intimal layer, through lesion progression to deep ulceration of plaque with penetration into media, to entrance of blood from aortic lumen into media and splitting of media with intramural haematoma. Haematoma formation may extend along the media, resulting in long-segment intramural haematoma.
Reproduced from Macura KJ, Corl FM, Fishman EK, Bluemke DA. Pathogenesis in acute aortic syndromes: aortic dissection, intramural hematoma, and penetrating atherosclerotic aortic ulcer. *AJR Am J Roentgenol.* © 2003 Aug;181(2), page 313, with permission from the American Journal of Roentgenology.

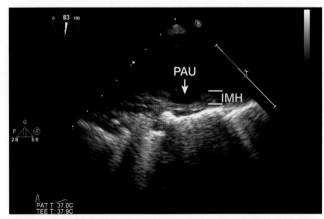

Figure 11.17 This long axis image of the descending aorta was recorded via transoesophageal echocardiography. A penetrating aortic ulcer (PAU) is shown (*arrow*). This appears as a 'pocket' or 'divot' within the aortic wall. There is associated intramural haematoma (IMH) which appears as a hypoechoic thickening of the aortic wall.

aorta; that is, the DeBakey types I and II. A type B dissection includes all other dissections that do not include the ascending aorta; that is, DeBakey type III.

Classification of Variants [11.1]

Another classification of aortic dissections has been proposed to account for iatrogenic and traumatic causes of aortic dissection and based on the fact that intramural haemorrhage, IMH and aortic PAU may be signs of evolving dissections or dissection subtypes. This classification therefore includes:

Class 1: classical aortic dissection (i.e. Stanford and DeBakey classifications)

Class 2: IMH

Class 3: limited dissection (limited intimal tear with eccentric bulge at tear site but without haematoma)

Class 4: penetrating atherosclerotic ulcer

Class 5: iatrogenic and traumatic dissection (e.g. coronary angiography or blunt chest injury)

Pathophysiology of Aortic Dissections

The postulated mechanisms of aortic dissection include weakening of the aortic wall by medial degeneration of abnormal connective tissues within the aortic wall or by excessive shear stresses resulting in IMH which eventually ruptures through the intima (Figure 11.20). Extension of an aortic dissection from its point of rupture occurs in both longitudinal and circumferential planes due to high pressure and pulsatile blood flow into the false lumen.

The risk factors associated with aortic dissections are listed in Table 11.5.

Echocardiography in Aortic Dissection

The role of echocardiography in aortic dissection includes:
- Identifying an aortic dissection,
- Assessment of LV systolic function,
- Identification of complications associated with an aortic dissection,
- Exclusion of differential diagnoses of aortic dissection.

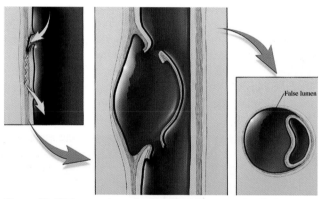

Figure 11.18 These schematics illustrate the events leading to aortic dissection from the formation of entrance tear and exit tear of intima to splitting of aortic media and formation of an intimal flap. Blood under pressure dissects the media longitudinally, and a double-channel aorta is formed with blood filling both the true and false lumens. Reproduced from Macura KJ, Corl FM, Fishman EK, Bluemke DA. Pathogenesis in acute aortic syndromes: aortic dissection, intramural hematoma, and penetrating atherosclerotic aortic ulcer. *AJR Am J Roentgenol*. © 2003 Aug;181(2), page 310, with permission from the American Journal of Roentgenology.

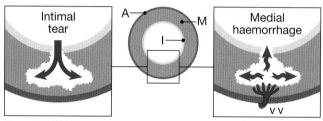

Figure 11.20 This schematic illustrates two proposed mechanisms of aortic dissection. **Left:** Aortic dissection begins with weakening of the aortic wall by medial degeneration (congenital or acquired disorders). This leads to an intimal tear that allows blood to enter the wall of the aorta. This results in the dissection of the media (M) and stripping of the intima (I) from the adventitia (A) in a longitudinal manner. The intima forms a boundary between the true and the false lumen. The medial dissection may continue both proximally and distally in the aorta. **Right:** Aortic dissection begins with excessive shear forces on the adventitia (A) caused by acute or chronic hypertension or trauma. This leads to rupture of the vasa vasorum (v v) within the aortic media which results in the development of an intramural haematoma. Medial haemorrhage then secondarily ruptures through the intima layer and creates the intimal tear and aortic dissection.

Figure 11.19 The DeBakey classification of aortic dissection includes three types. In Type I, the intimal tear usually originates in the proximal ascending aorta and the dissection involves the ascending aorta, the arch, and variable lengths of the descending and abdominal aorta. In Type II, the dissection is confined to the ascending aorta. In Type III, the dissection may be confined to the descending thoracic aorta (Type IIIa) or may extend into the abdominal aorta and iliac arteries (Type IIIb). The Stanford classification has two types. Type A includes all cases in which the ascending aorta is involved by the

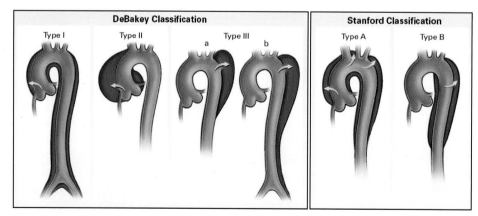

dissection, with or without involvement of the arch or the descending aorta. Type B includes cases in which the descending thoracic aorta is involved, with or without proximal (retrograde) or distal (anterograde) extension. Reproduced from Kouchoukos NT, Dougenis D. Surgery of the thoracic aorta. *N Engl J Med*. Jun 26;336(26), page 1878, © 1997 with permission from the Massachusetts Medical Society.

[11.1] Svensson LG, Labib SB, Eisenhauer AC, Butterly JR. Intimal tear without hematoma: an important variant of aortic dissection that can elude current imaging techniques. *Circulation*. 1999 Mar 16;99(10):1331-6.

Identifying an Aortic Dissection

An aortic dissection is identified by observing an intimal flap within the aortic root. On real-time imaging, this flap appears as a thin, undulating structure within the aortic lumen; colour flow Doppler imaging is also helpful in demonstrating the true and false lumens (Fig. 11.21). Other features that can be used to differentiate between the true and false lumens are listed in Table 11.6.

Importantly, in patients with a suspected aortic dissection, the imaging of the aorta from all possible acoustic windows should be attempted. This includes imaging from the right sternal edge as well as off-axis imaging (Fig. 11.22).

Table 11.5 Risk Factors for Development of Thoracic Aortic Dissection

Risk Factors for Development of Thoracic Aortic Dissection
Conditions associated with increased aortic wall stress
Hypertension, particularly if uncontrolled
Pheochromocytoma
Cocaine or other stimulant use
Weight lifting or other Valsalva manoeuvre
Trauma
Deceleration or torsional injury (e.g. motor vehicle crash, fall)
Coarctation of the aorta
Conditions associated with aortic media abnormalities
Genetic
Marfan syndrome
Ehlers-Danlos syndrome, vascular form
Bicuspid aortic valve (including prior aortic valve replacement)
Turner syndrome
Loeys-Dietz syndrome
Familial thoracic aortic aneurysm and dissection syndrome
Inflammatory vasculitides
Takayasu arteritis
Giant cell arteritis
Behçet arteritis
Other
Pregnancy
Polycystic kidney disease
Chronic corticosteroid or immunosuppression agent administration
Infections involving the aortic wall either from bacteremia or extension of adjacent infection

Reprinted from Hiratzka LF, Bakris GL, Beckman JA, et al. 2010 ACCF/AHA/AATS/ACR/ASA/SCA/SCAI/SIR/STS/SVM Guidelines for the Diagnosis and Management of Patients With Thoracic Aortic Disease: a report of the American College of Cardiology Foundation/American Heart Association Task Force on Practice Guidelines, American Association for Thoracic Surgery, American College of Radiology, American Stroke Association, Society of Cardiovascular Anesthesiologists, Society for Cardiovascular Angiography and Interventions, Society of Interventional Radiology, Society of Thoracic Surgeons, and Society for Vascular Medicine, *J Am Coll Cardiol*, Vol. 55 (14), page e61, © 2010, with permission from Elsevier.

> A Type A aortic dissection is a **medical emergency** because of the high mortality rates associated with this condition. Death is caused by proximal or distal extension of the dissection leading to acute severe AR, occlusion of major arch vessels and/or coronary arteries, rupture with exsanguination into the pleura or mediastinum, or rupture with cardiac tamponade.
> Importantly, there is no such thing as a stable Type A dissection. Therefore, identification of previously undiagnosed Type A aortic dissections should be immediately reported to the referring physician.

With transthoracic echocardiography an intimal flap may not be well seen in all cases of aortic dissection so it is important to be aware of other clues that may indicate the presence of an aortic dissection. For example, colour separation within the aortic lumen is a clue to the presence of an aortic dissection (Fig. 11.23). Other clues to a Type A aortic dissection are based on the identification of complications associated with this type of dissection. These clues include: (1) ascending aorta dilatation, (2) acute severe AR, (3) pericardial effusion, and/or (4) regional wall motion abnormalities (when the dissection involves a coronary artery). Therefore, when an intimal flap cannot be seen, the presence of aortic root dilatation associated with acute AR and/or a pericardial effusion are highly suggestive of a Type A aortic dissection.

> A normal TTE cannot exclude an aortic dissection; the sensitivity of TTE in the detection of aortic dissection is significantly lower than other imaging modalities such as TOE, CT and MRI. Therefore, if the clinical suspicion for an aortic dissection is high and TOE, CT or MRI are readily available, these imaging techniques are considered the method of choice for making the initial diagnosis. TOE, CT and MRI also have the added ability of localising aortic wall tears and assessing the extent of dissection.
> TTE, however, maintains an important role in the assessment of cardiac complications such as assessing the severity of AR, LV regional wall motion analysis and identifying pericardial effusion/tamponade.

Table 11.6 Features Differentiating True from False Lumens in Aortic Dissection

Characteristic	True Lumen	False Lumen
Shape (cross-section)	Oval or round	Crescentic
Flap curvature (cross-section)	Concave towards false lumen	Convex with acute angle between the dissection flap and the outer wall
Motion	Systolic expansion and diastolic collapse	Diastolic expansion
Flow	Forward flow into true lumen in systole	Reduced, absent or retrograde flow
Spontaneous echo contrast	Absent or low intensity	Common +/- pronounced
Thrombus	Minimal or none	Complete or partial thrombosis

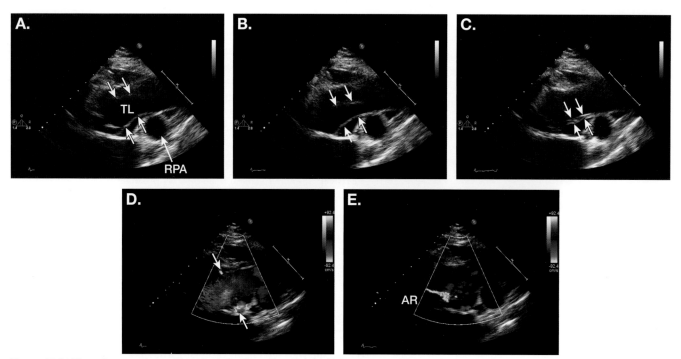

Figure 11.21 These images show a Type A aortic dissection. From a high parasternal long axis view (*top*) an intimal flap (*arrows*) is seen within the aortic lumen; the mobility of this flap is evident over the systolic **(A)**, early diastolic **(B)** and end-diastolic frames **(C)**. Observe that there is almost total collapse of the true lumen (TL) in diastole. Colour Doppler imaging shows flow into the false channels during systole (*arrows*) **(D)**; aortic regurgitation (AR) during diastole is also noted **(E)**. RPA = right pulmonary artery.

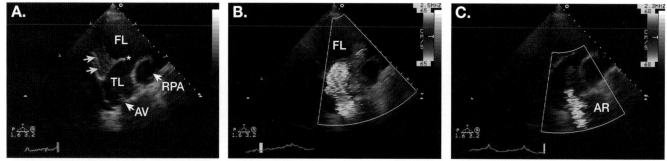

Figure 11.22 These images were recorded from the right sternal edge in a patient with a chronic Type A dissection. The 2D image **(A)** shows a massively dilated ascending aorta; the entry site between the true lumen (TL) and the false lumen (FL) is seen (*); the FL is also lined with thrombus (*yellow arrows*). The colour Doppler images highlight filling of the TL in systole **(B)** and aortic regurgitation (AR) in diastole **(C)**; low velocity flow is also seen within the FL confirming a communication between the TL and FL **(B)**. AV = aortic valve; RPA = right pulmonary artery.

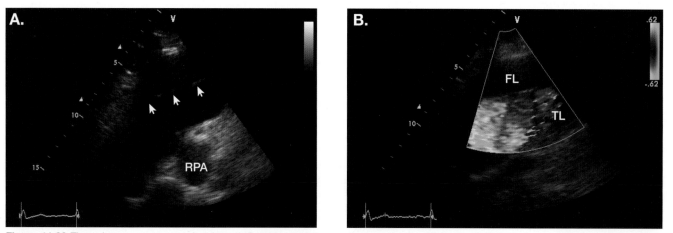

Figure 11.23 These images were recorded from the suprasternal long axis view. On the 2D image (*left*) there is a suggestion of a possible intimal flap within the aortic lumen (*arrows*). The colour flow image (*right*) shows colour separation which confirms that this faint linear echo is a dissection flap and is not an imaging artefact; observe the colour filling of the true lumen (TL) with no colour within the false lumen (FL). RPA = right pulmonary artery.

Not all linear structures within the aortic lumen are intimal flaps. Imaging artefacts as a result of reverberation or mirror artefacts may also mimic an intimal flap leading to a false-positive diagnosis of an aortic dissection. Differentiation between artefacts and a true dissection flap is based on several observations (Table 11.7 and Fig 11.24).

Occasionally, the left brachiocephalic (innominate) vein which courses transversely and superior to the aortic arch may appear quite prominent and may be confused with an aortic dissection flap. Verification that the structure superior to the aortic arch is in fact the left brachiocephalic vein can be achieved by attempting to follow this vessel into its long axis and to identify its connection with the superior vena cava (SVC) (Fig. 11.25).

Assessment of Left Ventricular Systolic Function

A Type A aortic dissection can also cause an acute myocardial infarction (AMI) and/or ischaemic chest pain due to coronary artery dissection or obstruction to the coronary artery ostium by the dissection flap. Therefore, regional wall motion abnormalities (RWMA) may be detected in these situations. Left ventricular systolic function and regional wall motion analysis is assessed by both M-mode and 2D echocardiography in the traditional manner (see Chapters 2 and 5).

Identification of Complications Associated with Aortic Dissection

Aortic Regurgitation

A Type A aortic dissection is an important cause of acute AR. Several mechanisms for AR in Type A aortic dissections have been described (see Fig. 7.49). These mechanisms include: (1) incomplete closure of a normal aortic valve due to ST junction dilatation; (2) aortic valve prolapse due to extension of the dissection into the aortic root which disrupts normal leaflet attachments to the aortic wall; (3) prolapse of the dissection flap through normal aortic valve leaflets that disrupts leaflet coaptation; (4) asymmetrical dissection where pressure from the dissecting haematoma may depress one leaflet below the line of closure of the other two leaflets; and (5) loss of annular support or tearing of the leaflets themselves may render the valve incompetent. The severity of AR is evaluated by indirect spectral and colour Doppler methods +/- quantitative methods as described in Chapter 7.

Myocardial Ischaemia or Infarction

As mentioned above, Type A aortic dissections can also cause an AMI and/or ischaemic chest pain. Therefore, the identification of RWMAs indicates coronary artery involvement. The pattern of RWMA can also predict which coronary artery is involved. Regional wall motion analysis is assessed in the traditional manner (see Chapter 5).

Pericardial Effusion and Tamponade

Pericardial effusions are frequently seen in acute Type A aortic dissections. Effusions occur due to transudation or oozing of fluid into the pericardial space; these effusions are considered to be haemodynamically insignificant. However, when there is free rupture into the pericardium cardiac tamponade with haemodynamic compromise ensues rapidly. Cardiac tamponade is the most common cause of death in aortic dissection and therefore, tamponade physiology in the setting of an acute Type A aortic dissection warrants prompt and urgent surgical repair.

Determination of cardiac tamponade physiology is assessed in the usual manner (see Chapter 12).

Differential Diagnosis of Aortic Dissection

The signs and symptoms of an aortic dissection may be associated with a number of aetiologies. Therefore, echocardiography has an important role in the differential diagnosis of these causes. Other causes of cardiac chest pain that can be diagnosed or identified by echocardiography include acute coronary syndrome, AMI, pericarditis, and acute pulmonary embolism. The echocardiographic features of these conditions are discussed in Chapter 5.

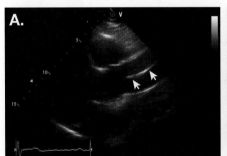 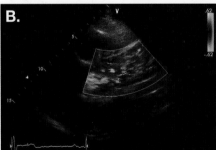 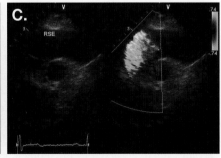

Figure 11.24 From a high parasternal long axis view **(A)** an apparent intimal flap (*arrows*) is seen within the aortic lumen. However, colour Doppler imaging shows complete filling of the aortic lumen during systole **(B)**. Further imaging from the right sternal edge (RSE) failed to identify the 'flap' within the aortic lumen and colour flow Doppler again confirmed complete filling of the lumen during systole **(C)**. This 'flap' was deemed to be a mirror artefact whereby the anterior aortic wall acted as a mirror; this resulted in the right ventricular wall being 'mirrored' within the aortic lumen.

Table 11.7 Methods for differentiating Artefacts from True Aortic Dissection Flaps

Observations	Aortic Dissection	Artefact
'Flap' imaged from multiple planes	Yes	Not usually (artefacts tend to be seen in only 1 imaging plane)
'Flap' motion independent of surrounding structures	Yes	No (follows motion of structure creating the artefact)
'Flap' contained within aortic lumen	Yes	Often extends beyond aortic lumen
Differential flow on either side of 'flap' via colour Doppler	Yes	No (colour is seen on both sides of 'flap'; colour separation is not seen)

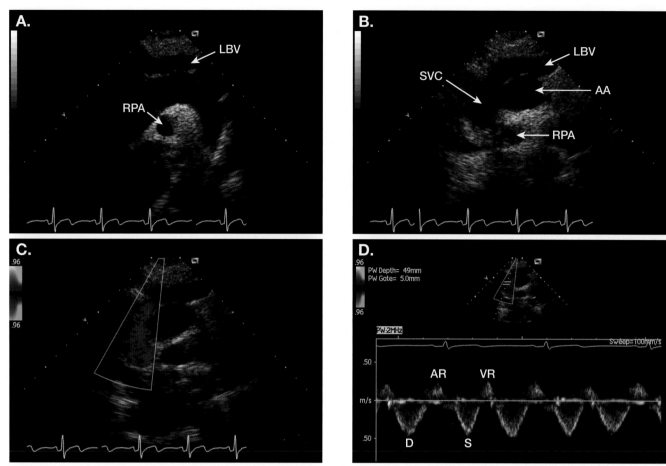

Figure 11.25 From the suprasternal view, the left brachiocephalic vein (LBV) can often be seen traversing superior to the aortic arch **(A)**. By rotating the transducer anti-clockwise, it is often possible to connect the LBV with the superior vena cava (SVC) **(B)**. Colour flow Doppler imaging can be used to confirm that this vein drains into the SVC **(C)**.Spectral Doppler can be used to demonstrate the characteristic venous flow profile of the LBV as it drains into the SVC **(D)**. AA = aortic arch; AR = atrial flow reversal; D = diastolic forward flow; RPA = right pulmonary artery; S = systolic forward flow; VR = ventricular flow reversal.

Traumatic Aortic Injury

Traumatic aortic injury (TAI), also referred to as traumatic aortic disruption, traumatic aortic rupture or aortic transection, is caused by the rapid acceleration or deceleration of the body which occurs most commonly during a motor vehicle accident. Other causes of TAI include direct blows to the chest, falls from great heights, sporting and industrial injuries, and kicks by animals. The pathophysiological features leading to TAI are illustrated in Figure 11.26.

TAI typically occurs at the point of fixation of the aorta with other structures. Most commonly this point is at the aortic isthmus because it is here that the ascending aorta and arch becomes relatively fixed to the thoracic cage by the pleural reflections, the intercostal arteries, and the left subclavian artery. Other sites of trauma include the ascending aorta, the aortic arch, the distal descending thoracic aorta and the abdominal aorta. The diagnosis of aortic trauma is achieved by aortography, CT, MRI or TOE (Fig. 11.27).

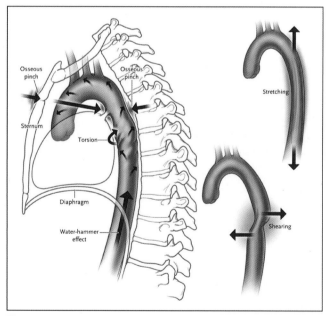

Figure 11.26 This schematic illustrates the possible mechanisms of blunt aortic injury; these mechanisms include stretching, shearing, torsion, a "water-hammer" effect (which involves simultaneous occlusion of the aorta and a sudden elevation in blood pressure), and the "osseous pinch" effect from entrapment of the aorta between the anterior chest wall and the vertebral column. Most injuries probably involve a combination of forces.

Reproduced from Neschis DG, Scalea TM, Flinn WR, Griffith BP. Blunt Aortic Injury. *N Engl J Med.* Oct 16;359(16), page 1709, © 2008 with permission from the Massachusetts Medical Society.

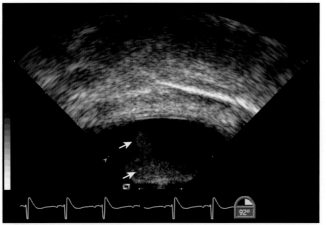 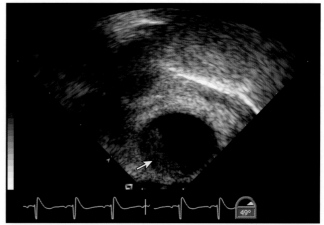

Figure 11.27 These images were recorded via transoesophageal echocardiography in a patient with suspected traumatic aortic injury following a motor vehicle accident. Longitudinal (*left*) and short axis (*right*) imaging planes are shown. Observe the appearance of a broad based mobile soft tissue mass attached to the posteromedial wall of the descending thoracic aorta (*arrows*); no clearly defined intimal surface is shown. The appearances were considered most consistent with a partial thickness traumatic injury of the descending thoracic aorta with associated thrombus attached to the abnormal ruptured intimal surface.

Key Points

Anatomy of the Aorta
* Aortic walls consist of three layers: tunica intima, tunica media and tunica adventitia
* The thoracic aorta is the section of aorta above the diaphragm; it includes 5 segments: (1) aortic root, (2) ascending aorta, (3) aortic arch, (4) aortic isthmus and (5) descending thoracic aorta
* The abdominal aorta is the section of aorta below the diaphragm; it includes 2 segments: (1) suprarenal segment and (2) infrarenal segment

2D Imaging and Measurements of the Aorta
* Imaging of various segments of the aorta can be achieved from:
  - all standard acoustic windows
  - additional windows including the high left parasternal view, right parasternal long axis (when the aorta is dilated) and posterior imaging through a left pleural effusion
* Aortic measurements are performed at end-diastole via the leading edge to leading edge technique (exception is the descending aorta which is measured inner edge to inner edge)
* LVOT is measured at mid-systole via the inner edge to inner edge technique

Aortic Aneurysms
* *Definition:* dilatation of all layers of the aorta 1.5 times greater than the normal arterial diameter
* *Types:* saccular (spherical outpouching), fusiform (spindle-shaped) and pseudoaneurysms (false aneurysm)
* *Location:* thoracic aorta, thoracoabdominal aorta (thoracic aneurysms extending into the abdomen), and abdominal aorta
* *Most common location:* abdominal aorta (infrarenal)
* *Aetiology:* most common causes of true aneurysms include medial degeneration, atherosclerosis, arteritis; rarely, mycotic aneurysms can form due to a primary infection of the aorta
* *Complications:* include rupture, aortic dissection, thrombus formation and embolism, vascular obstruction, and AR secondary to annular dilatation

Role of Echo in Aortic Aneurysms
* Identifying the presence and site of an aortic aneurysm
* Measuring the size of aortic aneurysm
* Assessing the severity of associated aortic regurgitation

Sinus of Valsalva Aneurysms (SVA)
* *Definition:* rare congenital anomaly where there is dilatation of a single sinus of Valsalva
* *Types:* right SVA (most common), non-coronary SVA, left SVA (very rare)
* *Associated lesions:* common anomalies include bicuspid aortic valves, VSD (right SVA); less common anomalies include pulmonary stenosis, coarctation, and atrial septal defect
* *Complications:* include fistulous communication between the aorta and another site (depends on the type of SVA); SVA in conjunction with a VSD can lead to aortic valve prolapse and AR; other complications of unruptured SVA include RVOT obstruction, conduction abnormalities and myocardial ischaemia/infarction

(continued over...)

Key Points (continued)

Role of Echo in SVA
- Determine the type/location of the SVA
- Establish the size of the SVA
- Identify associated lesions and complications

Acute Aortic Syndromes (AAS)
- *Definition:* A spectrum of life-threatening aortic emergencies caused by non-traumatic acute aortic injury. These conditions include aortic dissection, intramural haematoma (IMH) and penetrating atherosclerotic ulcer (PAU)
- *IMH:* the presence of blood or haemorrhage within the media of the aortic wall but there is no intimal tear; accounts for 10-30% of AAS; the characteristic echocardiographic feature of IMH is circular or crescentic thickening of the aortic wall > 5 mm
- *PAU:* an ulcerating atherosclerotic lesion that 'blisters' and erodes through the elastic lamina of the aortic wall and into the intima; accounts for < 5% of AAS; best diagnosed by CT or MRI; on TOE, appears in as a crater-like outpouching of the aortic intima with jagged edges

Aortic Dissections
- *Definition:* most common cause of AAS accounting for approximately 80%-90% of all cases
- *Classification:* DeBakey or Stanford classification based on the location of the dissection:
  - DeBakey Type I involves both the ascending aorta and arch, Type II is confined to the ascending aorta, while Type III begins in the descending aorta
  - Stanford Type A dissection includes all dissections involving the ascending aorta, Type B dissection includes all other dissections that do not include the ascending aorta

Role of Echo in Aortic Dissections:
- Identifying an aortic dissection (based on the detection of an intimal flap within the aorta)
- Assessment of LV systolic function
- Identification of complications associated with an aortic dissection (e.g. AR, pericardial effusion, RWMA)
- Exclude differential diagnosis of aortic dissection

Traumatic Aortic Injury
- *Aetiology:* most commonly caused by rapid acceleration or deceleration of the body during a motor vehicle accident. Other causes include direct blows to the chest, falls from great heights, sporting and industrial injuries, and kicks by animals
- *Site:* most common site of aortic injury is at the aortic isthmus
- *Diagnosis:* usually made by aortography, CT, MRI or TOE rather than by TTE

Further Reading (listed in alphabetical order)

Anatomy of the Aorta

Anderson RH. Clinical anatomy of the aortic root. *Heart.* 2000 Dec;84(6):670-3.

Ho SY. Structure and anatomy of the aortic root. *Eur J Echocardiogr.* 2009 Jan;10(1):i3-10.

Imaging of the Aorta

Evangelista A, Flachskampf FA, Erbel R, Antonini-Canterin F, Vlachopoulos C, Rocchi G, Sicari R, Nihoyannopoulos P, Zamorano J; European Association of Echocardiography; Document Reviewers:, Pepi M, Breithardt OA, Plonska-Gosciniak E. Echocardiography in aortic diseases: EAE recommendations for clinical practice. *Eur J Echocardiogr.* 2010 Sep;11(8):645-58.

Aortic Aneurysms

Booher AM, Eagle KA. Diagnosis and management issues in thoracic aortic aneurysm. *Am Heart J.* 2011 Jul;162(1):38-46.e1.

Hiratzka LF, Bakris GL, Beckman JA, Bersin RM, Carr VF, Casey DE Jr, Eagle KA, Hermann LK, Isselbacher EM, Kazerooni EA, Kouchoukos NT, Lytle BW, Milewicz DM, Reich DL, Sen S, Shinn JA, Svensson LG, Williams DM; 2010 ACCF/AHA/AATS/ACR/ASA/SCA/SCAI/SIR/STS/SVM Guidelines for the diagnosis and management of patients with thoracic aortic disease. A Report of the American College of Cardiology Foundation/American Heart Association Task Force on Practice Guidelines, American Association for Thoracic Surgery, American College of Radiology, American Stroke Association, Society of Cardiovascular Anesthesiologists, Society for Cardiovascular Angiography and Interventions, Society of Interventional Radiology, Society of Thoracic Surgeons, and Society for Vascular Medicine. *J Am Coll Cardiol.* 2010 Apr 6;55(14):e27-e129.

Ring WS. Congenital Heart Surgery Nomenclature and Database Project: aortic aneurysm, sinus of Valsalva aneurysm, and aortic dissection. *Ann Thorac Surg.* 2000 Apr;69(4 Suppl):S147-63.

Sinus of Valsalva Aneurysms

Feldman DN, Roman MJ. Aneurysms of the sinuses of Valsalva. *Cardiology.* 2006;106(2):73-81.

Ott DA. Aneurysm of the sinus of Valsalva. *Semin Thorac Cardiovasc Surg Pediatr Card Surg Annu.* 2006:165-76.

Acute Aortic Syndromes and Aortic Dissection

Erbel R, Alfonso F, Boileau C, Dirsch O, Eber B, Haverich A, Rakowski H, Struyven J, Radegran K, Sechtem U, Taylor J, Zollikofer C, Klein WW, Mulder B, Providencia LA; Task Force on Aortic Dissection, European Society of Cardiology. Diagnosis and management of aortic dissection. *Eur Heart J.* 2001 Sep;22(18):1642-81.

Meredith EL, Masani ND. Echocardiography in the emergency assessment of acute aortic syndromes. *Eur J Echocardiogr.* 2009 Jan;10(1):i31-9.

Nienaber CA, Powell JT. Management of acute aortic syndromes. *Eur Heart J.* 2011 Aug 2.

Vilacosta I, Román JA. Acute aortic syndrome. *Heart.* 2001 Apr;85(4):365-8.

Traumatic Aortic Injury

Neschis DG, Scalea TM, Flinn WR, Griffith BP. Blunt aortic injury. *N Engl J Med.* 2008 Oct 16;359(16):1708-16.

Khalil A, Helmy T, Porembka DT. Aortic pathology: aortic trauma, debris, dissection, and aneurysm. *Crit Care Med.* 2007 Aug;35(8 Suppl):S392-400.

Pericardial Disease

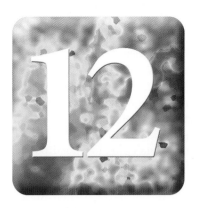

Anatomy and Function of the Pericardium

Pericardial Layers

The normal pericardium encloses the heart and covers the proximal segments of the great vessels arising from the heart. The pericardium is 1- 2 mm thick and consists of two "sacs": (1) an outer sac or fibrous pericardium and (2) a double-layered inner sac or serous pericardium (Fig. 12.1 and 12.2). The fibrous pericardium is a sac made of tough connective tissue that surrounds the heart. It is bounded to the central tendon of the diaphragm inferiorly and is attached to the posterior surface of the sternum via the sternopericardial ligaments anteriorly; it is also adherent to the mediastinal pleura. Via these anchorage points, the pericardium secures the position of the heart within the thoracic cavity; that is, the pericardium acts as a 'cardiac seat belt'.

The serous pericardium is a closed sac within the fibrous pericardium. It consists of two layers: the visceral and parietal layers. Although the visceral and parietal pericardia are histologically different they are continuous so that the visceral pericardium 'reflects' to become the parietal pericardium. The visceral (inner) layer consists of a thin layer of mesothelial cells closely adherent to the surface of the heart; this layer is also known as the epicardium. This inner layer is reflected onto the surface of the outer fibrous layer which forms the parietal pericardium. The parietal (outer) layer lines the internal surface of the fibrous pericardium and consists of collagenous fibrous tissue and elastic fibrils. As such this layer is thicker than the visceral pericardium.

Between the visceral and parietal layers is the pericardial space which contains approximately 10-30 mL of ultrafiltrate of plasma.

Pericardial Sinuses

As stated above, the visceral layer of the serous pericardium reflects to form the parietal layer. Therefore, there are two 'reflections' that meet to close the serous pericardial sac. These reflections are situated around the systemic and pulmonary venous inflows and around the great vessels. At these points where the visceral and parietal pericardia are continuous with one another, the pericardial sinuses are located. The pericardial sinuses are extensions of the pericardial cavity; therefore, fluid can accumulate within these sinuses.

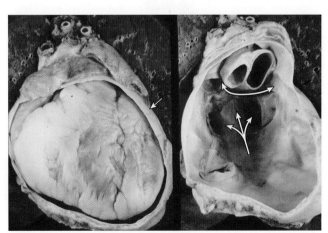

Figure 12.2 These pathological specimens show the anatomy of the pericardium with the heart in-situ (*left*) and with the heart removed (*right*). Observe that the outer fibrous pericardium is relatively thick-walled (about 1 mm). The two layers of the serous pericardium include the visceral layer which covers the surface of the heart and the parietal layer which lines the fibrous pericardium. On the left specimen, the fibrous pericardium has been cut away to show the parietal layer (*arrow*). The space between the visceral and the parietal layers denotes the pericardial cavity. With the heart removed the visceral pericardium is seen posteriorly around the great vessels. The three-headed arrow identifies the oblique sinus and the two-headed arrow indicates the transverse sinus.

By permission of Mayo Foundation for Medical Education and Research. All rights reserved. Courtesy of William D. Edwards, MD.

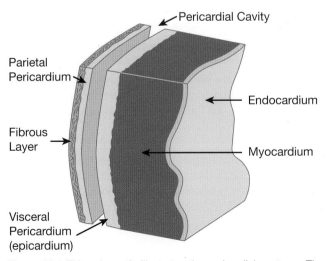

Figure 12.1 This schematic illustrates the pericardial anatomy. The pericardium consists of two sacs: the outer fibrous pericardium and the double-layered inner serous pericardium. The two layers of the serous pericardium are the visceral and the parietal layers. Between these two layers is the pericardial cavity.

There are two pericardial sinuses: the transverse sinus and the oblique sinus (Fig. 12.2 and 12.3). The transverse sinus is a tunnel-like structure which is situated anterior to the superior vena cava (SVC) and posterior to the ascending aorta and pulmonary trunk above the left atrium (LA); this is where the aorta and pulmonary artery leave the heart. The oblique pericardial sinus is an inverted J-shaped, cul-de-sac located superior and posterior to the LA; this is where the SVC, inferior vena cava (IVC) and pulmonary veins enter the heart. The two pericardial sinuses are not continuous; that is, the oblique sinus is separated from the transverse sinus superiorly by the double reflection of serous pericardium which connects the left and right upper pulmonary veins. Importantly, it should be noted that the pericardium does not cover the entire heart. In particular, the posterior portion of the LA is not totally covered by the pericardium (Fig. 12.4).

Function of the Pericardium

There are a number of functions of the pericardium including:
1. stabilisation of the heart's position within the thoracic cavity; this is achieved by virtue of its ligamentous attachments,
2. protection of the heart from infection from adjoining structures; this is accomplished by anatomically isolating the heart from the rest of the mediastinum and from the lungs and pleural spaces,
3. acting as a lubricant to reduce friction between the heart and surrounding structures; this allows the normal rotation and translation of the heart during the cardiac cycle,
4. limiting acute distension of the heart and preventing over filling of the heart; this is achieved by the non-distensible nature of the pericardium, and
5. facilitation of the interaction and coupling of the ventricles and atria.

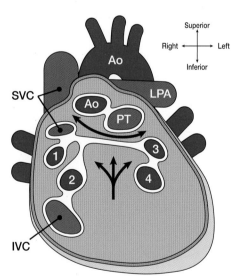

Figure 12.3 The heart is removed and the posterior part of the pericardium is viewed from in front. The transverse sinus (*2-headed arrow*) is limited by a pericardial reflection between the upper pulmonary veins (1 and 3) and the pulmonary trunk (PT). The oblique sinus (*3-headed arrow*) is bounded by an irregular continuous line that begins at the inferior vena cava (IVC), extends up to the right lower pulmonary vein (2), and turns to the left across the left atrium to the left upper and left lower pulmonary veins (3 and 4, respectively).The white areas indicate the bare regions between the serous pericardial reflections. Ao = aorta; LPA = left pulmonary artery; SVC = superior vena cava; 1 = right upper pulmonary vein.

In particular, this latter function explains the concept of ventricular interdependence or interaction. Ventricular interdependence describes the relationship between the size, shape, and compliance of one ventricle with the other. That is, changes to the size, shape, pressure and volume of one ventricle influences the size, shape, pressure and volume of the other. For example, as the right atrium (RA) and right ventricle (RV) fill during normal inspiration, there is a slight increase in RV chamber size. As the pericardium limits the ability of chambers to expand beyond a certain point, this then results in a very slight reduction in both left ventricular (LV) size and LV filling. This concept is especially important when considering cardiac tamponade and constrictive pericarditis.

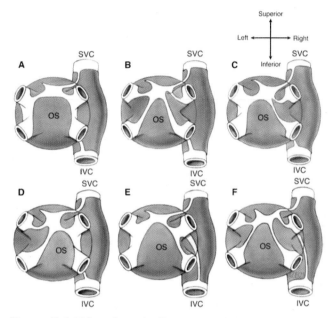

Figure 12.4 This schematic illustrates variations in pericardial covering as seen from the posterior view of the left atrium (LA). The four pulmonary veins, the inferior vena cava (IVC) and superior vena cava (SVC) are also shown. White areas indicate the uncovered areas between reflections of the serous pericardium; that is, the white areas indicate areas that are not covered by the pericardium. The most common anatomic variant is B. OS = oblique sinus.
Reproduced from D'Avila A, Scanavacca M, Sosa E, Ruskin JN, Reddy VY. Pericardial anatomy for the interventional electrophysiologist. *J Cardiovasc Electrophysiol*, Apr;14(4): page 425, © 2003 John Wiley and Sons with permission.

Pericardial Cysts

Pericardial cysts are rare, benign structural abnormalities of the pericardium that result from a defect in the embryonic development of the pericardium. Patients are usually asymptomatic. However pericardial cysts have been associated with chest discomfort or rhythm disturbances. These patients often present for echocardiography because of a distortion of the cardiac silhouette on the chest x-ray.

Most commonly, pericardial cysts are located in the right costophrenic angle. However, cysts may also be found at the left costophrenic angle, the hilum or the superior mediastinum. Importantly, pericardial cysts do not communicate with the pericardium.

On 2D echocardiography, pericardial cysts can be identified by their position and their echo-free appearance. Cysts appear as round or elliptical echo-free structures adjacent to a cardiac chamber; most often cysts appear adjacent to the RA (Fig. 12.5).

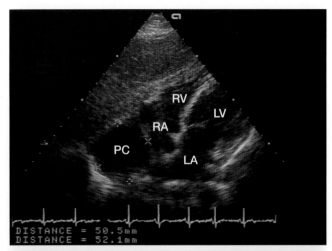

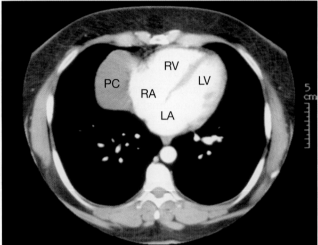

Figure 12.5 The subcostal 4-chamber view shows a large echolucent "mass" adjacent to the right atrium (RA) (*top*). The appearance and position of this mass is characteristic of a pericardial cyst. The computer tomography scan confirms the presence of a large pericardial cyst at the right costophrenic angle; this cyst appears as a gray "bubble" adjacent to the right atrium (*bottom*). LA = left atrium; LV = left ventricle; PC = pericardial cyst; RV = right ventricle.

Congenitally Absent Pericardium

Congenital absence of the pericardium or pericardial agenesis is a very rare, benign condition that is more common in men than women (male:female ratio is 3:1). Approximately 30% of patients also have other associated congenital cardiac anomalies such as atrial septal defect, bicuspid aortic valve, patent ductus arteriosus or tetralogy of Fallot. Congenital absence of the pericardium may be partial or complete. Complete absence is less common than partial absence which is usually left-sided. Complications of partial absence may include herniation and entrapment of a cardiac chamber.

Patients with partial or complete pericardial agenesis often present for echocardiography because of an abnormal ECG or chest x-ray. The characteristic echocardiographic features of congenital absence of the pericardium include: (1) unusual echocardiographic windows, (2) abnormal interventricular septal (IVS) motion, (3) cardiac hypermobility, (4) abnormal swinging motion of the heart and (5) apparent right-sided heart enlargement.

In particular, due to the unusual orientation of the heart within the chest the usual acoustic windows are typically higher and more laterally located than normal and the orientation of the images appears peculiar (Fig. 12.6). For example, from the apical 4-chamber view, the heart has been described as having an inverted 'teardrop' appearance whereby the atria are elongated and the ventricles are relatively bulbous.

Acute Pericarditis

Pericarditis refers to inflammation of the pericardium. The most common causes of acute pericarditis are viral infection and unknown causes (idiopathic).

The diagnosis of acute pericarditis is based on the major clinical manifestations of the disease which include characteristic chest pain and ECG findings as well as a pericardial friction rub on auscultation. Characteristic chest pain is usually exaggerated by inspiration, coughing and by being in a lying position and decreased when sitting upright or leaning forward. Characteristic ECG changes include widespread ST-segment elevation with the ST-segments concaving upwards. A pericardial friction rub is considered highly specific for acute pericarditis; this rub is described as a scratching, grating sound (like 'squeaky leather').

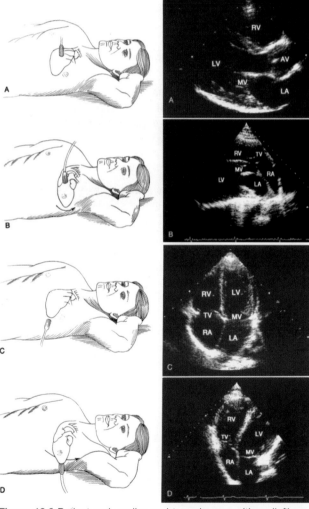

Figure 12.6 Patient and cardiac and transducer positions (*left*) and corresponding two-dimensional echocardiographic images (*right*) are shown. **A**, Normal parasternal long axis study. **B**, Parasternal long axis study shows congenital absence of pericardium. The arrow on the left image represents cardiac rotation. **C**, Normal apical 4-chamber study. **D**, Apical 4-chamber study shows congenital absence of pericardium. Arrow on the left image represents cardiac rotation. AV = aortic valve; LA = left atrium; LV = Left ventricle; MV = mitral valve; RA= right atrium; RV= right ventricle; TV = tricuspid valve.

Adapted from Connolly HM, Click RL, Schattenberg TT, Seward JB, Tajik AJ. Congenital absence of the pericardium: echocardiography as a diagnostic tool, *J Am Soc Echocardiogr*, Vol. 8 (11), page 89, © 1995, with permission from Elsevier.

The echocardiographic examination in patients with acute pericarditis is often entirely normal. However, pericardial effusions of any size and/or pericardial thickening with or without a pericardial effusion may be seen. Importantly, because a normal pericardial thickness is only between 1-2 mm, the detection of pericardial thickening is difficult. In addition, the accurate measurement of pericardial thickness is limited by the spatial resolution of the ultrasound machine.

While the finding of pericardial thickening and/or a pericardial effusion supports the diagnosis of acute pericarditis, the absence of these abnormalities does not exclude it. Therefore, the diagnosis of pericarditis is primarily a clinical, not an echocardiographic, diagnosis.

Pericardial Effusions

Aetiology

Pericardial effusion, which is the abnormal accumulation of fluid within the pericardial cavity, can occur due to inflammation of the pericardium (pericarditis), infection, radiation, autoimmune diseases, trauma, neoplasms and various medications (Table 12.1).

Types of Pericardial Effusion

Pericardial effusions can also be classified as transudative, exudative, haemorrhagic or malignant.

Transudative effusions result from either an increase in capillary hydrostatic pressure or a decrease in osmotic pressure inside blood vessels. This fluid is an ultrafiltrate of plasma and appears colourless, clear, and 'watery'. The most common cause of transudative effusions is congestive heart failure.

Exudative effusions occur due to increased capillary permeability or decreased lymphatic resorption; this results in 'oozing' of extravascular fluid into the pericardial cavity. This fluid contains proteins, cells, and other serum constituents. Exudative effusions most commonly occur secondary to infection in which case this condition is then are referred to as pericardial empyema or purulent pericarditis.

Haemorrhagic effusions contain red bloody fluid and occur when blood leaks into the pericardial cavity.

Malignant effusions may occur due to obstruction of the lymphatic drainage of the heart, a fluid-secreting malignancy or fluid accumulation caused by metastatic spread. Malignant effusions are often blood stained.

Pathophysiology of Pericardial Effusions

The pathophysiological consequences of pericardial effusions are dependent upon both the size of the effusion and the rate of its accumulation. For example, the normal compliant pericardium can stretch to accommodate slowly accumulating pericardial effusions without a significant rise in the intrapericardial pressure or haemdynamic compromise. In this instance, even large pericardial effusions can be present without haemodynamic compromise. Conversely, a rapidly accumulating effusion can be relatively small but cause a rapid rise in intrapericardial pressure which compresses cardiac chambers resulting in cardiac tamponade (see Cardiac Tamponade section later in this chapter).

Echocardiography in Pericardial Effusions

Echocardiography is the procedure of choice for the diagnosis and detection of pericardial effusions. In particular, echocardiography is useful in:
- detecting and sizing of pericardial effusions,
- determining the possible aetiology of pericardial effusions,
- differentiation of pericardial effusion from pleural effusions and other structures/pathologies,
- echo-guided pericardiocentesis.

Detection and Sizing of Pericardial Effusions

The echocardiographic appearance of pericardial effusions is dependent on the type and aetiology of the effusion (see the following section). However, as most pericardial effusions are transudative, effusions typically appear as echo-free spaces around the heart (Fig. 12.7). The size of the pericardial effusion can be roughly estimated based on the dimensions of the pericardial space (Fig. 12.8 and Table 12.2).

As mentioned above, the pericardium does not cover the posterior aspect of the LA. As a result most pericardial effusions, even when large, terminate at the left AV groove. For example, from the parasternal long axis view the effusion is not visible posterior to the LA. When the effusion is of a significant size, the pericardial sinuses can also often be observed from the parasternal long axis view (Fig. 12.9).

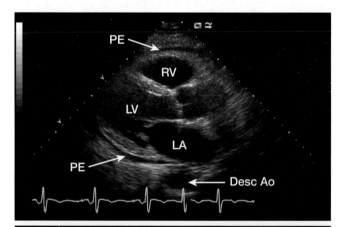

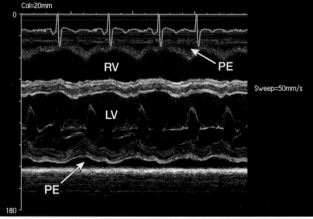

Figure 12.7 This 2D parasternal long axis image shows a small pericardial effusion (PE) anterior to the right ventricle (RV) and posterior to the left ventricle (LV). The corresponding M-mode trace with the cursor placed through the ventricles also displays the pericardial space posterior to the LV and anterior to the RV; observe that the space posterior to the LV is present throughout the cardiac cycle. Desc Ao = descending aorta; LA = left atrium.

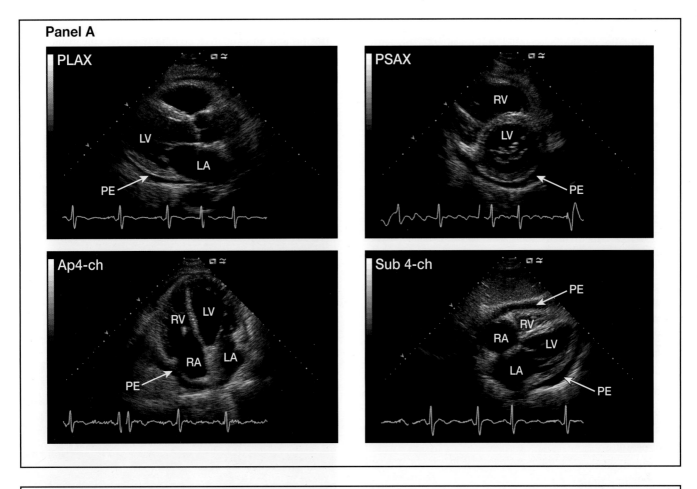

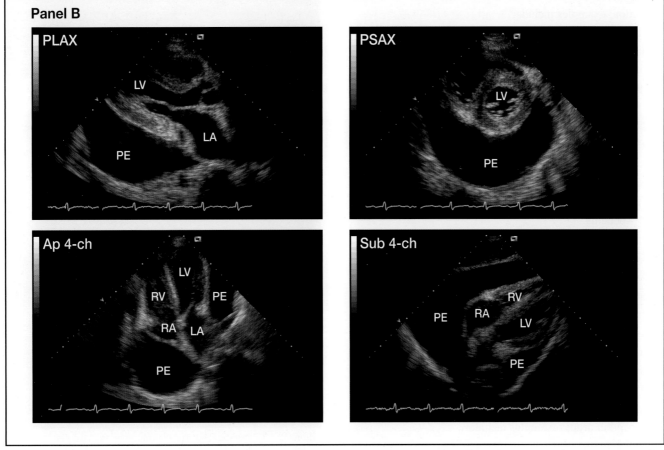

Figure 12.8 A small to moderate-sized pericardial effusion (**Panel A**) and a large pericardial effusion (**Panel B**) are shown. Images were recorded from the parasternal long axis (PLAX), the parasternal short axis (PSAX), the apical 4-chamber (Ap 4-ch) and the subcostal 4-chamber (Sub 4-ch) views. LA = left atrium; LV = left ventricle; PE = pericardial effusion; RA = right atrium; RV = right ventricle.

Aetiology of the Pericardial Fluid

The aetiology of the pericardial fluid can sometimes be suspected based on the echogenic properties or appearance of the effusion. For example, most transudative effusions appear relatively echo-free (anechoic) while exudative and haemorrhagic effusions are not entirely echo-free (variable echogenicity) and organised pericardial haematomas are characterised by a homogeneous and 'speckled' appearance (Fig. 12.10). The appearance of the haematoma, however, is dependent upon the chronicity of the collection. For example, in the acute setting, the haematoma appears essentially echo-free; then as the haematoma clots it becomes more heterogeneous in appearance with hypoechoic spaces noted within the collection (Fig. 12.11). The homogeneous and 'speckled' appearance occurs once the clot becomes organised.

Table 12.1 Aetiology of Pericardial Effusions

Most Common Causes of Pericardial Effusions
Idiopathic (unknown cause)
Acute Pericarditis
Radiation therapy
Cardiac disorders; examples include:
• Acute myocardial infarction
• Congestive heart failure
• Myocarditis
• Aortic dissection
• Free wall rupture
Infection; examples include:
• Viral
• Bacterial
• Fungal
Autoimmune diseases/responses; examples include:
• Rheumatic diseases (e.g. systemic lupus erythematosus, rheumatoid arthritis, systemic scleroderma)
• Rheumatic fever
• Postmyocardial infarction syndrome (Dressler's syndrome)
Metabolic disorders; examples include:
• Renal insufficiency (uraemia)
• Myxoedema
Trauma; examples include:
• Blunt
• Penetrating
• Iatrogenic (e.g. catheter and pacemaker perforations, cardiopulmonary resuscitation, post-thoracic surgery)
Neoplasms; examples include:
• Primary tumours (e.g. rhabdomyosarcoma, teratoma, fibroma, lipoma, leiomyoma)
• Secondary metastatic tumours (e.g. lung carcinoma, breast carcinoma, leukaemia and lymphoma)
Prescription drugs; examples include:
• Radiation therapy or chemotherapy drugs
• Antihypertensive (e.g. hydralazine, minoxidil), antiarrhythmic (e.g. procainamide, phenytoin), anticoagulants, antibiotics (e.g. isoniazid), methysergide

The presence of fibrinous strands within the pericardial effusion and an exudative coating over the epicardium may be seen in tuberculosis, malignant and bacterial effusions. Fibrinous strands appear as multiple linear or band-like structures extending across the pericardial space while an exudative coating is described as 'shaggy' echo densities overlying the epicardium (Fig. 12.12). Fibrinous strands may also be seen in long-standing or recurrent pericardial effusions.

Table 12.2 Sizing of Pericardial Effusion (PE) by Echocardiography

PE Size	Echo-Free Space*
Physiological	< 5 mm; seen in systole only
Trivial	< 5 mm; seen over systole and diastole
Small	< 10 mm
Moderate	10-20 mm
Large	> 20 mm

* Measured from the parasternal short axis view at the level of the papillary muscles at end-diastole.

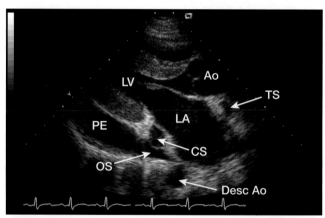

Figure 12.9 This parasternal long axis view of the left ventricle shows a moderate-sized pericardial effusion (PE). Observe that the effusion is anterior to the descending thoracic aorta (DescAo). In addition, the two pericardial sinuses can also be appreciated from this image: the transverse sinus (TS) lies posterior to the aortic root and anterior to the left atrium (LA) while the oblique sinus (OS) lies posterior to the LA and anterior to the DescAo. The OS should not be confused with the coronary sinus (CS) which lies within the atrioventricular groove. Ao = aorta; LV = left ventricle.

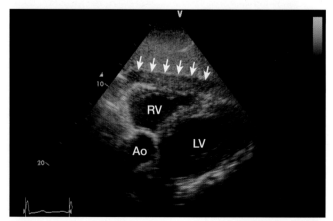

Figure 12.10 This subcostal view was recorded from a patient following a stab wound to the chest. Observe that the pericardium contains echo-dense material with a 'speckled' or 'mottled' appearance (*arrows*). This appearance is consistent with organised haematoma.

For the serial evaluation of the size of pericardial effusions, measurements should be performed from the same imaging views, at the same anatomic site, and at the same stage of the cardiac cycle. Furthermore, loculated or localised effusions may occur when pericardial adhesions confine the fluid to a limited space. This is especially common following cardiac surgery where loculation of fluid tends to accumulate anterior and lateral to the RA. In these situations, the criteria used to determine the size of the effusion are less helpful.

Differentiation of Pericardial Effusion from Pleural Effusions and Other Structures/Pathologies

Pleural effusions, especially left pleural effusions, can be mistaken for pericardial effusions. The distinction between a left pleural effusion and a pericardial effusion is based on the anatomical relationship of the fluid to the descending thoracic aorta. The pericardium does not cover the descending thoracic aorta; therefore, left pleural effusions appear posterior to the descending aorta while pericardial effusions appear anterior to the descending aorta.

The parasternal long axis view is the best view for determining if the effusion is pleural or pericardial (Fig. 12.13). From this view, a pericardial effusion is seen anterior to the descending thoracic aorta while a left pleural effusion is seen posterior to the descending aorta. Not infrequently, pericardial and pleural effusions may co-exist in the same patient; in this situation, fluid can be seen on both sides of the descending aorta (Fig. 12.14). The recognition of a pleural effusion may also be assisted by the identification of the wedge-shape, collapsed lung within the pleural effusion (Fig. 12.14).

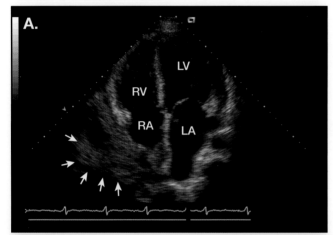

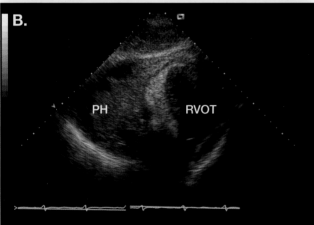

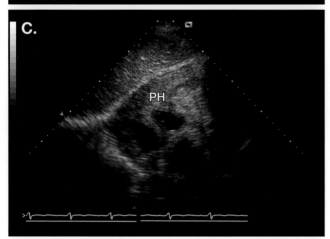

Figure 12.11 A localised pericardial haematoma lateral to the right atrial (RA) free wall in a patient following cardiac surgery is seen from the apical 4-chamber (**A**) and subcostal short axis (**B** & **C**) views. Observe the non-uniform echogenicity of the haematoma; this suggests that the haematoma is at various stages of organisation. PH = pericardial haematoma; LA= left atrium; LV = left ventricle; RV = right ventricle; RVOT = right ventricular outflow tract.

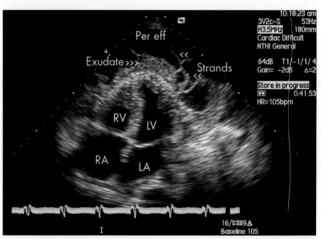

Figure 12.12 This apical 4-chamber view from a patient with tuberculous pericardial effusion shows multiple fibrin strands as linear or band-like structures crossing the pericardial space or protruding from the epicardium or parietal pericardium and exudates. LA = left atrium; LV = left ventricle; Per eff = pericardial effusion; RA = right atrium; RV = right ventricle.
Reproduced from George S, Salama AL, Uthaman B, Cherian G. Echocardiography in differentiating tuberculous from chronic idiopathic pericardial effusion. *Heart*. Nov;90(11), page 1339, © 2004 with permission from BMJ Publishing Group Ltd.

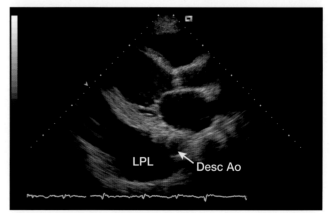

Figure 12.13 This parasternal long axis view of the left ventricle demonstrates the position of fluid with respect to the descending thoracic aorta (Desc Ao). Note that the fluid appears posterior to the descending aorta indicating that a left pleural effusion (LPL) is present.

Pleural fluid is an excellent transmitter of ultrasound and, therefore, creates a unique acoustic window for imaging the heart. To image the heart using a left pleural effusion, the patient is placed in a sitting position or rolled into a right lateral decubitus position; the transducer is then placed on the patient's back near the lower border of the left scapula. From this acoustic window it is possible to image the heart from posterior to anterior (Fig. 12.15).

Other anatomic and pathologic structures may also mimic a pericardial effusion. These structures as well as the characteristic features which can help distinguish them from pericardial effusions are summarised in Table 12.3; echocardiographic examples as shown in figures 12.16-12.20. In addition, a giant LA or a dilated coronary sinus may also lead to a misdiagnosis of a loculated pericardial effusion.

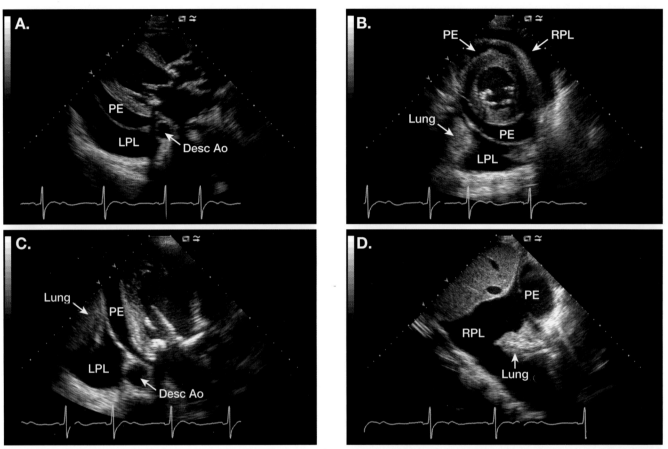

Figure 12.14 Bilateral pleural effusions and a pericardial effusion are shown from the parasternal long axis (**A**), the parasternal short axis (**B**), the apical long axis (**C**), and subcostal short axis (**D**) views. Note that the left pleural effusion (LPL) is located posterior to the descending thoracic aorta (Desc Ao) while the pericardial effusion (PE) is located anterior to the descending thoracic aorta. The pericardiopleural interface between these two effusions appears as a well-defined linear band. A right pleural effusion (RPL) is also present. Collapsed lungs can also be appreciated within the pleural effusions.

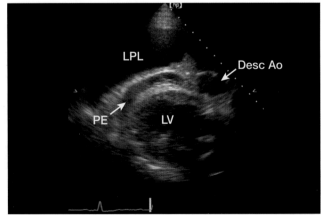

Figure 12.15 This image was recorded with the patient rolled into a right lateral decubitus position and with the transducer placed on the patient's back just below the left scapula. The large left pleural effusion (LPL) provides an acoustic window to the heart. A small pericardial effusion (PE) is also seen. Desc Ao = descending aorta; LV = left ventricle.

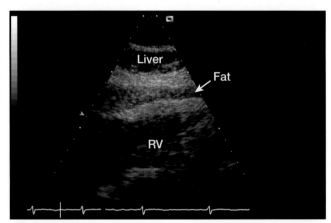

Figure 12.16 This zoomed view recorded from the subcostal 4-chamber view shows a layer of epicardial fat over the anterior right ventricle (RV). Observe the characteristic speckled or granular appearance of this fat.

Table 12.3 Mimics of Pericardial Effusions

Example	Distinguishing Echo Features
Epicardial Fat (Fig. 12.16)	• Speckled or granular appearance consistent with a soft tissue density • Most prominent anterior to the right ventricle • Best viewed from the parasternal long axis and subcostal 4-chamber view • Note: this appearance is very similar to organised haematoma but with epicardial fat there is a lack of abnormal tethering of underlying cardiac motion.
Left Ventricular (LV) Pseudoaneurysm (Fig. 12.17)	• Appears as an echo-free space adjacent to the LV • Can be differentiated from pericardial effusions by the identification of to-and-fro flow between the pseudoaneurysm and the ventricle via spectral and colour Doppler imaging
Ascites (Fig. 12.18)	• Appears as a large echo-free space around and in between the abdominal viscera • Identification of the falciform ligament differentiates ascites from pericardial effusions; this ligament appears as a sharp, thin band perpendicular to the abdominal wall and diaphragm • Best viewed from the subcostal 4-chamber view
Descending Thoracic Aortic Aneurysms (Fig. 12.19)	• In cross-section these aneurysms appear as echo-free circular structures posterior to the LA. • Differentiation of this aneurysm from a loculated pericardial effusion is achieved by rotating the transducer 90^0 to open this vessel up into its long axis.
Hiatus Hernia (Fig. 12.20)	• A hiatus hernia, which is the protrusion of a portion of the upper stomach through the diaphragm, can appear as an echo-free space posterior to the heart. • Can be differentiated from a loculated pericardial effusion by confirming a connection of this echo-free space with the gastrointestinal tract; this is accomplished by asking the patient to swallow a carbonated beverage. The appearance of gaseous bubbles within this 'space' confirms its connection with the stomach.

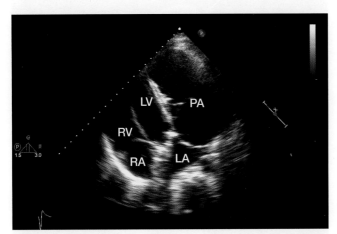
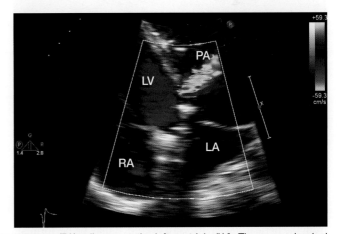

Figure 12.17 The apical 4-chamber view (*left*) shows a massive pseudoaneurysm (PA) adjacent to the left ventricle (LV). The zoomed apical 4-chamber view with colour Doppler imaging confirms the communication between the LV and this pseudoaneurysm (*right*). A prosthetic mitral valve is also present. LA = left atrium; RA = right atrium; RV = right ventricle.

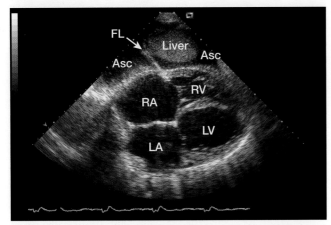
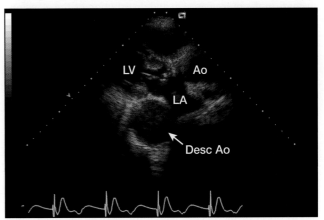

Figure 12.18 This subcostal 4-chamber view was recorded in a patient with congestive heart failure and ascites. Ascites (Asc) appears as an echo-free space between the liver and the heart and diaphragm. The falciform ligament (FL) which attaches to the liver on one side and the diaphragm on the other appears as a curvilinear band (*arrow*) within the ascitic fluid. LA = left atrium; LV = left ventricle; RA = right atrium; RV = right ventricle.

Figure 12.19 This slightly off-axis parasternal long axis view shows a large aneurysm of the descending thoracic aorta (Desc Ao) posterior to the left atrium (LA). Ao = ascending aorta; LV= left ventricle.

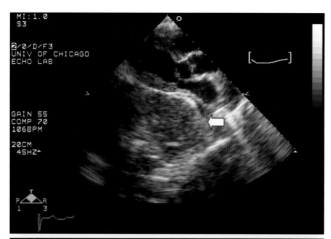

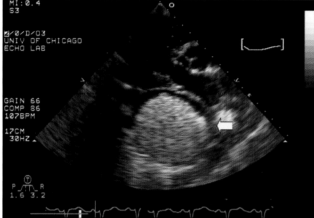

Figure 12.20 A mass posterior to the left atrium (*arrow*) is noted from the parasternal long axis view (*top*). Following the ingestion of a carbonated beverage mixed with 1.5 mL of activated Definity contrast media this mass became well delineated (*bottom*); thus confirming the suspicion that this extracardiac mass was a hiatus hernia.
Reprinted from Smelley M, Lang RM. Large Mass Impinging on the Left Atrium: Diagnostic Value of a New Cocktail, *J Am Soc Echocardiogr*, Vol. 20(12), page 1414.e6, © 2007 with permission from Elsevier.

Pericardiocentesis

Pericardiocentesis is a procedure whereby fluid is aspirated from the pericardial cavity via a needle. It may be performed: (1) when there is a large pericardial effusion, (2) to relieve cardiac tamponade, or (3) to obtain fluid for analysis.

The role of echocardiography in this procedure is to:

1. confirm the presence, size and distribution of the effusion,
2. identify the ideal puncture site and trajectory angle for needle entry,
3. confirm the needle location within the pericardial cavity,
4. reassess the amount of residual fluid following the procedure.

In particular, the ideal site and trajectory angle for needle entry is based on: (1) the shortest distance from the body surface to the pericardial effusion where fluid accumulation is maximal, and (2) a straight trajectory path that avoids vital structures such as the liver, myocardium and lungs.

Most commonly, pericardiocentesis is performed from the subcostal and para-apical locations (Fig. 12.21). The injection of a small volume of saline can be performed to confirm the location of the needle within the pericardial space (Fig. 12.22). This is especially important if a bloody fluid return is noted following needle insertion.

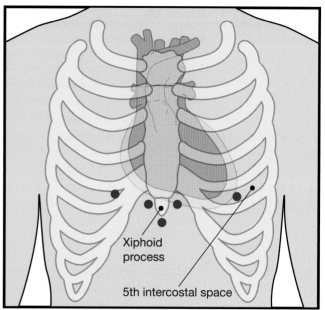

Figure 12.21 The red dots on this schematic indicate the commonly selected locations for pericardiocentesis.

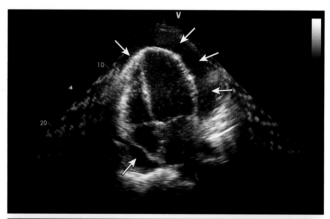

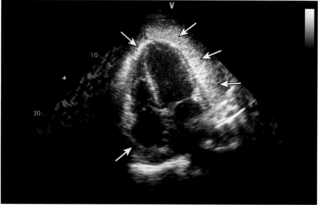

Figure 12.22 The apical 4-chamber view shows a large circumferential pericardial effusion (*top, arrows*). Following the injection of agitated saline through the pericardiocentesis needle opacification of the pericardial space is demonstrated confirming the intrapericardial position of the needle (*bottom, arrows*).

Important Note: Aortic dissection is a major contra-indication for pericardiocentesis due to the risk of intensified bleeding and extension of the dissection [12.1].

[12.1] Maisch B, Seferović PM, Ristić AD, Erbel R, Rienmüller R, Adler Y, Tomkowski WZ, Thiene G, Yacoub MH; Task Force on the Diagnosis and Management of Pericardial Diseases of the European Society of Cardiology. Guidelines on the diagnosis and management of pericardial diseases executive summary; The Task force on the diagnosis and management of pericardial diseases of the European Society of Cardiology. *Eur Heart J.* 2004 Apr;25(7):591 & 603.

Cardiac Tamponade

Cardiac tamponade occurs when there is an increase in the intrapericardial pressure (IPP) due to accumulation of an effusion, blood, clots, pus, gas or combinations of these within the pericardium. This ultimately leads to compression of the heart, impeded diastolic filling of both ventricles, systemic and pulmonary congestion, and a decreased stroke volume and cardiac output.

Pathophysiology of Cardiac Tamponade

In order to understand the pathophysiological changes that occur with cardiac tamponade, consideration of the transmural pressures, changes in right and left heart filling with respiration, and ventricular interdependence is required.

Transmural Filling Pressures

The transmural filling pressure describes the difference in pressure between the inside and the outside of a walled structure. Therefore, for the heart the transmural filling pressure (TMFP) can be used to describe the pressure difference between the intracavity pressure (ICP) and the IPP. In the normal situation, the intrathoracic pressure (ITP) is transmitted to the pericardial sac so the IPP is approximately the same as the negative (subatmospheric) ITP. Therefore, as the ICP is usually positive, there is a positive TMFP which is higher than the ICP. This positive TMFP maintains the shape of the cardiac chambers and prevents them from collapsing at end-diastole when the ICP falls to zero (Fig. 12.23).

With cardiac tamponade, the IPP is increased. As the IPP rises, the ICP also rises in an attempt to maintain a positive TMFP and an adequate cardiac output. However, further increases in the IPP result in a fall in the TMFP which will result in impeded diastolic filling of the heart and a subsequent reduction in cardiac output. When the TMFP becomes negative there is collapse (compression) of the cardiac chambers (Fig. 12.24).

Right and Left Heart Filling with Respiration

In the normal situation, there is augmentation of right heart filling with inspiration, a decrease in right heart filling with expiration, and minimal variation in left heart filling with respiration.

During inspiration, as the diaphragm descends there is an increase in the intraabdominal pressure (IAP) and a reduction in the ITP which leads to an augmentation of systemic venous return and increased filling of the right heart. With expiration, the opposite occurs so as the diaphragm ascends, there is an increase in the ITP and a decrease in the IAP which leads to a reduction in the systemic venous return and a decrease in right heart filling.

There is minimal variation in left heart filling with respiration. This is because changes in ITP are transmitted to both the pericardial sac (and the cardiac chambers) and the pulmonary veins to the same degree (Fig. 12.25, top). For instance, as the ITP decreases with inspiration the IPP and ICP also decrease to the same degree; and as the pulmonary veins are also contained within the thoracic cavity, the decrease in ITP is also reflected in the pulmonary veins to the same degree. Likewise with expiration, as the ITP increases so does the IPP, ICP and pulmonary venous pressure to the same degree. Therefore, the effective filling gradient (EFG) of the left heart changes only slightly during respiration. This slight respiratory variation in the left heart EFG is based on changes in right heart filling with inspiration as described above. In particular, increased RV filling during inspiration causes the IVS to bow slightly to the left; as a result there is a slight inspiratory reduction in LV filling and LV stroke volume as well as a slight inspiratory fall in the systemic arterial pressure (< 10 mm Hg).

In the case of tamponade, the normal respiratory changes described above are accentuated. That is, with inspiration left heart filling is decreased more than normal and right heart filling is increased more than normal. These changes occur because the IPP is increased. Therefore, the normal decline in the ITP during inspiration is not fully transmitted to the pericardial sac and to the cardiac chambers; however, the ITP decline is transmitted to the pulmonary veins as normal. As a result, the increased IPP means that the ICP does not fall as it should but because the pulmonary venous pressure falls

> The effective filling gradient (EFG) is calculated as the difference between the pulmonary capillary wedge pressure (PCWP) and the intrapericardial pressure (IPP). This value is almost the same as the diastolic gradient between the pulmonary veins and the ventricular cavity. Therefore, the EFG essentially reflects the driving pressure from the lungs across the pulmonary veins and into the left heart.

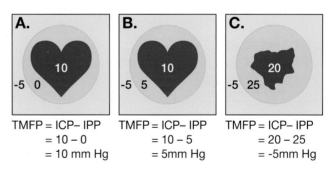

A.	B.	C.
TMFP = ICP– IPP	TMFP = ICP– IPP	TMFP = ICP– IPP
= 10 – 0	= 10 – 5	= 20 – 25
= 10 mm Hg	= 5mm Hg	= -5mm Hg

Figure 12.24 This schematic illustrates the changes to transmural filling pressures (TMFP) with increasing intrapericardial pressure (IPP). **Panel A:** IPP is zero and the intracardiac pressure (ICP) is 10 mm Hg; the resultant TMFP, which is the difference between the ICP and the IPP, is 10 mm Hg. Cardiac output and diastolic filling are maintained. **Panel B:** IPP is slightly positive at 5 mm Hg and ICP is 10 mmHg; the resultant TMFP is 5 mm Hg. This results in a decrease in both the cardiac output and diastolic filling. **Panel C:** IPP is more positive at 25 mm Hg and despite the increase in ICP to 20 mm Hg, the resultant TMFP is -5 mm Hg. This results in a negative TMFP and subsequent collapse of the cardiac chambers.

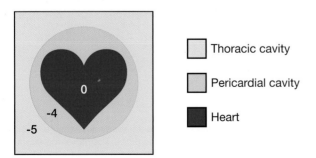

Thoracic cavity

Pericardial cavity

Heart

Figure 12.23 The transmural filling pressure (TMFP) is the difference between the intracavity pressure (ICP) and the intrapericardial pressure (IPP). In this schematic the ICP is 0 and the IPP is -4 so the TMFP is 4 mm Hg. Therefore, even when the ICP is 0 there is a positive TMFP which prevents the cardiac chambers from collapsing.

normally the EFG of the left heart is significantly reduced during inspiration (Fig. 12.25, bottom). Furthermore, this reduction in left heart filling during inspiration results in a leftward shift of the IVS which enhances right heart filling during inspiration. In addition, the decrease in LV volume with inspiration results in a decrease in LV stroke volume and this leads to pulsus paradoxus which is an abnormal drop in systolic arterial pressure (> 10 mm Hg) during inspiration.

Ventricular Interdependence

As the ventricles are confined within the pericardium and share a common IVS, any changes to the size, shape, pressure and volume of one ventricle affects the size, shape, pressure and volume of the other ventricle. This is referred to as ventricular interdependence or ventricular interaction.

In the normal situation, ventricular interaction is minimal. As stated above, with inspiration increased RV filling only slightly reduces LV filling which leads to a slight decrease in cardiac output and a slight decrease in the systemic arterial pressure.

In cardiac tamponade, there is exaggerated motion of the IVS during respiration; this is referred to as enhanced ventricular interdependence (interaction). This exaggerated IVS motion occurs due to the increased IPP which limits the normal 'expansion' of the ventricles during diastolic filling. This means that the ventricles have to compete with one another for a limited 'space' within the pericardial sac. Therefore, increased right heart filling during inspiration shifts the IVS to the left which impedes LV filling. During expiration, increased left heart filling shifts the IVS to the right which impedes RV filling.

Echocardiography in Cardiac Tamponade

Strictly speaking, the diagnosis of cardiac tamponade is a clinical diagnosis and echocardiographic abnormalities alone should not be used to establish the diagnosis of tamponade. However, echocardiographic findings can support the diagnosis

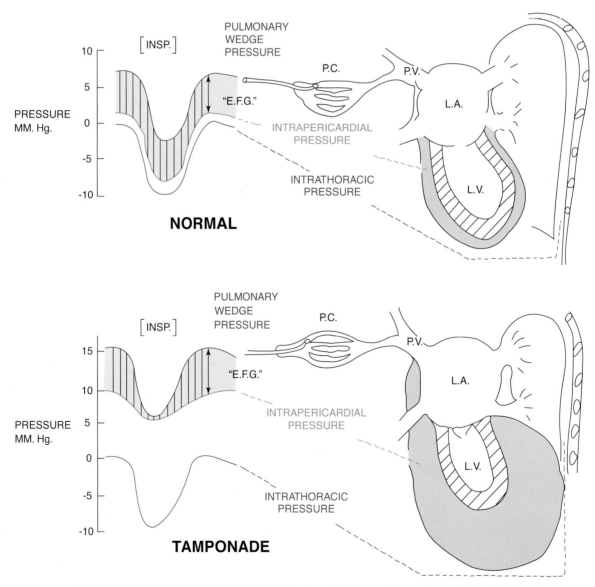

Figure 12.25 The top half of this schematic illustrates the normal situation in which the respiratory changes in the intrathoracic pressure (ITP) are transmitted (to the same degree) to the pericardial sac and the pulmonary veins (P.V.) and pulmonary capillaries (P.C.). Therefore, the effective filling gradient (E.F.G.) of the left ventricle (L.V.) changes only slightly during respiration. The bottom half of this schematic illustrates the situation in cardiac tamponade, in which the respiratory changes in the ITP are transmitted (to the same degree) to the P.V. and P.C. However, because the intrapericardial pressure is elevated the ITP is poorly transmitted to the pericardial sac. Therefore, the E.F.G. of the left ventricle is significantly reduced during inspiration (INSP.). L.A. = left atrium.
Adapted from Sharp JT, Bunnell IL, Holland JF, Griffith GT, Greene DG, Hemodynamics during induced cardiac tamponade in man, *American Journal of Medicine*, Vol. 29(4), page 641, © 1960, with permission from Elsevier.

of suspected cardiac tamponade, especially when the clinical diagnosis is equivocal. Echocardiographic signs of cardiac tamponade include:

- a swinging heart within a large pericardial effusion,
- collapse of the cardiac chambers,
- plethora of the inferior vena cava (IVC),
- exaggerated respiratory variation in diastolic filling,
- enhanced ventricular interaction,
- a reduction in the LV stroke volume.

Swinging Heart

A "swinging heart" refers to the free floating motion of the heart within a large pericardial effusion with the heart only anchored in place by the pulmonary veins. This motion accounts for the finding of electrical alternans on the ECG (Fig. 12.26). A "swinging heart" in conjunction with chamber collapse is a good indicator of the presence of cardiac tamponade.

Caveat

The appearance of a swinging heart in isolation is neither sensitive nor specific for tamponade. This highlights the important fact that it is not the volume of pericardial fluid that causes cardiac tamponade, it is the IPP as well as the degree of pericardial constraint that causes tamponade physiology. The pericardium is relatively noncompliant. As a result there is a nonlinear relationship between intrapericardial volume (IPV) and IPP. Therefore, when the elastic limit of the pericardial space is reached, any additional increases in the IPV will result in large increases in IPP leading to cardiac tamponade (Fig. 12.27). For example, in the acute setting, a small volume of fluid accumulating rapidly can quickly exceed the elastic limit of the pericardial space resulting in a marked elevation of IPP and subsequent cardiac tamponade.

Causes of a sudden and rapid accumulation of pericardial fluid include iatrogenic cardiovascular perforations, chest trauma, post cardiac surgery, a Type A aortic dissection with rupture, or following an acute myocardial infarction with rupture. Slowly accumulating effusions are encountered with malignancies.

Collapse of the Cardiac Chambers

Definitive echocardiographic signs of cardiac tamponade include late ventricular diastolic or early ventricular systolic inversion of the RA and early diastolic collapse of the RV.

RA collapse or inversion is seen when the IPP exceeds the RA pressure; this usually occurs during atrial relaxation, immediately following atrial contraction, when the RA pressure is at its lowest point. RA collapse or inversion is therefore seen during late ventricular diastole or early ventricular systole. RA collapse is best appreciated from the apical 4-chamber view (Fig. 12.28).

RV collapse occurs when the IPP exceeds the RV pressure; this usually occurs during early to mid diastole when the RV pressure is at its lowest point. RV diastolic collapse (RVDC) is best appreciated from the parasternal long axis view or the

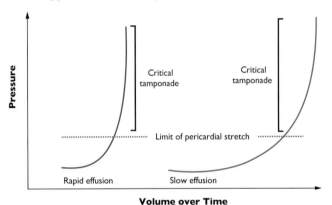

Figure 12.27 Pericardial pressure–volume curves are illustrated. In the left panel, a rapid accumulation of pericardial fluid first reaches the limit of the pericardial reserve volume (the initial flat segment) and then quickly exceeds the limit of pericardial stretch, causing a steep rise in intrapericardial pressure (IPP), which becomes even steeper as smaller increments in fluid cause a disproportionate increase in the IPP. In the right panel, a slower accumulation takes longer to exceed the limit of pericardial stretch, because there is more time for the pericardium to stretch and for compensatory mechanisms to become activated. Reproduced from Spodick D. Acute cardiac tamponade. *New Engl J Med.* Aug 14;349(7), page 685, © 2003 with permission from the Massachusetts Medical Society.

Figure 12.26 The 12-lead electro-cardiogram (ECG) reveals sinus tachycardia with low voltage and electrical alternans (**Panel A**). Electrical alternans appears as a variation in the amplitude +/- the direction of alternate QRS complexes (especially apparent in leads I, II, aVR, and V4-V6). Echocardiographic images shown were obtained during consecutive cardiac cycles and these images demonstrate a dramatic change (nearly 90 degrees) in the position of the heart from one beat (**Panel B**) to the next (**Panel C**). This swinging motion of the heart toward and away from the chest wall is responsible for the electrical alternans on the ECG. LV = left ventricle; PE = pericardial effusion; PL = pleural effusion; RVOT = right ventricular outflow tract. Reproduced from Longo MJ, Jaffe CC. Images in Clinical Medicine: Electrical Alternans. *New Engl J Med.* Dec 30;341(27), page 2060, © 1999 with permission from the Massachusetts Medical Society.

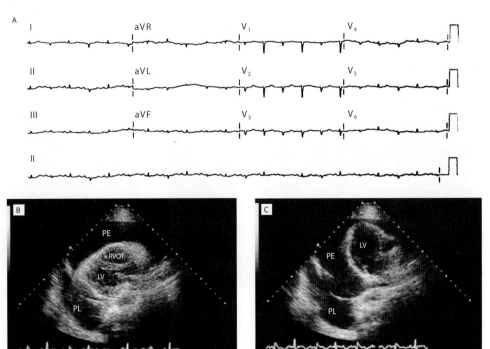

subcostal 4-chamber view (Fig. 12.29). M-mode echocardiography is especially helpful in determining the precise timing and duration of RVDC (Fig. 12.29, bottom).

The collapse of right heart chambers is exaggerated during expiration when right heart filling is reduced. RA inversion lasting more than one-third of the cardiac cycle and/or RVDC lasting more than one-third of diastole improves the specificity for cardiac tamponade.

Diastolic collapse of the left heart chambers is uncommon. LA collapse is seen in only 25% of patients with cardiac tamponade; when present however, this finding is highly specific for tamponade. LV diastolic collapse (LVDC) is infrequently seen because of the relatively high LV pressures. However, LVDC may be seen when there is a loculated effusion or with pulmonary hypertension (see below).

Caveat

RA and/or RV diastolic collapse may be absent even in the presence of cardiac tamponade. This may occur when there are loculated effusions over the left heart chambers as seen in postoperative patients (Fig. 12.30) or in patients with pulmonary hypertension. In particular, in patients with pulmonary hypertension, the right heart chambers may not collapse despite the presence of increased IPP. This is because right heart chamber collapse occurs when the pressure in the pericardium exceeds the intracardiac pressure so when the right heart pressures are significantly elevated collapse may not occur despite the presence of cardiac tamponade. In this situation, collapse of the left heart chambers may be seen instead (Fig. 12.31).

Plethora of the Inferior Vena Cava

In spontaneously breathing patients with suspected cardiac tamponade, a dilated IVC with a lack of inspiratory collapse is a sign of haemodynamic compromise. Plethora of the IVC reflects impaired systemic venous return to the RA caused by RA pressure elevation and/or RA compression that occurs secondary to increased IPP.

Caveat

A dilated IVC with a lack of inspiratory collapse reflects an elevation in central venous pressures. Therefore, this sign is not specific for cardiac tamponade as a dilated IVC with a lack of respiratory collapse is also seen when there is RV

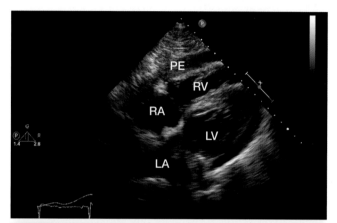

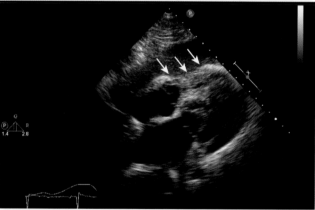

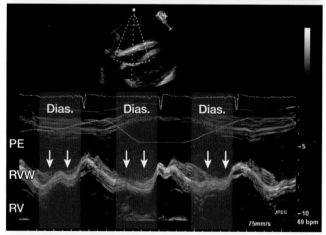

Figure 12.29 These images were recorded from the subcostal 4-chamber view in a patient with cardiac tamponade. Observe that in early systole the shape and contour of the right ventricle (RV) appears normal (*top*). However during early diastole there is significant collapse of the RV (*arrows*) (*middle*). The M-mode trace on the bottom also confirms diastolic collapse of the RV wall (RVW) (*arrows*). Dias. = diastole; LA = left atrium; LV = left ventricle; PE = pericardial effusion; RA = right atrium.

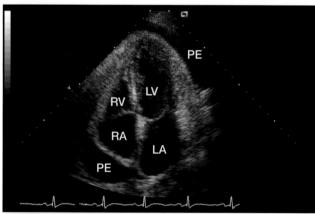

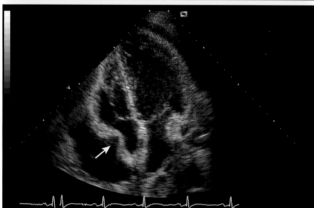

Figure 12.28 These two images were recorded in a patient with cardiac tamponade. Observe that in early diastole the shape and contour of the right atrium (RA) appears normal (*top*). However during early ventricular systole there is inversion of the RA wall (*arrow*) (*bottom*). LA = left atrium; LV = left ventricle; PE = pericardial effusion; RV = right ventricle.

failure and when RA pressure is elevated due to other causes. Furthermore, dilatation of the IVC is seen in patients on positive pressure ventilation.

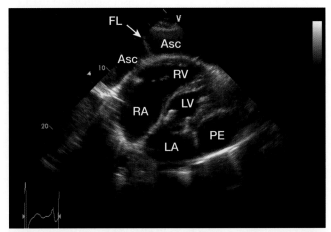

Figure 12.30 From the subcostal 4-chamber view, a loculated pericardial effusion (PE) causing diastolic collapse of the left ventricle is seen. This patient had a mitral valve replacement 5 days prior to this examination. Ascites (Asc) is also present; this appears as an echo-free space anterior to the heart. Ascites can be differentiated from a PE based on the appearance of the falciform ligament (FL).
LA = left atrium; LV = left ventricle; RA = right atrium; RV = right ventricle.

Table 12.4 Summary of Spectral Doppler Findings associated with Cardiac Tamponade *

Inspiration (1st beat)	Expiration (1st beat)
↓ **LV filling:**	↑ **LV filling:**
• Mitral: ↓ E	• Mitral: ↑ E
• PV: ↓ D	• PV: ↑ D
• IVRT: ↑	• IVRT: ↓
↑ **RV filling:**	↓ **RV filling:**
• Tric.: ↑ E	• Tric.: ↓ E
• HV: normal ↑ S & D	• HV: ↓, absent or reversed D; ↑ AR
• SVC: normal ↑ or reduced S & D (S dominant) +/- lack of inspiratory ↑ in D	• SVC: ↓ D (absent D = severe tamponade); ↑ AR

* These respiratory changes are exaggerated relative to normal.
AR = atrial reversal velocity; D = diastolic forward flow velocity; E = early diastolic velocity; HV = hepatic venous flow; IVRT = isovolumic relaxation time; PV = pulmonary venous flow; S = systolic forward flow; SVC = superior vena caval flow; Tric. = tricuspid.

The negative predictive values for RA inversion, RV collapse and IVC plethora in patients with cardiac tamponade are exceptionally high. This means that the absence of these signs virtually excludes the presence of cardiac tamponade.

Exaggerated Respiratory Variations in Diastolic Filling

Exaggerated respiratory variation in diastolic filling can be confirmed via spectral Doppler profiles of the left and right heart. A summary of these changes is listed in Table 12.4 and illustrated in Figure 12.32; the significance of these respiratory variations is listed in Table 12.5.

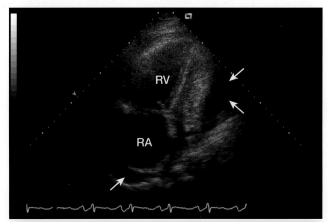

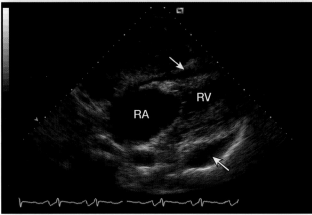

Figure 12.31 These images were recorded from a patient with pulmonary arterial hypertension. From the apical 4-chamber view (*top*) and the subcostal 4-chamber view (*bottom*), a pericardial effusion is seen (*arrows*). Observe that there is diastolic collapse of the left ventricle while the right heart chambers are not compromised because the right heart pressures are significantly elevated. RA = right atrium; RV = right ventricle.

Table 12.5 Percentage Change from Inspiration to Expiration in Normals, Cardiac Tamponade and Effusion with No Tamponade *

Pt. Group	IVRT		Mitral E velocity		Tricuspid E velocity	
	No.	ms	No.	cm/s	No.	cm/s
Normal	19	4 ± 6	18	-1 ± 5	14	7 ± 5
Tamponade	10	39 ± 19^	15	- 37 ± 13^	6	77 ± 37^
Eff-no tamponade	12	4 ± 5	11	0 ± 9	9	15 ± 11#

*Percentage inspiratory change is calculated as: [(inspiratory value - expiratory value) ÷ expiratory value] × 100%. A positive value indicates an increase during inspiration compared with expiration while a negative value represents a decrease during inspiration compared with expiration. Values are mean ± one standard deviation.
^ p<0.05 vs. all other groups; # p<0.05 difference from normal.
Eff = effusion; IVRT = isovolumic relaxation time; No. = number of patients; Pt. = patient.
Source: Burstow DJ, Oh JK, Bailey KR, Seward JB, Tajik AJ. Cardiac Tamponade: Characteristic Doppler Observations. *Mayo Clin Proc.* 1989 Mar;64(3):312-24.

Transmitral Inflow

In the normal situation, there is minimal variation of the peak E velocity over the respiratory cycle (Fig. 12.33, left). In cardiac tamponade, the EFG between the pulmonary veins and the left heart is significantly reduced during inspiration while with expiration diastolic filling of the left heart increases due to a rise in the EFG with secondary rightward shift of the IVS. These changes are reflected on the transmitral inflow signal as a reduction in the peak early diastolic (E) velocity on the first beat of inspiration and an increase in the peak E velocity on the first beat

of expiration (Fig. 12.33, right). A reduction in the transmitral E velocity > 30% with inspiration compared with expiration is consistent with cardiac tamponade. Furthermore, the isovolumic relaxation time (IVRT), which is the time interval between aortic valve closure and mitral valve opening, is prolonged on the first beat of inspiration in patients with cardiac tamponade. This is explained by the fact that in cardiac tamponade, the reduction in diastolic filling gradient with inspiration causes the mitral valve to open later than normal and this is reflected as prolongation of the IVRT. An increase in the IVRT > 20% during inspiration compared with expiration is consistent with cardiac tamponade.

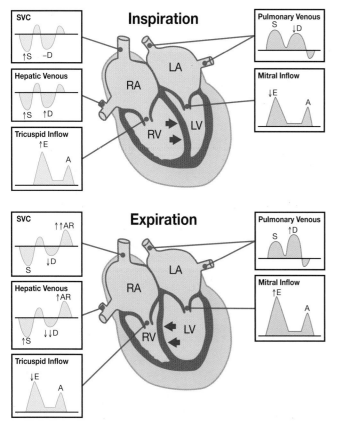

Figure 12.32 The schematic above illustrates the respiratory changes in Doppler flow profiles associated with cardiac tamponade. Note that during inspiration filling of the right heart is enhanced at the expense of left heart filling; during expiration, the opposite occurs. See text for further details. Based on Illustrations by the Mayo Clinic. A = velocity following atrial contraction; AR = atrial reversal velocity; D = diastolic forward flow velocity; E = early diastolic velocity; S = systolic forward flow velocity; SVC = superior vena cava.

Respirometer Display

The respirometer is typically displayed such that an upward deflection represents inspiration and a downward deflection represents expiration.

Calculation of Percentage Respiratory Change

When assessing the percentage change (%Δ) between inspiratory and expiratory values, the velocity (or time in the case of the IVRT) is measured on the first beat of inspiration and the first beat of expiration. So %Δ is derived as:

$$\%\Delta = (1st\ expiration - 1st\ inspiration) \div 1st\ expiration$$

Via this calculation, when the %Δ is a positive value, this reflects a decrease in the measured inspiratory parameter of x% compared with expiration. When the %Δ is a negative value, this reflects an increase in the measured inspiratory parameter of x% compared with expiration.

Eg: if the transmitral E velocity on the first beat of inspiration is 65 cm/s and 95 cm/s on the first beat of expiration then:

$$\%\Delta = (1st\ expiration - 1st\ inspiration) \div 1st\ expiration$$
$$= (95 - 65) \div 95$$
$$= 30\%$$

So there is a 30% reduction in the transmitral E velocity on the 1st beat of inspiration compared with the 1st beat of expiration, or more simply a 30% respiratory variation. Likewise, if the transtricuspid E velocity on the first beat of inspiration is 80 cm/s and 55 cm/s on the first beat of expiration then:

$$\%\Delta = (1st\ expiration - 1st\ inspiration) \div 1st\ expiration$$
$$= (55 - 80) \div 55$$
$$= -45\%$$

So there is a 45% increase in the transtricuspid E velocity on the 1st beat on inspiration compared with the 1st beat of expiration, or more simply a 45% respiratory variation.

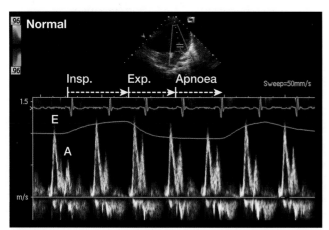

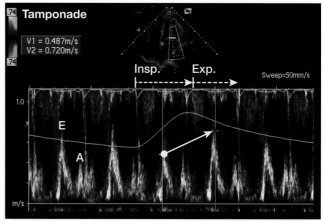

Figure 12.33 The normal transmitral inflow profile shows minimal variation in the peak E velocity over the respiratory cycle (*left*). The transmitral profile in cardiac tamponade shows a significant decrease in the peak E velocity during inspiration compared with expiration (*right*). In this example the inspiratory E velocity (V1) is 48.7 cm/s and the expiratory E velocity (V2) is 72 cm/s. The percentage change = [(72- 48.7) ÷ 72] x 100 = 32%. Therefore, there is a 32% respiratory variation. Insp. = inspiration; Exp. = expiration.

Transtricuspid Inflow

In the normal situation, the peak E velocity increases during inspiration with a normal respiratory variation usually less than 25% (Fig. 12.34, left). In cardiac tamponade, venous return to the right heart chambers is accentuated during inspiration while with expiration diastolic filling of the right heart is decreased due to the rightward shift of the IVS. These changes are reflected on the transtricuspid inflow signal as an increase in the peak E velocity during inspiration and a decrease in the peak E velocity on the first beat of expiration (Fig. 12.34, right). An increase in transtricuspid E velocity > 60% during inspiration compared with expiration is consistent with cardiac tamponade.

Venous Inflow

The respiratory changes reflected in the pulmonary venous flow profiles parallel the changes seen in the transmitral inflow profile. Therefore, in the normal situation, there is minimal variation of the peak D velocity over the respiratory cycle (Fig. 12.35, left). In cardiac tamponade, the pulmonary venous flow profile displays a decrease in the peak D velocity with inspiration compared with the peak D velocity at expiration (Fig. 12.35, right).

In the normal hepatic venous profile there are four waveforms: diastolic forward flow (D), systolic forward flow (S), atrial flow reversal (AR) and ventricular flow reversal (VR) (Fig. 12.36, left). Normally, the S velocity is higher than the D velocity and there is a slight increase in forward flow velocities during inspiration. The AR and VR velocities during inspiration or expiration are < 20% of the forward flow velocities; the AR velocity is slightly higher with expiration. In cardiac tamponade these changes are accentuated; with inspiration there is a slight increase in forward flow velocities while with expiration there is a marked decrease in hepatic venous D velocity plus a significant increase in the AR velocity (Fig. 12.36). In very severe cases, the D velocity may be totally absent or even reversed.

The SVC flow profile also shows similar expiratory changes as the hepatic venous flow profile. Therefore, in the normal SVC profile there is a slight increase in forward flow velocities during inspiration while during expiration there is a slight increase in the atrial reversal (AR) velocity (Fig. 12.37, left). In cardiac tamponade, respiratory changes in the SVC flow profile are variable and the variations in these flow profiles can be useful in determining the "severity" of tamponade (Fig. 12.37, middle and right).

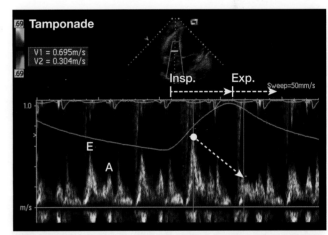

Figure 12.34 The normal transtricuspid inflow profile shows an inspiratory E velocity that is slightly greater than the expiratory E velocity (*left*). Typically, the transtricuspid E velocity can increase as much as 25% during inspiration compared with expiration. The transtricuspid inflow profile in cardiac tamponade shows a significant increase in the peak E velocity during inspiration compared with expiration (*right*). In this example, the inspiratory E velocity (V1) is 69.5 cm/s and the expiratory E velocity (V2) is 30.4 cm/s. The percentage change = [(30.4 - 69.5) ÷ 30.4] x 100 = -128%. Therefore, there is a128% respiratory variation. Insp. = inspiration; Exp. = expiration.

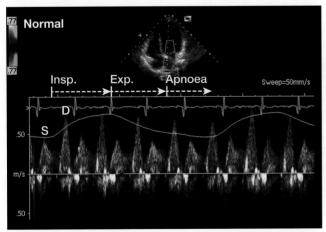
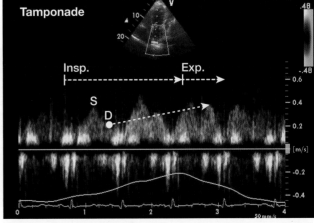

Figure 12.35 The normal pulmonary venous flow profile shows minimal variation in the peak diastolic (D) velocity over the respiratory cycle (*left*). The pulmonary venous flow profile in cardiac tamponade shows a significant decrease in the peak D velocity during inspiration compared with expiration (*right*). In this example there is a significant decrease in the D velocity on the first beat of inspiration compared with the D velocity on the first beat of expiration. Insp. = inspiration; Exp. = expiration; S = systolic forward flow velocity.

Enhanced Ventricular Interaction

In cardiac tamponade, the IVS shifts leftward during inspiration and this enhances filling of the right heart but at the expense of left heart filling. During expiration the opposite occurs; the IVS shifts rightwards and this enhances filling of the left heart at the expense of the right heart filling. This shifting of the IVS during respiration is referred to as enhanced ventricular interdependence.

Enhanced ventricular interdependence is reflected on the transmitral, transtricuspid and venous flow profiles as described above. In addition, enhanced ventricular interdependence can also be appreciated from the M-mode trace through the right and left ventricles (Fig. 12.38).

Reduction in Left Ventricular Stroke Volume

As mentioned above, variations in left heart filling due to an abnormal EFG results in the leftward shift of the IVS during inspiration which decreases the LV volume. This leads to a decrease in LV stroke volume during inspiration. Evidence of a decreased stroke volume can be seen as a decrease in the transmitral inflow velocities and the LV outflow tract (LVOT) velocities. In addition, the LVOT stroke volume can also be calculated from the LVOT diameter and the LVOT velocity time integral (see Chapter 1, Table 1.3).

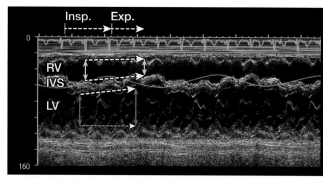

Figure 12.38 Enhanced ventricular interaction is displayed on this M-mode trace through the right and left ventricles. Observe that with inspiration the interventricular septum (IVS) shifts towards the left ventricle (LV). This results in an increase in the right ventricular (RV) cavity size and a decrease in the LV cavity size. On expiration the opposite occurs; the IVS shifts towards the RV so the RV size decreases and the LV cavity size increases. Insp. = inspiration; Exp. = expiration.

While the emphasis is placed on the identification of characteristic respiratory variations in the transmitral, transtricuspid and venous flow profiles, respiratory variations can also be seen on the LVOT, transaortic and transpulmonary valve flow profiles in patients with cardiac tamponade. LVOT and transaortic profiles will show a decrease in the peak velocity during inspiration compared with expiration while the transpulmonary valve profile will show an increase in the peak velocity during inspiration compared with expiration.

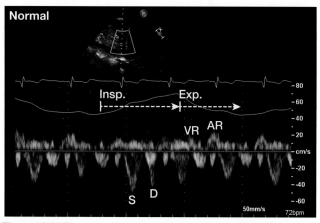

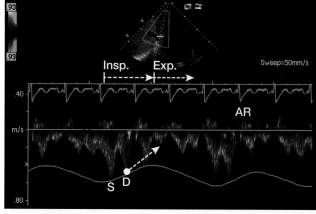

Figure 12.36 The normal hepatic venous profile consists of four waveforms: diastolic forward flow (D), systolic forward flow (S), atrial flow reversal (AR) and ventricular flow reversal (VR) (*left*). Observe that during inspiration there is a slight increase in forward flow velocities (S > D) while during expiration there is a slight increase in the AR velocity. The hepatic venous profile in cardiac tamponade shows a significant decrease in the D with expiration as well as an increase in the AR velocity on expiration (*right*). Insp. = inspiration; Exp. = expiration.

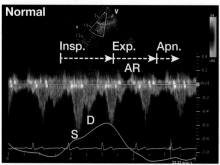
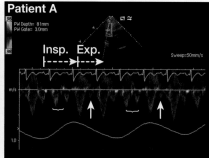
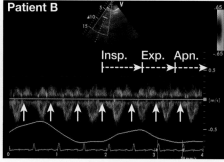

Figure 12.37 The normal SVC profile consists of three waveforms: diastolic forward flow (D), systolic forward flow (S), and atrial flow reversal (AR) (*left*). Observe that during inspiration there is a slight increase in forward flow (S and D) velocities while during expiration there is a slight increase in the AR velocity. The SVC profile in cardiac tamponade is variable; two traces are shown from two different patients. In patient A there is a loss of the normal inspiratory increase in SVC flow (*brackets*) and a loss of the expiratory diastolic (D) velocity (*arrows, middle*). In patient B there is complete loss of D velocity (*arrows, right*). Cardiac tamponade in patient B is more "severe" than patient A as there is a significant decrease in right heart filling over the entire respiratory cycle. Insp. = inspiration; Exp. = expiration.

Challenges in Cardiac Tamponade

Chronic Obstructive Pulmonary Disease

Abnormal respiratory variations in transmitral and transtricuspid inflow profiles are also seen in patients with chronic obstructive pulmonary disease (COPD). In patients with COPD exaggerated increases in the respiratory variation of these flow profiles occur due to exaggerated respiratory changes in the intrathoracic pressures.

Therefore, in COPD patients who also have a pericardial effusion it may be difficult to determine if the respiratory variations in the transmitral and transtricuspid inflow velocities are due to COPD alone or due to cardiac tamponade. In this situation, the evaluation of the SVC flow profile can be useful. In patients with COPD the intrapleural pressure becomes more negative during inspiration; as a result the RA pressure decreases more than usual and this leads to augmentation of SVC forward flow velocities ≥ 20 cm/s (Fig. 12.39, top). In patients with cardiac tamponade the SVC flow profile shows a loss of the normal inspiratory increase in SVC flow (especially diastolic forward flow) (Fig. 12.39, bottom). Furthermore, the respiratory variations in flow profiles associated with COPD are usually seen throughout respiration rather than just on the first beat of inspiration or the first beat of expiration.

Ventilated Patients

Patients with cardiac tamponade on positive pressure ventilators will have respiratory variations in Doppler flow profiles opposite to the changes described above. This is because positive pressure ventilators essentially push air into the lungs with inspiration, so during inspiration the ITP increases rather than decreases. Therefore, with cardiac tamponade the transmitral peak E velocity on the first beat of inspiration increases compared with the peak E velocity on the first beat of expiration while the transtricuspid peak E velocity decreases with the first beat of inspiration compared with the peak E velocity on the first beat of expiration.

Low Pressure Cardiac Tamponade

Low pressure cardiac tamponade (LPCT) refers to cardiac tamponade in the setting of low ICP and low IPP. LPCT is seen in patients with intravascular fluid depletion which occurs as a result of haemorrhage, advanced malignancy, or hypovolemia. The typical clinical findings associated with cardiac tamponade are absent in most of these patients. LPCT can be identified by echocardiography based on the presence of RA collapse, RVDC and the characteristic respiratory variations in the spectral Doppler profiles associated with cardiac tamponade.

Pleural Effusions causing Cardiac Tamponade Physiology

Cardiac tamponade physiology can occur in the setting of large pleural effusion. In this situation, there is an increase in the ITP which is transmitted to the pericardial sac and the resultant increase in IPP can produce tamponade-like physiology. Therefore, on the echocardiographic examination RVDC as well as characteristic respiratory variations in the spectral Doppler profiles consistent with cardiac tamponade may be seen.

The importance of recognising this phenomenon lies in the treatment strategy; for example, in patients who have both pleural and pericardial effusions, drainage of the pleural effusion instead of the pericardial effusion may be sufficient to eliminate any associated haemodynamic compromise.

Constrictive Pericarditis

Aetiology of Constrictive Pericarditis

Constrictive pericarditis (CP) occurs when there is inflammation, thickening, scarring, and/or calcification of the pericardium and fusion of the visceral and parietal pericardial layers (Fig. 12.40). The aetiology of CP is listed in Table 12.6. Tuberculosis is the most common cause of CP worldwide while pericardial 'injury' due to cardiac surgery and radiation therapy are the most common causes of CP in developed countries.

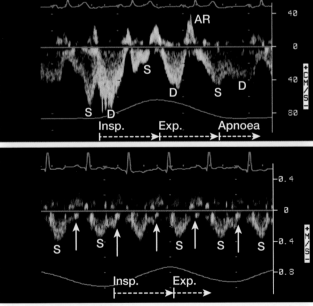

Figure 12.39 The superior vena cava (SVC) flow profile typical of chronic obstructive pulmonary disease shows marked augmentation of the SVC forward flow velocities with inspiration (*top*). The SVC flow profile characteristic of cardiac tamponade displays a loss of the normal inspiratory increase in SVC flow (*bottom*); a total loss of diastolic forward flow is also present (*arrows*). AR = atrial reversal; Insp. = inspiration; Exp. = expiration; D = diastolic forward flow; S = systolic forward flow.

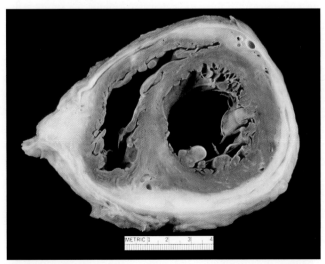

Figure 12.40 This gross pathological specimen of constrictive pericarditis shows a markedly thickened but non-calcified pericardium; fibrosis and adhesion of the pericardial layers can also be appreciated. By permission of Mayo Foundation for Medical Education and Research. All rights reserved. Courtesy of William D. Edwards, MD.

Table 12.6 **Aetiology of Constrictive Pericarditis**

Common Causes	Less Common Causes	Rare Causes

• Idiopathic (unknown)
• Infectious:
  - Bacterial; e.g. tuberculosis
  - Viral
• Radiation-induced (thoracic and mediastinal radiation therapy)
• Postsurgical (any procedure in which the pericardium is opened, manipulated, or damaged)
	• Infectious (fungal)
	• Neoplasms (e.g. breast and lung carcinomas, lymphomas, melanoma and mesothelioma)
	• Uremia
	• Connective tissue disorders (e.g. rheumatoid arthritis, systemic lupus erythematosus and scleroderma)
	• Drug-induced
	• Trauma
	• Post myocardial infarction (i.e. post-Dressler syndrome)
		• Toxic or metabolic
		• Intrapericardial instrumentation (e.g. epicardial pacemaker or automated implantable cardiac defibrillator)
		• Hereditary
		• Chemical trauma
		• Chylopericardium

Source: Sidney DS, et al. Constrictive Pericarditis. Medscape Reference, accessed on 23 December 2011; http://emedicine.medscape.com/article/157096-clinical#a0218.

Pathophysiology of Constrictive Pericarditis

The encasement of the heart within a rigid and noncompliant pericardial sac results in a fixed total intrapericardial volume and subsequent 'restricted' diastolic filling of the heart.

In particular, in early diastole there is rapid filling of the ventricles as per normal; however, in mid diastole there is rapid termination of diastolic flow. This occurs when the limits of pericardial compliance are reached so the pericardium can stretch no further. Due to the fixed total intrapericardial volume, this effect occurs almost simultaneously in all four cardiac chambers. The resultant haemodynamic hallmark of this condition is equalization of end-diastolic pressures in all four cardiac chambers. On the cardiac catheterization pressure trace, its effects appear as a characteristic 'dip-and-plateau' or 'square root' sign (Fig 12.41).

In addition, due to the isolation of the heart by the constrictive pericardial shell, the normal respiratory variations in ITP are not transmitted to the cardiac chambers. This dissociation between the ITP and the ICP results in haemodynamic effects similar to cardiac tamponade. That is, there are accentuated respiratory variations of ventricular filling as well as enhanced ventricular interaction.

Echocardiographic Features of Constrictive Pericarditis

As for the assessment of cardiac tamponade, echocardiography provides useful information that can support or suggest the diagnosis of CP. Characteristic echocardiographic findings associated with CP are summarised in Table 12.7. Many of these M-mode and 2D echocardiographic findings are difficult to appreciate or are neither sensitive nor specific for the diagnosis of CP. However, identification of exaggerated respiratory variations in diastolic filling and evidence of enhanced ventricular interaction are very useful in supporting the diagnosis of CP. In addition, evidence of annulus paradoxus and annulus reversus as seen on Doppler tissue imaging (DTI) are also valuable in the diagnosis of CP.

Exaggerated Respiratory Variations in Diastolic Filling

Accentuated respiratory changes in left and right heart filling occur due to dissociation between ITP and ICP caused by the constrictive pericardial shell. The mechanisms for these changes are essentially the same as already described for cardiac tamponade. Accentuated respiratory changes are reflected on the transmitral, transtricuspid, pulmonary venous and hepatic venous flow profiles (Fig. 12.42).

Kussmaul's sign and a pericardial knock are two clinical signs that manifest as a result of the pathophysiological effects of constrictive pericarditis (CP). Kussmaul's sign refers to the paradoxical rise in venous pressure with distension of the jugular veins during inspiration. This sign is not specific for CP as this sign is also seen in other conditions where there is severe right heart failure. A pericardial knock refers to the high pitched heart sound occurring in early diastole which occurs when rapid ventricular filling is abruptly halted by the constricting pericardium. A pericardial knock is a specific but insensitive indicator of CP.

Constrictive Pericarditis versus Cardiac Tamponade

Both constrictive pericarditis (CP) and cardiac tamponade restrict or impede ventricular diastolic filling resulting in accentuated respiratory changes in right and left heart filling as well as increased ventricular interaction. However, despite these similarities there are important pathophysiological differences between CP and cardiac tamponade. The distinctive differences between these two entities are summarised below.

	Constrictive Pericarditis	Cardiac Tamponade
Haemodynamic consequence	Dissociation between the ITP and ICP due to isolation of the heart by the constrictive pericardial shell	Dissociation between the ITP and ICP due to ↑ IPP which impedes the transmission of ITP to the pericardial sac and the heart
Diastolic filling	Early diastolic filling is rapid; restricted ventricular filling occurs in mid-to-late diastole	Restricted filling occurs progressively over the entire diastolic period
Systemic venous return	Variable; prominent D velocities with a brief flow duration noted during baseline apnoea (reflects rapid early filling of the RV which is then rapidly abbreviated by the rigid pericardium)	Variable; D velocities less prominent and abbreviated compared with CP which become progressively diminished with increasing tamponade (reflects progressive pan-diastolic compression)

The significance of these respiratory variations is listed in Table 12.8. Importantly, the calculation of the percentage change (%Δ) is derived as the difference between values

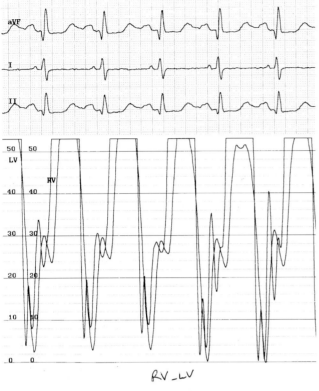

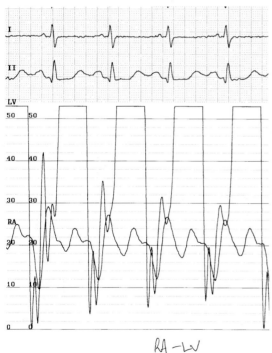

Figure 12.41 These pressure traces were recorded in a patient with constrictive pericarditis. The simultaneous right ventricular (RV) and left ventricular (LV) pressure tracings show diastolic equalization of pressures in both ventricles (*top*); the simultaneous right atrial (RA) and LV pressure tracings also show diastolic equalization of pressures in both chambers (*bottom*). Also observe the characteristic 'dip and plateau' or 'square root' sign of the diastolic ventricular pressure trace; this appears as a prominent downward deflection (dip) followed by a rapid diastolic pressure rise that remains high throughout the remainder of diastolic period (plateau).

measured at expiration and inspiration divided by the expiratory value (see page 358). An inspiratory decrease of the transmitral E velocity on the first beat of inspiration compared with the first beat of expiration of ≥ 25%, and an inspiratory increase of the transtricuspid E velocity on the first beat of inspiration compared with the first beat of expiration of > 40% are consistent with CP. Furthermore, an expiratory increase in hepatic venous AR velocity of ≥ 25% of forward flow velocity is also a characteristic feature of CP[12.2].

In addition to the characteristic respiratory variations in spectral Doppler flow profiles, the transmitral and transtricuspid inflow profiles also display features characteristic of restrictive ventricular filling. These characteristics include an increased E/A ratio (> 2) and a short deceleration time (< 160 m/s). In the setting of CP, restrictive filling occurs due to pericardial constraint rather than as a consequence of increased myocardial stiffness.

Enhanced Ventricular Interaction

Evidence of enhanced ventricular interaction associated with CP is based on the respiratory variations in Doppler traces described above. Furthermore, in CP the inspiratory leftward shift of the IVS due to decreased LV filling and the rightward shift of the IVS due to decreased RV filling creates a characteristic 'bouncing' motion of the IVS over the respiratory cycle. This septal bounce as well as the variation in RV and LV chamber dimensions during respiration is best appreciated with 2D real-time imaging from the apical 4-chamber view as well as on the M-mode trace through the right and left ventricles (Fig. 12.43).

Annulus Paradoxus and Annulus Reversus

Doppler tissue imaging (DTI) also has an important role in the diagnosis of CP. As discussed in Chapter 3, the transmitral E to DTI e' ratio has a positive relationship with LV filling pressures; that is, the higher the E/e' ratio, the higher the LV filling pressures. However, in CP the medial DTI e' velocity is usually preserved or even increased despite the presence of increased LV filling pressures. Therefore, in patients with CP, there is an inverse relationship between the E/e' ratio and LV filling pressures. That is, despite high LV filling pressures, the E/e' ratio is normal or low. This is 'paradoxical' to what is seen with primary myocardial disease and for this reason, the term 'annulus paradoxus' has been proposed to describe the relationship between a 'low' E/e' ratio and the elevated LV filling pressures in patients with CP.

Furthermore, in the normal individual, the lateral e' velocities of both the mitral and tricuspid annuli are higher than the medial e' velocity (Fig. 12.44, top). However, in CP the lateral e' velocities are lower than the medial e' velocity (Fig. 12.44, bottom). As this is the reverse of what is seen normally, the term 'annulus reversus' has been coined to describe this finding.

The mechanism for annulus paradoxus and annulus reversus in CP has been attributed to: (1) tethering of the adjacent fibrotic and scarred pericardium which impedes the diastolic longitudinal motion of the lateral annulus, and (2) a compensatory increase in the diastolic longitudinal motion of the medial mitral annulus.

[12.2] Oh JK, Hatle LK, Seward JB, Danielson GK, Schaff HV, Reeder GS, Tajik AJ. Diagnostic role of Doppler echocardiography in constrictive pericarditis. *J Am Coll Cardiol.* 1994 Jan;23(1):154-62.

Table 12.7 Echocardiographic Findings associated with Constrictive Pericarditis

Echocardiographic Finding	Mechanism
M-mode Signs	
Multiple parallel echoes posterior to left ventricle (LV)	Pericardial thickening
Interventricular septal (IVS) notching in early diastole or with atrial contraction	Transient and sudden shift of IVS due to asymmetric right and left ventricular filling that causes rapid changes in the transmural pressure between the right and left ventricles at these phases in the cardiac cycle
Diastolic flattening of LV posterior wall (PW)	PW motion is terminated abruptly in mid-diastole when the limit of the constricting pericardium is reached (reflects the plateau seen on the haemodynamic pressure waveform)
Sharp downward motion of posterior aortic root in early diastole	Rapid early ventricular filling
Premature pulmonic valve opening	Increased mid-diastolic RV pressure which exceeds pulmonary artery diastolic pressure
2D Echocardiographic Findings	
Increased echogenicity of the pericardium	Pericardial thickening
Absence of pericardial slippage	Thickened pericardium tethered to heart
Inferior vena cava plethora	Elevated right atrial pressure
IVS bounce	Exaggerated ventricular interdependence (leftward IVS shift with inspiration and rightward IVS shift with expiration)
Doppler Echocardiographic Findings	
Restrictive filling transmitral inflow (E/A ratio > 2, DT < 160 ms)	Restrictive filling due to rapid increase in LV diastolic pressure with termination of flow in mid-diastole when the limit of the constricting pericardium is reached
Accentuated respiratory variation in transmitral, transtricuspid, pulmonary venous and hepatic venous flow profile	Dissociation of intrathoracic pressure from intracardiac pressure
Annulus paradoxus	Pericardial constriction limits lateral expansion of the ventricles during diastole which results in increased longitudinal myocardial motion of the medial annulus
Annulus reversus (DTI medial mitral e' velocity > lateral mitral e' velocity)	Exaggerated longitudinal motion of IVS to compensate for limited motion of the lateral annulus due to adhesion of the constricting pericardium

Table 12.8 Percentage Change from Expiration to Inspiration in Normal, Constrictive Pericarditis and Restrictive Cardiomyopathy*

Pt. Group	No.	IVRT	Mitral E velocity	Tricuspid E velocity
		ms	cm/s	cm/s
Normal	20	2 ± 3	-4 ± 4	14 ± 9
Constrictive Pericarditis	7	$50 \pm 14^\wedge$	-33 ± 9 ^	$44 \pm 22^\wedge$
Restrictive Cardiomyopathy	12	4 ± 7	-3 ± 4	17 ± 16

* Percent change of expiratory to inspiratory values.
Values are mean ± one standard deviation. ^ $p<0.05$ versus restrictive cardiomyopathy and normal
IVRT = isovolumic relaxation time; No. = number patients; Pt. = patient.
Source: Hatle LK, Appleton CP, Popp RL. Differentiation of constrictive pericarditis and restrictive cardiomyopathy by Doppler echocardiography. *Circulation*. 1989 Feb;79(2):357-70.

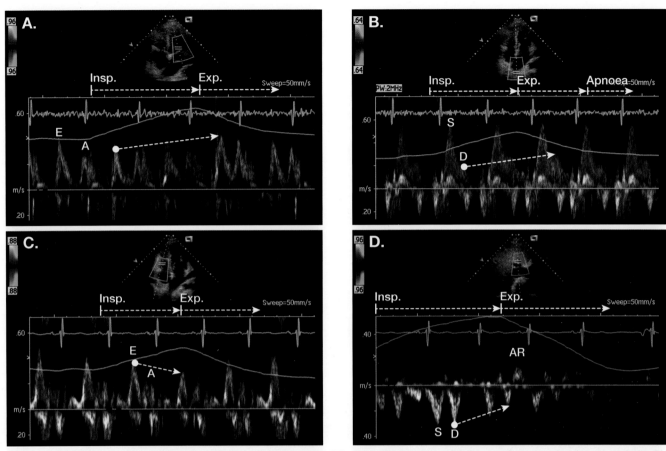

Figure 12.42 Transmitral **(A)**, pulmonary venous **(B)**, transtricuspid **(C)**, and hepatic venous **(D)** flow profiles recorded from a patient with constrictive pericarditis are shown. Observe that on the first beat of inspiration the transmitral peak early diastolic (E) velocity and pulmonary venous peak diastolic (D) velocity decrease when compared with the velocities on the first beat of expiration while the transtricuspid peak E velocity and hepatic venous peak D velocity are increased on the first beat of inspiration when compared with the velocities on the first beat of expiration. Also observe the marked increase in the hepatic venous atrial reversal (AR) velocity with expiration.
Insp. = inspiration; Exp. = expiration; A = velocity with atrial contraction; S = systolic forward flow.

Pitfalls in Echocardiographic Diagnosis of Constrictive Pericarditis

Chronic Obstructive Pulmonary Disease

As for cardiac tamponade the characteristic transmitral and transtricuspid inflow profiles associated with CP are also seen in patients with COPD. Recall that COPD causes exaggerated increases in the respiratory variation of these flow profiles due to exaggerated respiratory changes in the intrathoracic pressures. The evaluation of the SVC flow profile can be useful in distinguishing COPD from CP.

As stated above COPD results in the intrapleural pressure becoming more negative during inspiration; as a result the RA pressure decreases more than usual and this leads to augmentation of SVC forward flow velocities ≥ 20 cm/s (Fig. 12.45, top). In patients with CP the SVC flow profile shows minimal variation in forward flow velocities with respiration (Fig. 12.45, bottom).

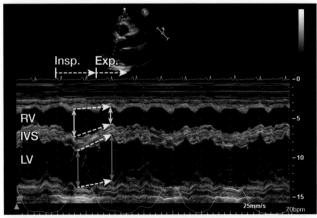

Figure 12.43 Enhanced ventricular interaction is displayed on this M-mode trace through the right and left ventricles. Observe that with inspiration the interventricular septum (IVS) shifts towards the left ventricle (LV). This results in an increase in the right ventricular (RV) cavity size and a decrease in the LV cavity size. On expiration the opposite occurs; the IVS shifts towards the RV so the RV size decreases and the LV cavity size increases. On real-time 2D imaging the IVS displays a characteristic septal bounce. Insp. = inspiration; Exp. = expiration.

Technical Tips

Septal Bounce: On real-time 2D imaging septal bounce associated with constrictive pericarditis is best observed from the apical 4-chamber view. Remember that this septal bounce occurs due to variations in RV and LV cavity size with respiration. Therefore, in order to appreciate this septal bounce, 5-10 beat loops should be digitally acquired.

Doppler Tissue Imaging: due to respiratory variations in the e' at both annuli an average of all absolute values throughout one respiratory cycle should be calculated. Due to the tethering effect of the lateral mitral annulus the E/e' ratio should be calculated using the medial e' rather than the lateral e' velocity.

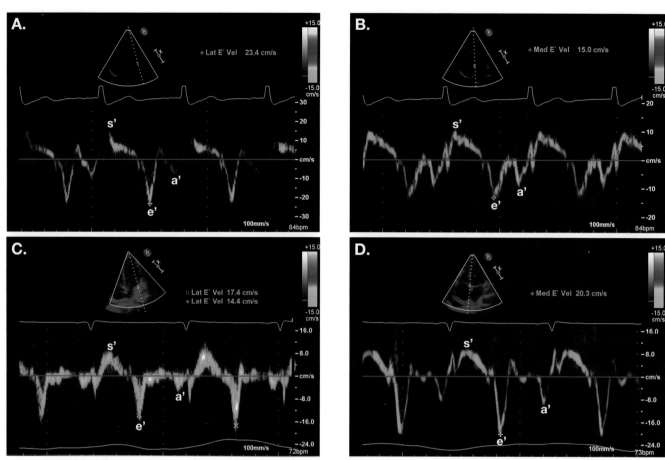

Figure 12.44 The normal relationship of the early diastolic myocardial velocities (e') between the lateral and medial mitral annuli are shown (*top*). Observe that in the normal situation the lateral e' velocity **(A)** is higher than the medial e' velocity **(B)**. The reversed relationship between the lateral e' and medial e' velocities is shown in constrictive pericarditis (*bottom*). Observe that in constrictive pericarditis the medial e' velocity is higher **(D)** than the lateral e' velocity **(C)**. a' = myocardial velocity at atrial contraction; s' = systolic myocardial velocity.

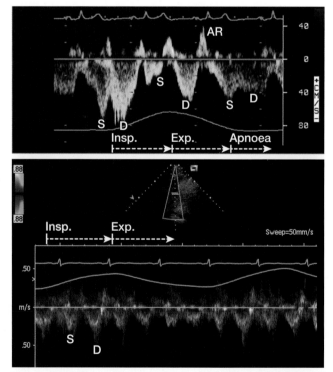

Figure 12.45 The superior vena cava (SVC) flow profile typical of chronic obstructive pulmonary disease shows marked augmentation of the SVC forward flow velocities with inspiration (*top*). The SVC flow profile characteristic of constrictive pericarditis displays minimal respiratory variation in systolic forward flow velocity from inspiration to expiration (*bottom*).

Insp. = inspiration; Exp. = expiration; D = diastolic forward flow; S = systolic forward flow.

Constrictive Pericarditis without Respiratory Variation

The echocardiographic findings characteristic of CP are based on exaggerated respiratory variations in the transmitral, transtricuspid, pulmonary venous and hepatic venous flow profiles. However, not all patients with CP demonstrate these respiratory variations. For example, an absence of exaggerated respiratory variations may occur when there is localised CP, when there is a combination of restrictive cardiomyopathy and CP, or when there is a marked elevation in atrial pressures.

In particular, if the LA pressure is markedly increased, 'unmasking' of the typical respiratory variations associated with CP may be achieved by decreasing LA pressure (preload reduction). One method of preload reduction is to change the patient position from supine to a standing or sitting position (Fig. 12.46).

Ventilated Patients

As in cardiac tamponade, patients with CP on positive pressure ventilators will have respiratory variations in Doppler velocities opposite to the changes described above. This is because ITP changes associated with positive pressure ventilation are the opposite of the ITP seen with spontaneous breathing. So as the ventilated patient inspires, the ITP increases rather than decreases. Therefore, with CP the transmitral peak E velocity on the first beat of inspiration increases compared to the peak E velocity on the first beat of expiration while the transtricuspid peak E velocity decreases with the first beat of inspiration compared to the peak E velocity on the first beat of expiration.

Table 12.9 Echocardiographic Features Distinguishing Constrictive Pericarditis from Restrictive Cardiomyopathy

Echocardiography Finding	Constrictive Pericarditis	Restrictive Cardiomyopathy
Pericardial thickening	Present (or absent)	Absent
Degree of atrial dilatation	Mild	Moderate - marked
Ventricular systolic function (ejection fraction)	Normal	Normal (decreased at end-stage disease)
Interventricular septal bounce	Present	Absent
Restrictive filling profiles ^	Present	Present ^^
Increased respiratory variation of mitral and tricuspid inflow velocities	Present (may be absent in certain conditions*)	Absent
Hepatic venous flow	↑ AR reversal with expiration	↑ AR velocity with inspiration
Medial e' velocity	Normal or increased (≥ 8 cm/s)	Decreased (< 8 cm/s)
Medial e' vs. lateral e' velocity	Medial e' > Lateral e'	Medial e' < Lateral e'
E/e' ratio#	Normal or decreased (< 8)	> 15
Flow propagation velocity	≥ 100 cm/s	< 45 cm/s

^ Defined from the transmitral inflow profile as an increased E velocity, a decreased A velocity, an E/A ratio > 2, and shortened deceleration time (< 160 ms)
^^ Doppler profiles can vary between abnormal relaxation, pseudonormal or restrictive filling.
* Absent respiratory variations when there is localised CP, a combination of restrictive cardiomyopathy and CP, or a marked elevation in atrial pressures.
# This ratio is calculated using the medial e' velocity

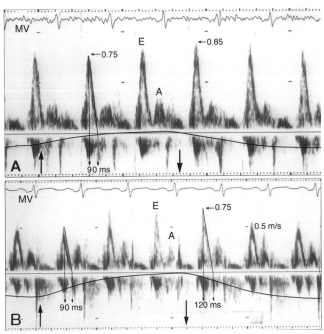

Figure 12.46 Pulsed-wave Doppler echocardiographic recordings of transmitral inflow at baseline with the patient in left lateral decubitus position **(A)** and repeated a few minutes after baseline study with patient in upright position **(B)** are shown. The respirometer recording is displayed at the bottom of each trace; upward and downward deflections indicate the onset of inspiration and expiration, respectively. The baseline trace shows an inspiratory mitral E velocity of 0.75 m/s (second beat) and a slightly increased expiratory velocity 0.85 m/s (fourth beat); the individual Doppler velocity pattern is restrictive, with a short deceleration time (90 ms), a small A velocity (0.25 m/s), and an increased E/A ratio. The Doppler study with the patient in upright position shows a decrease in the mitral E velocity during both inspiration (0.50 m/s) and expiration (0.75 m/s), with significant respiratory variation noted (>33%). The velocity pattern remained restrictive, with a respiratory variation in the deceleration time.
From Oh JK, Tajik AJ, Appleton CP, Hatle LK, Nishimura RA, Seward JB. Preload reduction to unmask the characteristic Doppler features of constrictive pericarditis. A new observation. *Circulation*, Feb 18;95(4), page 796-9, © 1997, Lippincott, Williams & Wilkins, with permission.

Constrictive Pericarditis versus Restrictive Cardiomyopathy

The characteristic clinical and physiologic presentation of patients with CP may be identical to that of patients with restrictive cardiomyopathy (RCM). As a result, CP is often clinically indistinguishable from RCM. Importantly, CP is a treatable cause of diastolic heart failure and, therefore, identification of this disorder is crucial as most symptoms can be reversed by surgical pericardiectomy.

Echocardiography is a valuable tool in the differentiation between CP and RCM. In particular, spectral Doppler, colour Doppler M-mode and DTI can be used to differentiate between these two entities (Table 12.9).

The echocardiographic evaluation of restrictive cardiomyopathy is discussed in detail in Chapter 6.

Effusive-Constrictive Pericarditis

Effusive-constrictive pericarditis is characterised by the presence of a pericardial effusion in conjunction with constrictive physiology. This entity is likely to represent an intermediate transition from acute pericarditis with pericardial effusion to CP.

The characteristic echocardiographic features of effusive-constrictive pericarditis include: (1) a small to moderate-sized pericardial effusion, (2) evidence of fibrinous strands within the pericardial space, and (3) classic spectral Doppler features of CP (Fig. 12.47).

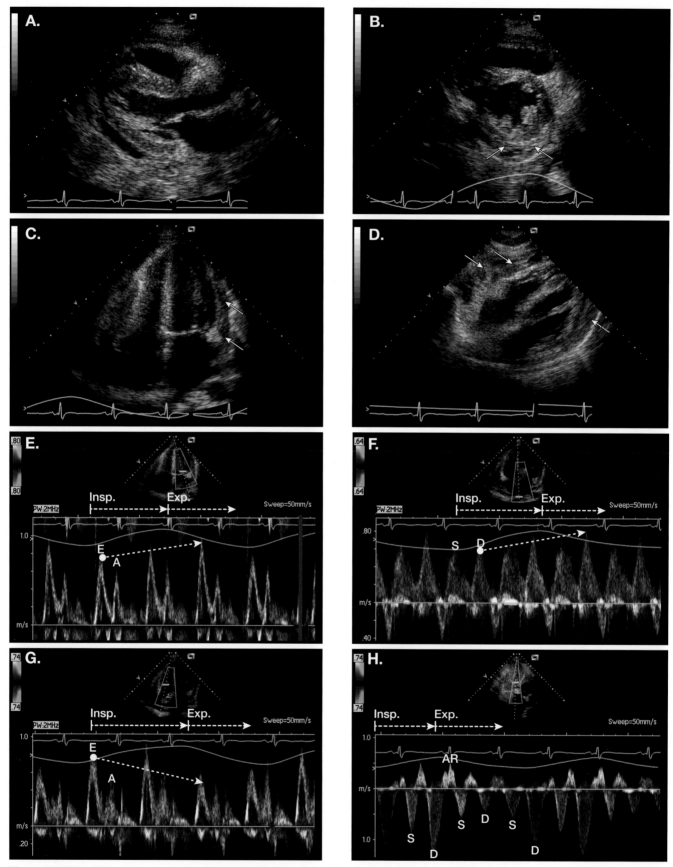

Figure 12.47 The 2D images recorded from the parasternal long axis **(A)**, the parasternal short axis **(B)**, the apical 4-chamber **(C)** and subcostal 4-chamber **(D)** views show a small-moderate pericardial effusion; semi-solid material and fibrinous strands are also noted within the pericardial space (*arrows*). The spectral Doppler findings are consistent with constrictive pericarditis. On the transmitral inflow profile the peak E velocity on the first beat of inspiration is decreased compared to expiration **(E)**; on the pulmonary venous profile there is a decrease in the D velocity on the first beat of inspiration compared to expiration **(F)**; on the transtricuspid inflow profile the peak E velocity on expiration is significantly decreased when compared to the first beat of inspiration **(G)**; on the hepatic venous profile there is an increase in forward flow velocities with inspiration and a marked decrease in diastolic forward flow as well as a marked increase in the atrial reversal velocity on the first beat of expiration **(H)**. The constellation of 2D and Doppler findings are consistent with effusive-constrictive pericarditis.

Key Points

Anatomy of the Pericardium
- Pericardium is 1- 2 mm thick and consists of an outer sac (fibrous pericardium) and a double-layered inner sac (serous pericardium)
- Serous pericardium has 2 layers: the parietal layer and visceral layer (known as the epicardium)
- Pericardial space contains approximately 10-30 mL of ultrafiltrate of plasma
- There are 2 pericardial sinuses: (1) transverse sinus which is anterior to the SVC and posterior to the ascending aorta and pulmonary trunk and (2) oblique sinus which is superior and posterior to the LA

Functions of the Pericardium
- Stabilisation of the heart within the thoracic cavity
- Protection of the heart from infection from adjoining structures
- Acting as a lubricant to reduce friction between the heart and surrounding structures
- Limiting acute distension of the heart and preventing over filling of the heart
- Facilitation of the interaction and coupling of the ventricles and atria (basis of ventricular interaction)

Pericardial Cysts
- Rare anomaly resulting from a defect in the embryonic development of the pericardium
- Most commonly located in the right costophrenic angle
- *Echocardiographic appearance:* round or elliptical echo-free structures adjacent to a cardiac chamber (usually the RA)

Absent Pericardium
- Very rare congenital anomaly; associated congenital cardiac anomalies include atrial septal defect, bicuspid aortic valve, patent ductus arteriosus, or tetralogy of Fallot
- May be complete or partial absence; complete absence less common than partial (usually left-sided)
- *Echocardiographic characteristics:* (1) unusual echocardiographic windows, (2) cardiac hypermobility, (3) abnormal interventricular septal motion, (4) abnormal swinging motion of the heart, and (5) apparent right-sided heart enlargement

Acute Pericarditis
- *Definition:* inflammation of the pericardium
- *Aetiology:* most commonly caused by a viral infection or due to unknown causes
- *Diagnosis:* based on clinical manifestations such as characteristic chest pain and ECG findings, and a pericardial friction rub on auscultation
- *Echocardiographic findings:* may be entirely normal, may have a pericardial effusion, may have pericardial thickening +/- a pericardial effusion; the diagnosis is clinical rather than echocardiographic

Pericardial Effusions: Basic Concepts
- *Definition:* presence of an abnormal accumulation of fluid within the pericardial cavity
- *Aetiology:* numerous causes including inflammation of the pericardium (pericarditis), infection, radiation, autoimmune diseases, trauma, neoplasms and medications
- *Types:* transudative (ultrafiltrate of plasma), exudative (extravascular fluid), haemorrhagic (blood) or malignant (obstruction of the lymphatic drainage, fluid-secreting malignancy, or fluid accumulation due to metastatic spread)
- *Pathophysiology:* dependent on the size and rate of accumulation of effusions

Role of Echocardiography in Pericardial Effusions
- Detection and sizing of pericardial effusions
- Determining the aetiology of pericardial effusions (e.g. transudative versus haemorrhagic)
- Differentiation of pericardial effusion from pleural effusions and other structures/pathologies
- Echo-guided pericardiocentesis. The role of echocardiography in this procedure is to:
  - confirm the presence, size and distribution of the effusion
  - identify the ideal puncture site and trajectory angle for needle entry
  - confirm the location of the needle within the pericardial cavity
  - reassess the amount of residual fluid following the procedure

Cardiac Tamponade: Basic Concepts
- *Pathophysiology:*
  - TMFP (difference between ICP and IPP) becomes less positive as IPP increases; when IPP exceeds ICP cardiac compression (collapse) occurs
  - An increased IPP results in decreased left heart filling, a decrease in LV stroke volume and pulsus paradoxus; a leftward shift of the IVS with inspiration also results in a further increase right heart filling
  - Exaggerated IVS motion causes enhanced ventricular interdependence

(continued over...)

Key Points (continued)

Echocardiography in Cardiac Tamponade

Supports the diagnosis of suspected cardiac tamponade by looking for the following signs:

- Swinging heart: not specific or sensitive
- Plethora of the inferior vena cava (IVC): not specific or sensitive
- Collapse of the cardiac chambers: RA inversion > 1/3 of the cardiac cycle and/or RV collapse > 1/3 of diastole improves the specificity for cardiac tamponade
- Exaggerated respiratory variation in diastolic filling (%Δ = (1st expiration − 1st inspiration) ÷ 1st expiration):
  ○ Inspiration compared with expiration:
    - ↓ transmitral E velocity (> 30%)
    - ↑ IVRT (> 20%)
    - ↓ pulmonary venous D velocity
    - ↑ transtricuspid E velocity (> 60%)
  ○ Hepatic venous and SVC flow profiles with expiration:
    - ↓ hepatic venous D velocity
    - ↑ hepatic venous AR velocity
    - Loss of SVC D velocity
- Signs of enhanced ventricular interaction
- Respiratory variation in spectral Doppler flow profiles as above
- Reciprocal changes in LV and RV cavity size over respiratory cycle
- Reduction in the LV stroke volume

Constrictive Pericarditis (CP): Basic Concepts

- *Definition:* inflammation, thickening, scarring, and/or calcification of the pericardium and fusion of the visceral and parietal pericardial layers
- *Aetiology:* most common cause in developed countries is pericardial injury (post cardiac surgery and radiation therapy); most common cause worldwide is tuberculosis
- *Pathophysiology:* encasement of the heart within a rigid and noncompliant pericardial sac results in:
  - a fixed total cardiac volume and subsequent 'restricted' diastolic filling of the heart
  - equalization of end-diastolic pressures in all four cardiac chambers
  - dissociation between the ITP and the ICP results in haemodynamic effects similar to cardiac tamponade (see above)

Echocardiographic Features of CP

- Exaggerated respiratory variation in diastolic filling (almost identical to cardiac tamponade)
- Signs of enhanced ventricular interaction (as for cardiac tamponade; characteristic septal bounce)
- Annulus paradoxus (high LV filling pressures indicated by low E/e' ratio)
- Annulus reversus (lateral e' velocity < medial e' velocity)
- Findings above plus a flow propagation velocity ≥ 100 ms valuable in differentiating CP from restrictive cardiomyopathy

Effusive-Constrictive Pericarditis:

- *Definition:* presence of a pericardial effusion in conjunction with constrictive physiology
- *Echocardiographic findings:* (1) small to moderate-sized pericardial effusion, (2) evidence of fibrinous strands within the pericardial space, and (3) classic Doppler features of CP

Further Reading (listed in alphabetical order)

Pericardial Anatomy

Lachman N, Syed FF, Habib A, Kapa S, Bisco SE, Venkatachalam KL, Asirvatham SJ. Correlative anatomy for the electrophysiologist, Part I: the pericardial space, oblique sinus, transverse sinus. *J Cardiovasc Electrophysiol.* 2010 Dec;21(12):1421-6.

Pericardial Disease (General)

Bahlmann E, Cramariuc D, Gerdts E, Gohlke-Baerwolf C, Nienaber CA, Abbas AE, Appleton CP, Liu PT, Sweeney JP. Congenital absence of the pericardium: case presentation and review of literature. *Int J Cardiol.* 2005 Jan;98(1):21-5.

Connolly HM, Click RL, Schattenberg TT, Seward JB, Tajik AJ. Congenital absence of the pericardium: echocardiography as a diagnostic tool. *J Am Soc Echocardiogr.* 1995 Jan-Feb;8(1):87-92.

Ivens EL, Munt BI, Moss RR. Pericardial Disease: What The General Cardiologist Needs To Know. *Heart.* 2007 Aug;93(8):993-1000

Khandaker MH, Espinosa RE, Nishimura RA, et al. Pericardial Disease: Diagnosis and Management. *Mayo Clin Proc.* 2010;85:572-593

Klein AL, Abbara S, Agler DA, Appleton CP, Asher CR, Hoit B, Hung J, Garcia MJ, Kronzon I, Oh JK, Rodriguez ER, Schaff HV, Schoenhagen P, Tan CD, White RD. American society of echocardiography clinical recommendations for multimodality cardiovascular imaging of patients with pericardial disease: endorsed by the society for cardiovascular magnetic resonance and society of cardiovascular computed tomography. *J Am Soc Echocardiogr.* 2013 Sep;26(9):965-1012.

Little WC, Freeman GL. Pericardial Disease. *Circulation.* 2006 Mar 28;113(12):1622-32. (Erratum in: *Circulation.* 2007 Apr 17;115(15):e406).

Maisch B, Seferovi PM, Risti AD, Erbel R, Rienmüller R, Adler Y, Tomkowski WZ, Thiene G, Yacoub MH; Task Force on the Diagnosis and Management of Pericardial Diseases of the European Society of Cardiology. Guidelines on the diagnosis and management of pericardial diseases executive summary; The Task force on the diagnosis and management of pericardial diseases of the European Society of Cardiology. *Eur Heart J.* 2004 Apr;25(7):587-610.

Silvestry FE, Kerber RE, Brook MM, Carroll JD, Eberman KM, Goldstein SA, Herrmann HC, Homma S, Mehran R, Packer DL, Parisi AF, Pulerwitz T, Seward JB, Tsang TS, Wood MA. Echocardiography-guided interventions. *J Am Soc Echocardiogr.* 2009 Mar;22(3):213-31. (Erratum in: *J Am Soc Echocardiogr.* 2009 Apr;22(4):336)

Tsang TS, Freeman WK, Sinak LJ, Seward JB. Echocardiographically guided pericardiocentesis: evolution and state-of-the-art technique. *Mayo Clin Proc.* 1998 Jul;73(7):647-52.

Cardiac Tamponade

Appleton CP, Hatle LK, Popp RL. Cardiac tamponade and pericardial effusion: respiratory variation in transvalvular flow velocities studied by Doppler echocardiography. *J Am Coll Cardiol.* 1988 May;11(5):1020-30.

Burstow DJ, Oh JK, Bailey KR, Seward JB, Tajik AJ. Cardiac Tamponade: Characteristic Doppler Observations. *Mayo Clin Proc.* 1989 Mar;64(3):312-24.

Goldstein JA. Cardiac Tamponade, Constrictive Pericarditis, and Restrictive Cardiomyopathy. *Curr Probl Cardiol.* 2004 Sep;29(9):503-67.

Kopterides P, Lignos M, Papanikolaou S, Papadomichelakis E, Mentzelopoulos S, Armaganidis A, Panou F. Pleural effusion causing cardiac tamponade: report of two cases and review of the literature. *Heart Lung.* 2006 Jan-Feb;35(1):66-7.

Roy CL, Minor MA, Brookhart MA, Choudhry NK. Does this patient with a pericardial effusion have cardiac tamponade? *JAMA.* 2007 Apr 25;297(16):1810-8.

Sagristà-Sauleda J, Angel J, Sambola A, Alguersuari J, Permanyer-Miralda G, Soler-Soler J. Low-pressure cardiac tamponade: clinical and hemodynamic profile. *Circulation.* 2006 Aug 29;114(9):945-52.

Spodick D. Pathophysiology of Cardiac Tamponade. *Chest.* 1998 May;113(5):1372-8

Spodick DH. Acute cardiac tamponade. *N Engl J Med.* 2003 Aug 14;349(7):684-90.

Traylor JJ, Chan K, Wong I, Roxas JN, Chandraratna PA. Large pleural effusions producing signs of cardiac tamponade resolved by thoracentesis. *Am J Cardiol.* 2002 Jan 1;89(1):106-8.

Tsang TS, Oh JK, Seward JB, Tajik AJ. Diagnostic value of echocardiography in cardiac tamponade. *Herz.* 2000 Dec;25(8):734-40.

Constrictive Pericarditis

Boonyaratavej S, Oh JK, Tajik AJ, Appleton CP, Seward JB. Comparison of mitral inflow and superior vena cava Doppler velocities in chronic obstructive pulmonary disease and constrictive pericarditis. *J Am Coll Cardiol.* 1998 Dec;32(7):2043-8.

Choi JH, Choi JO, Ryu DR, Lee SC, Park SW, Choe YH, Oh JK. Mitral and tricuspid annular velocities in constrictive pericarditis and restrictive cardiomyopathy: correlation with pericardial thickness on computed tomography. *JACC Cardiovasc Imaging.* 2011 Jun;4(6):567-75.

Dal-Bianco JP, Sengupta PP, Mookadam F, Chandrasekaran K, Tajik AJ, Khandheria BK. Role of echocardiography in the diagnosis of constrictive pericarditis. *J Am Soc Echocardiogr.* 2009 Jan;22(1):24-33.

Hatle LK, Appleton CP, Popp RL. Differentiation of constrictive pericarditis and restrictive cardiomyopathy by Doppler echocardiography. *Circulation.* 1989 Feb;79(2):357-70.

Oh JK, Hatle LK, Seward JB, Danielson GK, Schaff HV, Reeder GS, Tajik AJ. Diagnostic role of Doppler echocardiography in constrictive pericarditis. *J Am Coll Cardiol.* 1994 Jan;23(1):154-62.

Reuss CS, Wilansky SM, Lester SJ, Lusk JL, Grill DE, Oh JK, Tajik AJ. Using mitral 'annulus reversus' to diagnose constrictive pericarditis. *Eur J Echocardiogr.* 2009 May;10(3):372-5.

Veress G, Ling LH, Kim KH, Dal-Bianco JP, Schaff HV, Espinosa RE, Melduni RM, Tajik JA, Sundt TM 3rd, Oh JK. Mitral and tricuspid annular velocities before and after pericardiectomy in patients with constrictive pericarditis. *Circ Cardiovasc Imaging.* 2011 Jul;4(4):399-407.

Infective Endocarditis and Cardiac Masses

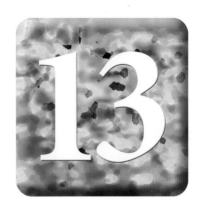

Infective Endocarditis

Infective endocarditis (IE) is a complex disease that occurs when the endothelial lining of the heart and valves becomes infected with microorganisms such as bacteria and fungus.

Pathogenesis of IE

The endothelial lining of the heart and cardiac valves is generally resistant to bacterial or fungal infection. However, when there is endothelial damage, microorganisms may adhere to the platelet and fibrin deposits which have formed as part of the healing process. This in turn produces a vegetation which is a clump of infection composed of platelets, fibrin, microorganisms, and inflammatory cells (Fig. 13.1). On gross examination, vegetations appear as grey, pink, or brown lesions (Fig. 13.2); these lesions are often friable.

IE is typically associated with underlying congenital or acquired heart disease whereby endothelial damage occurs from abrasions or from the impact of high velocity jets on the intracardiac valves or endocardium. IE however may also occur on normal intracardiac valves, on prosthetic heart valves, or on intracardiac devices such as pacemakers and defibrillators, ventricular assist devices, or indwelling catheters. Patients at risk for IE are listed in Table 13.1.

Common bacterial organisms that cause IE include Streptococci (oral viridans, beta-haemolytic, Group D streptococci), Staphylococci (aureus and epidermidis), and Enterococci (faecalis, faecium). Less common bacterial organisms causing IE include HACEK gram-negative bacteria [13.1] and fungal organisms such as Candida, Histoplasma and Aspergillus.

> Not all vegetations are due to infection. Non-infective vegetations of cardiac valves, also known as non-bacterial thrombotic endocarditis (NBTE), are associated with various conditions such as connective tissue disorders, autoimmune disorders and hypercoagulable states. In particular, non-infective valvular vegetations (verrucous or marantic vegetations or Libman-Sacks endocarditis) are a characteristic cardiac manifestation of the autoimmune disease systemic lupus erythematosus (see Chapter 14). In contrast to IE, NBTE does not destroy the cardiac valves.

Of these, the most common IE organism is oral viridans streptococci while Staphylococcus aureus (S. aureus) is the leading a cause of acute IE. In particular, S. aureus can infect structurally normal valves and is associated with higher rates of complications such as aggressive valve destruction and systemic embolic events.

Clinical Diagnosis of Infective Endocarditis

The clinical diagnosis of IE is based on the Modified Duke Criteria which include clinical, microbiological and echocardiographic criteria (Table 13.2). Clinically, IE is suspected in patients presenting with fever (often associated with chills, poor appetite and weight loss), a new regurgitant heart murmur, known underlying cardiac disease, bacteraemia, a new conduction disturbance, embolic events of unknown origin, and/or sepsis of unknown origin. Cutaneous/mucosal manifestations such Roth spots, Osler nodes, Janeway lesions, splinter haemorrhages and petechiae may be infrequently present in patients with IE (Table 13.3). These cutaneous/mucosal signs occur due to septic microemboli, necrotic microabscesses, or vascular and immunological phenomena. Importantly, these signs are not exclusively associated with IE and may be seen in other disorders.

The clinical hallmark for the diagnosis of IE is positive blood cultures. However, blood culture-negative endocarditis (BCNE), defined as endocarditis in which no causative microorganism can be grown in a blood culture, is not uncommon. Causes for BCNE include antibiotic administration prior to blood culture sampling or infection by organisms difficult to culture via conventional methods.

Echocardiography also has an important role in the diagnosis of IE and in the detection of complications, surveillance during therapy and follow-up of patients post-therapy. These roles are discussed in the following section.

Echocardiography in Infective Endocarditis

The aims of the echocardiographic examination in IE include:
• Aid in the diagnosis of IE
• Assess the functional abnormalities of the valve(s) affected
• Assess the secondary consequences of the valvular disease
• Identify complications of IE
• Surveillance during and after therapy.

[13.1] HACEK bacteria consists of Haemophilus species, Aggregatibacter (formerly Actinobacillus) actinomycetemcomitans, Cardiobacterium hominis, Eikenella corrodens, and Kingella species.

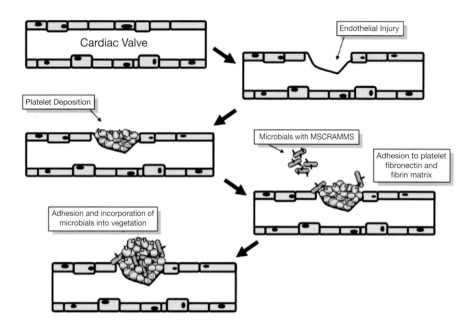

Figure 13.1 The steps in the development of the endocarditis lesion. The cardiac valve is represented by schematic top left. Endothelial injury results in platelet deposition. Adherence of microbials to the platelets occurs via MSCRAMMS (microbial surface components recognizing adhesive matrix molecules) on the microorganism and the fibronectin receptor on the platelet. Adherence also occurs between the microorganism and fibrin matrix. Eventually the microorganism becomes progressively incorporated into the vegetation and multiplies.
Reproduced from Bashore TM, Cabell C, Fowler V Jr. Update on infective endocarditis. *Curr Probl Cardiol.* Vol. 31(4), page 281, © 2006, with permission from Elsevier.

Table 13.1 **Patients at Risk for Infective Endocarditis ***

High-moderate Risk	Negligible Risk #
• Prosthetic heart valves • Valve repair using prosthetic materials • Previous infective endocarditis • Complex congenital heart disease (e.g. single-ventricles, transposition of the great arteries, tetralogy of Fallot) • Post-operative palliative shunts, conduits, or other prostheses • Other congenital cardiac valve malformations, particularly bicuspid aortic valves • Acquired valvular dysfunction (e.g., rheumatic heart disease) • Hypertrophic cardiomyopathy (latent or resting obstruction) • Mitral valve prolapse with mitral regurgitation and/or thickened leaflets	• Isolated secundum atrial septal defect • Surgical or percutaneous repair of atrial septal defect, ventricular septal defect, or patent ductus arteriosus (more than 6 months after operation) • Mitral valve prolapse without regurgitation or thickened leaflets on echocardiography • Physiological, functional, or innocent heart murmurs, including patients with aortic valve sclerosis • Trivial valvular regurgitation by echocardiography without structural abnormality and in the absence of a murmur

* Based on recommendations for endocarditis prophylaxis
# no greater risk than the general population
Based on data from Nishimura RA, Carabello BA, Faxon DP, Freed MD, Lytle BW, O'Gara PT, O'Rourke RA, Shah PM, Bonow RO, Carabello BA, Chatterjee K, de Leon AC Jr, Faxon DP, Freed MD, Gaasch WH, Lytle BW, Nishimura RA, O'Gara PT, O'Rourke RA, Otto CM, Shah PM, Shanewise JS, Smith SC Jr, Jacobs AK, Buller CE, Creager MA, Ettinger SM, Krumholz HM, Kushner FG, Lytle BW, Nishimura RA, Page RL, Tarkington LG, Yancy CW Jr. ACC/AHA 2008 guideline update on valvular heart disease: focused update on infective endocarditis: a report of the American College of Cardiology/American Heart Association Task Force on Practice Guidelines: endorsed by the Society of Cardiovascular Anesthesiologists, Society for Cardiovascular Angiography and Interventions, and Society of Thoracic Surgeons. *Circulation.* 2008 Aug 19;118(8):887-96.

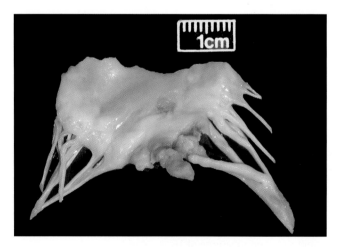

Figure 13.2 This gross pathological specimen is of an excised anterior mitral leaflet with vegetations on the leaflet and cords from infective endocarditis. The vegetations appear as brownish lumps or clusters on the valve and cords.
Reproduced from Veinot JP. Native Valve Pathology. *Surgical Pathology Clinics.* Vol. 5, page 339, © 2012, with permission from Elsevier.

Table 13.2 Modified Duke Criteria for Diagnosis of Infective Endocarditis

Definite IE
Pathologic criteria:
• Microorganisms demonstrated by culture or histologic examination of a vegetation, a vegetation that has embolised, or an intracardiac abscess specimen; OR
• Pathologic lesions; vegetation or intracardiac abscess confirmed by histologic examination showing active endocarditis
Clinical criteria:
• 2 major criteria; OR
• 1 major criterion and 3 minor criteria; OR
• 5 minor criteria
Possible IE
• 1 major criterion and 1 minor criterion; OR
• 3 minor criteria
Rejected
• Firm alternate diagnosis explaining evidence of IE; OR
• Resolution of IE syndrome with antibiotic therapy for <4 days; OR
• No pathologic evidence of IE at surgery or autopsy, with antibiotic therapy for <4 days; OR
• Does not meet criteria for possible IE, as above
Definition of Major Criteria
Blood culture positive for IE
• Typical microorganisms consistent with IE from 2 separate blood cultures:
- Viridans streptococci, Streptococcus bovis, HACEK group, Staphylococcus aureus; OR
- Community-acquired enterococci, in the absence of a primary focus; OR
• Microorganisms consistent with IE from persistently positive blood cultures, defined as follows:
- At least 2 positive cultures of blood samples drawn >12 hours apart; OR
- All of 3 or a majority of >4 separate cultures of blood (with first and last sample drawn at least 1 hour apart)
• Single positive blood culture for Coxiella burnetii or antiphase I IgG antibody titer >1:800
Evidence of endocardial involvement
• Echocardiogram positive for IE
- TOE recommended in patients with prosthetic valves, rated at least "possible IE" by clinical criteria, or complicated IE [paravalvular abscess]; TTE as first test in other patients; definition of positive echocardiogram:
○ Oscillating intracardiac mass on valve or supporting structures, in the path of regurgitant jets, or on implanted material in the absence of an alternative anatomic explanation; OR
○ Abscess; OR
○ New partial dehiscence of prosthetic valve
• New valvular regurgitation (Worsening or changing of pre-existing murmur not sufficient)
Definition of Minor Criteria
• Predisposition: predisposing heart condition or intravenous drug use
• Fever: temperature >38.0°C (100.4°F)
• Vascular phenomena: major arterial emboli, septic pulmonary infarcts, mycotic aneurysm, intracranial haemorrhage, conjunctival haemorrhages, and Janeway lesions
• Immunologic phenomena: glomerulonephritis, Osler nodes, Roth spots, and rheumatoid factor
• Microbiological evidence: positive blood culture but does not meet a major criterion# OR serological evidence of active infection with organism consistent with IE
• Echocardiographic minor criteria eliminated*

IE = infective endocarditis; TOE = transoesophageal echocardiography; TTE = transthoracic echocardiography.
# Excludes single positive cultures for coagulase-negative staphylococci and organisms that do not cause endocarditis.
* Previously used minor criterion "echocardiogram consistent with IE but not meeting major criterion" should be eliminated, given widespread use of TOE.
Adapted from Li JS, Sexton DJ, Mick N, Nettles R, Fowler VG Jr, Ryan T, Bashore T, Corey GR. Proposed modifications to the Duke criteria for the diagnosis of infective endocarditis. *Clin Infect Dis.* © 2000 Apr;30(4), pages 636 & 637, reproduced with permission of Oxford University Press.

Table 13.3 Peripheral Signs associated with Infective Endocarditis

Peripheral Sign	Description
Roth spots	Oval-shaped, white-centred retinal haemorrhages seen on funduscopic examination
Osler nodes	Painful, erythematous nodules most commonly found on the pads of the fingers and toes
Janeway lesions	Non-tender, erythematous and nodular lesions most commonly found on the palms of hands and soles of feet
Splinter haemorrhages	Small, linear haemorrhages under the finger and/or toe nails
Petechiae	Reddish-brown, pinpoint, haemorrhagic spots on the skin, conjunctivae, or oral mucosa

Diagnosis of IE

As described in the Modified Duke criteria for the diagnosis of IE, a positive echocardiogram is a major criterion which identifies endocardial involvement (see Table 13.2). A positive echocardiogram is one in which there is evidence of vegetations, abscess formation or new partial dehiscence of a prosthetic valve; other echocardiographic evidence of IE includes pseudoaneurysms, leaflet perforation, valve aneurysms and fistula (Table 13.4).

Vegetations

As stated above, a vegetation is an infected mass composed of a collection of platelets, fibrin, microorganisms, and inflammatory cells. The characteristic 2D echocardiographic feature of a vegetation is a hypermobile, echogenic mass (or masses) that exhibit independent, high frequency motion. Vegetations may be attached to native and/or prosthetic valves, other endocardial structures, or implanted intracardiac material. Typically the acoustic properties of 'new' vegetations are similar to myocardium while 'healed' vegetations appear more echogenic. Vegetation size and shape is also variable with large, bulky vegetations being more often associated with fungal endocarditis.

Vegetations tend to form at sites where blood flow injury is most likely to occur. Therefore, vegetations are located on the upstream side of the infected valve. For example, vegetations are typically attached to the atrial surface of atrioventricular (AV) valves, on the ventricular surface of the semilunar valves, and on the right ventricular (RV) side of a ventricular septal defect (VSD) (Fig. 13.3). Satellite vegetations or jet lesions may also be present along the infected flow path. For example, with mitral valve IE and mitral regurgitation (MR), jet lesions may be seen on the left atrial (LA) wall; with aortic valve IE and aortic regurgitation (AR), jet lesions may be seen on the anterior mitral valve leaflet; and with IE of a VSD, jet lesions may be seen on the septal tricuspid valve leaflet. Vegetations may also be attached to prosthetic valves, indwelling catheters or pacemaker leads (Fig. 13.4). In prosthetic valves, IE usually begins on the sewing ring and often extends outside the valvular apparatus, resulting in prosthetic valve dehiscence and abscess formation; in bioprosthetic valves, the leaflet tissue may also be infected.

M-mode echocardiography is especially useful in displaying the high frequency motion of the vegetation (Fig. 13.5). However, it is important to note that not all vegetations display independent, high frequency motion; that is, vegetations may be fixed and non-oscillating. Furthermore, other structures and masses besides vegetations may also display independent, high frequency motion.

Importantly, there are a number of 'mimickers' of vegetations. Examples include anatomic structures such as Lambl's excrescences, valvular strands, ruptured cords, myxomatous valves and Chiari network or Eustachian valves. Other 'masses' that may be confused with vegetations include thrombus, myxomas, calcification, sclerosis, papillary fibroelastomas, non-infective vegetations (marantic endocarditis), and imaging artefacts. Differentiation between vegetations and other structures/masses is based on a number of echocardiographic characteristics which are described in Table 13.5. In addition, consideration of the echocardiographic findings in the clinical context is extremely helpful in determining if a 'mass' is a vegetation. For example, the absence of: (1) vasculitic/embolic phenomena; (2) central venous access or pacing wires; (3) recent intravenous drug use; (4) a prosthetic valve; and (5) positive blood cultures indicates a zero probability that the transthoracic echocardiogram (TTE) will show evidence of IE [13.2].

Table 13.4 Anatomic and Echocardiographic Definitions of Infective Endocarditis

	Surgery/Necropsy	Echocardiography
Vegetation	Infected mass attached to an endocardial structure, or on implanted intracardiac material	Oscillating or non-oscillating intracardiac mass on valve or other endocardial structures, or on implanted intracardiac material
Abscess	Perivalvular cavity with necrosis and purulent material not communicating with the cardiovascular lumen	Thickened, non-homogeneous perivalvular area with echodense or echolucent appearance
Pseudoaneurysm	Perivalvular cavity communicating with the cardiovascular lumen	Pulsatile perivalvular echo-free space, with colour-Doppler flow detected
Perforation	Interruption of endocardial tissue continuity	Interruption of endocardial tissue continuity traversed by colour-Doppler flow
Fistula	Communication between two neighbouring cavities through a perforation	Colour-Doppler communication between two neighbouring cavities through a perforation
Valve aneurysm	Saccular outpouching of valvular tissue	Saccular bulging of valvular tissue
Dehiscence of a prosthetic valve	Dehiscence of the prosthesis	Paravalvular regurgitation identified by TTE/TEE, with or without rocking motion of the prosthesis

TEE = transesophageal echocardiography; TTE = transthoracic echocardiography.
Reproduced from Habib G, Hoen B, Tornos P, Thuny F, Prendergast B, Vilacosta I, Moreillon P, de Jesus Antunes M, Thilen U, Lekakis J, Lengyel M, Müller L, Naber CK, Nihoyannopoulos P, Moritz A, Zamorano JL; ESC Committee for Practice Guidelines. Guidelines on the prevention, diagnosis, and treatment of infective endocarditis (new version 2009): the Task Force on the Prevention, Diagnosis, and Treatment of Infective Endocarditis of the European Society of Cardiology (ESC). Endorsed by the European Society of Clinical Microbiology and Infectious Diseases (ESCMID) and the International Society of Chemotherapy (ISC) for Infection and Cancer. *Eur Heart J.* © 2009 Oct;30(19): page 2380,with permission of Oxford University Press.

[13.2] Greaves K, Mou D, Patel A, Celermajer DS. Clinical criteria and the appropriate use of transthoracic echocardiography for the exclusion of infective endocarditis. *Heart.* 2003 Mar;89(3):273-5.

Table 13.5 **Echocardiographic Characteristics of Likely and Unlikely Vegetations**

	Likely Vegetation	**Unlikely Vegetation**
Texture	Reflectance of myocardium (grey)	Hyper-reflective (white or 'echobright' consistent with calcium)
Location	Upstream side of valves; along jet pathway; on prosthetic material	Downstream side of valve
Motion	Independently mobile, high frequency	Fixed and immobile
Shape	Irregular and lobulated, may be multiple	Filamentous or 'stringy', discrete nodule, narrow base of attachment
Accompanying abnormalities	Regurgitation (valvular, paravalvular, or via perforation), abscess and pseudoaneurysm, fistulae, prosthetic dehiscence, valve aneurysm	None (i.e. lack of accompanying turbulent flow or regurgitation)

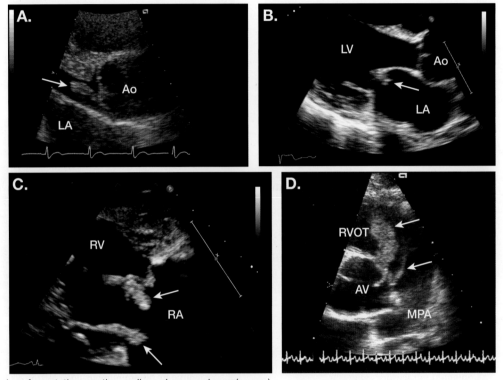

Figure 13.3 Examples of vegetations on the cardiac valves are shown (*arrows*).
A: A vegetation on the non-coronary cusp of the aortic valve recorded from a zoomed parasternal long axis view; B: A vegetation on the anterior mitral leaflet recorded from a zoomed parasternal long axis view; C: Vegetations on the anterior and posterior tricuspid leaflets recorded from a zoomed parasternal long axis view of right ventricular inflow; D: Pulmonary valve vegetations recorded from a zoomed parasternal short axis view. Observe that the site for mitral and tricuspid valve vegetations is on the atrial side of the valve while the site for aortic and pulmonary valve vegetations is on the ventricular side of the valves.
Ao = aorta; AV = aortic valve; LA = left atrium; LV = left ventricle; MPA = main pulmonary artery; RA = right atrium; RV = right ventricle; RVOT = right ventricular outflow tract.

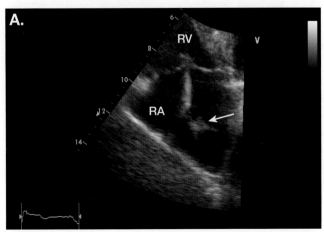
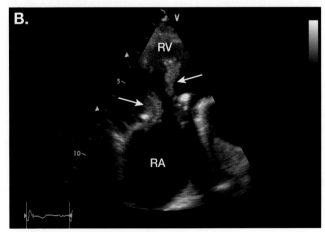

Figure 13.4 Examples of vegetations on a pacemaker lead (*left*) and on a prosthetic tricuspid valve (*right*) are shown (*arrows*). Both images are recorded from zoomed apical 4-chamber views in two different patients. RA = right atrium; RV = right ventricle.

Technical Tips

When performing an echocardiogram of patients with suspected IE, careful attention to image optimisation is crucial. In particular, all cardiac valves and intracardiac devices should be assessed on zoom-mode using the highest possible transducer frequency with the focal zone placed at the level of the cardiac valves and/or intracardiac devices; all of these manipulations improve spatial resolution. In addition, optimisation of images by adjusting the compression and contrast of the images may also be helpful in distinguishing vegetations from other cardiac structures. Finally, slow angulation and tilting through the valves/devices from all possible views should be performed to ensure that all aspects of these 3D structures are evaluated.

Abscesses

An abscess is a complication of IE where there is extension and penetration of the infection to surrounding tissues. Abscesses contain phlegmon (a purulent exudate or pus) and do not communicate with the circulation. Abscesses generally form in the perivalvular region and they are most commonly associated with prosthetic valve and aortic valve IE. In particular, with aortic valve IE, abscesses may form in the anterior aortic root or at the mitral-aortic intervalvular fibrosa (MAIF).

The characteristic echocardiographic features of an abscess include a perivalvular cavity or thickening of the valvular annulus or adjacent myocardium that appears heterogeneous or non-homogeneous (Fig. 13.6); on colour Doppler imaging there is no evidence of internal flow. In the early stages of formation, abscesses may be difficult to detect as only a mild thickening of the infected area is apparent. Abscesses can be further complicated by the progression to pseudoaneurysms and/or the formation of fistulas.

New Dehiscence of a Prosthetic Valve

Recall that prosthetic valve dehiscence (PVD) refers to the partial separation of the prosthetic sewing ring from the native valve annulus (see Chapter 10). In the case of IE, PVD occurs due to weakening of the infected native valve annulus resulting in 'pulling away' of the prosthetic valve from the annulus. The characteristic 2D echocardiographic appearance of PVD is "rocking" of the prosthetic valve at an angle far in excess of its normal excursion. Evidence of an echo-free space between the prosthetic valve and native valve annulus with associated paravalvular regurgitation is another clue to PVD. Therefore, prosthetic valve IE can be suspected in the presence of new PVD and/or paravalvular regurgitation even in the absence of vegetations or abscess formation.

Other Echocardiographic Findings Suggestive of IE

Additional echocardiographic findings suggestive of IE include the presence of other perivalvular complications such as pseudoaneurysms and fistulas, leaflet perforation, cordal rupture, valve aneurysms, and significant valvular dysfunction (regurgitation and/or obstruction). As stated above, pseudoaneurysms and fistulas may occur as a further complication of abscess formation. In particular, the MAIF is prone to the formation of pseudoaneurysms and perforations secondary to aortic valve IE. In this situation, extension of the infection occurs due to contiguous spread or due to the infected

AR jet striking the subvalvular structures (Fig. 13.7). On the echocardiographic examination, a pseudoaneurysm appears as a pulsatile, echo-free space with evidence of flow into this cavity which confirms a communication between the cavity and the circulation (Fig. 13.8). Fistulous communications can also occur when weakened and necrotic tissue breaks through

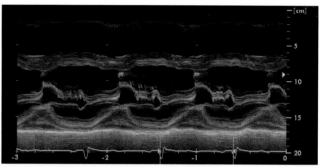

Figure 13.5 This M-mode trace was recorded through the mitral valve in a patient with anterior mitral leaflet endocarditis. Observe the high frequency vibration of the anterior mitral leaflet; this is a characteristic feature of vegetations.

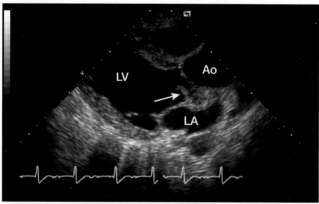

Figure 13.6 This image was acquired from a parasternal long axis view in a patient with aortic valve endocarditis. Observe the aortic valve vegetation (*arrow*) as well as a large perivalvular abscess between the aorta (Ao) and the left atrium (LA). Observe that the abscess appears heterogeneous. LV = left ventricle.

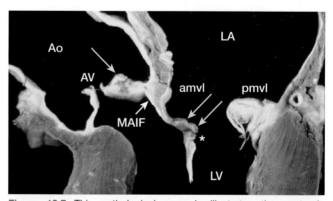

Figure 13.7 This pathological example illustrates the anatomic relationship between the aortic root (Ao) and the aortic valve (AV) to the mitral-aortic intervalvular fibrosa (MAIF) and the anterior mitral valve leaflet (amvl). The MAIF is defined as the junction between the left half of the non-coronary cusp and the adjacent third of the left coronary cusp of the aortic valve and the anterior mitral leaflet. Observe that in this case of active infective endocarditis there are vegetations on the non-coronary cusp of the aortic valve and the anterior mitral leaflet (*yellow arrows*); a perforation of the anterior mitral valve is also present (*). LA = left atrium; LV = left ventricle; pmvl = posterior mitral valve leaflet. By permission of Mayo Foundation for Medical Education and Research. All rights reserved. Courtesy of William D. Edwards, MD.

a valve annulus resulting in a direct communication between cardiac chambers or a cardiac chamber and great vessel (Fig. 13.9). In particular, rupture of an aortic abscess may result in fistulous tracks between the aorta and the right atrium (RA), the aorta and the LA, and the aorta and the RV.

Valve aneurysms occur as a consequence of valvular infection resulting in the weakening of the valve tissue and the loss of the elastic components of the valve. On the 2D echocardiographic examination, a valve aneurysm appears as a localised bulging of the valve (Fig. 13.10). A complication of valve aneurysms is leaflet perforation (Fig. 13.11).

Pseudoaneurysm versus Abscess
On the 2D echocardiographic examination, abscesses and pseudoaneurysms may both appear as perivalvular cavities. However, abscess cavities tend to appear non-pulsatile and heterogeneous with no communication between the cavity and the circulation noted on the colour Doppler examination. A pseudoaneurysm, on the other hand, appears as a pulsatile echo-free space with intracavity flow and communication between the cavity and the circulation evident on the colour Doppler examination.

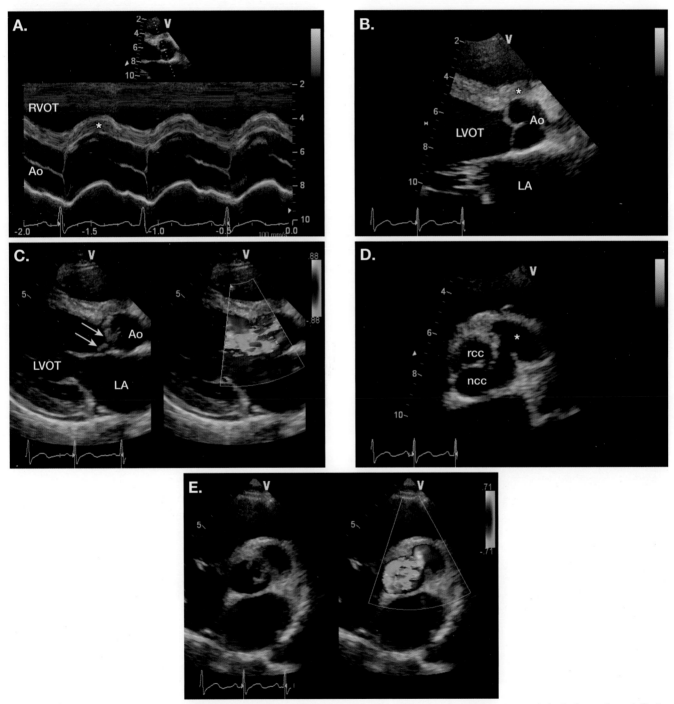

Figure 13.8 This series of images was recorded from a patient with aortic valve endocarditis and a pseudoaneurysm anterior to the aortic root. On the M-mode trace recorded through the aorta (A) and on the 2D image (B), thickening of the anterior aortic wall (*) is noted; this appearance is consistent with pus or phlegmon. With slight posterior tilting (C), multiple large echodensities consistent with vegetations are seen attached to the aortic valve which prolapses into the left ventricular outflow tract (*arrows*); associated severe aortic regurgitation is also evident on colour flow Doppler imaging. From the parasternal short axis view (D), the aortic valve appears trileaflet and there appears to be total destruction of the left coronary cusp of the aortic valve; in addition a large echolucent cavity is seen anterior and to the left of the aortic root (*). On colour flow Doppler imaging, communication between this cavity and the aorta is noted (E); this appearance is consistent with a pseudoaneurysm. Ao = aorta; LA = left atrium; LV = left ventricle; LVOT = left ventricular outflow tract; ncc = non-coronary cusp ; rcc = right coronary cusp; RVOT = right ventricular outflow tract.

In particular, perforation of the anterior mitral leaflet may occur secondary to aortic valve IE whereby the infected AR jet infects the anterior mitral leaflet. On the echocardiographic examination, leaflet perforation is identified by a focal defect within the leaflet with the regurgitant jet passing through this defect (Fig. 13.12).

> Leaflet perforation should be suspected when the regurgitant jet is located away from the site of leaflet coaptation.

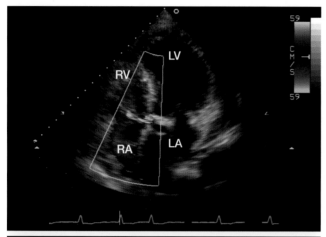

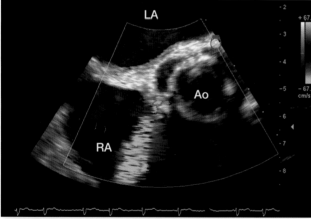

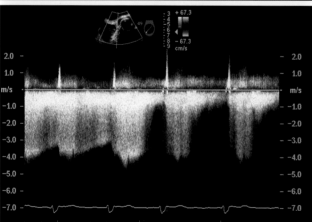

Figure 13.9 A fistulous communication between the aorta and the right atrium (RA) is suspected from the apical 4-chamber image where abnormal flow from the aorta to the RA is seen (*top*). On the corresponding transoesophageal echocardiogram, an echolucent cavity was noted around the aortic root (Ao) with fistulous flow between this cavity and the RA noted on colour flow imaging (*middle*). Via continuous-wave Doppler, high velocity, continuous flow was also observed confirming a shunt from the higher pressure aorta to the lower pressure RA (*bottom*). LA = left atrium; LV = left ventricle; RV = right ventricle.

TTE versus TOE

It is well recognised that the sensitivity for detecting vegetations and complications associated with IE is significantly greater via transoesophageal echocardiography (TOE) compared with TTE. This is because TOE images the heart via the oesophagus. As a result, TOE avoids interfaces such as the lungs, the chest wall and the bony structures of the rib cage and sternum; this allows superior imaging of the cardiac valves. Furthermore, due to the close relationship between the oesophagus and the heart, higher frequency transducers can be utilised which enhances spatial and temporal resolution and, therefore, allows the detection of very small lesions. In addition, the LA surface of prosthetic mitral valves, which is virtually always obscured via TTE, can be readily inspected by TOE so the detection of prosthetic mitral IE is greater. However, despite the obvious superiority of TOE over TTE, TTE is still considered the first choice imaging test in patients with suspected IE. This is because TTE is a non-invasive examination that may establish the diagnosis of IE without the need for TOE; moreover, TTE has the ability to provide additional useful information regarding ventricular function and valvular haemodynamics.

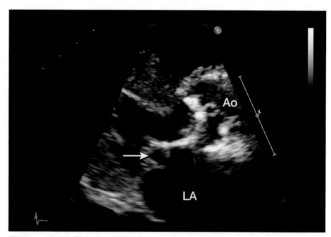

Figure 13.10 This image was recorded from a zoomed parasternal long axis view. Observe the saccular or pouch-like bulging of tissue on the anterior mitral leaflet (*arrow*); this appearance is consistent with a valve aneurysm secondary to infective endocarditis. Rupture of this aneurysm can lead to perforation of the leaflet. Ao = aorta; LA = left atrium.

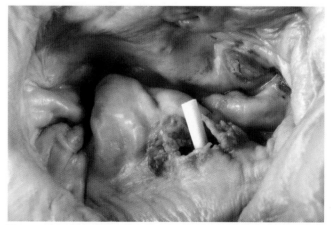

Figure 13.11 This gross pathological specimen shows perforation of a myxomatous mitral valve (clinically mitral valve prolapse) secondary to infective endocarditis.
By permission of Mayo Foundation for Medical Education and Research. All rights reserved. Courtesy of William D. Edwards, MD.

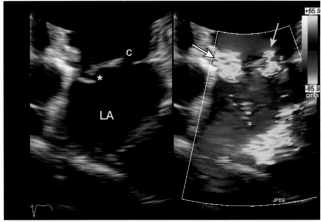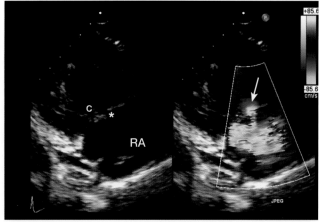

Figure 13.12 Two examples of leaflet perforation from two different patients are shown. The image on the left was recorded from a zoomed apical 4-chamber view. On the 2D image, a tissue defect is noted in the anterior mitral leaflet (*); on the corresponding colour Doppler image regurgitant flow through this defect is observed (*white arrow*). Observe that valvular regurgitation is also present at the site of leaflet coaptation (c) (*yellow arrow*). The image on the right was recorded from a parasternal long axis view of right ventricular inflow. On the 2D image, a tissue defect is noted in the anterior tricuspid leaflet (*) adjacent to the site of leaflet coaptation (c). On the corresponding colour Doppler image regurgitant flow through this defect is observed (*white arrow*). These appearances are consistent with leaflet perforation.
LA = left atrium; RA = right atrium.

Figure 13.13 illustrates an algorithm showing the role of echocardiography in the diagnosis and assessment of IE. Based on this algorithm, when IE is clinically suspected, TTE is performed first. Additional imaging using TOE is indicated: (1) in the setting of prosthetic valves or intracardiac devices; (2) when TTE image quality is suboptimal; and (3) when the TTE study is negative and the clinical suspicion for IE is high. TOE is not immediately warranted in cases where the TTE is negative, where image quality is excellent, when prosthetic devices are absent, and when there is a low pre-test probability for IE. However, in cases where TOE is performed and the initial examination is negative but the clinical level of suspicion for IE remains high, repeat TOE should be performed within 7–10 days. This is especially important in the setting of prosthetic valves where small vegetations or early peri-annular infection may be missed on the initial study. Importantly, in certain clinical situations where the clinical level of suspicion for IE is high and urgent diagnosis is required (for example, patients in septic and/or cardiogenic shock), an initial echocardiographic assessment via TOE rather than via TTE is considered appropriate [13.3].

Assess Functional Abnormalities of Affected Valve(s) and Assess Secondary Consequences of Valvular Disease

As previously stated, underlying congenital or acquired valve disease is one of the precursors of endothelial damage and subsequent IE. Therefore, echocardiography also has a role in the identification of pre-existing or underlying structural heart disease. In addition, as IE can result in valvular obstruction and/or regurgitation, echocardiography has an important role in assessing the degree of obstruction and/or regurgitation and in the evaluation of the secondary consequences of these lesions. Assessment of the degree and severity of valvular obstruction and/or regurgitation as well as the evaluation of

chamber dimensions, ventricular systolic function and the estimation of the pulmonary pressures are performed in the standard manner (see Chapters 7-10). In particular, evidence of acute, severe regurgitation may be apparent when there is rapid and aggressive destruction of the valve.

Identify Complications of IE

Three of the most common and severe complications of IE include: (1) heart failure, (2) perivalvular extension of the infection, and (3) embolic events. Heart failure in IE occurs due to significant valve dysfunction caused by leaflet destruction, leaflet perforation, and/or cordal rupture with flail leaflets which leads to significant valvular regurgitation. Perivalvular extension of the infection refers to the formation of abscess cavities, pseudoaneurysms and fistulas as described above. In addition, if the abscess extends into the conduction tissue located in the interventricular septum (IVS), conduction abnormalities such as first-, second-, and third-degree heart block may result.

An embolic event associated with IE is another important complication of IE. The risk of embolism is highest during the first 2 weeks of antibiotic therapy and is greater for mitral valve IE than aortic valve IE. Several echocardiographic and clinical parameters have been associated with increased risk of embolism. Clinical parameters identifying patients at risk of embolism include: (1) infection with specific microorganisms such as Staphylococci, Streptococcus bovis, and Candida species, (2) previous embolic events, and (3) biological markers. Echocardiographic parameters associated with an increased risk of embolism relate to the size, location, and mobility of the vegetation [13.4-13.5]. In particular, large mobile vegetations (>10 mm), vegetations located on the mitral valve, increasing size of the vegetation while antibiotic therapy is given and multivalvular infection identify patients at high-risk for embolic events.

[13.3] Sedgwick JF, Burstow DJ. Update on echocardiography in the management of infective endocarditis. *Curr Infect Dis Rep.* 2012 Aug;14(4):373-80.
[13.4] Thuny F, Di Salvo G, Belliard O, Avierinos JF, Pergola V, Rosenberg V, Casalta JP, Gouvernet J, Derumeaux G, Iarussi D, Ambrosi P, Calabró R, Riberi A, Collart F, Metras D, Lepidi H, Raoult D, Harle JR, Weiller PJ, Cohen A, Habib G. Risk of embolism and death in infective endocarditis: prognostic value of echocardiography: a prospective multicenter study. *Circulation.* 2005 Jul 5;112(1):69-75.
[13.5] Prendergast BD, Tornos P. Surgery for infective endocarditis: who and when? *Circulation.* 2010 Mar 9;121(9):1141-52.

Importantly, patients with refractory heart failure in combination with severe valvular regurgitation, infection extension with abscess or fistula formation, embolism with vegetations >10 mm or no embolism but vegetations >15 mm are recommended for emergent or urgent surgery [13.6].

Other less common complications of IE include purulent pericarditis, coronary obstruction due to vegetation embolism, coronary compression, or ostial occlusion by large vegetations, and myocarditis secondary to myocardial abscess formation.

Surveillance During and After Therapy

The frequency of repeat surveillance studies is dependent on factors such as the clinical presentation, the type of organism, initial echocardiographic findings, and the presence of prosthetic valves and intracardiac devices. For example, in patients with a Streptococcal infection, native valves and no valvular dysfunction, weekly TTE may be appropriate while in patients with a Staphylococcal infection, prosthetic valves and perivalvular regurgitation, twice weekly TOE studies may be required [13.7].

Following antibiotic therapy, echocardiography can be utilised to assess possible recurrence of infection which is higher in patients with prosthetic valve IE, perivalvular extension, and intravenous drug usage. In addition, heart failure is also higher in patients with persisting periannular infection and valve regurgitation while the need for surgery is higher in patients with persisting periannular infection and valve regurgitation. Likewise, the need for surgery is higher in these patients as well. Therefore, TTE is recommended prior to discharge (for subsequent comparison) and at 1, 3, 6 and 12 months after discharge and the completion of therapy [13.8].

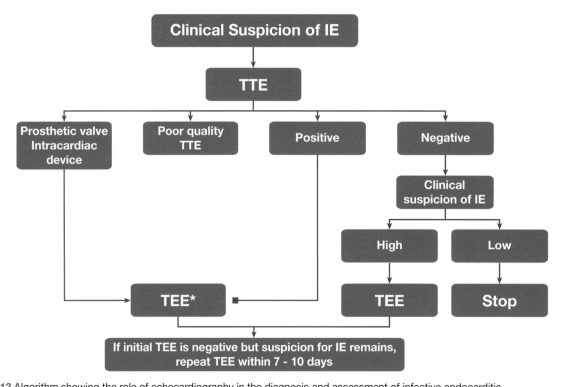

Figure 13.13 Algorithm showing the role of echocardiography in the diagnosis and assessment of infective endocarditis.
IE = infective endocarditis; TTE = transthoracic echocardiography; TEE = transoesophageal echocardiography.
*TEE is not mandatory in isolated right-sided native valve IE with good quality TTE examination and unequivocal echocardiographic findings.
Reproduced from Habib G, Hoen B, Tornos P, Thuny F, Prendergast B, Vilacosta I, Moreillon P, de Jesus Antunes M, Thilen U, Lekakis J, Lengyel M, Müller L, Naber CK, Nihoyannopoulos P, Moritz A, Zamorano JL; ESC Committee for Practice Guidelines. Guidelines on the prevention, diagnosis, and treatment of infective endocarditis (new version 2009): the Task Force on the Prevention, Diagnosis, and Treatment of Infective Endocarditis of the European Society of Cardiology (ESC). Endorsed by the European Society of Clinical Microbiology and Infectious Diseases (ESCMID) and the International Society of Chemotherapy (ISC) for Infection and Cancer. *Eur Heart J.* © 2009 Oct;30(19): page 2379, with permission of Oxford University Press.

[13.6] Habib G, Hoen B, Tornos P, Thuny F, Prendergast B, Vilacosta I, Moreillon P, de Jesus Antunes M, Thilen U, Lekakis J, Lengyel M, Müller L, Naber CK, Nihoyannopoulos P, Moritz A, Zamorano JL; ESC Committee for Practice Guidelines. Guidelines on the prevention, diagnosis, and treatment of infective endocarditis (new version 2009): the Task Force on the Prevention, Diagnosis, and Treatment of Infective Endocarditis of the European Society of Cardiology (ESC). Endorsed by the European Society of Clinical Microbiology and Infectious Diseases (ESCMID) and the International Society of Chemotherapy (ISC) for Infection and Cancer. *Eur Heart J.* 2009 Oct;30(19):2369-413.
[13.7] Sedgwick JF, Burstow DJ. Update on echocardiography in the management of infective endocarditis. *Curr Infect Dis Rep.* 2012 Aug;14(4):373-80.
[13.8] Habib G, Badano L, Tribouilloy C, Vilacosta I, Zamorano JL, Galderisi M, Voigt JU, Sicari R, Cosyns B, Fox K, Aakhus S; European Association of Echocardiography. Recommendations for the practice of echocardiography in infective endocarditis. *Eur J Echocardiogr.* 2010 Mar;11(2):202-19.

Cardiac Tumours

A tumour or neoplasm can be defined as any new or abnormal growth in which cell multiplication is uncontrolled and progressive. Tumours can be classified as benign or malignant; the criteria for distinguishing between benign and malignant tumours are listed in Table 13.6. The nomenclature for benign and malignant tumours is generally based on the cell of origin with the suffix "-oma" being added for benign tumours and the suffix of "-sarcoma" being added for malignant tumours. For example, a benign tumour arising from striated muscle is called a rhabdomyoma while a malignant tumour arising from striated muscle is called a rhabdomyosarcoma.

Tumours of the heart include benign primary cardiac tumours, malignant primary cardiac tumours, metastatic (secondary) cardiac tumours and extracardiac tumours. Approximately 75% of primary cardiac tumours are benign (Table 13.7). Malignant tumours account for the remaining 25% of primary cardiac tumours. Secondary cardiac tumours are about 20- to 40-fold more common than primary cardiac tumours. Each type of cardiac tumour can usually be identified by its location and characteristic echocardiographic appearance; however, in some situations it will not be possible to determine the exact type of tumour especially when the location and echocardiographic appearances are atypical. It is beyond the scope of this chapter to cover all cardiac tumours; therefore, only the more commonly encountered tumours are discussed.

Cardiac Myxomas

Myxomas are the most common benign cardiac tumours in the adult population. The characteristic location and morphological features of these tumours are described in Table 13.7. Myxomas may be familial and inherited as an autosomal dominant disease known as Carney complex. This syndrome is characterised by multiple myxomas (cardiac and extracardiac), abnormal skin pigmentation, endocrine tumours or overactivity, and schwannomas.

The characteristic echocardiographic features of myxomas are based on the appearance, location, site of attachment and mobility of the tumour. Typically, myxomas appear globular and finely speckled; occasionally an echolucent area may be identified within the tumour representing haemorrhage or liquefaction necrosis. Importantly, these tumours do not invade the underlying myocardium or adjacent cardiac

structures. Myxomas are most commonly seen within the LA with a stalk attachment to the interatrial septum in the region of the fossa ovalis (Fig. 13.14). LA myxomas are usually quite mobile and may prolapse through the mitral valve causing functional mitral stenosis. The presence and degree of obstruction can be assessed on the colour and spectral Doppler examination (Fig. 13.15).

The majority of myxomas are usually solitary tumours within the LA; however they may be multiple and may occur in other cardiac chambers. In addition, recurrence of myxomas has been reported following surgical resection; recurrence may occur due to inadequate or incomplete resection, inheritance (familial type), totipotent multicentricity (another tumour arising from a different site), or metastatic recurrence (in this case myxoma is not benign).

Papillary Fibroelastomas

Papillary fibroelastomas (PFE) are the most common tumours of the cardiac valves and the second most common primary cardiac tumours in adults. The characteristic location and morphological features of these tumours are described in Table 13.7. These tumours are most commonly located on the aortic valve and the mitral valves; PFE are less commonly seen on the pulmonary and tricuspid valves and are infrequently seen on other cardiac structures (see Fig. 13.39). These tumours also have characteristic sea anemone-like fronds that become more pronounced after immersion in normal saline.

On the echocardiographic examination, PFE characteristically appear as small, round, homogeneous masses attached to the valve (Fig. 13.16). Most commonly, PFE are attached to the valve via a stalk and therefore they display highly mobile and independent motion. PFE have also been described as having a "pom-pom" appearance as stated above. Aortic PFE are usually seen on the aortic aspect of the aortic cusps while mitral PFE are typically seen on the atrial aspect of the mitral leaflets; however, PFE may also be seen on the ventricular aspect of the valves.

> Distinction between PFE and vegetations can be difficult; consideration of the clinical history will be helpful in differentiating between these two masses.

Table 13.6 Distinction between Benign and Malignant Tumours

Characteristics	Benign	Malignant
Cell characteristics*	Well-differentiated	Well-differentiated to poorly or undifferentiated (anaplastic)
Rate of growth	Usually slow growing; may come to a standstill or regress	Usually rapid growing but may be slow growing
Local invasion	Well-circumscribed or encapsulated Freely mobile in relation to adjacent structures Do not invade or infiltrate surrounding normal tissues	Poorly circumscribed, indistinct irregular shape Not encapsulated Fixed to adjacent structures Locally invasive, infiltrating surrounding tissue
Metastasis	Do not metastasize	Frequently metastasize; spread occurs via: (1) direct seeding of body cavities or surfaces, (2) lymphatic spread, or (3) haematogenous spread

* Well-differentiated tumours are composed of cells resembling the mature normal cells of the tissue of origin of the neoplasm while poorly differentiated or undifferentiated (or anaplastic) tumours have primitive-appearing, unspecialised cells.

Table 13.7 Commonly Encountered Benign Primary Cardiac Tumours

Type of Tumour	Pathological Example	Characteristics
Myxoma (most common primary cardiac tumour in adults)	Large LA Myxoma (*arrow*) 	**Most Common Location** • LA attached to IAS at fossa ovalis • Less common in RA, ventricles **Morphological Features** • Usually solitary (may be multiple) • Ovoid and gelatinous; regular smooth surface • Attached via a narrow base (pedicle or stalk) • Range in size from 1-15 cm (average 5-6 cm) • Calcification, fibrosis, haemorrhage, necrosis common; heterogeneous composition consisting of haemorrhagic, necrotic, and cystic areas; calcific areas may also be observed
Papillary fibroelastoma (PFE) (most common tumour of cardiac valves)	Resected PFE (*left*), multiple PFE attached to rheumatic mitral valve and cords (*right*) 	**Most Common Location** • Aortic and mitral valves • Less common on pulmonary and tricuspid valves **Morphological Features** • Usually solitary • Small gelatinous polyps with multiple fronds • Rarely exceeds 1 cm diameter • Attached to the endocardium by a short pedicle or stalk
Lipomas & lipomatous hypertrophy of IAS	Pericardial lipoma & lipomatous hypertrophy of IAS 	**Most Common Location of Lipomas** • Subepicardial, subendocardial, intramyocardial **Morphological Features of Lipomas** • Homogeneous fatty encapsulated tumours • Broad based • Variable size (larger in subepicardium) **Morphological Features of Lipomatous Hypertrophy of IAS** • Involves limbus of fossa ovalis • Spares valve of fossa ovalis
Rhabdomyoma (most common cardiac tumour in children; associated with tubular sclerosis)	Multiple rhabdomyomas (*arrows*) 	**Most Common Location** • LV and/or RV myocardium; outflow tracts; AV valves **Morphological Features** • Frequently multiple • White-grey to yellow, flesh lesions • Well-circumscribed, non-infiltrative • Range in size from few mm to several cm • Spontaneous regression in size, number or both is common
Fibroma	LV Fibroma (*arrow*) 	**Most Common Location** • LV and ventricular septum **Morphological Features** • Usually solitary • Firm and white • Well-circumscribed • Tightly adherent to adjacent myocardium • Almost always intramural • Range in size from 1-10 cm • Do not regress spontaneously

AV = atrioventricular; IAS = interatrial septum; LA = left atrium; LV = left ventricle; RA = right atrium; RV = right ventricle

Photos by permission of Mayo Foundation for Medical Education and Research. All rights reserved. Courtesy of William D. Edwards, MD.

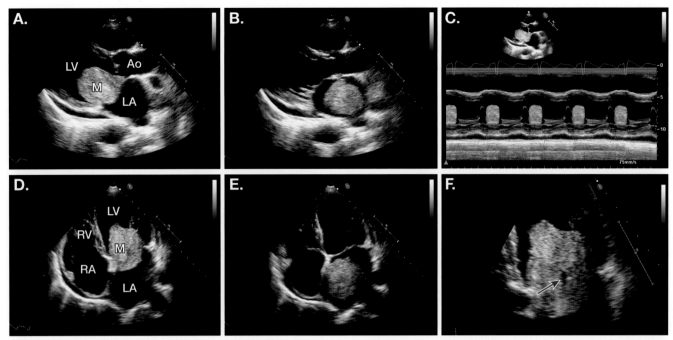

Figure 13.14 This series of images shows a very large myxoma (M) within the left atrium (LA). The images on the top were recorded from the parasternal long axis view and the images on the bottom were recorded from the apical 4-chamber view. The myxoma appears well circumscribed and has a speckled appearance. Also observe that during diastole, this myxoma prolapses through the mitral valve (A and D); during systole the myxoma returns to the LA where it is attached to the interatrial septum (B and E). On the M-mode trace recorded at the level of the mitral leaflet tips, the myxoma can be seen to occlude the mitral orifice in late diastole (C). On the zoomed apical 4-chamber view, a small central cystic area is also noted within the myxoma (*arrow*) (F). Ao = aorta; LV = left ventricle; RA = right atrium; RV = right ventricle.

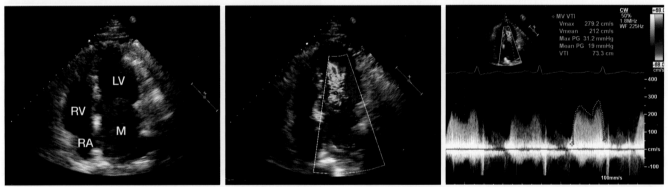

Figure 13.15 From the apical 4-chamber view, a very large homogeneous mass consistent with a myxoma (M) can be seen filling the left atrium (LA) (*left*). On colour flow imaging during diastole, turbulent flow across the mitral valve and into the left ventricle (LV) is apparent (*middle*). Continuous-wave Doppler confirms that this mass is causing significant obstruction to LV inflow with a mean pressure gradient between the LA and LV measured at 19 mmHg (*right*).

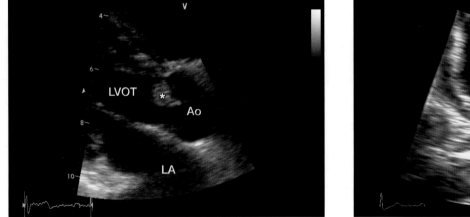
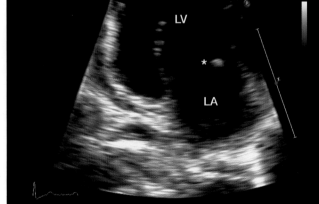

Figure 13.16 These images were recorded from a zoomed parasternal long axis view and a zoomed off-axis apical 4-chamber view in two different patients. Observe the small, round, homogenous mass (*) attached to the ventricular aspect of the right coronary cusp of the aortic valve (*left*) and attached to the atrial aspect of the posterior mitral valve (*right*). The appearance of these masses is consistent with a papillary fibroelastoma (PFE). Observe that the mitral PFE is attached via a short stalk while the aortic PFE has a broad-based attachment. Ao = aorta; LA = left atrium; LV = left ventricle; LVOT = left ventricular outflow tract.

Lipoma

Lipomas are benign tumours of the lipoctyes ('fat' cells) of adipose tissue. The characteristic location and morphological features of these tumours are described in Table 13.7.

Lipomatous hypertrophy of the interatrial septum (LHIAS) is a separate, non-neoplastic condition that may be mistaken for an intracardiac tumour. LHIAS is the result of the accumulation of excess adipose tissue within the interatrial septum with sparing of the fossa ovalis membrane.

On the echocardiographic examination, lipomas appear as echo-bright, homogenous masses within any chamber or within the myocardium (Fig. 13.17). LHIAS appears as thickening of the superior and inferior ends of the interatrial septum with sparing of the fossa ovalis membrane; this leads to the characteristic 'dumb-bell' or 'hour-glass' appearance of the interatrial septum (Fig. 13.18).

Rhabdomyoma

Rhabdomyomas are benign tumours of striated muscle and are the most common cardiac tumours in children. The characteristic location and morphological features of these tumours are described in Table 13.7. Rhabdomyomas are commonly associated with tuberous sclerosis which is an autosomal dominant syndrome characterised by hamartomas, epilepsy, and characteristic skin lesions.

Echocardiographically, rhabdomyomas appear as well circumscribed, homogenous masses with acoustic properties similar to the myocardium. Commonly, multiple masses are seen (Fig. 13.19). Careful interrogation of the outflow and inflow tracts is required as these tumours may cause obstruction to these regions.

Fibroma

Fibromas are benign connective tissue tumours and are the second most common cardiac tumours in children. The characteristic location and morphological features of these tumours are described in Table 13.7.

The typical echocardiographic appearance of a fibroma is a discrete, well demarcated echogenic mass within the ventricular wall, IVS, or at the ventricular apex (Fig. 13.20). When located within the IVS, these tumours may mimic hypertrophic cardiomyopathy or ventricular septal hypertrophy.

Malignant Primary Cardiac Tumours

Primary malignant tumours are extremely rare. The vast majority of these malignant primary tumours are sarcomas. Other less commonly encountered malignant primary cardiac tumours include lymphomas and mesotheliomas.

Of the sarcomas, angiosarcomas are the most common. These malignant vascular tumours are infiltrative into adjacent tissues and appear soft and haemorrhagic on gross examination (Fig. 13.21). Angiosarcomas are most commonly seen within the right heart, especially the RA, or within the pericardium. Other cardiac sarcomas include rhabdomyosarcomas (malignant tumours of striated muscle), leiomyosarcomas (malignant tumours of smooth muscles), liposarcomas (malignant tumour of fat cells), osteosarcomas (malignant tumours of the bone), fibrosarcomas and malignant fibrous histiocytomas (malignant tumours of connective tissue).

The echocardiographic features of malignant tumours include: (1) a mass with wide and poorly defined attachments to the myocardium or with invasive and destructive characteristics, (2) a mass with a large and irregular shape, especially if found in more than one cardiac chamber, (3) a mass with non-homogeneous (heterogeneous) soft tissue appearance,

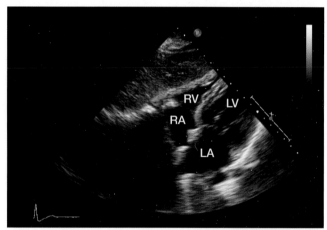

Figure 13.18 This subcostal 4-chamber view shows the characteristic features of lipomatous hypertrophy of the interatrial septum (IAS). Observe the marked thickening of the IAS with sparing of the fossa ovalis; this is frequently described as having a dumb-bell appearance.

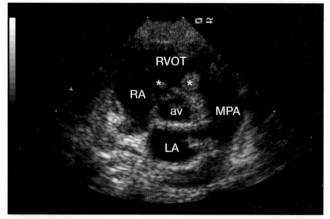

Figure 13.19 This parasternal short axis view shows two circular masses within the right ventricular outflow tract (RVOT) (*). The appearances of these masses, which have an appearance similar to the myocardium, are consistent with rhabdomyomas. av = aortic valve; LA = left atrium; MPA = main pulmonary artery; RA = right atrium.

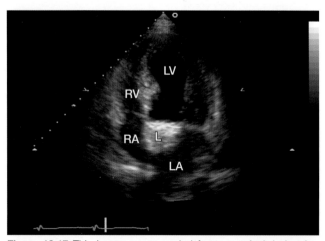

Figure 13.17 This image was recorded from an apical 4-chamber view. Observe the large, echo-bright, homogenous mass within the left atrium (LA). The appearance of this mass is consistent with a lipoma (L). LV = left ventricle; RA = right atrium; RV = right ventricle.

and (4) evidence of pericardial involvement (Fig. 13.22) [13.9].

Secondary (Metastatic) Cardiac Tumours

As previously stated, metastatic cardiac tumours are far more common than primary cardiac tumours of the heart. The most common malignant tumours that infiltrate or metastasize to the heart include melanomas, bronchogenic carcinomas (lung cancer), breast carcinomas, leukaemias, renal cell carcinomas, and lymphomas. Secondary cardiac tumours may be epicardial (majority), myocardial or endocardial (Fig. 13.23).

Metastatic tumours spread to the heart by: (1) haematogenous spread (melanomas, leukaemia), (2) direct extension from contiguous structures (mediastinal lymphomas), (3) lymphatic spread (bronchogenic and breast carcinomas), or (4) intracavity extension via the vena cava (renal cell carcinomas) (Fig 13.24) or pulmonary veins (lung cancer). Depending on the size and location, these tumours can cause various cardiac complications such as obstruction to left or right ventricular inflow or outflow tracts, pericardial effusion, and cardiac encasement resulting in constriction. On the echocardiographic examination, the features of metastatic tumours will appear similar to malignant primary tumours.

Carcinoid tumours are also rare, metastatic tumours that cause cardiac lesions. In particular, secretion of substances from metastatic carcinoid tumours results in the deposition of fibrous plaques on right-sided cardiac valves, leading to thickening, shortening, and retraction of tricuspid and pulmonic valves (see Chapter 9).

Contrast agents may also be useful in differentiating between benign and malignant tumours, or between tumours and thrombus. In particular, highly vascular or malignant tumours display a greater enhancement compared with surrounding myocardium; tumours with a poor blood supply, such as myxomas, appear hypoenhanced compared with surrounding myocardium; while thrombi are generally avascular and therefore show no enhancement.

Mulvagh SL, Rakowski H, Vannan MA, Abdelmoneim SS, Becher H, Bierig SM, Burns PN, Castello R, Coon PD, Hagen ME, Jollis JG, Kimball TR, Kitzman DW, Kronzon I, Labovitz AJ, Lang RM, Mathew J, Moir WS, Nagueh SF, Pearlman AS, Perez JE, Porter TR, Rosenbloom J, Strachan GM, Thanigaraj S, Wei K, Woo A, Yu EH, Zoghbi WA. American Society of Echocardiography Consensus Statement on the Clinical Applications of Ultrasonic Contrast Agents in Echocardiography. *J Am Soc Echocardiogr.* 2008 Nov;21(11):1179-201.

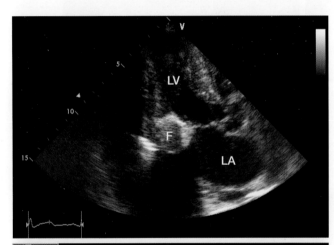

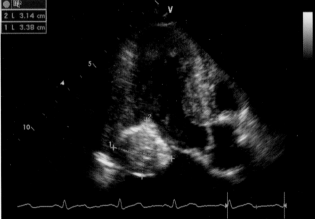

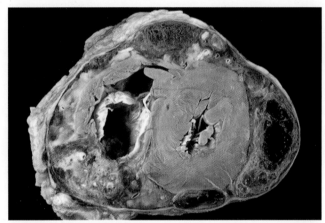

Figure 13.21 This gross pathological specimen shows an angiosarcoma with pericardial and right atrial involvement. The heart is sectioned in a short-axis plane through the ventricles with the parietal pericardium attached. Observe the large angiosarcoma at the right atrioventricular junction. A metastasis is present along the anterior aspect of the left ventricle. Clotted blood fills the pericardial sac due to erosion of malignant vessels in the angiosarcoma.
By permission of Mayo Foundation for Medical Education and Research. All rights reserved. Courtesy of William D. Edwards, MD.

Figure 13.20 These images were recorded from an apical long axis view. A large fibroma (F), measuring 3.1 x 3.4 cm, is present. Observe that this benign tumour appears as an echogenic, well demarcated mass within the posterior wall of the left ventricle (LV); the fibroma also casts a large acoustic shadow. LA = left atrium.

[13.9] Auger D, Pressacco J, Marcotte F, Tremblay A, Dore A, Ducharme A. Cardiac masses: an integrative approach using echocardiography and other imaging modalities. *Heart.* 2011 Jul;97(13):1101-9.

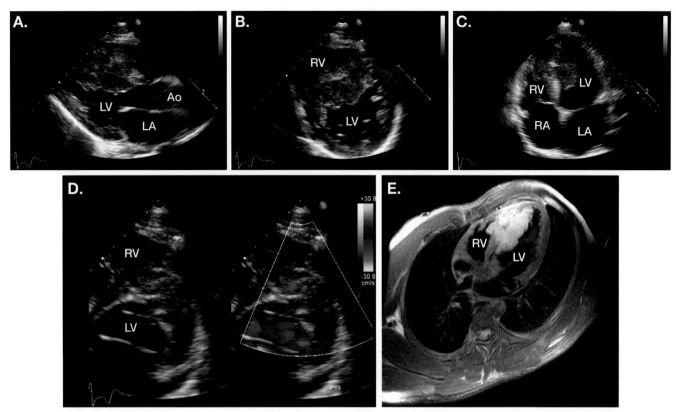

Figure 13.22 This series of images was recorded from a patient with a malignant cardiac tumour. From the parasternal long axis (A), the parasternal short axis (B) and the apical 4-chamber (C) views, a complex, echogenic mass is noted within the interventricular septum (IVS). There is extension of this mass from the mid to distal IVS, into the right ventricular (RV) and left ventricular (LV) cavities. Low velocity flow within this mass is also noted on colour flow imaging which suggests that this mass may be vascularized (D). On cardiac magnetic resonance imaging, a large 'aggressive' lesion within the mid to distal IVS with extension into the RV and LV cavities is also demonstrated (E). The appearance of this mass is consistent with malignant infiltration; possibly a primary angiosarcoma or a primary cardiac lymphoma.

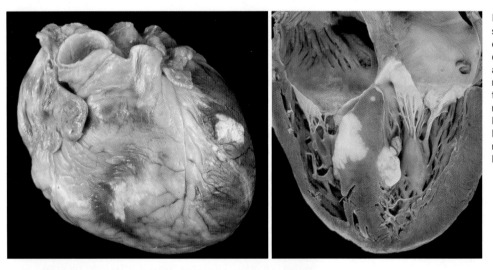

Figure 13.23 These gross pathological specimens show examples of an epicardial metastasis from a breast carcinoma (*left*) and both myocardial and endocardial metastases from a renal cell carcinoma (*right*). Metastatic tumours generally appear as white nodules.

By permission of Mayo Foundation for Medical Education and Research. All rights reserved. Courtesy of William D. Edwards, MD.

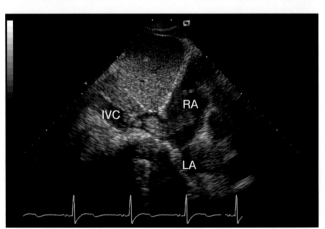

Figure 13.24 This subcostal image was acquired from a patient with known renal cell carcinoma. A large soft tissue mass is noted within the inferior vena cava (IVC) with intracavity extension into the right atrium (RA). On real-time imaging, this mass was seen to prolapse through the tricuspid valve during diastole. LA = left atrium.

Intracardiac Thrombus

There are three primary risk factors or predisposing conditions which influence the formation of thrombus: (1) endothelial injury [abnormal walls], (2) haemodynamic changes [abnormal blood flow], and (3) blood hypercoagulability [abnormal blood constituents]. These three predisposing conditions are referred to as Virchow's Triad.

Endothelial damage in the heart may occur due to atherosclerosis, myocardial infarction, trauma and inflammation. Endothelial dysfunction is also a predisposing factor for thrombus formation. Causes of endothelial dysfunction include hypertension, bacterial toxins, hypercholesterolemia, radiation, and cigarette smoking. Thrombus formation due to endothelial damage or dysfunction occurs due to: (1) platelet activators which promote platelet adhesion to the injured site, (2) exposure of tissue factor on the injured endothelium which initiates the coagulation cascade, and (3) depletion of natural antithrombotic agents.

Abnormal blood flow includes turbulent flow and stasis. Turbulence contributes to thrombus formation by causing endothelial injury or dysfunction as well as by producing local pockets of stasis. Stasis is the major contributor to thrombus formation. Stasis or turbulence promote thrombus formation by: (1) bringing platelets close to the endothelial surface, (2) allowing the accumulation of clotting factors in the injured region, and (3) promoting endothelial cell activation which leads to a prothrombotic state.

Hypercoagulability refers to an alteration in blood coagulation that leads to thrombosis. Hypercoagulable states can be divided into primary (genetic) and secondary (acquired) categories. Examples of high risk secondary hypercoagulable states include prolonged bed rest or immobilisation, post myocardial infarction, atrial fibrillation and mechanical prosthetic valves.

The most common causes for, and locations of, intracardiac thrombus are listed in Table 13.8; pathological examples are shown in Figure 13.25. Importantly, cardiac tumours and IE are also potential sources of thrombus.

Table 13.8 Intracardiac Thrombus by Aetiology and Location

Cardiac "Condition"	Common Location of Thrombus
Myocardial infarction (MI)	Site of infarcted myocardium (anterior MI > posterior MI) Ventricular aneurysms (true and pseudoaneurysms)
Dilated cardiomyopathy	Any cardiac chamber (most common within LV followed by RV, RAA and LAA) Right heart thrombus almost always in association with left heart thrombus
Endomyocardial fibrosis (EMF) Hypereosinophilic syndrome	Apices of both ventricles (characteristic) Inflow tracts of both ventricles (less common)
Mitral stenosis	LA (LAA and/or body of LA) RA (less common) Ventricles rare (unless coexistent systolic dysfunction)
Atrial fibrillation	LAA
Pulmonary thromboembolic disease	RA and/or RV (migratory thrombus) Main pulmonary artery and branches LA and/or LV (paradoxical emboli across PFO)
Prosthetic valves*	Prosthetic discs or leaflets LA (MVR)

* Especially mechanical valves with subtherapeutic anticoagulation.
LA = left atrium; LAA= left atrial appendage; LV = left ventricle; MVR = mitral valve replacement; PFO = patent foramen ovale; RA = right atrium; RAA = right atrial appendage; RV = right ventricle.

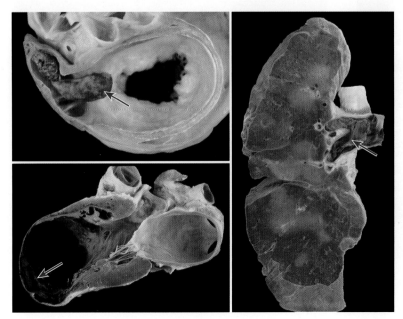

Figure 13.25 These gross pathological specimens show intracardiac thrombus within the left atrial appendage (*top, left*) and within an aneurysm at the left ventricular apex (*bottom, left*). An acute pulmonary embolism within the right pulmonary artery and its branches is also shown (*right*).
By permission of Mayo Foundation for Medical Education and Research. All rights reserved. Courtesy of William D. Edwards, MD.

Left Ventricular Thrombus

Left ventricular thrombus (LVT) occurs in regions of blood stasis or low velocity blood flow. Therefore, LVT is typically located at sites where there is an underlying regional wall motion abnormality. The most common location for LVT is at the LV apex following an anterior myocardial infarction. On 2D echocardiography, LVT generally appears as a discrete homogeneous mass that is contiguous with, but distinct from, the underlying endocardium and is seen in at least two imaging planes (Fig. 13.26-13.27). The appearance of LVT is variable in that it may be fixed and laminated, or pedunculated and mobile. LVT may also appear heterogeneous which is consistent with variable stages of clotting within the thrombus; this appearance is more consistent with acute or fresh thrombus.

As discussed in Chapter 5, poor image quality may mask LV thrombus (especially at the apex) and in these situations the use of colour flow Doppler imaging at a low Nyquist limit or the injection of intravenous contrast agents may be very useful in determining the presence or absence of thrombus (see Fig. 13.27 and Fig. 5.26 and 5.27).

Left Atrial Thrombus

As for LVT, left atrial thrombus (LAT) is most common where there is stasis of blood flow; therefore, LAT is most often associated with mitral valve stenosis, LA enlargement, and atrial fibrillation (AF). Normally, LA contraction prevents the formation of thrombus within the LA; however, when there is LA dysfunction or ineffective atrial contraction, the LA is

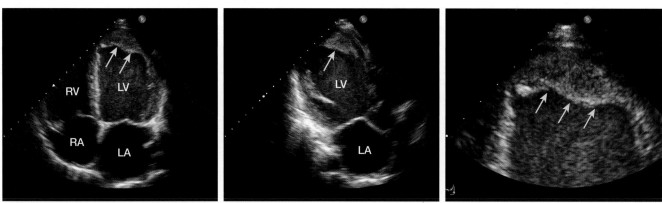

Figure 13.26 These images were recorded from a patient with a dilated cardiomyopathy. A large crescentic mural thrombus is seen within the left ventricular apex and extending along the anteroseptal wall (*arrows*). Images are recorded from the apical 4-chamber (*left*), apical long axis (*middle*) and zoomed apical 4-chamber (*right*) views. LA = left atrium; LV = left ventricle; RA = right atrium; RV = right ventricle.

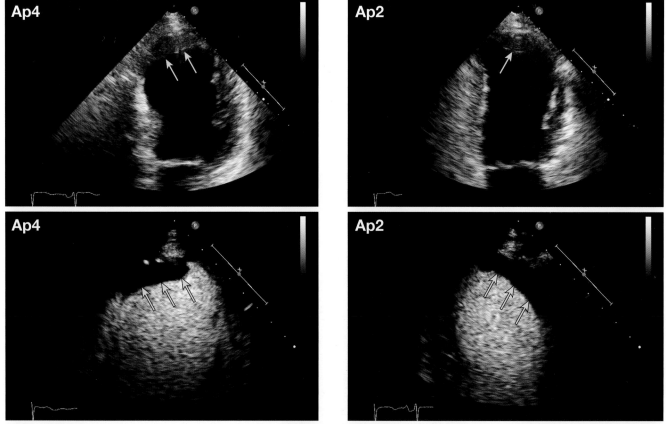

Figure 13.27 These images were recorded from the apical 4-chamber (Ap4) and apical 2-chamber (Ap2) views in a patient with a previous anterior myocardial infarction and an apical aneurysm. On the routine echocardiogram, a suspicious area at the left ventricular (LV) apex is noted (*arrows*) (*top images*). Following the administration of intravenous contrast a large, mural thrombus was clearly delineated at the LV apex, extending around the mid anterior wall (dark area within the LV apex) (*bottom images*).

prone to thrombus formation especially within the left atrial appendage (LAA).

Transthoracic views that best image the LAA include the parasternal short axis view, the apical 4-chamber view, the apical 2-chamber view, and the subcostal 4-chamber view (Fig. 13.28). Therefore, when LAT is suspected, careful interrogation of the LAA from these views is necessary.

On 2D imaging, LAT appears as an echogenic, homogeneous mass within the LAA or body of the LA (Fig 13.29). As for LVT, the appearance of LAT is variable in that it may be fixed and laminated, or pedunculated and mobile.

Importantly, in the setting of a negative TTE, LAT cannot be excluded. Therefore, when it is important to exclude LAT such as prior to cardioversion for AF or prior to mitral balloon valvuloplasty for mitral stenosis, then TOE is indicated.

Prosthetic Valve Thrombosis

Prosthetic valve thrombosis (PVT) is a potential and serious complication of prosthetic valves (see Chapter 10). PVT is significantly more common with mechanical valves than bioprosthetic valves and is also more common with mitral than aortic valves. When a thrombus forms around the prosthetic valve, it frequently interferes with valvular function. For example, in the presence of PVT the prosthetic discs may be stuck closed resulting in significant obstruction or stuck open resulting in significant regurgitation. Furthermore, in patients with mitral prosthetic valves and AF, thrombus may also form within the LAA due to stasis of blood flow.

Echocardiographic evidence of PVT includes: (1) increased transprosthetic velocities and pressure gradients compared

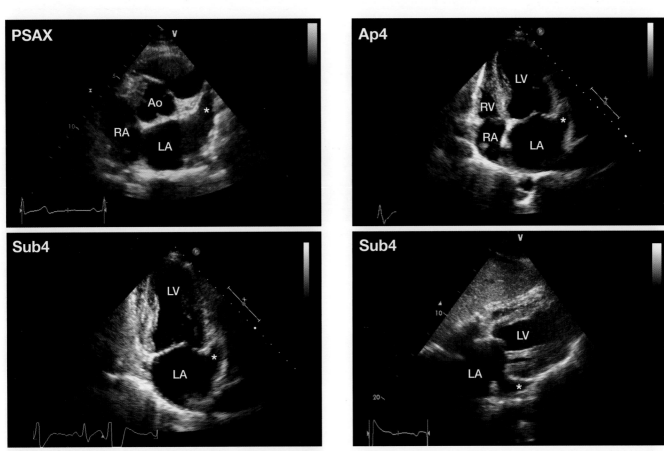

Figure 13.28 The left atrial appendage (*) is best imaged from the parasternal short axis (PSAX), the apical 4-chamber (Ap4), the apical 2-chamber (Ap2) and the subcostal 4-chamber (Sub4) views. Images are recorded from different patients.
Ao = aorta; LA = left atrium; LV = left ventricle; RA = right atrium; RV = right ventricle.

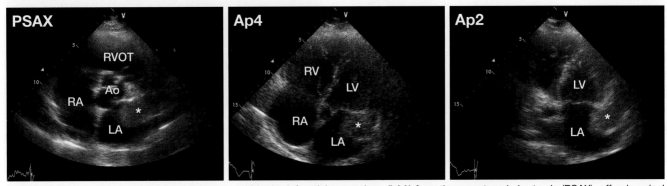

Figure 13.29 A large echogenic mass (*) is seen within the left atrial appendage (LAA) from the parasternal short axis (PSAX), off-axis apical 4-chamber (Ap4), and off-axis apical 2-chamber (Ap2) views. This mass extends from the LAA into the left atrial (LA) cavity. The LA is mildly dilated and atrial fibrillation is present. The appearance of this mass is consistent with a LAA thrombus.
Ao = aorta; LA = left atrium; LV = left ventricle; RA = right atrium; RV = right ventricle; RVOT = right ventricular outflow tract.

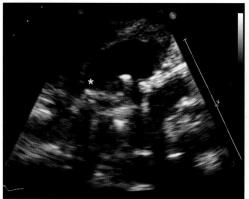
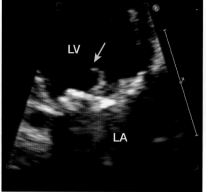
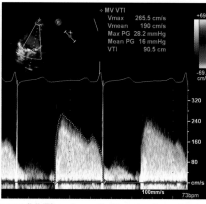

Figure 13.30 These images were recorded from a patient with a 27 mm St Jude mitral valve replacement (MVR) and prosthetic valve thrombosis. Observe on the 2D image recorded from the parasternal short axis that the medial disc (*) of the bileaflet tilting disk valve is stuck closed (*left*). On a zoomed apical 2-chamber view (Ap2) a soft tissue mass is seen projecting from the posterior MVR annulus into the left ventricular (LV) cavity (arrow) (*middle*). The mean gradient across the MVR via continuous-wave Doppler is 16 mmHg (*right*).

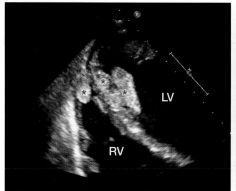
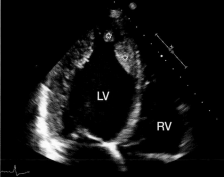
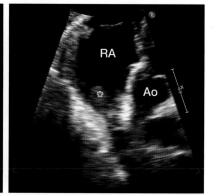

Figure 13.31 These images were acquired from a patient with a dilated cardiomyopathy. Multiple intracardiac thrombi (*) are noted within the left ventricle (LV), right ventricle (RV) and the right atrial (RA) appendage. Images are recorded from an RV focused apical 4-chamber view (*left*), a reversed apical 4-chamber view (*middle*) and a zoomed subcostal 4-chamber view with anterior tilt (*right*). Ao = aorta.

with the baseline study or compared with established normal values, (2) a reduced EOA compared with the baseline study or compared with established normal values, (3) reduced or absent prosthetic leaflets/disc mobility, and/or (4) the visualisation of echogenic material around the prosthetic valve (Fig. 13.30).

Also, as discussed in Chapter 10, serial Doppler studies have an important role in determining the duration and the efficacy of thrombolytic therapy in PVT.

Right Heart Thrombus

Formation of thrombus in the right heart is much less common than in the left heart. However, right heart thrombus may occur in the RA and/or RV when there is stagnation of blood for any reason; thrombus may also form on pacing leads or indwelling catheters in the right heart chambers.

Thrombus in the right heart is more likely to originate from deep vein thrombus (DVT) where the DVT has embolised and has become entangled within the tricuspid valve apparatus. This type of thrombus is referred to as migratory thrombus. Pulmonary thromboembolic (PTE) disease may also result in thrombus formation within the right and left pulmonary artery branches. PTE disease is a form of occlusive pulmonary vascular disease that may be acute or chronic and it is one of the causes of pulmonary arterial hypertension.

On the echocardiographic examination, right heart thrombus has a similar appearance to left heart thrombus in that it

appears as an echogenic, homogeneous mass which may be fixed and laminated, or pedunculated and mobile (Fig 13.31). In particular, migratory thrombi are usually highly mobile and display a snake-like or popcorn-like appearance on real-time imaging (Fig. 13.32).

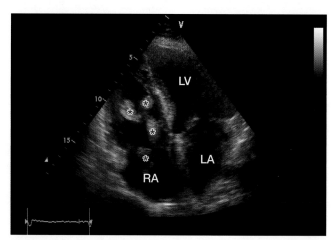

Figure 13.32 This image was recorded from an apical 4-chamber view in a patient with an acute pulmonary embolism. Observe the extensive thrombus within the right heart (*). On real-time imaging, these thrombi were bouncing around within the right heart creating a 'popcorn' appearance. In this clinical setting, the most likely origin of these thrombi is migratory deep vein thrombosis. LA = left atrium; LV = left ventricle; RA = right atrium.

Paradoxical Embolism across a PFO

Paradoxical embolism occurs when right heart or venous thrombus embolises across an intracardiac defect such as a patent foramen ovale (PFO). Recall that in foetal development, the foramen ovale provides a vital communication between the RA and LA allowing oxygen-rich blood from the maternal placenta to pass to the left heart to oxygenate the developing foetal brain. Following birth, the LA pressure exceeds the RA pressure and this leads to closure of the foramen ovale by the flap valve of the fossa ovalis which is located on the LA side of the interatrial septum (IAS).

In about 25-30% of the population there is a PFO but as long as the LA pressure exceeds RA pressure, the PFO remains closed by the flap valve. However, when the RA pressure exceeds the LA pressure, right-to-left shunting across the PFO may occur. Therefore, if there is thrombus within the right heart, this thrombus may paradoxically embolise across the PFO into the LA and left heart.

The definitive diagnosis of paradoxical embolism requires detection of thrombus lodged within the PFO (Fig. 13.33). However, when an actual thrombus crossing a PFO or other intracardiac defect is not seen, the diagnosis of paradoxical embolism may be suspected when there is: (1) a systemic embolism without an apparent source in the left heart or proximal arterial tree, (2) evidence of venous thrombus or pulmonary embolus as an embolic source, and (3) evidence of a PFO with right-to-left shunting.

Importantly, when a shunt across the region of the fossa ovalis cannot be seen and a PFO is clinically suspected, especially in the setting of a cerebral ischaemic event of uncertain origin in a young person, then a saline contrast bubble study is indicated (Fig. 13.34).

Spontaneous Echo Contrast

Spontaneous echo contrast (SEC) is seen within the heart when there is low blood flow or blood stasis. In this situation, the velocity of blood flow decreases which allows the red blood cells (RBCs) to overcome shear forces that normally separate them. This leads to rouleaux formation whereby RBCs become stacked one on top of another to form aggregates of RBCs. When this effect occurs, the potential size of the individual reflectors increases so that they are easily detected via ultrasound imaging. The characteristic appearance of RBC aggregates is a smoke-like appearance or swirling motion of blood flow within a cardiac chamber (Fig. 13.35). Importantly, SEC is considered to be a precursor for thrombus formation.

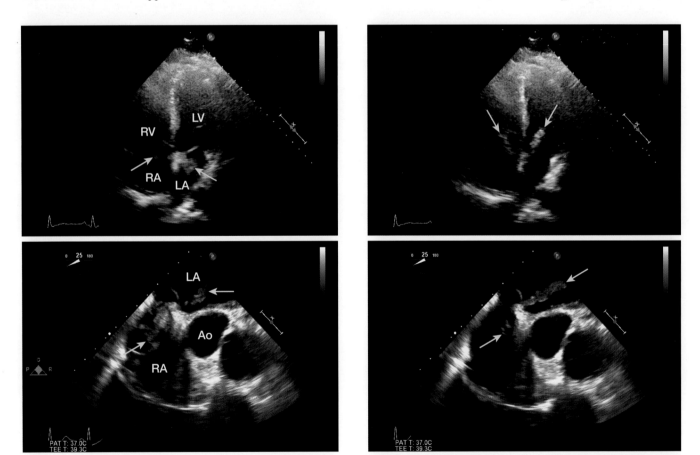

Figure 13.33 These images were recorded from a patient with an acute pulmonary embolism. The transthoracic images were recorded from the apical 4-chamber view (*top*). Observe the large echogenic masses within the right atrium (RA) and left atrium (LA) (*arrows*) which prolapse across the tricuspid and mitral valves into the right and left ventricles during diastole (*top right*). The corresponding transoesophageal images (TOE) are also shown (*bottom*). From these images it is apparent that there is thrombus extension from the RA across a patent foramen ovale (PFO) into the LA consistent with a paradoxical embolism across the PFO. Also observe that the interatrial septum bows from right to left on the TOE images suggesting that the RA pressure is greater than the LA pressure. Ao = aorta; LV = left ventricle; RV = right ventricle.

Protocol for Performing Agitated Saline Bubble Study for PFO

Supplies required:

1 x 3-way stop cock
1 x 18 or 20 gauge cannula with plastic tube extension
1 x tourniquet
4 x 10 mL boluses of saline
2 x 10 mL luer lock syringes

Step 1: Determine the best echocardiographic view for imaging the atrial septum and the right and left atria (apical 4-chamber or parasternal short axis views are best; avoid the subcostal 4-chamber view as bubbles in RA may shadow the LA).

Step 2: Determine whether prospective or retrospective capture will be used and set long loop capture (10 beat loop recommended).

Step 3: Insert an 18-20 gauge cannula into a vein in the antecubital fossa of the left or right arm and attach the 3-way stopcock.

Step 4: Connect both syringes to stopcock.

Step 5: Mix 1 mL of blood, 0.5 mL of air and 8.5 mL of saline into one syringe.

Step 6: With stopcock closed, prepare solution by rapidly agitating between the two syringes at least 5-10 times.

Step 7: Open stopcock and rapidly inject solution into patient's vein.

Step 8: Acquire digital loop on injection: for prospective capture, click store and count 10 beats; for retrospective capture, count 10 beats and then click store.

Positive test: Bubbles/contrast appear within the left heart within 3 beats after opacification of RA.

If negative at rest: If no shunt is noted at rest then the Valsalva manoeuvre or a cough should be performed by the patient to transiently increase the RA pressure. Note that the Valsalva is released as the contrast enters the RA.

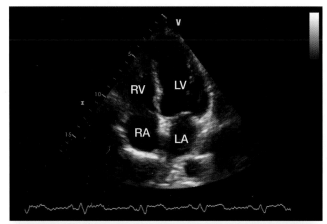

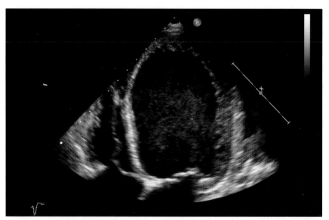

Figure 13.35 On this apical 4-chamber image, a smoke-like appearance is noted within the left ventricular cavity. On real-time imaging, swirling of this smoke was seen which is characteristic of low velocity blood flow.

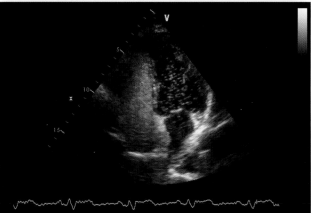

Figure 13.34 A saline bubble study was performed in this 51 year old patient who had suffered a stroke. Images from the apical 4-chamber view pre- and post-agitated saline bubble study are shown (*top* and *bottom*, respectively). Observe that following the injection of agitated saline, microbubbles can be seen opacifying the right heart chambers with bubbles also seen in the left heart chambers confirming the presence of a right-to-left shunt across a patent foramen ovale. LA = left atrium; LV = left ventricle; RA = right atrium; RV = right ventricle.

Normal Anatomy Simulating Cardiac Masses

There are several normal (or variants of normal) anatomic structures that may simulate intracardiac masses; these include RA structures, LA structures, valve excrescences, atrial septal aneurysms, ventricular muscle bands and false tendons. These structures can be differentiated from intracardiac tumours and thrombus by their characteristic echocardiographic appearance and their anatomic position and relationships within the heart. Some of the more commonly encountered structures are discussed below.

Right Atrial Structures

There are a number of normal structures within the RA that can simulate intracardiac masses especially when these structures become prominent (Fig. 13.36). In particular, the crista terminalis, the eustachian ridge and the eustachian valve are frequently seen on the echocardiographic examination. These structures can be differentiated from intracardiac tumours and thrombus by their characteristic echocardiographic appearance and position within the RA.

The crista terminalis is a C-shaped, fibromuscular ridge that extends along the posterolateral wall from the orifice of the superior vena cava (SVC) down to the orifice of the inferior vena cava (IVC), effectively dividing the trabeculated RA appendage from the posterior smooth-walled RA cavity. When prominent, this muscular ridge can protrude into the RA cavity and on the echocardiographic examination it may resemble an intracardiac mass, such as a tumour or thrombus (Fig. 13.37).

The eustachian ridge (or sinus septum) runs across the inferior border of the RA and separates the orifice of the IVC from the coronary sinus. The eustachian ridge is commonly seen in the

parasternal long axis view of the RV inflow and should not be confused with an intracardiac mass (Fig. 13.38). This ridge of tissue is also sometimes referred to as the RA 'Q-Tip' sign based on its echocardiographic appearance which is similar to a Q-tip (cotton bud).

The eustachian valve, or the valve of the IVC, is a remnant of the embryonic right valve of the sinus venosus. It arises from the orifice of the IVC and attaches to the IAS around the region of the fossa ovalis. In the foetal circulation, the eustachian

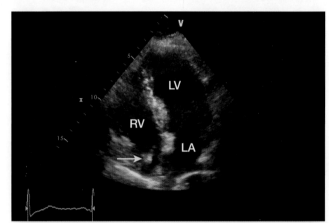
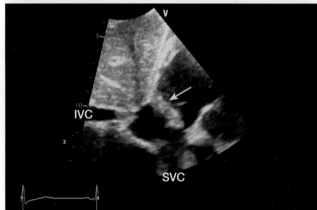

Figure 13.37 From the apical 4-chamber view, a prominent linear structure (arrows) is noted within the right atrium (RA) (top). From the subcostal short axis view, this prominent linear structure extends from the junction of the superior vena cava (SVC) and RA to the inferior vena cava (IVC) (bottom). Based on the appearance and location, this structure is consistent with a prominent crista terminalis. LA = left atrium; LV = left ventricle; RV = right ventricle.

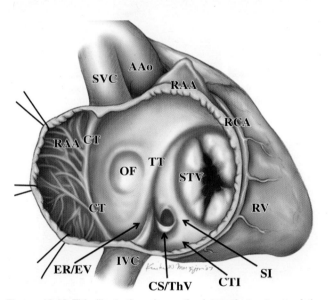

Figure 13.36 This illustration shows the internal structures of the right atrium as seen from a right anterior oblique view.
AAo = ascending aorta; CS = coronary sinus; CT = crista terminalis; CTI = cavotricuspid isthmus; EV = eustachian valve; ER = eustachian ridge; EV = eustachian valve; IVC = inferior vena cava; OF = oval fossa; RAA = RA appendage; RCA = right coronary artery; RV = right ventricle; SI = septal isthmus; STV = septal tricuspid valve; SVC = superior vena cava; ThV = thebesian valve; TT = tendon of Todaro.
Reproduced from Saremi F, Pourzand L, Krishnan S, Ashikyan O, Gurudevan SV, Narula J, Kaushal K, Raney A. Right atrial cavotricuspid isthmus: anatomic characterization with multi-detector row CT. Radiology. © 2008 Jun;247(3), page 660, with permission from the Radiological Society of North America and Farhood Saremi, MD, Professor of Radiology, University of California.

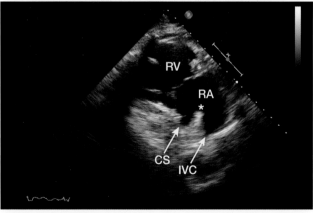

Figure 13.38 From the parasternal long axis of the right ventricular (RV) inflow view, the eustachian ridge is frequently seen (*) between the inferior vena cava (IVC) and the coronary sinus (CS). This appearance is sometimes referred to as the Q-tip sign of the right atrium (RA).

valve helps to direct oxygenated blood from the IVC toward the foramen ovale and into the LA to ensure that oxygen-rich blood reaches the developing foetal brain. Typically, the eustachian valve regresses during childhood but can persist into adulthood. The Chiari network is a fenestrated variant of the eustachian valve; therefore, the embryonic origin and

location of this network is essentially the same as that of the eustachian valve. The fenestrated Chiari network is more extensive than a eustachian valve and appears as a 'web-like' or 'lace-like' membrane (Fig. 13.39). On echocardiographic examination, the eustachian valve and Chiari network are best seen from the parasternal long axis of the RV inflow tract, the parasternal short axis, the apical 4-chamber and the subcostal views. The eustachian valve appears as a mobile linear structure stretching from the orifice of the IVC to the IAS while the Chiari network appears more 'wildly' mobile and whip-like (Fig. 13.40). When prominent, these structures may be confused with a RA tumour or thrombus.

Left Atrial Structures

Normal structures of the LA such as pectinate muscles and the bulbous partition between the LAA and the left upper pulmonary vein may also simulate intracardiac masses (Fig. 13.41). These structures can be differentiated from intracardiac tumours and thrombus by their characteristic echocardiographic appearance and position.

Pectinate muscles are prominent parallel ridges of atrial muscle that are located within the LAA; the characteristic projections of pectinate muscles resemble the teeth of a comb which accounts for the origin of their name. Most commonly pectinate muscles are only imaged via TOE (Fig. 13.42).

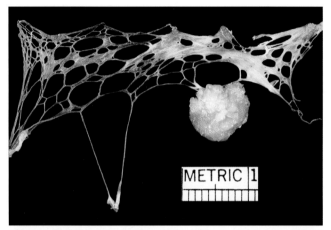

Figure 13.39 This is a very nice pathological specimen of a Chiari network. Observe the extensive 'web-like' appearance of this structure. A papillary fibroelastoma is also arising from this network. By permission of Mayo Foundation for Medical Education and Research. All rights reserved. Courtesy of William D. Edwards, MD.

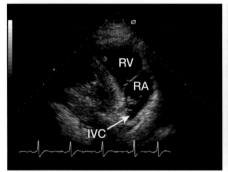 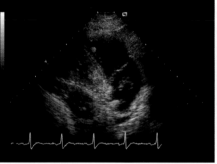 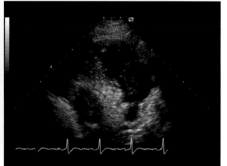

Figure 13.40 This series of images was recorded from the parasternal long axis of the right ventricular (RV) inflow view. Observe the echogenic structure within the right atrium (RA) in close proximity to the orifice of the inferior vena cava (IVC). Also note the undulating motion of the structure over the cardiac cycle. This appearance is consistent with a Chiari network.

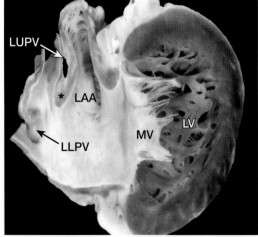

Figure 13.41 This pathological specimen shows the anatomy of the left atrium (LA). Observe the pectinate muscles within the left atrial appendage (LAA). Also observe the fold in the LA wall (*) that separates the orifice of the left upper pulmonary vein (LUPV) and the LAA.
LLPV = left lower pulmonary vein; LV = left ventricle; MV = mitral valve. Photo reproduced from Ho S Y and Ernst S. Anatomy for Cardiac Electrophysiologists - A Practical Handbook (Figure 8.8), © 2012 with permission from Cardiotext Publishing, Minneapolis USA.

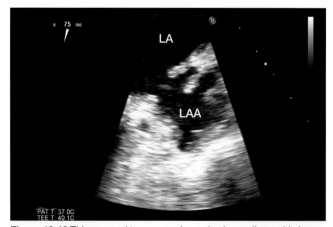

Figure 13.42 This zoomed transoesophageal echocardiographic image shows the left atrial appendage (LAA). Observe the projections into the cavity of the LAA. These projections represent prominent pectinate muscles.

When prominent, these atrial muscles may protrude into the LAA mimicking thrombi. Pectinate muscles can be differentiated from thrombi by their parallel ridge-like appearance, their relatively small size, and the absence of independent mobility (that is, pectinate muscles move with the LA wall and not independent of it).

The bulbous partition between the LAA and the left upper pulmonary vein may also appear prominent on the echocardiographic examination (Fig. 13.43). This ridge of tissue is referred to as the 'Q-Tip' sign based on its echocardiographic appearance which is similar to a Q-tip (cotton bud). This ridge of tissue is also referred to as the 'Coumadin' or 'Warfarin' ridge because this anatomic variant is often misidentified as a thrombus resulting in the subsequent administration of anticoagulation therapy with warfarin (Coumadin). The Coumadin ridge can be differentiated from thrombus or a myxoma based on its lack of mobility and its characteristic location.

Atrial Septal Aneurysm

An atrial septal aneurysm (ASA) refers to a localized, out-pouching of the IAS at the level of the fossa ovalis and this is frequently associated with a PFO (Fig. 13.44). On 2D echocardiography, an ASA may be confused with pathology when seen from the parasternal long axis view of the RV inflow.

However, diagnosis of an ASA can be easily made from the apical 4-chamber or subcostal 4-chamber views. From these views, an ASA appears as a thin linear bulge in the IAS that moves with the cardiac and respiratory cycles. An ASA is defined as having a basal width ≥ 15 mm and protruding beyond the plane of the residual atrial septum ≥ 15 mm (Fig. 13.45). As the LA pressure is usually slightly higher than the RA pressure, the aneurysm usually protrudes into the RA (Fig. 13.46, left); however, when the RA pressure exceeds LA pressure the ASA bulges into the LA (Fig. 13.46, right).

Importantly, an ASA with a PFO may be associated with an increased risk of embolic events and thrombus. Therefore, in the setting of a cerebral ischaemic event and when an ASA is identified and when a PFO cannot be detected on the routine echocardiogram, a saline contrast bubble study is indicated (Fig. 13.47).

Ventricular Muscle Bands and False Tendons

The moderator band is a prominent muscular trabeculation that traverses the RV at the level of the RV apex. The moderator band becomes more prominent when there is RV hypertrophy or heavy RV trabeculation. On 2D echocardiography, the moderator band is seen as a thick, echodense band extending from the lower IVS across the RV cavity to the RV free wall.

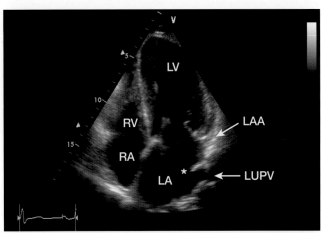
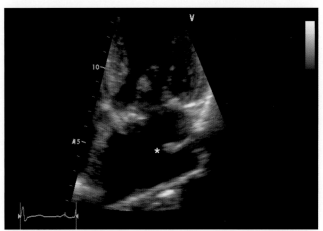

Figure 13.43 These images recorded from the apical 4-chamber view (unzoomed and zoomed views) show a prominent linear structure protruding into the left atrial (LA) cavity (*). This ridge of tissue structure is a normal anatomic structure which separates the left atrial appendage (LAA) from the left upper pulmonary vein (LUPV). This structure is often referred to as the Q-tip sign or the Coumadin or Warfarin ridge (see text for further details). LV = left ventricle; RA = right atrium; RV = right ventricle.

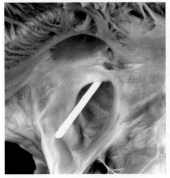
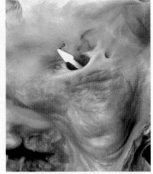

Figure 13.44 An atrial septal aneurysm (ASA) with a patent foramen ovale (PFO) is shown from the right atrial aspect (*left*) and from the left atrial (LA) aspect (*right*). The white probe demonstrates the PFO. The ASA is bulging towards the LA.
By permission of Mayo Foundation for Medical Education and Research. All rights reserved. Courtesy of William D. Edwards, MD.

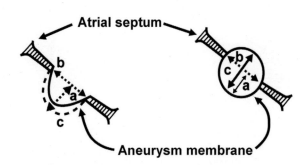

Figure 13.45 An atrial septal aneurysm may be defined as: (1) protrusion of the atrial septum or part of it at least 1.5 cm beyond the plane of the atrial septum (a ≥ 1.5 cm) or phasic excursion during the cardiorespiratory cycle exceeding 1.5 cm (c ≥ 1.5 cm), and (2) protrusion of the base of the aneurysm ≥ 1.5 cm in diameter (b).
Reproduced from Hanley PC, Tajik AJ, Hynes JK, Edwards WD, Reeder GS, Hagler DJ, Seward JB. Diagnosis and classification of atrial septal aneurysm by two-dimensional echocardiography: report of 80 consecutive cases. *J Am Coll Cardiol*. Vol. 6(6), page 1371, © 1985, with permission from Elsevier.

The moderator band is best seen from the apical 4-chamber view (see Fig. 13.46).

False tendons, also known as pseudotendons, aberrant bands, accessory cords or 'heart strings', are fibrous structures that traverse the LV cavity. These tendons may be multiple or single and they may pass between the papillary muscle and IVS, between the two papillary muscles, from the LV free wall to the IVS, or between two points of the LV free wall (Fig. 13.48). On 2D echocardiography, false tendons appear as thin, linear structures that course across the LV cavity (Fig. 13.49). As for the moderator band in the RV, these false tendons are best seen from the apical 4-chamber view.

False tendons and moderator bands may mimic thrombus or tumours; they can be differentiated from pathology by: (1) the identification of an echo-free space on each side of the structure, (2) a constant motion of the structure during the cardiac cycle, and (3) the presence of normal ventricular wall motion adjacent to the structure.

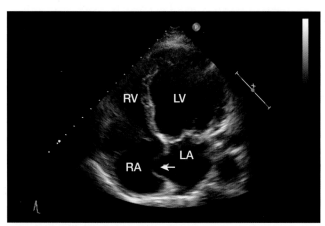
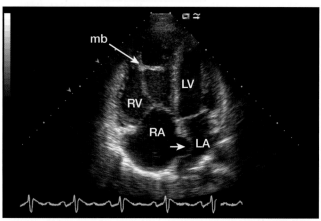

Figure 13.46 These apical 4-chamber views were recorded from two different patients with an atrial septal aneurysm (ASA). In the image on the left, the ASA bulges into the right atrium (RA); this suggests that the left atrial (LA) pressure is greater than the RA pressure. In the image on the right, the ASA bulges into the LA; this suggests that the RA pressure is greater than the LA pressure. Also observe the prominent moderator band (mb) in the right ventricle (RV) in the right image. LV = left ventricle.

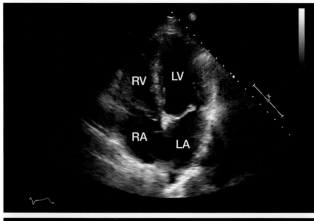
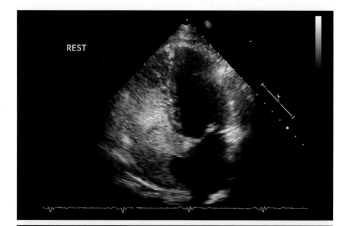
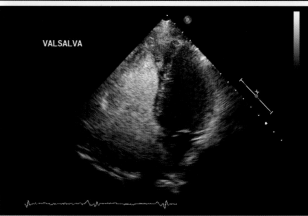
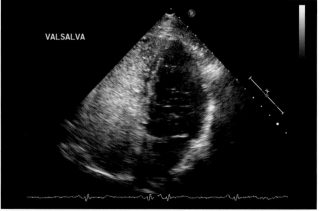

Figure 13.47 A saline bubble study was performed in this 61 year old patient who had suffered a stroke. From the apical 4-chamber view, an atrial septal aneurysm (ASA), bowing left-to-right can be seen (*top left*). On the resting agitated saline bubble study, microbubbles can be seen opacifying the right heart chambers and the ASA is nicely defined but no bubbles are seen within the left heart (*top right*). On the agitated saline bubble study with the Valsalva manoeuvre, the ASA can be seen to bow towards the left atrium (LA) indicating an increase in the right atrial (RA) pressure (*bottom left*). On the release of the Valsalva, microbubbles can be seen to fill the left heart chambers confirming the presence of a right-to-left shunt across a patent foramen ovale (*bottom right*). LV = left ventricle; RV = right ventricle.

Figure 13.48 These pathological specimens show the various locations of left ventricular false tendons (*arrows*).
A: Two false tendons from postero-medial papillary muscle (PM) to ventricular septum (VS).
B: False tendons between both the anterolateral (AL) and posteromedial (PM) papillary muscles and the ventricular septum (VS).
C: False tendons between the papillary muscle (PM) and the ventricular septum (VS) and between the left ventricular free wall (LVFW) and the ventricular septum (VS) and the papillary muscle (PM).
D: False tendons between the left ventricular free wall (LVFW) and the ventricular septum (VS) and papillary muscle (PM).
By permission of Mayo Foundation for Medical Education and Research. All rights reserved. Courtesy of William D. Edwards, MD.

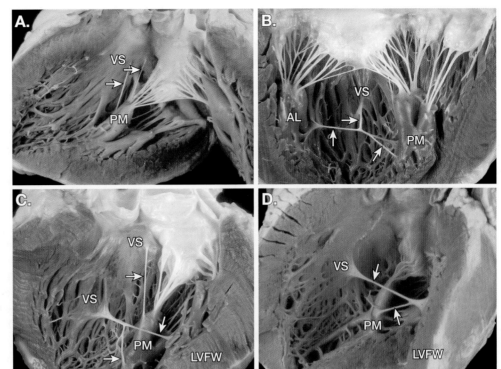

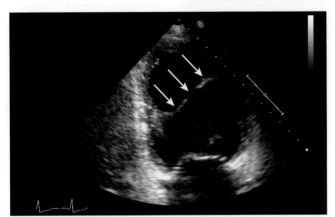

Figure 13.49 This apical 2-chamber view displays a false tendon stretching across the left ventricular cavity from the papillary muscle to the anterior wall (*arrows*).

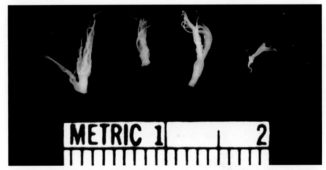

Figure 13.50 Resected Lambl's excrescences of the aortic valve are shown. Observe the frond-like appearance of these excrescences. By permission of Mayo Foundation for Medical Education and Research. All rights reserved. Courtesy of William D. Edwards, MD.

Valve Excrescences

Valve excrescences are fine filamentous strands or fronds that occur along the line of valve closure (Fig. 13.50). They may be seen on the ventricular side of the aortic and pulmonary valves (Lambl's excrescences) and on the atrial side of the mitral and tricuspid leaflets. These excrescences are thin (up to 1.5 mm wide), elongated (up to 10 mm long), and are frequently multiple [13.10]. Giant Lambl's excrescences may also occur when multiple adjacent excrescences adhere to one another.

On 2D echocardiography, valve excrescences appear as fine, linear mobile strands either attached to the valve closure zone or arising from the free borders of the leaflets (Fig. 13.51). While these filaments are more apparent on TOE, they may be seen on TTE when image quality is exceptionally good. Distinction between valve excrescences and valvular vegetations is based on the patient's clinical presentation as well as the characteristic fine, strand-like appearance of these excrescences.

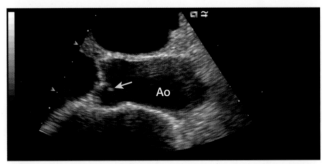

Figure 13.51 This zoomed high parasternal long axis view of the aortic valve and ascending aorta (Ao) shows a Lambl's excrescence attached to the non-coronary cusp of the aortic valve (*arrow*).

Extracardiac masses may also simulate intracardiac masses; these include pectus excavatum, the spine, the stomach, a hiatus hernia, and pericardial and bronchogenic cysts. Foreign bodies such as indwelling catheters, central lines, pacing wires, sutures and percutaneous closure devices can also be mistaken for intracardiac tumours and/or thrombus.

[13.10] Roldan CA, Shively BK, Crawford MH. Valve excrescences: prevalence, evolution and risk for cardioembolism. *J Am Coll Cardiol*. 1997 Nov 1;30(5):1308-14.

Imaging Artefacts Simulating Cardiac Masses

There are several imaging artefacts that may simulate cardiac masses. Imaging artefacts most likely to simulate cardiac masses are those artefacts which result in added echoes; these artefacts include beam width, slice thickness, grating lobe, range ambiguity, and reverberation artefacts. These artefacts are most apparent in echo-free cavities and should be suspected when 'masses' appear to cross tissue planes and organ boundaries, when 'masses' cannot be seen from multiple orthogonal windows, and/or when 'masses' display a motion that is separate from the heart.

Beamwidth Artefacts

The beamwidth is determined by the transducer frequency, the focal zone position and the aperture of the transducer element. Typically, the beamwidth ranges from less than 1 mm to more than 15 mm depending upon these variables. Echoes are generated from reflectors lying within the full width of the ultrasound beam and echoes will continue to be generated as long as a reflector remains within the beamwidth. Therefore, a strong reflector to the side of an echo-free cavity may appear within this cavity and create the appearance of a 'mass' (Fig. 13.52).

Slice Thickness Artefacts

Ultrasound beams are three-dimensional consisting of a beam width, a beam length and a slice thickness. The slice thickness (or elevation plane) of the ultrasound beam is perpendicular (90 degrees) to the main imaging plane. Any structure detected within the thickness of the ultrasound beam including structures in front of or behind the main imaging plane will be detected and echoes will be generated. The ultrasound machine assumes that these echoes have originated from the central part of the imaging plane and, therefore, will 'compress' these echoes into the 2D image (Fig. 13.53). Therefore, echoes generated from

structures in front of or behind the main imaging plane may appear within an echo-free cavity and create the appearance of a 'mass'. Rotating the transducer 90 degrees will usually identify the true origin of a slice thickness artefact (Fig. 13.54).

Grating Lobe Artefacts

Secondary beams of ultrasound energy also exist outside of the main beam. In electronic array transducers these secondary beams (grating lobes) are caused by diffraction effects. Grating lobes have the capacity of transmitting and receiving ultrasound energy just like the main beam. Therefore, structures interrogated by these secondary beams may generate energy strong enough to return to the transducer and be recorded. Echoes detected from these secondary beams are all assumed to have originated from the centre of the main beam. This results in echoes being added to the display (Fig. 13.55). Generally, echoes produced from secondary beams have much lower amplitudes than main beam echoes.

Grating lobe artefacts are commonly seen as linear structures within an echo-free cavity (Fig. 13.56).

Range Ambiguity Artefacts

In order to unambiguously display echoes, sufficient time must be allowed for an echo to return to the transducer before the next pulse is emitted. In particular, it is assumed that for each pulse, all echoes are received before the next pulse is emitted. Range ambiguity artefacts occur when a second pulse

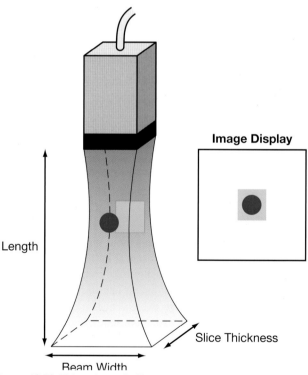

Figure 13.53 This schematic illustrates the production of a slice thickness artefact. Observe that the ultrasound beam is three-dimensional (3D) and includes a length, a width and a slice thickness (shown to the left). The red circle is located in front of the main imaging plane and the blue square is located behind the main imaging plane; however, both structures are still within the slice thickness of the ultrasound beam. Because these structures are within the slice thickness of the beam, they will generate echoes. All echoes within the slice thickness of the 3D ultrasound beam are then "collapsed" to produce a 2D image. As a result the displayed image is composed of echoes that have originated from the main imaging plane as well as those that have arisen from structures in front of and behind the main imaging plane (shown right).

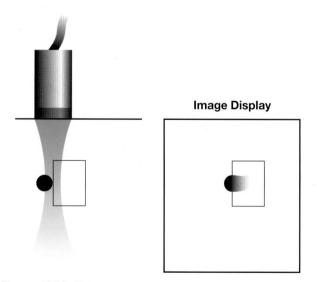

Figure 13.52 This schematic illustrates the production of a beamwidth artefact where a strong reflector to the side of an echo-free cavity appears within this cavity. Observe that when the strong reflector is detected at the edge of the ultrasound beam, an echo will be generated. Because the ultrasound machine assumes that this strong reflector has originated from the central axis of the beam it is placed as such. With this type of beamwidth artefact, the structure generating the artefact will always be imaged adjacent to the artefact. This artefact is most apparent in echo-free cavities.

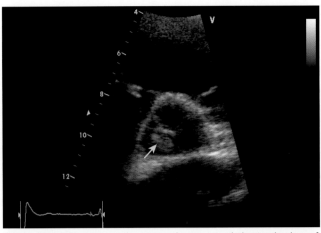 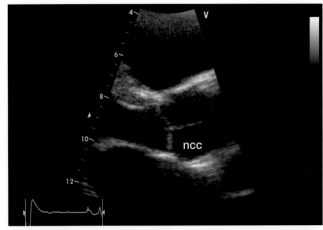

Figure 13.54 Observe on the zoomed parasternal short axis view of the aortic valve that there is an apparent 'mass' on the non-coronary cusp (ncc) of the aortic valve (*left; arrow*). However from the parasternal long axis view this 'mass' is not evident (*right*). As this 'mass' is only seen in one imaging plane, it is an artefact. The likely origin of this slice thickness artefact is the 'belly' of the aortic valve which has been detected behind the main beam and has been compressed onto the 2D image.

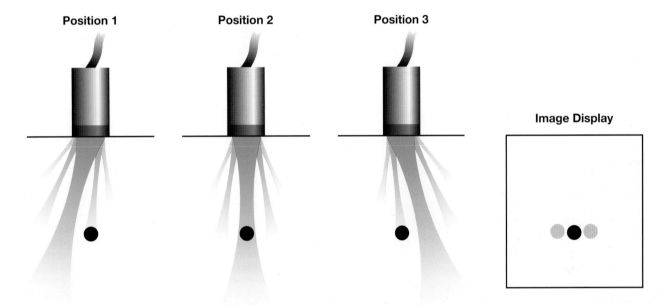

Figure 13.55 This schematic illustrates the production of grating lobe artefacts. The main beam is coloured orange while the secondary beams (grating lobes) are coloured blue. Observe the single dot in the centre of the main beam (position 2). As the beam sweeps to the left (position 1), the dot is detected by the secondary beam and is registered as though it has originated from the main beam. The same effect occurs as the beam sweeps to the right (position 3). On the image display, echoes originating from the main beam and the secondary beams are detected. This results in additional echoes appearing to the side of the real structure. The brightness of echoes arising from the secondary beams is much less than for those arising from the main beam because the intensity of secondary beams is much weaker than that of the main beam. This effect is most obvious in echo-free cavities.

is emitted before an echo returns from the first pulse. In this instance, the ultrasound machine will assume that a returning echo has originated from the most recently emitted pulse when, in fact, it may have originated from the previously emitted pulse. In other words, if an echo from pulse 1 is received after pulse 2 is emitted; the ultrasound machine will assume that the echo was generated from pulse 2. Since the depth of a reflector on the image display is determined by the time taken for a signal to return to the transducer, this echo will be placed closer to the transducer than it really is (Fig. 13.57).

Range ambiguity artefacts most commonly occur when the ultrasound beam passes through a structure that has very low attenuation and a structure outside the field of view is detected and displayed within the field of view (Fig. 13.58).

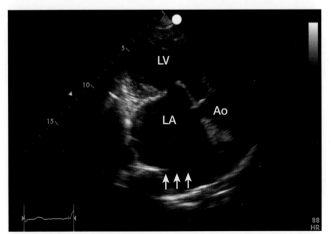

Figure 13.56 This apical long axis view shows a grating lobe artefact originating from the left atrial (LA) wall; this appears as a linear structure within the left atrium (*arrows*). Ao = aorta; LV = left ventricle.

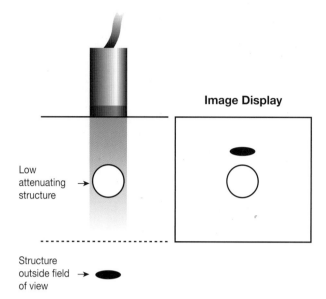

Figure 13.57 This schematic illustrates the formation of a range ambiguity artefact. As the ultrasound beam passes through a low attenuating structure, deeper structures outside the field of view are detected by the ultrasound beam. This is because the intensity of the ultrasound beam is not as attenuated as expected so sufficient intensity remains within the ultrasound beam. When echoes returning from the structure outside the field of view return to the transducer after transmission of the next pulse, then this structure will be placed on the image display as though the echoes have originated from the most recently sent pulse.

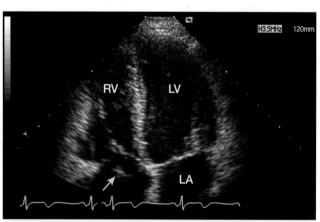

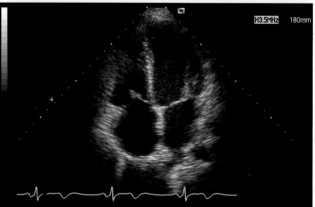

Figure 13.58 In the apical 4-chamber view at a shallow image depth an apparent 'mass' is seen within the cavity of the right atrium (arrow) (top). This is a range ambiguity artefact where the likely origin of this 'mass' is the roof of the atrium. Observe that this 'mass' is not seen at a greater image depth (bottom).
LA = left atrium; LV = left ventricle; RV = right ventricle.

Reverberation Artefacts

Reverberation artefacts can occur when there are two closely spaced interfaces orientated perpendicular to the ultrasound beam. When the ultrasound beam encounters an interface with a large acoustic mismatch some of the energy is returned to the transducer and some of the energy is re-reflected from this interface. This 'bouncing' of the ultrasound beam between two interfaces can occur multiple times resulting in the display of structures multiple times (Fig. 13.59).

Most commonly, reverberation artefacts are related to mechanical prosthetic valves. These artefacts are usually easily recognised by their linear appearance and the equal spacing between each linear echo (Fig. 13.60).

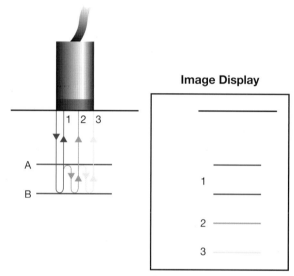

Figure 13.59 This schematic illustrates the formation of reverberation artefacts. When an ultrasound beam encounters two closely spaced, highly reflective interfaces (A and B), part of the ultrasound beam will be reflected back to the transducer from each interface (returning signal 1). However, part of the beam reflected from interface B is reflected a second time at interface A and back to interface B before returning to the transducer (returning signal 2). 'Bouncing' of the ultrasound beam between these two interfaces is again repeated before returning to the transducer (returning signal 3). On the image display, echoes reflected back to the transducer from interfaces A and B appear at the correct depth (position 1). However, because the second reflection takes longer to return to the transducer, it is positioned deeper than the real reflector B (position 2). The distance between positions 1 and 2 on the image display is equal to the distance between interfaces A and B. Likewise, because the third reflection takes longer to return to the transducer, it is positioned deeper than the real reflector (position 3). The distance between positions 2 and 3 on the image display is equal to the distance between interfaces A and B. The brightness of the reverberations progressively weakens throughout the field of view as the intensity of the ultrasound beam weakens each time it is re-reflected.
Note: The ultrasound beam paths are shown side-by-side to show how reverberation artefacts are produced; however, in reality, the ultrasound beam travels down and back along a single path.

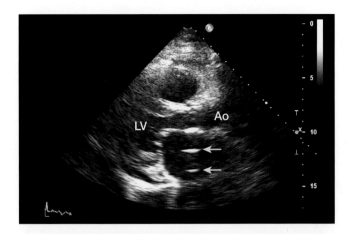

Figure 13.60 This parasternal long axis view shows multiple linear structures within the left atrium (*arrows*) which arise from the prosthetic aortic valve. Observe that these reverberation artefacts are equally spaced and become progressively weaker in intensity throughout the image depth. Ao = aorta; LV = left ventricle.

Key Points

Infective Endocarditis (IE): Basic Concepts
- IE occurs when the endothelial lining of the heart and valves becomes infected with mircoorganisms such as bacteria and fungus
- IE is typically associated with underlying congenital or acquired heart lesions; however, IE may also occur on normal intracardiac valves, on prosthetic heart valves or on intracardiac devices
- Common bacterial organisms that cause IE include Streptococci, Staphylococci, and Enterococci; less common organisms include HACEK gram-negative bacteria and fungal organisms
- The clinical diagnosis of IE is based on the Modified Duke Criteria which consist of clinical, microbiological and echocardiographic criteria

Role of Echo in IE
- Aid in the diagnosis of IE with a positive echo:
  - Positive echo = evidence of vegetations, abscess formation or new partial dehiscence of a prosthetic valve
  - Other echocardiographic evidence of IE includes pseudoaneurysms, leaflet perforation, valve aneurysms and fistula
- Assess the functional abnormalities of the valve(s) affected
- Assess the secondary consequences of the valvular disease
- Identify complications of IE
- Surveillance during and after therapy

Cardiac Tumours: Basic Concepts
- Tumours may be benign or malignant
- Nomenclature for benign and malignant tumours is based on the cell of origin with the suffix "-oma" added for benign tumours and the suffix of "-sarcoma" added for malignant tumours
- Tumours of the heart include benign primary tumours (75% of primary tumours), malignant primary cardiac tumours (25% of primary tumours), metastatic (secondary) cardiac tumours (20-40 fold more common than primary tumours) and extracardiac tumours
- In most cases, tumours can be identified based on their location and characteristic echocardiographic appearances

(continued over...)

Key Points (continued)

Echo Features of Cardiac Tumours
- Myxoma:
  - globular and finely speckled
  - most common within LA attached to IAS via a pedicle or stalk
  - usually highly mobile
  - may cause obstruction to LV inflow when large
- Papillary Fibroelastomas:
  - small, round, homogeneous masses attached to the valve
  - display a 'pom-pom' appearance
  - usually seen on aortic aspect of AV and on the ventricular side of the MV
- Lipoma and LHIAS:
  - Lipoma: echo-bright, homogenous mass
  - LHIAS: thickening of superior and inferior ends of IAS with sparing of the fossa ovalis membrane; creates a 'dumb-bell' or 'hour-glass' appearance
- Rhabdomyoma:
  - well circumscribed, homogenous masses
  - acoustic properties similar to myocardium
  - frequently multiple
- Fibroma:
  - discrete, well demarcated echogenic mass within ventricular wall, IVS, or at the ventricular apex
  - may mimic hypertrophic cardiomyopathy or ventricular septal hypertrophy
- Malignant Tumours:
  - wide and poorly defined attachments into the myocardium or with invasive and destructive characteristics
  - a mass with a large and irregular shape, especially if found in more than one cardiac chamber
  - inhomogeneous soft tissue appearance
  - evidence of pericardial involvement

Intracardiac Thrombus: Basic Concepts
- Basic concepts: 3 primary risk factors or predisposing conditions (Virchow's triad) influence thrombus formation: (1) endothelial injury, (2) haemodynamic changes, and (3) blood hypercoagulability
- Most common sites for intracardiac thrombus formation are sites of low blood flow (stasis) or on mechanical prosthetic heart valves (subtherapeutic anticoagulation)
- Most common source for right heart thrombus is an embolised DVT

Echo Features of Intracardiac Thrombus
- Left heart thrombus:
  - discrete homogeneous mass that is contiguous with, but distinct from, the underlying endocardium
  - may be fixed and laminated, or pedunculated and mobile
- Prosthetic valve thrombosis: suspect when:
  - increased velocities and pressure gradients compared with the baseline study or established normal values
  - a reduced EOA compared with the baseline study or established normal values
  - reduced or absent prosthetic leaflets/disc mobility; and/or
  - echogenic material around the prosthetic valve is seen
- Right heart thrombus:
  - similar appearance to left heart thrombus
  - migratory thrombus is usually highly mobile (snake-like or popcorn-like appearance on real-time imaging)
- Paradoxical embolism:
  - definitive diagnosis when thrombus seen lodged within the PFO
  - when not definitive, suspect when there is: (1) a systemic embolism without an apparent source in the left heart or proximal arterial tree, (2) evidence of venous thrombus or pulmonary embolus as an embolic source, and (3) evidence of a PFO with right-to-left shunting; saline bubble study may be required to confirm PFO.
- Spontaneous echo contrast (SEC):
  - smoke-like swirling blood flow within a cardiac chamber; precursor for thrombus

Key Points (continued)
Normal Anatomy Simulating Cardiac Masses • Includes RA structures (crista terminalis, eustachian ridge, eustachian valve, Chiari network), LA structures (pectinate muscles, 'Coumadin' ridge), valve excrescences, atrial septal aneurysms and ventricular muscle bands and false tendons • These structures can be differentiated from intracardiac tumours and thrombus by their characteristic echocardiographic appearance and their anatomic position and relationships within the heart
Imaging Artefacts • Imaging artefacts that can simulate cardiac masses include beam width, slice thickness, grating lobe, range ambiguity, and reverberation artefacts • These artefacts are most apparent in echo-free cavities and should be suspected when 'masses' appear to cross tissue planes and organ boundaries, when 'masses' cannot be seen from multiple orthogonal windows, and/or when 'masses' display a motion that is separate from the heart

Further Reading (listed in alphabetical order)

Infective Endocarditis

Bashore TM, Cabell C, Fowler V Jr. Update on infective endocarditis. *Curr Probl Cardiol.* 2006 Apr;31(4):274-352.

Habib G, Badano L, Tribouilloy C, Vilacosta I, Zamorano JL, Galderisi M, Voigt JU, Sicari R, Cosyns B, Fox K, Aakhus S; European Association of Echocardiography. Recommendations for the practice of echocardiography in infective endocarditis. *Eur J Echocardiogr.* 2010 Mar;11(2):202-19.

Habib G, Hoen B, Tornos P, Thuny F, Prendergast B, Vilacosta I, Moreillon P, de Jesus Antunes M, Thilen U, Lekakis J, Lengyel M, Müller L, Naber CK, Nihoyannopoulos P, Moritz A, Zamorano JL; ESC Committee for Practice Guidelines. Guidelines on the prevention, diagnosis, and treatment of infective endocarditis (new version 2009): the Task Force on the Prevention, Diagnosis, and Treatment of Infective Endocarditis of the European Society of Cardiology (ESC). Endorsed by the European Society of Clinical Microbiology and Infectious Diseases (ESCMID) and the International Society of Chemotherapy (ISC) for Infection and Cancer. *Eur Heart J.* 2009 Oct;30(19):2369-413.

Li JS, Sexton DJ, Mick N, Nettles R, Fowler VG Jr, Ryan T, Bashore T, Corey GR. Proposed modifications to the Duke criteria for the diagnosis of infective endocarditis. *Clin Infect Dis.* 2000 Apr;30(4):633-8.

Sedgwick JF, Burstow DJ. Update on echocardiography in the management of infective endocarditis. *Curr Infect Dis Rep.* 2012 Aug;14(4):373-80.

Thuny F, Di Salvo G, Belliard O, Avierinos JF, Pergola V, Rosenberg V, Casalta JP, Gouvernet J, Derumeaux G, Iarussi D, Ambrosi P, Calabró R, Riberi A, Collart F, Metras D, Lepidi H, Raoult D, Harle JR, Weiller PJ, Cohen A, Habib G. Risk of embolism and death in infective endocarditis: prognostic value of echocardiography: a prospective multicenter study. *Circulation.* 2005 Jul 5;112(1):69-75.

Tingleff J, Egeblad H, Gøtzsche CO, Baandrup U, Kristensen BO, Pilegaard H, Pettersson G. Perivalvular cavities in endocarditis: abscesses versus pseudoaneurysms? A transesophageal Doppler echocardiographic study in 118 patients with endocarditis. *Am Heart J.* 1995 Jul;130(1):93-100.

Tornos P, Gonzalez-Alujas T, Thuny F, Habib G. Infective endocarditis: the European viewpoint. Curr Probl Cardiol. 2011 May;36(5):175-222

Cardiac Tumours

Bruce CJ. Cardiac tumours: diagnosis and management. *Heart* 2011 Jan;97(2):151-60.

McAllister HA Jr, Hall RJ, Cooley DA. Tumors of the heart and pericardium. *Curr Probl Cardiol.* 1999 Feb;24(2):57-116

Sun JP, Asher CR, Yang XS, Cheng GG, Scalia GM, Massed AG, Griffin BP, Ratliff NB, Stewart WJ, Thomas JD. Clinical and echocardiographic characteristics of papillary fibroelastomas: a retrospective and prospective study in 162 patients. *Circulation.* 2001 Jun 5;103(22):2687-93.

Intracardiac Thrombus

Esposito R, Raia R, De Palma D, Santoro C, Galderisi M. The role of echocardiography in the management of the sources of embolism. *Future Cardiol.* 2012 Jan;8(1):101-14.

Marriott K, Manins V, Forshaw A, Wright J, Pascoe R. Detection of right-to-left atrial communication using agitated saline contrast imaging: experience with 1162 patients and recommendations for echocardiography. *J Am Soc Echocardiogr.* 2013 Jan;26(1):96-102.

Pepi M, Evangelista A, Nihoyannopoulos P, Flachskampf FA, Athanassopoulos G, Colonna P, Habib G, Ringelstein EB, Sicari R, Zamorano JL, Sitges M, Caso P. Recommendations for echocardiography use in the diagnosis and management of cardiac sources of embolism: European Association of Echocardiography (EAE) (a registered branch of the ESC). *Eur J Echocardiogr.* 2010 Jul;11(6):461-76.

Waller BF, Rohr TM, McLaughlin T, Grider L, Taliercio CP, Fetters J. Intracardiac thrombi: frequency, location, etiology, and complications: a morphologic review—Parts I - V. *Clin Cardiol.* 1995 Aug;18(8):477-9; Sep;18(9):530-4; Oct;18(10):587-90; Nov;18(11):669-74; Dec;18(12):731-4.

Normal Variants

Luetmer PH, Edwards WD, Seward JB, Tajik AJ. Incidence and distribution of left ventricular false tendons: an autopsy study of 483 normal human hearts. *J Am Coll Cardiol.* 1986 Jul;8(1):179-83.

Mügge A, Daniel WG, Angermann C, Spes C, Khandheria BK, Kronzon I, Freedberg RS, Keren A, Denning K, Engberding R, et al. Atrial septal aneurysm in adult patients. A multicenter study using transthoracic and transesophageal echocardiography. Circulation. 1995 Jun 1;91(11):2785-92.

Philip S, Cherian KM, Wu MH, Lue HC. Left ventricular false tendons: echocardiographic, morphologic, and histopathologic studies and review of the literature. *Pediatr Neonatol.* 2011 Oct;52(5):279-86.

Roldan CA, Shively BK, Crawford MH. Valve excrescences: prevalence, evolution and risk for cardioembolism. *J Am Coll Cardiol.* 1997 Nov 1;30(5):1308-14.

Systemic Diseases with Cardiac Manifestations

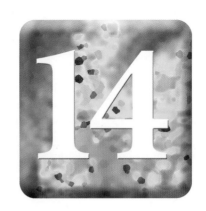

Introduction

Systemic diseases may be defined as disease processes that affect a number of tissues and/or organ systems, or diseases that affect the body as a whole. A large number of these systemic diseases can affect the cardiovascular system by causing morphologic, functional and/or haemodynamic abnormalities. Patients diagnosed with certain systemic diseases may be referred for an echocardiographic examination to determine if cardiac manifestations of the disease are present. Therefore, knowledge of the various cardiac findings associated with these diseases is important so that the sonographer is aware of what to 'look for' on the examination. Importantly, echocardiographic findings are often not diagnostic of the disease; for example, a common echocardiographic feature of hereditary connective tissue disorders is dilatation of the aorta but dilatation of the aorta cannot identify the specific hereditary connective tissue disorder. On the other hand, some systemic diseases display classic echocardiographic features; for example, carcinoid syndrome is associated with a characteristic thickening and retraction of the tricuspid valve leaflets.

In addition, the diagnosis of systemic diseases is important because some systemic diseases such as Fabry disease are potentially treatable and in other systemic diseases such as cardiac sarcoidosis early detection is crucial to help prevent sudden death.

It is beyond the scope of this chapter to include every systemic disease that affects the heart. The selected systemic diseases discussed within this chapter, along with the cardiac manifestations of these diseases, are listed in Table 14.1. Furthermore, only a brief overview of the echocardiographic findings associated with each systemic disease is included. For specific details regarding various echocardiographic appearances, measurements, and methods of quantification, readers should refer to the relevant chapters.

Systemic Rheumatic Diseases

Systemic rheumatic diseases are autoimmune inflammatory conditions with multi-organ involvement. These disorders are characterised by inflammation, degeneration, or metabolic derangement of connective tissues. The aetiology of these disorders is unknown; however, genetic, immunological and/or environment factors have been implicated.

Cardiac involvement in systemic rheumatic diseases may involve all of the cardiac structures; this includes the cardiac valves, the conduction system, the myocardium and endocardium, the pericardium, and the coronary arteries. Selected systemic rheumatic diseases are discussed below.

Ankylosing Spondylitis
Overview
'Spondylitis' refers to an inflammatory disorder of the vertebra. Ankylosing spondylitis (AKS) is a chronic and progressive inflammatory connective tissue disorder that primarily involves the vertebral and sacroiliac joints. This disease is diagnosed based on the clinical hallmark of the condition which is inflammatory back pain. The pain is of insidious onset which is worse in the morning and improves with exercise. Patients are more commonly male (male-to-female ratio ≈ 2:1 to 3:1) with the peak age of onset between 20 and 30 years. "Juvenile" AKS may occur in individuals less than 16 years of age.

The inflammatory process associated with AKS results in several cardiovascular manifestations as listed in Table 14.1. In particular, aortitis resulting in dilatation of the aorta is the most common finding of this condition. In addition, subaortic fibrosis can result in thickening of the aortomitral junction which creates a 'subaortic bump'. This subaortic bump causes retraction and decreased mobility of the anterior mitral leaflet which may lead to asymmetric or incomplete mitral leaflet coaptation and subsequent mitral regurgitation (MR).

Echocardiographic Findings
The echocardiographic examination in patients with AKS may show:
• aortic root dilatation
• aortic valve sclerosis with mild to moderate aortic regurgitation (AR)
• mild to moderate MR
When present, a subaortic bump at the base of the anterior mitral valve is best seen via transoesophageal echocardiography (TOE) (Fig. 14.1)

Rheumatoid Arthritis
Overview
Rheumatoid arthritis (RA) is a multisystem, autoimmune disease of unknown aetiology. The clinical hallmark feature of this condition is persistent inflammation of a synovial (joint-lining) membrane of the small joints of the hands and

Table 14.1 Selected Systemic Diseases and Cardiac Manifestations associated with these Diseases

Disorder	Cardiac Manifestations
Systemic Rheumatic Diseases	
Ankylosing Spondylitis	Aortitis (aortic root dilatation) (most common cardiac lesion) Aortic valvulitis +/- aortic regurgitation Subaortic fibrosis Conduction disorders
Rheumatoid Arthritis	Pericarditis (most common cardiac lesion) Constrictive pericarditis Valvular heart disease (aortic and/or mitral regurgitation, stenosis rare) Coronary artery disease Myocarditis Restrictive cardiomyopathy (due to secondary amyloidosis) Pulmonary vascular disease (pulmonary hypertension) Conduction system disease
Systemic Scleroderma	Pericarditis Constrictive pericarditis Valvular disease Myocarditis Coronary artery disease Systemic hypertension Pulmonary hypertension (due to pulmonary vascular disease) Conduction or rhythm disturbances
Systemic Lupus Erythematosus	Pericarditis (most common cardiac lesion) Constrictive pericarditis Valvular disease (e.g. Libman-Sacks endocarditis) Coronary artery disease (arteritis) Myocarditis Pulmonary vascular disease (pulmonary hypertension) Conduction system disease
Hereditary Connective Tissue Disorders	
Marfan Syndrome	Aortic regurgitation (secondary to aortic root dilatation) Aortic root and ascending aorta dilatation (most commonly at sinuses of Valsalva) Type A aortic dissection Descending thoracic aorta dilatation and dissection (uncommon) Main pulmonary artery dilatation (in absence of pulmonary valve stenosis) Mitral annular calcification (< 40 yrs of age) Mitral valve prolapse +/- mitral regurgitation
Ehlers-Danlos Syndrome, Type IV	Aortic regurgitation (secondary to aortic root dilatation) Aortic root dilatation and aortic aneurysms (most commonly at sinuses of Valsalva) Aortic valve prolapse +/- aortic regurgitation Mitral valve prolapse +/- mitral regurgitation

Loeys-Dietz Syndrome	Aortic dissection (in absence of a dilated aorta)
	Aortic regurgitation
	Aortic root dilatation and aortic aneurysms (most commonly at sinuses of Valsalva)
	Aneurysms of ascending and/or descending aorta (less common)
	Mitral valve prolapse +/- mitral regurgitation
	Congenital lesions:
	  • bicuspid aortic valve
	  • atrial septal defect
	  • patent ductus arteriosus

Table 14.1 Selected Systemic Diseases and Cardiac Manifestations associated with these Diseases (continued)

Disorder	Cardiac Manifestations
Endocrine Disorders	
Carcinoid Syndrome	Tricuspid valve disease (severe regurgitation and mild tricuspid stenosis, most common) Pulmonary valve disease (severe regurgitation and mild stenosis) Intramyocardial carcinoid metastasis (very rare)
Phaeochromocytoma	Systemic hypertension (most common) Acute myocarditis (uncommon) Dilated cardiomyopathy (uncommon) Hypertrophic cardiomyopathy Takotsubo cardiomyopathy Myocardial ischaemia Ventricular arrhythmias or other conduction disturbances
Diabetes Mellitus	Coronary artery disease (most common) Systemic hypertension Congestive heart failure Diastolic heart failure
Haemolytic Disorders	
Hypereosinophilic Syndrome	Dilated or restrictive cardiomyopathy Endomyocardial fibrosis Mural thrombi Valvular dysfunction (atrioventricular valves) Congestive heart failure Pulmonary hypertension ('primary' or secondary) Thrombembolic events (e.g. stroke or transient ischaemic attack, peripheral embolism, and/or pulmonary embolism)
Infiltrative Diseases	
Amyloidosis	Congestive heart failure Restrictive cardiomyopathy (late stage) Increased left ventricular wall thickness ('pseudohypertrophy') Pericardial effusion Valve leaflet thickening Conduction disturbances
Sarcoidosis	Congestive heart failure Dilated or restrictive cardiomyopathy Conduction disturbances and arrhythmias (most commonly complete heart block) Sudden death (from ventricular arrhythmia) Pulmonary hypertension ('primary' or secondary)
Storage Disorders	
Fabry disease	Concentric left ventricular hypertrophy (most common) Congestive heart failure Restrictive cardiomyopathy (rare) Myocardial ischaemia and infarction Valvular disease (mitral and aortic) Conduction system abnormalities
Haemochromatosis	Congestive heart failure Dilated cardiomyopathy Restrictive cardiomyopathy (advanced stage)
Hereditary Neuromuscular Diseases	
Friedreich's Ataxia	Hypertrophic cardiomyopathy (concentric and asymmetric) Dilated cardiomyopathy (late stage) Conduction system abnormalities
Duchenne's Muscular Dystrophy	Dilated cardiomyopathy Conduction system abnormalities

Figure 14.1 (A) This longitudinal transoesophageal echocardiography (TOE) view from a normal volunteer demonstrates normal aortic root walls (*small arrows*), noncoronary cusps (ncc) and right coronary cusps (rcc), aorto-mitral junction (*arrow*) and normal mobility of the anterior mitral leaflet (aml). **(B)** This TOE view from a patient with ankylosing spondylitis demonstrates moderate thickening of the aortic root predominantly of the posterior wall (*small arrows*) extending to the basal anterior mitral leaflet, forming a subaortic bump *(arrows)* and markedly decreasing its mobility (elbow sign). Mild mitral regurgitation was demonstrated. LA = left atrium; LV = left ventricle.
Reprinted from Roldan CA, Chavez J, Wiest PW, Qualls CR, Crawford MH. Aortic root disease and valve disease associated with ankylosing spondylitis, *J Am Coll Cardiol*, Vol. 32(5), page 1400, © 1998 with permission from Elsevier.

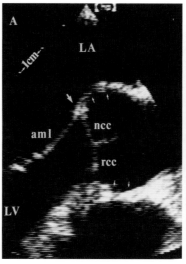
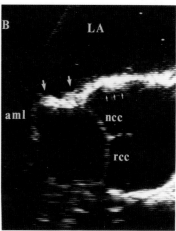

feet. This disease is diagnosed based on clinical manifestations. These clinical symptoms, present for at least 6 weeks, include morning stiffness of the joints lasting more than an hour, arthritis of three or more joint areas, arthritis of hand joints, or symmetrical arthritis; rheumatoid subcutaneous nodules may also be noted. This condition is more common in women than men (female-to-male ratio ≈ 2:1 to 3:1) with the peak age of onset between 50 and 75 years.

Cardiovascular manifestations commonly associated with RA are listed in Table 14.1. The most common cardiac manifestation is pericardial involvement. In addition, coronary artery disease (CAD) may occur due to accelerated atherosclerosis as a result of chronic inflammation and endothelial dysfunction; less commonly, CAD may occur due to coronary arteritis of the epicardial and small or medium sized intramyocardial arteries. Valvular heart disease in RA is produced by an acute, chronic or recurrent inflammatory process that leads to fibrosis of the leaflets, annulus and sub-valvular apparatus and the formation of nodules on the valve leaflets (Fig. 14.2). The aortic and mitral valves are most commonly affected by RA. Less commonly, nodules may be seen at the papillary muscle tips, atrial or ventricular endocardium, or on the aortic root wall.

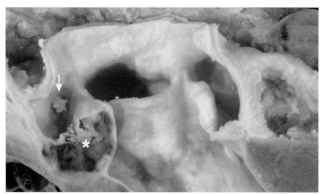

Figure 14.2 This gross pathological specimen shows an open aortic valve from a patient with rheumatoid arthritis. There is marked thickening of the semilunar leaflets with no fusion of the commissures. The right coronary sinus is partially filled with friable and bloody material (*asterisk*). A small vegetation is also seen (*arrow*).
Reproduced from Killinger LC, Gutierrez PS. Clinicopathologic session. Case 5/2001 - Heart failure and insufficiency of the aortic and mitral valves in a 68-year-old woman with rheumatoid arthritis. Arq Bras Cardiol. Vol.77(4), page 376, (c) 2001 with permission from Professor Alfredo J Mansur (Session Editor). Colour image kindly provided by Dr. Vera Demarchi Aiello, Laboratory of Pathology, Heart Institute (InCor), University of Sao Paulo School of Medicine, Brazil.

Echocardiographic Findings

Echocardiographic findings in RA are dependent on the level and extent of cardiac structure involvement. As mentioned above, pericardial involvement is most common; therefore, pericardial effusions +/- pericardial thickening are often seen. Valvular involvement appears as diffuse or localised sclerosis or thickening of the mitral and aortic leaflets with varying degrees of mitral and aortic regurgitation. In addition, valvular nodules may be seen. These nodules appear as homogenous, small (4–12 mm) oval-shaped lesions with well-defined borders; nodules are typically located at the basal or mid portions of the aortic and/or mitral valve leaflets (Fig. 14.3). Due to the superior resolution of TOE, these nodules are often better appreciated via this imaging modality.

Other abnormalities that may be seen on the echocardiographic examination include:

- left ventricular (LV) systolic dysfunction,
- regional wall motion abnormalities (RWMA) when there is associated CAD,
- signs of pulmonary hypertension; for example, increased tricuspid regurgitant velocity,
- features of a restrictive cardiomyopathy (see Amyloidosis below).

Systemic Scleroderma

Overview

Scleroderma is an autoimmune disease whereby excessive collagen accumulates in the skin, blood vessels, joints, skeletal muscles, and/or other organs including the heart. This condition is much more commonly seen in women (female-to-male ratio ≈ 4:1 to 9:1) with the peak age of onset between 30 and 50 years.

There are two major forms of scleroderma: (1) localised scleroderma and (2) systemic scleroderma (SSc). Localised scleroderma only affects the skin and there is no internal organ involvement whereas SSc is a multisystem disorder with multiple organ involvement.

SSc is further divided into two major clinical variants based on the extent of skin involvement. In the limited cutaneous type of SSc, skin changes are limited to the face and distal portion of the extremities, and the heart is generally spared. In the diffuse cutaneous type of SSc, there is symmetric fibrosis of the skin of the face, trunk, and extremities and involvement of the kidney, lung, and heart.

The initial diagnosis of SSc is based on the characteristic finding of skin thickening in association with Raynaud's phenomenon. A number of other diagnostic tests can then be performed to confirm the diagnosis.

Cardiac manifestations of SSc are listed in Table 14.1. The most common cardiac manifestation of this disease is pericardial involvement. Other cardiac manifestations occur secondary to other organ diseases (for example, renal or lung disease) or due to myocardial fibrosis, autonomic neuropathy, or small coronary vessel disease. In particular, CAD may occur due to endothelial damage of small coronary arteries. Myocardial ischaemia or infarction and myocardial dysfunction may then occur as a result of CAD or due to myocardial fibrosis or impaired vasodilation.

Importantly, pulmonary arterial hypertension (PAH) is an important complication of SSc and is a major cause of morbidity and mortality in these patients. PAH in SSc can result from intrinsic pulmonary artery disease or from interstitial fibrosis.

Echocardiographic Findings

Echocardiographic findings associated with SSc depend upon the level and extent of cardiac involvement. As mentioned above, pericardial involvement is most common; therefore, pericardial effusions +/- pericardial thickening are often seen. Due to the association of myocarditis, CAD and myocardial ischaemia with SSc, a careful evaluation of LV systolic function, including regional wall motion analysis, and LV diastolic function is required.

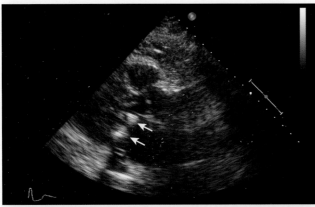

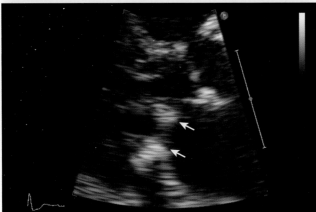

Figure 14.3 These images were recorded from a patient with rheumatoid arthritis. The parasternal long axis view *(top)* and the zoomed view of the mitral valve *(bottom)* demonstrate nodules located within the mid portion of the mitral leaflets *(arrows)*. These nodules appear as oval, echogenic lesions and are characteristic of valvular nodules associated with rheumatic arthritis. Observe that the tips of the mitral leaflets appear normal.

As PAH is a major cause of morbidity and mortality in SSc, estimation of the right ventricular systolic pressure (RVSP) via Doppler echocardiography and the evaluation of other signs of pulmonary hypertension is important in these patients. In particular, echocardiographic screening for PAH is usually recommended for all patients with SSc.

Other abnormalities that may be seen on the echocardiographic examination include:

- increased LV wall thickness (due to systemic hypertension)
- valvular disease (mild sclerosis of the mitral or aortic valves without significant regurgitation).

Systemic Lupus Erythematosus

Overview

Systemic lupus erythematosus (SLE) is a chronic multisystem, autoimmune disorder that results in a chronic or recurrent inflammatory disease predominately affecting the musculoskeletal and mucocutaneous systems.

There is a geographical and ethnic variation in SLE. For example, in the United States of America, the prevalence of the disease is higher among Asian, African, Caribbean, and Hispanic Americans compared with Americans of European decent; and in New Zealand, the prevalence of SLE is higher in Polynesians than in Caucasians. In addition, while this disease is more common in women than men, the female-to-male ratio varies according to age. For example, in adults, especially in women of child-bearing age, the ratio ranges from 7:1 to 15:1, while in 'older' individuals such as post-menopausal women, the ratio is ≈ 8:1.

The diagnosis of this disease is based on a positive antinuclear antibody (ANA) and the other clinical findings such as fever, joint pain and a malar rash ('butterfly', erythematous rash over the cheeks and nasal bridge).

Cardiac manifestations associated with SLE are listed in Table 14.1. The most common cardiac manifestation of this disease is pericardial involvement. In addition, CAD due to SLE is thought to occur due to an autoimmune vascular injury that predisposes the coronary arteries to atherosclerotic plaque formation. Valvular disease, which is also commonly encountered in SLE, occurs due to an autoimmune response resulting in an acute, chronic, or recurrent inflammation of the valve leaflets. Valvular abnormalities associated with SLE include leaflet thickening, valvular regurgitation, and valvular masses or vegetations; the mitral valve is most commonly affected.

Valvular vegetations associated with SLE are referred to as Libman-Sacks endocarditis. Libman-Sacks endocarditis, also known as verrucous, marantic, or nonbacterial thrombotic endocarditis, is almost exclusively found on the left-sided cardiac valves, especially the mitral valve. On gross inspection, these vegetations appear as wart-like (verrucous), reddish-tan lesions, usually less than 1 cm^2 in size, on the free edges or closure lines of cardiac valves (Fig. 14.4). When present on the mitral valve, these lesions are usually seen on the atrial side of the mitral valve. When present on the aortic valve, these vegetations are typically seen on the ventricular side or aortic side of the aortic valve. Importantly, extensive lesions can deform the valve leading to significant valvular regurgitation.

Echocardiographic Findings

As mentioned above, pericardial involvement is most common; therefore, pericardial effusions +/- pericardial thickening are often seen. Valvular thickening and valvular regurgitation are also commonly seen. When present, Libman-Sacks vegetations appear as heterogeneous, echogenic lesions that are round with irregular borders and usually less than 1 cm² in size (Fig. 14.5); lesions are attached to the atrial surface of the mitral valve and the aortic or ventricular side of the aortic valve and display no independent motion.

> Libman-Sacks vegetations can be found in approximately 1 in 10 patients (or 10% of patients) with SLE. The most frequently involved valve is the mitral valve followed by the aortic valve. Patients who have Libman-Sacks vegetations have a longer disease duration and higher disease activity. Furthermore, these patients are at greater risk of cerebral ischaemic events than those without these lesions.
>
> **Source:** Moyssakis I, Tektonidou MG, Vasilliou VA, Samarkos M, Votteas V, Moutsopoulos HM. Libman-Sacks endocarditis in systemic lupus erythematosus: prevalence, associations, and evolution. *Am J Med.* 2007 Jul;120(7):636-42.

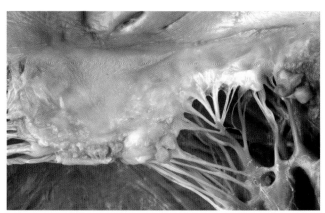

Figure 14.4 This gross pathological specimen from a patient with systemic lupus erythematosus shows Libman-Sacks endocarditis of the mitral valve. Observe the characteristic multiple wart-like, tan masses on the atrial side of the valve; these lesions may occur along the free edge or closing edge of the mitral valve, the ventricular aspect of the leaflets, or on the tendinous cords.
By permission of Mayo Foundation for Medical Education and Research. All rights reserved. Courtesy of William D. Edwards, MD.

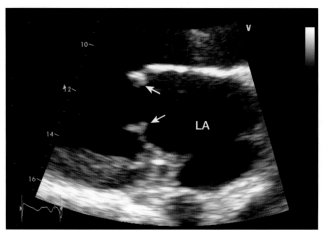

Figure 14.5 Libman–Sacks vegetations of the mitral valve are shown on a zoomed parasternal long axis view. Observe the nodular, echogenic masses on the left atrial (LA) side of the anterior and posterior mitral leaflets (*arrows*).

Other cardiac abnormalities that may be detected on the echocardiographic examination include:
- signs of pulmonary hypertension (for example, increased tricuspid regurgitant velocity),
- RWMA secondary to myocardial infarction.

> **Libman-Sacks versus Infective Endocarditis**
> Patients with SLE may have some clinical features consistent with infective endocarditis (IE); therefore, Libman-Sacks endocarditis may be confused with IE. Libman-Sacks endocarditis can be differentiated from IE based on the echocardiographic features of the lesion as cited below. It is important to note, however, that IE can coexist with Libman-Sacks vegetations.
>
> | | Infective Endocarditis | Libman-Sacks Endocarditis |
> |---|---|---|
> | Location | Almost always located at the line of leaflet closure | Predominantly located near the leaflet base |
> | Appearance | Usually homogeneous soft tissue density | Usually heterogeneous echodensity with central regions of high reflectance suggesting connective tissue or even calcific density |
> | Mobility | Vibratory or rotatory motion at least partly independent of the motion of the valve | Do not display independent motion; masses exactly parallel motion of related leaflet |
>
> **Source:** Roldan CA, Shively BK, Lau CC, Gurule FT, Smith EA, Crawford MH. Systemic lupus erythematosus valve disease by transesophageal echocardiography and the role of antiphospholipid antibodies. *J Am Coll Cardiol.* 1992 Nov 1;20(5):1127-34.

Hereditary Connective Tissue Disorders

As the name suggests, connective tissue disorders are diseases featuring abnormalities involving the connective tissues, most commonly collagen and elastin. There are more than 200 disorders that affect connective tissues including systemic rheumatic diseases as discussed above. This section focuses on selected hereditary connective tissue disorders.

Hereditary connective tissue disorders are diagnosed based on physical findings and the identification of the causative genetic mutation (Table 14.2). In particular, these syndromes are autosomal-dominant diseases; this means that the offspring of an affected parent have a 50% risk of inheriting the disease (Fig. 14.6). Therefore, echocardiographic examinations are frequently requested for all first-degree relatives of patients with hereditary connective tissue syndromes.

The most common cardiovascular manifestation of these disorders is dilatation of the aorta.

Marfan Syndrome

Overview

Marfan syndrome (MFS) is the most common of the hereditary connective tissue disorders. This syndrome is characterised by skeletal, cardiovascular and ocular features (Table 14.2). Approximately 75% of cases are familial (inherited as an autosomal dominant trait) while 25% of cases are sporadic (that is, the mutation occurs spontaneously and may be associated with older paternal age).

The diagnosis of this syndrome is based on the family history, clinical findings and identification of the defective gene. Clinical findings are based on the Ghent criteria which identifiy major and minor manifestations in a number of organ systems including the skeletal, ocular, cardiovascular, pulmonary, dura, and integumentary systems [14.1].

Cardiac manifestations of MFS are listed in Table 14.1. In particular, a loss of elastic tissue in the aortic wall results in medial degeneration which weakens the aortic walls leading to aortic dilatation and aortic aneurysms (mostly at the level of the sinuses of Valsalva), and possible type A aortic dissections.

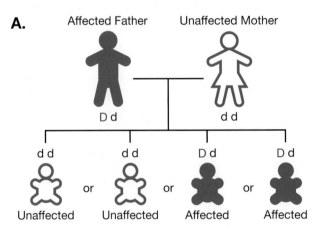

A.

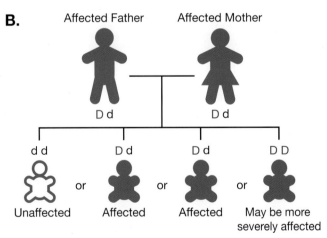

B.

Figure 14.6 These schematics illustrate the mode of inheritance of autosomal dominant disorders. **Panel A** shows how the disorder may be passed on when one parent has the autosomal dominant faulty gene. In this situation, there is a 50% chance that the child will inherit the faulty gene and will therefore be affected by, or be predisposed to developing the disease. **Panel B** shows how the disease may be passed on when both parents have the autosomal dominant faulty gene. In this situation, there is a 75% chance that the child will inherit the faulty gene from one parent and will therefore be affected by, or be predisposed to developing the disease. There is also a 25% chance that the child will inherit the faulty gene from both parents. In this case, the child may be more severely affected by the disease. **D** = faulty dominant gene, **d** = unaffected or normal gene.

Echocardiographic Findings

Echocardiography has a very important role in the assessment of MFS. In particular, characteristic echocardiographic features of a dilated aorta in conjunction with mitral valve prolapse (MVP) are often associated with this syndrome (Fig. 14.7). Most importantly, careful and accurate measurements of the aortic dimensions are required. Annual echocardiographic examinations are recommended for all patients with MFS to monitor the size of the aortic root and the annual rate of growth of the aortic dimensions. If the maximal aortic diameter is 4.5 cm or greater, or if the aortic diameter shows significant growth from baseline, more frequent review is required.

Echocardiography is also valuable in the:
- assessment of the degree of MR (secondary to MVP),
- assessment of the aetiology and degree of AR (secondary to aortic root dilatation),
- identification of dilatation of the main pulmonary artery (in the absence of pulmonary valve stenosis),
- identification of mitral annular calcification (< 40 yrs of age),
- diagnosis of a type A aortic dissection.

Ehlers-Danlos Syndrome

Overview

Ehlers-Danlos syndrome (EDS) refers to a group of inherited, connective tissue disorders that are characterised by joint hypermobility, cutaneous fragility and hyperextensibility.

There are more than 10 different types of disorders associated with EDS. The type that is most relevant with respect to cardiovascular involvement is EDS type IV, the vascular type of EDS. This type of EDS is defined by four features: (1) facial acrogeria (emaciated face with prominent cheekbones and sunken cheeks), (2) translucent skin with highly visible subcutaneous vessels on the trunk and lower back, (3) easy bruising, and (4) severe arterial, digestive and uterine complications.

The diagnosis of this syndrome is based on the family history, clinical features and identification of the defective gene.

The pathophysiology and, therefore, the cardiovascular manifestations of EDS type IV are very similar to MFS; these manifestations are listed in Table 14.1.

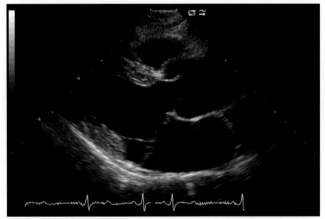

Figure 14.7 This image was recorded from a parasternal long axis view in a patient with Marfan syndrome. Observe that there is effacement of the aorta with aortic root dilatation (the aortic root measured 4.5 cm). Bileaflet mitral valve prolapse is also noted on this systolic frame.

[14.1] Loeys BL, Dietz HC, Braverman AC, et al. The revised Ghent nosology for the Marfan syndrome. *J Med Genet.* 2010 Jul;47(7):476-85.

Echocardiographic Findings

The most common echocardiographic findings associated with EDS, type IV include:

- Aortic root dilatation +/- AR,
- Aortic valve prolapse +/- AR,
- Mitral valve prolapse +/- MR,
- Aortic aneurysm at the sinus of Valsalva,
- Type A aortic dissection.

Loeys-Dietz Syndrome

Overview

The Loeys-Dietz syndrome (LDS) is an inherited, autosomal dominant aortic aneurysm syndrome with widespread systemic involvement. Importantly, individuals with this syndrome have a high risk of aneurysm and dissection throughout the arterial tree.

LDS is typically characterised by the triad of: (1) hypertelorism (wide-set eyes), cleft palate or bifid uvula, (2) arterial/aortic aneurysms, and (3) arterial tortuosity.

LDS is classified into two types based on the presence or absence of craniofacial characteristics. Type 1, the most common type, displays these craniofacial characteristics while in type 2 these craniofacial characteristics are absent.

Individuals with LDS also have other clinical features. For example type 1 LDS has skeletal features similar to MFS while type 2 LDS has skin features similar to EDS type IV.

The diagnosis of this syndrome is based on the family history, clinical features and identification of the defective gene.

The cardiovascular manifestations of LDS are very similar to MFS and EDS type IV; these manifestations are listed in Table 14.1. An important difference between LDS and MFS and EDS type IV is that cardiovascular disease in LDS is more aggressive and widespread.

Echocardiographic Findings

An important complication of LDS is aortic dissection which can occur *without* marked aortic dilatation. Furthermore, aortic dissection or rupture commonly occurs in childhood. Therefore, due to the aggressive nature of this syndrome, aortic imaging is required at frequent intervals, usually every 6 months, to monitor the status and growth of the ascending aorta.

Other common echocardiographic findings associated with LDS include:

- aortic root dilatation and aortic aneurysms (most commonly at the sinuses of Valsalva)
- ascending and/or descending aortic aneurysms (less common)
- AR (secondary to aortic root dilatation)
- mitral valve prolapse +/- MR.

In addition, certain congenital lesions are more frequently seen in LDS patients than in a normal population [14.2]. These lesions include a bicuspid aortic valve, atrial septal defects and patent ductus arteriosus.

An important and often lethal complication of Marfan syndrome (MFS) and Loeys-Dietz syndrome (LDS) is Type A aortic dissection. For this reason, elective surgical repair of the dilated aortic root/ascending aorta is recommended:

- in MFS: when the aorta reaches 5 cm, when there is rapid growth of the aorta (> 0.5 cm per year), when there is a family history of aortic dissections, or the presence of significant aortic regurgitation
- in LDS: when the aortic diameter is ≥ 4.2 cm by TOE (internal diameter) or 4.4 to 4.6 cm or greater by CT imaging and/or MRI (external diameter).

Source: Hiratzka LF, Bakris GL, Beckman JA, et al. 2010 ACCF/AHA/AATS/ACR/ASA/SCA/SCAI/SIR/STS/SVM guidelines for the diagnosis and management of patients with thoracic aortic disease. *J Am Coll Cardiol.* 2010 Apr 6;55(14):e27-e129.

Table 14.2 Genetic Defects and Common Clinical Features of Selected Hereditary Connective Tissue Disorders

Disorder	Genetic Defect	Common Clinical Features
Marfan Syndrome	FBN1 mutations	Skeletal features: • Arachnodactyly (abnormally long and thin digits) • Dolichostenomelia (long limbs relative to trunk length) • Pectus (chest wall) deformities; e.g. pectus excavatum & pectus carinatum • Kyphoscoliosis (front-to-back and side-to-side curvature of the spinal column) • Dolichocephaly (head is disproportionately long and narrow) Ectopia lentis (Abnormal position of the lens of the eye) Dural ectasia (widening or ballooning of the dural sac surrounding the spinal cord)
Ehlers-Danlos Syndrome, Type IV	COL3A1 mutations	Thin, translucent skin Friable tissues Gastrointestinal rupture Rupture of gravid uterus Rupture of medium-sized to large arteries
Loeys-Dietz Syndrome	TGFBR2 or TGFBR1 mutations	Bifid uvula or cleft palate Hypertelorism (wide-set eyes) Craniosynostosis (abnormal head shape) Skeletal features similar to Marfan syndrome Arterial tortuosity Aneurysms and dissections of other arteries

COL3A1 = procollagen type III, alpha 1 gene; FBN1 = fibrillin -1 gene; TGFBR1 = genetic mutation to transforming growth factor receptor Type I; TGFBR2 = genetic mutation to transforming growth factor receptor Type II gene.

[14.2] Van Hemelrijk C, Renard M, Loeys B. The Loeys-Dietz syndrome: an update for the clinician. *Curr Opin Cardiol.* 2010 Nov;25(6):546-5

Endocrine Disorders

Endocrine disorders may be subdivided into three groups: (1) endocrine gland hyposecretion (leading to hormone deficiency), (2) endocrine gland hypersecretion (leading to hormone excess), and (3) endocrine gland tumours (benign or malignant). Importantly, tumours of endocrine glands resulting in carcinoid syndrome and phaeochromocytoma, and endocrine gland hyposecretion such as diabetes mellitus are associated with cardiac manifestations; these disorders are discussed below.

Carcinoid Syndrome

Overview

Carcinoid tumours are neuroendocrine tumours that usually arise from the gastrointestinal tract and, rarely, from other sites such as the bronchus, biliary tract, pancreas, ovaries or testes. Carcinoid symptoms typically occur between the fifth and seventh decades of life with males and females being equally affected.

Carcinoid syndrome is most commonly caused by metastatic carcinoid tumours which secrete excessive amounts of the hormone serotonin. This syndrome is characterised clinically by: (1) cutaneous flushing of head and neck, (2) diarrhoea, and (3) bronchoconstriction causing asthma-like attacks. The diagnosis of metastatic carcinoid syndrome is based on the presence of elevated levels of the serotonin metabolite 5-hydroxyindoleacetic acid (5-HIAA) in a 24-hour urine sample.

Carcinoid heart disease is reported in approximately 50-60% of all patients with carcinoid syndrome with right heart disease being severe in 25% of patients. The cardiac manifestations of this disorder are listed in Table 14.1. The postulated pathogenesis of cardiac involvement is related to increased

> The majority of carcinoid tumours arise from the appendix. However, these tumours are neither invasive nor metastatic and, therefore, they do not cause the carcinoid syndrome.

circulating quantities of serotonin. These substances form thick, pearly white plaque-like deposits on the endocardial surfaces of the tricuspid and pulmonary valves and the endocardium (Fig. 14.8). These plaques cause the right-sided valves to become thickened, retracted and rigid. Therefore, the valve becomes both stenotic and regurgitant; the tricuspid valve is most commonly affected. Intramyocardial metastases also rarely occur. Because the humoral substances are inactivated by the lungs, cardiac lesions of the left side of the heart are rare unless there is a right-to-left shunt present.

Echocardiographic Findings

On the 2D examination, the tricuspid valve has a characteristic appearance where the leaflets appear thickened and retracted; as a result the valve remains in a fixed semi-open position throughout the cardiac cycle (Fig. 14.9). Due to the incomplete coaptation of the tricuspid leaflets during systole, severe tricuspid regurgitation (TR) is present on colour Doppler imaging (Fig. 14.10). The continuous-wave spectral Doppler signal of severe TR also shows a characteristic profile (Fig. 14.11).

When there is pulmonary valve involvement, the pulmonary valve will appear similar to the tricuspid valve (Fig. 14.12). That is, the pulmonary leaflets appear thickened, retracted and remain in a fixed semi-open position throughout the cardiac cycle. The colour Doppler examination will show moderate to severe pulmonary regurgitation (PR); mild pulmonary stenosis is also usually present.

Due to volume overloading of the right heart chambers secondary to severe TR +/- PR, moderate to marked dilatation of the right heart chambers as well as abnormal interventricular septal motion will be seen.

Left heart involvement in carcinoid syndrome is uncommon. However, evidence of mitral and/or aortic valve thickening should alert the sonographer to a possible patent foramen ovale (PFO) with right-to-left shunting. The presence of a PFO can be confirmed by an agitated saline contrast study (Fig. 14.13).

A metastatic tumour embedded within the myocardium is rarely seen (Fig. 14.14).

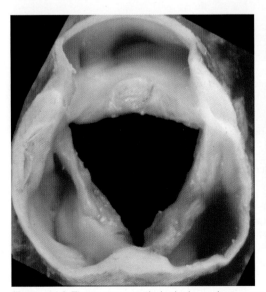
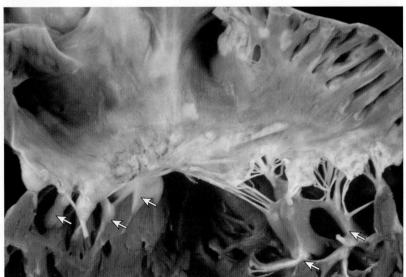

Figure 14.8 These gross pathological specimens are from two different patients with carcinoid syndrome. Observe that the leaflets of the pulmonary valve *(left)* and tricuspid valve *(right)* are thickened and retracted. Also observe the characteristic endocardial plaques that appear as thick, white deposits associated with the tricuspid valve *(arrows)*. By permission of Mayo Foundation for Medical Education and Research. All rights reserved. Courtesy of William D. Edwards, MD.

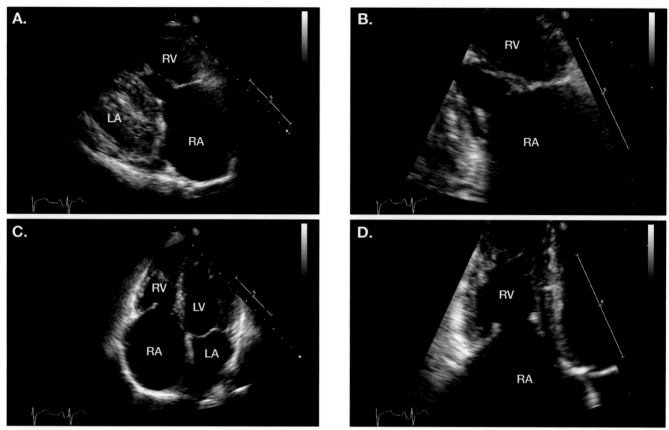

Figure 14.9 Images show the characteristic features of carcinoid tricuspid valve disease as seen from a parasternal long axis view of the right ventricular inflow **(A)**, a zoomed parasternal long axis view of right ventricular inflow **(B)**, an apical 4-chamber view **(C)** and a zoomed apical 4-chamber view **(D)**. Observe on these systolic frames that the tricuspid valve leaflets appear thickened and retracted and are in a fixed, semi-open position. LA = left atrium; LV = left ventricle; RA = right atrium; RV = right ventricle.

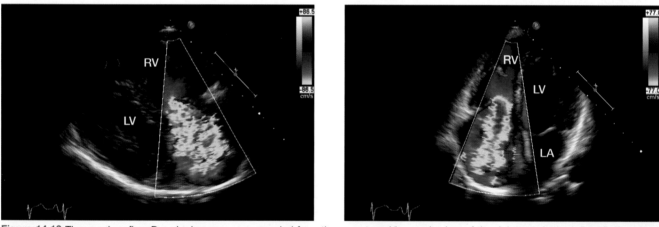

Figure 14.10 These colour flow Doppler images were recorded from the parasternal long axis view of the right ventricular inflow (*left*) and the apical 4-chamber view (*right*). Observe that there is severe tricuspid regurgitation (TR) into a dilated right atrium. TR occurs due to incomplete coaptation of the valve during systole. LA = left atrium; LV = left ventricle; RV = right ventricle.

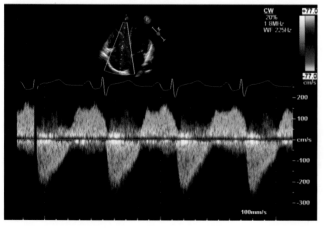

Figure 14.11 This continuous-wave Doppler signal of tricuspid regurgitation (TR) shows the characteristic features of severe TR. Observe that: **(1)** the intensity of the TR signal is strong which indicates that there is a large number of red blood cells moving within the Doppler beam during systole; **(2)** there is a "V cut-off" sign which reflects a rapid decline in the pressure gradient between the right ventricle and the right atrium (RA) in late systole which is caused by a significant increase in the RA pressure due to severe TR; and **(3)** there are increased forward flow velocities which are caused by an increased stroke volume (SV) across the tricuspid valve during diastole. In particular, the increased SV through the valve during diastole occurs because this SV includes the 'normal' volume returning to the RA from the vena cava and coronary sinus plus the regurgitant volume that leaked across the valve in systole. However, it is important to note that increased velocities may also occur with carcinoid tricuspid valve disease because of coexisting tricuspid stenosis.

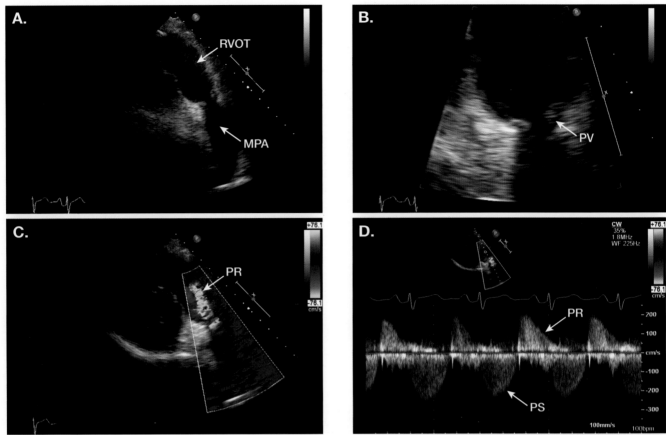

Figure 14.12 These images were recorded from a patient with features of carcinoid pulmonary valve disease. From the unzoomed and zoomed views recorded from the parasternal long axis view of the right ventricular outflow tract (RVOT), the pulmonary valve (PV) appears thickened, fixed, and retracted **(A and B)**. The colour Doppler image recorded from the parasternal long axis view of the RVOT during diastole demonstrates the turbulent pulmonary regurgitant (PR) jet **(C)**. The continuous-wave Doppler trace recorded across the pulmonary valve shows mild pulmonary stenosis (PS) as well as PR **(D)**. Observe that the PR signal has a short deceleration time which reflects a rapid decline in the pressure gradient between the pulmonary artery and the right ventricle (RV) during diastole which is caused by a significant increase in the RV diastolic pressure due to severe PR.

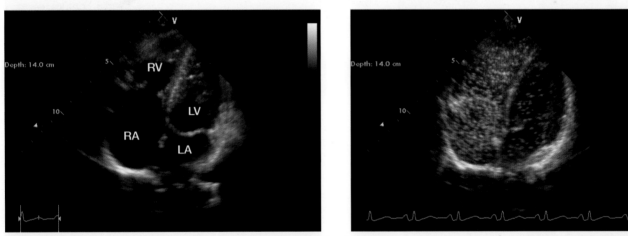

Figure 14.13 The apical 4-chamber view recorded in systole shows the characteristic appearance of a carcinoid tricuspid valve with thickened and retracted leaflets (*left*). Mitral involvement was also suspected so an agitated saline contrast study was performed; the appearance of contrast bubbles within the left heart confirmed the presence of a right-to-left shunt across a patent foramen ovale (*right*).

Phaeochromocytoma

Overview

Phaeochromocytoma is a rare and generally benign, catecholamine-secreting tumour of chromaffin cells. The majority of tumours (85-90%) are located within the adrenal medulla of the adrenal glands (Fig. 14.15). Approximately 10% of tumours are located outside the kidneys (extra-adrenal paraganglia); cardiac phaeochromocytomas are extremely rare. Although phaeochromocytomas may occur at any age, they are most common in the fourth to fifth decades of life with males and females being equally affected. The diagnosis of phaeochromocytomas is based on the detection of increased levels of catecholamines in the blood and urine.

The majority of patients with phaeochromoctyma will have systemic hypertension which may be persistent or paroxysmal. In particular, a life-threatening cardiovascular manifestation of phaeochromocytoma includes a hypertensive crisis which results from a rapid and massive release of catecholamines from the tumour. Other cardiac manifestations of this disorder are listed in Table 14.1; these disorders mostly occur as a result of high levels of circulating catecholamines.

Echo Examination

Most patients with phaeochromocytomas will have a normal echocardiogram. However, abnormal findings may include:

• concentric left ventricular hypertrophy (LVH) (secondary to systemic hypertension)

• RWMA (secondary to myocardial infarction)

• echocardiographic features of dilated, hypertrophic or Takotsubo cardiomyopathies.

As mentioned above primary cardiac phaeochromocytomas are extremely rare. However, when present these tumours may be identified based on their characteristic echocardiographic appearance. Cardiac tumours tend to be located at the base of the heart (that is, along the atrioventricular groove or near the origin of great arteries), they are well-circumscribed and are round or ovoid in shape, and the tumours have a homogeneous or fine granular appearance (Fig. 14.16).

Diabetes Mellitus

Overview

Diabetes mellitus (DM) refers to a group of metabolic disorders characterised by chronic hyperglycaemia and other abnormalities in carbohydrate, fat and protein metabolism that arise as a result of defects in insulin secretion, insulin

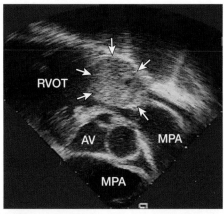

Figure 14.14 This transoesophageal echocardiogram was performed on a patient with carcinoid syndrome. This image shows a well circumscribed mass within the wall of the right ventricular outflow tract (RVOT) causing significant RVOT obstruction. This appearance is consistent with an intramyocardial carcinoid metastasis. AV = aortic valve; MPA = main pulmonary artery.

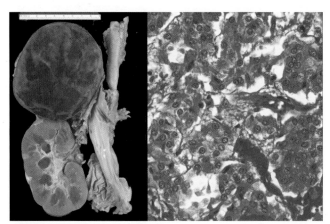

Figure 14.15 The gross pathological specimen shows a very large phaeochromocytoma of the adrenal gland which appears superior to the kidney (left). The histology specimen of the phaeochromocytoma reveals characteristic nests (zellballen) of tumour cells (right). By permission of Mayo Foundation for Medical Education and Research. All rights reserved. Courtesy of William D. Edwards, MD.

action, or a combination of both. The effects of DM include long-term damage, dysfunction and failure of various organs. There are three main types of diabetes:

1. Type 1 diabetes mellitus (T1DM): results from insulin deficiency due to a destruction of pancreatic β-cells by either an autoimmune mechanism or an unknown cause. T1DM mostly occurs in young patients and is usually detected before 30 years of age. This type of DM is also known as insulin-dependent diabetes mellitus (IDDM) or juvenile diabetes.

2. Type 2 diabetes mellitus (T2DM): is the most common type of DM which occurs due to a combination of decreased insulin secretion and decreased insulin sensitivity (insulin resistance). T2DM is frequently associated with obesity and decreased physical activity. This type of DM is also known as non-insulin dependent diabetes mellitus (NIDDM). As the onset of this type of DM typically occurs in patients over 40 years of age, it is also referred to as adult-onset diabetes mellitus (AODM). However, it should be noted that this type of DM is increasingly being diagnosed in children and adolescents.

3. Gestational diabetes mellitus (GDM): is defined as glucose intolerance with the first onset or first recognition occurring during pregnancy.

The diagnosis of T1DM and T2DM is based on clinical features and laboratory tests such as a fasting plasma glucose test and urine blood sugar levels.

The cardiac manifestations of DM are listed in Table 14.1. Importantly, CAD is the leading cause of morbidity and mortality in DM.

Insulin is a hormone that is secreted by β-cells of the pancreatic islets of Langerhans. Insulin contributes to carbohydrate, fat, and protein metabolism; in particular, insulin facilitates glucose entry into muscle, adipose and several other tissues. In diabetes mellitus, a decreased production of insulin or a reduction in the effectiveness of insulin results in the failure or a decrease of glucose absorption into the cells. This leads to increased blood glucose levels which leads to the formation of advanced glycation end products (AGEs). These AGEs cause inflammatory conditions of the vasculature and contribute to the accelerated development of atherosclerosis.

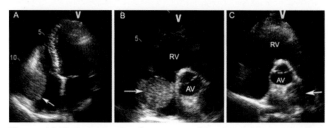

Figure 14.16 An example of a rare cardiac phaeochromocytoma is shown from the apical 4-chamber view (A) and from the parasternal short axis views at the aortic valve level (B and C). From the apical 4-chamber view, a tumour is seen near the right atrioventricular groove (arrow). From the parasternal short axis view the tumour (arrow) appears encapsulated (B). Another tumour (arrow) was located between the aortic root, left atrium roof and pulmonary artery (C). AV = aortic valve; RV = right ventricle.
Reproduced from Li L, Zhu W, Fang L, Zeng Z, Miao Q, Zhang C, Fang Q. Transthoracic Echocardiographic Features of Cardiac Pheochromocytoma: A Single-Institution Experience. *Echocardiography*. Feb;29(2): page 155, © 2012 John Wiley and Sons with permission.

Echocardiographic Findings

Echocardiography has an important role in the assessment of patients with DM. In particular, echocardiography is able to:
• assess LV systolic function,
• identify RWMAs associated with CAD,
• identify increased LV wall thickness due to systemic hypertension,
• evaluate diastolic dysfunction.

In addition, stress echocardiography in patients with DM is useful for risk stratification, investigating inducible ischaemia and for the assessment of myocardial viability.

Haematologic Disorders

Haematologic diseases are disorders which primarily affect the blood. An example of a haematologic disorder with cardiac manifestations is hypereosinophilic syndrome; this disorder is discussed below.

Hypereosinophilic Syndrome

Overview

Hypereosinophilic syndromes (HES) are a group of rare disorders characterised by persistent overproduction of eosinophils which is not due to other underlying diseases known to cause increases in eosinophils. HES is usually diagnosed between the ages of 20 to 50 years. Several variants of HES have been identified based on clinical features and specific aetiological abnormalities with certain variants almost exclusively seen in males (myeloproliferative variants) while other variants affect males and females equally.

The criteria for the diagnosis of HES include: (1) sustained eosinophilia ($> 1.5 \times 10^9$ eosinophils/L) for more than six months or documented on at least two occasions, (2) an absence of other causes of eosinophilia (such as parasitic infection, allergic diseases, drug-induced or chemical-induced eosinophilia, eosinophilic pneumonias or malignancies), and (3) signs and symptoms of multiple organ involvement (such as heart failure, gastrointestinal dysfunction, central nervous system abnormalities, fever or weight loss).

Cardiac involvement in HES is a major cause of morbidity and mortality. It generally develops in three stages:

1. The acute necrotic stage is characterised by eosinophilic infiltration of the endocardium and myocardium.

2. The thrombotic stage follows the acute stage with the formation of mural thrombi on the surfaces of the denuded myocardium, often involving the apices of both ventricles and the ventricular surfaces of the atrioventricular (AV) valves (Fig. 14.17); thromboembolism may occur during this stage.

3. The fibrotic stage results in the replacement of thrombus by fibrosis. Endomyocardial fibrosis causes a restrictive or dilated cardiomyopathy; when the AV valves are involved valvular regurgitation ensues.

Löeffler's Endocarditis
Obliteration of the ventricular apices by infiltrating eosinophils is also referred to as Löeffler's endocarditis. However, the cases first described by Wilhelm Löeffler in 1932 were of eosinophilic pneumonia caused by a parasitic infection rather than due to idiopathic HES.

The cardiac manifestations of HES are listed in Table 14.1. In particular, pulmonary hypertension may occur due to primary eosinophilic infiltration of lung parenchyma or secondary to left heart disease. Thromboembolic events may occur secondarily to the presence of intracardiac thrombus.

Echocardiographic Findings

Echocardiographic findings associated with HES include:
• endocardial thickening and fibrous (that is, endomyocardial fibrosis),
• mural thrombus of the ventricular apices with apical obliteration (Fig. 14.18),
• thickening, adhesion and tethering of the posterior mitral leaflet to the LV wall,
• significant MR due to restricted motion of the posterior mitral leaflet as above,
• features of restrictive cardiomyopathy.

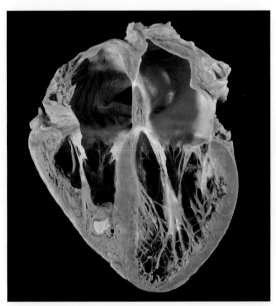

Figure 14.17 This is a gross pathological specimen of a heart from a patient with hypereosinophilic syndrome. Observe the thrombus within the apex of the right ventricle and the fibrosis/thrombus associated with the posterior mitral leaflet. By permission of Mayo Foundation for Medical Education and Research. All rights reserved. Courtesy of William D. Edwards, MD.

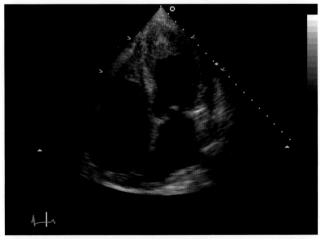

Figure 14.18 This image was recorded from the apical 4-chamber view during systole. Observe the abnormal "filling in" of the apices of both the right and left ventricles. This appearance is a characteristic feature of hypereosinophilic syndrome with apical obliteration occurring due to thrombus formation.

Hypereosinophilic Syndrome versus Tropical Endomyocardial Fibrosis

Endomyocardial fibrosis (EMF) can occur in idiopathic hypereosinophilic syndrome (HES) as well as in a condition referred to a 'Tropical EMF'. The differences between these two conditions are based on several variables as listed below.

	Tropical EMF	HES
Aetiology	Unknown; possible causes include infectious agents, allergy, malnutrition and toxic agents	Unknown; characterised by overproduction of eosinophils
Geography	High prevalence in tropical regions of sub-Saharan Africa, South Asia, and South America	Cases mostly occur in temperate countries
Age and Sex	Affects children of both sexes equally In adults, women are affected twice as often as men	Incidence in the 4th decade and usually affects more men than women
Pattern of Ventricular Involvement	Mainly affects the right ventricle	Affects either ventricle

Sources: Bukhman G, Ziegler J, Parry E. Endomyocardial fibrosis: still a mystery after 60 years. *PLoS Negl Trop Dis.* 2008 Feb 27;2(2):e97; Kleinfeldt T, Nienaber CA, Kische S, Akin I, Turan RG, Körber T, Schneider H, Ince H. Cardiac manifestation of the hypereosinophilic syndrome: new insights. *Clin Res Cardiol.* 2010 Jul;99(7):419-27; Marijon E, Jani D, Ou P. Endomyocardial fibrosis: progression to restricted ventricles and giant atria. *Can J Cardiol.* 2006 Nov;22(13):1163-4.

Infiltrative Disorders

Infiltrative disorders are conditions where there is diffusion or accumulation of abnormal substances within cells or tissues. The deposition of abnormal substances within the heart can lead to increased ventricular wall thickness or chamber enlargement with secondary wall thinning. In particular, infiltrative disorders result in progressive diastolic dysfunction and a restrictive cardiomyopathy.

Infiltrative disorders discussed in this section include amyloidosis and sarcoidosis. Disorders such as Fabry disease and Friedreich ataxia may also be considered as infiltrative disorders; these disorders are discussed elsewhere.

Amyloidosis

Overview

Amyloidosis is an infiltrative disease that is characterised by the deposition of amyloid fibrils in the extracellular space of various tissues. The deposition of these amyloid fibrils may be localised to one specific site or, most commonly, deposits are systemic occurring throughout the body.

Amyloidosis may be acquired or inherited. Numerous amyloid precursors, which are capable of forming amyloid fibrils,

have been identified and these precursor amyloid proteins are used to classify amyloidosis. Examples of the systemic forms of amyloidosis are listed in Table 14.3. The age of onset of amyloidosis is related to the type of amyloidosis. For example, acquired amyloidosis typically occurs in adults over 40 years of age while senile amyloidosis occurs in patients over 80 years of age. However, acquired AA amyloidosis may also be seen in children with severe juvenile rheumatoid arthritis; this is the only type of systemic amyloidosis that occurs in children.

Cardiac amyloidosis occurs when amyloid proteins are deposited between cardiac myocytes. The diagnosis of this condition is made by endomyocardial biopsy (Fig. 14.19, right). The cardiac manifestations of cardiac amyloidosis are listed in Table 14.1. In particular, infiltration of these abnormal, waxy, insoluble fibrils within the myocardium leads to a marked thickening of the left and right ventricular walls (Fig. 14.19, left). As a result the myocardium becomes rigid and non-functioning. This leads to increased ventricular stiffness which impedes ventricular filling and a subsequent restrictive cardiomyopathy ensues. In fact, cardiac amyloidosis is the most common cause of restrictive cardiomyopathy in the developed countries.

Echocardiographic Findings

The characteristic echocardiographic findings associated with cardiac amyloidosis include:
- increased thickness of the LV and right ventricular (RV) walls,
- normal or small LV cavity size (may become dilated in later stages of the disease),
- normal LVEF (may decrease in later stages of the disease),
- diastolic dysfunction (variable pattern),
- granular, 'ground-glass' or 'sparkling' appearance of the myocardium,
- biatrial enlargement,
- thickened papillary muscles,
- diffuse valvular thickening with mild regurgitation,
- small to moderate pericardial effusion.

In particular, increased ventricular wall thickness occurs due to amyloid infiltration of the myocardium (Fig. 14.20). It is important to note that this increased wall thickening is not the same as hypertrophy (see 'Increased LV Wall Thickness versus LV Hypertrophy' information box). Furthermore, the myocardial appearance associated with cardiac amyloidosis is not pathognomonic; for example, the 'ground-glass' or 'sparkling' appearance of the myocardium can also be seen in other conditions and this appearance is also commonly encountered with harmonic imaging in normal individuals who exhibit good quality images.

The characteristic haemodynamic feature of cardiac amyloidosis is diastolic dysfunction. Therefore, a thorough Doppler assessment of diastolic function is important in these patients. Importantly, while cardiac amyloidosis is the most common cause of restrictive cardiomyopathy in the developed countries, not all cases of amyloidosis produce restrictive haemodynamics. Diastolic function abnormalities may vary between an abnormal relaxation pattern to a pseudonormal profile to a restrictive filling profile and have been shown to relate to disease progression.

Increased LV Wall Thickness versus LV Hypertrophy

Increased LV wall thickness is not synonymous with LV hypertrophy (LVH). This is illustrated in patients with cardiac amyloidosis where there is increased LV wall thickness due to infiltration rather than hypertrophy. 2D echocardiography is unable to distinguish between increased LV wall thickness due to cardiac amyloidosis from LVH associated with hypertensive disease and hypertrophic cardiomyopathy (HCM). However, differentiation between cardiac amyloidosis, true LVH and HCM is important as the treatments for these conditions differ. Therefore, the ECG is especially useful in distinguishing increased LV wall thickness due to infiltration from true hypertrophy. With cardiac amyloidosis, low or normal voltages are seen on the ECG, whereas the ECG in patients with LVH or HCM will have increased QRS voltages consistent with hypertrophy. Also, a pseudo-infarction pattern, usually involving the precordial ECG leads (V1-V3) or in the inferior leads (II, III, and aVF), may also be noted in patients with cardiac amyloidosis.

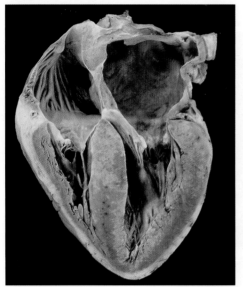
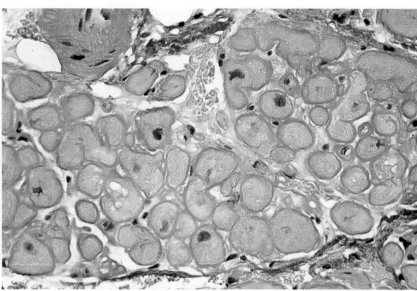

Figure 14.19 The gross pathological specimen of the heart from a patient with cardiac amyloidosis shows amyloid infiltration (pale areas of the myocardium) with thickened left ventricular walls (*left*). The corresponding histology specimen shows a sulfated Alcian blue (SAB) stain which stains amyloid deposits green and myocytes yellow-orange (*right*). By permission of Mayo Foundation for Medical Education and Research. All rights reserved. Courtesy of William D. Edwards, MD.

Table 14.3 Types of Systemic Amyloidosis: Precursor Amyloid Protein, Underlying Disease and Clinical Features

Type	Precursor Amyloid Protein	Underlying Disease	Clinical Features
Acquired AL amyloidosis (Primary amyloidosis)	Kappa or lambda immunoglobulin light chain (L)	Monoclonal plasma cell dyscrasia (plasma cell tumour)	Arthropathy **Cardiomyopathy** Nephropathy Carpal tunnel syndrome Enteropathy Glossomegaly Hepatopathy Neuropathy Splenomegaly
Acquired AA amyloidosis (Secondary amyloidosis)	Serum amyloid A protein (SAA)	Chronic inflammation	Autonomic neuropathy **Cardiomyopathy** Enteropathy Nephropathy
Acquired Aβ2M amyloidosis (Dialysis amyloidosis)	β2-microglobulin	Longstanding dialysis	Arthropathy Carpal tunnel syndrome
Acquired ATTR amyloidosis (Senile amyloidosis)	Transthyretin (TTR)	Advanced age (>80 years, predominantly male)	**Cardiomyopathy**
Hereditary ATTR amyloidosis (Familial amyloidosis)	Transthyretin (TTR)	Inherited (autosomal dominant)	**Cardiomyopathy** Nephropathy Peripheral neuropathy Vitreous opacities

Additional Notes: Cardiomyopathy has recently been associated with some apolipoprotein AI mutations leading to AApoAI amyloidosis. AA or secondary amyloidosis is associated with chronic inflammatory diseases such as rheumatoid arthritis.

Source: Groningen Unit for Amyloidosis Research & Development (GUARD) n.d., accessed 21 January 2012, http://www.amyloid.nl/classification.htm, reproduced with permission from Dr. Bouke Hazenberg, Assistant Professor Rheumatology, University of Groningen, Netherlands.

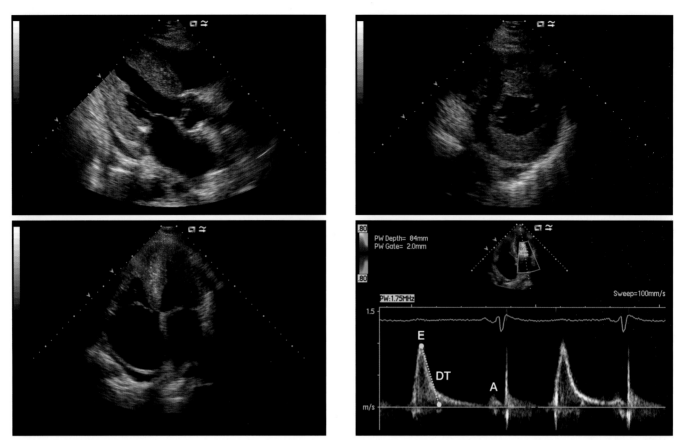

Figure 14.20 These echocardiographic images were recorded from a patient with cardiac amyloidosis. The 2D echocardiographic images recorded from the parasternal long axis view (*top, left*), the parasternal short axis (*top, right*) and from the apical 4-chamber view (*bottom, left*) show characteristic features of cardiac amyloid. These features include normal sized ventricles, a markedly increased left ventricular wall thickness, biatrial dilatation and a small pericardial effusion. The transmitral Doppler inflow profile reveals a restrictive filling pattern with a prominent early diastolic (E) velocity, a rapid deceleration time (DT) and a very small atrial contraction (A) velocity (*bottom, right*).

Sarcoidosis

Overview

Sarcoidosis is an infiltrative, granulomatous disease of unknown aetiology that can affect multiple organs such as the lungs, lymph nodes, liver, spleen, skin, parotid glands and the heart. There is geographic and ethnic variation of cardiac involvement in sarcoidosis. For example, this disease is more common in Japan, Scandinavia and Ireland and is more common in African-American populations.

Primary cardiac involvement is uncommon but when present noncaseating granulomas occur within the right and left ventricles, interventricular septum, papillary muscles, atria, conduction system and pericardium (Fig. 14.21). In particular, healing granulomas result in scarring, fibrosis, and thinning of ventricular walls. Secondary cardiac involvement may also present in patients with pulmonary involvement. In these patients, diffuse pulmonary fibrosis may result in right heart failure and pulmonary hypertension.

The cardiac manifestations of this disorder are listed in Table 14.1. The presence or absence of cardiac manifestations is dependent upon the amount of myocardium replaced by granulomas, the amount of ventricular scarring and the location of the granulomas or scars within the heart.

Diagnosis of cardiac sarcoidosis is confirmed by myocardial biopsy; however, due to patchy cardiac infiltration a false-negative result may occur. Therefore, other diagnostic criteria including the identification of proven extracardiac sarcoidosis and a combination of major or minor diagnostic criteria have been described by the Japanese Society of Sarcoidosis and Other Granulomatous Disorders [14.3].

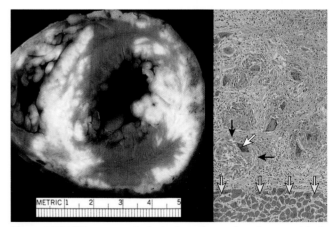

Figure 14.21 This gross pathological specimen of cardiac sarcoidosis shows scattered white areas in the myocardium (*left*). These patchy, white areas represent coalescing granulomas and scar tissue typical of cardiac sarcoidosis. The corresponding histology specimen (*right*) reveals noncaseating granulomas (*black arrows*) and a multinucleated giant cell (*white arrow*); the normal myocardial border is shown by the yellow arrows.

By permission of Mayo Foundation for Medical Education and Research. All rights reserved. Courtesy of William D. Edwards, MD.

[14.3] Soejima K, Yada H. The work-up and management of patients with apparent or subclinical cardiac sarcoidosis: with emphasis on the associated heart rhythm abnormalities. *J Cardiovasc Electrophysiol.* 2009 May;20(5):578-83.

Echocardiographic Findings

The echocardiographic findings associated with cardiac sarcoidosis are non-specific. As stated above, cardiac manifestations, and therefore echocardiographic features of this disorder, are dependent upon the degree of cardiac involvement. Abnormalities that can be detected in patients with cardiac sarcoidosis include:

* ventricular wall thickening or thinning (thickening due to granulomatous expansion or thinning due to fibrosis),
* RWMA,
* normal or dilated chamber dimensions,
* normal or impaired ventricular systolic function,
* diastolic dysfunction.

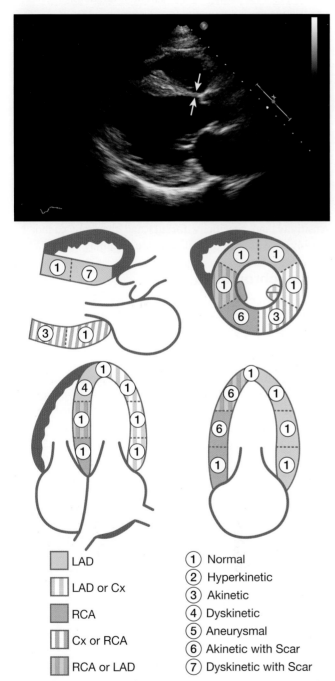

LAD

LAD or Cx

RCA

Cx or RCA

RCA or LAD

① Normal
② Hyperkinetic
③ Akinetic
④ Dyskinetic
⑤ Aneurysmal
⑥ Akinetic with Scar
⑦ Dyskinetic with Scar

Figure 14.22 The parasternal long axis view of a patient with cardiac sarcoidosis is shown (*top*). Observe that the basal septum shows marked thinning (*arrows*). The regional wall motion analysis for this patient is also shown (*bottom*); these abnormalities are not consistent with the expected coronary artery supply. Cx = left circumflex coronary artery territory; LAD = left anterior descending artery territory; LCA = left coronary artery territory; RCA = right coronary artery territory.

Although the echocardiographic features of cardiac sarcoidosis are non-specific, this disease should be suspected when there are RWMA in non-coronary distribution areas or RWMA in the absence of CAD and/or myocardial infarction. These 'atypical' RWMA reflect the patchy nature of sarcoid infiltration of the heart. A characteristic but uncommon finding in cardiac sarcoidosis is thinning of the basal anterior septum (Fig. 14.22). In addition, in patients with pulmonary involvement it is important to determine the presence or absence of pulmonary hypertension.

Storage Disorders

Storage disorders are conditions that cause the body to absorb too much of a substance from the diet or occur when the body is unable to breakdown dietary substances. The resultant accumulation of an abnormal amount of these substances within the body's cells and tissues can result in organ damage. Storage disorders discussed in this section include Fabry disease and haemochromatosis.

Fabry Disease

Overview

Fabry disease (FD), also known as Anderson-Fabry disease, is an X-linked recessive disorder whereby the defective gene causing the disease is passed on by a female carrier and/or an affected father (Fig. 14.23). As an X-linked disease, this disorder is most commonly expressed in affected males; however, carrier females may also express this disease but they typically have a more benign presentation.

FD is a rare lysosomal storage disorder which occurs due to a deficiency or absence of the enzyme α-galactosidase A. The lack of this lysosomal enzyme results in excessive accumulation of intracellular neutral glycosphingolipids within the tissues and vascular endothelium (Fig. 14.24). The organs primarily affected include the skin, kidneys, heart and the cerebrovascular system. Atypical variants of FD include a cardiac variant and a renal variant; these variants are identified when the disease is confined to the heart or to the kidneys.

Cardiac manifestations in patients with FD are very common (see Table 14.1); typically occuring in the forth decade of life. In particular, concentric LVH is a characteristic finding associated with this disorder. Myocardial ischaemia in FD may occur due to endothelial dysfunction of the coronary arteries and/or secondary to an increased oxygen demand of hypertrophied myocardium. Valvular disease may occur due to lipid deposition and fibrosis of valvular tissue.

FD is diagnosed based on endomyocardial biopsy, measurement of plasma α galactosidase A activity and/or genetic testing.

> LVH associated with Fabry disease (FD) can be misdiagnosed as hypertrophic cardiomyopathy. Distinction between these two diseases is important as the treatment strategies for each disease differ; in particular, patients with FD can be successfully treated with enzyme replacement therapy. Echocardiography is not useful in differentiating between these two diseases, although asymmetric hypertrophy with significant LV outflow tract obstruction is not typically seen in FD. Cardiac magnetic resonance imaging may be helpful in identifying FD based on a unique pattern of myocardial gadolinium hyperenhancement.

A.

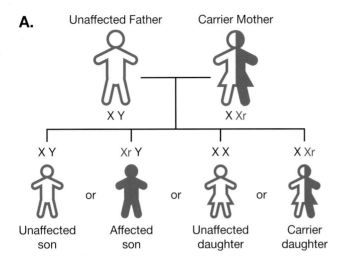

B.

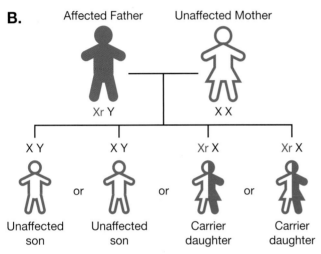

C.

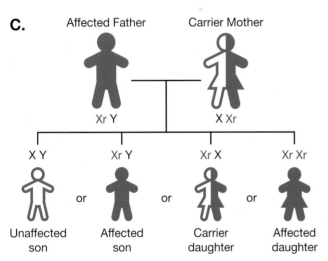

Figure 14.23 These schematics illustrate the mode of inheritance of X-linked recessive disorders. **Panel A:** shows how a disorder may be passed on from an unaffected father and a carrier mother to their children. In this situation, there is 50% chance that each son will inherit the faulty gene and will therefore be affected by the disease; there is a 50% probability that each daughter will become a carrier of the disease. **Panel B:** with an affected father and an unaffected mother, all daughters will inherit the faulty gene and become carriers of the disease but the sons will not inherit the faulty gene so the sons will not be affected. **Panel C:** with the female carrier and an affected father, there is 50% chance that each son will inherit the faulty gene and will therefore be affected by the disease; there is a 50% probability that each daughter will either become a carrier of the disease or inherit the disease.

X = X chromosome, Xr = X chromosome with faulty recessive gene, Y = Y chromosome.

Echocardiographic Findings

The echocardiographic findings associated with FD are non-specific. The most common echocardiographic features seen in patients with FD are concentric LVH and diastolic dysfunction. Other echocardiographic abnormalities that may be seen include:

- right ventricular hypertrophy (RVH); this is usually seen in conjunction with LVH,
- biatrial dilatation,
- aortic root dilatation,
- valvular thickening (aortic and mitral valves +/- associated regurgitation),
- mitral valve prolapse,
- RWMA (in the setting of myocardial infarction),
- restrictive cardiomyopathy (rare).

Additional echocardiographic signs that have been reported in FD include thinning of the posterior wall due to replacement fibrosis and the binary endocardial appearance (Fig. 14.25). The binary endocardial appearance (or binary sign) refers to the appearance of an apparent two-layered myocardium; that is, there is a hyperechogenic endocardium with a hypoechogenic space between the endocardium and the rest of the myocardium. This appearance is thought to be caused by the increased deposition of glycosphingolipids in the subendocardial layers of the myocardium. While the binary sign has been reported as an echocardiographic hallmark of FD; subsequent studies have found that this sign lacks sensitivity and specificity for FD and therefore cannot be reliably used as an echocardiographic screening tool for FD.

Haemochromatosis

Overview

Haemochromatosis is an iron metabolism disorder or an iron storage disease which is characterised by the accumulation of excessive iron within the cells of various organs. Two forms of haemochromatosis have been recognised: (1) a hereditary or primary form and (2) a secondary or acquired form.

Hereditary or primary haemochromatosis is an autosomal recessive disorder; therefore, the individual must inherit

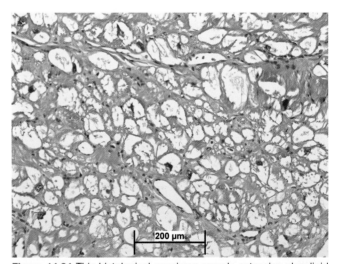

Figure 14.24 This histological specimen reveals extensive glycolipid inclusion vacuoles (hematoxylin and eosin stain ×200). The presence of glycolipid deposits within these vacuoles is characteristic of Fabry disease. By permission of Mayo Foundation for Medical Education and Research. All rights reserved. Courtesy of William D. Edwards, MD.

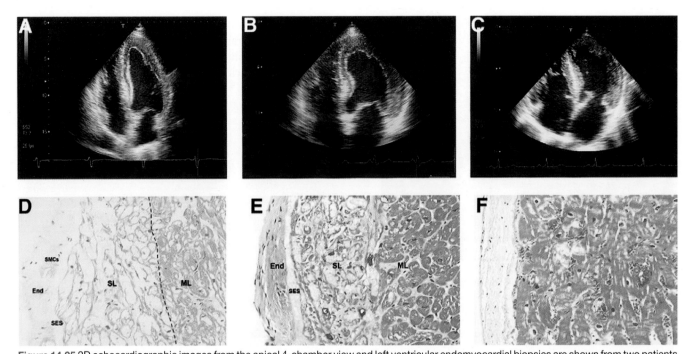

Figure 14.25 2D echocardiographic images from the apical 4-chamber view and left ventricular endomyocardial biopsies are shown from two patients with Fabry disease cardiomyopathy with left ventricular hypertrophy (**A,D** and **B,E,** respectively) and a patient with left ventricular hypertrophy due to hypertrophic cardiomyopathy **(C,F)**. Comparison of the three echocardiographic frames reveals the presence of a binary appearance of left ventricular endocardial border in the two Fabry patients **(A,B)**. This hyperechogenic layer reflects the glycosphingolipids compartmentalization involving a thickened endocardium (End) with enlarged and engulfed smooth muscle cells (SMCs), a subendocardial empty space (SES), and a prominent involvement of subendocardial myocardial layer (SL), while the middle layer (ML) appears partially spared **(D,E)**. The echocardiographic pattern was absent in the hypertrophic cardiomyopathy patient **(C)**, despite a similar thickening of the endocardium **(F)**.
Reproduced from Pieroni M, Chimenti C, De Cobelli F, Morgante E, Del Maschio A, Gaudio C, Russo MA, Frustaci A. Fabry's disease cardiomyopathy: echocardiographic detection of endomyocardial glycosphingolipid compartmentalization, *J Am Coll Cardiol*, Vol 47(8), page 1667, © 2006, with permission from Elsevier.

a faulty copy of the gene from both parents to express this disease (Fig. 14.26). The cause of this form of haemochromatosis is unknown with men being more commonly affected than women (male-to-female ratio ≈ 1.8:1 to 3:1). Haemochromatosis usually becomes apparent after 40 years of age in men and after 50 years of age in women. In this form of the disease there is an abnormal increase in iron absorption which leads to iron overload in tissues.

Secondary or acquired haemochromatosis usually is the result of another disease or condition that causes iron overload. For example, iron overload may occur in patients with chronic liver disease, as the result of multiple blood transfusions in patients with chronic anaemia or thalassemia major, or from excess iron in the diet.

The organs most commonly affected by excessive iron include the liver, heart, pancreas and pituitary. In the heart, intracellular deposition of iron occurs within the ventricles, especially within the subepicardium, subendocardium, papillary muscles, and less commonly within the myocardium and atria (Fig. 14.27).

The diagnosis of myocardial iron deposition can be made via T2 star (T2*) cardiovascular magnetic resonance imaging. Other diagnostic tests for haemochromatosis include blood tests (demonstrating elevated serum transferrin saturation and elevated serum ferritin) and liver function tests. A liver biopsy is the definitive test for identifying iron overload. Genetic testing can be performed to diagnose hereditary haemochromatosis.

Echocardiographic Findings

The echocardiographic findings associated with haemochromatosis are non-specific. The most common echocardiographic feature is that of a dilated cardiomyopathy. Due to dilatation of the cardiac chambers, varying degrees of AV valve regurgitation may result (Fig. 14.28). Diastolic function is also abnormal; restrictive physiology may be seen in the advanced stage of the disease.

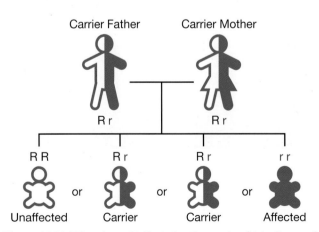

Figure 14.26 This schematic illustrates the mode of inheritance of autosomal recessive disorders. When both parents are unaffected genetic carriers for the disease, there is a 25% chance for the child to inherit both copies of the faulty gene. In this situation, the child will be affected by the disease. In addition, there is a 50% chance that a child will inherit the faulty gene and they will therefore become a genetic carrier for the disease. r = faulty recessive gene, R = unaffected or normal gene.

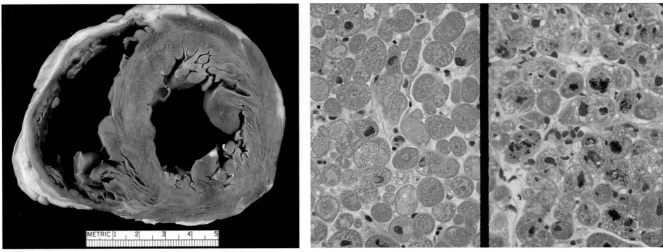

Figure 14.27 The gross pathological specimen of a heart from a patient with haemochromatosis shows a reddish-orange appearance of the myocardium that occurs due to excessive iron accumulation within myocytes (*left*). Also observe the dilatation of both ventricles. Haemochromatosis is an iron storage disease and not an infiltrative disease; its clinical manifestation is as dilated cardiomyopathy and not as restrictive cardiomyopathy. The corresponding histology specimen shows a haematoxylin and eosin stain on the left and an iron stain on the right (*right*). Observe that iron within the myocardium appears as blue deposits on the iron stain.
By permission of Mayo Foundation for Medical Education and Research. All rights reserved. Courtesy of William D. Edwards, MD.

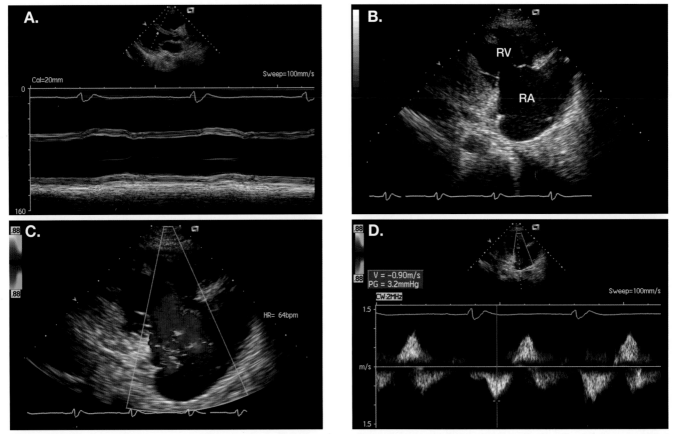

Figure 14.28 These images were recorded from a patient with haemochromatosis secondary to thalassaemia major. The M-mode trace recorded through the left ventricle (LV) demonstrates poor LV systolic function **(A)**; the fractional shortening was calculated at 14%. From the parasternal long axis of the right ventricular inflow, marked dilatation of the right heart chambers is seen; observe that the tricuspid valve fails to coapt on this systolic frame **(B)**. The colour flow Doppler image shows low velocity, 'wide-open' or 'free' tricuspid regurgitation **(C)**. The continuous-wave Doppler signal of tricuspid regurgitation confirms the presence of low velocity systolic flow **(D)**; this indicates that there is almost no pressure gradient between the right ventricle and the right atrium during systole.

Hereditary Neuromuscular Diseases

Neuromuscular disorders include a large group of diseases that affect any part of the central and peripheral nervous system resulting in impaired muscle function. While neuromuscular diseases may be acquired, most of these diseases are genetic in origin. Neuromuscular disease can be classified depending on the primary location of the pathology; for example, these diseases can be classified as muscular dystrophies, neuromuscular junction diseases, peripheral nerve disease, mitochondrial myopathies or motor neuron diseases. The disorders discussed in this section include Friedreich's ataxia and Duchenne muscular dystrophy.

Friedreich's Ataxia

Overview

Friedreich's ataxia (FRDA) is an autosomal recessive degenerative neuromuscular disease; therefore, the individual must inherit a faulty copy of the gene from both parents (see Fig. 14.26). This neuromuscular disease produces spinal cerebellar ataxia and primarily affects the central nervous system, spinal cord, peripheral nerves, pancreas and heart.

The major clinical manifestations of FRDA include neurologic features such as skeletal muscle weakness and progressive limb ataxia, loss of reflexes, slurred speech (dysarthria), cardiac features such as cardiomyopathy and pancreatic disorders such as diabetes mellitus.

FRDA generally becomes apparent in early childhood (between the ages of 6 and 9 years) or during adolescence (between the ages of 12 and 15 years); patients may also present in adulthood but usually before 25 years of age. The diagnosis of FRDA is based upon clinical findings and can be confirmed by genetic testing.

Cardiac involvement in FRDA is very common. Cardiac manifestations of this disorder are listed in Table 14.1. Complications relating to cardiac dysfunction and pulmonary infections are a common cause of death in these patients.

Echocardiographic Findings

The echocardiographic features in patients with FRDA include:
• concentric LVH with normal systolic function,
• increased thickening of papillary muscles,
• diastolic dysfunction (abnormal relaxation).

Less commonly, asymmetric septal hypertrophy (with or without left ventricular outflow tract obstruction) or a dilated cardiomyopathy may be seen. In particular, the presence of dilated cardiomyopathy in these patients is associated with a poor prognosis.

Duchenne Muscular Dystrophy

Overview

Muscular dystrophies, or dystrophinopathies, are progressive hereditary degenerative diseases of skeletal muscles which occur due to an absence or deficiency of the protein dystrophin. These dystrophies include Duchenne muscular dystrophy and Becker muscular dystrophy. X-linked dilated cardiomyopathy is also a rare type of muscular dystrophy with rapidly progressive cardiomyopathy but almost no skeletal muscle impairment.

These muscular dystrophies are X-linked recessive disorders; therefore, they are almost exclusively seen in males (see Fig. 14.23). Symptoms relating to these disorders first appear in early childhood.

Duchenne Muscular Dystrophy (DMD) is the most common childhood muscular dystrophy. The diagnosis of DMD is based on genetic testing or muscle biopsy.

Cardiac involvement in DMD occurs in all patients older than 18 years old. Cardiac manifestations of this disorder are listed in Table 14.1. In particular, in the heart the loss of dystrophin leads to cardiac cell death which leads to fibro-collagenous scar tissue formation and myocardial fibrosis. As a result, a dilated cardiomyopathy develops; thinning and stretching of fibrotic regions leads to segmental myocardial scarring.

The median life expectancy of patients with DMD is around 35 years of age with death occurring due to respiratory or cardiac failure.

Echocardiographic Findings

The echocardiographic features in patients with DMD include:
• dilated cardiomyopathy,
• RWMA (due to fibrosis and myocardial scarring; most commonly seen in the inferior, inferolateral, and anterolateral segments of the LV).

Key Points (Diseases listed in alphabetical order)		
Disease	**Description**	**Echo features include:**
Amyloidosis	An infiltrative disease that is characterised by the deposition of amyloid fibrils in the extracellular space of various tissues including the heart.	• Increased LV and RV wall thickness • Small or normal LV and RV cavity size • Normal or decreased LV systolic function • Biatrial dilatation • Diastolic dysfunction (variable) • Small pericardial effusion • Diffuse vavular thickening with mild regurgitation
Ankylosing Spondylitis (AKS)	A chronic, inflammatory connective tissue disorder primarily involving the vertebral and sacroiliac joints; this inflammatory process also affects the connective tissues of the heart.	• Aortic root dilatation • Aortic valve sclerosis with mild-moderate AR • Mild-moderate MR (2^0 to subaortic involvement)
(continued over...)		

Key Points (Diseases listed in alphabetical order, continued)		
Disease	**Description**	**Echo features include:**
Carcinoid Syndrome	Carcinoid heart syndrome occurs due to the secretion of excessive amounts of serotonin from metastatic carcinoid tumours.	• Thickened, retracted tricuspid +/- pulmonary leaflets • Severe TR/PR and mild tricuspid/pulmonary stenosis • RV volume overload • Thickening of left-sided valve (in setting of PFO)
Diabetes Mellitus (DM)	A group of metabolic disorders characterised by chronic hyperglycaemia due to defects in insulin secretion, insulin action, or a combination of both; leads to long-term organ damage and dysfunction.	• RWMA (2^0 to CAD or myocardial infarction) • LVH (2^0 to systemic hypertension) • Diastolic dysfunction
Duchenne Muscular Dystrophy (DMD)	The most common X-linked recessive muscular dystrophy; loss of dystrophin leads to cardiac cell death.	• Dilated cardiomyopathy • RWMA (most commonly in inferior, inferolateral, and anterolateral segments)
Ehlers-Danlos Syndrome (EDS), Type IV	This type of EDS is an inherited, connective tissue disorder with cardiac manifestations.	• Aortic root dilatation +/- AR • Aortic valve prolapse • Mitral valve prolapse +/- MR • Aortic aneurysm at the sinuses of Valsalva • Type A aortic dissection
Fabry Disease (FD)	A rare X-linked recessive, lysosomal storage disorder resulting in excessive accumulation of glycosphingolipids within tissues including the heart.	• Concentric LVH +/- RVH • Diastolic dysfunction • Biatrial dilatation • Aortic root dilatation • Thickening of aortic and mitral valves +/- associated regurgitation • Mitral valve prolapse +/- MR • RWMA (2^0 to CAD or myocardial infarction) • Restrictive cardiomyopathy (rare)
Friedreich's Ataxia (FRDA)	An autosomal recessive neuromuscular degenerative disease that produces spinal cerebellar ataxia and primarily affects the central nervous system, spinal cord, peripheral nerves, pancreas and heart.	• Concentric LVH • Increased thickening of papillary muscles • Diastolic dysfunction (abnormal relaxation) • Dilated LV with systolic dysfunction (advanced stage) • Asymmetric septal hypertrophy, with or without left ventricular outflow tract obstruction (less common)
Haemochromatosis	An iron metabolism disorder or an iron storage disease characterised by the accumulation of excessive iron within the cells of various organs.	• Dilated LV with decreased systolic function • AV valve regurgitation (2^0 to ventricular dilatation) • Diastolic dysfunction; restrictive diastolic filling (advanced stage)
Hypereosinophilic Syndrome (HES)	Characterised by a persistent overproduction of eosinophils; cardiac involvement occurs due to endocardial and myocardial necrosis, thrombosis and fibrosis.	• Endocardial thickening and fibrous • Mural ventricular apical thrombus (apical obliteration) • Posterior mitral leaflet adhesion/tethering to LV wall • Significant MR (2^0 to above) • Restrictive cardiomyopathy
Loeys-Dietz Syndrome (LDS)	An inherited, autosomal dominant aortic aneurysm syndrome.	• Aortic root dilatation and aortic aneurysms • Ascending and/or descending aortic aneurysms (less common) • Type A aortic dissection • AR (2^0 to aortic root dilatation) • Mitral valve prolapse +/- MR
Marfan Syndrome (MFS)	The most common hereditary connective tissue disorder which is characterised by skeletal, cardiovascular and ocular features.	• Dilatation of the aortic root and ascending aorta • AR (2^0 to annular dilatation) • Mitral valve prolapse +/- MR • Dilatation main pulmonary artery • Type A aortic dissection
Phaeochromocytoma	A rare and usually benign, catecholamine-secreting tumour most commonly located within the adrenal glands; cardiac manifestations occur due to high levels of circulating catecholamines.	• Concentric LVH (2^0 to systemic hypertension) • RWMA (2^0 to CAD or myocardial infarction) • Dilated, hypertrophic or Takotsubo cardiomyopathies

Key Points (Diseases listed in alphabetical order, continued)		
Disease	**Description**	**Echo features include:**
Rheumatoid Arthritis (RA)	RA is a systemic rheumatic, autoimmune disease of unknown aetiology that is characterised by persistent inflammation of a synovial membrane of the small joints of the hands and feet.	• Pericardial effusion (most common) • Diffuse aortic and mitral valve thickening +/- AR and MR • Valvular nodules (located at the basal or mid portions of the aortic and/or mitral valve leaflets) • LV systolic dysfunction • RWMA (when associated CAD) • Signs of pulmonary hypertension • restrictive cardiomyopathy (when secondary amyloidosis)
Sarcoidosis	Sarcoidosis is an infiltrative, granulomatous disease of unknown aetiology that can affect multiple organs such as the lungs, lymph nodes, liver, spleen, skin, parotid glands and the heart.	• RWMA (non-coronary distribution) • Thinning or thickening of ventricular walls (e.g. thinning of basal anterior septum) • Normal or dilated cardiac chambers • Normal or impaired systolic function • Diastolic dysfunction • Pulmonary hypertension (pulmonary involvement)
Systemic Lupus Erythematosus (SLE)	SLE is a chronic multisystem, autoimmune disorder that results in a chronic or recurrent inflammatory disease that predominately affects the musculoskeletal and mucocutaneous systems.	• Pericarditis (most common) • Libman-Sacks endocarditis • RWMA (secondary to myocardial infarction) • Valvular thickening with associated regurgitation • Pulmonary hypertension
Systemic Scleroderma (SSc)	Scleroderma is an autoimmune disease whereby excessive connective tissue accumulates in the skin, blood vessels, joints, skeletal muscle, and/or other organs including the heart.	• Pericardial effusion (most common) • RWMA (secondary to CAD, myocardial infarction) • Pulmonary hypertension • Valvular sclerosis

Further Reading (listed in alphabetical order)

General

Alizad A, Seward JB. Echocardiographic features of genetic diseases: part 1. Cardiomyopathy. *J Am Soc Echocardiogr.* 2000 Jan;13(1):73-86.

Alizad A, Seward JB. Echocardiographic features of genetic diseases: part 2. Storage disease. J Am Soc Echocardiogr. 2000 Feb;13(2):164-70.

Alizad A, Seward JB. Echocardiographic features of genetic diseases: part 4. Connective tissue. *J Am Soc Echocardiogr.* 2000 Apr;13(4):325-30.

Click RL, Olson LJ, Edwards WD, Miller FA, Khandheria BK, Seward JB, Tajik AJ. Echocardiography and systemic diseases. *J Am Soc Echocardiogr.* 1994 Mar-Apr;7(2):201-16.

Nihoyannopoulos P, Dawson D. Restrictive cardiomyopathies. *Eur J Echocardiogr.* 2009 Dec;10(8):iii23-33.

Seward JB, Casaclang-Verzosa G. Infiltrative cardiovascular diseases: cardio-myopathies that look alike. *J Am Coll Cardiol.* 2010 Apr 27;55(17):1769-79.

Systemic Rheumatic Diseases

Evangelista A, Flachskampf FA, Erbel R, Antonini-Canterin F, Vlachopoulos Bourré-Tessier J, Huynh T, Clarke A, Bernatsky S, Joseph L, Belisle P, Pineau C. Features associated with cardiac abnormalities in systemic lupus erythematosus. *Lupus.* 2011;20(14):1518-25.

Lautermann D, Braun J. Ankylosing spondylitis--cardiac manifestations. Clin Exp Rheumatol. 2002 Nov-Dec;20(6 Suppl 28):S11-5.

Pagnoux C, Guillevin L. Cardiac involvement in small and medium-sized vessel vasculitides. *Lupus.* 2005;14(9):718-22.

Roldan CA. Valvular and coronary heart disease in systemic inflammatory diseases: Systemic Disorders in heart disease. *Heart.* 2008 Aug;94(8):1089-101.

Sarzi-Puttini P, Atzeni F, Gerli R, Bartoloni E, Doria A, Barskova T, Matucci-Cerinic M, Sitia S, Tomasoni L, Turiel M. Cardiac involvement in systemic rheumatic diseases: An update. *Autoimmun Rev.* 2010 Oct;9(12):849-52.

Turiel M, Sitia S, Atzeni F, Tomasoni L, Gianturco L, Giuffrida M, De Gennaro Colonna V, Sarzi-Puttini P. The heart in rheumatoid arthritis. *Autoimmun Rev.* 2010 Apr;9(6):414-8.

Hereditary Connective Disorders

Ammash NM, Sundt TM, Connolly HM. Marfan syndrome-diagnosis and management. *Curr Probl Cardiol.* 2008 Jan;33(1):7-39.

Cañadas V, Vilacosta I, Bruna I, Fuster V. Marfan syndrome. Part 1: pathophysiology and diagnosis. Nat Rev Cardiol. 2010 May;7(5):256-65.

Germain DP. Ehlers-Danlos syndrome type IV. Orphanet J Rare Dis. 2007 Jul 19;2:32.

Loeys BL, Schwarze U, Holm T, Callewaert BL, Thomas GH, Pannu H, De Backer JF, Oswald GL, Symoens S, Manouvrier S, Roberts AE, Faravelli F, Greco MA, Pyeritz RE, Milewicz DM, Coucke PJ, Cameron DE, Braverman AC, Byers PH, De Paepe AM, Dietz HC. Aneurysm syndromes caused by mutations in the TGF-beta receptor. *N Engl J Med.* 2006 Aug 24;355(8):788-98.

Endocrine Disorders

Li L, Zhu W, Fang L, Zeng Z, Miao Q, Zhang C, Fang Q. Transthoracic Echocardiographic Features of Cardiac Pheochromocytoma: A Single-Institution Experience. *Echocardiography.* 2012 Feb;29(2):153-7.

Li YW and Aronow WS. Diabetes Mellitus and Cardiovascular Disease. *J Clinic Experiment Cardiol.* 2011 2(1):1-9.

Osranek M, Bursi F, Gura GM, Young WF Jr, Seward JB. Echocardiographic features of pheochromocytoma of the heart. *Am J Cardiol.* 2003 Mar 1;91(5):640-3.

Palaniswamy C, Frishman WH, Aronow WS. Carcinoid Heart Disease. *Cardiol Rev.* 2012 Feb 6.

Pellikka PA, Tajik AJ, Khandheria BK, Seward JB, Callahan JA, Pitot HC, Kvols LK. Carcinoid heart disease. Clinical and echocardiographic spectrum in 74 patients. *Circulation.* 1993 Apr;87(4):1188-96.

Prejbisz A, Lenders JW, Eisenhofer G, Januszewicz A. Cardiovascular manifestations of phaeochromocytoma. *J Hypertens.* 2011 Nov;29(11):2049-60.

(continued over...)

Haemolytic Disorders

Kleinfeldt T, Nienaber CA, Kische S, Akin I, Turan RG, Körber T, Schneider H, Ince H. Cardiac manifestation of the hypereosinophilic syndrome: new insights. Clin Res Cardiol. 2010 Jul;99(7):419-27.

Ogbogu PU, Rosing DR, Horne MK 3rd. Cardiovascular manifestations of hypereosinophilic syndromes. *Immunol Allergy Clin North Am.* 2007 Aug;27(3):457-75.

Ommen SR, Seward JB, Tajik AJ. Clinical and echocardiographic features of hypereosinophilic syndromes. *Am J Cardiol.* 2000 Jul 1;86(1):110-3.

Infiltrative Diseases

Dubrey SW, Hawkins PN, Falk RH. Amyloid diseases of the heart: assessment, diagnosis, and referral. *Heart.* 2011 Jan;97(1):75-84.

Youssef G, Beanlands RS, Birnie DH, Nery PB. Cardiac sarcoidosis: applications of imaging in diagnosis and directing treatment. *Heart.* 2011 Dec;97(24):2078-87.

Storage Disorders

Linhart A, Elliott PM. The heart in Anderson-Fabry disease and other lysosomal storage disorders. *Heart.* 2007 Apr;93(4):528-35.

O'Mahony C, Elliott P. Anderson-Fabry disease and the heart. Prog *Cardiovasc Dis.* 2010 Jan-Feb;52(4):326-35.

Hereditary Neuromuscular Diseases

Dutka DP, Donnelly JE, Nihoyannopoulos P, Oakley CM, Nunez DJ. Marked variation in the cardiomyopathy associated with Friedreich's ataxia. *Heart.* 1999 Feb;81(2):141-7.

Hermans MC, Pinto YM, Merkies IS, de Die-Smulders CE, Crijns HJ, Faber CG. Hereditary muscular dystrophies and the heart. *Neuromuscul Disord.* 2010 Aug;20(8):479-92.

Introduction to Congenital Heart Disease

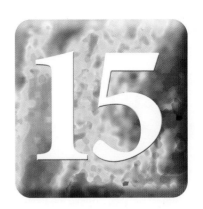

Introduction

Congenital heart disease (CHD) includes a broad spectrum of congenital heart malformations that include simple shunt lesions such as atrial and ventricular septal defects and very complex lesions such as a criss-cross heart with discordant atrioventricular (AV) valves, a double outflow right ventricle (RV) and transposition of the great arteries (TGA). It is beyond the scope of this chapter to cover all types of CHD so only selected anomalies that are more likely to be encountered in an adult echocardiographic laboratory will be covered. CHD is also associated with a number of genetic syndromes; selected genetic syndromes associated with CHD are listed in Appendix 5. Appendix 6 provides a quick reference list of the various palliative and corrective surgical operations performed for various types of CHD.

In the simplest of terms, CHD can be classified as shunt lesions, obstructive lesions and cyanotic lesions. Table 15.1 lists the "Top 3" lesions in each category and each of these lesions is discussed within this chapter. Note that less commonly encountered congenital heart lesions such as cor triatriatum and Ebstein's anomaly have also been briefly covered in Chapters 7 and 9, respectively; these lesions will not be discussed further within this chapter.

Shunt Lesions

Atrial Septal Defects

An atrial septal defect (ASD) is a congenital heart lesion where there is a communication between the left atrium (LA) and the right atrium (RA); ASDs comprise approximately 10% of congenital heart lesions.

In an ASD blood is usually shunted left-to-right as the pressure within the LA is normally slightly higher than the pressure in the RA. Due to this left-to-right shunting, there is an increased volume of blood into the right heart and this leads to the subsequent dilatation of the RA, the RV and the pulmonary artery (PA). The degree of right heart dilatation is essentially dependent upon the degree of shunting across the ASD as well as the pressure differences between the left and right atria. In order to appreciate the aetiology for each type of ASD it is important to first understand the embryological development of the atrial septum, the sinus venosus and the sinus horns.

Embryology
Normal Development of the Atrial Septum
Complete formation of the interatrial septum (IAS) requires contributions from three structures: (1) the primum atrial septum, (2) the secundum atrial septum, and (3) the endocardial cushions (Fig. 15.1). This complex, staged formation of the IAS ensures that there is always a communication between the RA and LA throughout foetal development. This communication is required for two important reasons: (1) the foetal lungs are inactive so diverting blood flow to the LA minimises blood flow to the lungs, and (2) this ensures that oxygen-rich blood reaches the developing foetal brain and heart musculature. So in the foetal circulation, oxygenated blood from the maternal placenta travels to the developing foetal heart via the inferior vena cava (IVC). Upon entering the RA, the eustachian valve (valve of the IVC) directs the majority of blood across the foramen ovale into the LA.

Sinus Venosus and Sinus Horns
The sinus venosus is derived from the venous system of the embryo and initially consists of a small transverse sinus, the right sinus horn and the left sinus horn. This structure receives the venous return and drains into the primitive common atrium through a central orifice called the sinuatrial orifice. In the early stages of development, the sinus venosus is bilaterally symmetrical and the right and left horns of the sinus venosus are the same size (Fig. 15.2 left). As development continues, significant modifications occur to the primitive systemic venous system. In particular, left-to-right shunting of blood between the left and right systemic venous systems results in the regression of some left-side channels and the progressive enlargement of the right venous channels (Fig 15.2 right).

Table 15.1 **Introduction to Congenital Heart Disease**

Shunt Lesions	Obstructive Lesions	Cyanotic Lesions
• Atrial septal defects	• Pulmonary stenosis	• Tetralogy of Fallot
• Ventricular septal defects	• Congenital aortic stenosis	• Transposition of the great arteries
• Patent ductus arteriosus	• Coarctation of the aorta	• Tricuspid atresia

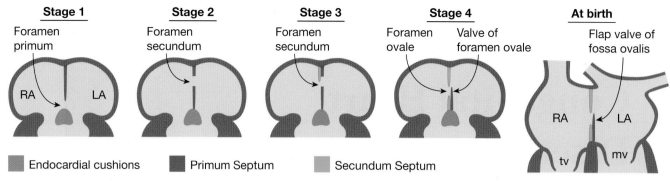

Figure 15.1 These schematics illustrate the formation of the interatrial septum (IAS). **Stage 1:** The primum septum is the first of two atrial septa to form. It arises from the roof of the common atrium and grows inferiorly towards the endocardial cushions. Between the lower margin of the primum septum and the endocardial cushions is the foramen primum. **Stage 2:** As the primum septum grows inferiorly, the foramen primum decreases in size and eventually closes; however, before the primum septum fuses with the endocardial cushions, perforations appear in the upper part of this septum to form another opening known as the foramen secundum. **Stage 3:** The secundum septum is the second atrial septum to form. This septum grows inferiorly from the right side of the primum septum and gradually overlaps the foramen secundum but does not completely cover this opening; the oval opening that remains is the foramen ovale. The foramen ovale is held open as the right atrial (RA) pressure is higher than the left atrial (LA) pressure and this ensures right-to-left flow of oxygenated blood from the inferior vena cava into the LA and left ventricle (LV). **Stage 4:** With continued development, the upper primum septum disappears and the remaining lower part of the primum septum becomes the valve of the foramen ovale. **At birth:** There is an increase in pulmonary blood flow resulting in an increase in pulmonary venous flow to the LA and a subsequent increase in LA pressures. At the same time, there is an increase in the systemic vascular resistance and a decline in the RA pressure and pulmonary vascular resistance. So now the pressure in the LA exceeds that of the RA. This increased LA pressure pushes the valve of the foramen ovale against the secundum septum effectively closing the foramen ovale. Over time, fusion between the primum and secundum atrial septa occurs resulting in an oval-shaped depression in the IAS is known as the fossa ovalis; the valve of the foramen ovale becomes the flap valve over the fossa ovalis. mv = mitral valve; tv = tricuspid valve.

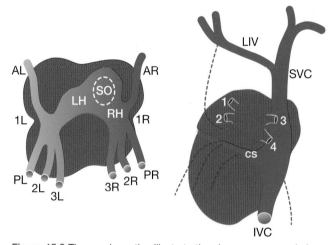

Figure 15.2 These schematics illustrate the sinus venosus and sinus horns from the posterior aspect in the early foetal heart (*left*) and in the fully developed heart (*right*). Observe that in early foetal heart development the venous system is symmetrical. Three main paired venous systems drain into the right horn (RH) and left horn (LH) of the sinus venosus where blood then enters the primitive common atrium via the sinuatrial orifice (SO).

The three main paired venous systems include: the right and left common cardinal veins (1R and 1L), the right and left umbilical veins (2R and 2L), and the right and left vitelline veins (3R and 3L). The common cardinal veins also receive blood from the anterior right and anterior left cardinal veins (AR and AL) and from the posterior right and posterior left cardinal veins (PR and PL). Note that the pulmonary veins are not yet developed at this stage. In the fully developed heart the right horn of the sinus venosus persists as a part of the right atrium while the anterior right cardinal vein (AR) and the right common cardinal vein (1R) form the superior vena cava (SVC). The inferior vena cava (IVC) is formed by the right vitelline vein (3R) while the posterior right cardinal vein (PR) becomes the azygos vein; the right umbilical vein (2R) completely degenerates. The majority of the left veins also degenerate (*dashed lines*); in particular, the left vitelline vein (3L), the left umbilical vein (2L) and the posterior left cardinal vein (PL) all disappear. The left sinus horn regresses and loses its connection with the anterior left cardinal vein (AL); a remnant of the left sinus horn and the adjacent left common cardinal vein (1L) remain as the coronary sinus (CS) and the oblique vein of the left atrium. The anterior left cardinal vein (AL) anastomoses with the anterior right cardinal vein (AR) to form the left innominate vein (LIV). The four pulmonary veins are also now present: 1 = left upper pulmonary vein; 2 = left lower pulmonary vein; 3 = right upper pulmonary vein; 4 = right lower pulmonary vein.

In addition, there is regression of the left sinus horn with the persistence of the proximal left horn which contributes to the formation of the coronary sinus. The coronary sinus, which drains the cardiac veins into the RA, traverses the posterior left atrioventricular canal.

Types of ASD

There are four types of ASD (Fig. 15.3) and each of these is often associated with other congenital heart lesions (Table 15.2); more than one type of ASD may be present. A patent foramen ovale (PFO) which is a remnant of the normal foetal circulation also allows shunting between the two atria.

An ostium primum (1^0) ASD accounts for about 15% of all ASDs. These defects, also referred to as partial AV canal defects, are located in the inferior portion of the IAS near the primitive foramen primum. This type of ASD occurs when there is failure of the septum primum to fuse with the endocardial cushions or when there is deficiency of endocardial cushion tissue. Due to the close proximity of this ASD to the AV canal, this defect is often associated with abnormalities of the endocardial cushions and of the AV valves.

An ostium secundum ($2°$) ASD is the most common type of ASD accounting for approximately 80% of all ASDs. These defects are located in the region of the fossa ovalis and are caused by excessive cell death or resorption of the septum primum or inadequate development of the septum secundum.

Sinus venosus (SV) and coronary sinus (CS) ASDs also result in a communication between the LA and RA; however, unlike the 2^0 and 1^0 ASDs, these defects do not occur due to malformation of the IAS. Instead, these defects occur due to maldevelopment of the sinus venosus and sinus horns. The SV ASD occurs due to an error in the incorporation of the sinus venosus chamber into the RA. There are two types of SV ASD: a superior defect and an inferior defect. The superior SV ASD is located superiorly near the SVC and accounts for approximately 5% of all ASDs. The inferior SV ASD is located near the IVC; this type of ASD is rare accounting for less than 2%

of all ASDs. As illustrated in Figure 15.2, there is a close anatomical relationship between the SVC and IVC and the right pulmonary veins. This explains why SV ASDs are usually associated with anomalous connection of the right pulmonary veins. In particular, the superior SV ASD is usually associated with anomalous connection of some or all of the right pulmonary veins to the SVC or the RA while the inferior SV ASD is associated with anomalous pulmonary venous drainage of the right lower pulmonary vein into the RA.

The CS ASD is the least common of all ASDs. This defect occurs when there is improper development of the wall between the LA and the coronary sinus. This defect may be fenestrated or totally absent ("unroofed" coronary sinus). A CS ASD results in a direct communication between the LA and the coronary sinus; the coronary sinus then drains into the RA. This defect is commonly associated with a persistent left SVC to the coronary sinus.

Role of Echocardiography in ASD

When assessing a patient with an ASD, it is important to:
• determine the type of defect
• estimate the anatomic size of the defect
• determine the shunt direction
• estimate the haemodynamic significance of the shunt
• estimate the right ventricular systolic pressure (pulmonary artery systolic pressure)
• identify any associated lesions.

ASD Type and Shunt Direction

The ASD type is based on its anatomic location. For example, a 2^0 ASD is seen in the region of the fossa ovalis (Fig. 15.4) while a 1^0 ASD is seen inferior towards the AV valves (Fig. 15.5).

The best views for imaging a 2^0 ASD are views in which the IAS is orientated perpendicular to the ultrasound beam; these views include the subcostal 4-chamber and subcostal short axis views. Images recorded from an off-axis para-apical 4-chamber view and right parasternal position may also be useful for interrogating the IAS. When the defect is large, it may also be seen from the parasternal short axis and the apical 4-chamber views.

The best views for imaging a 1^0 ASD include the apical 4-chamber and subcostal 4-chamber views as these views nicely show the cardiac crux. With a 1^0 ASD, the AV valves are attached to the interventricular septum (IVS) at the same level; that is, the normal apical displacement of the septal tricuspid valve leaflet is absent.

SV ASDs are very difficult to detect via transthoracic echocardiography (TTE) in the adult patient. When attempting to image a superior SV ASD, the best windows include the apical and subcostal windows with anterior tilting of the transducer (Fig. 15.6).

As for SV ASDs, CS ASDs are also very difficult to detect via TTE in the adult patient. The best windows for attempting to image these defects include the apical and subcostal windows with posterior tilting of the transducer (Fig. 15.7). A CS ASD may also be suspected when the coronary sinus appears dilated in the apical 4-chamber view (with posterior tilt) but from the parasternal long axis view a dilated coronary sinus is not evident because the coronary sinus is 'unroofed' (Fig. 15.8).

The shunt direction across an ASD is identified via colour flow imaging (CFI). Most commonly, the LA pressure is higher than the RA pressure so the shunt direction is from left-to-right (see Fig. 15.4-7). However, when there is a marked increase in the right heart pressures shunting may be reversed (right-to-left) or bidirectional (Fig. 15.9).

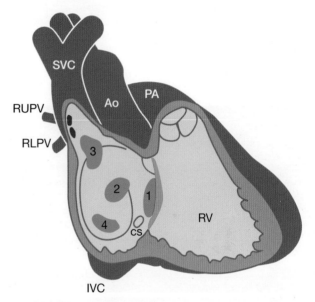

Figure 15.3 This schematic illustrates an ostium primum atrial septal defect (ASD) (1), an ostium secundum ASD (2), a superior sinus venosus ASD (3), and an inferior sinus venosus ASD (4). A coronary sinus ASD which occurs when there is a defect between the posterior left atrial wall and the coronary sinus is not shown.
Ao = aorta; CS = coronary sinus; IVC = inferior vena cava; PA = pulmonary artery; RLPV = right lower pulmonary vein; RUPV = right upper pulmonary vein; RV = right ventricle; SVC = superior vena cava.

Table 15.2 Atrial Septal Defect (ASD): Incidence and Associated Cardiac Lesions

Type of ASD	Incidence of All ASD	Associated Cardiac Lesions
Ostium primum	≈ 15%	"Cleft" anterior leaflet of mitral valve Atrioventricular canal defect
Ostium secundum	≈ 80%	Usually isolated; maybe associated with mitral valve prolapse and/or pulmonary stenosis
Sinus venosus: Superior type Inferior type	≈ 5% < 1%	Anomalous pulmonary venous drainage
Coronary sinus	< 1%	Persistent left superior vena cava Total anomalous pulmonary venous drainage

2D echocardiographic interrogation for an ASD from the apical 4-chamber view only is not advised as "drop-out" of the IAS in the region of the fossa ovalis is very common in this view. This "drop-out" artefact occurs because from this view the ultrasound beam is parallel to the thinnest portion of the septum. As a result there is poor backscatter of echoes from this relatively thin structure so little or no sound is reflected back to the transducer. In particular, a 2^0 ASD can be falsely diagnosed from this view due to "drop-out" of echoes in the area of the fossa ovalis.

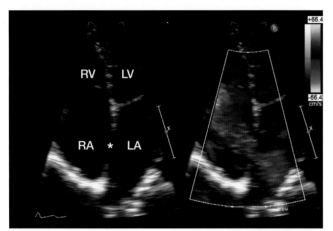

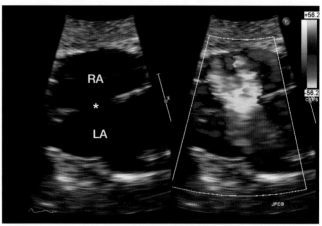

Figure 15.4 These images show a large secundum (2^0) atrial septal defect (ASD). Images are recorded from a zoomed apical 4-chamber view (*left*) and a zoomed subcostal 4-chamber view (*right*). Observe that this defect is located in the middle of the atrial septum in the region of the fossa ovalis (*). Colour flow Doppler images confirm the presence of a left-to-right shunt across this defect; this appears as red flow towards the transducer. LA = left atrium; LV = left ventricle; RA = right atrium; RV = right ventricle.

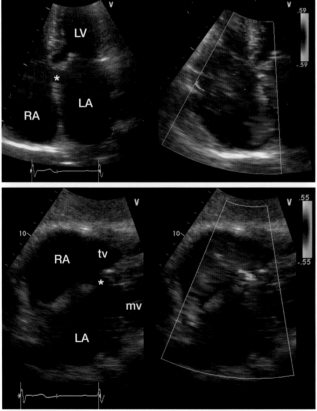

Figure 15.5 These images show a large primum (1^0) atrial septal defect (ASD). Images are recorded from a zoomed apical 4-chamber view (*top*) and a zoomed subcostal 4-chamber view (*bottom*). Observe that this ASD is located in the lower aspect of the atrial septum close to the atrioventricular valves (*). Colour flow Doppler images confirm the presence of a left-to-right shunt across this defect; this appears as red flow towards the transducer.

LA = left atrium; LV = left ventricle; mv = mitral valve; RA = right atrium; RV = right ventricle; tv = tricuspid valve.

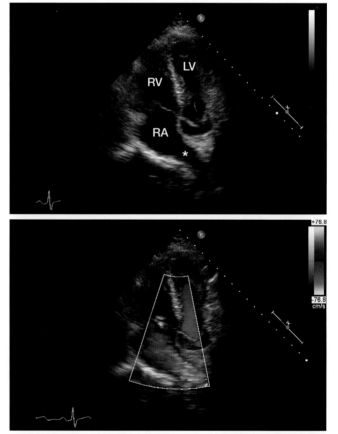

Figure 15.6 These images recorded from an apical 5-chamber view show a superior sinus venosus atrial septal defect (ASD). Observe that this ASD is located in the superior aspect of the atrial septum (*). The colour flow Doppler image confirms the presence of a left-to-right shunt across this defect; this appears as red flow towards the transducer.

LV = left ventricle; RA = right atrium; RV = right ventricle.

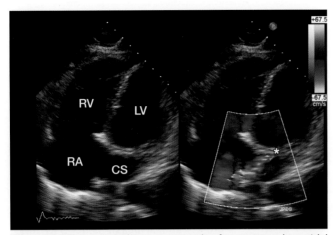

Figure 15.7 This image shows an example of a coronary sinus atrial septal defect (ASD). Observe that there is marked dilatation of the coronary sinus (CS) and left-to-right shunting can be seen in the region of the coronary sinus ostium (*); as flow is directed away from the transducer, this appears as blue flow.
LV = left ventricle; RA = right atrium; RV = right ventricle.

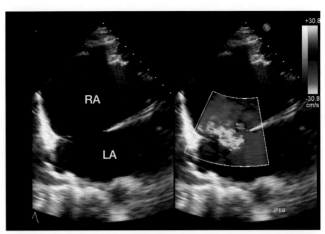

Figure 15.9 This zoomed subcostal 4-chamber view shows a large secundum atrial septal defect (ASD) with right-to-left shunting across the defect which appears as blue flow away from the transducer.
LA = left atrium; RA = right atrium.

Patient 1

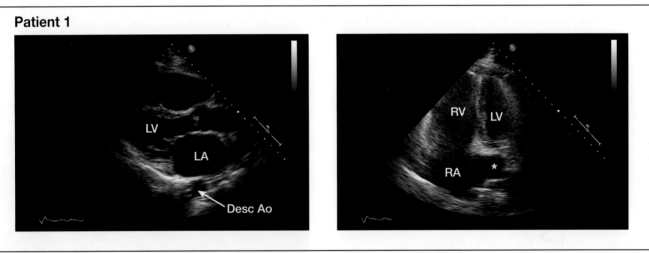

Patient 2

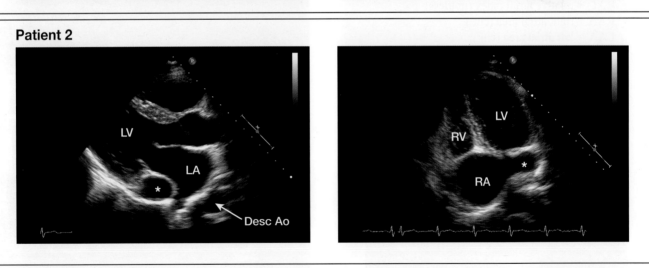

Figure 15.8 Patient 1 is the same patient as in Figure 15.7; this patient has a coronary sinus atrial septal defect (ASD). Patient 2 has a dilated coronary sinus (CS) due to a persistent left superior vena cava (LSVC). Observe that in the apical 4-chamber views with posterior tilt, the CS (*) is dilated in both patients (*right images*). However, in the parasternal long axis views, the dilated CS (*) is only noted in patient 2 (*bottom left*). In patient 1 (CS ASD), the expected dilated CS channel is not seen (*top left*); this appearance is consistent with an unroofed CS or CS ASD.

Anatomic Size of ASDs

Using 2D echocardiography, it is also possible to measure the anatomical size of the ASD. Importantly, ASDs are often oblong or elliptical in shape and this is best appreciated via 3D echocardiography (Fig. 15.10). Therefore, via 2D echocardiography these ASDs should be measured in two orthogonal planes (Fig. 15.11). CFI may also be useful in identifying the borders of a defect.

Haemodynamic Significance of ASDs

The haemodynamic significance of an ASD can be estimated based on the degree of right heart dilatation and quantification of the shunt ratio.

As previously stated, left-to-right shunting across an ASD leads to right heart volume overload and subsequent dilatation of the right heart chambers. The degree of right heart dilatation provides a clue as to the haemodynamic significance of the shunt. For example, mild right heart chamber dilatation suggests a small shunt while marked right heart chamber dilatation suggests a significant shunt. In addition, marked RV volume overload leads to diastolic flattening of the IVS which is best appreciated from the parasternal short axis view. Importantly, RV volume overload and RV pressure overload both result in RV dilatation and flattening of the IVS. Distinction between volume overload and pressure overload is based on the phase of the cardiac cycle in which flattening of the IVS is most predominant (see Fig. 2.4).

Another clue to the presence of an ASD is when the RA appears larger than the LA. In particular, a relative atrial index (RAI) > 0.92 should alert the sonographer to the presence of a possible ASD[15.1]. The RAI is simply calculated as the ratio of the RA and LA areas traced from the apical 4-chamber view:

Equation 15.1

$$RAI = RAA \div LAA$$

where   RAI   = relative atrial index (unitless)
        RAA   = right atrial area (cm²)
        LAA   = left atrial area (cm²)

Calculation of the QP:QS shunt ratio is based on stroke volume calculations (see Chapter 1). In the case of an ASD, the QP estimates the volume of blood flow to the lungs while QS estimates the volume of blood flow to the body (Fig. 15.12). Most commonly, the QP:QS ratio is calculated from the left ventricular outflow tract (LVOT) stroke volume [QS]

and the right ventricular outflow tract (RVOT) stroke volume [QP] (Fig. 15.13).

Equation 15.2

$$QS = CSA_{LVOT} \times VTI_{LVOT}$$

where   QS   = stroke volume to the body (mL)
        CSA_{LVOT} = cross-sectional area of the LVOT (cm²)
        VTI_{LVOT} = velocity time integral of the LVOT (cm)

Equation 15.3

$$QP = CSA_{RVOT} \times VTI_{RVOT}$$

where   QP   = stroke volume to the lungs (mL)
        CSA_{RVOT} = cross-sectional area of the RVOT (cm²)
        VTI_{RVOT} = velocity time integral of the RVOT (cm)

The QP:QS shunt ratio is derived as the ratio of the pulmonary venous SV and the systemic SV:

Equation 15.4

$$QP:QS = QP \div QS$$

where   QP   = stroke volume to the lungs (mL)
        QS   = stroke volume to the body (mL)

A QP:QS shunt ratio of 1.5:1 indicates the presence of a haemodynamically significant shunt. The limitations of stroke volume calculations are detailed in Chapter 1.

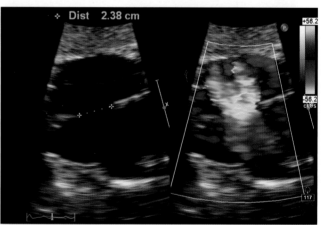

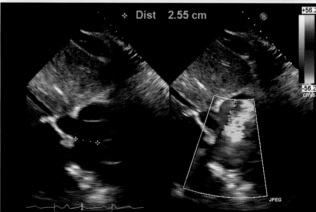

Figure 15.11 These images show the measurement of a 2⁰ atrial septal defect from the subcostal 4-chamber and subcostal short axis views. Colour flow imaging is used to assist in the identification of the defect borders.

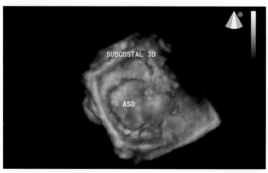

Figure 15.10 This 3D echocardiographic image acquired from a subcostal window shows a large 2⁰ atrial septal defect (ASD). Observe that the defect is D-shaped rather than circular.

[15.1] Kelly NF, Walters DL, Hourigan LA, Burstow DJ, Scalia GM. The relative atrial index (RAI)--a novel, simple, reliable, and robust transthoracic echocardiographic indicator of atrial defects. *J Am Soc Echocardiogr.* 2010 Mar;23(3):275-81.

Figure 15.12 This schematic illustrates the volumetric flow through the systemic and pulmonary venous circulations as seen with an atrial septal defect (ASD). Volumetric flow is depicted as cylinders. Observe that there is shunting from the left atrium (LA) to the right atrium (RA) via the ASD. This leads to a greater volume of blood flow to the pulmonary circulation compared with that to the systemic circulation (QP > QS). Observe that the QP (flow to the lungs) can be calculated using the stroke volumes derived at the tricuspid valve (tv), the right ventricular outflow tract (RVOT), or the main pulmonary artery (MPA); while QS (flow to the body) can be calculated using the stroke volume derived at the mitral valve (mv), the left ventricular outflow tract (LVOT), or the ascending aorta (Asc Ao). Most commonly, the shunt ratio is calculated from the stroke volumes measured at the LVOT and RVOT.

IVC = inferior vena cava; LV = left ventricle; Pul. veins = pulmonary veins; RV = right ventricle; SVC = superior vena cava.

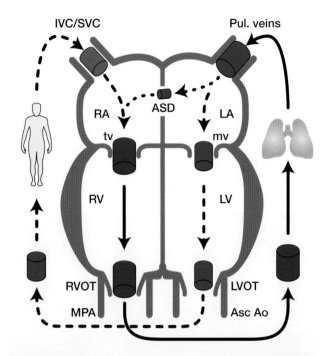

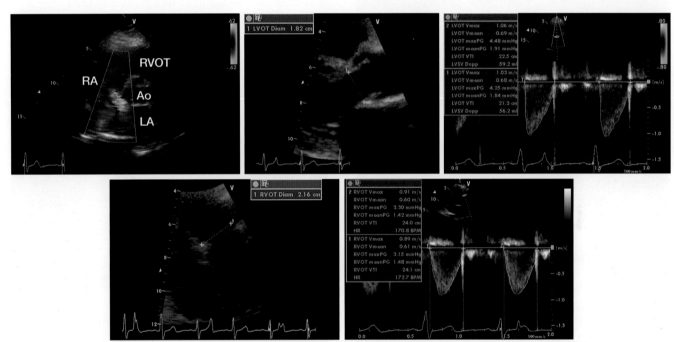

Figure 15.13 From the parasternal short axis view, an ostium secundum atrial septal defect is seen (*top left*). The QS (systemic stroke volume) or the volume of blood to the body is estimated from the left ventricular outflow tract (LVOT) diameter and the LVOT velocity time integral (VTI). The LVOT diameter is measured from a zoomed parasternal long axis view at mid-systole with the callipers placed from the inner edge of the junction between the anterior aortic wall and the interventricular septum to the inner edge of the junction between the posterior aortic wall and the anterior leaflet of the mitral valve (*top middle*). From an apical 5-chamber view, the LVOT VTI is traced from the pulsed-wave Doppler signal with a 2-4 mm sample volume placed 0.5 cm proximal to the aortic valve (*top right*). The QS is calculated as:

$$QS = CSA \times VTI$$
$$= (0.785 \times 1.82^2) \times 21.9$$
$$= 57\ mL$$

The QP (pulmonary stroke volume) or the volume of blood to the lungs is estimated from the right ventricular outflow tract (RVOT) diameter and the RVOT VTI. The RVOT diameter is measured from the zoomed parasternal long axis view of the RVOT at mid-systole with the callipers placed from the inner edge to the inner edge of the RVOT (*bottom left*). From the parasternal short axis view, the RVOT VTI is traced from the pulsed-wave Doppler signal with a 2-4 mm sample volume placed 0.5 cm proximal to the pulmonary valve (*bottom right*). The QP is calculated as:

$$QP = CSA \times VTI$$
$$= (0.785 \times 2.16^2) \times 24.0$$
$$= 88\ mL$$

The QP:QS is then derived as:

$$QP:QS = QP \div QS$$
$$= 88 \div 57$$
$$= 1.5$$

Ao = aorta; LA = left atrium; RA = right atrium.

Estimation of RVSP

In the presence of an ASD it is also important to estimate the right ventricular systolic pressure (RVSP). Recall that an ASD results in volume overload and/or pressure overload of the right heart and this can lead to pulmonary vascular injury and pulmonary hypertension. Therefore, the estimation of the pressure to the lungs is extremely important in patients with an ASD. The RVSP is estimated from the tricuspid regurgitant (TR) velocity in the standard manner and in the absence of RVOT obstruction and/or pulmonary stenosis, the RVSP is equal to the pulmonary artery systolic pressure (PASP).

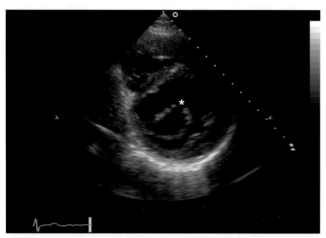

Figure 15.14 From this diastolic frame recorded from the parasternal short axis view, a cleft in the anterior leaflet of the mitral valve is seen (*).

Associated Lesions

As listed in Table 15.2, ASDs are commonly associated with other cardiac lesions and therefore, the echocardiographic examination should attempt to confirm or exclude these lesions. A common associated finding of a 1^0 ASD is a 'cleft' anterior leaflet of the mitral valve. This is best seen in the parasternal short axis view in diastole (Fig. 15.14). On real-time imaging, a cleft mitral leaflet has the appearance of 'two hands clapping'. Mitral regurgitation (MR) is frequently found with a 'cleft' mitral leaflet so assessment of the severity of MR is also important.

2^0 ASDs are usually isolated lesions; however, mitral valve prolapse and/or pulmonary valve stenosis may also be present. Therefore, when there is a 2^0 ASD, a thorough interrogation of the mitral and pulmonary valves is required.

As illustrated in Figure 15.3, the right pulmonary veins are in close proximity to the SVC so in the presence of a superior SV ASD, partial anomalous connection of the right pulmonary veins into the RA or SVC is common. Pulmonary venous drainage is usually difficult to assess by TTE and transoesophageal echocardiography (TOE) is usually required to confirm the drainage of all four pulmonary veins.

With a CS ASD, an associated persistent left superior vena cava (LSVC) is common. As illustrated in Figure 15.3, there is an embryologic connection between the left anterior cardinal vein (LACV), the left common cardinal vein (LCCV) and the left horn of the sinus venosus. Normally, the left sinus horn regresses and loses its connection with the LACV; a

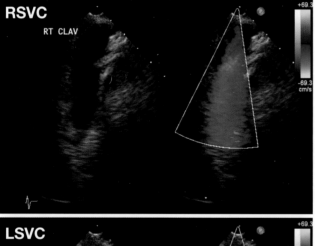

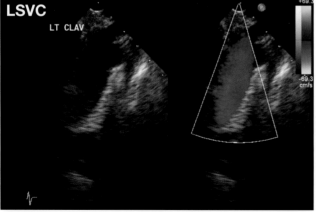

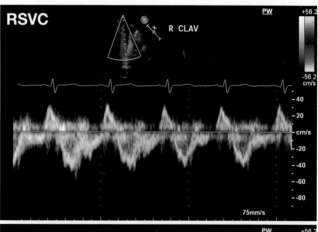

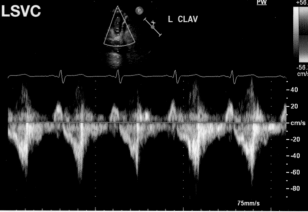

Figure 15.15 Images of a normal right superior vena cava (RSVC) and a persistent left superior vena cava (LSVC) are shown (*top and bottom, respectively*). Images for the right SVC are acquired from the right supraclavicular fossa while images of the LSVC are obtained from the left supraclavicular fossa. From these windows, the normal right SVC is imaged as a vertical vein to the right of the aortic arch while a persistent LSVC is imaged as a vertical vein to the left of the aortic arch. Colour flow Doppler imaging is extremely useful in identifying these vessels; flow within the vena cava appears as blue continuous flow away from the transducer. Pulsed-wave spectral Doppler can also be used to confirm the presence of venous flow away from the transducer (*right images*).

remnant of the left sinus horn and the adjacent LCCV remains as the coronary sinus. In the case of a CS ASD there is also a maldevelopment of the left venous structures such that the LACV persists as the LSVC which drains into the coronary sinus. One method for confirming the presence of a persistent LSVC is to image the LSVC from the left supraclavicular fossa similar to the manner in which the right SVC is imaged from the right supraclavicular fossa (Fig. 15.15).

Patent Foramen Ovale (PFO)

As previously mentioned, the foramen ovale provides a vital communication between the RA and LA during foetal development. Following birth, an increase in LA pressure leads to closure of the foramen ovale by the flap valve of the fossa ovalis. However, in about 25-30% of the population the

foramen ovale remains patent resulting in a small interatrial shunt in the region of the fossa ovalis; this is a PFO.

The definitive echocardiographic diagnosis of a PFO is based on identifying the separation of the flap valve of the fossa ovalis from the IAS. This is difficult to assess by TTE and is better seen by TOE (Fig. 15.16). On TTE, a PFO is usually detected via CFI as a small left-to-right shunt in the region of the fossa ovalis; this is best seen from the subcostal views (Fig. 15.17). An elevation in RA pressure can cause right-to-left shunting across a PFO and detection of a PFO in this situation is very important as this may lead to a paradoxical embolism (see Chapter 13 Paradoxical Embolism across a PFO).

A **persistent LSVC** may also occur as a variant of normal anatomy and its presence may be suspected when a dilated coronary sinus is seen from the standard parasternal long axis view. A persistent LSVC can be confirmed by imaging a vertical vein to the left of the aortic arch (see Fig 15.15) or by performing a saline contrast bubble study (see figures below)

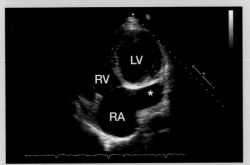

From this apical 4-chamber view with posterior tilt, a dilated coronary sinus (CS) is evident (*). LV = left ventricle; RA = right atrium; RV = right ventricle.

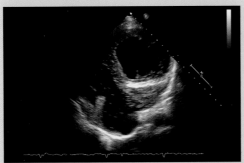

Following the saline contrast injection into the left antecubital vein, there is early opacification of the CS prior to contrast enhancement of other right-sided chambers.

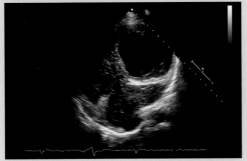

Following opacification of the CS, contrast enhancement of the RA and RV is observed.

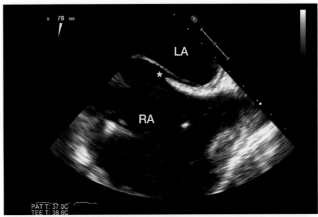

Figure 15.16 This transoesophageal echocardiographic image shows a patent foramen ovale (PFO). The PFO is evident by the appearance of a gap between the flap valve of the fossa ovalis and the atrial septum (*). LA = left atrium; RA = right atrium.

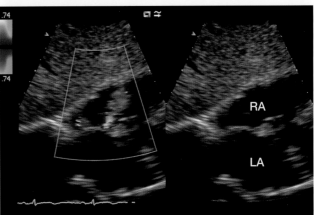

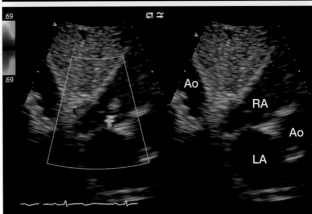

Figure 15.17 These images were recorded from the subcostal 4-chamber view (*top*) and the subcostal short axis view (*bottom*). Observe the left-to-right shunt across the atrial septum in the region of the fossa ovalis. This appearance is consistent with a patent foramen ovale. Ao = aorta; LA = left atrium; RA = right atrium.

> When a PFO is clinically suspected and a shunt across the region of the fossa ovalis cannot be detected, then a saline contrast bubble study is indicated. Please refer to Chapter 13 Paradoxical Embolism across a PFO.

Ventricular Septal Defects

A ventricular septal defect (VSD) is a congenital lesion where there is a communication between the left and right ventricles. VSDs account for approximately 20-25% of all congenital heart lesions.

With a VSD blood is usually shunted left-to-right as the pressure within the left ventricle (LV) is normally much higher than the pressure in the RV. Due to this left-to-right shunting, there is an increased volume of blood flow to the lungs, which in turn leads to an increase in the pulmonary venous return into the left heart. Therefore, in the presence of a significant left-to-right shunt across a VSD, there is dilatation of the left heart chambers. Dilatation of the right heart chambers may also occur when there is associated pulmonary hypertension. In order to appreciate the aetiology for each type of VSD it is important to first understand the embryological development of the IVS.

Embryological Development of the IVS

As for the formation of the IAS, the formation of the IVS is also quite complex. In particular, there are four distinct segments of the definitive IVS and each segment develops at different stages (Fig. 15.18). This complex staged formation of the IVS ensures that there is proper alignment of the AV valves with the respective ventricles and that the great arteries arise from their proper ventricles. As a result, in the fully developed heart, there are four major components of the IVS (Fig. 15.19). The muscular IVS forms the bulk of the IVS and includes the inlet, trabecular, and outlet (infundibular) components. The inlet septum separates the tricuspid and mitral valves and extends from the septal tricuspid leaflet to the distal cordal attachments of the tricuspid valve. The outlet (infundibular) septum separates the right and left ventricular outflow tracts and extends up to the pulmonary valve. The trabecular IVS is the largest part of the muscular IVS, extending from the inlet septum out to the apex and up to the outlet septum. The membranous septum accounts for a small section of the IVS; it is located at the base of the heart between the inlet and outlet components of the muscular septum and below the right and non-coronary cusps of the aortic valve. The septum between the insertion of the septal tricuspid leaflet and the anterior mitral leaflet represents the atrioventricular septum, because it lies between the RA and the LV.

Types of VSD

There are four types of VSD (Fig. 15.20) and these defects are named based on their anatomic location within the IVS. The perimembranous VSD is located beneath the aortic valve bordering the septal tricuspid leaflet and inferior to the crista supraventricularis. This defect is the most common type of VSD accounting for approximately 80% of all VSDs. These defects are also referred to as paramembranous, membranous or infracristal VSDs.

Muscular VSDs are the most common defects in infancy but as many of these defects spontaneously close; overall, they account for only about 20% of all VSDs. Muscular VSDs are located anywhere along the trabecular septum and they are bordered only by muscle. Muscular VSDs can be classified as anterior (anterior to the septal band), mid-muscular (posterior to the septal band), apical (inferior to the moderator band), and posterior (beneath the septal tricuspid leaflet). Muscular VSDs may also be multiple.

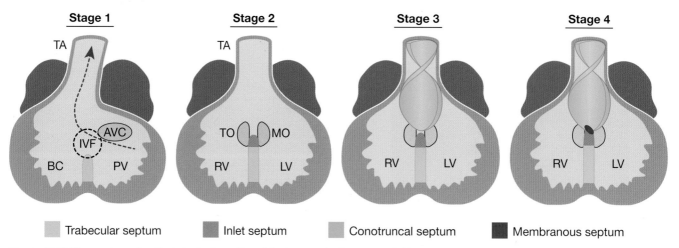

Figure 15.18 These schematics illustrate the formation of the interventricular septum (IVS). Note that the bulbus cordis (BC) becomes the definitive right ventricle (RV) and the primitive ventricle (PV) becomes the definitive left ventricle (LV). **Stage 1:** The trabecular IVS is the first to form, it grows from the apex towards the base of the heart. However, before this septum reaches the atrioventricular canal (AVC), it stops. This is because at this stage of development the truncus arteriosus (TA) only communicates with the bulbus cordis so blood flow from the primitive ventricle travels to the truncus arteriosus via the interventricular foramen (IVF). If fusion of the trabecular septum with the AVC occurred too soon the primitive ventricle would be shut off from the truncus arteriosus. **Stage 2:** As the truncus arteriosus moves to a central position and the AVC also shifts centrally to then divide into the tricuspid and mitral orifices (TO and MO), trabeculations from the inlet region form the inlet IVS which grows into the ventricular cavity perpendicular to the trabecular IVS. The fusion of these two septa forms the bulk of the muscular IVS. **Stage 3:** The conotruncal septum grows in a spiral direction and divides the truncus arteriosus into the aorta and pulmonary artery and the conus cordis into the right and left ventricular outflow tracts; thus, the outlet end of this septum forms the outlet muscular septum. This septum fuses with the endocardial cushions, the trabecular IVS and the inlet IVS. **Stage 4:** When there is complete division of the truncus arteriosus into the aorta and pulmonary trunk, the membranous IVS forms. Formation of the membranous IVS results in the complete closure of the interventricular foramen.
Note: The ventricular septum is a complex curved structure; however, for simplicity the formation of the IVS is illustrated in a two-dimensional plane.

Inlet VSDs result from deficiency of the inlet septum; these defects are located posterior and inferior to the membranous IVS beneath the tricuspid and mitral valves. An inlet VSD, also referred to as an AV canal type defect, accounts for approximately 5% of all VSDs.

A supracristal VSD occurs due to deficiency in the IVS above and anterior to the crista supraventricularis; these defects are located anterior to the membranous IVS and beneath the semilunar valves. Supracristal VSDs are also referred to as outlet, infundibular, conal, doubly committed or subarterial defects; they account for approximately 5% of all VSDs.

VSDs usually occur as isolated lesions. However, VSDs are often components of other more complex congenital cardiac anomalies such as tetralogy of Fallot (see below). Also VSDs often coexist with patent ductus arteriosus (PDA) or coarctation of the aorta. Furthermore, with a perimembranous or supracristal VSD, aortic regurgitation (AR) may occur due to distortion or incomplete support of the aortic valve cusps or annulus (see Fig. 7.43).

Role of Echocardiography in VSD
When assessing a patient with a VSD, it is important to:
- determine the type of defect
- estimate the anatomic size of the defect
- determine the shunt direction
- estimate the haemodynamic significance of the shunt
- estimate the RVSP.

VSDs Type and Shunt Direction
The VSD type is based on its anatomic location as well as the echocardiographic view in which the defect is seen. In particular, perimembranous and outlet VSDs can be differentiated from the parasternal short axis view (Fig. 15.21) while inlet VSDs and perimembranous VSDs can be differentiated from the apical views (Fig. 15.22).

The formation of aneurysmal tissue along the RV side of a perimembranous VSD is often seen (Fig. 15.23). On real-time imaging, aneurysmal tissue displays a characteristic 'windsock' appearance. The progressive development of aneurysmal tissue often leads to spontaneous closure of these defects.

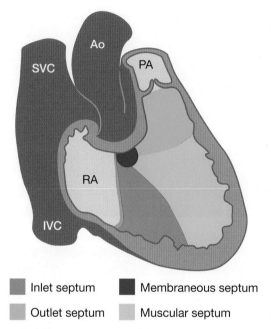

Figure 15.19 Four components of the interventricular septum are shown from a right ventricular aspect. See text for details.
Ao = aorta; IVC = inferior vena cava; PA = pulmonary artery; RA = right atrium; SVC = superior vena cava.

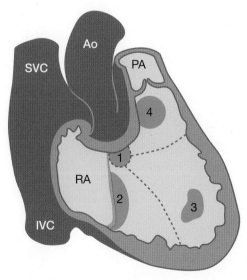

Figure 15.20 This schematic illustrates the four types of ventricular septal defect (VSD) from a right ventricular aspect: 1 = perimembranous VSD; 2 = inlet VSD; 3 = muscular VSD; 4 = supracristal or outlet VSD.
Ao = aorta; IVC = inferior vena cava; PA = pulmonary artery; RA = right atrium; SVC = superior vena cava.

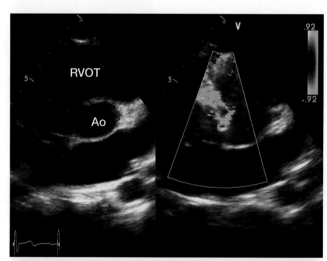

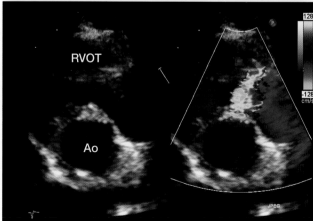

Figure 15.21 The parasternal short axis view can be used to differentiate between a perimembranous and a supracristal (outlet) VSD. A perimembranous VSD is located between 9 and 12 o'clock (top) while an outlet or supracristal VSD is located between 12 and 3 o'clock (bottom). Observe on the colour Doppler images flow through both VSDs is left-to-right; this appears as turbulent flow towards the transducer. Ao = aorta; RVOT = right ventricular outflow tract.

Muscular VSDs may occur anywhere along the muscular septum. When small, these defects may be difficult to detect via 2D imaging alone and CFI may be required to identify these VSDs (Fig. 15.24).

CFI also confirms the shunt direction as well as the phase of the cardiac cycle in which the shunt occurs (see Fig. 15.22-24). Most commonly, the LV systolic pressure is much higher than the RV systolic pressure so left-to-right shunting is most obvious during systole. In addition, when the LV diastolic pressure exceeds the RV diastolic pressure, left-to-right shunting during diastole may also be observed (Fig. 15.24).

When there is a marked increase in the right heart pressures, as seen with Eisenmenger's syndrome, shunting may be bidirectional or reversed (Fig. 15.25).

Anatomic Size of VSDs

Measurement of the anatomical size of the VSD is possible via 2D echocardiography (Fig. 15.26) and via CFI (see Fig. 15.28). Importantly, with a perimembranous VSD, the aortic valve may be sucked into the defect (see Fig. 7.43); as a result, the defect appears smaller and may be more difficult to detect.

Haemodynamic Significance of VSDs

The haemodynamic significance of a VSD can be estimated via calculation of the shunt ratio. In the case of a VSD, the QP estimates the volume of blood flow to the lungs or returning from the lungs while QS estimates the volume of blood flow to the body or returning from the body (Fig. 15.27). Calculation of the QP:QS ratio for a VSD is performed in the same manner as for calculation of the QP:QS in an ASD (Fig. 15.28).

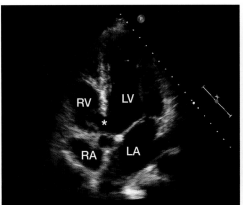
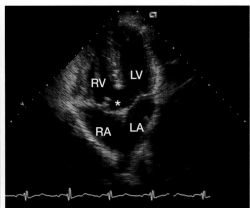

Figure 15.22 The apical views can be used to differentiate between a perimembranous and an inlet ventricular septal defect (VSD). Perimembranous VSDs are more anterior and are therefore seen in an apical 5-chamber view (*left*) while inlet VSDs are more inferior and posterior so these defects are seen in the apical 4-chamber view (*right*). Defects are indicated by the asterisk (*).
LA = left atrium; LV = left ventricle; RA = right atrium; RV = right ventricle.

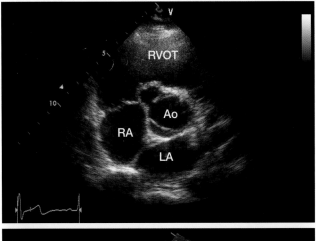
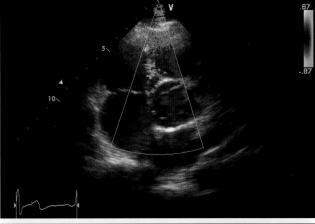
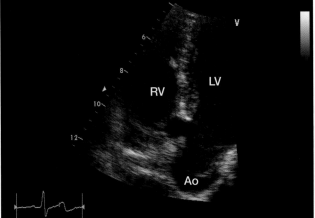
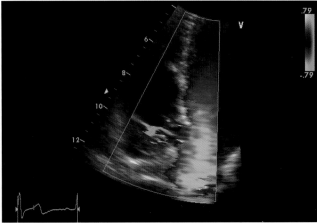

Figure 15.23 Aneurysmal tissue formation on the right ventricular (RV) side of a perimembranous ventricular septal defect is shown from a parasternal short axis view (*top images*) and a zoomed apical 5-chamber view (*bottom images*). Observe on the colour Doppler images that flow 'tunnels' through the defect from left-to-right. Ao = aorta; LA = left atrium; LV = left ventricle; RA = right atrium; RVOT = right ventricular outflow tract.

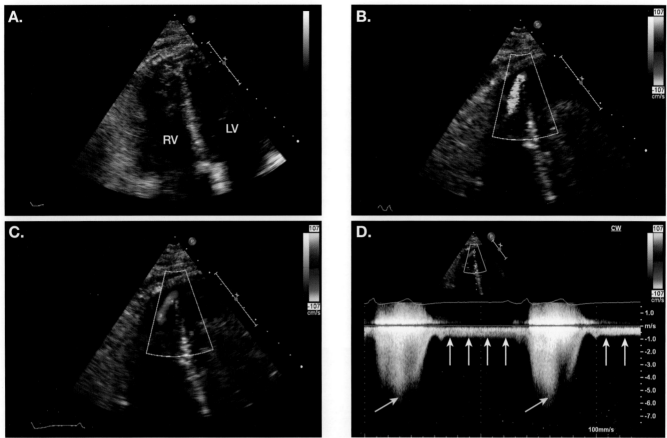

Figure 15.24 These images, recorded from the apical 4-chamber view, show a small apical ventricular defect (VSD). This defect is difficult to detect on 2D imaging (A). However, colour flow Doppler imaging clearly delineates left-to-right shunting across this defect in systole (B) as well as in diastole (C). The corresponding continuous-wave (CW) Doppler trace (D) confirms the presence of a high velocity gradient between the left ventricle (LV) and right ventricle (RV) during systole (*yellow arrows*) and a low velocity gradient between the ventricles during diastole (*white arrows*).
LV = left ventricle; RV = right ventricle.

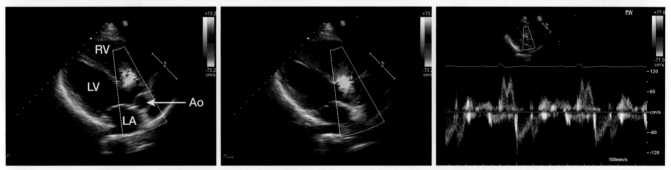

Figure 15.25 These images, recorded from an off-axis parasternal long axis view, show an Eisenmenger ventricular septal defect (VSD). Bidirectional shunting from left-to-right (red flow) and from right-to-left (blue flow) is shown on the colour Doppler images (*left and middle*). The corresponding pulsed-wave (PW) Doppler trace (*right*) also confirms the presence of bidirectional shunting from left-to-right (above the zero baseline) and from right-to-left (below the zero baseline). Ao = aorta; LA = left atrium; LV = left ventricle; RV = right ventricle.

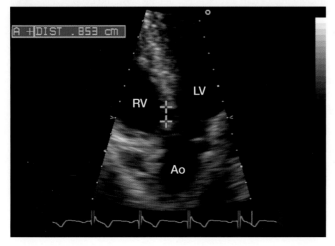

Figure 15.26 This image shows the measurement of a perimembranous ventricular septal defect from a zoomed apical 5-chamber 2D image.
Ao = aorta; LV = left ventricle; RV = right ventricle.

Figure 15.27 This schematic illustrates the volumetric flow through the systemic and pulmonary venous circulations as seen with a ventricular septal defect (VSD). Volumetric flow is depicted as cylinders. Observe that there is shunting from the left ventricle (LV) to the right ventricle (RV) via the VSD. This leads to a greater volume of blood flow to the pulmonary circulation compared with that to the systemic circulation (QP > QS). Observe that the volumetric flow across the right ventricular outflow tract (RVOT), main pulmonary artery (MPA) and the mitral valve (mv) is the same; this is the QP (flow to/from the lungs). Also observe that the volumetric flow across the left ventricular outflow tract (LVOT), the ascending aorta (AscAo) and the tricuspid valve (tv) is the same; this is the QS (flow to/from the body). Therefore, QP can be calculated using the RVOT, MPA or the mitral valve; while QS can be calculated using the LVOT, ascending aorta or the tricuspid valve. Most commonly, the shunt ratio is calculated from the stroke volumes measured at the LVOT and RVOT.

Also note that due to the increased volume of blood returning to the left heart from the lungs, the left heart tends to be dilated in the presence of a VSD.

IVC = inferior vena cava; LA = left atrium; Pul. veins = pulmonary veins; RA = right atrium; SVC = superior vena cava.

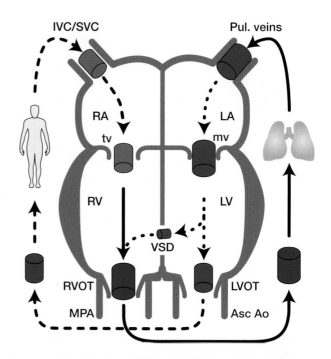

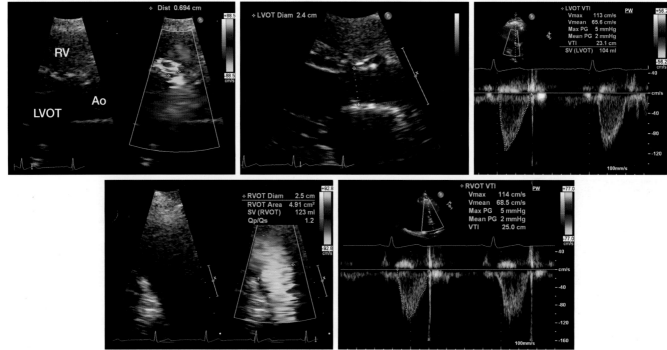

Figure 15.28 From a zoomed parasternal long axis view, a perimembranous ventricular septal defect measuring approximately 7 mm is seen (*top left*). The QS (systemic stroke volume) or the volume of blood to the body is estimated from the left ventricular outflow tract (LVOT) diameter and the LVOT velocity time integral (VTI). The LVOT diameter is measured from a zoomed parasternal long axis view at mid-systole with the callipers placed from the inner edge of the junction between the anterior aortic wall and the interventricular septum to the inner edge of the junction between the posterior aortic wall and the anterior leaflet of the mitral valve (*top middle*). From an apical 5-chamber view, the LVOT VTI is traced from the pulsed-wave Doppler signal with a 2-4 mm sample volume placed 0.5 cm proximal to the aortic valve (*top right*). The QS is calculated as:

$$QS = CSA \times VTI$$
$$= (0.785 \times 2.4^2) \times 23$$
$$= 104 \ mL$$

The QP (pulmonary stroke volume) or volume of blood to the lungs is estimated from the right ventricular outflow tract (RVOT) diameter and the RVOT VTI. The RVOT diameter is measured from a zoomed parasternal long axis view of the RVOT at mid-systole with the callipers placed from the inner edge to the inner edge of the RVOT (bottom left). Colour flow Doppler imaging has been used to help identify the RVOT borders. From the parasternal short axis view, the RVOT VTI is traced from the pulsed-wave Doppler signal with a 2-4 mm sample volume placed 0.5 cm proximal to the pulmonary valve (bottom right). The QP is calculated as:

$$QP = CSA \times VTI$$
$$= (0.785 \times 2.5^2) \times 25$$
$$= 123 \ mL$$

The QP:QS is then derived as:

$$QP:QS = QP \div QS$$
$$= 123 \div 104$$
$$= 1.2$$

Ao = aorta; RV = right ventricle.

Therefore, the QS can be calculated from the LVOT stroke volume while the QP is calculated from the RVOT stroke volume (see Equations 15.2, 15.3 and 15.4).

A QP:QS shunt ratio of 1.5:1 indicates the presence of a haemodynamically significant shunt. The limitations of stroke volume calculations are detailed in Chapter 1.

Estimation of RVSP

As for ASDs, estimation of the RVSP is also important when there is a VSD. This is because VSDs can cause pulmonary vascular injury and subsequent pulmonary hypertension due to increased volume overload and/or pressure overload to the pulmonary circulation. The RVSP can be estimated from the TR velocity in the standard manner or it can also be estimated from the peak VSD velocity. Recall that the peak systolic velocity across a VSD reflects the pressure difference between the LV and RV in systole. Therefore, from

the VSD velocity and from an estimation of the systolic blood pressure, it is possible to estimate the RVSP (Fig. 15.29) (also see Chapter 4, Estimation of Pulmonary Artery Pressures, Equations 4.16-4.17). Also remember that in the absence of RVOT obstruction and/or pulmonary stenosis, the RVSP is equivalent to the PASP.

Gerbode Defect

A Gerbode defect or an AV septal defect is another type of VSD that results in a LV-to-RA shunt. This defect occurs within the AV septum (Fig. 15.30). These defects may be acquired or congenital. Acquired defects may occur secondary to infective endocarditis of a VSD, or may result from trauma, acute myocardial infarction, or an aortic valve replacement.

On echocardiographic examination, a Gerbode defect is identified by detecting a shunt from the LV to the RA (Fig. 15.31). Importantly, the jet velocity across this defect should not be confused with the TR velocity. The systolic velocity through a Gerbode defect will be very high as this jet reflects the pressure difference between the LV and the RA during systole; therefore, if this jet is mistaken for the TR velocity, the RVSP will be significantly overestimated.

Atrioventricular Canal Defect

An atrioventricular canal defect (AVCD), also known as atrioventricular septal defect (AVSD) or endocardial cushion defect, accounts for approximately 3% of all CHDs. In order to appreciate this defect, it is important to first review the embryological development of the IAS, the IVS and the AV canal. As illustrated in Figure 15.18, the common AV canal divides into the right and left orifices which eventually form

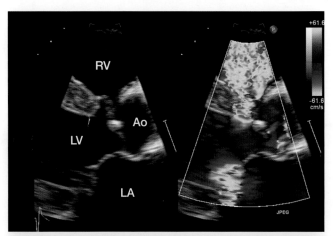

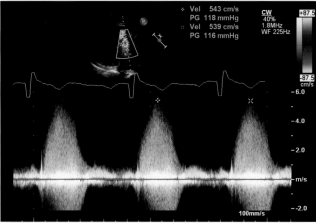

Figure 15.29 From a zoomed parasternal long axis view, a perimembranous ventricular septal defect (VSD) is apparent (*top*); mitral valve prolapse and mitral regurgitation are also evident. Via continuous-wave Doppler the peak systolic VSD velocity is measured at 5.4 m/s (*bottom*). This systolic VSD velocity reflects the pressure difference between the LV and the RV in systole. Using the simplified Bernoulli equation ($4V^2$), the VSD velocity can be converted to a pressure gradient. Therefore, if the VSD velocity is measured and the LV systolic pressure (LVSP) is known then the RVSP can be estimated. In the absence of aortic stenosis or LVOT obstruction, the LVSP can be estimated from the systolic blood pressure (SBP). The SBP at the time of the study was 140 mm Hg, therefore, the RVSP in this example is:

$$RVSP = SBP - 4\,V_{VSD}^2$$
$$= 140 - 4\,(5.4)^2$$
$$= 140 - 117$$
$$= 23\ mm\ Hg$$

Ao = aorta; LA = left atrium; LV = left ventricle; RV = right ventricle.

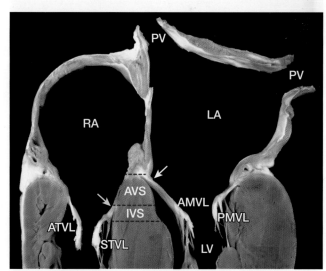

Figure 15.30 This gross pathological specimen illustrates normal anatomical relationships. Observe that the septal tricuspid valve leaflet (STVL) (*yellow arrow*) is 'lower' than the insertion of the anterior mitral valve leaflet (AMVL) (*white arrow*). As a result a portion of the ventricular septum lies between the right atrium and the left ventricle. This is the atrioventricular septum, and the AV node is located along the right atrial aspect of this septum. When this portion of the septum is congenitally absent, the mitral annulus will "drop" to the same level as the tricuspid annulus; the result will be an interatrial communication. In the partial form of AV septal defect this communication is referred to as a primum atrial septal defect.
ATVL = anterior tricuspid valve leaflet; LA = left atrium; PMVL = posterior mitral valve leaflet; PV = pulmonary vein.
By permission of Mayo Foundation for Medical Education and Research. All rights reserved. Courtesy of William D. Edwards, MD.

the tricuspid and mitral orifices. Septation is initiated by the growth of two endocardial cushions which appear at the superior and inferior borders of the common AV canal. The endocardial cushions also contribute to the formation of the primum IAS, the membranous IVS, the septal leaflet of the tricuspid valve and the anterior leaflet of the mitral valve. AVCD occurs when there is maldevelopment or malfusion of the superior and inferior endocardial cushions. There

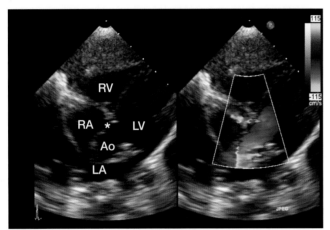

Figure 15.31 This image recorded from the subcostal 5-chamber view shows a Gerbode defect (*). On colour flow imaging, a shunt from the left ventricle (LV) to the right atrium (RA) is evident. Ao = aorta; LA = left atrium; RV = right ventricle.

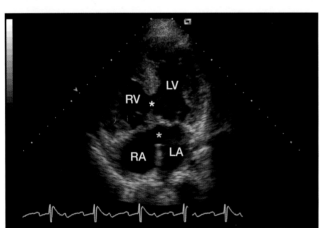

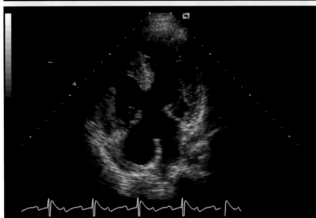

Figure 15.32 These apical 4-chamber images show a complete atrioventricular (AV) canal defect in systole (*top*) and diastole (*bottom*). Observe that there is a large common AV valve, a large inlet ventricular septal defect (*white* *) and a large 1⁰ atrial septal defect (*yellow* *). Observe that during diastole when the common AV valve opens there is a large 'hole' in the centre of the heart.
LA = left atrium; LV = left ventricle; RA = right atrium; RV = right ventricle.

are several types of AVCD depending on the degree of maldevelopment of the endocardial cushions.

Complete AVCD is characterised by a 1⁰ ASD, an inlet VSD and a large common AV valve. More than 75% of patients with complete AVCD have Down syndrome (see Appendix 5). A partial AV canal defect is characterised by a 1⁰ ASD and a cleft anterior mitral valve leaflet (see Atrial Septal Defects). AVCD is also associated with other congenital heart lesions such as tetralogy of Fallot.

The best echocardiographic views for identifying complete AVCD include the apical 4-chamber view (Fig. 15.32) and the subcostal 4-chamber view as these views best evaluate the cardiac crux. Echocardiography is also useful in assessing the severity of AV valve regurgitation, the degree and direction of intracardiac shunting, LV and RV systolic function, and estimation of the PA pressures.

Patent Ductus Arteriosus

In the foetal heart, the ductus arteriosus (DA), which is derived from the distal portion of the left sixth aortic arch, provides an arterial connection between the upper descending aorta and the PA. This communication is essential in foetal circulation. In the foetal heart, the lungs are inactive and the pulmonary vascular resistance is high so the DA serves to redirect the majority of blood away from the developing lungs into the descending aorta. Following birth, the DA spontaneously closes within 72 hours. The obliterated ductus arteriosus forms the ligamentum arteriosum.

A patent ductus arteriosus (PDA) occurs when there is a persistent communication between the distal main PA (near the origin of the left PA) and the descending aorta (just distal to the left subclavian artery) (Fig. 15.33). PDAs comprise approximately 10% of CHDs at birth; PDAs are associated with a number of congenital heart defects but they may occur in isolation.

Role of Echocardiography in PDA

The role of echocardiography in a PDA includes to:
- establish the diagnosis
- determine the shunt direction
- estimate the haemodynamic significance of the shunt
- estimate the PASP.

Diagnosis of a PDA and Shunt Direction

A PDA is best imaged from a high parasternal long axis view of the PA ('ductal' view), a high parasternal short axis view of the PA bifurcation, or from the suprasternal long axis view with slight counter-clockwise rotation (Fig. 15.34). In the adult patient, 2D imaging of the PDA is difficult, especially if it is of a small calibre, so CFI is often required to identify this defect. On the colour flow Doppler examination, PDA flow appears continuous. This is because normally the aortic pressure exceeds the PA pressure during systole and diastole. However, when there is Eisenmenger's physiology, shunting may be absent (equalisation of pressures) or reversed (PA pressure exceeds aortic pressure). From the above-mentioned views, PDA flow is typically directed towards the transducer.

Haemodynamic Significance of a PDA

The haemodynamic significance of a PDA can be estimated based on the calculation of the QP:QS shunt ratio. In the case of a PDA, the QP estimates the volume of blood flow returning from the lungs while QS estimates the volume of blood flow returning from the body (Fig. 15.35). Most commonly, QP is calculated using the stroke volume derived from the LVOT which determines the stroke volume returning from the lungs and QS is calculated using the stroke volume derived from the RVOT which determines the stroke volume returning from the body (Fig. 15.36). Importantly, this is the opposite to the manner in which the QP:QS shunt ratio is calculated for an ASD or a VSD.

> **Technical Tip**
>
> When using the calculation package on ultrasound machines for the QP:QS shunt ratio, it is assumed that the stroke volume measured from the LVOT is the QS and that the stroke volume measured from the RVOT is the QP. This is not the case in the presence of a PDA whereby the LVOT stroke volume is the QP (blood flow returning from the lungs) and the RVOT stroke volume is the QS (blood flow returning from the body).

A QP:QS shunt ratio of 1.5:1 indicates the presence of a haemodynamically significant shunt. The limitations of stroke volume calculations are detailed in Chapter 1.

Estimation of PASP

In the presence of a PDA, the PASP can be estimated from the peak systolic PDA velocity. Recall that the peak systolic velocity across a PDA reflects the systolic pressure difference between the aorta and PA. Therefore, from the systolic PDA velocity and from an estimation of the systolic blood pressure, it is possible to estimate the PASP (Fig. 15.37) (also see Chapter 4, Estimation of Pulmonary Artery Pressures, Equations 4.18).

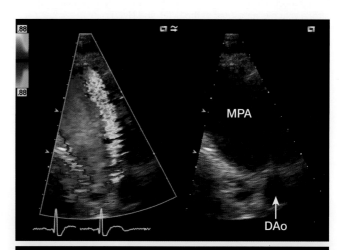

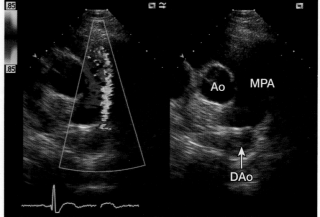

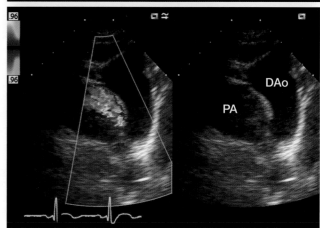

Figure 15.34 These images show a patent ductus arteriosus (PDA) recorded from a high parasternal long axis view of the pulmonary artery (PA) (*top*), a high parasternal short axis view of the PA bifurcation (*middle*), and a suprasternal window (*bottom*). The colour flow Doppler images confirm shunting across the PDA from the descending aorta (DAo) to the main pulmonary artery (MPA); this appears as red flow towards the transducer. Ao = aorta.

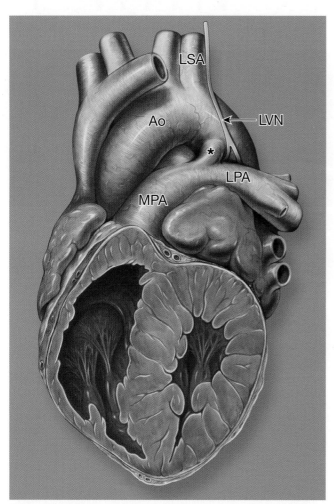

Figure 15.33 This schematic illustrates a patent ductus arteriosus (PDA). The PDA (*) is an arterial communication between the distal main pulmonary artery (MPA), near the origin of the left pulmonary artery (LPA), and the descending aorta (Ao), just distal to the left subclavian artery (LSA). The left vagus nerve (LVN) is also shown. Reproduced from
https://en.wikipedia.org/wiki/File:Heart_patent_ductus_arteriosus.jpg
Patrick J. Lynch; illustrator; C. Carl Jaffe; MD; cardiologist Yale University Center for Advanced Instructional Media. Medical Illustrations by Patrick Lynch, generated for multimedia teaching projects by the Yale University School of Medicine, Center for Advanced Instructional Media, 1987-2000.

Figure 15.35 This schematic illustrates the volumetric flow through the systemic and pulmonary venous circulations in a patent ductus arteriosus (PDA). Volumetric flow is depicted as cylinders. Observe that there is shunting from the descending aorta (Ao) to the pulmonary artery via the PDA. This results in a greater volume of blood flow to the pulmonary circulation compared with that to the systemic circulation (QP > QS). Observe that the volumetric flow across the right ventricular outflow tract (RVOT), the main pulmonary artery (MPA) and the tricuspid valve (tv) is the same; this represents the volumetric flow returning from the body (QS). Also observe that the volumetric flow across the left ventricular outflow tract (LVOT), the ascending aorta (AscAo) and the mitral valve (mv) is the same; this reflects the volumetric flow returning from the lungs (QP). Therefore, QP (volume returning from the lungs) can be calculated using the LVOT, ascending aorta (proximal to the PDA) or the mitral valve; while the QS (volume returning from the body) can be calculated using the RVOT, MPA (proximal to the PDA) or the tricuspid valve. Most commonly, the shunt ratio is calculated from the stroke volumes measured at the LVOT and RVOT.

Also note that due to the increased volume of blood returning to the left heart from the lungs, the left heart tends to be dilated in the presence of a PDA.

IVC = inferior vena cava; LA = left atrium; LV = left ventricle; Pul. veins = pulmonary veins; RA = right atrium; RV = right ventricle; SVC = superior vena cava.

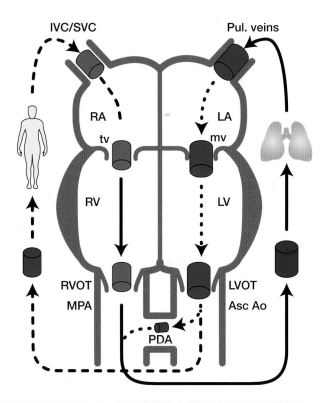

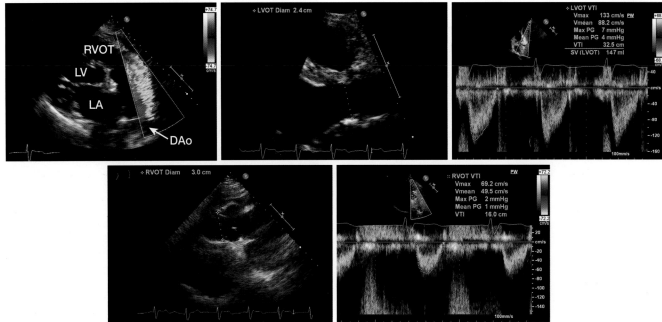

Figure 15.36 From an off-axis parasternal long axis view of the right ventricular outflow tract (RVOT), a patent ductus arteriosus is seen (*top left*). The QP (pulmonary stroke volume) or the volume of blood flow ***returning from the lungs*** is estimated from the left ventricular outflow tract (LVOT) diameter and the LVOT velocity time integral (VTI). The LVOT diameter is measured from a zoomed parasternal long axis view at mid-systole with the callipers placed from the inner edge of the junction between the anterior aortic wall and the interventricular septum to the inner edge of the junction between the posterior aortic wall and the anterior leaflet of the mitral valve (*top middle*). From an apical 5-chamber view, the LVOT VTI is traced from the pulsed-wave Doppler signal with a 2-4 mm sample volume placed 0.5 cm proximal to the aortic valve (*top right*). The QP is calculated as:

QP   = CSA x VTI
           = (0.785 x 2.4^2) x 32.5
           = 147 mL

The QS (systemic stroke volume) or the volume of blood flow ***returning from the body*** is estimated from the right ventricular outflow tract (RVOT) diameter and the RVOT VTI. The RVOT diameter is measured from a zoomed high parasternal long axis view of the RVOT at mid-systole with the callipers placed from the inner edge to the inner edge of the RVOT (bottom left). From the parasternal short axis view, the RVOT VTI is traced from the pulsed-wave Doppler signal with a 2-4 mm sample volume placed 0.5 cm proximal to the pulmonary valve (bottom right). The QS is calculated as:

QS   = CSA x VTI
           = (0.785 x 3.0^2) x 16
           = 113 mL

The QP:QS is then derived as:

QP:QS   = QP ÷ QS
             = 147 ÷ 113
             = 1.3

DAo = descending aorta; LA = left atrium; LV = left ventricle.

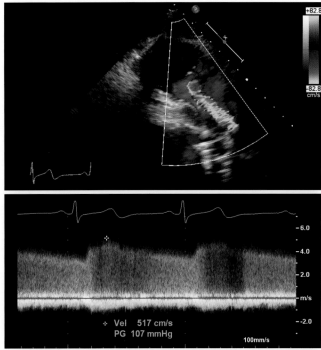

Figure 15.37 From a parasternal long axis view of the right ventricular outflow tract, a patent ductus arteriosus (PDA) is apparent (*top*). Via continuous-wave Doppler the peak systolic PDA velocity is measured at 5.2 m/s (*bottom*). This systolic PDA velocity reflects the systolic pressure difference between the aorta (Ao) and the pulmonary artery (PA). Using the simplified Bernoulli equation ($4V^2$), the PDA velocity can be converted to a pressure gradient. Therefore, if the systolic PDA velocity is measured and the systolic blood pressure (SBP) is known then the PASP can be estimated. The SBP at the time of the study was measured at 135 mm Hg, therefore, the PASP in this example is:

$$PASP = SBP - 4\ V_{PDA}^2$$
$$= 135 - 4\ (5.17)^2$$
$$= 135 - 107$$
$$= 28\ mm\ Hg$$

Closure Devices for Intracardiac Shunts

Mid-muscular and perimembranous VSDs, 2° ASDs and PDAs may be closed by transcatheter (percutaneous) closure devices (Fig. 15.38). For these procedures, echocardiography has an important role in patient selection, monitoring and guiding the procedure, assessing the end result, and detection of post-procedure complications. In particular, prior to device closure of an ASD or VSD, TOE is used to ensure that there are sufficient tissue rims to allow for safe anchoring of the device and that there will be an adequate distance between the device and other surrounding cardiac structures. In addition prior to percutaneous ASD closures, TOE is employed to ensure that pulmonary venous connections are normal. TOE is also utilised to monitor and guide the procedure. Following the procedure, TTE is used to confirm that the device is well seated and to detect the degree of any residual shunting (Fig. 15.39).

TTE may also be used to detect rare device complications such as device embolisation, partial dehiscence, cardiac perforation, device erosion, or thrombus formation (Fig. 15.40-15.42). In particular, erosion of the device through cardiac structures may occur when an oversized device rubs against the cardiac walls with each cardiac cycle while device embolisation may occur with smaller devices and insufficient tissue rims.

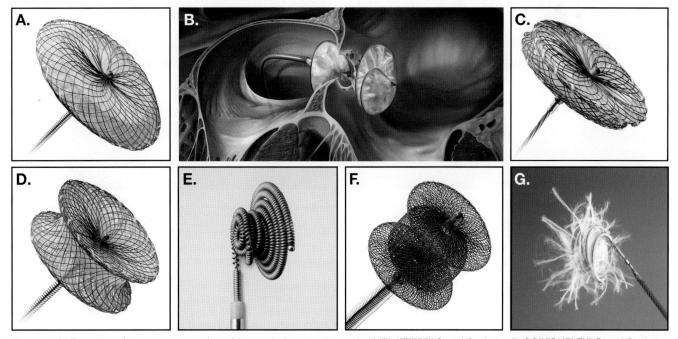

Figure 15.38 Examples of percutaneous occluder/closure devices are shown. A: AMPLATZER™ Septal Occluder; B: GORE® HELEX® Septal Occluder; C: AMPLATZER™ Membranous VSD Occluder; D: AMPLATZER™ Muscular VSD Occluder; E: Nit-Occlud® PDA; F: AMPLATZER™ Duct Occluder II Additional Sizes; G: Flipper® PDA Closure Detachable Coil.

AMPLATZER and St. Jude Medical are trademarks of St. Jude Medical, Inc. or its related companies. Images A, C, D and F reprinted with permission of St. Jude Medical™, ©2013 All rights reserved. Image B reprinted with permission of W. L. Gore & Associates, Inc. Flagstaff, AZ. Image E reprinted with permission of the pfm medical ag, Köln, Germany. Permission for use of Image G granted by Cook Medical Incorporated, Bloomington, Indiana.

Panel A

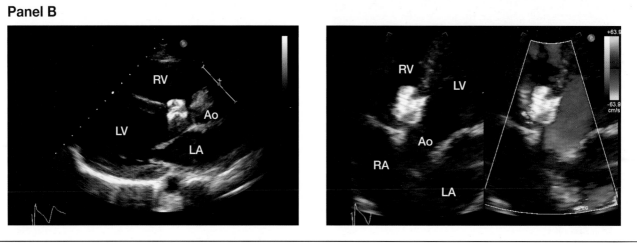

Panel B

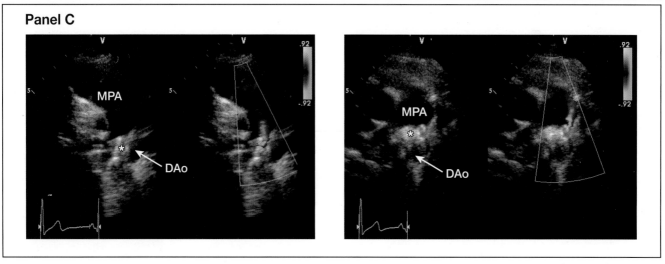

Panel C

Figure 15.39 These images show examples of various occluder devices for an atrial septal defect (ASD), a ventricular septal defect (VSD) and a patent ductus arteriosus (PDA).

Panel A: A 22 mm AMPLATZER™ Atrial Septal Occluder closing a secundum ASD is in-situ. Images are recorded from a low parasternal short axis view. Observe that the device appears well seated with both fully deployed discs on the appropriate sides of the septum (*left*). On the colour Doppler image, trivial intradevice flow is noted (*right*).

Panel B: An 8 mm AMPLATZER™ Ventricular Septal Occluder closing a perimembranous VSD is in-situ. From an off axis parasternal long axis view, the device appears well seated with both fully deployed discs on the appropriate sides of the septum (*left*). On the colour Doppler image acquired from a zoomed apical 5-chamber view, trivial left-to-right shunting at the superior aspect of the device is noted (*right*).

Panel C: A PDA coil closing a PDA is in-situ. Images are recorded from the parasternal long axis view of the right ventricular outflow tract (*left*) and the parasternal short axis view (*right*). The PDA coil device appears well seated (*). A trivial degree of residual left-to-right shunting is noted on the colour Doppler images; this appears as red flow towards the transducer.

Ao = aorta; DAo = descending aorta; MPA = main pulmonary artery; LA = left atrium; LV = left ventricle; RA = right atrium; RV = right ventricle.

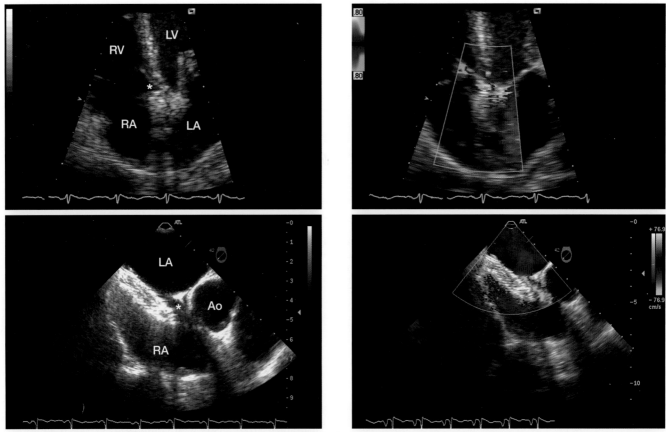

Figure 15.40 A 34 mm atrial septal occluder device is in-situ. On the transthoracic images, recorded from zoomed apical 4-chamber views, apparent separation of the device from the plane of the atrial septum at the anterosuperior margin is noted (*) (*top left*). On the corresponding colour Doppler image, residual left-to-right shunting at this margin is detected; this appears as red flow towards the transducer (*top right*). On the transoesophageal echocardiogram, partial dehiscence of the device anteriorly and superiorly, adjacent to the aortic root and superior vena cava was confirmed (*) (*bottom left*). On the corresponding colour Doppler image, a moderate degree of continuous left-to-right shunting across this defect was observed; this appears as blue flow away from the transducer (*bottom right*). Ao = aorta; LA = left atrium; LV = left ventricle; RA = right atrium; RV = right ventricle.

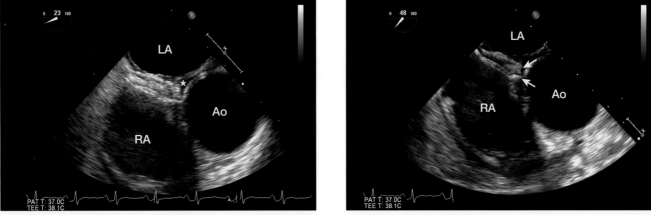

Figure 15.41 A patent foramen ovale (PFO) occluder device is in-situ. Transoesophageal echocardiographic images are shown. Observe that a very small localised pericardial effusion within the transverse sinus is evident (*). On closer inspection, the PFO occluder device is seen to protrude through the cardiac wall into this pericardial space (*arrows*) (*right*). These features are consistent with device erosion and cardiac perforation. Ao = aorta; LA = left atrium; RA = right atrium.

Device erosion is a serious and potentially life threatening complication of percutaneous atrial septal occluder (ASO) devices. Clues to the presence of ASO device erosion include:

- new cardiac symptoms of pericardial pain, dyspnoea, or cardiac tamponade;
- device size and geometry in relation to atrial size, particularly if the device extends more than 90% across the atrial septum;
- relationship of the device to the aorta and posterior LA wall, especially if the device is in contact with these structures;
- pre-implantation deficient superior-anterior rim;
- presence of pericardial fluid adjacent to the device, even if trivial, especially with confirmed haemopericardium;
- transoeosophgeal echocardiographic or computed tomography evidence of disc protrusion into or through the atrial/aortic wall.

Reference: Ivens E, Hamilton-Craig C, Aroney C, Clarke A, Jalali H, Burstow DJ. Early and late cardiac perforation by Amplatzer atrial septal defect and patent foramen ovale devices. *J Am Soc Echocardiogr.* 2009 Sep;22(9):1067-70.

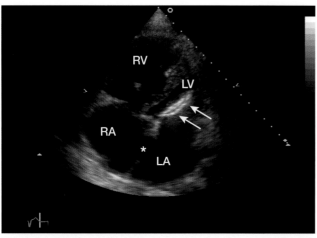 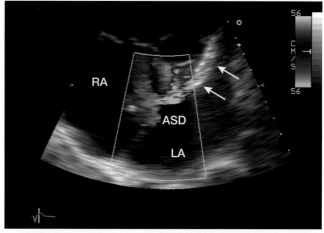

Figure 15.42 From an off-axis apical 4-chamber view, an atrial septal occluder (ASO) device has dislodged and embolised to the left heart where it is lodged across the mitral valve (*arrows*) (*left*); the large atrial septal defect (*) and marked right atrial (RA) and right ventricular (RV) dilatation are also obvious. From a zoomed view with colour flow imaging, left-to-right shunting across the atrial septal defect (ASD) is apparent (*right*); the dislodged ASO device is also seen (*arrows*). LA = left atrium; LV = left ventricle.

Obstructive Lesions

Pulmonary Stenosis

Congenital pulmonary stenosis (PS) may occur at the valve level (valvular PS), below the pulmonary valve (subvalvular PS or infundibular stenosis), above the pulmonary valve (supravalvular PS), at the main PA branches (branch stenosis) and/or within the peripheral pulmonary arteries (peripheral stenosis). Valvular PS is the most common site of congenital PS and accounts for approximately 10% of congenital heart lesions. Congenital PS is associated with a number of congenital and genetic syndromes (see Appendix 5).

The role of echocardiography in congenital PS includes:
- determining the site and severity of obstruction
- assessing RV size and systolic function
- estimating the PASP.

The comprehensive echocardiographic assessment of PS is described in detail in Chapter 9 and will not be discussed further.

Congenital Aortic Stenosis

As for congenital PS, congenital aortic stenosis (AS) may also occur at multiple levels including at the valve level (valvular AS), below the aortic valve (subvalvular AS), or above the aortic valve (supravalvular AS). Valvular AS is the most common site of congenital AS and accounts for approximately 70% of patients with congenital AS. There are also a number of congenital heart lesions associated with congenital AS (Table 15.3).

Valvular AS

Congenital causes of valvular AS include bicuspid and unicuspid aortic valves. These valve morphologies have been previously discussed in Chapter 7 (Aortic Valve Stenosis). To summarise, a unicuspid aortic valve (UAV) is a very rare lesion that occurs when there is fusion between two of the three developing aortic valve cusps or fusion of all three developing cusps resulting in an abnormal valve with a solitary opening. UAVs may be acommissural or unicommissural (see Fig. 7.9).

A bicuspid aortic valve (BAV), which occurs in approximately 1-2% of the general population, may be categorised as those with a raphe and those without a raphe (see Fig. 7.10).

The orientation of BAVs is variable (Fig. 15.43). The most common site of a raphe is between the right and left coronary cusps (≈ 85% of cases) followed by fusion between the right and non coronary cusps (≈ 15% of cases); fusion between the left and non coronary cusps is rare. A BAV without a raphe is less common than a BAV with a raphe; these 'true' BAVs account for only 10% of all BAVs. Typically a true BAV has near-equal sized cusps with commissures located anteriorly and posteriorly or medially and laterally.

The role of echocardiography in UAV and BAV includes:
- identifying valvular morphology
- assessment of LV size and systolic function
- determining the degree of any associated LV hypertrophy
- estimating the severity of stenosis.

Importantly, the diagnosis of a UAV and a BAV is made from the parasternal short axis view by identifying the number of commissural attachments to the aortic root during systole.

Table 15.3 Common CHDs associated with Congenital AS

Level	Associated Lesions
Valvular AS (BAV)	CoAo (50% of CoAo have BAV) ASD VSD PDA Common in Shone syndrome*
Subvalvular AS (Fixed)	CoAo PDA VSD Part of Shone syndrome*
Supravalvular AS	ASD PDA VSD CoAo PA stenosis (valvular or branch stenosis) Coronary artery anomalies

* Shone syndrome is comprised of a series of left heart obstructive lesions including supravalvular mitral ring, parachute mitral valve, subaortic stenosis and coarctation of the aorta.
AS = aortic stenosis; ASD = atrial septal defect; BAV = bicuspid aortic valve; CoAo = coarctation of the aorta; PA = pulmonary artery; PDA = patent ductus arteriosus; VSD = ventricular septal defect

Technical Tips for the Diagnosis of a BAV

Systole not Diastole

The diagnosis of a BAV with a raphe is best made from the PSAX view in systole. This is because during diastole when the valve is closed the BAV may mimic a normal trileaflet valve (*below left*). During systole the orifice of the BAV appears oval and only two commissures can be seen extending to the aortic root (*below right*).

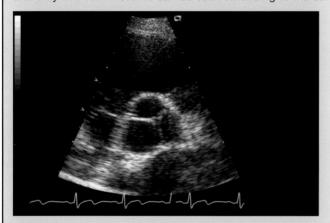
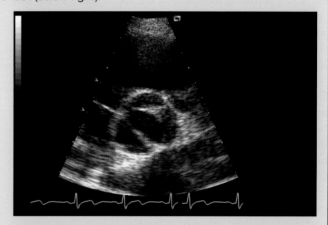

Eccentric Closure of the Aortic Valve

A BAV with a raphe often results in unequal cusp size due to fusion of two cusps which effectively creates one larger cusp. Therefore during diastole the valve does not close in the centre of the aortic root. From the parasternal long axis (PLAX) view this appears as eccentric closure of the valve. This appearance can be appreciated on M-mode (*below left*) and 2D imaging (*below right*).

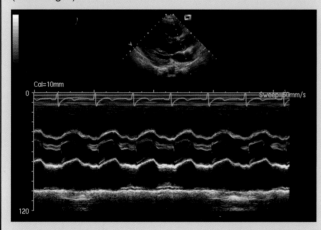
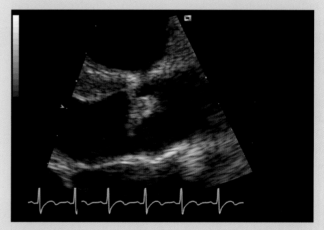

Diastolic Prolapse & Systolic Doming of the Aortic Valve (PLAX)

From the PLAX view diastolic prolapse of the aortic valve (*below left*) and systolic doming of the valve *(below right)* are also clues to the presence of a BAV. In particular, with a BAV the narrowing occurs at the tips of the aortic leaflets which results in the characteristic systolic doming of the valve.

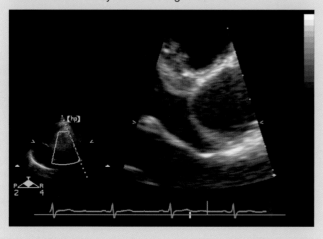
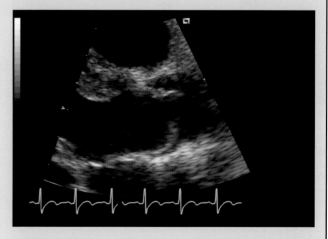

For example, an acommissural UAV, where there are no commissural attachments to the aortic root, has a 'volcano' appearance while a unicommissural UAV in which there is only one commissural attachment to the aortic root displays a characteristic eccentric orifice opening during systole (see Fig 7.12). A BAV is identified by the appearance of only two commissural attachments to the aortic root (see Fig. 7.13). The comprehensive echocardiographic assessment of AS which may be associated with a UAV or a BAV is described in detail in Chapter 7 and will not be discussed further.

Subvalvular AS

Subvalvular AS refers to obstruction proximal to or just below the aortic valve; that is, obstruction occurs on the LVOT side of the valve. Subvalvular AS accounts for approximately 30% of congenital AS cases and may occur as a fixed obstruction or a dynamic obstruction (Fig. 15.44). Fixed obstruction may be in the form of a discrete fibrous membrane, a fibromuscular ridge, or a circumferential, tunnel-like narrowing. Dynamic obstruction is most commonly associated with hypertrophic cardiomyopathy where there is asymmetric septal hypertrophy (ASH) which causes systolic anterior motion (SAM) of the anterior mitral valve into the LVOT during systole (see Chapter 6, Hypertrophic Cardiomyopathy).

On the echocardiographic examination, subvalvular AS can be diagnosed by identifying the subaortic membrane, the fibromuscular ridge or tunnel, or SAM of the anterior mitral leaflet. Importantly, as a subaortic membrane is often quite thin, this structure is best identified from the apical views where the membrane is orientated perpendicular to the ultrasound beam (Fig. 15.45). CFI is especially valuable in identifying the level of stenosis while continuous-wave (CW) Doppler is used to determine the pressure gradient across the obstruction. Aortic regurgitation (AR) is also frequently seen with subaortic AS.

Supravalvular Aortic Stenosis

Supravalvular AS refers to obstruction distal to or above the aortic valve; that is, obstruction occurs on the aortic side of the valve. This is the least common type of congenital AS accounting for about 5% of congenital AS cases. Three morphological types of supravalvular stenosis have been described: (1) an hourglass deformity (most common), (2) a fibrous membrane with central orifice, and (3) a diffusely hypoplastic ascending aorta (Fig. 15.46). Supravalvular AS is most often encountered in patients with William syndrome (see Appendix 5).

On the echocardiographic examination, supravalvular AS is best identified by imaging the ascending aorta from the parasternal long axis view, a high parasternal long axis view, the suprasternal window and/or from the right sternal edge (Fig. 15.47-15.48). As for subvalvular AS, CFI is especially valuable in identifying the level of obstruction while CW Doppler is used to determine the pressure gradient across the narrowing.

Coarctation of the Aorta

Coarctation of the aorta (CoAo) is characterised by a discrete narrowing of the descending thoracic aorta, just distal to the left subclavian artery and adjacent to the ligamentum arteriosum (Fig. 15.49). Anatomic variations to CoAo include the location of the narrowing and the type of narrowing; for example, CoAo may occur as a long segment stenosis or diffuse hypoplasia and rarely the coarctation may be located in the ascending or abdominal aorta. CoAo accounts for about 6–8% of patients with CHD. CoAo is also associated with a number of congenital heart lesions (Table 15.4) and genetic syndromes (see Appendix 5).

In order to appreciate the possible causes for CoAo and to appreciate the various segments of the aorta, it is first important to review the embryological development of the aortic arches.

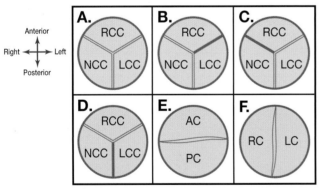

Figure 15.43 Various orientations of bicuspid aortic valves (BAV) compared with a normal trileaflet valve are illustrated based on the parasternal short axis view of the aortic valve. A = Normal trileaflet aortic valve with a non-coronary cusp (NCC), a right coronary cusp (RCC) and a left coronary cusp (LCC); B = BAV with a raphe between the RCC and LCC; C = BAV with a raphe between RCC and NCC; D = BAV with a raphe between LCC and NCC; E = true BAV with an anterior cusp (AC) and posterior cusp (PC); F = true BAV with a right cusp (RC) and a left cusp (LC). In the BAV with a raphe the most common site of cuspal fusion is between the RCC and LCC (B), followed by fusion between the RCC and NCC (C); LCC and NCC fusion is rarely seen (D).

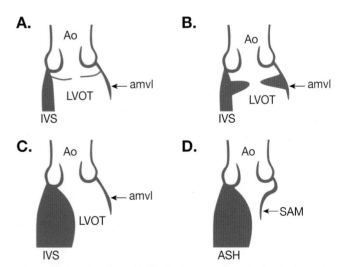

Figure 15.44 This schematic illustrates examples of subvalvular aortic stenosis (AS). A: a discrete fibrous membrane located underneath the aortic valve; B: a discrete fibromuscular ridge of muscular tissue within the left ventricular outflow tract (LVOT); C: a fibromuscular tunnel with septal hypertrophy and a thickened anterior mitral valve leaflet (amvl); D: dynamic subvalvular AS secondary to asymmetric septal hypertrophy (ASH) and systolic anterior motion (SAM) of the amvl into the LVOT. Ao = aorta; IVS = interventricular septum.

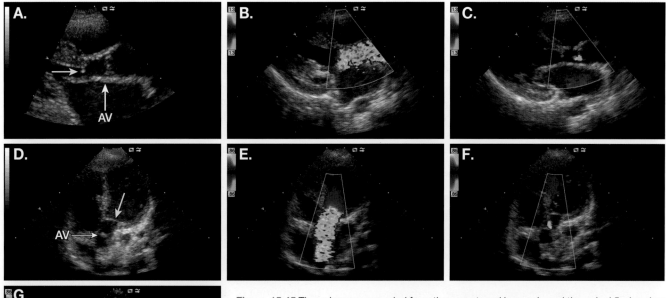

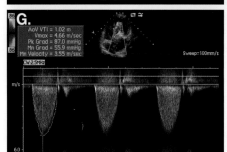

Figure 15.45 These images recorded from the parasternal long axis and the apical 5-chamber views show a subaortic membrane with significant left ventricular outflow tract (LVOT) obstruction. The subaortic membrane appears as a linear structure below the aortic valve (AV) (*yellow arrows*) (A & D). On the colour Doppler images, turbulence is noted within the LVOT at the site of the membrane during systole (B & E); trace aortic regurgitation is also noted during diastole (C &F). Via continuous-wave Doppler, the maximum pressure gradient across the LVOT is 87 mmHg and the mean pressure gradient is 56 mmHg (G).

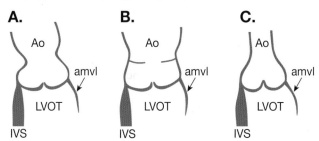

Figure 15.46 This schematic illustrates examples of supravalvular AS A: an hour-glass type with dysplasia of the aortic wall immediately above the aortic cusps; B: a membranous type where a thin membrane or fibrous diaphragm with a central orifice is located immediately above the aortic valve; C: tubular or diffuse type where there is uniform, diffuse hypoplasia of the ascending aorta.

amvl = anterior mitral valve leaflet; Ao = ascending aorta; IVS = interventricular septum; LVOT = left ventricular outflow tract.

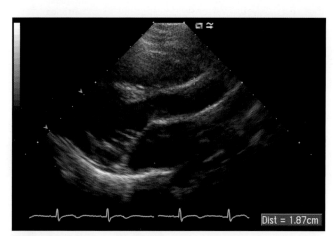

Figure 15.47 This parasternal long axis view was recorded from an adult patient with William syndrome. Mild hypoplasia of the ascending aorta is noted.

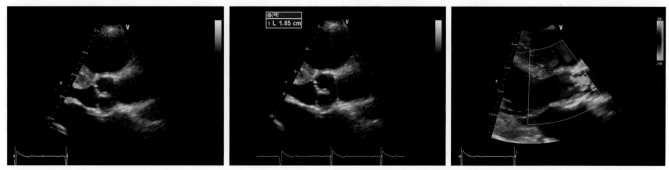

Figure 15.48 These images recorded from a high parasternal long axis view show an hourglass deformity of the ascending aorta (*left*). The aorta measured at the sinotubular junction is 1.7 cm (*middle*). On colour Doppler imaging, turbulent flow is noted at the narrowed site (*right*).

Embryology of the Aortic Arches

Embryologically, the definitive aorta is formed by various parts of the truncus arteriosus, the aortic sac, the aortic arches and the dorsal aortas (Fig. 15.50). In the early stages of foetal heart development, the dilated distal end of the truncus arteriosus connects to the aortic sac which then communicates with the bilateral dorsal aortas by a series of six pairs of aortic arches. Initially, the aortic arch system exhibits early symmetry similar to the paired primitive venous system as previously described (see Sinus Venosus and Sinus Horns). As for the primitive venous system, the aortic arch system is also greatly modified and gradually loses its original symmetry as development continues. In particular, the ascending aorta is formed by segments of the truncus arteriosus and the aortic sac while the aortic arch is formed by segments of the aortic sac, the 4th left aortic arch and the left dorsal aorta; the descending thoracic aorta is formed by the left dorsal aorta (see Fig. 15.50 Stage 3). The fate and evolution of the aortic arches and other related structures are summarised in Table 15.5.

Aetiology of CoAo

The underlying mechanism leading to CoAo is not fully known; however, two concepts have been proposed: (1) the ectopic ductal tissue theory and (2) the reduced-flow (haemodynamic) theory.

In the ectopic ductal tissue theory, it is postulated that during the formation of the aortic arch, muscle tissue of the ductus arteriosus 'invades' the wall of the aorta just distal to the aortic isthmus. Then when the ductus arteriosus contracts at birth, the ductal muscle in the aorta also contracts forming a shelf or indentation in the descending thoracic aorta opposite to the insertion site of the ductus arteriosus.

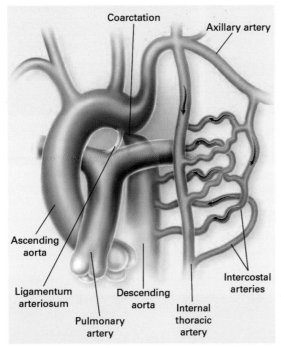

Figure 15.49 This schematic illustrates a severe coarctation of the aorta. The descending thoracic aorta and its branches are perfused by collateral channels from the axillary and internal thoracic arteries through the intercostal arteries (*arrows*).
Reproduced from Brickner ME, Hillis LD, Lange RA. Congenital heart disease in adults. First of two parts. *N Engl J Med.* Jan 27;342(4), page 261, © 2000 with permission from the Massachusetts Medical Society.

Table 15.4 Common CHDs associated with CoAo

Associated Lesions
BAV (50% of CoAo have BAV)
Congenital AS (any level)
VSD
PDA
Part of Shone syndrome *

* Shone syndrome is comprised of a series of left heart obstructive lesions including supravalvular mitral ring, parachute mitral valve, subaortic stenosis and coarctation of the aorta.
AS = aortic stenosis; BAV = bicuspid aortic valve; CoAo = coarctation of the aorta; PDA = patent ductus arteriosus; VSD = ventricular septal defect.

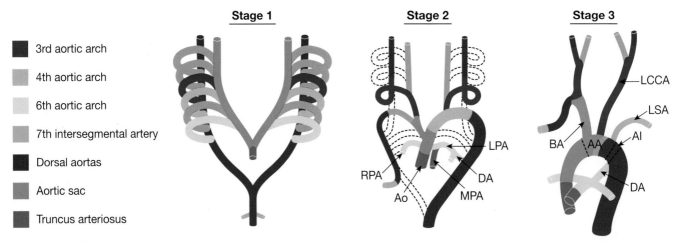

Figure 15.50 These schematics illustrate the formation of the aorta from the truncus arteriosus, the aortic sac, the aortic arches and the dorsal aortas. **Stage 1:** The aortic sac and truncus arteriosus communicate with the paired dorsal aortas via six pairs of aortic arches. The paired aortic arches do not all appear at the same time but are shown in this manner for simplicity. **Stage 2:** As development continues, the 1st and 2nd aortic arches essentially disappear leaving only small portions which develop into the small arteries of the head, neck and ear. The 5th pairs of aortic arches never develop in most foetuses. The remaining pairs of aortic arches regress and change directions. Note that at this stage of development, the truncus arteriosus forms the proximal aorta (Ao) and main pulmonary artery (MPA) while the proximal portion of the right and left 6th arches develop into the right and left pulmonary arteries (RPA and LPA) and the distal portion of left 6th arch forms the ductus arteriosus (DA). **Stage 3:** At this stage of development, the aortic arch (AA) is now fully formed and includes segments of the aortic sac, the 4th left aortic arch and left dorsal aorta. The brachiocephalic artery (BA) is formed by the right aortic sac, the left common carotid artery (LCCA) is formed by the left 3rd aortic arch and the left subclavian artery (LSA) is formed by the left 7th intersegmental artery. Note that the aortic isthmus (AI) is the portion of the aorta between the LSA and the DA.

In the reduced-flow theory, it is hypothesised that the coarctation occurs due to reduced flow in the aortic isthmus during foetal life. Recall that the aortic isthmus is the portion of the aorta between the left subclavian artery and the ductus arteriosus. In the foetal circulation blood flow into the ascending aorta is mostly directed towards the upper body while blood flow from the PA into the ductus arteriosus and descending thoracic aorta is directed to the lower body (Fig. 15.51); as a result there is little blood flow into the aortic isthmus and therefore the aortic isthmus is normally a little narrower than the aorta either side of it. Following closure of the ductus arteriosus, the aortic isthmus normally enlarges until it is the same diameter as the aorta on each side of it. However, if this enlargement does not occur then the narrowing persists as a coarctation.

While these two theories might explain CoAo at the region of the ductus arteriosus, these theories do not explain why CoAo occurs at other sites of the aorta.

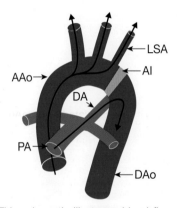

Figure 15.51 This schematic illustrates blood flow direction in the aorta and pulmonary artery during foetal life. Observe that blood flow from the ascending aorta (AAo) is mostly directed to supply the upper body while blood flow from the pulmonary artery (PA) is directed across the ductus arteriosus (DA) to the descending thoracic aorta (DAo) to supply the lower body. As a result there is little blood flow across the aortic isthmus (AI) which is located between the left subclavian artery (LSA) and the ductus arteriosus (DA).

Role of Echocardiography in CoAo

The primary role of echocardiography in CoAo is to:
- establish the diagnosis
- estimate the severity of the coarctation
- assess the LV size, wall thickness and systolic function
- evaluate the aortic valve morphology.

Echocardiography also has an important role in assessing the aorta post coarctation repair.

Establish the Diagnosis

The diagnosis of CoAo is based on visualisation of a shelf-like narrowing of the aorta or a tissue ridge extending into the aortic lumen. The site of CoAo is most commonly opposite the ligamentum arteriosus. Therefore, the CoAo is best visualised from the suprasternal window (Fig. 15.52-15.53, Fig 4.14.). CFI is also extremely useful in identifying turbulent flow at the site of the coarctation.

Estimation of Coarctation Severity

The severity of CoAo can be estimated by measuring the peak velocity and maximum pressure gradient across the narrowing (Fig. 15.53). Recall that the maximum pressure gradient is determined by the application of the simplified Bernoulli equation:

Equation 15.5

$$\Delta P = 4V^2$$

where ΔP = the pressure difference between 2 points (mm Hg)
  V = peak velocity between 2 points (m/s)

However, there are two important limitations of this simplified equation in the assessment of CoAo. Application of the simplified Bernoulli equation excludes the velocity proximal to the coarctation; therefore, when this proximal velocity is elevated ($\geq$ 1.2 m/s) calculation of the pressure gradient will be overestimated as this proximal velocity is ignored in the simplified Bernoulli equation. In this instance, the "corrected" pressure gradient should be estimated.

Table 15.5 Summary of the Fate of the Aortic Arches and Other Related Structures

	Left	Right
Truncus arteriosus	Aortic root	Pulmonary artery root
Aortic Sac	Proximal segment of aortic arch	Right brachiocephalic artery
Aortic Arches I	Left maxillary artery and portion of left external carotid artery	Right maxillary artery and portion of right external carotid artery
II	Regresses rapidly, small portion remaining forms left stapedial and hyoid arteries	Regress rapidly, small portion remaining forms right stapedial and hyoid arteries
III	Left common carotid artery Proximal portion of left internal carotid arteries	Right common carotid artery Proximal portion of right internal carotid arteries
IV	Definitive aortic arch	Proximal right subclavian artery
V	Does not develop	Does not develop
VI	Proximal portion develops into left pulmonary artery Distal portion develops into the ductus arteriosus	Proximal portion develops into right pulmonary artery Distal portion degenerates
7th Intersegmental Arteries	Left subclavian artery	Distal part of right subclavian artery (in conjunction with right dorsal aorta)
Dorsal Aortas	Distal aortic arch and descending aorta Distal portion of left internal carotid artery	Right subclavian artery Distal portion of right internal carotid artery

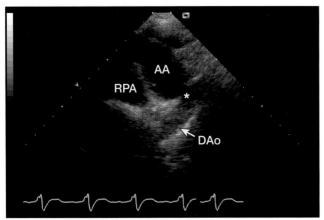
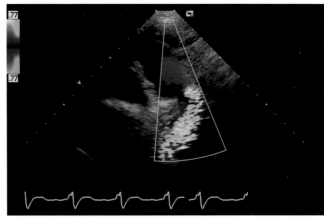

Figure 15.52 These images were recorded from the suprasternal window. The views are slightly off-axis in an attempt to better visualise the descending thoracic aorta (DAo). The 2D image shows a "shelf" in the descending thoracic aorta (*) which denotes the area of the coarctation (*left*). Colour flow Doppler imaging confirms the presence of turbulent flow through this region (*right*).
AA = aortic arch; RPA = right pulmonary artery.

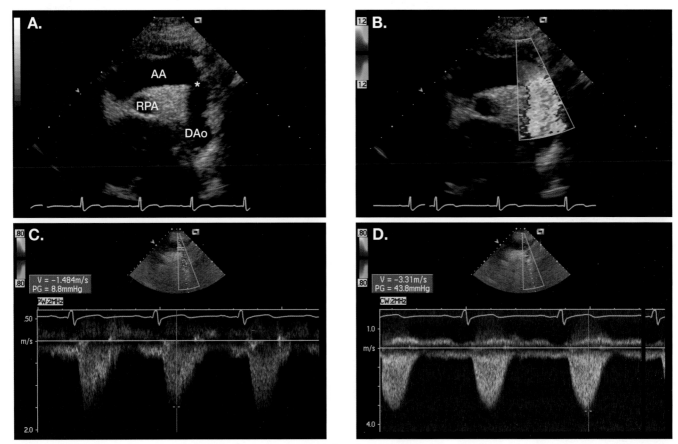

Figure 15.53 These images were recorded from the suprasternal window. A: On the 2D image a discrete narrowing of the descending thoracic aorta (DAo) is noted (*). B: The colour flow Doppler image confirms the presence of turbulent flow through the narrowed region. C: Via pulsed-wave (PW) Doppler the peak velocity proximal to the coarctation is measured at 1.5 m/s yielding a maximum pressure gradient of 9 mm Hg. D: Via continuous-wave (CW) Doppler, the peak velocity across the coarctation is measured at 3.3 m/s yielding a maximum pressure gradient of 44 mm Hg. The corrected pressure gradient across the coarctation is 35 mm Hg (see Eq. 15.6).
AA = aortic arch; RPA = right pulmonary artery.

Assessment of the descending thoracic aorta in the adult patient can be extremely challenging and this may lead to false positive and false negative diagnoses of CoAo.

False positive results may occur when the aorta is imaged from an oblique plane leading to the appearance of a 'pseudo-shelf'. Therefore, care should be taken to ensure that the descending thoracic aorta is appropriately 'opened out'; this is achieved by slight transducer rotations and angulations. False negative results may occur due to inability to image the distal descending thoracic aorta so the coarctation site is not imaged.

The incidence of false positive and false negative results may be reduced by ensuring that both colour flow imaging and continuous-wave Doppler are used to interrogate the descending thoracic aorta.

The "corrected" pressure gradient is determined by application of the "expanded" Bernoulli equation (Fig. 15.53):

Equation 15.6

$$\Delta P_C = \Delta P_{CoAo} - \Delta P_{prox}$$

where ΔP_C = corrected maximum pressure gradient (mm Hg)
ΔP_{CoAo} = maximum pressure gradient across the coarctation (mm Hg)
ΔP_{prox} = maximum pressure gradient proximal to the coarctation (mm Hg)

In the presence of significant collateral blood flow or a large PDA with left-to-right shunting, flow across the coarctation is reduced. For example, when a collateral circulation develops, blood flow is diverted to the internal thoracic and intercostal arteries; thus, blood flow effectively bypasses the coarctation (see Fig. 15.49). Likewise, when there is a large PDA with left-to-right shunting, blood flow is shunted from the aorta to the PA so blood flow across the coarctation is diminished. Therefore, in these two situations as blood flow across the coarctation is reduced, the pressure gradient across the coarctation will also be decreased and the severity of the coarctation may be underestimated.

The shape of the spectral Doppler signal across the coarctation is also very useful in the assessment of coarctation severity.

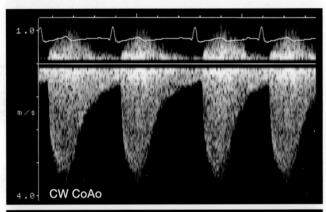

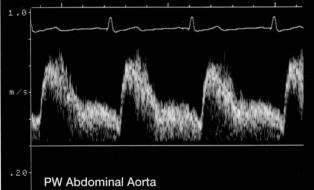

Figure 15.54 These spectral Doppler traces were recorded from a patient with a severe coarctation of the aorta (CoAo). The continuous-wave (CW) Doppler trace recorded from the suprasternal window shows a continuous pressure gradient across the coarctation over both systole and diastole (*top*). The pulsed-wave (PW) Doppler trace recorded from the abdominal aorta (Abdo Ao) also shows a continuation of forward flow throughout diastole (*bottom*). These features are characteristic of a severe coarctation.

In severe CoAo, there is a persistent pressure gradient across the narrowing over both systole and diastole (Fig. 15.54 and Fig. 4.14). On the CW Doppler trace, this appears as a characteristic 'diastolic tail' or 'saw-tooth' pattern. In addition, with a severe CoAo diastolic flow continuation may also be noted on the pulsed-wave (PW) Doppler signal recorded from within the abdominal aorta. In particular, this abdominal aortic flow profile may be especially useful in identifying a significant coarctation when the descending thoracic aorta cannot be adequately imaged from the suprasternal window.

Assessment of LV Size, Wall Thickness and Systolic Function
Left ventricular size, wall thickness and systolic function can be assessed by both M-mode and 2D echocardiography in the traditional manner (see Chapter 2). In particular, patients with a significant CoAo may develop LV hypertrophy secondary to chronic LV pressure overload. Recall that CoAo is an identifiable cause of secondary systemic hypertension (see Chapter 4, Systemic Hypertension). Therefore, in the presence of increased LV wall thickness a careful interrogation of the aorta should be performed to exclude coarctation.

Aortic Valve Morphology
Approximately 50% of patients with CoAo also have a BAV. Therefore, assessment of aortic valve morphology is also important in these patients. In particular, if a BAV is present, measurements of the maximum and mean pressure gradients across the BAV, calculation of the aortic valve area, an assessment of AR severity and measurements of aortic dimensions are also required.

Assessment Post Coarctation Repair
Repair of CoAo can be performed percutaneously or surgically. Percutaneous dilatation of the coarctation region can be achieved via balloon angioplasty. Surgical repair techniques include resection of the coarctation with an end-to-end anastomosis or the use of a subclavian flap or synthetic patch aortoplasty.

The echocardiographic assessment post coarctation repair includes an assessment of LV size, systolic function and wall thickness as well as an evaluation of the coarctation repair site. In addition, the examination should attempt to identify potential post-operative complications such as re-coarctation and the formation of an aortic aneurysm at the site of the coarctation repair. These post-operative complications, however, are best evaluated by other imaging techniques such as cardiac magnetic resonance imaging (CMR).

Three categories of aortic arch remodelling have also been described by CMR post-surgical coarctation repair[15.2]. These geometric shapes are labelled based on similarities between the aortic arch post-operative shapes with architectural styles: (1) the Gothic arch has an angular geometry, (2) the Crenel arch has a rectangular shape, and (3) the Romanesque arch has a smooth rounded shape similar to normal arch anatomy. An example of a Gothic aortic arch seen on TTE is shown in Figure 15.55. In particular, assessment of Doppler velocities across this type of aortic arch remodelling is often difficult due to the acute angle of the arch so parallel alignment with flow is not possible.

[15.2] Ou P, Bonnet D, Auriacombe L, Pedroni E, Balleux F, Sidi D, Mousseaux E. Late systemic hypertension and aortic arch geometry after successful repair of coarctation of the aorta. *Eur Heart J.* 2004 Oct; 25(20):1853-9.

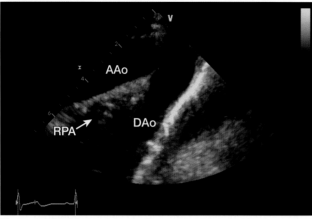

Figure 15.55 This suprasternal image was recorded from a patient with a coarctation repair. Observe that the aortic arch geometry is quite deformed. In particular, the aortic arch has a marked angular shape which is consistent with a Gothic aortic arch.
AAo = ascending aorta; DAo = descending thoracic aorta; RPA = right pulmonary artery.

Cyanotic Lesions

Cyanotic CHD occurs when deoxygenated blood enters the systemic circulation due to right-to-left or bidirectional shunting, or malposition of the great arteries. There are a vast number of cyanotic CHDs (Table 15.6). It is beyond the scope of this section to cover each of these defects; so selected cyanotic CHDs discussed in this section include tetralogy of Fallot (TOF), dextro-transposition of the great arteries (d-TGA) and tricuspid valve atresia (TVA). As these cyanotic defects are first diagnosed at birth or during infancy, only a brief review of the anatomy of each lesion will be discussed and emphasis will be placed on the surgical repair and postoperative echocardiographic assessment of these defects.

Embryology of the Conotruncal Septum

Before discussing lesions such as TOF and d-TGA, it is first important to understand the embryological septation of the great arteries and the ventricular outflow tracts. There are a number of theories regarding this septation although the outcome is the same; that is, the RVOT and LVOT are separated from one another and the truncus arteriosus is divided into the aorta and PA.

Table 15.6 Examples of Cyanotic CHDs

Congenital Defect	Brief Description
Double outlet right ventricle (DORV)	Both the PA and aorta arise from the morphologic RV; cyanosis occurs as deoxygenated blood is ejected from the RV into the aorta and systemic circulation
Ebstein's anomaly	Displacement of septal tricuspid valve into RV; cyanosis occurs when there is right-to-left shunting of deoxygenated blood across a PFO or ASD to the left heart and systemic circulation
Eisenmenger's Syndrome	Bidirectional or right-to-left shunting of deoxygenated blood across pre-existing shunt lesions such as a large ASD, VSD, PDA, AVCD, or AP window
Hypoplastic left heart syndrome (HLHS)	Marked hypoplasia of LV and ascending aorta; cyanosis occurs due to right-to-left shunting of deoxygenated blood across the PDA to the aorta and systemic circulation
Interrupted aortic arch	Complete loss of luminal communication between ascending and descending thoracic aorta; cyanosis occurs due to right-to-left shunting across the PDA to the aorta and systemic circulation
Pulmonary atresia +/- intact ventricular septum	Absent pulmonary valve; with an intact septum cyanosis occurs due to right-to-left shunting of deoxygenated blood across an ASD; with a VSD cyanosis occurs due to right-to-left shunting of deoxygenated blood across the VSD to the aorta and systemic circulation
Tetralogy of Fallot (TOF)*	Includes 4 congenital cardiac lesions: RVOT obstruction, overriding aorta, VSD, and RV hypertrophy; cyanosis occurs when deoxygenated blood is shunted across the VSD and to the overriding aorta and the systemic circulation
Total anomalous pulmonary venous connection (TAPVC)*	Abnormal connection or drainage of all 4 pulmonary veins into systemic veins; cyanosis occurs due to mixing of the pulmonary venous return with the systemic venous return, deoxygenated blood is then shunted right-to-left across an ASD to the left heart and to the systemic circulation
Transposition of the great arteries - dextro (TGA)*	Aorta arises from morphological RV and PA arises from morphological LV; systemic and pulmonary circulations run in parallel; cyanosis occurs as deoxygenated blood circles from body to the right heart to the aorta and to the body
Tricuspid valve atresia (TVA)*	Absent tricuspid valve; cyanosis occurs due to right-to-left shunting of deoxygenated blood across the ASD to the left heart and to the systemic circulation
Truncus arteriosus*	A persistent truncus arteriosus gives rise to both PA and aorta; cyanosis occurs due to right-to-left shunting of deoxygenated blood across a VSD to the left heart and to the systemic circulation
Univentricular heart	Single ventricle physiology: RV or LV is missing or hypoplastic; includes double inlet left ventricle (DILV), HLHS, a common ventricle and TVA; cyanosis occurs due to mixing of oxygenated and deoxygenated blood within the single ventricle which delivers deoxygenated blood to the systemic circulation

* These defects are referred to as the 5 "T's" of cyanotic heart disease
AP = aorticopulmonary; ASD = atrial septal defect; AVCD = atrioventricular canal defect; LA = left atrium; LV = left ventricle; PA = pulmonary artery; PDA = patent ductus arteriosus; PFO = patent foramen ovale; RV = right ventricle; RVOT = right ventricular outflow tract; VSD = ventricular septal defect.

One theory regarding this septation is based on the development of a single conotruncal (aorticopulmonary) septum which arises from two tissue ridges or swellings within the aortic sac which grow together and fuse to form this septum. This septum then grows inferiorly and superiorly spiralling in opposite directions to divide the truncus arteriosus into the aorta and PA and the conus cordis into the RVOT and LVOT. In addition, the distal end of this septum forms the outlet IVS (see Fig. 15.18). Ultimately the conotruncal septum will fuse with the endocardial cushions, the trabecular IVS and the inlet IVS. Importantly, the spiralling of this septum ensures the normal anatomic relationship of the great arteries such that the aorta is positioned posterior and leftward and arises from the LV while the PA is positioned anterior and rightward and arises from the RV (Fig. 15.56).

Abnormalities in the development of the conotruncal septum lead to defects involving the outflow tracts and the great arteries. The most common conotruncal defects include TOF, transposition of the great arteries (TGA), double outlet RV and truncus arteriosus. TOF and TGA are discussed below.

Tetralogy of Fallot

TOF is a conotruncal septal anomaly that results when there is anterior and superior deviation of the outlet IVS. This leads to a malalignment of the outlet IVS compared with the rest of the muscular IVS as well as an unequal division of the ventricular outflow tracts and the great arteries. As a result four different cardiac abnormalities develop (Fig. 15.57):

(1) a large malalignment VSD: this occurs as the conotruncal septum and the trabecular and inlet IVS do not line up and connect,

(2) an over-riding aorta: anterior displacement of the conotruncal septum leads to the rightward shift of the aorta so the aorta straddles the VSD and therefore opens over both the RV and LV,

(3) narrowing and obstruction of the RVOT: this results from "crowding" of the subpulmonary outflow by muscular and fibrous tissues of the abnormal outlet IVS; obstruction may occur as narrowing of the RVOT (infundibulum), stenosis or hypoplasia of the pulmonary valve, hypoplasia of the main PA and/or branch pulmonary arteries, or a combination of these,

(4) RV hypertrophy: this occurs as a compensatory mechanism to the increased RV pressures caused by RVOT obstruction.

There are also several anatomic variants of TOF and a number of associated congenital heart lesions (Table 15.7). In addition, TOF is also linked with several congenital and genetic syndromes (see Appendix 5).

As illustrated in Figure 15.57, TOF causes cyanosis when deoxygenated blood is shunted right-to-left across the VSD to the aorta and systemic circulation. Therefore, the aorta receives deoxygenated blood from the RV and oxygenated blood from the LV. The degree of mixing, and therefore cyanosis, is essentially dependent upon the severity of RVOT obstruction. That is, the more severe the RVOT obstruction, the more blood is shunted from the RV across the VSD and into the aorta and therefore the greater the degree of cyanosis.

On echocardiographic examination, TOF is diagnosed by identifying the four abnormalities associated with this lesion (Fig. 15.58). In particular, the malalignment VSD is visualised from the parasternal long axis, the parasternal short axis, the apical 5-chamber and the subcostal views; the overriding of

Table 15.7 **Anatomic Variants and Common CHDs associated with Tetralogy of Fallot (TOF)**

Anatomic Variants
TOF + pulmonary atresia
TOF + an absent pulmonary valve
TOF + a DORV
TOF + AVCD
Associated Lesions
Right aortic arch
Coronary artery anomalies
ASD
Additional VSDs

ASD = atrial septal defect; AVCD = atrioventricular canal defect; DORV = double outlet right ventricle; VSD = ventricular septal defect.

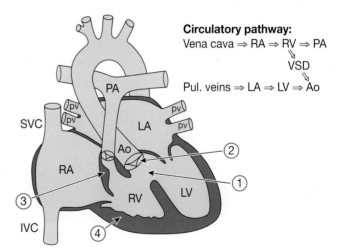

Circulatory pathway:
Vena cava ⇒ RA ⇒ RV ⇒ PA
⇘
VSD
⇘
Pul. veins ⇒ LA ⇒ LV ⇒ Ao

Figure 15.57 This schematic illustrates the anatomy of TOF which is characterised by: (1) a large malalignment ventricular septal defect (VSD), (2) an aorta that overrides the left and right ventricles, (3) obstruction of the right ventricular outflow tract (RVOT), and (4) right ventricular hypertrophy (RVH). The circulatory pathway in TOF is also shown. Observe that oxygenated blood returns to the left atrium (LA) via the pulmonary veins (pv) and then passes to the left ventricle (LV) while deoxygenated blood from the inferior vena cava (IVC) and superior vena cava (SVC) enters the right atrium (RA) and flows to the right ventricle (RV). From the RV, blood is ejected through the narrowed RVOT to the pulmonary artery (PA) and is also shunted across the VSD; mixed deoxygenated and oxygenated blood is then ejected out the aorta (Ao). Deoxygenated blood to the systemic circulation results in cyanosis.

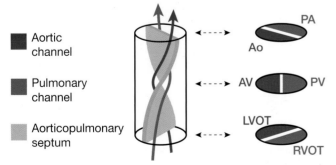

Aortic channel

Pulmonary channel

Aorticopulmonary septum

Figure 15.56 This schematic illustrates the spiral septation of the truncus arteriosus by the conotruncal septum. As a result of this process the pulmonary artery (PA) and aorta (Ao) spiral around one another and this ensures that the pulmonary artery arises from the right ventricle (RV) and that the aorta arises from the left ventricle (LV). AV = aortic valve; LVOT = left ventricular outflow tract; PV = pulmonary valve; RVOT = right ventricular outflow tract.

the aorta is best seen from the parasternal long axis and apical 5 chamber views; RVOT obstruction is best assessed from the parasternal long axis of RVOT and parasternal short axis views; while RV hypertrophy can be assessed from the parasternal, apical and subcostal views. CFI is useful in assessing the direction of shunting across the VSD and for determining the site of RVOT obstruction. The maximum and mean pressure gradients across the RVOT are measured via CW Doppler.

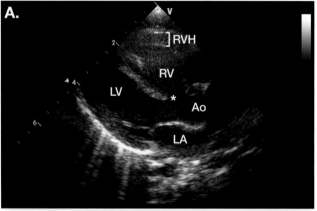

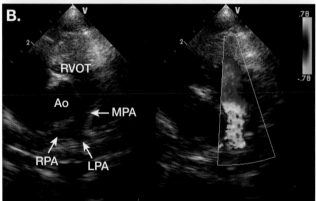

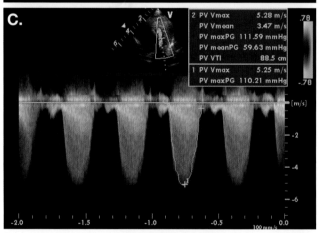

Figure 15.58 These images show the classic echocardiographic features of TOF. A: From the parasternal long axis view, a malalignment ventricular septal defect (*) and an overriding aorta (Ao) are seen; right ventricular hypertrophy (RVH) is also apparent. B: From the parasternal short axis view hypoplasia of the main pulmonary artery (MPA) and the pulmonary artery branches is evident. The colour Doppler image confirms the presence of turbulent blood flow across the hypoplastic MPA. C: Via continuous-wave Doppler, the peak velocity across this narrowing is 5.3 m/s yielding a maximum pressure gradient of 110 mm Hg with a mean pressure gradient of 60 mm Hg. LA = left atrium; LPA = left pulmonary artery; LV = left ventricle; RPA = right pulmonary artery; RV = right ventricle; RVOT = right ventricular outflow tract.

Surgical Repair and Post-Operative Assessment

Palliative repairs for TOF are rarely performed as a complete repair is preferable in most cases. However, palliative procedures may be performed when the anatomy is not yet amenable to total repair. Palliative procedures include a pulmonary valvotomy or a systemic-to-PA shunt (see Appendix 6).

Complete surgical repair is achieved by a patch closure of the VSD and relief of the RVOT obstruction, which sometimes includes RVOT widening via a transannular patch (Fig. 15.59). The primary role of the echocardiographic examination in the post-operative assessment of TOF repair includes the:

- evaluation of the IVS for residual defects across the VSD patch
- estimation of pulmonary regurgitation (PR) severity
- assessment of the RVOT for aneurysms (secondary to the outflow tract patch)
- detection of persistent RVOT obstruction and, if present, to determine the site and severity of obstruction
- assessment of LV and RV size and systolic function
- measurement of the aortic root (progressive dilatation is common)
- evaluation of the presence and severity of AR (secondary to aortic root dilatation).

The most common post-operative complications of TOF repair include RV failure, severe PR and persistent RVOT obstruction.

The RV is almost always dilated post-TOF repair and some degree of systolic dysfunction is also usually present. Therefore, a comprehensive evaluation of the RV size and systolic function should be performed (see Chapter 2). Advanced echocardiographic modalities such as strain imaging have also been investigated for the assessment of RV function and these techniques may provide more sensitive measures for detecting RV dysfunction [15.3].

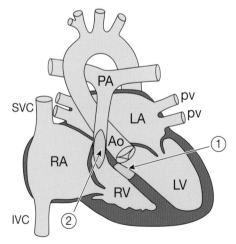

Figure 15.59 This schematic illustrates a TOF repair which includes: (1) a patch repair of the ventricular septal defect and (2) a transannular patch of the right ventricular outflow tract (RVOT). This surgical repair re-establishes the normal cardiac connections and intracardiac circulation, and relieves the RVOT obstruction.
Ao = aorta; IVC = inferior vena cava; LA = left atrium; LV = left ventricle; PA = pulmonary artery; pv = pulmonary vein; RA = right atrium; RV = right ventricle; SVC = superior vena cava.

[15.3] Scherptong RW, Mollema SA, Blom NA, Kroft LJ, de Roos A, Vliegen HW, van der Wall EE, Bax JJ, Holman ER. Right ventricular peak systolic longitudinal strain is a sensitive marker for right ventricular deterioration in adult patients with tetralogy of Fallot. Int J Cardiovasc Imaging. 2009 Oct;25(7):669-76.

The severity of PR is assessed in the usual manner as described in detail in Chapter 9. Importantly, severe or 'free' PR can be easily missed. This is because the PR jet has a low velocity so PR flow appears laminar on CFI; in addition, the PR duration may be very brief, appearing in early diastole only (Fig. 15.60).

A persistent RVOT obstruction is assessed by determining the level of obstruction using CFI and by measuring the maximum and mean pressure gradients across the obstruction via CW Doppler. It is also important to remember that in the presence of RVOT obstruction, the RVSP estimated from the TR velocity is not the same as the PASP. The RVSP is only the same as the PASP in the absence of RVOT obstruction. When there is RVOT obstruction, the RVSP will be greater than the PASP. So

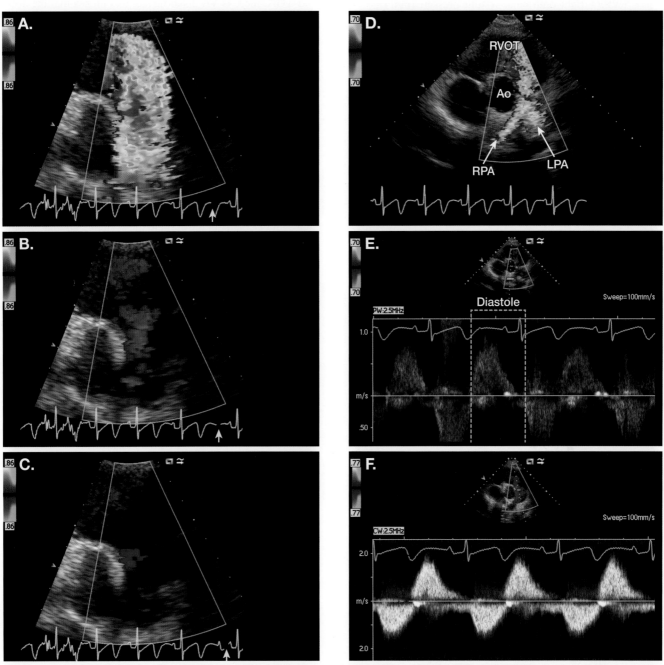

Figure 15.60 These images were recorded from a patient with 'free' or 'wide-open' pulmonary regurgitation (PR) following a TOF repair. The series of colour Doppler images (*top*) were recorded from a zoomed parasternal short axis view (PSAX) of the right ventricular outflow tract (RVOT). A: In this early diastolic frame, severe PR is evident by the PR jet filling the RVOT. B: In this mid diastolic frame, the PR jet is less apparent; this is because the pressure difference between the pulmonary artery (PA) and right ventricle (RV) has decreased due to an increase in the RV diastolic pressure. C: In this late diastolic frame, the PR jet is totally absent; this early termination of the PR jet prior to the end of diastole occurs when there is equalisation between the PA and RV diastolic pressures. D: In this diastolic still frame image recorded from the unzoomed PSAX view, diastolic flow reversal is observed within the main pulmonary artery and from the level of the right and left pulmonary artery branches; this appears as red flow towards the transducer. E: This pulsed-wave (PW) Doppler signal was recorded with the sample volume placed within the right pulmonary artery (RPA); diastolic flow reversal is confirmed by the appearance of flow above the zero baseline during diastole. F: This continuous-wave (CW) Doppler trace demonstrates a strong PR signal intensity compared with forward flow and a rapid deceleration slope of the PR signal which reaches the zero baseline before the end of diastole; early termination of the PR signal indicates an equalisation of diastolic pressures between the PA and RV.

Ao = aorta; LPA = left pulmonary artery.

in the presence of RVOT obstruction, the PASP is derived from the RVSP and the pressure gradient across the RVOT. In most situations, the PASP via Doppler can be estimated as:

Equation 15.7

$$PASP = RVSP - mPG$$

where PASP = pulmonary artery systolic pressure (mm Hg)
      RVSP = right ventricular systolic pressure (mm Hg)
      mPG = mean pressure gradient across RVOT (mm Hg)

In patients with very severe or critical RVOT obstruction, which is identified by a rounded, mid-systolic peaking signal (see Fig. 9.53), the PASP is estimated as:

Equation 15.8

$$PASP_C = RVSP - MIPG$$

where $PASP_C$ = pulmonary artery systolic pressure in critical
        RVOT obstruction (mm Hg)
     RVSP = right ventricular systolic pressure (mm Hg)
     MIPG = maximum instantaneous pressure gradient
            across the RVOT (mm Hg)

Formation of the Primitive Heart Tube and the Cardiac Loop

Initially, the primary heart appears as a straight tube within the pericardial cavity. As development continues dilatations and constrictions appear along this tube (below left). These dilatations will ultimately form the various chambers and great vessels of the heart. As the heart continues to grow, it loops and bends upon itself (below right). This looping and bending occurs because the superior and inferior ends of the heart tube are "anchored" and the bulbus cordis and primitive ventricle grow faster than the rest of the heart. Normally, the outer curvature of the C-shaped bulboventricular loop points towards the right side of the body so this is referred to as a dextral-loop or d-loop. As a result of normal cardiac looping the bulbus cordis is displaced inferiorly, anteriorly and to the right; the primitive ventricle is displaced to the left; the truncus arteriosus moves slightly rightward; and the common atrium and sinus venosus move posterior and superior to the bulbus cordis and the primitive ventricle. Note that eventually the bulbus cordis will become the definitive RV, the primitive ventricle will become the definitive LV, the common atria will become the RA and LA, and the truncus arteriosus will divide into the aorta and PA.

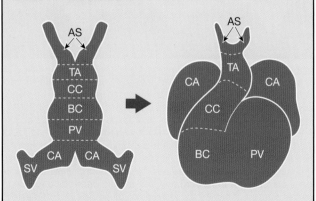

AS = aortic sac; TA = truncus arteriosus; CA = common atria; CC = conus cordis; BC = bulbus cordis; PV = primitive ventricle; SV = sinus venosus.

---

d-Transposition of the Great Arteries

In the normal heart, there is atrioventricular (AV) and ventriculoarterial (VA) concordance. AV concordance refers to the fact that the LA connects to a morphological LV and the RA connects to a morphological RV while VA concordance refers to the fact that the LV connects to the aorta and the RV connects to the PA.

In d-TGA, there is VA discordance; this means that the aorta arises from the morphological RV while the PA arises from the morphological LV. In d-TGA, also commonly referred to as dextro-TGA, simple TGA or complete TGA, the primitive heart tube loops to the right (dextral looping) so that the RV is positioned normally on the right side. However, the conotruncal septum fails to grow in its normal spiral course and instead runs straight down. As a result, the aorta is anterior and rightward and arises from the morphological RV while the PA is posterior and leftward and arises from the morphological LV. The consequence of this lesion is that the systemic and pulmonary circulations run in parallel (Fig. 15.61). That is, the aorta receives deoxygenated blood from the RV which circulates to the body and then returns to the RA and RV and is then again ejected out the aorta to the systemic circulation; the PA receives oxygenated blood from the LV which circulates to the lungs and then returns to the LA and LV and is then again ejected out the PA to the pulmonary circulation. Therefore, in order to survive, a communication between the atria (via a PFO) and/or a PDA must exist. d-TGA is also associated with other congenital heart lesions (Table 15.8) as well as a number of congenital and genetic syndromes (see Appendix 5).

On the echocardiographic examination, d-TGA is diagnosed from the parasternal long axis view by demonstrating the side-by-side or parallel alignment of the aorta (seen anteriorly)

Circulatory pathway:
Vena cava ⇒ RA ⇒ RV ⇒ Ao
           ⇑   ⇑
           PFO   PDA
           ⇑   ⇑
Pul. veins ⇒ LA ⇒ LV ⇒ PA

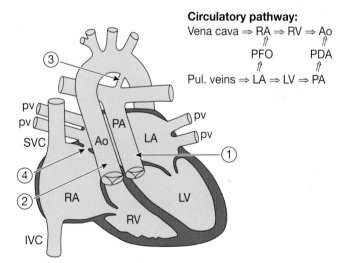

Figure 15.61 This schematic illustrates the anatomy of d-TGA which is characterised by ventriculoarterial discordance: (1) the pulmonary artery (PA) arises from the morphological left ventricle (LV) and (2) the aorta arises from the morphological right ventricle (RV). In addition, for survival, there must be shunting of oxygenated blood to the systemic circulation via: (3) a patent ductus arteriosus (PDA) and/or (4) a patent foramen ovale (PFO). The circulatory pathway in d-TGA is also shown. Observe that oxygenated blood returns to the left atrium (LA) via the pulmonary veins (pv) and then passes to the left ventricle (LV) and then to the pulmonary artery (PA) while deoxygenated blood from the inferior vena cava (IVC) and superior vena cava (SVC) enters the right atrium (RA) and flows to the right ventricle (RV) and is then ejected into the aorta (Ao). Cyanosis occurs as deoxygenated blood is ejected into the systemic circulation.

and the PA (seen posteriorly) (Fig. 15.62, top). From the parasternal short axis view both great vessels are seen in their short axis with the aorta again seen anterior to the PA (Fig. 15.62, bottom).

In particular, the normal 'sausage-circle' appearance of the great arteries is absent from the parasternal short axis view and this further assists the diagnosis of d-TGA. The initial diagnosis of d-TGA should also include an assessment of the patency of the ductus arteriosus and of the foramen ovale as well as an assessment of the coronary artery anatomy. Coronary artery anatomy is especially important for the arterial switch operation where the coronary arteries are transferred to the neo-aorta (see Surgical and Post-Operative Assessment below). Abnormal origins of the coronary arteries and/or an anomalous course of these arteries may increase the risk of the arterial switch operation.

Surgical Repair and Post-Operative Assessment

Palliative procedures such as a balloon atrial septostomy may be performed in infants when the PFO is inadequate and the PDA has closed or in anticipation of duct closure which will occur spontaneously. The balloon atrial septostomy is commonly performed under echocardiographic guidance. Echocardiography is used to ensure that the inflated balloon is within the LA, and not across the mitral valve, prior to jerking the inflated balloon back across the IAS. Echocardiography is also useful in evaluating the efficiency of the septostomy; that is, the size of the resultant 'hole' in the IAS and degree of shunting through this defect.

Corrective surgeries used for d-TGA include the atrial switch and arterial switch operations; a Rastelli operation is performed for d-TGA + a VSD + significant PS.

Atrial Switch Operations

The atrial switch operations were the first successful procedures performed for the correction of d-TGA. There are two atrial switch operations: the Mustard and Senning repairs. The surgical technique for each operation varies but essentially the outcome is the same. That is, at the atrial level the systemic venous return is baffled to the systemic venous atrium (SVA), across the mitral valve, to the LV and then ejected to the PA; the pulmonary venous blood is returned to the pulmonary venous atrium (PVA), across the tricuspid valve, to the RV and ejected to the aorta (Fig. 15.63). Therefore, via this procedure deoxygenated blood from the vena cava is directed to the SVA; from the SVA blood then travels to the LV and is ejected into the PA where it then travels to the lungs to be oxygenated. Oxygenated blood then returns to the pulmonary veins and is directed to the PVA; from the PVA blood travels to the RV where it is ejected into the aorta and to the body. As a result, the circulation is corrected.

Table 15.8 **Common CHDs associated with d-TGA**

Associated Lesions
VSD
Pulmonary outflow tract obstruction
CoAo
Aortic arch hypoplasia
Variations in coronary artery origin and course

CoAo = coarctation of the aorta; VSD = ventricular septal defect.

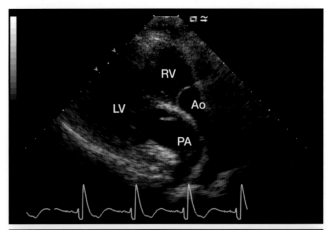

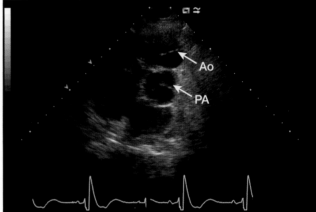

Figure 15.62 These images show the characteristic echocardiographic appearance of d-TGA. The parasternal long axis view shows the characteristic parallel alignment of the aorta (Ao) and pulmonary artery (PA) as seen in d-TGA (*top*). Observe that the aorta is anterior to the pulmonary artery which courses posteriorly. The parasternal short axis image shows the typical orientation of the great arteries in d-TGA (*bottom*). Observe that the aorta is anterior to the PA and the normal 'sausage-circle' arrangement (the PA in its long axis [sausage] and the aorta in its short axis [circle]) is absent.
LV = left ventricle; RV = right ventricle.

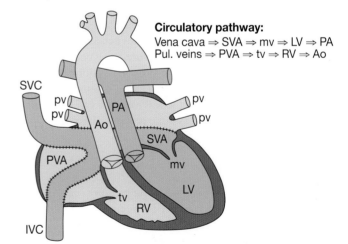

Circulatory pathway:
Vena cava ⇒ SVA ⇒ mv ⇒ LV ⇒ PA
Pul. veins ⇒ PVA ⇒ tv ⇒ RV ⇒ Ao

Figure 15.63 This schematic illustrates the atrial switch operation for d-TGA. An atrial baffle diverts deoxygenated blood from both the superior vena cava (SVC) and the inferior vena cava (IVC) to the systemic venous atrium (SVA). From the SVA deoxygenated blood crosses the mitral valve (mv) to the morphological left ventricle (LV) where it is then ejected to the pulmonary artery (PA) to be oxygenated in the lungs. Oxygenated blood from the lungs returns to pulmonary veins (pv) where it is diverted to the pulmonary venous atrium (PVA). From the PVA oxygenated blood travels across the tricuspid valve (tv) to morphological right ventricle (RV) where blood is then ejected to the aorta (Ao).

The primary role of the echocardiographic examination in the atrial switch operations includes the:

- assessment of intra-atrial channel patency
- assessment of RV and LV size and systolic function
- evaluation of TR severity and
- estimation of PASP.

The echocardiographic appearance of the Mustard and Senning operations appears very similar. The pulmonary venous and IVC intra-atrial channels are best assessed from the apical 4-chamber view while the SVC channel may be imaged from an off-axis parasternal long axis view (Fig. 15.64). Most commonly, the SVC channel cannot be well visualised by TTE in adult patients.

The most common post-operative complications for the atrial switch operations include baffle leaks and obstruction, RV failure, and significant TR. Baffle leaks can be detected by CFI (Fig. 15.65); a baffle leak is equivalent to an ASD. Baffle obstruction can also be detected via CFI and spectral Doppler (Fig. 15.66). In particular, severe baffle obstruction may be considered when the peak Doppler velocities across the baffle are ≥ 2 m/s [15.4].

RV dilatation and systolic dysfunction are extremely common post an atrial switch operation. Recall that in this situation the morphological RV is actually the systemic ventricle. The RV is not meant to sustain systemic pressures so this leads to RV dilatation and RV systolic dysfunction. Therefore, a comprehensive evaluation of the RV size and systolic function should be performed (see Chapter 2). Advanced echocardiographic modalities such as strain imaging may also be used to quantify RV function [15.5].

Varying degrees of TR are also common following the atrial switch operation. TR occurs due to annular dilatation and the high RVSP. In particular, the tricuspid valve is not 'designed' to sustain high pressures; therefore, TR may result due to the systemic pressures generated by the systemic RV. The severity of TR is assessed in the usual manner; the comprehensive echocardiographic assessment of TR is described in detail in Chapter 9.

It is also important to remember that the TR velocity cannot be used to estimate the PASP in the atrial switch as the RV gives rise to the aorta and not the PA; therefore, the RVSP estimated from the TR velocity reflects the systemic systolic pressure. Estimation of the PASP, however, can be determined in the presence of MR. Recall that the MR velocity can be used to estimate the left ventricular systolic pressure (LVSP):

Equation 15.7

$$LVSP = 4V_{MR}^2 + LAP$$

where LVSP = left ventricular systolic pressure (mm Hg)

$4V_{MR}^2$ = pressure gradient between the left ventricle and left atrium during systole (m/s)

    LAP = left atrial pressure (mm Hg)

Also recall that the LV gives rise to the PA (pulmonic ventricle); therefore, in the absence of LVOT obstruction or AS, the LVSP is equal to the PASP.

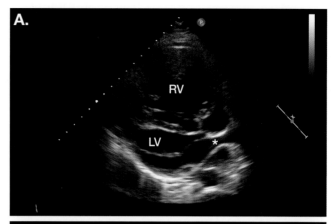

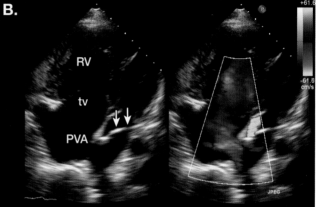

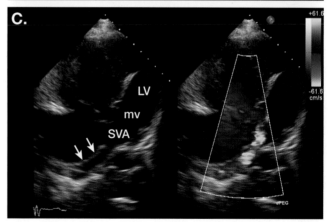

Figure 15.64 These images were recorded in a patient with a Senning's repair for d-TGA.

A: This is an off-axis parasternal long axis view with posterior tilt and slight medial angulation. From this view, the superior vena cava (SVC) channel can be seen (*). This channel runs almost parallel to the posterior aortic wall.

B: From the standard apical 4-chamber view, the intra-atrial baffle (arrows) can be seen channelling pulmonary venous blood to the pulmonary venous atrium (PVA), across the tricuspid valve (tv), into the morphological right ventricle (RV); this oxygenated blood is then ejected to the aorta. The corresponding colour Doppler image confirms patency of this channel; this is evident by laminar flow within this channel.

C: With slight posterior tilting, the inferior vena cava (IVC) channel can be seen (arrows). This channel baffles blood to the systemic venous atrium (SVA), across the mitral valve (mv), into the morphological left ventricle (LV); this deoxygenated blood is then ejected to the pulmonary artery. The corresponding colour Doppler image shows laminar flow through this channel confirming its patency.

[15.4] Vick GW 3rd, Murphy DJ Jr, Ludomirsky A, Morrow WR, Morriss MJ, Danford DA, Huhta JC. Pulmonary venous and systemic ventricular inflow obstruction in patients with congenital heart disease: detection by combined two-dimensional and Doppler echocardiography. *J Am Coll Cardiol.* 1987 Mar;9(3):580-7.

[15.5] Diller GP, Radojevic J, Kempny A, Alonso-Gonzalez R, Emmanouil L, Orwat S, Swan L, Uebing A, Li W, Dimopoulos K, Gatzoulis MA, Baumgartner H. Systemic right ventricular longitudinal strain is reduced in adults with transposition of the great arteries, relates to subpulmonary ventricular function, and predicts adverse clinical outcome. *Am Heart J.* 2012 May;163(5):859-66.

Arterial Switch Operation

The arterial switch operation (Jatene procedure) is now considered the method of choice for the correction of d-TGA. This operation restores the normal anatomic relationship between the ventricles and the great arteries (Fig. 15.67). This procedure involves transection of the great arteries above their respective roots and detachment of the coronary arteries, including a 'button' of the aortic wall, from the aorta. The great arteries are then switched and reattached so the distal end of the transected aorta is connected to the original pulmonary root to create the neo-aorta and the distal end of the transected pulmonary trunk is connected to the original aortic root to create the neo-PA. The coronary 'buttons' are then implanted to the neo-aorta. In addition, this surgical technique may include bringing the PA and its branches forward so these arteries are anterior to the aorta (the LeCompte Manoeuvre). Following this manoeuvre, the ascending aorta then lies under and posterior to the PA bifurcation.

The primary role of the echocardiographic examination in the arterial switch operation includes the:

- assessment of LV systolic function and exclusion of regional wall motion abnormalities (RWMAs)
- evaluation of the PA and aorta (especially at the anastomosis sites and the PA bifurcation)
- determination of the presence and degree of neo-aortic regurgitation.

Importantly, the presence of LV systolic dysfunction and RWMAs is suggestive of myocardial ischaemia due to problems associated with the re-implantation of the coronary arteries. Therefore, a careful evaluation of LV systolic function in required post-arterial switch operations.

Variable degrees of neo-aortic regurgitation may also be seen post-arterial switch. Recall that following this operation, the valve of the neo-aorta is actually the morphological pulmonary valve and the morphological pulmonary valve is not designed to be a high-pressure valve. As a result, this valve may become incompetent.

The most common complications of the arterial switch operation include narrowing at the arterial anastomosis sites and narrowing of the PA branches. In particular, supravalvular PS can develop due to inadequate growth at the neo-pulmonary anastomosis site. Branch PS may also occur following the LeCompte manoeuvre whereby the branch pulmonary arteries are 'stretched' into their anterior position over the aorta; this results in narrowing of the vessel lumen. The PA branches are best evaluated from the suprasternal window where they can be seen straddling the aorta (Fig. 15.68).

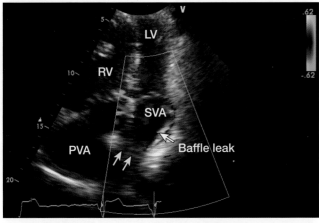

Figure 15.65 This zoomed apical 4-chamber view shows the pulmonary venous channel and the intra-atrial baffle (*yellow arrows*) in a Mustard's repair for d-TGA. Observe that an intra-atrial baffle leak is present resulting in pulmonary venous flow leaking across the baffle into the systemic venous atrium (SVA). LV = left ventricle; PVA = pulmonary venous atrium; RV = right ventricle.

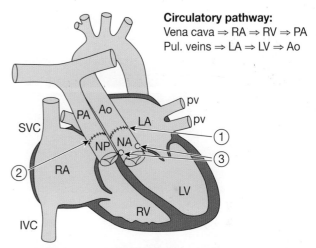

Circulatory pathway:
Vena cava ⇒ RA ⇒ RV ⇒ PA
Pul. veins ⇒ LA ⇒ LV ⇒ Ao

Figure 15.67 This schematic illustrates the arterial switch operation for d-TGA: (1) the aorta (Ao) is transected, switched and reattached so the proximal end of the 'new' aorta becomes the neo-aorta (NA); (2) the pulmonary artery (PA) is transected, switched and reattached so the proximal end of the 'new' pulmonary artery becomes the neo-pulmonary artery (NP); (3) the coronary arteries are also detached and reimplanted into the neo-aorta. Also note in this illustration that the PA and its branches are brought forward (LeCompte manoeuvre) and the distal aorta is moved posteriorly.
IVC = inferior vena cava; LA = left atrium; LV = left ventricle; pv = pulmonary veins; RA = right atrium; RV = right ventricle; SVC = superior vena cava.

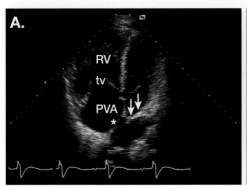
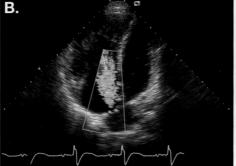
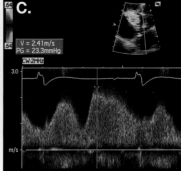

Figure 15.66 These apical images in a Senning's repair for d-TGA show baffle obstruction to the pulmonary venous channel. A: This apical 4-chamber image shows the intra-atrial baffle (*arrows*) which channels pulmonary venous blood into the pulmonary venous atrium (PVA), across the tricuspid valve (tv), into the morphological right ventricle (RV). A ridge of tissue extends into this channel (*). B: On colour flow Doppler imaging, turbulent flow is noted confirming the presence of baffle obstruction. C: Via continuous-wave (CW) Doppler, the peak velocity across this obstruction was 2.4 m/s.

Rastelli Operation

The Rastelli operation is performed when there is d-TGA with a large VSD and significant PS. This operation involves patching of the VSD to baffle blood flow from the LV across to the aorta and the insertion of a RV-to-PA valved conduit (Fig 15.69). The Rastelli operation is not unique to d-TGA + VSD + PS; this operation may also be performed for truncus arteriosus, pulmonary atresia with a VSD, or a double outlet RV with PS. The primary role of the echocardiographic examination post Rastelli operation includes:

• assessment of LV and RV size and systolic function
• evaluation of the conduit for stenosis and/or regurgitation
• interrogation of the VSD patch for residual defects
• assessment of the LVOT for residual obstruction.

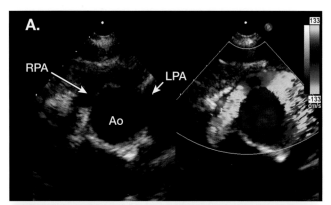

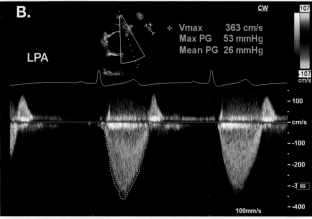

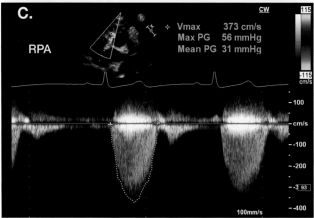

Figure 15.68 These suprasternal images were recorded following an arterial switch operation which included the LeCompte manoeuvre. A: From the 2D image, the aorta (Ao) is seen in cross section posterior to the pulmonary artery and the right pulmonary artery (RPA) and left pulmonary artery (LPA) branches are seen straddling the aorta. The corresponding colour Doppler image reveals turbulence is within the RPA and the LPA. B & C: Via continuous-wave (CW) Doppler the peak velocity across the LPA is 3.63 m/s and the peak velocity across the RPA is 3.73 m/s.

The most common post-operative complications of the Rastelli operation include conduit degeneration, stenosis and incompetence of the conduit valve, and residual LVOT obstruction. Echocardiographic examples of a normal LVOT tunnel, LVOT tunnel narrowing, and a residual VSD are shown in Figures 15.70-15.72.

Congenitally Corrected Transposition of the Great Arteries

Recall that in the normal heart, there is AV and VA concordance. When there is AV discordance and VA discordance, blood from the LA enters the morphological RV via a tricuspid valve and blood is ejected into the aorta while blood from the RA enters the morphological LV via a mitral valve and blood is ejected into the PA (Fig. 15.73). Therefore, the ventricles are inverted and the great arteries are transposed. However, as a result of this 'double' discordance, the circulation is correct even though the anatomy is not; therefore, this congenital anomaly is referred to as congenitally corrected transposition of the great arteries (cc-TGA).

Importantly, isolated cc-TGA is NOT a cyanotic heart lesion. However, this lesion is discussed in this section to distinguish cc-TGA from d-TGA.

cc-TGA is also commonly referred to as ventricular inversion or levo-TGA (l-TGA); the latter term refers to the fact that the primitive heart tube loops to the left instead of to the right so the ventricles are inverted with the morphological RV on the left and the morphological LV on the right. In addition to this abnormal looping, development of the conotruncal septum is also abnormal such that the aorta is abnormally positioned anterior and to the left of the PA.

Importantly, cc-TGA rarely occurs in isolation and other cardiac abnormalities are present in more than 90% of cases (Table 15.9). Anatomical repair of cc-TGA can be achieved by a double switch operation (see Appendix 6); in patients with cc-TGA + a VSD + significant PS, a Senning procedure along with a Rastelli procedure may be performed to restore normal anatomic connections.

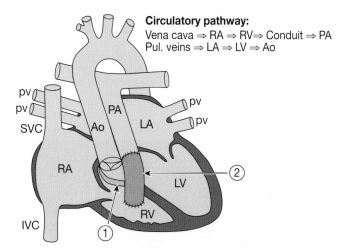

Figure 15.69 This schematic illustrates the Rastelli operation for d-TGA with a ventricular septal defect (VSD) and significant pulmonary stenosis: (1) a VSD patch is positioned to baffle blood flow from the left ventricle (LV) to the aorta (Ao) and (2) a valved conduit is inserted between the right ventricle (RV) and the pulmonary artery (PA). Observe that the circulation is essentially normalised via this procedure.
IVC = inferior vena cava; LA = left atrium; LV = left ventricle; pv = pulmonary vein; RA = right atrium; SVC = superior vena cava.

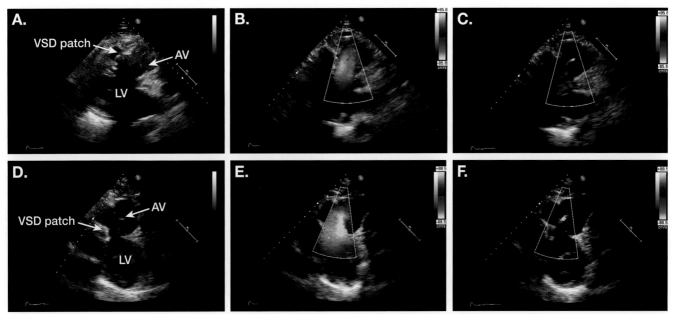

Figure 15.70 These images were acquired post the Rastelli Procedure for d-TGA + VSD + PS. Images were acquired from the parasternal long axis view (*top*) and the parasternal short axis view (*bottom*). Observe that the ventricular septal defect (VSD) patch creates a tunnel to the LVOT; this tunnel appears widely patent. On the colour Doppler images, laminar flow is observed through the LVOT tunnel during systole (*middle images*) with trace aortic regurgitation noted during diastole (*right images*). AV = aortic valve; LV = left ventricle.

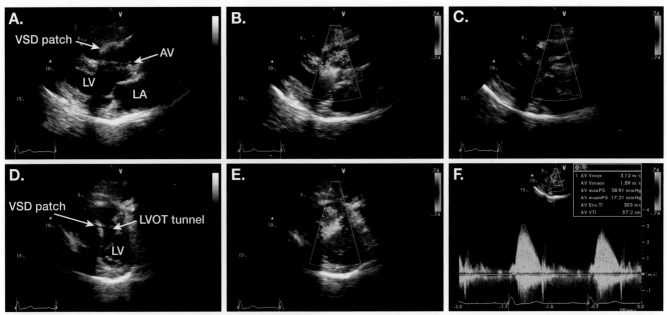

Figure 15.71 These images, post the Rastelli Procedure for d-TGA + VSD + PS, show obstruction through the LVOT tunnel. Images were acquired from the parasternal long axis view (*top*) and the parasternal short axis view (*bottom*). LVOT tunnel narrowing is most apparent on the colour Doppler images acquired during systole (*middle images*). Mild aortic regurgitation is also noted during diastole (*top right*). Via continuous-wave (CW) Doppler the peak velocity through the LVOT is 3.1 m/s yielding a maximum pressure gradient of 39 mm Hg and a mean pressure gradient of 17 mm Hg (*bottom right*). AV = aortic valve; LA = left atrium; LV = left ventricle.

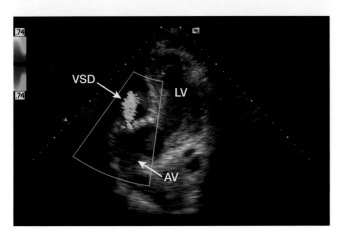

Figure 15.72 This apical 5-chamber image was acquired from a patient post the Rastelli Procedure for d-TGA + VSD + PS. A small residual ventricular septal defect (VSD) can be seen at the aortic end of the VSD patch. Also observe the distal position of the aortic valve (AV) within the left ventricular outflow tract tunnel: the VSD might be easily missed if colour Doppler interrogation was 'limited' to the left ventricular (LV) end of the VSD patch.

On echocardiographic examination, cc-TGA is diagnosed by recognising that the septal insertion of the left-sided AV valve is more apically positioned compared with the septal insertion of the right-sided AV valve (Fig. 15.74). This anatomical relationship of the septal insertions of the AV valves identifies the left-sided AV valve as the tricuspid valve and the right-sided AV valve as the mitral valve. Furthermore, as the tricuspid valve always leads to a morphologic RV and as the mitral valve always leads to a morphologic LV, identifying the AV valves also identifies the ventricles. Other clues to identifying a morphologic RV include the presence of characteristic coarse ventricular trabeculations and the moderator band within the ventricle.

In cc-TGA, the great arteries are transposed and parallel so the aorta is abnormally positioned anterior and to the left of the PA. As a result, on-axis images from the parasternal long axis view are not possible and this may provide the first clue to the presence of abnormal cardiac connections.

As cc-TGA rarely occurs in isolation particular attention should be given to identifying other associated congenital heart lesions such as VSDs and abnormalities of the left-sided tricuspid valve such as Ebstein's anomaly (Fig. 15.75).

An important complication of cc-TGA relates to the fact that the morphological RV is actually the systemic ventricle. As previously stated, the RV is not meant to support the systemic circulation and, therefore, the RV dilates and systolic function deteriorates. Likewise, TR is very common due to the systemic pressure load faced by this valve. TR is further exacerbated by dilatation of the tricuspid annulus as well as any morphological abnormalities of the valve.

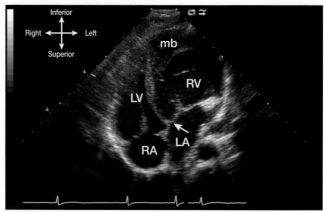

Figure 15.74 This apical 4-chamber image shows the characteristic features of cc-TGA. In relation to the cardiac crux, observe that the septal insertion of the left atrioventricular (AV) valve (*arrow*) is positioned more apically than the septal insertion of the right AV valve. This relationship identifies the left AV valve as the tricuspid valve. Therefore, the left-sided ventricle must be the morphological right ventricle (RV). The moderator band (mb) and a false tendon can also be seen within the RV. The right AV is the mitral valve and the right-sided ventricle is therefore the morphological left ventricle (LV).

Table 15.9 Common Congenital Heart Defects associated with cc-TGA

Associated Lesions
VSDs (usually perimembranous)
Pulmonary outflow tract obstruction (usually accompanied by a large VSD)
TV abnormalities (e.g. Ebstein's anomaly)
CoAo
Dextrocardia or mesocardia

CoAo = coarctation of the aorta; TV = tricuspid valve; VSD = ventricular septal defect.

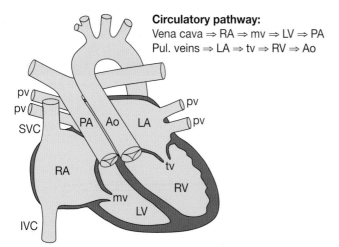

Circulatory pathway:
Vena cava ⇒ RA ⇒ mv ⇒ LV ⇒ PA
Pul. veins ⇒ LA ⇒ tv ⇒ RV ⇒ Ao

Figure 15.73 This schematic illustrates the anatomy of cc-TGA which is characterised by atrioventricular and ventriculoarterial discordance. The right atrium (RA) connects with the morphological left ventricle (LV) via the mitral valve (mv) and the LV gives rise to the pulmonary artery (PA). The left atrium (LA) connects with the morphological right ventricle (RV) via the tricuspid valve (tv) and the RV gives rise to the aorta (Ao). Therefore, the circulation is "congenitally corrected" with deoxygenated blood from the inferior vena cava (IVC) and superior vena cava (SVC) being directed to the PA via the discordant LV and oxygenated blood from the pulmonary veins (pv) being directed to the aorta via the discordant RV.

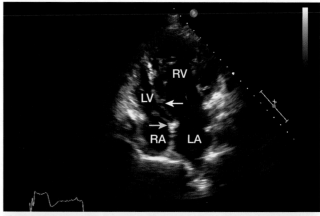

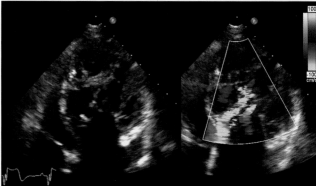

Figure 15.75 These apical 4-chamber images show cc-TGA with Ebstein's anomaly of the tricuspid valve. Observe the marked apical displacement of the septal insertion of the tricuspid valve, which is the left atrioventricular (AV) valve (*white arrow*) compared to the septal insertion of the mitral valve, which is the right AV valve (*yellow arrow*) (*top*). Also observe the coarse trabeculations of the right-sided ventricle which is the morphological right ventricle (RV). The image recorded at a shallower image depth also shows the coarse trabeculations of the morphological RV and the abnormal displacement of the septal tricuspid leaflet; associated tricuspid regurgitation (TR) is also evident (*bottom*). Observe that the origin of the TR jet assists in confirming the apical displacement of the tricuspid orifice.

Tricuspid Valve Atresia

Tricuspid valve atresia (TVA) is a cyanotic congenital heart lesion that is characterised by congenital agenesis or absence of the tricuspid valve (Fig. 15.76). As a result, there is no direct communication between the RA and the RV. Therefore, for survival there must be right-to-left shunting of the systemic venous return, at the atrial level, across a PFO or ASD. Most commonly, a small restrictive VSD, a small hypoplastic or rudimentary RV and a hypoplastic PA are also present. Cyanosis occurs because all of the systemic venous return is shunted right-to-left to the left heart and to the systemic circulation.

There are three main classifications of TVA based on the anatomic relationship of the great vessels and these main classifications are then sub classified depending on the presence or absence of a VSD and whether there is PS or pulmonary atresia (Table 15.10). Of these classifications, the most common type of TVA is Type Ib: TVA with normally related great arteries, a VSD and PS or pulmonary hypoplasia. In addition, TVA is associated with a number of additional CHDs including ASDs (present in all cases), RV hypoplasia, aortic or subaortic stenosis, CoAo or interrupted aortic arch and coronary artery anomalies.

On the echocardiographic examination, the definitive diagnosis of TVA is based on the absence of the tricuspid valve and the presence of an ASD and RV hypoplasia. TVA is best identified from the apical 4-chamber view (Fig. 15.77). The presence or absence of a VSD as well as the degree of RV hypoplasia can also be appreciated from this view. Furthermore, due to the various classifications of TVA and the number of congenital heart lesions that may be associated with TVA, an extensive evaluation of cardiac anatomy, valvular and ventricular function, and intracardiac haemodynamics is required.

Surgical Repair and Post-Operative Assessment

The surgical correction for TVA involves the creation of a Fontan circuit (Fig. 15.78). The original Fontan operation included a Glenn shunt and an atriopulmonary connection between the RA appendage and the main pulmonary artery (MPA). This operation has since undergone many modifications and has now been replaced by the total cavopulmonary connection (TCPC) operation where there is a bidirectional Glenn shunt or a hemi-Fontan (see Appendix 6) and either an intra-atrial (lateral) tunnel or an extracardiac conduit between the IVC and the PA. The intra-atrial or extracardiac conduit may also be fenestrated to allow shunting into the RA when the pulmonary vascular resistance is high.

The TCPC operation is usually performed in two stages: stage 1 is the bidirectional Glenn shunt or a hemi-Fontan and stage 2 is the intra-atrial tunnel or an extracardiac conduit between the IVC and the PA. Therefore, with this operation the RV is excluded from the circulation so the systemic venous return is channelled directly into the PA via the intra-atrial or extracardiac conduit. The Fontan circuit may also be described as having a "Push-Pull" physiology whereby the elevated central venous pressure (CVP) pushes blood into the lungs and the systemic LV pulls or sucks blood from the lungs during inspiration.

It is also important to note that the Fontan circuit is not unique to TVA and may be performed in any hearts that have a univentricular physiology or a single functional ventricle.

The echocardiographic assessment in the post-operative Fontan or TCPC patient includes the assessment of:
- LV size and systolic function
- the presence and severity of mitral regurgitation (MR)
- the anatomy and function of the Fontan circuit.

Assessment of the Fontan circuit includes evaluation of the Fontan connections, recognition of normal and abnormal CFI and spectral Doppler patterns within the vena cava, hepatic veins and tunnels, identification of baffle leaks and the exclusion of thrombus.

The intra-atrial (lateral) tunnel is best imaged from the apical 4-chamber view where the channel appears as a circle within the RA (Fig. 15.79). Imaging of the atriopulmonary connection and the extracardiac conduit connections is best attempted from a high right parasternal window; however, these connections are very difficult to image by TTE as many of the connections are retrosternal.

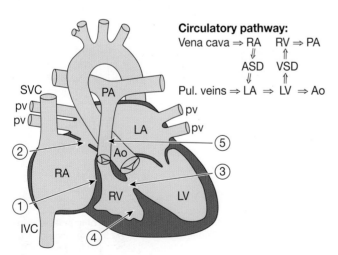

Circulatory pathway:

Vena cava ⇒ RA   RV ⇒ PA
⇓   ⇑
ASD   VSD
⇓   ⇑
Pul. veins ⇒ LA ⇒ LV ⇒ Ao

Figure 15.76 This schematic illustrates the anatomy of tricuspid valve atresia which is characterised by: (1) an absent tricuspid valve, (2) an atrial septal defect (ASD), (3) a small restrictive ventricular septal defect (VSD), (4) a hypoplastic right ventricle (RV) and (5) a hypoplastic pulmonary artery (PA). Observe that deoxygenated blood from the inferior vena cava (IVC) and superior vena cava (SVC) enters the right atrium (RA). From the RA, all of the systemic venous return is shunted right-to-left across the ASD where it mixes with oxygenated blood returning to the left atrium (LA) via the pulmonary veins (pv). From the LA, deoxygenated blood flows to the left ventricle (LV) where the majority of blood is ejected to the aorta (Ao) and the systemic circulation. A small portion of blood is shunted through the restrictive VSD to the diminutive RV where it is ejected through the hypoplastic PA to the lungs. As all of the systemic venous return is shunted to the left heart, there is marked cyanosis.

Table 15.10 Classifications of Tricuspid Valve Atresia

Anatomic Variants
Type I: TVA with normally related great arteries: Type Ia – intact IVS with pulmonary atresia Type Ib - small VSD with pulmonary stenosis/hypoplasia Type Ic - large VSD without pulmonary stenosis or atresia
Type II: TVA with d-TGA Type IIa - VSD with pulmonary atresia Type IIb - VSD with pulmonary stenosis/hypoplasia Type IIc – VSD without pulmonary stenosis or atresia
Type III: TVA with l-TGA or malposition of the great arteries other than d-TGA plus associated complex lesions (e.g. truncus arteriosus, AVCD, DORV)

AVCD = atrioventricular canal defect; d-TGA = dextro-transposition of the great arteries; DORV = double outlet right ventricle; IVS = interventricular septum; VSD = ventricular septal defect.

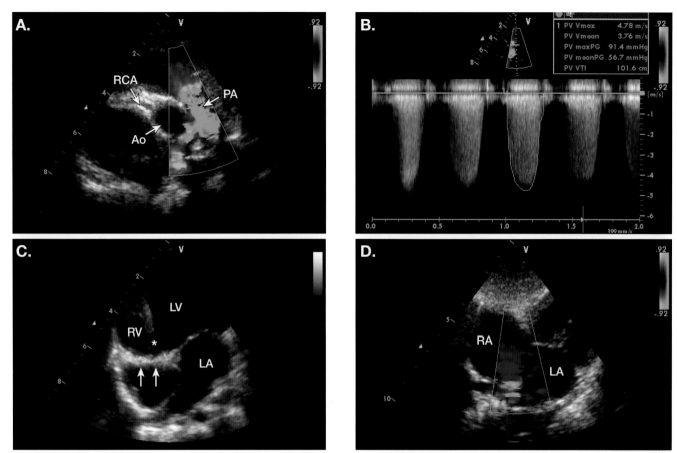

Figure 15.77 These images were recorded from an infant with tricuspid valve atresia (TVA) Type 1b (normally related great arteries with a small ventricular septal defect (VSD) and pulmonary stenosis). A: From the parasternal short axis view, the normal anatomical arrangement of the aorta (Ao) and pulmonary artery (PA) can be appreciated. Turbulent flow across the PA is also evident. B: Via continuous-wave (CW) Doppler, the peak velocity across the pulmonary valve is 4.8 m/s yielding a maximum pressure gradient of 91 mm Hg; the mean pressure gradient is 57 mm Hg. C: From the apical 4-chamber view, a small right ventricle (RV), a small ventricular septal defect (*) and an absent tricuspid valve (*arrows*) are noted. Observe that the interatrial septum (IAS) bows right-to-left consistent with elevated right atrial (RA) pressures. D: From the subcostal 4-chamber view, colour flow imaging shows right-to-left shunting across a restrictive atrial septal defect (ASD); this appears as turbulent flow directed away from the transducer. LA = left atrium; LV = left ventrcle; RCA = right coronary artery.

Figure 15.78 These schematics illustrate various types of the Fontan circuit.

A: The original Fontan operation with a Glenn shunt and an atriopulmonary connection: (1) the Glenn shunt consists of an anastomosis of the distal right pulmonary artery (RPA) to the superior vena cava (SVC); (2) the atriopulmonary connection is an anastomosis of the right atrial (RA) appendage to the proximal right pulmonary artery (RPA); (3) the atrial septal defect (ASD) is also closed; and

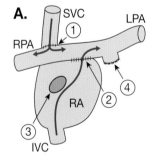
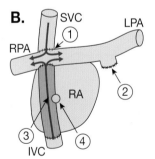
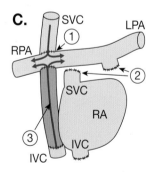

(4) the main pulmonary artery (MPA) is also transected and oversewn.

B: A bidirectional Glenn shunt (BGS) and an intra-atrial total cavopulmonary connection (lateral tunnel): (1) the BGS consists of an anastomosis of the SVC to the RPA; (2) the MPA is also transected and oversewn; (3) the tubular intra-atrial lateral tunnel channels blood from the inferior vena cava (IVC) to the RPA; (4) a fenestration within the lateral tunnel is also shown.

C: A BGS and an extracardiac total cavopulmonary connection: (1) the BGS consists of an anastomosis of the SVC to the RPA; (2) the MPA and the cardiac ends of SVC and IVC are transected and oversewn; (3) the tubular extracardiac total cavopulmonary connection channels from the IVC to the RPA.

> The Fontan operation has been referred to as both palliative and corrective. However, it is not truly corrective or palliative. It is not corrective due to the fact that anatomically there is still no RV and because there are many complications associated with this procedure. Likewise, this operation is not a palliative procedure as it provides more than just symptomatic relief; it also separates the systemic and pulmonary circuits. Therefore, this procedure may be referred to as an "orthoterminal correction"; that is, this operation results in adequate perfusion of the systemic and pulmonary capillary beds without repairing the underlying anatomical malformation.
> Reference: Sade RM. Orthoterminal correction of congenital cardiovascular defects. *Ann Thorac Surg* 1975;19:105-7.

Importantly, the Doppler patterns in each type of connection are different and the flow varies with respiration; therefore, the evaluation of signals requires knowledge of each type of connection as well as a careful analysis of these flow profiles over the respiratory cycle.

Potential complications of the Fontan operations that may be detected on the echocardiogram include ventricular dysfunction, pulmonary venous obstruction of the right pulmonary veins due to marked RA dilatation, systemic venous obstruction due to atriopulmonary connection stenosis, lateral tunnel stenosis, SVC stenosis, peripheral

PA stenosis, and/or RA and conduit thrombus. In particular, suspected RA thrombus and conduit thrombus, which may occur due to the low velocity flow within these areas, often requires TOE.

> Due to the complexity of the Fontan and TCPC operations, variations in surgical techniques as well as the number of complications associated with this procedure, it is highly recommended that follow-up echocardiograms be performed in tertiary centres with experience in imaging these patients.

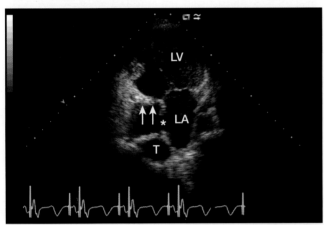 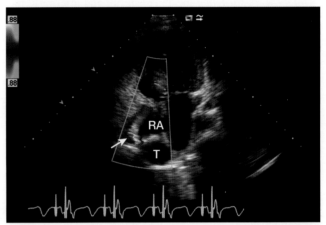

Figure 15.79 These apical 4-chamber images were recorded from a patient with tricuspid valve atresia and an intra-atrial lateral tunnel. The 2D image shows tricuspid atresia (*arrows*), an atrial septal defect (*) and the lateral tunnel (T) within the right atrium (RA) (*left*). On the corresponding colour Doppler image, the fenestration in this tunnel is shown (*arrow*); observe that this results in a shunt from the tunnel into the RA (*right*).

Key Points

Atrial Septal Defects (ASDs)
- *Ostium primum (1⁰ ASD):* account for ≈ 15% of all ASDs; located at inferior IAS in the region of the AV valves; associated lesions include "cleft" anterior leaflet of mitral valve, AVCD
- *Ostium secundum (2⁰ ASD):* account for ≈ 80% of all ASDs; located in the region of the fossa ovalis; usually isolated; may be associated with MVP and/or PS
- *Sinus venous (SV ASD):* 2 types: superior type (≈ 5% of all ASDs) located superiorly near the SVC; inferior type (< 1% of all ASDs) located inferiorly near the IVC; associated lesions include anomalous pulmonary venous drainage
- *Coronary sinus (CS ASD):* account for <1% of all ASDs; located between posterior wall of LA and coronary sinus; associated lesions include persistent LSVC

Role of Echo in ASDs:
- Determine the type of defect:
  - based on anatomic location
  - 2⁰ ASD: best seen in subcostal 4-chamber, subcostal short axis, para-apical views
  - 1⁰ ASD: best seen in apical 4-chamber and subcostal 4-chamber views
  - SV ASD: difficult to detect via TTE, best seen in apical and subcostal windows with anterior tilting of the transducer
  - CS ASD: difficult to detect via TTE, suspected when dilated coronary sinus seen in apical 4-chamber view (with posterior tilt) but not seen from parasternal long axis view (unroofed CS)
- Estimate the anatomic size of the defect:
  - measure in orthogonal imaging planes
- Determine the shunt direction:
  - via CFI; most commonly left-to-right; shunt reversal with Eisenmenger's syndrome
- Estimate the haemodynamic significance of the shunt:
  - indirect signs of significant shunt: dilatation of right heart; RA larger than LA (RAI > 0.92)
  - quantification via QP:QS calculation (QP derived from RVOT stroke volume and QS derived from LVOT stroke volume)
  - QP:QS shunt ratio ≥1.5:1 indicates haemodynamically significant shunt
- Estimate RVSP (PASP)
- Identify any associated lesions

(continued over...)

Key Points (continued)

Patent Foramen Ovale (PFO)
• Persistence of foetal communication between RA and LA
• Located at fossa ovalis, present in 25-30% population
• Definitive diagnosis: identification of separation of flap valve of fossa ovalis from IAS
• On TTE: best detected via CFI
• When clinically suspected but not detected, saline contrast bubble study is indicated

Ventricular Septal Defects (VSDs)
• *Perimembranous:* account for ≈ 80% of all VSDs; located beneath aortic valve bordering septal tricuspid leaflet and inferior to the crista supraventricularis
• *Muscular:* account for ≈ 20% of all VSDs; includes inlet, outlet and trabecular VSDs
• *Trabecular:* located anywhere along trabecular septum; bordered only by muscle
• *Inlet (AV canal-type):* located posterior and inferior to membranous IVS beneath tricuspid and mitral valves
• *Outlet (supracristal):* located anterior to membranous IVS and beneath semilunar valves
Role of Echo in VSDs:
• Determine the type of defect:
  - based on anatomic location and echo view in which defect seen
  - Perimembranous: seen in parasternal short axis view between 9 and 12 o'clock and apical 5-chamber view
  - Outlet: seen in parasternal short axis view between 12 and 3 o'clock
  - Inlet: seen in standard apical 4-chamber view
  - Trabecular: seen anywhere along muscular septum
• Estimate the anatomic size of the defect
• Determine the shunt direction:
  - via CFI; most commonly left-to-right; shunt reversal with Eisenmenger's syndrome
• Estimate the haemodynamic significance of the shunt:
  - quantification via QP:QS calculation (QP derived from RVOT stroke volume and QS derived from LVOT stroke volume)
  - QP:QS shunt ratio ≥1.5:1 indicates haemodynamically significant shunt
• Estimate the RVSP:
  - using TR velocity: $RVSP = 4V_{TR}^2 + RAP$
  - using VSD velocity: $RVSP = SBP - 4V_{VSD}^2$

Gerbode Defect
• Another type of VSD that results in a LV-to-RA shunt
• Located in the supravalvular segment of membranous IVS; i.e. within AV septum
• Congenital or acquired
• Identified by CFI with left-to-right shunting from LV to RA

Atrioventricular Canal Defect (AVCD)
• Occur due to maldevelopment or malfusion of superior and inferior endocardial cushions
• *Complete AVCD:* characterised by 1° ASD, an inlet VSD and a large common AV valve; > 75% of patients have Down syndrome
• *Partial AVCD:* characterised by 1° ASD and cleft anterior mitral valve leaflet
• AVCD is best identified from apical 4-chamber view
• Echo also useful in assessing severity of AV valve regurgitation, degree and direction of intracardiac shunting, LV and RV systolic function, and estimation of the PA pressures

Patent Ductus Arteriosus (PDA)
• Persistence of foetal communication between PA and aorta
• Located between distal main PA (near the origin of the left PA) and descending aorta (just distal to the left subclavian artery)
Role of Echo in PDAs:
• Establish the diagnosis and determine shunt direction:
  - PDA best imaged from high parasternal long axis view of PA ('ductal' view), high parasternal short axis view of PA bifurcation, or from suprasternal long axis view with slight counter-clockwise rotation
  - CFI shows continuous flow; most commonly left-to-right; shunt absence or reversal with Eisenmenger's syndrome
• Estimate the haemodynamic significance of the shunt:
  - quantification via QP:QS calculation
  - QP derived from LVOT stroke volume and QS derived from RVOT stroke volume: **NB:** QP:QS in PDA is opposite to calculation of QP:QS in ASDs and VSDs
  - QP:QS shunt ratio ≥1.5:1 indicates haemodynamically significant shunt
• Estimate the PASP:
  - using peak systolic PDA velocity: $SBP - 4V_{PDA}^2$

(continued over...)

Key Points (continued)

Closure Devices for ASDs, VSDs and PDA
- 2^0 ASDs, mid-muscular and perimembranous VSDs, and PDAs may be closed by transcatheter (percutaneous) closure devices
- Role of echo includes:
  - patient selection
  - monitoring and guiding the procedure
  - assessing the end result, and
  - detection of post-procedure complications

Congenital Pulmonary Stenosis (PS)
- May occur at:
  - valve level (valvular PS): most common site
  - below pulmonary valve (subvalvular PS or infundibular stenosis)
  - above pulmonary valve (supravalvular PS)
  - at main PA branches (branch stenosis)
  - and/or within the peripheral pulmonary arteries (peripheral stenosis)
- Role of echo:
  - Determining the site and severity of obstruction
  - Assessing RV size and systolic function
  - Estimating the PASP

Congenital Aortic Stenosis (AS)
- May occur at:
  - valve level (valvular AS): most common site; usually due to BAV or UAV
  - below aortic valve (subvalvular AS): may be dynamic as in HOCM or fixed in form of a discrete fibrous membrane, a fibromuscular ridge, or a circumferential, tunnel-like narrowing
  - above aortic valve (supravalvular AS): may be in form of an hourglass deformity (most common), a fibrous membrane with central orifice, or a diffusely hypoplastic ascending aorta
- Role of echo:
  - Determining the site and severity of obstruction
  - Assessment of LV wall thickness, LV size and systolic function

Coarctation of the Aorta
- A discrete narrowing of descending thoracic aorta, just distal to left subclavian artery and adjacent to ligamentum arteriosum
- Commonly associated with BAV ($\approx 50\%$ cases)
- Proposed mechanisms include ectopic ductal tissue theory and reduced-flow (haemodynamic) theory
- Role of echo:
  - Establish the diagnosis
  - Estimate the severity of coarctation
  - Assess the LV size, wall thickness and systolic function
  - Evaluate aortic valve morphology
  - Assessment post coarctation repair

Tetralogy of Fallot (TOF)
- Cyanotic heart lesion; characterised by 4 cardiac abnormalities: (1) large malalignment VSD, (2) narrowing and obstruction of the RVOT, (3) over-riding aorta, and (4) RV hypertrophy
- Echo diagnosis based on identifying 4 above-mentioned abnormalities
- Complete surgical repair includes a patch closure of the VSD, widening of the RVOT, and relief of RVOT obstruction
- Role of echo post-op TOF repair:
  - Evaluation of the IVS for residual VSDs
  - Estimation of PR severity
  - Assessment of RVOT for aneurysms
  - Detection of persistent RVOT obstruction and, if present, to determine the site and severity of obstruction
  - Assessment of RV and LV size and systolic function
  - Measurement of the aortic root (progressive dilatation is common)
  - Evaluation of presence and severity of AR (secondary to aortic root dilatation)
- Most common post-operative TOF repair complications include RV failure, severe PR and a persistent RVOT obstruction

(continued over...)

Key Points (continued)

Dextro-Transposition of the Great Arteries (d-TGA)
- Cyanotic heart lesion caused by VA discordance: i.e. aorta arises from morphological RV while PA arises from morphological LV
- Echo diagnosis based on identifying parallel alignment of aorta and PA from parasternal long axis view
- Corrective surgeries include atrial switch and arterial switch operations; a Rastelli operation is performed for d-TGA + a VSD + significant PS

Atrial Switch for d-TGA:
- Includes Mustard and Senning repairs
- At atrial level systemic venous return is baffled to systemic venous atrium, across mitral valve, to LV and then ejected to PA; pulmonary venous blood is returned to pulmonary venous atrium, across tricuspid valve, to RV and ejected to aorta
- Role of Echo in atrial switch:
  - Assessment of intra-atrial channel patency
  - Assessment of RV and LV size and systolic function
  - Evaluation of the severity of TR
  - Estimation of PASP
- Most common post-operative complications include baffle leaks and obstruction, RV failure (systemic ventricle), and significant TR (facing systemic pressures)

Arterial Switch for d-TGA:
- Method of choice for correction of d-TGA
- Restores normal anatomic relationship between ventricles and great arteries: aorta reconnected to morphological LV and PA reconnected to morphological RV
- Coronary arteries reimplanted to neoaorta, PA and its branches usually brought forward so anterior to aorta (LeCompte Manoeuvre)
- Role of Echo in arterial switch:
  - Assessment of LV systolic function and exclusion of RWMAs
  - Evaluation of PA and aorta (especially at anastomosis sites and PA bifurcation)
  - Determination of presence and degree of neo-aortic regurgitation

Rastelli operation for d-TGA + VSD + PS:
- Involves: (1) patching of the VSD to baffle blood flow from the LV across to the aorta and (2) the insertion of a RV-to-PA valved conduit
- Role of Echo post-Rastelli:
  - Assessment of LV and RV size and systolic function
  - Evaluation of conduit for stenosis and/or regurgitation
  - Interrogation of VSD patch for residual defects
  - Assessment of LVOT for residual obstruction

Congenitally Corrected-Transposition of the Great Arteries (cc-TGA)
- Characterised by AV discordance and VA discordance
- "Double discordance" means that circulation is correct: LA enters morphological RV via a tricuspid valve and blood is ejected into aorta while blood from RA enters morphological LV via a mitral valve and blood is ejected into PA
- Other cardiac abnormalities are present in more than 90% of cases
- Echo diagnosis based on identifying more apically positioned septal insertion of left-sided AV valve (tricuspid valve) compared with that of right-sided AV valve (mitral valve); best seen from apical 4-chamber view
- Most common complications include RV failure (systemic ventricle) and significant TR (facing systemic pressures)

Tricuspid Valve Atresia (TVA)
- Cyanotic heart lesion characterised by an absent tricuspid valve; for survival, right-to-left shunting of the systemic venous return, at the atrial level across a PFO or ASD, must be present
- Most commonly associated with a small restrictive VSD, a small hypoplastic or rudimentary RV and a hypoplastic PA
- Many anatomic variants: classified based on anatomic relationship of great vessels, presence or absence of a VSD, and whether there is PS or pulmonary atresia
- Echo diagnosis based on identifying absent tricuspid valve
- Corrective surgery is staged: stage 1 = bidirectional Glenn shunt or a hemi-Fontan and stage 2 = intra-atrial tunnel or extracardiac conduit between IVC and PA
- Role of echo post-op Fontan/TCPC repair:
  - Assessment of LV size and systolic function
  - Determine presence and severity of MR
  - Evaluate anatomy and function of Fontan circuit
- Potential complications detected by echo include ventricular dysfunction, pulmonary venous obstruction, systemic venous and/or RA/conduit thrombus
- Echo examinations in Fontan patients should be performed in tertiary centres with experience in imaging these patients

Further Reading (listed in alphabetical order)

Embryology

Abdulla R, Blew GA, Holterman MJ. Cardiovascular embryology. *Pediatr Cardiol.* 2004 May-Jun;25(3):191-200.

Anderson RH, Webb A, Brown NA, Lamers W, Moorman A. Development of the heart: (3) Formation of the ventricular outflow tracts, arterial valves, and intrapericardial arterial trunks. *Heart.* 2003 September; 89(9): 1110–1118.

Anderson RH, Webb A, Brown NA, Lamers W, Moorman A. Development of the heart: (2) Septation of the atriums and ventricles. *Heart.* 2003 August; 89(8): 949–958.

Moorman A, Webb S, Brown NA, Lamers W, Anderson RH Development of the Heart: (1) Formation Of The Cardiac Chambers And Arterial Trunks. *Heart.* 2003 July; 89(7): 806–814.

Congenital Heart Defects and Surgical Repairs

Adult Congenital Heart Disease. Edited by Carole A. Warnes. © 2009 American Heart Association.

Baumgartner H, Bonhoeffer P, De Groot NM, de Haan F, Deanfield JE, Galie N, Gatzoulis MA, Gohlke-Baerwolf C, Kaemmerer H, Kilner P, Meijboom F, Mulder BJ, Oechslin E, Oliver JM, Serraf A, Szatmari A, Thaulow E, Vouhe PR, Walma E; Task Force on the Management of Grown-up Congenital Heart Disease of the European Society of Cardiology (ESC); Association for European Paediatric Cardiology (AEPC); ESC Committee for Practice Guidelines (CPG). ESC Guidelines for the management of grown-up congenital heart disease (new version 2010). *Eur Heart J.* 2010 Dec;31(23):2915-57.

Brickner ME, Hillis LD, Lange RA. Congenital heart disease in adults. First of two parts. *N Engl J Med.* 2000 Jan 27;342(4):256-63

Brickner ME, Hillis LD, Lange RA.Congenital heart disease in adults. Second of two parts. *N Engl J Med.* 2000 Feb 3;342(5):334-42.

Gaca AM, Jaggers JJ, Dudley LT, Bisset GS 3rd. Repair of congenital heart disease: a primer-part 1. *Radiology.* 2008 Jun;247(3):617-31.

Gaca AM, Jaggers JJ, Dudley LT, Bisset GS 3rd. Repair of congenital heart disease: a primer--Part 2. *Radiology.* 2008 Jul;248(1):44-60.

Rhodes JF, Hijazi ZM, Sommer RJ. Pathophysiology of congenital heart disease in the adult, part II. Simple obstructive lesions. *Circulation.* 2008 Mar 4;117(9):1228-37.

Sommer RJ, Hijazi ZM, Rhodes JF Jr. Pathophysiology of congenital heart disease in the adult: part I: Shunt lesions. *Circulation.* 2008 Feb 26;117(8):1090-9.

Sommer RJ, Hijazi ZM, Rhodes JF. Pathophysiology of congenital heart disease in the adult: part III: Complex congenital heart disease. *Circulation.* 2008 Mar 11;117(10):1340-50.

Warnes CA. Transposition of the great arteries. *Circulation.* 2006 Dec 12;114(24):2699-709.

Wu JC, Child JS. Common congenital heart disorders in adults. *Curr Probl Cardiol.* 2004 Nov;29(11):641-700.

Closure Devices

Arzamendi D, Miró J. Percutaneous intervention in adult congenital heart disease. *Rev Esp Cardiol (Engl Ed).* 2012 Aug;65(8):690-9.

Gruenstein DH, Bass JL. Transcatheter device closure of congenital ventricular septal defects. Progress in Pediatric *Cardiology.* 2012 33(2): 131–141

Ivens E, Hamilton-Craig C, Aroney C, Clarke A, Jalali H, Burstow DJ. Early and late cardiac perforation by Amplatzer atrial septal defect and patent foramen ovale devices. *J Am Soc Echocardiogr.* 2009 Sep;22(9):1067-70.

Spies C, Cao Q-L, Hijazi ZM. Transcatheter closure of congenital and acquired septal defects. *Eur Heart J Suppl* (2010) 12 (suppl E): E24-E34.

Tobis J, Shenoda M. Percutaneous treatment of patent foramen ovale and atrial septal defects. *J Am Coll Cardiol.* 2012 Oct 30;60(18):1722-32.

Yared K, Baggish AL, Solis J, Durst R, Passeri JJ, Palacios IF, Picard MH. Echocardiographic assessment of percutaneous patent foramen ovale and atrial septal defect closure complications. Circ Cardiovasc Imaging. 2009 Mar;2(2):141-9. Arzamendi D, Miró J. Percutaneous intervention in adult congenital heart disease. *Rev Esp Cardiol (Engl Ed).* 2012 Aug;65(8):690-9.

Appendices

Appendix 1

Normal Haemodynamic Values for Selected Prosthetic Aortic Valves

Valve Type [Ref.]	Valve Size (mm)	Peak Gradient (mmHg)	Mean Gradient (mmHg)	Effective Orifice Area (cm²)
Allograft [1] (Homograft)	17-19	9.7 ± 4.2 (n=16)	4.2 ± 1.8 (n=16)	1.7 ± 0.3 (n=16)
	19-21	-	5.4 ± 0.9 (n=5)	-
	20-21	7.9 ± 4.0 (n=22)	3.6 ± 2.0 (n=22)	2.3 ± 0.4 (n=22)
	20-22	7.2 ± 3.0 (n=12)	3.5 ± 1.5 (n=12)	2.3 ± 0.5 (n=12)
	22	-	5.8 ± 3.2 (n=6)	2.0 ± 0.6 (n=6)
	22-23	5.6 ± 3.1 (n=12)	2.6 ± 1.4 (n=12)	2.5 ± 0.3 (n=12)
	22-24	-	5.6 ± 1.7 (n=26)	-
	24-27	6.2 ± 2.6 (n=7)	2.8 ± 1.1 (n=7)	2.7 ± 0.3 (n=7)
	26	-	6.8 ± 2.9 (n=6)	2.4 ± 0.7 (n=6)
	25-28	-	6.2 ± 2.5 (n=25)	-
ATS Open Pivot [1,2] (Bileaflet)	19	47.0 ± 12.6 (n=9)	25.3 ± 8.0 (n=9)	0.96 ± 0.18 (n=9)
	21	25.5 ± 6.1 (n=15)	14.4 ± 3.5 (n=15)	1.58 ± 0.37 (n=15)
	23	-	14.4 ± 4.9 (n =246)	1.7 ± 0.5 (n=139)
	25	-	11.3 ± 3.7 (n=240)	2.1 ± 0.7 (n=139)
	27	-	8.4 ± 3.7 (n=88)	2.5 ± 0.1 (n=76)
	29	-	8.0 ± 3.0 (n=24)	3.1 ± 0.8 (n=24)
ATS AP [1] (Bileaflet)	16	47.7 ± 12 (n=6)	27 ± 7.3 (n=6)	0.61 ± 0.09 (n=6)
	18	-	21.0 ± 1.8 (n=9)	1.2 ± 0.3 (n=9)
	20	21.4 ± 4.2 (n=21)	11.1 ± 3.5 (n=59)	1.3 ± 0.3 (n=59)
	22	18.7 ± 8.3 (n=41)	10.5 ± 4.5 (n=93)	1.7 ± 0.4 (n=91)
	24	15.1 ± 5.6 (n=27)	7.5 ± 3.1 (n=56)	2.0 ± 0.6 (n=56)
	26	-	6.0 ± 2.0 (n=7)	2.1 ± 0.4 (n=7)
Biocor Stentless [2] (Stentless)	21	35.97 ± 4.06 (n=45)	18 ± 4 (n=45)	-
	23	29.15 ± 8.28 (n=115)	18.64 ± 7.14 (n=115)	1.4 ± 0.5 (n=115)
	25	28.65 ± 6.6 (n=100)	17.72 ± 6.99 (n=100)	1.6 ± 0.38 (n=100)
	27	25.87 ± 2.81 (n=55)	18 ± 2.8 (n=55)	1.9 ± 0.46 (n=55)
Bjork-Shiley [1,2] (Single tilting disc)	19	46.0 (n=37)	26.67 ± 7.87 (n=37)	0.94 ± 0.19 (n=37)
	21	32.41 ± 9.73 (n=161)	18.64 ± 6.09 (n=161)	1.1 ± 0.3 (n=13)
	23	26.52 ± 9.67 (n=153)	14.5 ± 6.2 (n=153)	1.3 ± 0.3 (n=25)
	25	22.33 ± 7 (n=89)	13.3 ± 4.96 (n=89)	1.5 ± 0.4 (n=35)
	27	18.31 ± 8 (n=61)	10.41 ± 4.38 (n=61)	1.6 ± 0.3 (n=12)
	29	12 ± 8 (n=9)	7.67 ± 4.36 (n=9)	-

(continued over...)

Appendix 1 (continued)

Normal Haemodynamic Values for Selected Prosthetic Aortic Valves

Valve Type [Ref.]	Valve Size (mm)	Peak Gradient (mmHg)	Mean Gradient (mmHg)	Effective Orifice Area (cm²)
Carpentier-Edwards Standard [1] (Stented)	19	43.5 ± 12.7 (n=56)	25.6 ± 8.0 (n=56)	0.9 ± 0.2 (n=56)
	21	27.7 ± 7.6 (n=73)	17.3 ± 6.2 (n=73)	1.5 ± 0.3 (n=73)
	23	28.9 ± 7.5 (n=110)	16.1 ± 6.2 (n=111)	1.7 ± 0.5 (n=100)
	25	24.0 ± 7.1 (n=85)	12.9 ± 4.6 (n=97)	1.9 ± 0.5 (n=85)
	27	22.1 ± 8.2 (n=50)	12.1 ± 5.5 (n=56)	2.3 ± 0.6 (n=50)
	29	-	9.9 ± 2.9 (n=24)	2.8 ± 0.5 (n=24)
Carpentier-Edwards Pericardial [1] (Stented)	19	32.1 ± 3.4 (n=14)	24.2 ± 8.6 (n=14)	1.2 ± 0.3 (n=14)
	21	25.7 ± 9.9 (n=34)	20.3 ± 9.1 (n=34)	1.5 ± 0.4 (n=34)
	23	21.7 ± 8.6 (n=20)	13.0 ± 5.3 (n=20)	1.8 ± 0.3 (n=0)
	25	16.5 ± 5.4 (n=5)	9.0 ± 2.3 (n=5)	-
Carpentier-Edwards Supra-Annular [1] (Stented)	19	34.1 ± 2.7 (n=14)	-	1.1 ± 0.1 (n=14)
	21	28.0 ± 10.5 (n=26)	17.5 ± 3.8 (n=82)	1.4 ± 0.9 (n=74)
	23	25.3 ± 10.5 (n=43)	13.4 ± 4.5 (n=54)	1.6 ± 0.6 (n=80)
	25	24.4 ± 7.6 (n=34)	13.2 ± 4.8 (n=71)	1.8 ± 0.4 (n=60)
	27	16.7 ± 4.7 (n=6)	8.8 ± 2.8 (n=13)	1.9 ± 0.7 (n=13)
Cryolife-O'Brien [1] (Stentless)	19	-	9.0 ± 2.0 (n=47)	1.5 ± 0.3 (n=47)
	21	-	6.6 ± 2.9 (n=172)	1.7 ± 0.4 (n=146)
	23	-	6.0 ± 2.3 (n=158)	2.3 ± 0.2 (n=125)
	25	-	6.1 ± 2.6 (n=209)	2.6 ± 0.2 (n=169)
	27	-	4.0 ± 2.4 (n=144)	2.8 ± 0.3 (n=133)
Edwards SAPIEN [3] (Percutaneous)	23	21.4 ± 7.1 (n=16)	11.9 ± 4.2 (n=16)	1.47 ± 0.14 (n=16)
	26	15.8 ± 5.7 (n=32)	8.5 ± 3.1 (n=32)	1.82 ± 0.48 (n=32)
Hancock I [1,2] (Stented)	21	18.0 ± 6.0 (n=7)	12.0 ± 2.0 (n=7)	-
	23	19.09 ± 4.35 (n=14)	12.36 ± 3.82 (n=14)	-
	25	17.61 ± 3.13 (n=26)	11 ± 2.85 (n=26)	-
	27	18.11 ± 6.92 (n=20)	10 ± 3.46 (n=20)	-
Hancock II [1,2] (Stented porcine)	21	20 ± 4 (n=39)	14.8 ± 4.1 (n=17)	1.3 ± 0.4 (n=17)
	23	34.0 ± 13.0 (n=15)	16.6 ± 8.5 (n=8)	1.3 ± 0.4 (n=23)
	25	22.0 ± 5.3 (n=6)	10.8 ± 2.8 (n=15)	1.6 ± 0.4 (n=15)
	27	14 ± 3 (n=133)	10 ± 3.46 (n=26)	1.55 ± 0.18 (n=133)
	29	16.2 ± 1.5 (n=5)	8.2 ± 1.7 (n=5)	1.6 ± 0.2 (n=5)
MCRI On-X [1] (Bileaflet)	19	21.3 ± 10.8 (n=5)	11.8 ± 3.4 (n=5)	1.5 ± 0.2 (n=5)
	21	16.4 ± 5.9 (n=11)	9.9 ± 3.6 (n=11)	1.7 ± 0.4 (n=11)
	23	15.9 ± 6.4 (n=23)	8.6 ± 3.4 (n=30)	1.9 ± 0.6 (n=30)
	25	16.5 ± 10.2 (n=12)	6.9 ± 4.3 (n=22)	2.4 ± 0.6 (n=22)
Medtronic Advantage [1] (Bileaflet)	23	-	10.4 ± 3.1 (n=6)	2.2 ± 0.3 (n=6)
	25	-	9.0 ± 3.7 (n=14)	2.8 ± 0.6 (n=14)
	27	-	7.6 ± 3.6 (n=11)	3.3 ± 0.7 (n=11)
	29	-	6.1 ± 3.8 (n=5)	3.9 ± 0.7 (n=5)
Medtronic CoreValve [3] (Percutaneous)	26	15.5 ± 6.6 (n=40)	8.4 ± 3.8 (n=40)	1.78 ± 0.4 (n=40)
	29	17.7 ± 8.5 (n=58)	9.7 ± 5.3 (n=58)	1.94 ± 0.43 (n=58)

(continued over...)

Appendix 1 (continued)

Normal Haemodynamic Values for Selected Prosthetic Aortic Valves

Valve Type [Ref.]	Valve Size (mm)	Peak Gradient (mmHg)	Mean Gradient (mmHg)	Effective Orifice Area (cm²)
Medtronic Freestyle [1] (Stentless)	19	-	13.0 ± 3.9 (n=20)	-
	21	-	9.1 ± 5.1 (n=112)	1.4 ± 0.3 (n=112)
	23	11.0 ± 4.0 (n=10)	8.1 ± 4.6 (n=508)	1.7 ± 0.5 (n=498)
	25	-	5.3 ± 3.1 (n=492)	2.1 ± 0.5 (n=492)
	27	-	4.6 ± 3.1 (n=47)	2.5 ± 0.1 (n=47)
Medtronic-Hall [1] (Single tilting disc)	20	34.4 ± 13.1 (n=24)	17.1 ± 5.3 (n=24)	1.2 ± 0.5 (n=24)
	21	26.9 ± 10.5 (n=30)	14.1 ± 5.9 (n=30)	1.1± 0.2 (n=30)
	23	26.9 ± 8.9 (n=27)	13.5 ± 4.8 (n=27)	1.4 ± 0.4 (n=27)
	25	17.1 ± 7.0 (n=17)	9.5 ± 4.3 (n=17)	1.5 ± 0.5 (n=17)
	27	18.9 ± 9.7 (n=8)	8.7 ± 5.6 (n=8)	1.9 ± 0.2 (n=8)
Medtronic Intact [1,2] (Stented)	19	40.4 ± 15.4 (n=15)	24.5 ± 9.3 (n=15)	-
	21	40.9 ± 15.6 (n=16)	19.6 ± 8.1 (n=51)	1.6 ± 0.4 (n=34)
	23	32.7 ± 9.6 (n=36)	19.0 ± 6.1 (n=116)	1.6 ± 0.4 (n=87)
	25	29.7 ± 15.0 (n=16)	17.7 ± 7.9 (n=30)	1.7 ± 0.3 (n=12)
	27	25.27 ± 7.58 (n=16)	15.0 ± 3.94 (n=16)	2.2 ± 0.17 (n=16)
	29	31 (n=5)	15.6 ± 2.1 (n=5)	2.38 ± 0.54 (n=5)
Medtronic Mosaic Porcine [1] (Stented)	21	-	14.2 ± 5.0 (n=489)	1.4 ± 0.4 (n=385)
	23	23.8 ± 11.0 (n=20)	13.7 ± 4.8 (n=1043)	1.5 ± 0.4 (n=732)
	25	22.5 ± 10.0 (n=18)	11.7 ± 5.1 (n=665)	1.8 ± 0.5 (n=446)
	27	-	10.4 ± 4.3 (n=246)	1.9 ± 0.1 (n=161)
	29	-	11.1 ± 4.3 (n=41)	2.1 ± 0.2 (n=33)
Sorin Mitroflow [1,4] (Stented)	19	18.6 ± 5.3 (n=10)	13.1 ± 3.3 (n=10)	1.1 ± 0.2 (n=10)
	21	-	15.3 ± 5.4 (n=26)	1.44 ± 0.3 (n=26)
	23	-	12.4 ± 3.6 (n=27)	1.57 ± 0.3 (n=27)
	25	-	11.0 ± 4.2 (n=18)	2.03 ± 0.3 (n=18)
	27	-	12.4 ± 2.4 (n=5)	2.36 ± 0.4 (n=5)
Starr-Edwards [1,2] (Ball and cage)	21	29.0 (n=5)	-	1.0 (n=5)
	23	32.6 ± 12.8 (n=22)	22.0 ± 9.0 (n=22)	1.1 ± 0.2 (n=10)
	24	34.1 ± 10.3 (n=43)	22.1 ± 7.5 (n=43)	1.1 ± 0.3 (n=9)
	26	31.8 ± 9.0 (n=29)	19.7 ± 6.1 (n=29)	-
	27	30.8 ± 6.3 (n=14)	18.5 ± 3.7 (n=14)	-
	29	29.0 ± 9.3 (n=8)	16.3 ± 5.5 (n=8)	-
Stentless Porcine Xenograft [2] (Stentless)	21	14 ± 5 (n=3)	8.7 ± 3.5 (n=3)	1.33 ± 0.38 (n=3)
	22	16 ± 5.6 (n=3)	9.7 ± 3.7 (n=3)	1.32 ± 0.48 (n=3)
	23	13 ± 4.8 (n=4)	7.7 ± 2.3 (n=4)	1.59 ± 0.6 (n=4)
	24	13 ± 3.8 (n=3)	7.7 ± 2.2 (n=3)	1.0 ± 0.01 (n=3)
	25	11.5 ± 7.1 (n=6)	7.4 ± 4.5 (n=6)	2.13 ± 0.7 (n=6)
	26	10.7 (n=3)	7 ± 2.1 (n=3)	2.15 ± 0.2 (n=3)
St Jude Epic Supra [5] (Stented; supra-annular)	Annulus < 23	-	15.5 ± 4.5 (n=12)	1.6 ± 0.3 (n=12)
	Annulus 23-24	-	14.9 ± 6.4 (n=20)	1.7 ± 0.5 (n=20)
	Annulus > 24	-	17.6 ± 12.7 (n=14)	1.7 ± 0.5 (n=14)

(continued over...)

Appendix 1 (continued)

Normal Haemodynamic Values for Selected Prosthetic Aortic Valves

Valve Type [Ref.]	Valve Size (mm)	Peak Gradient (mmHg)	Mean Gradient (mmHg)	Effective Orifice Area (cm²)
St Jude Medical Standard [1,2] (Bileaflet)	19	42.0 ± 10.0 (n=151)	24.5 ± 5.8 (n=164)	1.5 ± 0.1 (n=113)
	21	25.7 ± 9.5 (n=299)	15.2 ± 5.0 (n=257)	1.4 ± 0.4 (n=112)
	23	25.28 ± 7.89 (n=236)	13.77 ± 5.33 (n=236)	1.6 ± 0.43 (n=236)
	25	22.57 ± 7.68 (n=169)	12.65 ± 5.14 (n=169)	1.93 ± 0.45 (n=169)
	27	19.85 ± 7.55 (n=82)	11.18 ± 4.82 (n=82)	2.35 ± 0.59 (n=82)
	29	17.72 ± 6.42 (n=18)	9.86 ± 2.9 (n=18)	2.81 ± 0.57 (n=18)
	31	16.0 (n=4)	10 ± 6 (n=4)	3.08 ± 1.09 (n=4)
St Jude Toronto [1] (Stentless)	21	22.6 ± 14.5 (n=49)	10.7 ± 7.2 (n=49)	1.3 ± 0.6 (n=49)
	23	16.2 ± 9.09 (n=179)	8.2 ± 4.7 (n=247)	1.6 ± 0.6 (n=224)
	25	12.7 ± 8.2 (n=419)	6.3 ± 4.1 (n=557)	1.8 ± 0.5 (n=571)
	27	10.1 ± 5.8 (n=520)	5.0 ± 2.9 (n=739)	2.0 ± 0.3 (n=747)
	29	7.7 ± 4.4	4.1 ± 2.4	2.4 ± 0.6
St Jude Trifecta [6] (Stented; supra-annular)	19	-	10.7 ± 4.6 (n=68)	1.41 ± 0.24 (n=68)
	21	-	8.1 ± 3.5 (n=160)	1.63 ± 0.29 (n=160)
	23	-	7.2 ± 2.8 (n=198)	1.81 ± 0.30 (n=198)
	25	-	6.2 ± 2.7 (n=136)	2.02 ± 0.32 (n=136)
	27	-	4.8 ± 2.0 (n=40)	2.20 ± 0.20 (n=40)
	29	-	4.7 ± 1.6 (n=15)	2.35 ± 0.22 (n=15)

References [Ref.]:

[1] Rajani R, Mukherjee D, Chambers JB. Doppler echocardiography in normally functioning replacement aortic valves: a review of 129 studies. *J Heart Valve Dis.* 2007 Sep;16(5):519-35.

[2] Rosenhek R, Binder T, Maurer G, Baumgartner H. Normal values for Doppler echocardiographic assessment of heart valve prostheses. *J Am Soc Echocardiogr.* 2003 Nov;16(11):1116-27.

[3] Spethmann S, Dreger H, Schattke S, Baldenhofer G, Saghabalyan D, Stangl V, Laule M, Baumann G, Stangl K, Knebel F. Doppler haemodynamics and effective orifice areas of Edwards SAPIEN and CoreValve transcatheter aortic valves. *Eur Heart J Cardiovasc Imaging.* 2012 Aug;13(8):690-6.

[4] Bleiziffer S, Eichinger WB, Hettich IM, Ruzicka D, Badiu CC, Guenzinger R, Bauernschmitt R, Lange R. Hemodynamic characterization of the Sorin Mitroflow pericardial bioprosthesis at rest and exercise. *J Heart Valve Dis.* 2009 Jan;18(1):95-100.

[5] Ruzicka DJ, Hettich I, Hutter A, Bleiziffer S, Badiu CC, Bauernschmitt R, Lange R, Eichinger WB. The complete supraannular concept: in vivo hemodynamics of bovine and porcine aortic bioprostheses. *Circulation.* 2009 Sep 15;120(11 Suppl):S139-45.

[6] St Jude Medical white paper: www.accessdata.fda.gov/cdrh_docs/pdf10/P100029c.pdf

Appendix 2

Normal Haemodynamic Values for Selected Prosthetic Mitral Valves

Valve Type [Ref.]	Valve Size (mm)	Peak E Velocity (m/s)	Mean Gradient (mmHg)	Pressure Half-time (ms)	Effective Orifice Area* (cm²)
ATS Open Pivot [1] (Bileaflet)	23	-	4.6 ± 0.9 (n=5)	-	1.6 ± 0.3 (n=5)
	25	-	5.4 ± 4.7 (n=3)	-	1.8 ± 0.5 (n=3)
	27	-	4.5 ± 0.9 (n=23)	-	2.9 ± 0.9 (n=23)
	29	-	3.7 ± 0.7 (n=71)	-	2.8 ± 0.3 (n=71)
	31-33	-	3.1 ± 0.2 (n=175)	-	2.9 ± 0.2 (n=175)
Bjork-Shiley [2] (Tilting disc)	23	1.7 (n=1)	-	115 (n=1)	-
	25	1.75 ± 0.38 (n=14)	6 ± 2 (n=14)	99 ± 27 (n=14)	1.72 ± 0.6 (n=14)
	27	1.6 ± 0.49 (n=34)	5 ± 2 (n=34)	89 ± 28 (n34)	1.81 ± 0.54 (n=34)
	29	1.37 ± 0.25 (n=21)	2.83 ± 1.27 (n=21)	79 ± 17 (n=21)	2.17 ± 0.64 (n=21)
	31	1.41 ± 0.26 (n=21)	2 ± 1.9 (n=21)	70 ± 14 (n=21)	-
Carpentier-Edwards [2] (Stented)	27	1.7 ± 0.3 (n=16)	6 ± 2 (n=16)	98 ± 28 (n=16)	-
	29	1.76 ± 0.27 (n=22)	4.7 ± 2 (n=22)	92 ± 14 (n=22)	-
	31	1.54 ± 0.15 (n=22)	4.4 ± 2 (n=22)	92 ± 19 (n=22)	-
	33	-	6 ± 3 (n=6)	93 ± 12 (n=6)	-
Carpentier-Edwards Perimount [3] (Stented)	25	1.7 ± 0.10 (n=3)	4.0 ± 1.00 (n=3)	67 ± 21.5 (n=3)	1.75 ± 0.53 (n=3)
	27	1.7 ± 0.27 (n=16)	6.3 ± 1.65 (n=16)	74 ± 20.6 (n=16)	1.88 ± 0.52 (n=16)
	29	1.8 ± 0.19 (n=16)	6.0 ± 1.41 (n=16)	76 ± 17.9 (n=16)	2.02 ± 0.57 (n=16)
	31	1.8 ± 0.20 (n=15)	5.5 ± 1.06 (n=15)	80 ± 21.8 (n=15)	2.09 ± 0.48 (n=15)
	33	1.7 ± 0.23 (n=7)	6.1 ± 1.86 (n=7)	77 ± 13.2 (n=7)	2.24 ± 0.97 (n=7)
Hancock I or not specified [2] (Stented)	27	-	5 ± 2 (n=3)	-	1.3 ± 0.8 (n=3)
	29	-	2.46 ± 0.79 (n=13)	115 ± 20 (n=13)	1.5 ± 0.2 (n=13)
	31	-	4.86 ± 1.69 (n=22)	95 ± 17 (n=22)	1.6 ± 0.2 (n=22)
	33	-	3.87 ± 2 (n=8)	90 ± 12 (n=8)	1.9 ± 0.2 (n=8)
Hancock II [3] (Stented)	25	1.7 ± 0.26 (n=3)	5.7 ± 3.21 (n=3)	73 ± 10.4 (n=3)	1.44 ± 0.59 (n=3)
	27	2.0 ± 0.31 (n=10)	6.8 ± 1.79 (n=10)	91 ± 16.9 (n=10)	1.51 ± 0.32 (n=10)
	29	1.9 ± 0.23 (n=18)	6.1 ± 1.75 (n=18)	69 ± 16.8 (n=18)	1.80 ± 0.69 (n=18)
	31	1.9 ± 0.56 (n=5)	6.8 ± 2.17 (n=5)	87 ± 16.2 (n=5)	1.58 ± 0.31 (n=5)
Lillehei-Kaster [2] (Tilting disc)	18	1.7 (n=1)	-	140 (n=1)	-
	20	1.7 (n=1)	-	67 (n=1)	-
	22	1.56 ± 0.09 (n=4)	-	94 ± 22 (n=4)	-
	25	1.38 ± 0.27 (n=5)	-	124 ± 46 (n=5)	-
Medtronic-Hall [2] (Tilting disc)	27	1.4 (n=1)	-	78 (n=1)	-
	29	1.57 ± 0.1 (n=5)	-	69 ± 15 (n=5)	-
	31	1.45 ± 0.12 (n=7)	-	77 ± 17 (n=7)	-
Medtronic Intact [2] (Stented)	29	1.6 ± 0.22 (n=3)	3.5 ± 0.51 (n=3)	-	-
	31	1.6 ± 0.26 (n=14)	4.2 ± 1.44 (n=14)	-	-
	33	1.4 ± 0.24 (n=13)	4 ± 1.3 (n=13)	-	-
	35	1.3 ± 0.5 (n=2)	3.2 ± 1.77 (n=2)	-	-
Medtronic Mosaic (Stented) [3]	25	2.1 ± 0.28 (n=4)	7.7 ± 1.53 (n=4)	76 ± 19.8 (n=4)	1.42 ± 0.29 (n=4)
	27	2.0 ± 0.28 (n=24)	5.9 ± 1.23 (n=24)	81 ± 18.9 (n=24)	1.62 ± 0.47 (n=24)
	29	2.0 ± 0.31 (n=29)	6.5 ± 2.18 (n=29)	77 ± 15.1 (n=29)	1.83 ± 0.68 (n=29)
	31	2.0 ± 0.32 (n=23)	6.0 ± 1.64 (n=23)	76 ± 12.1 (n=23)	1.70 ± 0.41 (n=23)
	33	1.9 ± 0.50 (n=6)	5.6 ± 1.82 (n=6)	65 ± 8.7 (n=6)	2.71 ± 0.77 (n=6)

(continued over...)

Appendix 2 (continued)

Normal Haemodynamic Values for Selected Prosthetic Mitral Valves

Valve Type [Ref.]	Valve Size (mm)	Peak E Velocity (m/s)	Mean Gradient (mmHg)	Pressure Half-time (ms)	Effective Orifice Area* (cm²)
Mitroflow [2] (Stented)	25	2.0 (n=1)	6.9 (n=1)	90 (n=1)	-
	27	1.5 (n=3)	3.07 ± 0.91 (n=3)	90 ± 20 (n=3)	-
	29	1.43 ± 0.29 (n=15)	3.5 ± 1.65 (n=15)	102 ± 21 (n=15)	-
	31	1.32 ± 0.26	3.85 ± 0.81	91 ± 22	-
Starr-Edwards [2] (Ball and cage)	26	-	10 (n=1)	-	-
	28	-	7 ± 2.75 (n=27)	-	-
	30	1.7 ± 0.3 (n=25)	6.99 ± 2.5 (n=25)	125 ± 25 (n=25)	-
	32	1.7 ± 0.3 (n=17)	5.08 ± 2.5 (n=17)	-	-
	34	-	5 (n=1)	-	-
St Jude Medical Standard [2] (Bileaflet)	23	1.5 (n=1)	4 (n=1)	160 (n=1)	1.0 (n=1)
	25	1.34 ± 1.12 (n=4)	2.5 ± 1 (n=4)	75 ± 4 (n=4)	1.35 ± 0.17 (n=4)
	27	1.61 ± 0.29 (n=16)	5 ± 1.82 (n=16)	75 ± 10 (n=16)	1.67 ± 0.17 (n=16)
	29	1.57 ± 0.29 (n=40)	4.15 ± 1.8 (n=40)	85 ± 10 (n=40)	1.75 ± 0.24 (n=40)
	31	1.59 ± 0.33 (n=41)	4.46 ± 2.22 (n=41)	74 ± 13 (n=41)	2.03 ± 0.32 (n=41)

* Effective orifice area via the continuity equation only.

References [Ref.]:

[1] ATS white paper: www.accessdata.fda.gov/cdrh_docs/pdf/P990046c.pdf

[2] Rosenhek R, Binder T, Maurer G, Baumgartner H. Normal values for Doppler echocardiographic assessment of heart valve prostheses. *J Am Soc Echocardiogr.* 2003 Nov;16(11):1116-27.

[3] Blauwet LA, Malouf JF, Connolly HM, Hodge DO, Evans KN, Herges RM, Sundt TM 3rd, Miller FA Jr. Comprehensive echocardiographic assessment of normal mitral Medtronic Hancock II, Medtronic Mosaic, and Carpentier-Edwards Perimount bioprostheses early after implantation. *J Am Soc Echocardiogr.* 2010 Jun;23(6):656-66.

Appendix 3

Normal Haemodynamic Values for Selected Prosthetic Tricuspid Valves

Valve Type [Ref.]	Valve Size (mm)	Peak E Velocity (m/s)	Mean Gradient (mmHg)	Pressure Half-time (ms)	Effective Orifice Area* (cm²)
Carpentier-Edwards Duraflex [1] (Stented)	27	1.5 ± 0.26 (n=13)	5.2 ± 1.69 (n=13)	130 ± 45.4 (n=13)	1.34 ± 0.22 (n=13)
	29	1.7 ± 0.27 (n=23)	6.0 ± 1.95 (n=23)	102 ± 26.5 (n=23)	1.54 ± 0.38 (n=23)
	31	1.0 ± 0.27 (n=36)	5.7 ± 1.67 (n=36)	115 ± 40.8 (n=36)	1.57 ± 0.39 (n=36)
	33	1.5 ± 0.26 (n=44)	5.6 ± 2.10 (n=44)	116 ± 39.7 (n=44)	1.69 ± 0.44 (n=44)
	35	1.5 ± 0.25 (n=61)	5.3 ± 1.61 (n=61)	83 ± 26.5 (n=61)	1.63 ± 0.38 (n=61)
Carpentier-Edwards Perimount [1] (Stented)	29	1.1 ± 0.21 (n=2)	2.0 ± 1.41 (n=2)	94 ± 2.8 (n=2)	2.16 ± 0.43 (n=2)
	31	1.2 ± 0.20 (n=3)	3.7 ± 1.53 (n=3)	74 ± 26.2 (n=2)	2.12 ± 0.53 (n=3)
	33	1.4 ± 0.21 (n=7)	3.9 ± 1.07 (n=7)	137 ± 53.0 (n=2)	1.93 ± 0.43 (n=7)
Hancock II [1] (Stented)	31	1.6 ± 0.19 (n=6)	5.7 ± 1.37 (n=6)	-	1.40 ± 0.21 (n=6)
	33	1.4 ± 0.28 (n=2)	5.5 ± 3.54 (n=2)	-	1.40 ± 0.59 (n=2)
	35	1.3 ± 0.32 (n=3)	5.3 ± 0.58 (n=3)	-	2.11 ± 0.23 (n=3)
Medtronic Mosaic [1] (Stented)	27	1.6 ± 0.17 (n=4)	5.5 ± 0.58 (n=4)	-	1.53 ± 0.16 (n=4)
	29	1.5 ± 0.26 (n=8)	6.0 ± 2.00 (n=8)	115 ± 13.4 (n=8)	1.96 ± 0.39 (n=8)
	31	1.5 ± 0.21 (n=24)	5.2 ± 1.43 (n=24)	144 ± 28.6 (n=24)	1.74 ± 0.52 (n=24)
	33	1.4 ± 0.19 (n=12)	4.3 ± 1.30 (n=12)	139 ± 56.5 (n=12)	2.00 ± 0.53 (n=12)
Starr-Edwards [2] (Ball and cage)	32	1.5 ± 0.44	4.0 ± 1.00	-	1.87 ± 0.33
	34	1.8 ± 0.28	5.7 ± 1.63	118 ± 32.9	1.81 ± 0.48
St Jude Biocor [1] (Stented)	29	1.6 (n=1)	6.0 (n=1)	-	2.84 (n=1)
	31	1.5 ± 0.34 (n=9)	5.1 ± 1.36 (n=9)	106 ± 48.5 (n=9)	1.67 ± 0.30 (n=9)
	33	1.3 ± 0.23 (n=26)	3.9 ± 1.20 (n=26)	125 ± 45.7 (n=26)	1.92 ± 0.50 (n=26)
St Jude Mechanical Standard [2] (Bileaflet)	27	1.1 ± 0.32 (n=7)	2.4 ± 1.27 (n=7)	77 ± 14.6 (n=4)	2.54 ± 0.64 (n=7)
	29	1.2 ± 0.21 (n=7)	2.6 ± 1.13 (n=7)	100 ± 35.2 (n=4)	2.20 ± 0.33 (n=7)
	31	1.4 ± 0.31 (n=20)	3.3 ± 1.21 (n=20)	81 ± 13.5 (n=14)	2.49 ± 0.45 (n=20)
	33	1.3 ± 0.22 (n=17)	3.2 ± 1.24 (n=17)	82 ± 18.8 (n=11)	2.46 ± 0.59 (n=17)

* Effective orifice area via the continuity equation.
Values are the means of 5 cardiac cycles for all Doppler measurements and calculations using Doppler measurements

References [Ref.]:
[1] Blauwet LA, Danielson GK, Burkhart HM, Dearani JA, Malouf JF, Connolly HM, Hodge DO, Herges RM, Miller FA Jr. Comprehensive echocardiographic assessment of the hemodynamic parameters of 285 tricuspid valve bioprostheses early after implantation. *J Am Soc Echocardiogr.* 2010 Oct;23(10):1045-1059, 1059.e1-2.
[2] Blauwet LA, Burkhart HM, Dearani JA, Malouf JF, Connolly HM, Hodge DO, Herges RM, Miller FA Jr. Comprehensive echocardiographic assessment of mechanical tricuspid valve prostheses based on early post-implantation echocardiographic studies. *J Am Soc Echocardiogr.* 2011 Apr;24(4):414-24.

Appendix 4

A. Normal Haemodynamic Values for Selected Prosthetic Pulmonary Valves

Valve Type	Size (mm)	Peak Velocity (m/s)	Mean Gradient (mmHg)
Aortic Allograft (n=3)	22.3 ± 1.2	2.5 ± 0.4	14.4 ± 3.4
Carpentier-Edwards (n=24)	26.5 ± 1.8	2.4 ± 0.5	12.1 ± 5.3
Hancock (n=3)	26.0 ± 3.0	2.4 ± 0.5	14.0 ± 5.7
Pulmonary Allograft (n=17)	24.2 ± 1.8	1.8 ± 0.6	8.4 ± 4.8
All valves (n=51)	-	2.2 ± 0.6	11.0 ± 5.1

Reference: Novaro GM, Connolly HM, Miller FA. Doppler hemodynamics of 51 clinically and echocardiographically normal pulmonary valve prostheses. *Mayo Clin Proc.* 2001 Feb;76(2):155-60.

B. Normal Haemodynamic Values for Prosthetic Pulmonary Valves based on Size

Valve Size* (mm)	Peak Velocity (m/s)	Maximum Gradient (mmHg)	Mean Gradient (mmHg)	Effective Orifice Area (cm²)
21 (n=2)	2.3 ± 0.28	22.0 ± 5.6	12.0 ± 2.8	1.5 ± 0.28
23 (n=9)	2.59 ± 0.28	27.6 ± 5.7	15.96 ± 3	1.45 ± 027
25 (n=25)	2.17 ± 0.39	20.2 ± 6.9	11.2 ± 4.1	1.66 ± 0.37
27 (n=4)	2.33 ± 0.36	21.2 ± 1.5	10.0 ± 0.8	2.0 ± 0.28

* includes 27 biologic valves and 13 mechanical valves

Reference: Sadeghpour A, Saadatifar H, Kiavar M, Esmaeilzadeh M, Maleki M, Ojaghi Z, Noohi F, Samiei N, Mohebbi A. Doppler echocardiographic assessment of pulmonary prostheses: a comprehensive assessment including velocity time integral ratio and prosthesis effective orifice area. *Congenit Heart Dis.* 2008 Nov-Dec;3(6):415-21.

Appendix 5

Selected Genetic Syndromes associated with Congenital Heart Disease

Syndrome Description	Incidence of Cardiac Anomalies	Most Common Cardiac Anomalies
DiGeorge Syndrome (Velocardiofacial Syndrome) **Aetiology:** • Chr 22 abnormality (deletion of the long arm of Chr 22 [22q11]) **Characteristic features (non-cardiac):** • Distinctive facial features; e.g. high and broad nasal bridge, long face, narrow palpebral fissures, micrognathia • Thymus aplasia/hypoplasia • Parathyroid aplasia/hypoplasia	≈ 75-85%	Conotruncal abnormalities: • truncus arteriosus • TOF Aortic arch anomalies; • interrupted aorta (type B) • right aortic arch
Down Syndrome (Trisomy 21) **Aetiology:** • Chr 21 abnormality (trisomy of Chr 21) **Characteristic features (non-cardiac):** • Distinctive facial features; e.g. flat facies, slanted eyelid fissures, small ears • Mental retardation	≈ 40-50%	• AVCD (most common) • VSD • ASD (1^0 &/or 2^0) • PDA • TOF
Foetal Alcohol Syndrome **Aetiology:** • Impaired growth, mental and physical birth defects associated with high levels of maternal alcohol consumption during pregnancy **Characteristic features (non-cardiac):** • Facial anomalies such as short palpebral fissures, thin upper lip, long, smooth philtrum • Prenatal or postnatal growth retardation (below 10th percentile for age/race) • Microcephaly	Uncertain	• VSD • ASD • TOF
Foetal Rubella Syndrome **Aetiology:** • Result of maternal infection and subsequent foetal infection with rubella virus **Characteristic features (non-cardiac):** • Deafness • Cataracts • Mental retardation with microcephaly and spastic diplegia	≈ 30-60%	• PDA • VSD • ASD • PS • TOF
Goldenhar Syndrome (Oculo-Auriculo-Vertebral Spectrum) **Aetiology:** • Unknown aetiology; possibly due to maldevelopment of the branchial arches **Characteristic features (non-cardiac):** • Ocular abnormalities • Ear malformations • Vertebral defects • Hemifacial microsomia	≈ 50-60%	• VSD • TOF • PDA • CoAo • D-TGA
Holt-Oram Syndrome (Heart-Hand Syndrome) **Aetiology:** • Inherited autosomal dominant disorder (mutations in TBX5 gene) **Characteristic features (non-cardiac):** • Upper limb deformities	≈ 80%	• ASD (usually 2^0) • VSD (usually muscular) • TOF • AVCD • Conduction defects

(continued over...)

Appendix 5 (continued)
Selected Genetic Syndromes associated with Congenital Heart Disease

Syndrome Description	Incidence of Cardiac Anomalies	Most Common Cardiac Anomalies
Noonan Syndrome **Aetiology:** • Inherited autosomal dominant disorder (mutations in PTPN11, SOS1, RAF1, KRAS, NRAS and BRAF genes) **Characteristic features (non-cardiac):** • Distinctive facial features (e.g. Low-set & posteriorly rotated ears, ocular hypertelorism) • Widely spaced nipples • Webbing of neck • Short stature • Developmental delay • Learning difficulties • Renal anomalies • Lymphatic malformations	≈ 80-90%	• PS (most common) • +/- branch PA stenosis • ASD • HCM • PDA
Turner Syndrome (XO syndrome) **Aetiology:** • Monosomy X (absence of an X chromosome); females only affected **Characteristic features (non-cardiac):** • Short stature • Webbed neck • Broad chest with wide spaced nipples • Gonadal dysgenesis	≈ 20-50%	• CoAo (most common) • BAV (most common) • AS • HLHS
William Syndrome (Williams–Beuren syndrome) **Aetiology:** • Chr 7 abnormality (deletion of genetic material Chr 7 [Del 7q11.23]) **Characteristic features (non-cardiac):** • Distinctive facial features (e.g. Elfin faces, prominent lips, long philtrum, small & widely spaced teeth) • Characteristic behaviour (e.g. "cocktail party" type personality) • Mental retardation	≈ 50-80%	• Supravalvular AS (most common) • PS • Branch PA stenosis

1^0 = primum; 2^0 = secundum; AS = aortic stenosis; ASD = atrial septal defect; AVCD = atrioventricular canal defect; Chr = chromosome; CoAo = coarctation of the aorta; D-TGA = dextro-transposition of the great arteries; HCM = hypertrophic cardiomyopathy; HLHS = hypoplastic left heart syndrome; PA = pulmonary artery; PAPVC = partial anomalous pulmonary venous connection; PDA = patent ductus arteriosus; PS = pulmonary stenosis; TOF = tetralogy of Fallot; VSD = ventricular septal defect

Other definitions:
Gonadal dysgenesis = underdevelopment or defective development of reproductive system
Hemifacial microsomia = asymmetrical underdevelopment of lower half of the face; primarily affecting ear, mouth and jaw
Hypertelorism = widely spaced eyes
Microcephaly = small head
Micrognathia = under-sized jaw
Palpebral fissures = separation between upper and lower eyelids
Philtrum = midline groove in the upper lip that runs from the top of the lip to the nose
Spastic diplegia = paralysis of corresponding parts on both sides of the body

Further Reading

Blue GM, Kirk EP, Sholler GF, Harvey RP, Winlaw DS. Congenital heart disease: current knowledge about causes and inheritance. *Med J Aust.* 2012 Aug 6;197(3):155-9.

Burd L, Deal E, Rios R, Adickes E, Wynne J, Klug MG. Congenital heart defects and fetal alcohol spectrum disorders. *Congenit Heart Dis.* 2007 Jul-Aug;2(4):250-5.

Fahed AC, Gelb BD, Seidman JG, Seidman CE. Genetics of congenital heart disease: the glass half empty. Circ Res. 2013 Feb 15;112(4):707-20.

Formigari R, Michielon G, Digilio MC, Piacentini G, Carotti A, Giardini A, Di Donato RM, Marino B. Genetic syndromes and congenital heart defects: how is surgical management affected? *Eur J Cardiothorac Surg.* 2009 Apr;35(4):606-14.

Marino B, Digilio MC. Congenital heart disease and genetic syndromes: specific correlation between cardiac phenotype and genotype. *Cardiovasc Pathol.* 2000 Nov-Dec;9(6):303-15.

Appendix 6

Part A - Selective Palliative Operations for Various Congenital Heart Lesions

These operations provide symptomatic relief and extend life but do not correct underlying pathophysiological defect; often an initial operation prior to complete repair.

Palliative Procedures to Increase Pulmonary Blood Flow		
Performed for pulmonary obstructions such as TOF, tricuspid atresia + PS, pulmonary atresia +/- VSD, single ventricle + PS, d-TGA + VSD + PS		
Procedure	**Illustrative Example**	**Brief Description**
Blalock-Taussig (BT) Shunt		**Classic:** End-to-side anastomosis between the right subclavian (or the innominate) and PA
		Modified: Gore-Tex graft between left subclavian artery and PA
Central Shunt		Anastomosis between ascending aorta and MPA via Gore-Tex graft
Potts Shunt		Side-to-side anastomosis between descending aorta and LPA No longer performed due to complications associated with this procedure
Waterston Shunt		Side-to-side anastomosis between ascending aorta and RPA No longer performed due to complications associated with this procedure

(continued over...)

Appendix 6 (continued)

Part A - Selective Palliative Operations for Various Congenital Heart Lesions (continued)

Palliative Procedures to Increase Pulmonary Blood Flow & Reduce Ventricular Workload		
Performed for tricuspid atresia and univentricular hearts; Stage 1 of total cavopulmonary connection; i.e. Fontan operation		
Procedure	**Illustrative Example**	**Brief Description**
Glenn Shunt		**Classic:** End-to-end anastomosis of SVC to RPA (RPA transected at PA end)
		Bidirectional: End-to-side anastomosis of SVC to RPA (RPA still connected to MPA)
Hemi-Fontan		Similar to Glenn shunt so there is an anastomosis between SVC and PA plus RA patch

Palliative Procedures to Increase Pulmonary & Aortic Blood Flow		
Performed for HLHS, aortic atresia, or AS with insufficient LV.		
Procedure	**Illustrative Example**	**Brief Description**
Norwood Procedure (Stage 1 of 3 for correction of HLHS*)		(1) Modified BT shunt: provides blood flow to PAs (2) removal of atrial septum: enhances blood flow from LA to RA (3) disconnection of pulmonary trunk from left and right pulmonary arteries and (4) creation of neoaorta by anastomosing aorta and pulmonary trunk: increases blood flow to aorta via neoaorta The RV = systemic pump

* Stage 2 of the surgical repair for HLHS involves performing a bidirectional Glenn shunt or a hemi-Fontan and takedown of the modified BT shunt (deoxygenated blood from SVC is routed directly to PA; mixture of oxygenated and deoxygenated blood is sent to the body via the anastomosed aorta and pulmonary trunk). Stage 3 is a complete Fontan reconstruction (see below).

(continued over...)

Appendix 6 (continued)

Part A - Selective Palliative Operations for Various Congenital Heart Lesions (continued)

Palliative Procedures to Increase Atrial Shunting		
Performed for d-TGA, tricuspid atresia or TAPVD with inadequate PFO.		
Procedure	**Illustrative Example**	**Brief Description**
Rashkind Balloon Septostomy		Deflated balloon catheter enters RA via IVC, crosses PFO into the LA; balloon then inflated and jerked across IAS Increases mixing of deoxygenated and oxygenated blood at atrial level. Most commonly performed under echo guidance

Palliative Procedures to Increase Blood Flow to Aorta		
Performed for systemic outflow tract obstruction + single ventricle (e.g. double inlet LV, tricuspid atresia with d-TGA, or d-TGA with a hypoplastic right heart)		
Procedure	**Illustrative Example**	**Brief Description**
Damus-Kaye-Stansel (DKS)		(1) PA is divided near its bifurcation and proximal PA is anastomosed to the side of ascending aorta using a patch; (2) pulmonary circulation re-established via modified Blalock-Taussig (MBT) shunt (shown), or a valved conduit from RV to distal MPA, or a bidirectional Glenn shunt or extracardiac Fontan procedure

Palliative Procedures to Decrease Pulmonary Blood Flow		
Performed for large left-to-right shunts with pulmonary over-circulation: e.g. large VSD, d-TGA, single ventricle, AV canal defects.		
Procedure	**Illustrative Example**	**Brief Description**
PA Band		Constrictive band around MPA Decreased pulmonary blood flow protects pulmonary bed from high pressures

(continued over...)

Appendix 6 (continued)
Part B - Corrective Operations for Various Congenital Heart Lesions
These operations are designed to return heart circulation to normal.

Corrective Procedures	Congenital Defect	Illustrative Example	Brief Description
Arterial Switch (Jatene)	d-TGA		Aorta and PA transected and reconnected to proper ventricles (1 & 2), coronaries reimplanted into neoaorta (NA) (3) Creates normal relationship between the ventricles and great arteries
Double Switch	CC-TGA		Atrial switch (Mustard or Senning) plus arterial switch Systemic venous blood is rerouted into RV and to PA (blue arrows); pulmonary venous return rerouted into LV and aorta (red arrows); coronaries reimplanted into neoaorta (NA) (yellow buttons) Creates normal relationship between the ventricles and great arteries
Fontan#	Single ventricle: examples • Tricuspid atresia • Pulmonary atresia with intact IVS • Double inlet LV		**Original:** Glenn shunt plus atriopulmonary connection between RA appendage and PA plus closure of ASD **Total cavopulmonary connection (TCPC):** bidirectional Glenn shunt or Hemi-Fontan (1) plus re-direction of systemic venous return to PA via intra-atrial lateral tunnel or an extracardiac conduit (2) Increases pulmonary blood flow via diversion of systemic venous return directly to PA (bypasses RV)
Mustard	d-TGA		Atrial switch using intra-atrial baffle made of pericardium Systemic venous blood is rerouted into SVA, LV and PA (blue arrows); pulmonary venous return rerouted into PVA, RV and aorta (red arrows) Directs oxygen-rich blood to body and deoxygenated blood to the lungs

(continued over...)

Appendix 6 (continued)

Part B - Corrective Operations for Various Congenital Heart Lesions
These operations are designed to return heart function to normal.

Corrective Procedures	Congenital Defect	Illustrative Example	Brief Description
Rastelli	• d-TGA + VSD + PS • Truncus arteriosus • Pulmonary atresia + VSD • Double outlet RV + PS or pulmonary atresia		(1) Creation of patch redirecting blood from LV through VSD and into aorta; (2) external valved conduit from RV to PA Increases pulmonary blood flow, re-establishes normal relationship between the ventricles and great arteries
Senning	d-TGA		Atrial switch using intra-atrial baffle derived from atrial septum and RA wall Systemic venous blood is rerouted into SVA, LV and PA (blue arrow); pulmonary venous return rerouted into PVA, RV and aorta (red arrow) Directs oxygen-rich blood to body and deoxygenated blood to the lungs
TOF Repair	TOF		(1) VSD patch closure; (2) widening of RVOT via infundibular resection, RVOT transannular patch, pulmonary valvotomy or valvectomy, or PV replacement Re-establish normal cardiac connections and relieve RVOT obstruction with increased pulmonary blood flow

\# The Fontan operation is not truly a correction operation due to the fact that anatomically there is still no RV and because of the many complications associated with this procedure. However, the Fontan operation is not a palliative procedure either because this operation provides more than just symptomatic relief; it also separates the systemic and pulmonary circuits. Therefore, this procedure may be referred to as an "orthoterminal correction" (Ref: Sade RM. Orthoterminal correction of congenital cardiovascular defects. Ann Thorac Surg 1975;19:105-7).

Abbreviations: Ao = aorta; AS = aortic stenosis; ASD = atrial septal defect; CC-TGA = congenitally corrected transposition of the great arteries (or L-TGA); d-TGA = dextro-transposition of the great arteries; HLHS = hypoplastic left heart syndrome; IAS = interatrial septum; IVC = inferior vena cava; LA = left atrium; LPA = left pulmonary artery; LV = left ventricle; MBT = modified Blalock-Taussig shunt; MPA = main pulmonary artery; mv = mitral valve; NPA = neo pulmonary artery; PA = pulmonary artery; PFO = patent foramen ovale; PS = pulmonary stenosis; PV = pulmonary valve; PVA = pulmonary venous atrium; RA = right atrium; RAA = right atrial appendage; RPA = right pulmonary artery; RV = right ventricle; RVOT = right ventricular outflow tract; SVC= superior vena cava; SVA = systemic venous atrium; TAPVD = total anomalous pulmonary venous drainage; TOF = tetralogy of Fallot; tv = tricuspid valve; VSD = ventricular septal defect.

Further reading:
Brickner ME, Hillis LD, Lange RA.Congenital heart disease in adults. Second of two parts. *N Engl J Med.* 2000 Feb 3;342(5):334-42.
Gaca AM, Jaggers JJ, Dudley LT, Bisset GS 3rd. Repair of congenital heart disease: a primer-part 1. *Radiology.* 2008 Jun;247(3):617-31.
Gaca AM, Jaggers JJ, Dudley LT, Bisset GS 3rd. Repair of congenital heart disease: a primer--Part 2. *Radiology.* 2008 Jul;248(1):44-60.
Joffs C, Sade RM. Congenital Heart Surgery Nomenclature and Database Project: palliation, correction, or repair? *Ann Thorac Surg.* 2000 Apr;69(4 Suppl):S369-72..
Yuan SM, Jing H. Palliative procedures for congenital heart defects. *Arch Cardiovasc Dis.* 2009 Jun-Jul;102(6-7):549-57.

Appendix 7

Echocardiographic Parameter Tables
This appendix provides a quick reference to specific echocardiographic-related tables included within this text. Tables are listed in alphabetical order by cardiac disease.

Echocardiographic Parameter Tables	Page
Aortic Regurgitation (AR)	
• Additional Echocardiographic Signs of Severe AR (Table 7.11)	211
• Qualitative Colour Doppler Parameters for Grading AR Severity (Table 7.7)	202
• Qualitative Spectral Doppler Parameters for Grading AR Severity (Table 7.9)	205
• Quantitative Methods for Grading AR Severity (Table 7.10)	208
Aortic Stenosis (AS)	
• Abnormal Stress Echo Measurements in Asymptomatic AS (Table 7.4)	195
• Differentiation between AS and MR Spectral Doppler Signals (Table 7.3)	187
• Recommendations for Classification of AS Severity (Table 7.1)	186
Cardiomyopathies	
• Classifications (Table 6.2)	146
• Diagnostic Criteria for ARVD/C (Table 6.14)	169
• Echocardiographic Parameters distinguishing Athlete's Heart from HCM (Table 6.12)	165
• Mimics of HCM (Table 6.11)	165
• Selected M-Mode and Doppler Indices for Dyssynchrony (Table 6.9)	156
Diseases of the Aorta	
• Absolute and Indexed Normal Values of Aortic Segments (Table 11.1)	328
• Aneurysms: Thresholds for Elective Intervention for Aortic Aneurysms based on Aortic Dimensions (Table 11.4)	332
• Dissection: Features Differentiating True from False Lumens in Aortic Dissection (Table 11.6)	337
• Dissection: Methods for differentiating Artefacts from True Aortic Dissection Flaps (Table 11.7)	339
dP/dt	
• Reference Limits and Partition Values (Table 2.8)	44
Infective Endocarditis	
• Anatomic and Echocardiographic Definitions (Table 13.4)	376
• Echocardiographic Characteristics of Likely and Unlikely Vegetations (Table 13.5)	377
• Modified Duke Criteria for Diagnosis of Infective Endocarditis (Table 13.2)	375
Intracardiac Pressures	
• Estimation from Doppler Velocities (Table 1.2)	6
• Estimation of RAP based on IVC Diameter and Collapse (Table 4.15)	101
• Normal Values (Figure 1.10)	7
Ischaemic Heart Disease	
• Complications of MI (Table 5.6)	126
• Stress Echo: Normal and Abnormal Responses (Table 5.4)	124
• Stress Echo: Viable versus Non-Viable Myocardium (Table 5.5)	125
• Takotsubo cardiomyopathy: Morphological LV Variants (Table 5.11)	139
• Takotsubo cardiomyopathy: Proposed Mayo Clinic criteria (Table 5.10)	138
• Differences between True Aneurysms and Pseudoaneurysms (Table 5.7)	130
Left Atrial Size	
• Reference Limits and Partition Values of LA and LV Size (Table 6.5)	148
Left Ventricular Diastolic Function	
• Assessment of LV Filling Pressures in Special Populations (Table 3.7)	78
• Clues to Pseudonormalisation of the Transmitral Inflow Profile (Table 3.4)	65
• Grading of Diastolic Function and Associated LVFP (Table 3.5)	77
• Normal Values for Doppler-Derived Diastolic Measurements (Table 3.3)	63
• Significance for Ratios in Identifying Increased LVFP (Table 3.6)	77
Left Ventricular Mass	
• Reference Limits and Partition Values (Table 4.7)	90
Left Ventricular Size	
• Reference Limits and Partition Values (Table 2.2)	32

(continued over...)

Appendix 7 (continued)

Echocardiographic Parameter Tables

This appendix provides a quick reference to specific echocardiographic-related tables included within this text. Tables are listed in alphabetical order by cardiac disease.

Echocardiographic Parameter Tables (continued)	Page
Left Ventricular Systolic Function	
• dP/dt Reference Limits and Partition Values (Table 2.8)	44
• Normal Values for Commonly Used Indices (Table 2.4)	36
• Reference Limits and Partition Values (Table 2.5)	39
Mitral Regurgitation (MR)	
• Qualitative Colour Doppler Parameters for Grading MR Severity (Table 8.9)	245
• Qualitative Spectral Doppler Parameters for Grading MR Severity (Table 8.10)	247
• Quantitative Methods for Grading Mitral Regurgitation Severity (Table 8.11)	249
• Selected Pre-Operative 2D Echo Predictors of Post-Operative Persistent or Recurrent MR (Table 8.8)	245
Mitral Stenosis (MS)	
• Echocardiographic Score for Severe MR Following Percutaneous Mitral Balloon Valvotomy by the Padial et al. Criteria (Table 8.3)	224
• Grading of Mitral Valve Characteristics by the Wilkins et al. Criteria (Table 8.2)	224
• Recommendations for Classification of MS Severity (Table 8.4)	225
Pericardial Diseases	
Constrictive Pericarditis:	
• % Change from Expiration to Inspiration in Normal, Constrictive Pericarditis and Restrictive Cardiomyopathy (Table 12.8)	364
• Echocardiographic Features Distinguishing Constrictive Pericarditis from Restrictive Cardiomyopathy (Table 12.9)	367
• Echocardiographic Findings associated with Constrictive Pericarditis (Table 12.7)	364
Effusions:	
• Mimics of Pericardial Effusions (Table 12.3)	351
• Sizing of Pericardial Effusion by Echo (Table 12.2)	348
Tamponade:	
• % Change from Inspiration to Expiration in Normals, Cardiac Tamponade and Effusion with No Tamponade (Table 12.5)	357
• Summary Spectral Doppler Findings associated with Cardiac Tamponade (Table 12.4)	357
Prosthetic Valves	
• DVI: Normal and Abnormal Doppler Velocity Indices (Table 10.7)	307
• Obstruction: Doppler Echocardiographic Criteria for Detection and Quantification of Prosthetic Aortic and/or Mitral Stenosis/Obstruction (Table 10.9)	310
• Obstruction: Doppler Echocardiographic Criteria for Detection of Prosthetic Tricuspid Stenosis (Table 10.10)	311
• Parameters for Differentiating Prosthetic Valve Thrombus from Pannus Formation (Table 10.12)	315
• PPM: Identification and Quantification of PPM in Aortic, Mitral and Tricuspid Prostheses (Table 10.8)	308
• Regurgitation: Qualitative and Quantitative Doppler Parameters for Grading Prosthetic Valve Regurgitation Severity (Table 10.11)	313
Pulmonary Hypertension (PHTN)	
• Clinical Classification of PHTN (Dana Point, 2008) (Table 4.9)	96
• Commonly used Doppler-estimates of Pulmonary Artery Pressures (Table 4.14)	99
• Selected Doppler Methods for Estimation of Pulmonary Vascular Resistance (Table 4.16)	106
• Echocardiographic Prognostic Variables in PAH (Table 4.18)	110
• Various Echocardiographic Signs suggesting PHTN (Table 4.17)	107
• Estimation of RAP based on IVC Diameter and Collapse (Table 4.15)	101
• Grades of Severity of PHTN based on RVSP/PASP (Table 4.13)	99
• PHTN based on TR peak velocity and PASP at rest (Table 4.12)	98
Pulmonary Regurgitation (PR)	
• Qualitative Doppler Parameters for Grading PR Severity (Table 9.8)	285
• Sensitivity, Specificity and Predictive Valves of Doppler Echo Variables for Detecting Severe PR (Table 9.9)	287
Pulmonary Stenosis (PS)	
• Recommendations for Classification of PS Severity (Table 9.6)	282
Right Atrium	
• Estimation of RAP based on IVC Diameter and Collapse (Table 4.15)	101
• Size: Normal values (Table 6.6)	148

(continued over...)

Appendix 7 (continued)

Echocardiographic Parameter Tables

This appendix provides a quick reference to specific echocardiographic-related tables included within this text. Tables are listed in alphabetical order by cardiac disease.

	Page
Right Ventricular Diastolic Function	
• Grading of RV Diastolic Function (Table 3.8)	82
Right Ventricular Dimensions	
• Normal Values for Various Indices (Table 2.9)	49
Right Ventricular Systolic Function	
• Normal Values for Commonly Used Indices (Table 2.11)	51
Systemic Diseases	
• Selected Systemic Diseases and Cardiac Manifestations associated with these Diseases (Table 14.1)	408
Systemic Hypertension	
• American Classification (Table 4.2)	88
• Australian Classification (Table 4.1)	88
• European Classification (Table 4.3)	88
Tricuspid Regurgitation (TR)	
• Qualitative Colour Doppler Parameters for Grading TR Severity (Table 9.3)	270
• Qualitative Spectral Doppler Parameters for Grading TR Severity (Table 9.4)	273
• Quantitative Parameters for Grading Tricuspid Regurgitation Severity (Table 9.5)	274
Tricuspid Stenosis (TS)	
• Findings Indicative of Haemodynamically Significant TS (Table 9.1)	262

Glossary

Statistical Terms

Negative predictive value: the proportion of patients with negative test results who are correctly diagnosed (e.g. healthy people correctly identified as healthy); calculated as the number of true negatives divided by the sum of the number of true negatives + number of false negatives

Positive predictive value: the proportion of patients with positive test results who are correctly diagnosed (e.g. sick people correctly identified as sick); calculated as the number of true positives divided by the sum of the number of true positives + number of false positives

Sensitivity: the proportion of actual positives which are correctly identified as such (e.g. percentage of sick people who are correctly identified as having the condition); calculated as the number of true positives divided by the sum of the number of true positives + number of false negatives

Specificity: the proportion of negatives which are correctly identified (e.g. percentage of healthy people who are correctly identified as not having the condition); calculated as the number of true negatives divided by the sum of the number of true negatives + number of false positives

Other Terms

A

Acute aortic syndrome (AAS): the spectrum of life-threatening aortic emergencies caused by non-traumatic acute aortic injury

Acute coronary syndrome (ACS): the spectrum of clinical presentations related to acute myocardial ischaemia

Afterload: load or tension against which the heart contracts to eject blood; e.g. aortic systolic pressure for the LV, pulmonary systolic pressure for the RV

Akinesis: absence of movement; absence of or minimal systolic myocardial thickening

Aortic Sclerosis: focal thickening and calcific changes of the aortic valve level without haemodynamic obstruction to blood flow; differentiated from aortic stenosis by the appearance of irregular and non-uniform thickening of the aortic valve leaflets; systolic motion of leaflets is either non-restrictive or only minimally restricted; on the spectral Doppler examination the peak velocity across a sclerotic valve is ≤ 2.5 m/s

Anomalous mitral arcade: a rare congenital malformation of the mitral apparatus characterised by enlarged papillary muscles connected to mitral leaflets by a typical fibrous tissue bridge

Anechoic: absence of echoes; appears echo-free or black

Aneurysmal: of aorta: dilatation involving all layers of the aorta 1.5 times greater than the normal arterial diameter; of blood vessels: localised balloon-like bulge of vessel wall; of chambers: constantly deformed segment throughout systole and diastole with outward movement bulging in systole

Annuloaortic ectasia: combination of ascending aortic aneurysm, dilatation of the sinuses of Valsalva, and dilatation of the aortic annulus

Annulus paradoxus: paradoxical relationship between the E/e' ratio and LV filling pressures; i.e. high LV filling pressures associated with low or normal E/e' ratio (as seen in constrictive pericarditis)

Annulus reversus: lateral e' velocities are lower than medial e' velocities (as seen in constrictive pericarditis)

Arterial switch: corrective surgery for d- transposition of the great arteries whereby the great arteries are transected and reattached to the proper ventricles and the coronary arteries are reimplanted into the neo-aorta; also referred to as the Jatene Arterial Switch

Arteritis: an inflammation of the arterial walls as a result of infection or an auto-immune response; results in medial destruction and subsequent aneurysm formation

Ataxia: lack of muscle coordination

Atrial switch: corrective surgery for d- transposition of the great arteries where at the atrial level systemic venous blood is rerouted into LV and pulmonary artery, and pulmonary venous return is rerouted into RV and aorta; atrial switch operations include the Mustard and Senning repairs

Atrioventricular concordance: normal anatomical relationship between the atria and ventricles; that is, the RA connects to the morphological RV and the LA connects to the morphological LV

Atrioventricular discordance: abnormal anatomical relationship between the atria and ventricles; that is, the RA connects to the morphological LV and the LA connects to the morphological RV

Axial resolution: ability of the ultrasound machine to detect echoes from two closely spaced reflectors at different depths along the axis of the beam and to display these reflectors as being separate

B

Barlow's disease: degenerative mitral valve disease where there are diffuse myxomatous changes and excess mitral leaflet tissue; cords are also thickened and elongated

Behçet's disease: a multisystemic and chronic relapsing inflammatory disorder characterised by the histopathologic finding of nonspecific vasculitis involving various-sized vessels in multiple organs

C

Cardiac tamponade: occurs when there is an increase in the intrapericardial pressure due to accumulation of an effusion, blood, clots, pus, gas or combinations of these within the pericardium; leads to compression of the heart, impeded diastolic filling of both ventricles, systemic and pulmonary congestion, and a decreased stroke volume and cardiac output

Cardiac output: volume of blood being pumped by the heart per minute; measured in litres per minute

Carney's complex: a hereditary syndrome characterised by multiple myxomas (cardiac and extracardiac), abnormal skin pigmentation, endocrine tumours or overactivity, and schwannomas

Cachexia: general physical wasting and malnutrition usually associated with chronic disease and cancer

Coandă effect: In echocardiography this effect refers to the tendency of a regurgitant jet to cling to the receiving chamber wall; thus, the jet appears smaller in area than a free jet

Contractile reserve (CR): the ability of the LV to increases its contractility during stress (exercise or dobutamine); CR is identified by an increase or improvement in the ejection fraction, stroke volume, or wall motion score when compared to resting values

Coronary artery steal: syndrome where blood is 'stolen' from one region of the coronary tree by another artery or chamber

Coronary flow reserve: The ability to increase coronary blood flow in response to vasoactive mechanisms

Cor triatriatum: a rare cardiac abnormality in which the left atrium is subdivided into two distinct chambers

Cor triatriatum dexter: a rare cardiac abnormality in which the right atrium is subdivided into two distinct chambers

Costophrenic angle: angle between the diaphragm (-phrenic) and the ribs (costo-)

Cyanosis: a bluish discoloration of skin and mucous membranes; Cyanosis can be secondary to cardiac, respiratory, hematologic and metabolic causes. Cyanotic congenital heart disease occurs when deoxygenated blood bypasses the lungs and enters the systemic circulation

D

Degassing phenomenon: refers to dissolved gases coming out of solution and arises when there is separation of carbon dioxide (CO_2) contained within blood following a transient drop in pressure; this phenomenon is commonly seen in patients with mechanical prosthetic valves

Dehiscence: of a prosthetic valve, referes to partial separation of sewing ring from native valve annulus

Dextrocardia: abnormal cardiac position in which the apex of the heart is pointed to the right instead of to the left; usually associated with situs inversus where the heart is a mirror image of normal

Dressler's syndrome: post-myocardial infarction syndrome or post-cardiac injury syndrome associated with pericarditis thought to occur as an immune system response to cardiac or pericardial injury

Dyskinesis: abnormal motion; myocardial walls or segments are thin during diastole and display outward movement or bulging during systole

E

Effacement: the gradual increase in the intraluminal diameter from the aortic annulus, through the sinuses of Valsalva and into the ascending aorta; that is, there is an absence of the normal distinctive sinotubular junction between the aortic root and the ascending aorta

Eccentric hypertrophy: an increased LV mass due to chamber dilatation rather than increased wall thickness

Echogenic (or hyperechoic): bright echoes

Echogenicity: refers to amplitude level of returning echoes; echo "brightness" is directly related to the acoustic properties of the tissue

Effective orifice area: haemodynamically-derived area of a narrowed orifice (stenotic or regurgitant)

Eisenmenger's syndrome: complication of large shunt lesions which leads to chronic pulmonary arterial hypertension, an elevated pulmonary vascular resistance and shunt reversal

Ejection fraction: the percentage of the ventricular end-diastolic volume that is ejected with systole

Electrical alternans: the beat-to-beat variation in the vector, amplitude, and duration of the ECG complexes; in cardiac tamponade, this phenomenon is caused by the pendulum-like motion of the swinging heart within a large pericardial effusion which changes the anatomical relationship of the heart to the ECG electrodes

Exudate: A fluid that has exuded out of a tissue or its capillaries due to injury or inflammation

F

Falciform ligament: a remnant of the umbilical vein of the foetus that attaches the liver to the anterior abdominal wall anteriorly and the diaphragm superiorly and also divides the liver into right and left lobes

Fontan circuit: diversion of systemic venous return directly to PA (bypasses RV) via an extracardiac conduit or intracardiac lateral tunnel (often fenestrated); also includes a bidirectional Glenn shunt

Fractional area change: the percentage change of the RV area following systole

Fractional shortening: the percentage change of the LV end-diastolic cavity dimension following systole

Frank-Starling law: in simple terms this law states that, within certain limits, by increasing the ventricular end-diastolic volume the ventricular wall stretches which in turn causes cardiac muscle to contract more forcefully resulting in an increased stroke volume during systole

Friable: easily crumbled or broken apart

Functional: secondary causes of valvular stenosis or regurgitation that occur when cardiac diseases or lesions "disrupt" otherwise anatomically normal valve leaflets

G

Giant cell arteritis (also known as temporal arteritis): an elastic vessel vasculitis involving the aorta and its secondary and tertiary branches

H

Hamartoma: a benign, focal malformation that resembles a neoplasm in the same tissue from which it grows

Heterogeneous: non-uniform echoes; echo level varies within the structure

Hibernating myocardium: type of viable myocardium where there is chronic LV regional dysfunction due to severe coronary artery disease and chronic ischaemia; complete or partial recovery of function occurs following coronary revascularisation

Hilum: of the lung: a wedge-shaped depression on the mediastinal surface of each lung where the bronchus, blood vessels, nerves, and lymphatics enter or leave the lung

Homogeneous: uniform echoes; echo level same throughout structure as tissues are acoustically similar

Hypokinesis: reduced motion; reduced myocardial thickening during systole

I

Iatrogenic: injuries or defects caused by surgery or diagnostic procedures

Inotropy (or contractility): the inherent strength of cardiac muscle and its ability to shorten with ventricular systole

Integumentary system: an organ system that protects the body from damage; includes the skin and other associated components such as hair, nails, and assorted glands

International normalized ratio (INR): measure of the time taken for blood to clot (the higher the INR, the longer it takes for blood to clot); for patients with mechanical prosthetic valves, the recommended INR is 3.0 +/- 0.5 (an INR ≤ 2.5 indicates inadequate anticoagulation)

K

Kussmaul sign: absence of normal jugular vein collapse or a paradoxical rise in the jugular column due to impaired venous return to the right heart on inspiration; associated severe right-sided congestive heart failure and constrictive pericarditis

L

Laplace law: describes the relationship between the tension or wall stress, intracavity pressure, radius, and thickness of a thinned-walled sphere; this law explains why a dilated ventricle requires more tension to generate the same pressure as a normal ventricle

Lateral resolution: ability of the ultrasound machine to detect echoes from two closely spaced reflectors positioned perpendicular to the axis of the ultrasound beam and to display these reflectors as being separate

LeCompte Manoeuvre: Surgical procedure in which the pulmonary artery is brought anterior to the aorta during an arterial switch procedure in patients with d-transposition of the great arteries

Low flow, low gradient aortic stenosis: low velocities in the presence of severe aortic stenosis due to either low flow in the setting of a normal LV ejection fraction (low flow due to a small LV size or severe mitral regurgitation) or low flow in the setting of a reduced LV ejection fraction

Lutembacher Syndrome: combination of acquired mitral stenosis and an acquired or congenital left-to-right shunt at atrial level

M

Malignant fibrous histiocytomas: malignant tumours arising from primitive mesenchymal cells and composed of spindle cells (fibroblasts), round (histiocytic) cells, pleomorphic giant cells and inflammatory cells

Mesocardia: abnormal cardiac position in which the apex of the heart is in the midline of the thorax instead of pointing to the left

McConnell sign: describes the presence of akinesis of the RV mid-free wall with preserved contractility or sparing of the RV apex; has a high accuracy for diagnosing massive pulmonary embolism

Myocardial performance index (MPI): a measure of "global" myocardial performance and incorporates both elements of systole and diastole; useful in conditions where systolic and diastolic dysfunction coexist

Myxoedema: severe hypothyroidism characterised by firm inelastic oedema, dry skin and hair, and loss of mental and physical vigor

O

Organic: primary causes of valvular stenosis or regurgitation that occur when there is an intrinsic anatomical abnormality of the valve and/or its supporting apparatus

Orthoterminal correction: describes surgical techniques designed to achieve adequate perfusion of the systemic and pulmonary capillary beds without repairing the underlying anatomical malformations

Ortner's syndrome (or cardiovocal syndrome): hoarseness of the voice occurring secondary to compression of the left recurrent laryngeal nerve against the pulmonary artery by marked LA dilatation

P

Palliative surgery: surgery for congenital heart diseases that provides symptomatic relief and extends life but does not correct underlying pathophysiological defect; often an initial operation prior to complete surgical repair of underlying defect

Pannus: abnormal layer of fibrous tissue; due to excessive scarring or keloid formation

Parachute Mitral Valve: characterised by unifocal attachment of the mitral valve cords to a single (or fused) papillary muscle; usually results in restricted the motion of the mitral leaflets due to associated short and thickened cords

Paradoxical low flow aortic stenosis: low velocities in the presence of severe aortic stenosis due to low flow in the setting of a normal LV ejection fraction where low flow occurs due to marked LV concentric remodelling and a small LV cavity size

Pericardiotomy: surgical incision of the pericardium

Plethora: excess of blood

Preload: refers to the muscle length (or muscle stretch) immediately prior to contraction (at end-diastole); commonly used indices to describe preload include end-diastolic volume end-diastolic pressure and/or atrial pressure

Prinzmetal's angina: rare type of angina thought to be caused by coronary spasm; angina is not related to exercise and often occurs between midnight and early morning, with the attacks usually occurring at the same time each day; also referred to as variant angina

Prosthesis-patient mismatch (PPM): occurs when a normally functioning prosthetic valve is too small in relation to the patient's body size; this leads to abnormally high transprosthetic gradients compared with the normal range for the valve subtype and size

Pulsus paradoxus: an exaggeration of the normal variation in the systemic arterial pressure during the inspiratory phase of respiration; that is, the drop in systolic arterial pressure during inspiration exceeds 10 mm Hg

Pseudo-aortic stenosis: reduced aortic valve area due to LV systolic dysfunction rather than severe aortic stenosis; differentiated from true severe aortic stenosis via dobutamine stress echocardiography

R

Raphe: A raphe is a seam or fibrous ridge of tissue between two cusps; a raphe is also known as a false commissure

Rastelli procedure: surgical repair for certain combinations of cyanotic congenital heart defects such as d- transposition of the great arteries + a ventricular septal defect (VSD) + pulmonary stenosis; involves the creation of a patch redirecting blood from LV through the VSD and into aorta as well as an external valved conduit from RV to PA

Raynaud's phenomenon: an abnormal response of the fingers and toes to cold whereby digits turn white, then blue and finally red after exposure to cold; this phenomenon is seen in patients with connective tissue disease

Refractory heart failure: advanced heart failure with marked symptoms at rest despite maximal medical therapy

Regurgitant fraction: the percentage of blood that regurgitates or leaks back through an incompetent valve

Regurgitant volume: the volume of blood that regurgitates or leaks back through an incompetent valve; measured in millilitres

Ross procedure: double valve replacement whereby the aortic valve is replaced by the patient's own pulmonary valve (autograft) and pulmonary valve is replaced with an allograft

S

Shone syndrome: consists of a series of four left heart obstructive lesions including: (1) supravalvular mitral membrane, (2) a parachute mitral valve, (3) subaortic stenosis and (4) aortic coarctation. A bicuspid aortic valve is also common

Spontaneous echo contrast (SEC): smoke-like swirling of blood within a cavity due to low velocity blood flow; precursor to thrombus formation

Stroke volume: volume of blood being pumped by the heart per beat; measured in millilitres

Stunned myocardium: type of viable myocardium where there is a persistence of LV regional dysfunction after transient coronary occlusion; recovery of wall motion abnormalities is delayed despite adequate reperfusion therapy or restoration of normal coronary flow

Schwannoma: a benign nerve sheath tumour composed of Schwann cells (supporting cells of the peripheral nervous system)

T

Takayasu arteritis (also known as pulseless disease): an idiopathic vasculitis of the elastic arteries, involving the aorta and its branches

TAPSE: Tricuspid annular plane systolic excursion; measure of RV longitudinal fibre shortening during ventricular systole

Totipotent multicentricity: totipotent cells have the ability to give rise to any cell type; multicentricity indicates multiple and independent sites of origin

Transudate: a fluid substance that has passed through a membrane or has been extruded from a tissue

Transmural filling pressure: the pressure difference between the intracavity pressure (ICP) and the intrapericardial pressure (IPP)

Tuberous sclerosis: a rare multi-system genetic disorder associated with benign tumour growths in the brain and in other vital organs such as the kidneys, skin and heart; associated cardiac tumours include rhabdomyomas

V

Vena contracta: narrowest part of a jet downstream from a narrowed orifice; created as blood streamlines through the narrowed orifice

Ventricular interdependence: describes the relationship between the size, shape, and compliance of one ventricle upon the other

Ventriculoarterial concordance: normal anatomical relationship between the ventricles and the great arteries; that is, the morphological RV connects to the PA and the morphological LV connects to the aorta

Ventriculoarterial discordance: abnormal anatomical relationship between the ventricles and the great arteries; that is, the morphological RV connects to the aorta and the morphological LV connects to the PA

Venturi effect: result of fluid pressure differentials that create a suction effect

Viable myocardium: dysfunctional myocardium that improves contractile function with restoration of an adequate coronary blood flow; classified as "stunned" or "hibernating"

W

Wall stress (or wall tension): the tension within the ventricular wall of the LV; determined by the pressure in the ventricle, the internal radius of the ventricle, and the thickness of the wall; expressed by Laplace's Law

Index

Page numbers followed by an 'A' refer to Appendices, page numbers followed by an 'f' refer to figures, page numbers followed by a 't' refer to a table